EASY CODER

2000 EDITION

BY

PAUL K. TANAKA, M.D., C.P.C.

Published by
Unicor Medical, Inc.
4160 Carmichael Rd.
Montgomery, AL 36106
(334) 260-8150

DISCLAIMER

Unicor's Easy Coder code book has been written for use with codes taken from the Federal Government. Information has been referenced from official Health Care Financing Administration (HCFA) material, and includes the same codes as those from Volumes 1 and 2, 1999, of the U.S. Department of Health and Human Services' official code books.

Unicor Medical, Inc. has made every reasonable effort to assure that the information contained in the Easy Coder is completely accurate. The ultimate responsibility for the correct assignment of diagnosis codes, however, falls upon the medical provider.

Unicor Medical, Inc. and its principals, employees, or staff neither explicitly nor implicitly warranty/guarantee that the contained codes, statements, or narratives are error-free. We disclaim any responsibility or liability if a dispute of payment based on codes from the book arises with any third party payor, nor do we bear any responsibility or liability as to any use of the book, either medically or otherwise.

Users of the book purchase the material without any warranty/guarantee of any kind, either expressed or implied, as to the fitness of the book for their use. Neither is any warranty/guarantee given for the consequences or results from Easy Coder's use.

Editing and Production:

Wanda K. Hamm, C.P.C.
Jean Rollings Jackson, C.P.C.
Becky Lobdell, R.R.A.
Richard D. Morris, C.P.C.
Shelley Walworth Richardson, R.R.A., C.P.C.
Rex A. Stanley, R.N., C.M.M., C.P.C.
Peter O. Tanaka, C.P.C.
Alyssa N. Vrocher

PREFACE

Unicor Medical, Inc. is the most innovative company in the field of medical coding. We have entirely reorganized the ICD-9 system in order to help produce fast, complete, and precise coding. Accurate ICD-9 coding not only helps to optimize reimbursement but also produces a savings in the amount of employee time and effort spent on the coding/reimbursement process. When used properly and in conjunction with all current coding and reimbursement guidelines, Easy Coder is an important investment in the future earnings of a practice or medical facility.

The purpose of Easy Coder is to help you: 1) find ICD-9 codes efficiently, 2) use multiple codes so that the complete nature of the encounter is fully described, and 3) ensure the specificity and accuracy of the codes selected so as to adequately justify the services involved, thereby optimizing reimbursements. Great care has been taken in this book to incorporate and follow HCFA guidelines, as well as third party payor regulations.

The rules to survive in the new coding climate are very complex, and mistakes are common and are costly for all parties involved. Not only does the physician pay for coding errors, but patients also suffer unjustly when services are not covered. *Remember, you communicate with carriers through numbers.* You must fully and accurately describe patient encounters numerically. Easy Coder will help you do just that. And just as your office is committed to providing quality medical care for your patients, Unicor Medical, Inc. stresses a sincere corporate commitment to assist you in every way possible.

THE UNICOR QUALITY GUARANTEE

We believe that your 2000 Easy Coder will be the fastest, easiest, and most accurate ICD-9 book you've ever used. You'll quickly become familiar with the innovative Easy Coder format when you read the *Introduction* on the following pages.

If you ever have a problem finding a code in Easy Coder, we'd be happy to help. Simply call us toll-free at 1-800-825-7421 between 8am and 5pm CST Monday through Friday. You'll speak with a member of our own coding staff who will quickly locate for you the code you need... at no charge whatsoever.

Complimentary coding support is provided exclusively for ICD-9 coding and exclusively for users of Unicor Medical products. Coding support for 2000 Easy Coder users extends from October 1, 1999 through October 1, 2000.

Please use the following unique identification number when you call:

CODING AUTHORIZATION NUMBER
116-3

INTRODUCTION

ICD-9 CM coding is the process of assigning a numerical code to a written description of a diagnosis, problem, condition, etc. You should code all the documented current diagnoses, including underlying diseases and secondary diagnoses.

Easy Coder is designed to do much of the coding analysis for you by providing a format for the codes that is logical and simple, by incorporating many basic rules within the format of the book, and by providing "help text" windows throughout the book. It is important, though, to consistently stay up to date on all the numerous rules and guidelines that help define which codes are acceptable under which circumstances.

One of the most important rules to remember has to do with the sequencing of codes. Sequencing in ICD-9 coding is determined by the intensity and acuity of service, the inherent DRG value, and the "level of service." The procedure indicated on the claim must be commensurate with the diagnosis or diagnoses indicated, and appropriate secondary diagnoses must be filed.

Proper sequencing of the diagnosis codes is of utmost importance. Occasionally, however, the rules for proper sequencing may seem confusing. AHA coding and sequencing guidelines were derived from inpatient data and are not necessarily logical in all cases when they are adapted to the outpatient rules of coding. Although these coding guidelines are far from perfect, they, nevertheless, are the guidelines by which many carriers now pay or reject claims.

The main rule to remember is the "reason rule," which says that the reason for the patient visit (encounter) is coded first. The only exception to the reason rule applies in the following situation: After study, the physician's major work and effort is directed toward a certain diagnosis or procedure different from the one the patient originally came in for. Then the diagnosis that required the greater amount of effort should be coded first.

Now that you know how important it is to understand coding rules, and you are familiar with the important "reason rule," it's time to explain how Easy Coder makes following these rules easier and makes coding more efficient.

FINDING THE DIAGNOSIS

The traditional system of categories and exclusions does not exist in Easy Coder. Easy Coder is completely alphabetical. Some diagnoses have their own singular listing, while others are listed under a main boldface heading along with all the other types, kinds, states, conditions, or possible locations associated with that heading. For example, when you look up arthritis alphabetically, you'll find that arthritis is a main heading and that indented under it is a list of all the different types of arthritis.

The most important element is this: Whether it is a singular listing or part of a list under a main boldface heading, *each and every diagnosis is listed with its own correct code* at ultimate specificity. You will never find an exclusion in Easy Coder. Just look up the diagnosis alphabetically, and you'll find the exact code. There are three (3) ways that a diagnosis may be listed:

1. By the key word in the diagnosis

Most diagnoses are listed under a "key word." The key word is the most important or most descriptive word in the diagnosis. The key word is the word that gives you the most information about the diagnosis. It's usually a noun or a noun derivative.

Often you'll find that a key word for one diagnosis is also the key word for several other related or similar diagnoses. In this case, the key word is a main boldface heading, and it is followed by an indented listing of the various diagnoses, which usually convey particular types, states, or possible locations.

Once you determine the key word, look for that word alphabetically, just as if you were using a dictionary. Here are some examples of diagnoses and their key words:

biliary cirrhosis

Cirrhosis would be the key word in this example, since it tells you more about the diagnosis than biliary does. The word biliary describes what type of cirrhosis; it is secondary information.

Since the key word for this diagnosis is cirrhosis, you would find the diagnosis under the alphabetical listing for cirrhosis.

hiatal hernia

Hernia would be the key word for his diagnosis, since it gives the most important descriptive information. Hiatal, of course, describes the type of hernia.

2. By the anatomical site

The second way that a diagnosis may be listed is under the anatomical site. A diagnosis will typically be listed by anatomical site if it is surgical in nature, or if the condition or disorder involved is rather non-descriptive, such as "injury." Here are just a few examples of diagnoses that are listed this way:

progressive atrophy of the iris-- found alphabetically under iris
deviated nasal septum-- found alphabetically under septum
congenital absence of an arm-- found alphabetically under arm

Please note that it is not uncommon for a diagnosis to be listed by the anatomical site as well as by a key word or exactly as it was written in the documentation. In standard code books, diagnoses are listed only one way. *In Easy Coder, however, most diagnoses are listed several ways so that the need for multiple searches and cross referencing is practically eliminated.* For example, congestive heart failure can be found alphabetically under congestive and CHF. Laceration of the eyeball can be found alphabetically under laceration and ocular.

3. Exactly as it is written in the patient's record

Many diagnoses are listed exactly as they are written in the patient's record or chart from which you're coding. In other words, you'll simply look for the diagnosis alphabetically by the first word in its description, just as if you were using a dictionary. Here are just a few examples of diagnoses that are listed by the first word in the description:

spinal cord compression-- found alphabetically under spinal (cord)
hypertensive retinopathy-- found alphabetically under hypertensive
myocardial infarction--found alphabetically under myocardial

Note that *one word diagnoses* and *discrete diagnoses* are always found alphabetically under the first word of the diagnosis, exactly as they are written in the documentation. Again, here are just a few of the many possible examples:

intertrigo--found alphabetically under intertrigo
fructose intolerance-- found alphabetically under fructose
idiopathic hypertrophic subaortic stenosis-- found alphabetically under idiopathic

Also note that most diagnoses can be found not only under their exact medical name, but also under any common name, abbreviation, and acronym. For instance:

temporomandibular joint disorder--found alphabetically under temporomandibular, and under its common abbreviation, TMJ
hepatomegaly--found alphabetically under hepatomegaly and under its common name, liver enlargement

Remember, a diagnosis will always be listed alphabetically, either by the first word in the diagnosis (exactly as it's documented in the record), by a key word in the diagnosis, or by the anatomical site involved. A diagnosis may have its own singular one-line listing, or it may be part of a comprehensive listing under a main heading.

Main headings are words or phrases that are in **boldface** type and that are followed by a list of indented entries. A main heading may be the key word or the anatomical site for several various types, kinds, states, or locations of related or similar diagnoses. These specific diagnoses are given in an indented list immediately below the main heading. The indented entries are specific choices for the main heading. Note that the main headings have been set up for coding ease, not for classification of medical terms.

FINDING THE CODE

Easy Coder is organized to give you all the codes you need for every diagnosis in just one step. To the left of every diagnosis is a code. If the code is not at ultimate specificity already, a menu follows. If you need to use a second code in order to completely code for all additional diagnoses or underlying diseases, you'll find the second code provided for you to the right of the diagnosis, or you'll be reminded to select the appropriate additional code in cases where several codes could be applicable.

Following are descriptions of the symbols and formats used to ensure that you have all the digits and all the correctly sequenced codes needed to fully code the diagnosis. Note that all of the following symbols and formats may be used in conjunction with one another and more than one can appear at a time; apply all the necessary ones that appear for any diagnosis.

1. Menus

You will always be able to tell when a code is not at ultimate specificity because the code number will be in boldface type and there will be a pound sign (#) in the location where the fourth or fifth digit should be. There will be also be a "menu," a selection of choices, immediately following. You should choose the appropriate description from the menu and then append the corresponding digit to the base code in order to obtain ultimate specificity.

If the bold code number is 3 digits long and has one # sign next to it, the choice from the menu will take the diagnosis to its ultimate 4th digit specificity.

If the bold code number is 4 digits long and has one # sign next to it, the appropriate choice from the menu will take the diagnosis to its ultimate 5th digit specificity.

If the bold code number is 3 digits long and has two # signs next to it, two menus will follow, and the choices together will take the diagnosis to its 5th digit ultimate specificity.

Here's an example:

Dx= benign hypertensive renal disease with renal failure

HYPERTENSIVE
403.## RENAL DISEASE
4th Digit: 403.
0. MALIGNANT
1. BENIGN
9. NOS
5th Digit: 403.
0. WITHOUT RENAL FAILURE
1. WITH RENAL FAILURE

To take the code for this diagnosis to ultimate specificity, you would first select choice "1" from the 4th digit menu, since the diagnosis indicates that the renal disease is benign. You then would select the "1" from the 5th digit menu, since the diagnosis does indicate renal failure. The code for this diagnosis, then, is 403.11 at ultimate specificity.

If the diagnosis were malignant hypertensive renal disease, the selection would be "0" from the first menu and "0" from the second menu. The code at ultimate specificity would be 403.00.

Note: In a very few cases, you will see a single menu that contains both 4th and 5th digits. Some of the choices in the menu will have only a 4th digit; others will have a 4th and a 5th digit. Simply make the appropriate selection from the menu, and assign the corresponding digit or digits.

Here's an example:

BACTERIAL INFECTION

041.9	NOS
041.85	AEROBACTER AEROGENES
041.82	BACILLUS FRAGILES
041.84	BACTEROIDES (FRAGILIS)
041.83	CLOSTRIDIUM PERFRINGENS
041.4	E COLI
041.81	EATON'S AGENT
041.3	FRIEDLANDER'S BACILLUS
041.84	GRAM-NEGATIVE ANAEROBES
041.85	GRAM-NEGATIVE BACTERIA NOS
041.5	H. INFLUENZAE
041.86	H. PYLORI (HELICOBACTER PYLORI)
041.3	KLEBSIELLA
041.85	MIMA POLYMORPHA
041.81	MYCOLPLASMA
041.81	PLEUROPNEUMONIA LIKE ORGANISMS
041.2	PNEUMOCOCCUS
041.6	PROTEUS (MIRABILIS) (MORGANII)
041.7	PSEUDOMONAS
041.85	SERRATIA
041.10	STAPHYLOCOCCUS UNSPECIFIED
041.11	STAPHYLOCOCCUS AUREUS
041.19	STAPHYLOCOCCUS OTHER
041.00	STREPTOCOCCUS
041.01	STREPTOCOCCUS GROUP A
041.02	STREPTOCOCCUS GROUP B
041.02	STREPTOCOCCUS GROUP C
041.04	STREPTOCOCCUS GROUP D
041.05	STREPTOCOCCUS GROUP G
041.09	STREPTOCOCCUS OTHER
041.89	OTHER SPECIFIED BACTERIA

The correct code for the organism E coli would be 041.4.

The correct code for the organism streptococcus, group D would be 041.04.

If there is only a 4th digit listed for your menu selection, then use just a 4th digit to take the code to ultimate specificity. If there are a 4th and a 5th digit listed, then append both digits to take the code to ultimate specificity.

2. "Use Additional Code(s)"

Sometimes more than one code is needed to correctly code a diagnosis. There are two conventions for referencing additional codes in Easy Coder. In the majority of cases, the additional code is listed in brackets to the right of the diagnosis. In some cases, when there are numerous codes that could be used as an additional code, and the selection of the correct additional code is dependent on what diagnoses were documented for the particular episode of care, a help box is provided reminding you to use the additional code that is correct for the encounter you are coding (if one is required). Remember, only code the diagnoses that are documented by the physician and that are relevant for that particular episode of care.

A. Additional Code in Brackets

Two codes

When a diagnosis requires a second code for an underlying disease or a secondary diagnosis, the appropriate second code may be listed in brackets to the right of the diagnosis. If both conditions inherent in the diagnosis are documented in the record, then the code in brackets is a mandatory part of correct coding for the particular diagnosis; it is not optional.

The relationship of the diagnosis to the codes is indicated by underlining. One code, either the code to the left of the diagnosis or the code in brackets to the right, will be underlined; also underlined will be part of the diagnosis description. *The code number that is underlined goes with the part of the diagnosis that is underlined. The code number that is not underlined goes with the part of the diagnosis that is not underlined.* Remember, though, underlining indicates correspondence only, not sequencing priority.

A code in a main heading

Easy Coder sometimes will list an additional code in brackets beside a main heading if that code may apply to all the diagnoses listed under that heading. The bracketed code, if used, would be sequenced after the primary code for the diagnosis.

Three codes

In some cases, a diagnosis requires two additional codes. In these cases, Easy Coder provides both of the additional codes to the right of the diagnosis. Both codes will be contained in brackets.

One of the three codes and one part of the diagnosis description will be underlined once. Another code and another part of the diagnosis description will be underlined twice. *The code with one underline goes with the part of the diagnosis with one underline. The code with two underlines goes with the part of the diagnosis with two underlines. Of course, the code that is not underlined goes with the part of the diagnosis that is not underlined.*

Sequencing

Any time Easy Coder gives you an additional code in brackets, it also puts the codes in order for sequencing. *Always sequence multiple codes from left to right.*

The code to the left of the diagnosis sequences first. The bracketed code immediately to the right of the diagnosis sequences second. If there are two bracketed codes located to the right of the diagnosis, the far-right code sequences third. The rule is easy: sequence left to right, regardless of which code is underlined, and regardless of which part of the diagnosis you actually looked up alphabetically. The work has already been done for you. Just sequence from left to right.

Here are some examples of additional codes in brackets. Remember, the underlining indicates the correspondence between the codes and the diagnosis. The sequencing is always done from left to right.

272.7 FABRY'S DISEASE WITH CEREBRAL DEGENERATION [330.2]

The correct codes and sequencing for the above listing would be as follows:

272.7 Fabry's Disease
330.2 cerebral degeneration

DEMENTIA OTHER CAUSES

294.8 DIALYSIS [E879.1]
985.8 DIALYSIS DUE TO ALUMINUM OVERLOAD [294.8] [E879.1]
293.9 DIALYSIS TRANSIENT [E879.1]

SPONDYLOSIS

WITH OSTEOPOROSIS [733.0#]

721.0 CERVICAL
721.1 CERVICAL WITH MYELOPATHY (CORD COMPRESSION)
721.3 LUMBAR

The correct codes and sequencing for the diagnosis cervical spondylosis with osteoporosis would be as follows:

721.0 cervical spondylosis
733.0# osteoporosis

Remember that if the diagnosis did not include osteoporosis, you would have used only the codes 721.0 for the cervical spondylosis.

Remember that any time there is a # sign following a code, you need to append at least one more digit from the associated menu(s) in order to gain ultimate specificity. However, for the sake of space and clarity, the menus for the notated codes above have not been listed out in these examples.

B. Additional Code Reminder Box

For some diagnoses, coding guidelines suggest that an additional code be used to show the specific complication, manifestation, disease, etc., if one is documented. In most of these cases, there are numerous additional codes that may be applicable; the choice of which code is correct for the particular episode of care you are coding can only be determined by the documentation of the diagnoses seen during that episode.

In these cases, when there is not a specific code indicated in brackets, there will be a help text box nearby to remind you that you should use an appropriate additional code. As its name suggests, the additional code should be sequenced after the primary diagnosis, unless otherwise specified.

Here is an example of a help box reminding you to use an additional code:

USE AN ADDITIONAL CODE TO FURTHER SPECIFY THE COMPLICATION OF ANESTHESIA OR OTHER SEDATION.

ANESTHESIA COMPLICATING LABOR & DELIVERY

668.9# COMPLICATION NOS
668.1# CARDIAC COMPLICATIONS
668.2# CENTRAL NERVOUS SYSTEM COMPLICATIONS
668.0# PULMONARY COMPLICATIONS
668.8# OTHER SPECIFIED COMPLICATIONS

5th Digit: 668.0-9

0. EPISODE OF CARE NOS OR N/A
1. DELIVERED
2. DELIVERED POSTPARTUM COMPLICATION
3. ANTEPARTUM COMPLICATION
4. POSTPARTUM COMPLICATION

The 668 code identifies that there is a complication, but it does not identify the specific complication. To show exactly what the complication is, you need to use an additional code. Since there can be numerous conditions that are complications of anesthesia (such as hypoxia, hyperpyrexia, various types of cardiac dysrhythmia, etc.), you must select the additional code that specifies what the exact complication was for the specific episode of care you are coding. As the name suggests, the additional code is sequenced after the primary code (unless otherwise noted).

If your documentation indicates that the patient experienced hypoxia in reaction to the anesthesia given during delivery, the correct codes and sequencing would be as follows:

668.0# pulmonary complication / anesthesia complicating labor and delivery
799.0 hypoxia

MORPHOLOGY CODES

Morphology codes, or "M" codes, are an adaptation of the International Classification of Diseases of Oncology. Published by the World Health Organization, "M" codes indicate the histological origin and the behavior of neoplasms.

M-codes consist of five digits. Histological origin or cell-type is indicated by the first four digits, while the fifth digit indicates behavior.

The fifth digit indicates the following behaviors:

/0 benign
/1 uncertain whether benign or malignant, borderline malignancy
/2 carcinoma in situ
    intraepithelial
    non-infiltrating
    non-invasive
/3 malignant, primary site
/6 malignant, secondary site or metastatic
/9 malignant, uncertain whether primary or metastatic

The morphology codes given include a fifth digit for the assumed behavior based on the cell-type. However, the patient's records and documentation may indicate a different behavior and therefore prompt the use of a different fifth digit. For example, a Leydig Cell Tumor unspecified is generally assumed to be malignant and would be assigned a morphology code of M8650/3. But if the supporting documents for the case you are coding indicate that the tumor is benign, the appropriate behavior code would be /0 and the correct M-code would be M8650/0. Generally speaking, the documented description of the neoplasm should decide the appropriate morphology code where applicable.

The M code is listed in Easy Coder to the right of the diagnosis description.

When a morphological diagnosis contains two qualifying adjectives, and the adjectives correspond to different M-codes, use the higher number. Most likely, the higher number is a more specific description. For example, a papillary carcinoma has a morphology code of M8050/3, while a papillary serous carcinoma has a morphology code of M8460/3. For the correct code for papillary serous carcinoma, you would choose the higher of the two morphology numbers and select M8460/3.

Note that the fifth digit of /9 is inapplicable in the context of ICD-9, since all malignant neoplasms are presumed to be primary (/3) or secondary (/6) according to the information on the medical record.

E-CODES

An E-code is an ICD-9 code that provides supplementary information concerning the external cause of an injury. E-codes do not indicate the injury itself, but rather why the injury occurred. E-codes can be used to show the environmental events, circumstances, conditions, or nature of the condition, and they help provide to the carrier a more detailed analysis of what happened to the patient that resulted in the current condition. E-codes are also very important for reporting purposes.

E-codes can be used in conjunction with any other code from 001-999, but they can not be used alone and they can not be assigned as the principal diagnosis. The only E-codes that are mandatory nationwide are E-codes that indicate drugs that have caused adverse effects during therapeutic use. Several states, however, now require the use of any and all E-codes when applicable.

E-codes are listed in the back of Easy Coder. The section is divided into logical and easy-to-use categories. An E-code directory is provided at the beginning of the E-code section. The directory tells you on what page you'll find the various categories.

Following is an example of correctly using E-codes.

Scenario: A patient suffers a hip contusion after slipping on a wet spot on the floor and falling at the factory where he works.

After coding the contusion as 924.01, you're ready to find the correct E-codes. First, you'll turn to the E-code directory at the beginning of the E-code section and find the appropriate category which, in this case, would be "falls." When you turn to the page referenced in the directory, you'll then see three types of falls, one involving falls between two levels, one involving a fall on just one level, and one for fall unspecified. Since the scenario says the man slipped on the floor, only one level is involved.

	FALLS FROM / INTO SAME LEVEL
E885	SLIPPING OR TRIPPING
E886.0	SPORTS (COLLISION)
E886.9	OTHER AND SPECIFIED COLLISION

For the scenario above, you would choose code E885 from the types of falls listed.

An injury code always sequences before an E-code, so you know that the 924.01 code comes first, followed by E885.

The correct sequenced codes for the above example are as follows:

924.01 hip contusion
E885 fall from/ into same level

SUMMARY

All diagnoses are listed alphabetically. A diagnosis may be a singular one-line listing or part of an indented list of diagnoses under a main heading.

Find the diagnosis by looking alphabetically for the key word, the anatomical site, or the first word in the diagnosis description. Remember, the diagnosis may be listed under its exact medical name, common name, abbreviation, or acronym. If a proper name (such as Refsum's, Coat's, etc.) is in the description, the diagnosis is usually listed under the proper name.

The key word is usually a noun or a noun-based derivative. It is the most descriptive or most important word in the diagnosis description-- the word that gives the most information about the diagnosis.

Many diagnoses are listed at least two different ways to avoid cross-referencing and multiple searches.

If a code is followed by a # sign, choose the appropriate selection from the corresponding menu to take the code to ultimate specificity.

If an additional code is given in brackets, underlining indicates correspondence between the code and the diagnosis description only. It does not indicate sequencing. Sequence multiple codes from left to right.

SYMBOLS & FORMATS

The **"#"** sign indicates that the ICD-9 code is not to the ultimate specificity. The appropriate 4th or 5th digit menu will immediately follow the diagnoses.

The **"[ ]"** are used to enclose a supplementary code. If the diagnosis with which the code corresponds is documented in the patient's record, the supplemental code must be used. This code must be sequenced secondarily.

An underline **"__________"** under a code number and part of a diagnosis description means that that code and that part of the description correspond. Likewise, a double-underlined code corresponds with the double-underlined part of the diagnosis description.

The **"( )"** are used to enclose other words that can be used interchangeably in the diagnosis description, and for words used to make the meaning of the description clearer.

The **"0"** in place of a code indicates that the code(s) for that particular description is listed under a synonym. There will be a description telling you where to find the appropriate diagnosis. You may not select a diagnosis with a code of 0.

0 AB (ABORTION) SEE 'ABORTION'

ABASIA/ASTASIA

307.9 ABASIA/ASTASIA
781.3 ATACTICA (CHOREIC) (PAROXYSMAL TREPIDENT) (SPASTIC) (TREMBLING) (TREPIDANS)
300.11 HYSTERICAL

270.0 ABDERHALDEN-KAUFMANN-LIGNAC SYNDROME

ABDOMEN, ABDOMINAL

793.6 ABNORMAL (X-RAY) (OTHER TEST OR STUDY)
902.0 AORTA INJURY
908.4 AORTA INJURY LATE EFFECT
787.3 BLOATING
787.3 DISTENTION (GASEOUS)
746.87 HEART
868.00 INJURY UNSPECIFIED SITE
902.9 INJURY BLOOD VESSEL NOS
908.1 INJURY LATE EFFECT
868.09 INJURY MULTIPLE OR OTHER SPECIFIED SITE
868.10 INJURY WITH OPEN WOUND UNSPECIFIED SITE
868.19 INJURY WITH OPEN WOUND MULTIPLE OR OTHER SPECIFIED SITE
789.3# MASS

5th Digit: 789.3

0. UNSPECIFIED SITE
1. UPPER RIGHT QUADRANT
2. UPPER LEFT QUADRANT
3. LOWER RIGHT QUADRANT
4. LOWER LEFT QUADRANT
5. PERIUMBILIC
6. EPIGASTRIC
7. GENERALIZED
9. OTHER SPECIFIED SITE (MULTIPLE)

346.2# MIGRAINE SYNDROME

5th Digit: 346.2

0. WITHOUT MENTION INTRACTABLE MIGRAINE
1. WITH INTRACTABLE MIGRAINE

756.79 MUSCLE DEFICIENCY SYNDROME
756.79 OBSTIPUM
789.0# PAIN

5th Digit: 789.0

0. UNSPECIFIED SITE
1. UPPER RIGHT QUADRANT
2. UPPER LEFT QUADRANT
3. LOWER RIGHT QUADRANT
4. LOWER LEFT QUADRANT
5. PERIUMBILIC
6. EPIGASTRIC
7. GENERALIZED
9. OTHER SPECIFIED SITE (MULTIPLE)

0 PREGNANCY SEE 'ECTOPIC PREGNANCY (RUPTURED) (UNRUPTURED)'
728.84 RECTUS DIASTASIS
665.8# RECTUS DIASTASIS COMPLICATING PREGNANCY

5th Digit: 665.8

0. EPISODE OF CARE NOS OR N/A
1. DELIVERED
2. DELIVERED WITH POSTPARTUM COMPLICATION
3. ANTEPARTUM COMPLICATION
4. POSTPARTUM COMPLICATION

756.79 RECTUS DIASTASIS CONGENITAL
789.4# RIGIDITY

5th Digit: 789.4

0. UNSPECIFIED SITE
1. UPPER RIGHT QUADRANT
2. UPPER LEFT QUADRANT
3. LOWER RIGHT QUADRANT
4. LOWER LEFT QUADRANT
5. PERIUMBILIC
6. EPIGASTRIC
7. GENERALIZED
9. OTHER SPECIFIED SITE (MULTIPLE)

ABDOMEN, ABDOMINAL (continued)

739.9 SEGMENTAL OR SOMATIC DYSFUNCTION
789.3# SWELLING

5th Digit: 789.3

0. UNSPECIFIED SITE
1. UPPER RIGHT QUADRANT
2. UPPER LEFT QUADRANT
3. LOWER RIGHT QUADRANT
4. LOWER LEFT QUADRANT
5. PERIUMBILIC
6. EPIGASTRIC
7. GENERALIZED
9. OTHER SPECIFIED SITE (MULTIPLE)

789.9 SYMPTOM OTHER
789.0# SYNDROME ACUTE
789.6# TENDERNESS

5th Digit: 789.0, 6

0. UNSPECIFIED SITE
1. UPPER RIGHT QUADRANT
2. UPPER LEFT QUADRANT
3. LOWER RIGHT QUADRANT
4. LOWER LEFT QUADRANT
5. PERIUMBILIC
6. EPIGASTRIC
7. GENERALIZED
9. OTHER SPECIFIED SITE (MULTIPLE)

756.70 WALL ANOMALY - NOS
756.71 WALL ANOMALY - PRUNE BELLY SYNDROME
756.79 WALL ANOMALY - OTHER
959.1 WALL INJURY
911.8 WALL INJURY OTHER AND NOS SUPERFICIAL
911.9 WALL INJURY OTHER AND NOS SUPERFICIAL - INFECTED

378.54 ABDUCENS NERVE DISORDER (ATROPHY) (PALSY)
951.3 ABDUCENS NERVE INJURY
277.3 ABERCROMBIE'S SYNDROME (AMYLOID DEGENERATION)
272.5 ABETALIPOPROTEINEMIA
790.91 ABG ABNORMAL
780.79 ABIONARCE
743.62 ABLEPHARON DEFORMITIES EYELID CONGENITAL

ABNORMAL TESTS, SYMPTOMS, SIGNS, OR ILL-DEFINED CONDITIONS MAY ALSO BE FOUND UNDER SPECIFIC DESCRIPTIONS. SEARCH., EKG, COMA, CHEST, X-RAY, ETC.

ABNORMAL

787.5 BOWEL SOUNDS
786.7 CHEST SOUNDS
793.1 CXR
787.7 FECES
796.5 FINDINGS ANTENATAL SCREENING
790.0 FINDINGS ANISOCYTOSIS
796.9 FINDINGS OTHER SPECIFIED
781.2 GAIT
781.0 HEAD MOVEMENTS
374.43 INNERVATION SYNDROME EYELID
781.0 INVOLUNTARY MOVEMENTS
524.5 JAW CLOSURE
786.7 PERCUSSION CHEST
781.9 POSTURE
796.1 REFLEX
786.4 SPUTUM (AMOUNT) (COLOR) (ODOR)
792.1 STOOL COLOR
524.5 SWALLOWING (MALOCCLUSION)
783.1 WEIGHT GAIN
783.2 WEIGHT LOSS

ABNORMAL BODY FLUIDS OR SUBSTANCES

792.3	AMNIOTIC FLUID
792.1	BLOOD OCCULT
792.0	CEREBROSPINAL
792.9	PERITONEAL
792.4	SALIVA
795.2	SALIVA IN CHROMOSOMAL ANALYSIS
792.2	SEMEN
792.2	SPERMATOZOA
792.1	STOOL
792.9	SYNOVIAL
792.9	VAGINAL
792.9	OTHER

ABNORMAL CULTURE

790.7	BLOOD
V08	HIV
795.3	NOSE
795.0	PAP SMEAR CERVIX (DYSKARYOTIC)
795.3	SKIN LESION NEC
792.0	SPINAL FLUID
795.3	SPUTUM
792.1	STOOL
795.3	THROAT
791.9	URINE
795.3	WOUND
795.3	NEC

ABNORMAL FUNCTION STUDIES - BRAIN

794.00	BRAIN UNSPECIFIED
794.01	ECHOENCEPHALOGRAM
794.02	EEG
794.09	OTHER BRAIN SCAN

ABNORMAL FUNCTION STUDIES - CARDIOPULMONARY

794.39	BALLISTOCARDIOGRAM
794.30	CARDIOVASCULAR UNSPECIFIED
794.39	CARDIOVASCULAR OTHER
794.31	EKG
794.39	PHONOCARDIOGRAM
794.2	PULMONARY
794.39	VECTORCARDIOGRAM

ABNORMAL FUNCTION STUDIES - NERVOUS SYSTEM

794.15	AUDITORY FUNCTION STUDIES
794.00	CENTRAL NOS
794.09	CENTRAL OTHER SPECIFIED
794.12	ELECTRO-OCULOGRAM (EOG)
794.17	EMG
794.11	ERG (RETINAL FUNCTION STUDIES)
794.10	NERVE STIMULATION UNSPECIFIED
794.14	OCULOMOTOR STUDIES
794.19	PERIPHERAL NERVES OTHER
794.11	RETINAL
794.16	VESTIBULAR FUNCTION STUDIES
794.13	VISUALLY EVOKED POTENTIAL

ABNORMAL FUNCTION STUDIES - OTHER

794.7	BASAL METABOLISM
794.9	BLADDER
794.9	BONE
794.4	KIDNEY
794.8	LIVER
794.9	PANCREAS
794.9	PLACENTAL
794.2	PULMONARY
794.4	RENAL
794.9	SPLEEN
794.5	THYROID
794.6	OTHER ENDOCRINE
794.9	OTHER

IF THERE IS A SPECIFIC CONDITION STATED IN THE MEDICAL RECORD, REMEMBER TO CODE THAT CONDITION (I.E. HYPOGLYCEMIA, HYPERKALEMIA, HYPERLIPIDEMIA, ETC.). ABNORMAL FINDINGS ARE TO BE USED ONLY WHEN THERE IS NO DEFINITIVE DIAGNOSIS.

ABNORMAL LAB TEST (BLOOD) NONSPECIFIC

790.99	NOS
790.99	ALBUMIN GLOBULIN RATIO
790.3	ALCOHOL LEVEL INCREASED
795.79	ANTIBODY NOS
790.91	ARTERIAL BLOOD GAS OR OTHER EXAM OF BLOOD
790.7	BACTEREMIA ANY KIND
790.92	BLEEDING TIME PROLONGED
790.6	BUN AND CREATINE ELEVATED
275.40	CALCIUM
790.6	CHEMISTRIES (EXCEPT ELECTROLYTES)
790.94	EUTHYROID SICK SYNDROME
790.2	GLUCOSE (GLUCOSE TOLERANCE)
795.79	IMMUNOLOGICAL OTHER (IMMUNOGLOBULINS)
790.5	OTHER ENZYMES PHOSPHATASE AMYLASE (ETC.)
276.8	POTASSIUM DEFICIENCY
276.7	POTASSIUM EXCESS
790.93	PSA (ELEVATED) PROSTATIC SPECIFIC ANTIGEN
790.0	RBC (RED BLOOD CELLS) VOLUME MORPHOLOGY
790.1	SED RATE ELEVATED
796.0	TOXICOLOGY
790.4	TRANSAMINASE OR LDH
790.8	VIREMIA ANY KIND
288.8	WHITE BLOOD CELL COUNT ELEVATED
288.0	WHITE BLOOD CELL COUNT LOW
288.9	WHITE BLOOD CELL DIFFERENTIAL
288.9	WHITE BLOOD CELL MORPHOLOGY
790.99	OTHER SPECIFIED

ABNORMAL RADIOLOGICAL STUDY

793.#	ECHOGRAM
793.#	THERMOGRAPHY
793.#	ULTRASOUND
793.#	X RAY

4th Digit: 793

- **0. SKULL AND HEAD**
- **1. LUNG FIELD**
- **2. OTHER INTRATHORACIC**
- **3. BILIARY TRACT**
- **4. GASTROINTESTINAL TRACT**
- **5. GENITOURINARY ORGANS**
- **6. ABDOMINAL AREA INCLUDING RETROPERITONEUM**
- **7. MUSCULOSKELETAL SYSTEM**
- **8. BREAST**
- **9. OTHER**

ABNORMAL URINALYSIS

791.4	BILIRUBINURIA
791.7	CELLS, CASTS
791.1	CHYLURIA
791.9	CRYSTALS OR OTHER
791.5	GLYCOSURIA, GLUCOSE
791.2	HEMOGLOBINURIA
791.6	KETONE ACETONE
791.3	MYOGLOBINURIA
791.0	PROTEINURIA ALBUMINURIA BENCE JONES
796.0	TOXICOLOGY

ABO INCOMPATIBILITY

773.1	CAUSING HEMOLYTIC DISEASE (FETUS) (NEWBORN)
773.1	FETUS OR NEWBORN
999.6	INFUSION OR TRANSFUSION REACTION
656.2#	MATERNAL AFFECTING MANAGEMENT OF MOTHER

5th Digit: 656.2

- **0. EPISODE OF CARE NOS OR N/A**
- **1. DELIVERED**
- **3. ANTEPARTUM COMPLICATION**

646.3# ABORTER HABITUAL WITH CURRENT PREGNANCY
5th Digit: 646.3
0. EPISODE OF CARE NOS OR N/A
1. DELIVERED
3. ANTEPARTUM COMPLICATION

629.9 ABORTER HABITUAL WITHOUT CURRENT PREGNANCY

ABORTION-REMOVAL OR EXTRACTION OF ALL OR PART OF PLACENTA OR MEMBRANE WITH OR WITHOUT AN IDENTIFIABLE FETUS WEIGHING LESS THAN 500 GRAMS OR OVER 22 WEEKS GESTATION. USE 644.21 EARLY ONSET DELIVERY, PREMATURE LABOR WITH ONSET OF DELIVERY BEFORE 37 WEEKS GESTATION.

SPONTANEOUS-OCCURS WITHOUT INSTRUMENTATION OR CHEMICAL INTERVENTION (634.##)

LEGALLY INDUCED-THERAPEUTIC OR ELECTIVE TERMINATION OF PREGNANCY (635.##)

ILLEGALLY INDUCED-AGAINST PROVISIONS OF STATE LAW OR REGULATORY REQUIREMENTS (WHEN A PATIENT HAS ABORTION PERFORMED OUTSIDE AND IS ADMITTED TO TREAT A COMPLICATION OR FOR COMPLETION) (636.#)

FAILED-PROCEDURE DOES NOT WORK, WOMAN IS STILL PREGNANT (638.#)

ABORTION

637.## UNSPECIFIED
638.# FAILED ATTEMPTED
636.## INDUCED - ILLEGALLY
635.## INDUCED - LEGALLY
4th Digit: 635, 636, 637, 638
0. WITH INFECTION
1. WITH DELAYED OR EXCESSIVE HEMORRHAGE
2. WITH DAMAGE TO PELVIC ORGANS OR TISSUE
3. WITH RENAL FAILURE
4. WITH METABOLIC DISORDER
5. WITH SHOCK
6. WITH EMBOLISM
7. WITH OTHER SPECIFIED COMPLICATIONS
8. WITH UNSPECIFIED COMPLICATION
9. UNCOMPLICATED
5th Digit: 635, 636, 637
0. UNSPECIFIED
1. INCOMPLETE
2. COMPLETE

632 MISSED <22 WEEKS
632 MISSED <22 WEEKS - WITH COMPLICATION DURING TREATMENT [**639.#**]
639.# MISSED <22 WEEKS - WITH COMPLICATION FOLLOWING TREATMENT
4th Digit: 639
0. GENITAL TRACT AND PELVIC INFECTION
1. DELAYED OR EXCESSIVE HEMORRHAGE
2. DAMAGE TO PELVIC ORGANS AND TISSUE
3. RENAL FAILURE
4. METABOLIC DISORDERS
5. SHOCK
6. EMBOLISM
8. OTHER SPECIFIED COMPLICATION
9. UNSPECIFIED COMPLICATION

639.0 SEPTIC
639.0 SEPTIC WITH SHOCK

ABORTION (continued)

634.## SPONTANEOUS <22 WEEKS
761.8 SPONTANEOUS <22 WEEKS - AFFECTING FETUS OR NEWBORN
635.## THERAPEUTIC
4th Digit: 634, 635
0. WITH INFECTION
1. WITH DELAYED OR EXCESSIVE HEMORRHAGE
2. WITH DAMAGE TO PELVIC ORGANS OR TISSUE
3. WITH RENAL FAILURE
4. WITH METABOLIC DISORDER
5. WITH SHOCK
6. WITH EMBOLISM
7. WITH OTHER SPECIFIED COMPLICATIONS
8. WITH UNSPECIFIED COMPLICATION
9. UNCOMPLICATED
5th Digit: 634, 635
0. UNSPECIFIED
1. INCOMPLETE
2. COMPLETE

640.0# THREATENED
5th Digit: 640.0
0. EPISODE OF CARE NOS OR N/A
1. DELIVERED
3. ANTEPARTUM COMPLICATION

759.89 ABRACHIOCEPHALIA
759.89 ABRACHIOCEPHALUS
283.9 ABRAMI'S DISEASE (ACQUIRED HEMOLYTIC JAUNDICE)

IF ABRASIONS ARE ASSOCIATED WITH AN UNDERLYING INJURY, SUCH AS A FRACTURE, CODE THE UNDERLYING INJURY ONLY. THE ABRASION IS INCIDENTAL TO THE INJURY.

ABRASION

919.0 SITE NOS
919.1 SITE NOS INFECTED
911.0 ABDOMINAL WALL
911.1 ABDOMINAL WALL INFECTED
916.0 ANKLE
916.1 ANKLE INFECTED
911.0 ANUS
911.1 ANUS INFECTED
912.0 ARM UPPER
912.1 ARM UPPER INFECTED
912.0 AXILLA
912.1 AXILLA INFECTED
911.0 BACK
911.1 BACK INFECTED
911.0 BREAST
911.1 BREAST INFECTED
911.0 BUTTOCK
911.1 BUTTOCK INFECTED
916.0 CALF
916.1 CALF INFECTED
910.0 CHEEK
910.1 CHEEK INFECTED
911.0 CHEST WALL
911.1 CHEST WALL INFECTED
918.2 CONJUNCTIVAL
918.1 CORNEA
910.0 EAR
910.1 EAR INFECTED
913.0 ELBOW
913.1 ELBOW INFECTED
918.9 EYE
918.0 EYELID AND PERIOCULAR AREA
910.0 FACE
910.1 FACE INFECTED

ABRASION (continued)

915.0	FINGER
915.1	FINGER INFECTED
911.0	FLANK
911.1	FLANK INFECTED
917.0	FOOT
917.1	FOOT INFECTED
913.0	FOREARM
913.1	FOREARM INFECTED
911.0	GROIN
911.1	GROIN INFECTED
910.0	GUM
910.1	GUM INFECTED
914.0	HAND
914.1	HAND INFECTED
917.0	HEEL
917.1	HEEL INFECTED
916.0	HIP
916.1	HIP INFECTED
911.0	INTERSCAPULAR REGION
911.1	INTERSCAPULAR REGION INFECTED
916.0	KNEE
916.1	KNEE INFECTED
911.0	LABIA
911.1	LABIA INFECTED
906.2	LATE EFFECT
916.0	LEG
916.1	LEG INFECTED
910.0	LIP
910.1	LIP INFECTED
919.0	MULTIPLE
919.1	MULTIPLE INFECTED
910.0	NECK
910.1	NECK INFECTED
910.0	NOSE
910.1	NOSE INFECTED
911.0	PENIS
911.1	PENIS INFECTED
911.0	PERINEUM
911.1	PERINEUM INFECTED
910.0	SCALP
910.1	SCALP INFECTED
912.0	SCAPULAR REGION
912.1	SCAPULAR REGION INFECTED
911.0	SCROTUM
911.1	SCROTUM INFECTED
912.0	SHOULDER
912.1	SHOULDER INFECTED
911.0	TESTIS
911.1	TESTIS INFECTED
916.0	THIGH
916.1	THIGH INFECTED
910.0	THROAT
910.1	THROAT INFECTED
915.0	THUMB
915.1	THUMB INFECTED
917.0	TOE
917.1	TOE INFECTED
911.0	TRUNK
911.1	TRUNK INFECTED
911.0	VAGINA
911.1	VAGINA INFECTED
911.0	VULVA
911.1	VULVA INFECTED
913.0	WRIST
913.1	WRIST INFECTED
919.0	OTHER SITES
919.1	OTHER SITES INFECTED

0 ABRIKOSSOV'S TUMOR BENIGN SITE SPECIFIED SEE 'BENIGN NEOPLASM' CONNECTIVE TISSUE M9580/0

0 ABRIKOSSOV'S TUMOR MALIGNANT SITE SPECIFIED SEE 'CANCER' CONNECTIVE TISSUE BY SITE M9580/3

641.2# ABRUPTIO PLACENTA

5th Digit: 641.2

- **0. EPISODE OF CARE NOS OR N/A**
- **1. DELIVERED**
- **3. ANTEPARTUM COMPLICATION**

762.1 ABRUPTIO PLACENTAE AFFECTING FETUS OR NEWBORN

> *WHEN CODING AN INFECTION, USE AN ADDITIONAL CODE, [041.#(#)], TO IDENTIFY THE ORGANISM. SEE 'BACTERIAL INFECTION'.*

ABSCESS

682.9	SITE NOS
567.2	ABDOMEN (ABDOMINAL CAVITY)
682.2	ABDOMINAL WALL
567.2	ABDOMINOPELVIC
474.9	ADENOID DISEASE NOS
474.10	ADENOID WITH TONSIL HYPERTROPHY
255.8	ADRENAL (CAPSULE) (GLAND)
522.5	ALVEOLAR (ORAL)
006.3	AMEBIC LIVER
566	ANAL REGIONS
682.6	ANKLE
682.3	ANTECUBITAL SPACE
540.1	APPENDIX WITH PERITONEAL ABSCESS
611.0	AREOLA
675.1#	AREOLA DUE TO PREGNANCY

5th Digit: 675.1

- **0. EPISODE OF CARE NOS OR N/A**
- **1. DELIVERED**
- **2. DELIVERED WITH POSTPARTUM COMPLICATION**
- **3. ANTEPARTUM COMPLICATION**
- **4. POSTPARTUM COMPLICATION**

682.3	ARM (ANY PART EXCEPT HAND)
447.2	ARTERY (WALL)
380.10	AUDITORY CANAL (EXTERNAL)
380.10	AURICLE (EAR)
380.10	AURICLE (EAR) STAPHYLOCOCCAL **[041.1#]**

5th Digit: 041.1

- **0. UNSPECIFIED**
- **1. AUREUS**
- **9. OTHER**

380.10 AURICLE (EAR) STREPTOCOCCAL **[041.0#]**

5th Digit: 041.0

- **0. NOS**
- **1. GROUP A**
- **2. GROUP B**
- **3. GROUP C**
- **4. GROUP D (ENTEROCOCCUS)**
- **5. GROUP G**
- **9. OTHER STREP**

682.3	AXILLA
682.2	BACK (ANY PART EXCEPT BUTTOCK)
616.3	BARTHOLIN'S GLAND (NONOBSTETRICAL)
595.89	BLADDER
006.8	BLADDER AMEBIC
730.0#	BONE ACUTE OR SUBACUTE
730.1#	BONE CHRONIC (OLD)
730.2#	BONE

5th Digit: 730.0-2

- **0. SITE NOS**
- **1. SHOULDER REGION**
- **2. UPPER ARM (ELBOW) (HUMERUS)**
- **3. FOREARM (RADIUS) (WRIST) (ULNA)**
- **4. HAND (CARPAL) (METACARPAL) (FINGERS)**
- **5. PELVIC REGION AND THIGH (HIP) (BUTTOCK) (FEMUR)**
- **6. LOWER LEG (FIBULA) (KNEE) (PATELLA) (TIBIA)**
- **7. ANKLE AND/OR FOOT (METATARSALS) (TOES) (TARSAL)**
- **8. OTHER (HEAD) (NECK) (RIB) (SKULL) (TRUNK)**
- **9. MULTIPLE**

ABSCESS (continued)

324.0 BRAIN
006.5 BRAIN AMEBIC
324.0 BRAIN CEREBELLAR
324.0 BRAIN CYSTIC
324.1 BRAIN INTRASPINAL
324.0 BRAIN OTOGENIC
013.3# BRAIN TUBERCULOUS

5th Digit: 013.3

0. NOS
1. LAB NOT DONE
2. LABS PENDING
3. MICROSCOPY POSITIVE (IN SPUTUM)
4. CULTURE POSITIVE - MICROSCOPY NEGATIVE
5. CULTURE NEGATIVE - MICROSCOPY POSITIVE
6. CULTURE AND MICROSCOPY NEGATIVE CONFIRMED BY OTHER METHODS

611.0 BREAST
680.2 BREAST CARBUNCLE
675.1# BREAST MATERNAL DUE TO PREGNANCY

5th Digit: 675.1

0. EPISODE OF CARE NOS OR N/A
1. DELIVERED
2. DELIVERED WITH POSTPARTUM COMPLICATION
3. ANTEPARTUM COMPLICATION
4. POSTPARTUM COMPLICATION

614.3 BROAD LIGAMENT ACUTE
614.4 BROAD LIGAMENT CHRONIC OR UNSPECIFIED
016.7# BROAD LIGAMENT TUBERCULOUS

5th Digit: 016.7

0. NOS
1. LAB NOT DONE
2. LABS PENDING
3. MICROSCOPY POSITIVE (IN SPUTUM)
4. CULTURE POSITIVE - MICROSCOPY NEGATIVE
5. CULTURE NEGATIVE - MICROSCOPY POSITIVE
6. CULTURE AND MICROSCOPY NEGATIVE CONFIRMED BY OTHER METHODS

528.3 BUCCAL CAVITY
597.0 BULBOURETHRAL GLAND
727.89 BURSA
682.5 BUTTOCK
372.20 CANTHUS

> *WHEN CODING AN INFECTION OF AN OSTOMY, USE AN ADDITIONAL CODE TO SPECIFY THE ORGANISM. SEE 'BACTERIAL INFECTION'*

569.61 CECOSTOMY WITH ABSCESS OF ABDOMEN [682.2]
013.3# CEREBELLAR (CEREBRAL) TUBERCULOUS

5th Digit: 013.3

0. NOS
1. LAB NOT DONE
2. LABS PENDING
3. MICROSCOPY POSITIVE (IN SPUTUM)
4. CULTURE POSITIVE - MICROSCOPY NEGATIVE
5. CULTURE NEGATIVE - MICROSCOPY POSITIVE
6. CULTURE AND MICROSCOPY NEGATIVE CONFIRMED BY OTHER METHODS

324.0 CEREBELLAR (EMBOLIC)
324.0 CEREBRAL (EMBOLIC)
616.0 CERVIX (STUMP) (UTERI)
682.0 CHEEK (EXTERNAL)
682.2 CHEST WALL
682.0 CHIN
363.00 CHOROID
364.3 CILIARY BODY
569.5 COLON (WALL)

ABSCESS (continued)

> *WHEN CODING AN INFECTION OF AN OSTOMY, USE AN ADDITIONAL CODE TO SPECIFY THE ORGANISM. SEE 'BACTERIAL INFECTION'*

569.61 COLOSTOMY WITH ABSCESS OF ABDOMEN [682.2]
372.00 CONJUNCTIVA
682.9 CONNECTIVE TISSUE NEC
370.55 CORNEAL
370.00 CORNEAL WITH ULCERATION
597.0 COWPER'S GLAND
522.5 DENTAL
522.5 DENTOALVEOLAR
681.9 DIGIT
380.10 EAR (EXTERNAL AUDITORY CANAL)
380.11 EAR (PINNA)
682.3 ELBOW

> *WHEN CODING AN INFECTION OF AN OSTOMY, USE AN ADDITIONAL CODE TO SPECIFY THE ORGANISM. SEE 'BACTERIAL INFECTION'*

569.61 ENTEROSTOMY WITH ABSCESS OF ABDOMEN [682.2]
604.0 EPIDIDYMIS
604.0 EPIDIDYMIS E. COLI [041.4]
604.0 EPIDIDYMIS HEMOPHILUS INFLUENZA [041.5]
604.0 EPIDIDYMIS KLEBSIELLA [041.3]
604.0 EPIDIDYMIS PNEUMOCOCCUS [041.2]
604.0 EPIDIDYMIS PNEUMONIAE [041.89]
604.0 EPIDIDYMIS PROTEUS [041.6]
604.0 EPIDIDYMIS PSEUDOMONAS [041.7]
604.0 EPIDIDYMIS STAPHYLOCOCCAL **[041.1#]**

5th Digit: 041.1

0. UNSPECIFIED
1. AUREUS
9. OTHER

604.0 EPIDIDYMIS STREPTOCOCCAL **[041.0#]**

5th Digit: 041.0

0. NOS
1. GROUP A
2. GROUP B
3. GROUP C
4. GROUP D (ENTEROCOCCUS)
5. GROUP G
9. OTHER STREP

604.0 EPIDIDYMIS OTHER SPECIFIED **[041.8#]**

5th Digit: 041.8

1. MYCOPLASMA, EATON'S AGENT, PPLO
2. BACILLUS FRAGILIS
3. CLOSTRIDIUM PERFRINGENS
4. OTHER ANAEROBES
5. AEROBACTER AEROGENES, MIMA POLYMORPHA, SERRATIA, (OTHER GRAM-NEGATIVE)
9. OTHER SPECIFIED BACTERIA

324.0 EPIDURAL (EMBOLIC) BRAIN
324.1 EPIDURAL (EMBOLIC) SPINAL
013.5# EPIDURAL SPINAL CORD TUBERCULOUS

5th Digit: 013.5

0. NOS
1. LAB NOT DONE
2. LABS PENDING
3. MICROSCOPY POSITIVE (IN SPUTUM)
4. CULTURE POSITIVE - MICROSCOPY NEGATIVE
5. CULTURE NEGATIVE - MICROSCOPY POSITIVE
6. CULTURE AND MICROSCOPY NEGATIVE CONFIRMED BY OTHER METHODS

478.79 EPIGLOTTIS
530.19 ESOPHAGUS
380.10 EXTERNAL EAR CANAL
324.9 EXTRADURAL - NOS
324.0 EXTRADURAL - BRAIN (EMBOLIC)
324.1 EXTRADURAL - SPINAL CORD (EMBOLIC)
360.00 EYE
373.13 EYELID

ABSCESS (continued)

682.0 FACE
614.2 FALLOPIAN TUBE
728.89 FASCIA
681.01 FELON
681.00 FINGER
681.01 FINGER FELON
681.02 FINGERNAIL
682.2 FLANK
682.7 FOOT (EXCEPT TOES)
682.3 FOREARM
682.0 FOREHEAD
575.0 GALLBLADDER (SEE ALSO 'CHOLECYSTITIS', ACUTE)

WHEN CODING AN INFECTION OF AN OSTOMY, USE AN ADDITIONAL CODE TO SPECIFY THE ORGANISM. SEE 'BACTERIAL INFECTION'

536.41 GASTROSTOMY WITH ABSCESS OF ABDOMEN [682.2]
523.3 GINGIVAL
682.5 GLUTEAL REGION
682.2 GROIN
682.4 HAND (EXCEPT FINGERS AND THUMB)
682.8 HEAD (EXCEPT FACE)
429.89 HEART
682.7 HEEL
682.6 HIP

WHEN CODING AN INFECTION OF AN OSTOMY, USE AN ADDITIONAL CODE TO SPECIFY THE ORGANISM. SEE 'BACTERIAL INFECTION'

569.61 ILEOSTOMY WITH ABSCESS OF ABDOMEN [682.2]
569.5 ILEUM
540.1 ILIAC FOSSA
682.2 ILIAC REGION
683 INGUINAL LYMPH GLAND OR NODE
682.2 INGUINAL REGION
540.1 INTESTINAL APPENDICEAL
569.5 INTESTINAL NONAPPENDICEAL
997.4 INTESTINAL POSTOPERATIVE
560.81 INTESTINAL WITH OBSTRUCTION ADHESIVE
324.0 INTRACRANIAL (EMBOLIC)
326 INTRACRANIAL (LATE EFFECTS)
324.1 INTRASPINAL
324.1 INTRASPINAL (SPINAL) (EMBOLIC)
364.3 IRIS
566 ISCHIORECTAL
682.0 JAW
526.4 JAW (ACUTE CHRONIC SUPPURATIVE)
682.0 JAW (SKIN)

WHEN CODING AN INFECTION OF AN OSTOMY, USE AN ADDITIONAL CODE TO SPECIFY THE ORGANISM. SEE 'BACTERIAL INFECTION'

569.61 JEJUNOSTOMY WITH ABSCESS OF ABDOMEN [682.2]
0 JOINT SEE 'ARTHRITIS OTHER SPECIFIED' PYOGENIC
590.2 KIDNEY
616.4 LABIA (MAJUS) (MINUS)
375.30 LACRIMAL (PASSAGES) (SAC)
375.00 LACRIMAL GLAND
373.31 LACRIMAL SYSTEM
478.79 LARYNX
682.6 LEG (EXCEPT FOOT)
528.5 LIP
597.0 LITTRE'S GLAND
572.0 LIVER
006.3 LIVER (AMEBIC)
513.0 LUNG
006.4 LUNG (AMEBIC)
513.0 LUNG (MULTIPLE)
683 LYMPH GLAND OR NODE
0 LYMPH GLAND SEE ALSO 'LYMPHADENITIS'
683 LYMPH LYMPHATIC GLAND OR NODE (ACUTE)

ABSCESS (continued)

0 MAMMARY GLAND SUBMAMMARY SEE 'ABSCESS' BREAST
383.00 MASTOID
383.01 MASTOID SUBPERIOSTEAL
513.1 MEDIASTINUM
567.2 MESENTERIC
567.2 MESENTERIC (SUPPURATIVE PERITONITIS)
682.2 MONS PUBIS
528.3 MOUTH
681.9 NAIL
478.1 NASAL SEPTUM
0 NASAL SINUS SEE 'SINUSITIS' CHRONIC
478.29 NASOPHARYNX
682.1 NECK
675.0# NIPPLE MATERNAL DUE TO PREGNANCY

5th Digit: 675.0
0. EPISODE OF CARE NOS OR N/A
1. DELIVERED
2. DELIVERED WITH POSTPARTUM COMPLICATION
3. ANTEPARTUM COMPLICATION
4. POSTPARTUM COMPLICATION

682.0 NOSE (EXTERNAL)
478.1 NOSE (INTERNAL)
478.1 NOSE (SEPTUM)
567.2 OMENTUM
681.02 ONYCHIA FINGER
681.11 ONYCHIA TOE
998.59 OPERATIVE WOUND
376.01 ORBIT
324.0 OTOGENIC (EMBOLIC)
526.4 PALATE - HARD
528.3 PALATE - SOFT
577.0 PANCREAS
523.3 PARADONTAL
614.3 PARAMETRIC PARAMETRIUM (ACUTE)
614.4 PARAMETRIC PARAMETRIUM (CHRONIC)
478.22 PARAPHARYNGEAL
681.02 PARONYCHIA FINGER
681.11 PARONYCHIA TOE
527.3 PAROTID (DUCT) (GLAND)
528.3 PAROTID REGION
682.2 PECTORAL REGION
614.3 PELVIC (FEMALE) ACUTE
614.4 PELVIC (FEMALE) CHRONIC OR UNSPECIFIED
567.2 PELVIC (MALE)
016.7# PELVIC TUBERCULOUS (FEMALE)

5th Digit: 016.7
0. NOS
1. LAB NOT DONE
2. LABS PENDING
3. MICROSCOPY POSITIVE (IN SPUTUM)
4. CULTURE POSITIVE - MICROSCOPY NEGATIVE
5. CULTURE NEGATIVE - MICROSCOPY POSITIVE
6. CULTURE AND MICROSCOPY NEGATIVE CONFIRMED BY OTHER METHODS

567.2 PELVIRECTAL
607.2 PENIS
566 PERIANAL
522.7 PERIAPICAL (TOOTH) (WITH SINUS)
522.5 PERIAPICAL (TOOTH) (WITHOUT SINUS)
540.1 PERIAPPENDICEAL
590.2 PERINEPHRIC
682.2 PERINEUM
523.3 PERIODONTAL

A

ABSCESS (continued)

730.3# PERIOSTEUM
5th Digit: 730.3
0. SITE NOS
1. SHOULDER REGION
2. UPPER ARM (ELBOW) (HUMERUS)
3. FOREARM (RADIUS) (WRIST) (ULNA)
4. HAND (CARPAL) (METACARPAL) (FINGERS)
5. PELVIC REGION AND THIGH (HIP) (BUTTOCK) (FEMUR)
6. LOWER LEG (FIBULA) (KNEE) (PATELLA) (TIBIA)
7. ANKLE AND/OR FOOT (METATARSALS) (TOES) (TARSALS)
8. OTHER (HEAD) (NECK) (RIB) (SKULL) (TRUNK) (VERTEBRAE)
9. MULTIPLE

566 PERIRECTAL (ANAL RECTAL REGIONS)
590.2 PERIRENAL (TISSUE)
567.2 PERITONEUM
998.59 PERITONEUM POSTOPERATIVE
475 PERITONSILLAR
614.2 PERITUBAL
593.89 PERIURETERAL
597.0 PERIURETHRAL
595.89 PERIVESICAL
478.29 PHARYNX
685.0 PILONIDAL (CYST) (FISTULA) (SINUS)
253.8 PITUITARY
510.9 PLEURA
510.0 PLEURA WITH FISTULA
682.6 POPLITEAL
998.59 POSTOPERATIVE
614.4 POUCH OF DOUGLAS (CHRONIC OR NOS)
016.7# POUCH OF DOUGLAS TUBERCULOUS
5th Digit: 016.7
0. NOS
1. LAB NOT DONE
2. LABS PENDING
3. MICROSCOPY POSITIVE (IN SPUTUM)
4. CULTURE POSITIVE - MICROSCOPY NEGATIVE
5. CULTURE NEGATIVE - MICROSCOPY POSITIVE
6. CULTURE AND MICROSCOPY NEGATIVE CONFIRMED BY OTHER METHODS

682.6 PREPATELLAR
601.2 PROSTATE
511.0 PULMONARY
566 RECTAL
566 RECTAL SUBMUCOSAL
590.2 RENAL AND PERINEPHRIC
363.00 RETINA
376.01 RETROBULBAR
567.2 RETROCECAL
567.2 RETROPERITONEAL
478.24 RETROPHARYNGEAL
566 RETRORECTAL
527.3 SALIVARY GLAND
682.8 SCALP
355.0 SCIATIC NERVE
379.09 SCLERAL
017.2# SCROFULOUS
5th Digit: 017.2
0. NOS
1. LAB NOT DONE
2. LABS PENDING
3. MICROSCOPY POSITIVE (IN SPUTUM)
4. CULTURE POSITIVE - MICROSCOPY NEGATIVE
5. CULTURE NEGATIVE - MICROSCOPY POSITIVE
6. CULTURE AND MICROSCOPY NEGATIVE CONFIRMED BY OTHER METHODS

ABSCESS (continued)

608.4 SCROTUM (SPERMATIC CORD)
608.0 SEMINAL VESICLE
478.1 SEPTUM (NASAL)
682.3 SHOULDER
597.0 SKENE'S DUCT OR GLAND
682.9 SKIN NEC
608.4 SPERMATIC CORD
013.5# SPINAL CORD (TUBERCULOUS)
5th Digit: 013.5
0. NOS
1. LAB NOT DONE
2. LABS PENDING
3. MICROSCOPY POSITIVE (IN SPUTUM)
4. CULTURE POSITIVE - MICROSCOPY NEGATIVE
5. CULTURE NEGATIVE - MICROSCOPY POSITIVE
6. CULTURE AND MICROSCOPY NEGATIVE CONFIRMED BY OTHER METHODS

289.59 SPLEEN
998.59 STITCH
324.9 SUBARACHNOID
324.0 SUBARACHNOID (BRAIN) (CEREBRAL)
567.2 SUBDIAPHRAGMATIC
324.9 SUBDURAL - NOS
324.0 SUBDURAL - BRAIN (INTRACRANIAL) (EMBOLIC)
324.1 SUBDURAL - SPINAL CORD (EMBOLIC)
013.3# SUBDURAL TUBERCULOUS - BRAIN
013.5# SUBDURAL TUBERCULOUS - SPINAL CORD
5th Digit: 013.3, 5
0. NOS
1. LAB NOT DONE
2. LABS PENDING
3. MICROSCOPY POSITIVE (IN SPUTUM)
4. CULTURE POSITIVE - MICROSCOPY NEGATIVE
5. CULTURE NEGATIVE - MICROSCOPY POSITIVE
6. CULTURE AND MICROSCOPY NEGATIVE CONFIRMED BY OTHER METHODS

567.2 SUBHEPATIC
528.3 SUBLINGUAL
527.3 SUBLINGUAL GLAND
682.0 SUBMANDIBULAR
527.3 SUBMANDIBULAR GLAND
682.0 SUBMAXILLARY
527.3 SUBMAXILLARY GLAND
682.0 SUBMENTAL (PYOGENIC)
527.3 SUBMENTAL GLAND
566 SUBMUCOSAL, RECTUM
567.2 SUBPHRENIC
998.59 SUBPHRENIC POSTOPERATIVE
682.2 SUBSCAPULAR
681.9 SUBUNGUAL
682.3 SUPRACLAVICULAR (FOSSA)
566 SUPRALEVATOR
682.0 TEMPLE REGION
727.89 TENDON
604.0 TESTIS
604.0 TESTIS E. COLI [041.4]
604.0 TESTIS HEMOPHILUS INFLUENZA [041.5]
604.0 TESTIS KLEBSIELLA [041.3]
604.0 TESTIS PNEUMOCOCCUS [041.2]
604.0 TESTIS PNEUMONIAE [041.89]
604.0 TESTIS PROTEUS [041.6]
604.0 TESTIS STAPHYLOCOCCAL [**041.1#**]
5th Digit: 041.1
0. UNSPECIFIED
1. AUREUS
9. OTHER

ABSCESS (continued)

604.0 TESTIS STREPTOCOCCAL [**041.0#**]

5th Digit: 041.0

0. NOS
1. GROUP A
2. GROUP B
3. GROUP C
4. GROUP D (ENTEROCOCCUS)
5. GROUP G
9. OTHER STREP

604.0 TESTIS OTHER SPECIFIED [**041.8#**]

5th Digit: 041.8

1. MYCOPLASMA, EATON'S AGENT, PPLO
2. BACILLUS FRAGILIS
3. CLOSTRIDIUM PERFRINGENS
4. OTHER ANAEROBES
5. AEROBACTER AEROGENES, MIMA POLYMORPHA, SERRATIA, (OTHER GRAM-NEGATIVE)
9. OTHER SPECIFIED BACTERIA

682.6 THIGH
510.9 THORAX
681.00 THUMB
254.1 THYMUS
681.10 TOE
681.11 TOE (ONYCHIA) (PARONYCHIA)
681.11 TOENAIL
529.0 TONGUE
522.5 TOOTH TEETH (ROOT)
478.9 TRACHEA

WHEN CODING AN INFECTION OF AN OSTOMY, USE AN ADDITIONAL CODE TO SPECIFY THE ORGANISM. SEE 'BACTERIAL INFECTION'

519.01 TRACHEOSTOMY WITH ABSCESS OF NECK [682.1]
682.2 TRUNK
614.2 TUBO OVARIAN
614.6 TUBO OVARIAN WITH ADHESIONS (POSTOPERATIVE) (POSTINFECTION)
608.4 TUNICA VAGINALIS
682.2 UMBILICUS
771.4 UMBILICUS (NEWBORN)
593.89 URETER
597.0 URETHRA
599.3 URETHRAL (CARUNCLE)
615.9 UTERUS - NOS
615.0 UTERUS - ACUTE
760.8 UTERUS - AFFECTING FETUS OR NEWBORN
615.1 UTERUS - CHRONIC
670.0# UTERUS - MAJOR MATERNAL DUE TO PREGNANCY (PUERPERAL)

5th Digit: 670.0

0. NOS
2. DELIVERED WITH POSTPARTUM COMPLICATION
4. POSTPARTUM COMPLICATION

364.3 UVEITIS
528.3 UVULA
623.2 VAGINA (CHRONIC) (POSTOPERATIVE) (POSTRADIATION)
616.10 VAGINA (WALL)
616.10 VAGINORECTAL
608.4 VAS DEFERENS
360.04 VITREOUS
478.5 VOCAL CORD
616.4 VULVA (NONOBSTETRICAL)
616.3 VULVOVAGINAL GLAND
682.4 WRIST

0 ABSENCE SEE ANATOMICAL SITE
117.7 ABSIDIA INFECTION

304.6# ABSINTHE ADDICTION

5th Digit: 304.6

0. NOS
1. CONTINUOUS
2. EPISODIC
3. IN REMISSION

291.81 ABSTINENCE ALCOHOL SYNDROME
292.0 ABSTINENCE DRUG SYNDROME
202.5# ABT-LETTERER-SIWE SYNDROME (ACUTE HISTIOCYTOSIS X) M9722/3

5th Digit: 202.5

0. UNSPECIFIED SITE, EXTRANODAL AND SOLID ORGAN SITES
1. LYMPH NODES OF HEAD FACE NECK
2. LYMPH NODES INTRATHORACIC
3. LYMPH NODES ABDOMINAL
4. LYMPH NODES AXILLA AND UPPER LIMB
5. LYMPH NODES INGUINAL REGION AND LOWER LIMB
6. LYMPH NODES INTRAPELVIC
7. SPLEEN
8. LYMPH NODES MULTIPLE SITES

WHEN THE CAUSE OF AN INJURY IS STATED TO BE ABUSE, MULTIPLE CODES SHOULD BE ASSIGNED, IF APPLICABLE, TO IDENTIFY ANY ASSOCIATED INJURIES. THEY ARE TO BE SEQUENCED IN THE FOLLOWING ORDER:

1. TYPE OF ABUSE - CHILD OR ADULT (995.5, 995.8)

2. TYPE OF INJURY

3. PERPETRATOR OF THE ABUSE - SEE E-CODE DIRECTORY 'ASSAULT' (E967)

4. NATURE OF THE ABUSE - SEE E-CODE DIRECTORY 'ASSAULT' (E904.0, E960-E966, E968)

ABUSE

995.8# ADULT (VICTIM)

5th Digit: 995.8

0. MALTREATMENT UNSPECIFIED
1. PHYSICAL, BATTERY
2. EMOTIONAL / PSYCHOLOGICAL (DEPRIVATION)
3. SEXUAL
4. NEGLECT (NUTRITIONAL), DESERTION
5. OTHER ABUSE AND NEGLECT, MULTIPLE FORMS

V61.12 ADULT COUNSELING - SPOUSAL (PARTNER) PERPETRATOR
V61.11 ADULT COUNSELING - SPOUSAL (PARTNER) V!CTIM
V62.83 ADULT COUNSELING - OTHER PERPETRATOR OF PHYSICAL / SEXUAL ABUSE NEC
V62.89 ADULT COUNSELING - OTHER VICTIM
995.84 ADULT DESERTION
V71.6 ADULT EVALUATION - BATTERY (ALLEGED)
V71.5 ADULT EVALUATION - SEXUAL (ALLEGED)
V15.4# ADULT HISTORY

5th Digit: V15.4

1. PHYSICAL ABUSE, RAPE
2. EMOTIONAL ABUSE, NEGLECT
9. OTHER PSYCHOLOGICAL TRAUMA

ABUSE (continued)

SUBSTANCE ABUSE DESCRIBES THE PRACTICE OF USING DRUGS OR ALCOHOL TO EXCESS WITHOUT REACHING THE STATE OF PHYSICAL DEPENDENCE. SUBSTANCE DEPENDENCE IS ADDICTION. DEPENDENCE INVOLVES THE LOSS OF CONTROL AND JUDGMENT AND/OR THE INABILITY TO USE IN MODERATION. DEPENDENCE IS MARKED BY COMPULSIVE PHYSICAL DEMANDS WHICH ARE TRIGGERED BY FURTHER INGESTION.

303.0# ALCOHOL - DEPENDENT
305.0# ALCOHOL - NONDEPENDENT
5th Digit: 303.0, 305.0
0. NOS
1. CONTINUOUS
2. EPISODIC
3. IN REMISSION

V65.42 ALCOHOL COUNSELING
V11.3 ALCOHOL HISTORY

WHEN THE CAUSE OF AN INJURY IS STATED TO BE ABUSE, MULTIPLE CODES SHOULD BE ASSIGNED, IF APPLICABLE, TO IDENTIFY ANY ASSOCIATED INJURIES. THEY ARE TO BE SEQUENCED IN THE FOLLOWING ORDER:

1. TYPE OF ABUSE - CHILD OR ADULT (995.5, 995.8)

2. TYPE OF INJURY

3. PERPETRATOR OF THE ABUSE - SEE E-CODE DIRECTORY 'ASSAULT' (E967)

4. NATURE OF THE ABUSE - SEE E-CODE DIRECTORY 'ASSAULT' (E904.0, E960-E966, E968)

995.5# CHILD (VICTIM)
5th Digit: 995.5
0. UNSPECIFIED
1. EMOTIONAL / PSYCHOLOGICAL (DEPRIVATION)
2. NEGLECT (NUTRITIONAL), DESERTION
3. SEXUAL
4. PHYSICAL
5. SHAKEN INFANT SYNDROME
9. OTHER ABUSE AND NEGLECT, MULTIPLE FORMS

V61.22 CHILD COUNSELING - PERPETRATOR PARENTAL CHILD ABUSE
V62.83 CHILD COUNSELING - OTHER PERPETRATOR OF PHYSICAL / SEXUAL ABUSE
V61.21 CHILD COUNSELING - VICTIM
995.52 CHILD DESERTION
V71.6 CHILD EVALUATION - BATTERY (ALLEGED)
V71.5 CHILD EVALUATION - SEXUAL (ALLEGED)
V15.4# CHILD HISTORY
5th Digit: V15.4
1. PHYSICAL ABUSE, RAPE
2. EMOTIONAL ABUSE, NEGLECT
9. OTHER PSYCHOLOGICAL TRAUMA

304.## DRUG - DEPENDENT (ADDICTION)
4th Digit: 304
0. OPIOID
1. BARBITURATE, SEDATIVES, AND TRANQUILIZERS WITH A SIMILAR EFFECT
2. COCAINE
3. CANNABIS
4. AMPHETAMINE TYPE
5. HALLUCINOGENIC
6. OTHER SPECIFIED
7. MIXED WITH OPIOID
8. MIXED
9. NOS

5th Digit: 304
0. NOS
1. CONTINUOUS
2. EPISODIC
3. IN REMISSION

ABUSE (continued)

SUBSTANCE ABUSE NONDEPENDENT DESCRIBES THE PRACTICE OF USING DRUGS OR ALCOHOL TO EXCESS WITHOUT REACHING THE STATE OF PHYSICAL DEPENDENCE.

305.## DRUG - NONDEPENDENT (ABUSE)
4th Digit: 305
0. ALCOHOL
2. CANNABIS
3. HALLUCINOGEN
4. BARBITURATE, SEDATIVE, OR HYPNOTIC WITH A SIMILAR EFFECT
5. OPIOID
6. COCAINE
7. AMPHETAMINE TYPE
8. ANTIDEPRESSANT TYPE
9. MIXED OR OTHER SPECIFIED

5th Digit: 305
0. NOS
1. CONTINUOUS
2. EPISODIC
3. IN REMISSION

V65.42 DRUG COUNSELING
V11.8 DRUG HISTORY

648.3# : CODE THE SPECIFIC MATERNAL DRUG ABUSE OR DEPENDENCE WITH AN ADDITIONAL CODE. SEE 'ABUSE' DRUG.

648.3# DRUG MATERNAL CURRENT (CO-EXISTENT) IN PREGNANCY
5th Digit: 648.3
0. EPISODE OF CARE UNSPECIFIED OR N/A
1. DELIVERED
2. DELIVERED WITH POSTPARTUM COMPLICATION
3. ANTEPARTUM COMPLICATION
4. POSTPARTUM COMPLICATION

655.5# DRUG MATERNAL IN PREGNANCY WITH SUSPECTED DAMAGE TO FETUS
5th Digit: 655.5
0. EPISODE OF CARE UNSPECIFIED OR N/A
1. DELIVERED
3. ANTEPARTUM COMPLICATION

V15.4# HISTORY (ADULT) (CHILD)
5th Digit: V15.4
1. PHYSICAL ABUSE, RAPE
2. EMOTIONAL ABUSE, NEGLECT
9. OTHER PSYCHOLOGICAL TRAUMA

0 SUBSTANCE SEE 'ABUSE', DRUG
V65.42 SUBSTANCE COUNSELING
305.1 TOBACCO NONDEPENDENT

313.83 ACADEMIC UNDERACHIEVEMENT DISORDER (EMOTIONAL DISTURBANCES OF CHILDHOOD OR ADOLESCENCE)

275.40 ACALCEROSIS
275.40 ACALCICOSIS
784.69 ACALCULIA NOS (AUDITORY) (VISUAL) (ORGANIC)

125.4 ACANTHOCHEILONEMA PERSTANS INFECTION
125.6 ACANTHOCHEILONEMA STREPTOCERCA INFECTION

530.89 ACANTHOSIS GLYCOGENIC ESOPHAGUS
701.2 ACANTHOSIS NIGRICANS ACQUIRED

ACARIASIS
133.9 NOS
133.8 DEMODEX FOLLICULORUM
133.0 SCABIES
133.8 OTHER SPECIFIED

333.99 ACATHISIA DUE TO DRUGS

ACCESSORY

755.56 CARPAL BONE
755.01 FINGERS
752.49 HYMEN
748.69 LOBE OF LUNG
756.82 MUSCLE ANOMALIES OTHER SPECIFIED CONGENITAL
757.6 NIPPLE
752.0 OVARY CONGENITAL
755.00 POLYDACTYLY, UNSPECIFIED DIGITS
755.02 TOES
744.1 TRAGUS CONGENITAL
753.4 URETER

ACCESSORY NERVE

352.4 ATROPHY
352.4 DISORDER
951.6 INJURY
352.4 NEURITIS

ACCOMMODATION

367.9 DISORDER
367.89 DISORDER DRUG INDUCED OR TOXIC
367.51 PARESIS
367.53 SPASM

V62.4 ACCULTURATION PROBLEM
718.6# ACETABULUM UNSPECIFIED INTRAPELVIC PROTRUSION

5th Digit: 718.6

0. SITE NOS
5. PELVIC REGION AND THIGH (HIP) (BUTTOCK) (FEMUR)

736.39 ACETABULUM WANDERING
791.6 ACETONURIA
286.3 AC GLOBULIN DEFICIENCY
286.7 AC GLOBULIN DEFICIENCY ACQUIRED
530.0 ACHALASIA (OF CARDIA)
255.2 ACHARD-THIERS (ADRENOGENITAL) SYNDROME

ACHILLES

726.71 TENDINITIS
727.81 TENDON CONTRACTURE
845.09 TENDON LACERATION
892.2 TENDON LACERATION (WITH OPEN WOUND)
727.67 TENDON RUPTURE NONTRAUMATIC

536.0 ACHLORHYDRIA
756.4 ACHONDROPLASIA CONGENITAL
709.00 ACHROMA CUTIS
368.54 ACHROMATOPSIA
316 ACHROMATOPSIA PSYCHOGENIC [368.54]
536.3 ACHYLIA GASTRICA NEUROGENIC
656.8# ACID BASE BALANCE ABNORMAL AFFECTING MANAGEMENT OF MOTHER

5th Digit: 656.8

0. EPISODE OF CARE UNSPECIFIED OR N/A
1. DELIVERED
3. ANTEPARTUM COMPLICATION

276.9 ACID BASE BALANCE DISORDER
276.4 ACID BASE BALANCE DISORDER MIXED (WITH HYPERCAPNIA)
536.8 ACID PEPTIC DISEASE
790.5 ACID PHOSPHATASE ABNORMAL BLOOD LEVEL
997.3 ACID PULMONARY ASPIRATION SYNDROME
668.0# ACID PULMONARY ASPIRATION SYNDROME - OBSTETRIC (MENDELSON'S)

5th Digit: 668.0

0. EPISODE OF CARE NOS OR N/A
1. DELIVERED
2. DELIVERED WITH POSTPARTUM COMPLICATION
3. ANTEPARTUM COMPLICATION
4. POSTPARTUM COMPLICATION

ACIDEMIA

276.2 NOS
270.6 ARGINOSUCCINIC
768.2 FETAL LIVEBORN - BEFORE ONSET OF LABOR
768.3 FETAL LIVEBORN - DURING LABOR
768.4 FETAL LIVEBORN - UNSPECIFIED AS TO TIME OF ONSET
270.7 PIPECOLIC

ACIDOPHIL

194.3 CARCINOMA SITE NOS
0 CARCINOMA SITE SPECIFIED SEE 'CANCER' BY SITE M8280/3
194.3 BASOPHIL CARCINOMA (MIXED) SITE NOS
0 BASOPHIL CARCINOMA (MIXED) SITE SPECIFIED SEE 'CANCER' BY SITE M8281/3

ACIDOSIS

276.2 NOS
656.8# FETAL AFFECTING MANAGEMENT OF MOTHER

5th Digit: 656.8

0. EPISODE OF CARE UNSPECIFIED OR N/A
1. DELIVERED
3. ANTEPARTUM COMPLICATION

770.8 FETAL AFFECTING NEWBORN
250.1# KETOACIDOSIS
250.3# KETOACIDOSIS WITH COMA

5th Digit: 250.1, 3

0. TYPE II, ADULT-ONSET, NON-INSULIN DEPENDENT (EVEN IF REQUIRING INSULIN), OR UNSPECIFIED; CONTROLLED
1. TYPE I, JUVENILE-ONSET OR INSULIN-DEPENDENT; CONTROLLED
2. TYPE II, ADULT-ONSET, NON-INSULIN DEPENDENT (EVEN IF REQUIRING INSULIN); UNCONTROLLED
3. TYPE I, JUVENILE-ONSET OR INSULIN-DEPENDENT; UNCONTROLLED

276.2 LACTIC
276.2 METABOLIC
775.7 METABOLIC NEWBORN (LATE)
588.8 RENAL TUBULAR
276.2 RESPIRATORY
276.4 RESPIRATORY COMPLICATED BY METABOLIC ACIDOSIS

CARCINOMAS AND NEOPLASMS SHOULD BE CODED BY SITE IF POSSIBLE. CODE BY CELL TYPE - "SITE NOS", IF AND ONLY IF A SITE IS NOT SPECIFIED IN THE DIAGNOSIS. OTHERWISE - REFER TO THE APPROPRIATE CATEGORY OF NEOPLASM FOR A MORE SPECIFIC CODE: SEE 'CANCER' 'CANCER METASTATIC', 'NEOPLASM UNCERTAIN BEHAVIOR', 'NEOPLASM UNSPECIFIED NATURE', OR 'BENIGN NEOPLASM'.

229.9 ACINAR CELL ADENOMA NOS
0 ACINAR CELL ADENOMA SITE SPECIFIED SEE 'BENIGN NEOPLASM', BY SITE M8550/0
199.1 ACINAR CELL CARCINOMA SITE NOS
0 ACINAR CELL CARCINOMA SITE SPECIFIED SEE 'CANCER' BY SITE M8550/3
238.9 ACINAR CELL TUMOR SITE NOS
0 ACINAR CELL TUMOR SITE SPECIFIED SEE 'NEOPLASM UNCERTAIN BEHAVIOR' BY SITE M8550/1

0 ACL (ANTERIOR CRUCIATE LIGAMENT) SEE 'ANTERIOR', CRUCIATE

ACNE

706.1 NOS
706.1 CONGLOBATA
706.1 CONJUNCTIVA
706.1 CYSTIC
695.3 ERYTHEMATOSA
706.0 FRONTALIS
706.0 NECROTICA
706.1 PUSTULAR

ACNE (continued)
695.3 ROSACEA
692.72 SUMMER
706.0 VARIOLIFORMIS
706.1 VULGARIS

993.2 ACOSTA'S DISEASE

ACOUSTIC
742.8 NERVE ABSENCE CONGENITAL
388.5 NERVE DEGENERATION (ATROPHY)
388.5 NERVE DISORDER
388.5 NEURITIS
094.86 NEURITIS (SYPHILITIC)
225.1 NEUROMA
388.11 TRAUMA (EAR) (EXPLOSIVE)

736.09 ACQUIRED DEFORMITY UPPER LIMB
736.89 ACQUIRED DEFORMITY ARM OR LEG OTHER NEC
0 ACQUIRED IMMUNE DEFICIENCY SYNDROME SEE 'AIDS'
740.0 ACRANIA CONGENITAL
117.4 ACREMONIUM FALCIFORME INFECTION
755.55 ACROCEPHALOSYNDACTYLY SYNDROME
756.0 ACROCEPHALY
443.89 ACROCYANOSIS

ACRODERMATITIS
701.8 ATROPHICANS CHRONICA
696.1 CONTINUA
686.8 ENTEROPATHICA

253.0 ACROMEGALY

ACROMIOCLAVICULAR
831.04 DISLOCATION CLOSED
831.14 DISLOCATION OPEN
739.7 REGION SEGMENTAL OR SOMATIC DYSFUNCTION
840.0 SEPARATION (RUPTURE) (TEAR) (LACERATION)
840.0 STRAIN (SPRAIN) (AVULSION) (HEMARTHROSIS)

ACROPARESTHESIA
443.89 NOS
443.89 SIMPLE (SCHULTZE'S TYPE)
443.89 VASOMOTOR (NOTHNAGEL'S TYPE)

300.29 ACROPHOBIA
710.1 ACROSCLEROSIS

ACTH
255.3 OVERPRODUCTION
255.3 OVERPRODUCTION ADRENAL
253.1 OVERPRODUCTION PITUITARY

ACTINIC
692.72 CHEILITIS
692.82 CHEILITIS CHRONIC DUE TO RADIATION
692.74 CHEILITIS CHRONIC NEC
692.89 DERMATITIS
692.82 DERMATITIS DUE TO ROENTGEN RAYS
692.82 DERMATITIS OTHER THAN SUN
692.70 DERMATITIS (SOLAR) (SUN)
692.72 DERMATITIS (SOLAR) (SUN) ACUTE
692.74 DERMATITIS (SOLAR) (SUN) CHRONIC
692.74 ELASTOSIS
692.73 GRANULOMA DUE TO SOLAR RADIATION
370.24 KERATITIS
702.0 KERATOSIS
702.0 KERATOSIS (SOLAR)
692.73 RETICULOID DUE TO SOLAR RADIATION

024 ACTINOBACILLUS MALLEI INFECTION

0 ACTINOMADURA SEE 'ACTINOMYCOSIS'
0 ACTINOMYCETALES SEE 'ACTINOMYCOSIS'

ACTINOMYCOSIS
039.9 UNSPECIFIED SITE
039.2 ABDOMINAL
039.3 CERVICOFACIAL
039.0 CUTANEOUS
039.3 EYELID [373.5]
039.4 MADURA FOOT
039.1 PULMONARY
039.1 THORACIC
039.8 OTHER SPECIFIED SITES

0 ACTINOMYCOTIC MYCETOMA SEE 'ACTINOMYCOSIS'

286.3 ACTIVATING FACTOR (BLOOD) DEFICIENCY

789.0# ACUTE ABDOMINAL SYNDROME
5th Digit: 789.0
0. UNSPECIFIED SITE
1. UPPER RIGHT QUADRANT
2. UPPER LEFT QUADRANT
3. LOWER RIGHT QUADRANT
4. LOWER LEFT QUADRANT
5. PERIUMBILIC
6. EPIGASTRIC
7. GENERALIZED
9. OTHER SPECIFIED SITE (MULTIPLE)

415.0 ACUTE COR PULMONALE

207.0# ACUTE ERYTHREMIC MYELOSIS M9840/3
5th Digit: 207.0
0. WITHOUT MENTION OF REMISSION
1. WITH MENTION OF REMISSION

446.1 ACUTE FEBRILE MUCOCUTANEOUS LYMPH NODE SYNDROME (MCLS)

648.9# ACUTE FEBRILE MUCOCUTANEOUS LYMPH NODE SYNDROME (MCLS) MATERNAL CURRENT (CO-EXISTENT) IN PREGNANCY [446.1]
5th Digit: 648.9
0. EPISODE OF NOS OR N/A
1. DELIVERED
2. DELIVERED WITH POSTPARTUM COMPLICATION
3. ANTEPARTUM COMPLICATION
4. POSTPARTUM COMPLICATION

363.15 ACUTE POSTERIOR MULTIFOCAL PLACOID PIGMENT EPITHELIOPATHY

997.5 ACUTE TUBULAR NECROSIS SPECIFIED AS DUE TO PROCEDURE

646.7# ACUTE YELLOW ATROPHY OF PREGNANCY (LIVER)
5th Digit: 646.7
0. EPISODE OF CARE NOS OR N/A
1. DELIVERED
3. ANTEPARTUM COMPLICATION

755.4 ADACTYLY LIMB NOS (CONGENITAL)
756.51 ADAIR-DIGHTON SYNDROME

170.# ADAMANTINOMA BONE AND ARTICULAR CARTILAGE M9310/0
4th Digit: 170
0. SKULL AND FACE
1. MANDIBLE
2. VERTEBRAL COLUMN
3. RIBS STERNUM CLAVICLE
4. SCAPULA LONG BONES UPPER LIMB
5. SHORT BONES UPPER LIMB
6. PELVIC BONES SACRUM COCCYX
7. LONG BONES LOWER LIMB
8. SHORT BONES LOWER LIMB
9. SITE NOS

426.9 ADAMS-STOKES (-MORGAGNI) SYNDROME (SYNCOPE WITH HEART BLOCK)

426.9 ADAMS-STOKES (SYNCOPE WITH HEART BLOCK) DISEASE

309.9 ADAPTATION REACTION NOS

ADD (ATTENTION DEFICIT DISORDER) - (ADULT) (CHILD)

314.00 NOS
314.00 INATTENTIVE
314.01 WITH HYPERACTIVITY / IMPULSIVENESS
314.8 WITH OTHER SPECIFIED MANIFESTATIONS

SUBSTANCE DEPENDENCE IS ADDICTION. DEPENDENCE INVOLVES THE LOSS OF CONTROL AND JUDGMENT AND/OR THE INABILITY TO USE IN MODERATION. DEPENDENCE IS MARKED BY COMPULSIVE PHYSICAL DEMANDS WHICH ARE TRIGGERED BY FURTHER INGESTION.

ADDICTION

303.0# ALCOHOL - ACUTE EPISODE
303.9# ALCOHOL - CHRONIC

5th Digit: 303.0, 9
0. NOS
1. CONTINUOUS
2. EPISODIC
3. IN REMISSION

304.## DRUG

4th Digit: 304
0. OPIOID
1. BARBITURATES, SEDATIVES, TRANQUILIZERS WITH SIMILAR EFFECT
2. COCAINE
3. CANNABIS
4. AMPHETAMINE TYPE
5. HALLUCINOGENIC
6. OTHER SPECIFIED
7. MIXED WITH OPIOID
8. MIXED
9. NOS

5th Digit: 304
0. NOS
1. CONTINUOUS
2. EPISODIC
3. IN REMISSION

ADDISON'S, ADDISONIAN

281.0 ANEMIA (PERNICIOUS)
255.4 CRISIS
255.4 DISEASE NOS
255.4 DISEASE WITH MYOPATHY [359.5]
701.0 KELOID
255.4 SYNDROME
017.6# TUBERCULOSIS

5th Digit: 017.6
0. NOS
1. LAB NOT DONE
2. LABS PENDING
3. MICROSCOPY POSITIVE (IN SPUTUM)
4. CULTURE POSITIVE - MICROSCOPY NEGATIVE
5. CULTURE NEGATIVE - MICROSCOPY POSITIVE
6. CULTURE AND MICROSCOPY NEGATIVE CONFIRMED BY OTHER METHODS

0 ADENITIS SEE 'LYMPHADENITIS'

CARCINOMAS AND NEOPLASMS SHOULD BE CODED BY SITE IF POSSIBLE. CODE BY CELL TYPE - "SITE NOS", IF AND ONLY IF A SITE IS NOT SPECIFIED IN THE DIAGNOSIS. OTHERWISE - REFER TO THE APPROPRIATE CATEGORY OF NEOPLASM FOR A MORE SPECIFIC CODE: SEE 'CANCER' 'CANCER METASTATIC', 'NEOPLASM UNCERTAIN BEHAVIOR', 'NEOPLASM UNSPECIFIED NATURE', OR 'BENIGN NEOPLASM'.

ADENOCARCINOMA

199.1 SITE NOS
0 SITE SPECIFIED SEE 'CANCER' BY SITE M8140/3
153.9 ADENOMATOUS POLYPOSIS COLI SITE NOS
0 ADENOMATOUS POLYPOSIS COLI SITE SPECIFIED SEE 'CANCER' BY SITE M8220/3

ADENOCARCINOMA (continued)

0 ALVEOLAR SITE SPECIFIED SEE 'CANCER' BY SITE M8251/3
173.# APOCRINE M8401/3

4th Digit: 173
0. LIP
1. EYELID CANTHUS
2. EAR (AURICLE) AURICULAR CANAL (EXTERNAL) (ACOUSTIC)
3. UNSPECIFIED PARTS OF FACE CHEEK (EXTERNAL) CHIN EYEBROW FOREHEAD NOSE (EXT) TEMPLE
4. SCALP AND NECK
5. TRUNK AXILLA BREAST (OR MASTECTOMY SITE) BUTTOCK GROIN PERIANAL SKIN PERINEUM UMBILICUS
6. UPPER LIMB SHOULDER
7. LOWER LIMB HIP
8. OTHER SPECIFIED SKIN SITES CONTIGUOUS OR OVERLAPPING UNDETERMINED POINT OF ORIGIN
9. SITE NOS

162.9 BRONCHIOLOALVEOLAR SITE NOS
0 BRONCHIOLOALVEOLAR SITE SPECIFIED SEE 'CANCER' BY SITE M8250/3

173.# CERUMINOUS M8420/3

4th Digit: 173
0. LIP
1. EYELID CANTHUS
2. EAR (AURICLE) AURICULAR CANAL (EXTERNAL) (ACOUSTIC) OR SITE UNSPECIFIED
3. UNSPECIFIED PARTS OF FACE CHEEK (EXTERNAL) CHIN EYEBROW FOREHEAD NOSE (EXT) TEMPLE
4. SCALP AND NECK
5. TRUNK AXILLA BREAST (OR MASTECTOMY SITE) BUTTOCK GROIN PERIANAL SKIN PERINEUM UMBILICUS
6. UPPER LIMB SHOULDER
7. LOWER LIMB HIP
8. OTHER SPECIFIED SKIN SITES CONTIGUOUS OR OVERLAPPING UNDETERMINED POINT OF ORIGIN

199.1 CLEAR CELL SITE NOS
0 CLEAR CELL SITE SPECIFIED SEE 'CANCER' BY SITE M8310/3

0 ENDOMETRIOID (BORDERLINE MALIGNANCY) SITE SPECIFIED SEE 'NEOPLASM UNCERTAIN BEHAVIOR', BY SITE M8381/1
183.0 ENDOMETRIOID (MALIGNANT) SITE NOS
0 ENDOMETRIOID (MALIGNANT) SITE SPECIFIED SEE 'CANCER' BY SITE M8381/3

220 ENDOMETRIOID SITE NOS
0 ENDOMETRIOID SITE SPECIFIED SEE 'BENIGN NEOPLASM' BY SITE M8381/0

199.1 FOLLICULAR SITE NOS
0 FOLLICULAR SITE SPECIFIED SEE 'CANCER' BY SITE M8330/3
193 FOLLICULAR (TRABECULAR TYPE) SITE NOS
0 FOLLICULAR (TRABECULAR TYPE) SITE SPECIFIED SEE 'CANCER' BY SITE M8332/3

193 FOLLICULAR (WELL DIFFERENTIATED TYPE) SITE NOS
0 FOLLICULAR (WELL DIFFERENTIATED TYPE) SITE SPECIFIED SEE 'CANCER' BY SITE M8331/3
234.9 IN SITU SITE NOS
0 IN SITU SITE SPECIFIED SEE 'CA IN SITU' BY SITE M8140/2
151.9 INTESTINAL TYPE SITE NOS
0 INTESTINAL TYPE SITE SPECIFIED SEE 'CANCER' BY SITE M8144/3
157.9 ISLET CELL AND EXOCRINE (MIXED) SITE NOS
0 ISLET CELL AND EXOCRINE (MIXED) SITE SPECIFIED SEE 'CANCER' BY SITE M8154/3

ADENOCARCINOMA (continued)

199.1 METASTATIC SITE NOS
0 METASTATIC SITE SPECIFIED SEE 'CANCER' BY SITE, METASTATIC M8140/6

199.1 MIXED CELL SITE NOS M8323/3
0 MIXED CELL SITE SPECIFIED SEE 'CANCER' BY SITE M8323/3

199.1 MUCIN PRODUCING SITE NOS
0 MUCIN PRODUCING SITE SPECIFIED SEE 'CANCER' BY SITE M8481/3

199.1 MUCINOUS SITE NOS
0 MUCINOUS SITE SPECIFIED SEE 'CANCER' BY SITE M8480/3

199.1 OXYPHILIC SITE NOS
0 OXYPHILIC SITE SPECIFIED SEE 'CANCER' BY SITE M8290/3

199.1 PAPILLARY SITE NOS
0 PAPILLARY SITE SPECIFIED SEE 'CANCER' BY SITE M8260/3

193 PAPILLARY AND FOLLICULAR SITE NOS
0 PAPILLARY AND FOLLICULAR SITE SPECIFIED SEE 'CANCER' BY SITE M8340/3

233.0 PAPILLARY NONINFILTRATING INTRADUCTAL SITE NOS
0 PAPILLARY NONINFILTRATING INTRADUCTAL SITE SPECIFIED SEE 'CA IN SITU' BY SITE M8503/2

199.1 SCIRRHOUS SITE NOS
0 SCIRRHOUS SITE SPECIFIED SEE 'CANCER' BY SITE M8141/3

199.1 SEBACEOUS SITE NOS
0 SEBACEOUS SITE SPECIFIED SEE 'CANCER' BY SITE M8400/3

220 SEROUS SITE NOS
0 SEROUS SITE SPECIFIED SEE 'BENIGN NEOPLASM' BY SITE M9014/0

199.1 SUPERFICIAL SPREADING SITE NOS
0 SUPERFICIAL SPREADING SITE SPECIFIED SEE 'CANCER' BY SITE M8143/3

173.# SWEAT GLAND M8400/3

4th Digit: 173

- **0. LIP**
- **1. EYELID CANTHUS**
- **2. EAR (AURICLE) AURICULAR CANAL (EXTERNAL) (ACOUSTIC)**
- **3. UNSPECIFIED PARTS OF FACE CHEEK (EXTERNAL) CHIN EYEBROW FOREHEAD NOSE (EXT) TEMPLE**
- **4. SCALP AND NECK**
- **5. TRUNK AXILLA BREAST (OR MASTECTOMY SITE) BUTTOCK GROIN PERIANAL SKIN PERINEUM UMBILICUS**
- **6. UPPER LIMB SHOULDER**
- **7. LOWER LIMB HIP**
- **8. OTHER SPECIFIED SKIN SITES CONTIGUOUS OR OVERLAPPING UNDETERMINED POINT OF ORIGIN**
- **9. SITE NOS**

199.1 TRABECULAR SITE NOS
0 TRABECULAR SITE SPECIFIED SEE 'CANCER' BY SITE M8190/3

199.1 TUBULAR SITE NOS
0 TUBULAR SITE SPECIFIED SEE 'CANCER' BY SITE M8262/3

199.1 VILLOUS SITE NOS
0 VILLOUS SITE SPECIFIED SEE 'CANCER' BY SITE M8262/3

194.1 WATER CLEAR CELL SITE NOS
0 WATER CLEAR CELL SITE SPECIFIED SEE 'CANCER' BY SITE M8322/3

ADENOCARCINOMA (continued)

CARCINOMAS AND NEOPLASMS SHOULD BE CODED BY SITE IF POSSIBLE. CODE BY CELL TYPE - "SITE NOS", IF AND ONLY IF A SITE IS NOT SPECIFIED IN THE DIAGNOSIS. OTHERWISE - REFER TO THE APPROPRIATE CATEGORY OF NEOPLASM FOR A MORE SPECIFIC CODE: SEE 'CANCER' 'CANCER METASTATIC', 'NEOPLASM UNCERTAIN BEHAVIOR', 'NEOPLASM UNSPECIFIED NATURE', OR 'BENIGN NEOPLASM'.

199.1 WITH CARTILAGINOUS AND OSSEOUS METAPLASIA SITE NOS
0 WITH CARTILAGINOUS AND OSSEOUS METAPLASIA SITE SPECIFIED SEE 'CANCER' BY SITE M8571/3

199.1 WITH APOCRINE METAPLASIA SITE NOS
0 WITH APOCRINE METAPLASIA SITE SPECIFIED SEE 'CANCER' BY SITE M8573/3

194.3 WITH SPINDLE CELL METAPLASIA SITE NOS
0 WITH SPINDLE CELL METAPLASIA SITE SPECIFIED SEE 'CANCER' BY SITE M8572/3

199.1 WITH SQUAMOUS METAPLASIA SITE NOS
0 WITH SQUAMOUS METAPLASIA SITE SPECIFIED SEE 'CANCER' BY SITE M8570/3

ADENOFIBROMA

220 SITE NOS
0 SITE SPECIFIED SEE 'BENIGN NEOPLASM', BY SITE

220 CLEAR CELL SITE NOS M8313/0
0 CLEAR CELL SITE SPECIFIED SEE 'BENIGN NEOPLASM' , BY SITE M8313/0

220 ENDOMETROID M8313/0
236.2 ENDOMETROID BORDERLINE MALIGNANCY M8381/1
183.0 ENDOMETROID MALIGNANT M8381/3

220 MUCINOUS SITE NOS M9015/0
0 MUCINOUS SITE SPECIFIED SEE 'BENIGN NEOPLASM' , BY SITE M8313/0

600 PROSTATE

220 SEROUS SITE NOS
0 SEROUS SITE SPECIFIED SEE 'BENIGN NEOPLASM', BY SITE

ADENOID

199.1 CYSTIC CARCINOMA SITE NOS
0 CYSTIC CARCINOMA SITE SPECIFIED SEE 'CANCER' BY SITE M8200/3
474.9 DISEASE
474.12 HYPERPLASIA (HYPERTROPHY) (ENLARGEMENT)
474.00 HYPERPLASIA (HYPERTROPHY) (ENLARGEMENT) WITH CHRONIC TONSILLITIS
474.02 HYPERPLASIA (HYPERTROPHY) (ENLARGEMENT) WITH CHRONIC TONSILLITIS AND ADENOIDITIS
474.10 HYPERPLASIA (HYPERTROPHY) (ENLARGEMENT) WITH TONSIL HYPERTROPHY (HYPERPLASIA)
959.09 INJURY
474.8 TAG
474.01 TAG INFECTED
474.2 VEGETATIONS

ADENOIDITIS

463 ACUTE
474.01 CHRONIC
474.02 CHRONIC WITH CHRONIC TONSILLITIS
474.01 CHRONIC WITH HYPERTROPHY (ADENOID) (TONSILLAR)
474.02 CHRONIC WITH HYPERTROPHY (ADENOID) (TONSILLAR) WITH CHRONIC TONSILLITIS

210.2 ADENOLYMPHOMA SITE NOS
0 ADENOLYMPHOMA SITE SPECIFIED SEE 'BENIGN NEOPLASM' BY SITE M8561/0

ADENOMA (SEE ALSO 'BENIGN NEOPLASM')

229.9 SITE NOS
0 SITE SPECIFIED SEE 'BENIGN NEOPLASM' BY SITE M8140/0

194.3 ACIDOPHIL BASOPHIL (MIXED) SITE NOS
0 ACIDOPHIL BASOPHIL (MIXED) SITE SPECIFIED SEE 'BENIGN NEOPLASM' BY SITE M8281/0

227.3 ACIDOPHIL SITE NOS
0 ACIDOPHIL SITE SPECIFIED SEE 'BENIGN NEOPLASM' BY SITE M8280/0

229.9 ACINAR CELL SITE NOS
0 ACINAR CELL SITE SPECIFIED SEE 'BENIGN NEOPLASM' BY SITE M8550/3

227.0 ADRENAL CORTICAL (CLEAR CELL TYPE) SITE NOS M8401/0
0 ADRENAL CORTICAL (CLEAR CELL TYPE) SITE SPECIFIED SEE 'BENIGN NEOPLASM' BY SITE M8373/0

227.0 ADRENAL CORTICAL (COMPACT CELL TYPE) SITE NOS
0 ADRENAL CORTICAL (COMPACT CELL TYPE) SITE SPECIFIED SEE 'BENIGN NEOPLASM' BY SITE M8371/0

227.0 ADRENAL CORTICAL (GLOMERULOSA CELL TYPE) SITE NOS
0 ADRENAL CORTICAL (GLOMERULOSA CELL TYPE) SITE SPECIFIED SEE 'BENIGN NEOPLASM' BY SITE M8374/0

227.0 ADRENAL CORTICAL (HEAVILY PIGMENTED VARIANT) SITE NOS
0 ADRENAL CORTICAL (HEAVILY PIGMENTED VARIANT) SITE SPECIFIED SEE 'BENIGN NEOPLASM' BY SITE M8372/0

227.0 ADRENAL CORTICAL (MIXED CELL TYPE) SITE NOS
0 ADRENAL CORTICAL (MIXED CELL TYPE) SITE SPECIFIED SEE 'BENIGN NEOPLASM' BY TYPE M8375/0

227.0 ADRENAL CORTICAL SITE NOS
0 ADRENAL CORTICAL SITE SPECIFIED SEE 'BENIGN NEOPLASM', BY SITE M8370/0

227.0 ALVEOLAR SITE NOS
0 ALVEOLAR SITE SPECIFIED SEE 'BENIGN NEOPLASM' BY SITE M8251/0

217 APOCRINE BREAST SOFT TISSUE (CONNECTIVE OR GLANDULAR TISSUE)

216.# APOCRINE SKIN M8401/0

4th Digit: 216

0. LIP (SKIN OF)
1. EYELID INCLUDING CANTHUS
2. EAR (EXTERNAL) (AURICLE) (PINNA)
3. FACE (CHEEK) (NOSE)
4. SCALP NECK
5. TRUNK BACK CHEST
6. UPPER LIMB INCLUDING SHOULDER
7. LOWER LIMB INCLUDING HIP
8. OTHER SPECIFIED SITES
9. SKIN NOS

229.9 BASAL CELL SITE NOS
0 BASAL CELL SITE SPECIFIED SEE 'BENIGN NEOPLASM' BY SITE M8147/0

227.3 BASOPHIL SITE NOS
0 BASOPHIL SITE SPECIFIED SEE 'BENIGN NEOPLASM' BY SITE M8300/0

211.5 BILE DUCT SITE NOS
0 BILE DUCT SITE SPECIFIED SEE 'BENIGN NEOPLASM' BY SITE M8160/0

235.7 BRONCHIAL SITE NOS
0 BRONCHIAL SITE SPECIFIED SEE 'NEOPLASM UNCERTAIN BEHAVIOR' BY SITE M8140/1

ADENOMA (SEE ALSO 'BENIGN NEOPLASM') (continued)

216.# CERUMINOUS

4th Digit: 216

0. LIP
1. EYELID CANTHUS
2. EAR (AURICLE) AURICULAR CANAL (EXTERNAL) (ACOUSTIC)
3. UNSPECIFIED PARTS OF FACE CHEEK (EXTERNAL) CHIN EYEBROW FOREHEAD NOSE (EXT) TEMPLE
4. SCALP AND NECK
5. TRUNK AXILLA BREAST BUTTOCK CHEST GROIN PERIANAL SKIN PERINEUM UMBILICUS
6. UPPER LIMB SHOULDER
7. LOWER LIMB HIP
8. OTHER SPECIFIED SKIN SITES CONTIGUOUS OR OVERLAPPING UNDETERMINED POINT OF ORIGIN

227.1 CHIEF CELL SITE NOS
0 CHIEF CELL SITE SPECIFIED SEE 'BENIGN NEOPLASM' BY SITE M8321/0

227.3 CHROMOPHOBE SITE NOS
0 CHROMOPHOBE SITE SPECIFIED SEE 'BENIGN NEOPLASM' BY SITE M8270/0

229.9 CLEAR CELL SITE NOS
0 CLEAR CELL SITE SPECIFIED SEE 'BENIGN NEOPLASM' BY SITE M8310/0

229.9 EMBRYONAL SITE NOS
0 EMBRYONAL SITE SPECIFIED SEE 'BENIGN NEOPLASM' BY SITE M8191/0

237.4 ENDOCRINE (MULTIPLE) SITE NOS
0 ENDOCRINE (MULTIPLE) SITE SPECIFIED SEE 'NEOPLASM UNCERTAIN BEHAVIOR' BY SITE M8360/1

238.9 ENDOMETRIOID (BORDERLINE MALIGNANCY) SITE NOS
0 ENDOMETRIOID (BORDERLINE MALIGNANCY) SITE SPECIFIED SEE 'NEOPLASM UNCERTAIN BEHAVIOR', BY SITE M8380/1

229.9 ENDOMETRIOID SITE NOS
0 ENDOMETRIOID SITE SPECIFIED SEE 'BENIGN NEOPLASM' BY SITE M8380/0

226 FOLLICULAR SITE NOS
0 FOLLICULAR SITE SPECIFIED SEE 'BENIGN NEOPLASM' BY SITE M8330/0

211.7 ISLET CELL SITE NOS
0 ISLET CELL SITE SPECIFIED SEE 'BENIGN NEOPLASM' BY SITE M8150/0

211.5 LIVER CELL SITE NOS
0 LIVER CELL SITE SPECIFIED SEE 'BENIGN NEOPLASM' BY SITE M8170/0

226 MACROFOLLICULAR SITE NOS
0 MACROFOLLICULAR SITE SPECIFIED SEE 'BENIGN NEOPLASM' BY SITE M8334/0

226 MICROFOLLICULAR SITE NOS
0 MICROFOLLICULAR SITE SPECIFIED SEE 'BENIGN NEOPLASM' BY SITE M8333/0

229.9 MIXED CELL SITE NOS
0 MIXED CELL SITE SPECIFIED SEE 'BENIGN NEOPLASM' BY SITE M8323/0

229.9 MONOMORPHIC SITE NOS
0 MONOMORPHIC SITE SPECIFIED SEE 'BENIGN NEOPLASM' BY SITE M8146/0

229.9 MUCINOUS SITE NOS
0 MUCINOUS SITE SPECIFIED SEE 'BENIGN NEOPLASM' BY SITE M8480/0

ADENOMA (SEE ALSO 'BENIGN NEOPLASM') (continued)

226 OXYPHILIC SITE NOS
0 OXYPHILIC SITE SPECIFIED SEE 'BENIGN NEOPLASM' BY SITE M8290/0
229.9 PAPILLARY (INTRACYSTIC) SITE NOS
0 PAPILLARY (INTRACYSTIC) SITE SPECIFIED SEE 'BENIGN NEOPLASM' BY SITE M8504/0
229.9 PAPILLARY SITE NOS
0 PAPILLARY SITE SPECIFIED SEE 'BENIGN NEOPLASM' BY SITE M8260/0
229.9 PLEOMORPHIC SITE NOS
0 PLEOMORPHIC SITE SPECIFIED SEE 'BENIGN NEOPLASM' BY SITE M8940/0
600 PROSTATE (BENIGN)
216.# SEBACEOUS
216.# SKIN APPENDAGE M8390/0
216.# SWEAT GLAND M8400/0

4th Digit: 216

0. LIP (SKIN OF)
1. EYELID INCLUDING CANTHUS
2. EAR (EXTERNAL) (AURICLE) (PINNA)
3. FACE (CHEEK) (NOSE)
4. SCALP NECK
5. TRUNK BACK CHEST
6. UPPER LIMB INCLUDING SHOULDER
7. LOWER LIMB INCLUDING HIP
8. OTHER SPECIFIED SITES
9. SKIN NOS

229.9 TRABECULAR SITE NOS
0 TRABECULAR SITE SPECIFIED SEE 'BENIGN NEOPLASM' BY SITE M8190/0
220 TUBULAR FEMALE SITE NOS
222.0 TUBULAR MALE SITE NOS
0 TUBULAR SITE SPECIFIED SEE 'BENIGN NEOPLASM' BY SITE M8211/0
229.9 TUBULOVILLOUS SITE NOS
0 TUBULOVILLOUS SITE SPECIFIED SEE 'BENIGN NEOPLASM' BY SITE M8263/0
238.9 VILLOUS SITE NOS
0 VILLOUS SITE SPECIFIED SEE 'NEOPLASM UNCERTAIN BEHAVIOR' BY SITE M8261/1
227.1 WATER CLEAR CELL SITE NOS
0 WATER CLEAR CELL SITE SPECIFIED SEE 'BENIGN NEOPLASM' BY SITE M8322/0

229.9 ADENOMATOID TUMOR SITE NOS
0 ADENOMATOID TUMOR SITE SPECIFIED SEE 'BENIGN NEOPLASM' BY SITE M9054/0
153.9 ADENOMATOUS POLYPOSIS COLI SITE NOS
0 ADENOMATOUS POLYPOSIS COLI SITE SPECIFIED SEE 'BENIGN NEOPLASM' BY SITE M8220/0
229.9 ADENOMYOMA SITE NOS
0 ADENOMYOMA SITE SPECIFIED SEE 'BENIGN NEOPLASM' BY SITE M8932/0
617.0 ADENOMYOSIS
785.6 ADENOPATHY (LYMPH GLANDS)
091.4 ADENOPATHY SYPHILIS SECONDARY
0 ADENOPATHY TUBERCULOUS SEE 'TUBERCULOSIS', LYMPH NODES
277.2 ADENOSINE DEAMINASE DEFICIENCY
199.1 ADENOSQUAMOUS CARCINOMA SITE NOS
0 ADENOSQUAMOUS CARCINOMA SITE SPECIFIED SEE 'CANCER' BY SITE M8560/3
0 ADENOTONSILITIS SEE 'TONSILITIS'

V01.7 ADENOVIRUS EXPOSURE
008.62 ADENOVIRUS GASTROENTERITIS
079.0 ADENOVIRUS INFECTION (INFECTING AGENT)

ADH (ANTIDIURETIC HORMONE SECRETION)

259.3 ECTOPIC SECRETION
259.3 INAPPROPRIATE SECRETION ECTOPIC
253.6 INAPPROPRIATE SECRETION NEUROHYPOPHYSICAL
253.6 SYNDROME

ADHESION, ADHESIVE

568.0 ABDOMINAL WALL
762.8 AMNION TO FETUS AFFECTING FETUS OR NEWBORN
658.8# AMNION TO FETUS COMPLICATING CHILDBIRTH

5th Digit: 658.8

0. EPISODE OF CARE NOS OR N/A
1. DELIVERED
3. ANTEPARTUM COMPLICATION

543.9 APPENDIX
0 ARACHNOID SEE 'ADHESION, ADHESIVE', MENINGEAL
381.89 AUDITORY TUBE
622.3 BAND CERVIX
568.0 BAND INTESTINE
568.0 BAND INTESTINE POSTOPERATIVE (POSTINFECTION)
560.81 BAND INTESTINE POSTOPERATIVE (POSTINFECTION) OBSTRUCTED
621.5 BAND UTERUS
576.8 BILE DUCT (ANY)
596.8 BLADDER (SPHINCTER)
568.0 BOWEL
568.0 BOWEL POSTOPERATIVE (POSTINFECTION)
560.81 BOWEL POSTOPERATIVE (POSTINFECTION) OBSTRUCTED
620.8 BROAD LIGAMENT
726.0 CAPSULITIS SHOULDER
423.1 CARDIAC
398.99 CARDIAC RHEUMATIC
568.0 CECUM
568.0 CECUM POSTOPERATIVE (POSTINFECTION)
560.81 CECUM POSTOPERATIVE (POSTINFECTION) OBSTRUCTED
622.3 CERVICOVAGINAL
752.49 CERVICOVAGINAL CONGENITAL
674.8# CERVICOVAGINAL MATERNAL DUE TO PREGNANCY

5th Digit: 674.8

0. EPISODE OF CARE NOS OR N/A
2. DELIVERED WITH POSTPARTUM COMPLICATION
4. POSTPARTUM COMPLICATION

622.3 CERVICOVAGINAL POSTPARTAL, OLD
622.3 CERVIX
622.3 CERVIX (BANDS) (OLD LACERATION)
622.3 CERVIX CICATRIX (POSTPARTUM)
624.4 CLITORIS
568.0 COLON
568.0 COLON POSTOPERATIVE (POSTINFECTION)
560.81 COLON POSTOPERATIVE (POSTINFECTION) OBSTRUCTED
576.8 COMMON DUCT
743.63 CONJUNCTIVA - CONGENITAL
372.63 CONJUNCTIVA - EXTENSIVE
372.62 CONJUNCTIVA - LOCALIZED
371.00 CORNEA - NOS
371.03 CORNEA - CENTRAL
743.43 CORNEA - CONGENITAL
743.42 CORNEA - CONGENITAL INTERFERING WITH VISION
371.01 CORNEA - MINOR
371.02 CORNEA - PERIPHERAL
575.8 CYSTIC DUCT
568.0 DIAPHRAGM (PERITONEAL)
560.81 DIAPHRAGM (PERITONEAL) POSTOPERATIVE (POSTINFECTION) OBSTRUCTED
568.0 DUODENUM
560.81 DUODENUM POSTOPERATIVE (POSTINFECTION) OBSTRUCTED

ADHESION, ADHESIVE (continued)

385.10 EAR MIDDLE
385.19 EAR MIDDLE - DRUM HEAD
385.11 EAR MIDDLE - DRUM HEAD TO INCUS
385.13 EAR MIDDLE - DRUM HEAD TO PROMONTORIUM
385.12 EAR MIDDLE - DRUM HEAD TO STAPES
385.19 EAR MIDDLE - OTHER ADHESIONS AND COMBINATIONS
608.89 EPIDIDYMIS
478.79 EPIGLOTTIS
381.89 EUSTACHIAN TUBE
743.63 EYE - CONJUNCTIVA CONGENITAL
372.63 EYE - CONJUNCTIVA EXTENSIVE
372.62 EYE - CONJUNCTIVA LOCALIZED
371.00 EYE - CORNEA NOS
371.03 EYE - CORNEA CENTRAL
743.43 EYE - CORNEA CONGENITAL
743.42 EYE - CORNEA CONGENITAL INTERFERING WITH VISION
371.01 EYE - CORNEA MINOR
371.02 EYE - CORNEA PERIPHERAL
360.89 EYE - GLOBE
364.70 EYE - IRIS
996.79 EYE - IRIS TO CORNEAL GRAFT
379.29 EYE - VITREOUS
374.46 EYELID
997.99 EYELID POSTOPERATIVE COMPLICATION
V45.69 EYELID SURGICALLY CREATED (STATUS)
755.11 FINGERS CONGENITAL
575.8 GALLBLADDER
568.0 GASTROINTESTINAL TRACT
568.0 GASTROINTESTINAL TRACT POSTOPERATIVE
560.81 GASTROINTESTINAL TRACT WITH OBSTRUCTION POSTOPERATIVE
568.0 ILEOCECAL
568.0 ILEOCECAL POSTOPERATIVE (POSTINFECTION)
560.81 ILEOCECAL POSTOPERATIVE (POSTINFECTION) OBSTRUCTED
568.0 ILEUM
568.0 ILEUM POSTOPERATIVE (POSTINFECTION)
560.81 ILEUM POSTOPERATIVE (POSTINFECTION) OBSTRUCTED
568.0 INTESTINE
568.0 INTESTINE POSTOPERATIVE
560.81 INTESTINE WITH OBSTRUCTION
0 INTESTINE WITH OBSTRUCTION AND HERNIA SEE 'HERNIA', BY SITE, INCARCERATED
0 INTESTINE WITH OBSTRUCTION AND HERNIA GANGRENOUS SEE 'HERNIA', BY SITE, GANGRENOUS
560.81 INTESTINE WITH OBSTRUCTION POSTOPERATIVE (POSTINFECTION)
0 JOINT SEE 'ANKYLOSIS'
593.89 KIDNEY
624.4 LABIUM (MINUS)
752.49 LABIUM (MAJUS) (MINUS) CONGENITAL
572.8 LIVER
511.0 LUNG
519.3 MEDIASTINUM
349.2 MENINGEAL (CEREBRAL) (SPINAL)
742.4 MENINGEAL CONGENITAL CEREBRAL
742.59 MENINGEAL CONGENITAL SPINAL
0 MENINGEAL TUBERCULOSIS SEE 'TUBERCULOSIS', MENINGES
568.0 MESENTERIC
568.0 MESENTERIC POSTOPERATIVE (POSTINFECTION)
478.1 NASAL OR INTRANASAL
355.9 NERVE NEC
355.0 NERVE SCIATIC
378.60 OCULAR MUSCLE
568.0 OMENTUM
751.4 OMENTUM ANOMALOUS CONGENITAL
568.0 OMENTUM POSTOPERATIVE (POSTINFECTION)

ADHESION, ADHESIVE (continued)

385.10 OTITIS
385.11 OTITIS - DRUM HEAD TO INCUS
385.13 OTITIS - DRUM HEAD TO PROMONTORIUM
385.12 OTITIS - DRUM HEAD TO STAPES
385.19 OTITIS - OTHER ADHESIONS AND COMBINATIONS
614.6 OVARY
614.6 OVARY POSTOPERATIVE (POSTINFECTION)
752.0 OVARY TO CECUM CONGENITAL
752.0 OVARY TO KIDNEY CONGENITAL
752.0 OVARY TO OMENTUM CONGENITAL
614.6 PARAUTERINE
614.6 PARAUTERINE POSTOPERATIVE (POSTINFECTION)
614.6 PAROVARIAN
614.6 PAROVARIAN POSTOPERATIVE (POSTINFECTION)
614.6 PELVIC PERITONEAL - FEMALE
614.6 PELVIC PERITONEAL - FEMALE POSTOPERATIVE (POSTINFECTION)
568.0 PELVIC PERITONEAL - MALE
568.0 PELVIC PERITONEAL - POSTOPERATIVE
560.81 PELVIC PERITONEAL - POSTOPERATIVE OBSTRUCTED
752.69 PENIS TO SCROTUM (POSTINFECTIONAL) (POSTOPERATIVE) (CONGENITAL)
568.0 PERIAPPENDICEAL
568.0 PERIAPPENDICEAL POSTOPERATIVE (POSTINFECTION)
560.81 PERIAPPENDICEAL POSTOPERATIVE (POSTINFECTION) OBSTRUCTED
423.1 PERICARDIUM
393 PERICARDIUM RHEUMATIC
017.9# PERICARDIUM TUBERCULOSUS [420.0]

5th Digit: 017.9

0. NOS
1. LAB NOT DONE
2 . LABS PENDING
3. MICROSCOPY POSITIVE (IN SPUTUM)
4. CULTURE POSITIVE - MICROSCOPY
5. CULTURE NEGATIVE - MICROSCOPY POSITIVE
6. CULTURE AND MICROSCOPY NEGATIVE CONFIRMED BY OTHER METHODS

575.8 PERICHOLECYSTIC
568.0 PERIGASTRIC
568.0 PERIGASTRIC POSTOPERATIVE (POSTINFECTION)
560.81 PERIGASTRIC POSTOPERATIVE (POSTINFECTION) OBSTRUCTED
602.8 PERIPROSTATIC
568.0 PERIRECTAL
568.0 PERIRECTAL POSTOPERATIVE (POSTINFECTION)
560.81 PERIRECTAL POSTOPERATIVE (POSTINFECTION) OBSTRUCTED
568.0 PERITONEAL
751.4 PERITONEAL - CONGENITAL
614.6 PERITONEAL - FEMALE
614.6 PERITONEAL - PELVIC, FEMALE
568.0 PERITONEAL - PELVIC, MALE
568.0 PERITONEAL - POSTOPERATIVE
614.6 PERITONEAL - POSTOPERATIVE, FEMALE
560.81 PERITONEAL - POSTOPERATIVE OBSTRUCTED
614.6 PERITONEAL - TO UTERUS
614.6 PERITONEAL - TO UTERUS POSTOPERATIVE (POSTINFECTION)
537.3 PERITONEAL - WITH DUODENAL OBSTRUCTION
560.81 PERITONEAL - WITH INTESTINAL OBSTRUCTION
614.6 PERITUBAL
614.6 PERITUBAL POSTOPERATIVE (POSTINFECTION)
596.8 PERIVESICAL

ADHESION, ADHESIVE (continued)

511.0 PLEURA PLEURITIC
012.0# PLEURAL TUBERCULOSIS
5th Digit: 012.0
0. NOS
1. LAB NOT DONE
2 . LABS PENDING
3. MICROSCOPY POSITIVE (IN SPUTUM)
4. CULTURE POSITIVE - MICROSCOPY
5. CULTURE NEGATIVE - MICROSCOPY POSITIVE
6. CULTURE AND MICROSCOPY NEGATIVE CONFIRMED BY OTHER METHODS

511.0 PLEUROPERICARDIAL
624.4 POSTPARTAL, OLD
605 PREPUCE
511.0 PULMONARY
568.0 PYLORUS
568.0 PYLORUS POSTOPERATIVE (POSTINFECTION)
560.81 PYLORUS POSTOPERATIVE (POSTINFECTION) OBSTRUCTED
478.29 ROSENMULLER'S FOSSA
355.0 SCIATIC NERVE
608.89 SEMINAL VESICLE
726.0 SHOULDER (JOINT) (CAPSULITIS)
726.2 SHOULDER SUBSCAPULAR
608.89 SPERMATIC CORD
752.8 SPERMATIC CORD CONGENITAL
349.2 SPINAL CANAL
355.9 SPINAL NERVE NEC
724.9 SPINAL NERVE ROOT SITE NOS
723.4 SPINAL NERVE ROOT CERVICAL
724.4 SPINAL NERVE ROOT LUMBOSACRAL
724.4 SPINAL NERVE ROOT THORACIC
568.0 STOMACH
568.0 STOMACH POSTOPERATIVE (POSTINFECTION)
560.81 STOMACH POSTOPERATIVE (POSTINFECTION) OBSTRUCTED
726.90 TENDONITIS SITE UNSPECIFIED
726.0 TENDONITIS SHOULDER
608.89 TESTICLE
755.13 TOES CONGENITAL
529.8 TONGUE
750.12 TONGUE CONGENITAL
519.1 TRACHEA
614.6 TUBO OVARIAN
614.6 TUBO OVARIAN POSTOPERATIVE (POSTINFECTION)
608.89 TUNICA VAGINALIS
593.89 URETER
598.2 URETHRA POSTOPERATIVE
763.89 UTERUS AFFECTING FETUS OR NEWBORN
654.4# UTERUS COMPLICATING CHILDBIRTH
5th Digit: 654.4
0. EPISODE OF CARE NOS OR N/A
1. DELIVERED
2. DELIVERED WITH POSTPARTUM COMPLICATION
3. ANTEPARTUM COMPLICATION
4. POSTPARTUM COMPLICATION

621.5 UTERUS (INTRAUTERINE)
614.6 UTERUS TO ABDOMINAL WALL
623.2 VAGINA (CHRONIC) (POSTOPERATIVE) (POSTRADIATION)

0 ADHESIVE SEE 'ADHESION, ADHESIVE'
379.46 ADIE (-HOLMES) (PUPIL) SYNDROME
272.8 ADIPOSIS DOLORA
278.00 ADIPOSITY
278.1 ADIPOSITY LOCALIZED
253.8 ADIPOSOGENITAL DYSTROPHY
253.8 ADIPOSOGENITAL SYNDROME

ADJUSTMENT REACTION

309.9 NOS
309.29 CULTURE SHOCK
309.1 DEPRESSIVE REACTION PROLONGED
309.22 EMANCIPATION DISORDER OF ADOLESCENCE AND EARLY ADULT LIFE
309.9 JUVENILE
309.81 POSTTRAUMATIC (CHRONIC)
309.81 POSTTRAUMATIC PROLONGED
309.21 SEPARATION ANXIETY
309.23 SPECIFIC ACADEMIC OR WORK INHIBITION
309.28 WITH ANXIETY AND DEPRESSION
309.24 WITH ANXIOUS MOOD
309.3 WITH CONDUCT DISTURBANCE DESTRUCTIVENESS
309.4 WITH MIXED DISTURBANCE OF EMOTIONS AND CONDUCTS
309.28 WITH MIXED EMOTIONAL FEATURES
309.82 WITH PHYSICAL SYMPTOMS
309.83 WITH WITHDRAWAL
309.89 OTHER

V68.81 ADMINISTRATIVE ENCOUNTER REFERRAL WITHOUT EXAM OR TREATMENT
V68.9 ADMINISTRATIVE ENCOUNTER UNSPECIFIED PURPOSE
V68.89 ADMINISTRATIVE ENCOUNTER OTHER SPECIFIED PURPOSE
379.8 ADNEXA DISORDER OTHER SPECIFIED (EYE)
V21.2 ADOLESCENCE
V61.29 ADOPTED CHILD PROBLEM (REASON FOR ENCOUNTER)
V68.89 ADOPTION - ENCOUNTER FOR ADMINISTRATIVE PURPOSES
V70.3 ADOPTION - MEDICAL EXAM

ADRENAL

759.1 ABERRANT CONGENITAL
255.8 ABSENCE (GLAND)
759.1 ABSENCE (GLAND) CONGENITAL
759.1 ACCESSORY CONGENITAL
255.3 ANDROGENIC OVERACTIVITY ACQUIRED BENIGN
255.4 ATROPHY
255.4 CALCIFICATION (CAPSULE) (GLAND)
194.0 CORTICAL CARCINOMA SITE NOS M8370/3
0 CORTICAL CARCINOMA SEE 'CANCER', BY SITE
255.4 CORTICAL CRISIS
255.4 CRISIS (CORTICAL)
255.9 DISORDER NOS
255.2 DISORDER ADRENOGENITAL
255.8 DISORDER SPECIFIED NEC
759.1 ECTOPIC GLAND CONGENITAL
255.8 FIBROSIS GLAND (SUBCUTANEOUS)
772.5 HEMORRHAGE PERINATAL
036.3 HEMORRHAGE SYNDROME
255.3 HYPERFUNCTION (CORTICAL) (ANDROGENIC)
255.6 HYPERFUNCTION (MEDULLOADRENAL)
255.8 HYPERPLASIA
255.0 HYPERPLASIA (DUE TO ACTH EXCESS)
255.2 HYPERPLASIA MALE WITH SEXUAL PRECOCITY
255.2 HYPERPLASTIC CONGENITAL
255.4 HYPOFUNCTION
255.4 INFARCTION
255.8 INFLAMMATION
868.01 INJURY (TRAUMATIC)
868.11 INJURY (TRAUMATIC) WITH OPEN WOUND INTO CAVITY
908.1 INJURY (TRAUMATIC) LATE EFFECT
255.4 INSUFFICIENCY - NOS
255.5 INSUFFICIENCY - MEDULLARY
036.3 INSUFFICIENCY - MEDULLARY MENINGOCOCCAL

ADRENAL (continued)

017.6# INSUFFICIENCY - TUBERCULOUS

5th Digit: 017.6

0. NOS
1. LAB NOT DONE
2. LABS PENDING
3. MICROSCOPY POSITIVE (IN SPUTUM)
4. CULTURE POSITIVE - MICROSCOPY NEGATIVE
5. CULTURE NEGATIVE - MICROSCOPY POSITIVE
6. CULTURE AND MICROSCOPY NEGATIVE CONFIRMED BY OTHER METHODS

036.3 MENINGOCOCCIC SYNDROME
229.9 REST TUMOR SITE NOS
0 REST TUMOR SITE SPECIFIED SEE 'BENIGN NEOPLASM' BY SITE M8671/0
255.8 OTHER SPECIFIED DISORDER

259.3 ADRENALIN ECTOPIC SECRETION
255.3 ADRENOCORTICAL SYNDROME
0 ADRENOCORTICOTROPIC SEE 'ACTH'
255.2 ADRENOGENITAL DISORDERS
255.2 ADRENOGENITAL FEMINIZING SYNDROME
760.79 ADRENOGENITAL IATROGENIC SYNDROME AFFECTING FETUS OR NEWBORN
255.2 ADRENOGENITAL SYNDROME (ACQUIRED) (CONGENITAL)
255.2 ADRENOGENITAL VIRILISM SYNDROME (ACQUIRED) (CONGENITAL)

WHEN THE CAUSE OF AN INJURY IS STATED TO BE ABUSE, MULTIPLE CODES SHOULD BE ASSIGNED, IF APPLICABLE, TO IDENTIFY ANY ASSOCIATED INJURIES. THEY ARE TO BE SEQUENCED IN THE FOLLOWING ORDER:

1. TYPE OF ABUSE - CHILD OR ADULT (995.5, 995.8)

2. TYPE OF INJURY

3. PERPETRATOR OF THE ABUSE - SEE E-CODE DIRECTORY 'ASSAULT' (E967)

4. NATURE OF THE ABUSE - SEE E-CODE DIRECTORY 'ASSAULT' (E904.0, E960-E966, E968)

ADULT

995.8# ABUSE (VICTIM)

5th Digit: 995.8

0. MALTREATMENT UNSPECIFIED
1. PHYSICAL, BATTERY
2. EMOTIONAL / PSYCHOLOGICAL (DEPRIVATION)
3. SEXUAL
4. NEGLECT (NUTRITIONAL), DESERTION
5. OTHER ABUSE AND NEGLECT, MULTIPLE FORMS

V61.12 ABUSE COUNSELING - SPOUSAL (PARTNER) PERPETRATOR
V61.11 ABUSE COUNSELING - SPOUSAL (PARTNER) VICTIM
V62.83 ABUSE COUNSELING - OTHER PERPETRATOR OF PHYSICAL/SEXUAL ABUSE NEC
V62.89 ABUSE COUNSELING - OTHER VICTIM
995.84 ABUSE DESERTION
V71.6 ABUSE EVALUATION - BATTERY (ALLEGED)
V71.5 ABUSE EVALUATION - SEXUAL (ALLEGED)
V15.4# ABUSE HISTORY

5th Digit: V15.4

1. PHYSICAL ABUSE, RAPE
2. EMOTIONAL ABUSE, NEGLECT
9. OTHER PSYCHOLOGICAL TRAUMA

995.81 MALTREATMENT SYNDROME

ADULT RESPIRATORY DISTRESS SYNDROME

507.0 ASSOCIATED WITH ASPIRATION PNEUMONIA
514 ASSOCIATED WITH HYPOSTATIC PNEUMONIA
518.81 ASSOCIATED WITH RESPIRATORY FAILURE - ACUTE IN OTHER CONDITIONS
518.84 ASSOCIATED WITH RESPIRATORY FAILURE - ACUTE AND CHRONIC IN OTHER CONDITIONS
518.83 ASSOCIATED WITH RESPIRATORY FAILURE - CHRONIC IN OTHER CONDITIONS
518.5 ASSOCIATED WITH SHOCK
518.82 ASSOCIATED WITH OTHER CONDITIONS
518.5 FOLLOWING TRAUMA AND SURGERY
518.5 TRAUMATIC OR POSTSURGICAL
518.82 OTHER SPECIFIED

IN ICD-9 TERMS, AN "ADVERSE EFFECT" IS A REACTION TO A SUBSTANCE PROPERLY ADMINISTERED, WHILE A "POISONING" IS A REACTION TO A SUBSTANCE IMPROPERLY ADMINISTERED. (IE. ACCIDENT, SUICIDE ATTEMPT, OR ASSAULT) ADVERSE EFFECTS ARE CODED WHEN THE PROPER ADMINISTRATION OF A DRUG RESULTS IN AN ADVERSE CONDITION. CODE THE RESULTANT CONDITION FIRST WITH AN ADDITIONAL E-CODE FROM 'DRUGS AND CHEMICALS' INDEX, 'THERAPEUTIC' COLUMN (E930-E949).

ADVERSE EFFECT

995.2 UNSPECIFIED TO DRUG, MEDICINAL, OR BIOLOGICAL SUBSTANCE (SEE ALSO TABLE OF DRUGS AND CHEMICALS, THERAPEUTIC)
909.5 DRUG (TO CORRECTLY ADMINISTERED SUBSTANCE) LATE EFFECT
994.8 ELECTRIC CURRENT (SHOCK)
909.4 ELECTRIC CURRENT (SHOCK) LATE EFFECT
994.5 EXERTION (EXCESSIVE)
909.4 EXERTION (EXCESSIVE) LATE EFFECT
994.4 EXPOSURE (EXHAUSTION)
909.4 EXPOSURE (EXHAUSTION) LATE EFFECT
994.2 HUNGER
909.4 HUNGER LATE EFFECT
692.82 INFRARED DERMATITIS
692.82 RADIATION DERMATITIS OR ECZEMA
692.82 RADIOACTIVE DERMATITIS
692.82 RADIOTHERAPY DERMATITIS
692.70 SUN DERMATITIS
692.82 ULTAVIOLET DERMATITIS
692.82 X-RAY DERMATITIS

0 ADVICE SEE 'COUNSELING'
560.1 ADYNAMIC ILEUS
753.22 ADYNAMIC URETER
993.0 AERO OTITIS MEDIA
909.4 AERO OTITIS MEDIA LATE EFFECT
008.2 AEROBACTER AEROGENES GASTROENTERITIS
041.85 AEROBACTER AEROGENES INFECTION OR ORGANISM
998.81 AERODERMECTASIA SURGICAL
993.3 AEROEMBOLISM
909.4 AEROEMBOLISM LATE EFFECT
306.4 AEROPHAGY CYCLICAL
993.1 AEROSINUSITIS
909.4 AEROSINUSITIS LATE EFFECT

309.1 AFFECTIVE DISORDER SEASONAL
V11.1 AFFECTIVE DISORDERS HISTORY
292.84 AFFECTIVE ORGANIC DRUG INDUCED SYNDROME
293.89 AFFECTIVE ORGANIC SYNDROME NEC
301.10 AFFECTIVE PERSONALITY DISORDER
296.90 AFFECTIVE PSYCHOSIS
296.99 AFFECTIVE PSYCHOSIS OTHER

537.89 AFFERENT LOOP SYNDROME NEC

AFIBRINOGENEMIA

286.6 ACQUIRED
639.1 POST ABORTION OR ECTOPIC/MOLAR PREGNANCY
666.3# POSTPARTUM
5th Digit: 666.3
0. NOS
2. DELIVERED WITH POSTPARTUM COMPLICATION
4. POSTPARTUM COMPLICATION

273.3 AFRICAN MACROGLOBULINEMIA SYNDROME
086.5 AFRICAN SLEEPING SICKNESS
082.1 AFRICAN TICK TYPHUS
115.1# AFRICAN HISTOPLASMOSIS
5th Digit: 115.1
0. UNSPECIFIED
1. MENINGITIS
2. RETINITIS
3. PERICARDITIS
4. ENDOCARDITIS
5. PNEUMONIA
9. OTHER SITE

> *AFTERCARE GENERALLY INCLUDES FITTING AND ADJUSTMENTS, CHECKING, CHANGING, CLEANSING, REMOVAL AND REPLACEMENT UNLESS OTHERWISE STATED.*

AFTERCARE

V58.9 NOS
V53.09 AUDITORY SUBSTITUTION DEVICE
V58.2 BLOOD TRANSFUSION
V53.02 BRAIN PACEMAKER (NEUROPACEMAKER)
V53.32 CARDIAC DEFIBRILLATOR AUTOMATIC IMPLANTABLE
V53.31 CARDIAC PACEMAKER
V53.39 CARDIAC DEVICE OTHER SPECIFIED
V56.1 CATHETER - DIALYSIS EXTRACORPOREAL
V56.2 CATHETER - DIALYSIS PERITONEAL
V58.82 CATHETER - NONVASCULAR NEC
V53.6 CATHETER - URINARY
V58.81 CATHETER - VASCULAR
V53.01 CEREBRAL VENTRICULAR (COMMUNICATING) SHUNT
V58.1 CHEMOTHERAPY MAINTENANCE
V53.1 CONTACT LENSES
V53.9 DEVICE NOS
V58.3 DRESSING CHANGE
V53.2 HEARING AID

> *ANTIBIOTICS, COUMADIN, DIGOXIN, CHEMOTHERAPY DRUGS, AND ANY OTHER DRUGS WITH A RISK OF ADVERSE REACTIONS ARE CONSIDERED TO BE HIGH-RISK MEDICATIONS. CODES V58.61, V58.62 AND V58.69 ARE TO BE USED TO IDENTIFY PATIENTS THAT ARE CURRENTLY BEING MONITORED WHILE TAKING HIGH RISK MEDICATION. CODE V67.51 IS TO BE USED TO IDENTIFY PATIENTS THAT HAVE COMPLETED HIGH RISK MEDICATION THERAPY.*

HIGH RISK MEDICATION

V58.62 ANTIBIOTICS - CURRENT THERAPY
V58.61 ANTICOAGULANT - CURRENT THERAPY
V67.51 ANTICOAGULANT - COMPLETED THERAPY
V58.69 OTHER - CURRENT THERAPY
V67.51 OTHER - COMPLETED THERAPY

AFTERCARE (continued)

V58.89 MEDICAL NEC
V53.02 NERVOUS SYSTEM DEVICE - PACEMAKER
V53.09 NERVOUS SYSTEM DEVICE - OTHER
V53.02 NEUROPACEMAKER (BRAIN) (PERIPHERAL NERVE) (SPINAL CORD)
V58.5 ORTHODONTIC
V53.4 ORTHODONTIC DEVICE

AFTERCARE (continued)

ORTHOPEDIC

V54.9 UNSPECIFIED
V54.8 CHANGE, CHECKING OR REMOVAL OF AN EXTERNAL DEVICE: (CAST) (EXTERNAL FIXATION) (KIRSCHNER WIRE) (SPLINT EXTERNAL) (TRACTION DEVICE)
V53.7 FITTING AND ADJUSTMENT OF A DEVICE: (BRACE) (CAST) (CORSET) (SHOES)
V54.0 REMOVAL INTERNAL FIXATION DEVICE: (FRACTURE PLATE) (PIN) (PLATES) (ROD) (SCREWS)
V54.8 OTHER SPECIFIED CARE

OSTOMY

V55.9 NOS
V55.4 CECOSTOMY
V55.3 COLOSTOMY
V55.5 CYSTOSTOMY
V55.4 ENTEROSTOMY
V55.1 GASTROSTOMY
V55.2 ILEOSTOMY
V55.4 JEJUNOSTOMY
V55.6 NEPHROSTOMY
V55.0 TRACHEOSTOMY
V55.6 URETEROSTOMY
V55.6 URETHROSTOMY
V55.4 OTHER DIGESTIVE
V55.6 OTHER URINARY
V55.8 OTHER SPECIFIED SITE

AFTERCARE (continued)

V66.7 PALLIATIVE
V53.02 PERIPHERAL NERVE PACEMAKER (NEUROPACEMAKER)
V58.49 POSTOPERATIVE NEC

PROSTHESIS

V52.9 NOS
V52.0 ARM
V52.4 BREAST
V52.3 DENTAL
V52.2 EYE
V52.1 LEG
V52.8 OTHER SPECIFIED

AFTERCARE (continued)

V58.0 RADIOTHERAPY
V53.09 SPECIAL SENSES DEVICE
V53.1 SPECTACLES
V53.02 SPINAL CORD PACEMAKER (NEUROPACEMAKER)
V58.3 SURGICAL DRESSINGS
V58.3 SUTURE REMOVAL
V58.81 VASCULAR CATHETER REMOVAL
V53.01 VENTRICULAR SHUNT (CEREBRAL) (COMMUNICATING)
V53.09 VISUAL SUBSTITUTION DEVICE
V53.8 WHEELCHAIR
V58.41 WOUND CLOSURE POSTOPERATIVE (PLANNED)
V58.49 OTHER SPECIFIED POSTSURGICAL
V58.89 OTHER SPECIFIED

AFTER CATARACT

366.50 NOS
366.53 OBSCURING VISION
366.52 OTHER NOT OBSCURING VISION

0 AGALACTIA SEE 'LACTATION' FAILURE

AGAMMAGLOBULINEMIA

279.00 NOS
279.2 AUTOSOMAL RECESSIVE
279.04 BRUTON'S TYPE
279.2 SWISS-TYPE
279.11 THYMIC (HYPOPLASIA) (DYSPLASIA)
279.04 X-LINKED
279.2 X-LINKED RECESSIVE

A

751.3 AGANGLIONOSIS CONGENITAL

ELDERLY MULTIGRAVIDA: SECOND OR MORE PREGNANCY IN A WOMAN WHO WILL BE 35 YEARS OF AGE OR OLDER AT EXPECTED DATE OF DELIVERY.

659.6# AGE ADVANCED MATERNAL COMPLICATING LABOR AND DELIVERY - ELDERLY MULTIGRAVIDA
5th Digit: 659.6
0. EPISODE OF CARE UNSPECIFIED OR N/A
1. DELIVERED
3. ANTEPARTUM COMPLICATION

ELDERLY PRIMIGRAVIDA: FIRST PREGNANCY IN A WOMAN WHO WILL BE 35 YEARS OF AGE OR OLDER AT EXPECTED DATE OF DELIVERY.

659.5# AGE ADVANCED MATERNAL COMPLICATING LABOR AND DELIVERY - ELDERLY PRIMIGRAVIDA
5th Digit: 659.5
0. EPISODE OF CARE UNSPECIFIED OR N/A
1. DELIVERED
3. ANTEPARTUM COMPLICATION

YOUNG MATERNAL AGE: PREGNANCY IN FEMALE WHO IS LESS THAN 16 YEARS OLD AT EXPECTED DATE OF DELIVERY.

659.8# AGE YOUNG MATERNAL COMPLICATING LABOR AND DELIVERY
5th Digit: 659.8
0. EPISODE OF CARE UNSPECIFIED OR N/A
1. DELIVERED
3. ANTEPARTUM COMPLICATION

AGENESIS
742.8 ACOUSTIC NERVE
751.8 DIGESTIVE ORGAN (S) OR TRACT (COMPLETE) (PARTIAL)
751.2 DIGESTIVE ORGAN (S) OR TRACT (LOWER)
750.8 DIGESTIVE ORGAN (S) OR TRACT (UPPER)
747.89 DUCTUS ARTERIOSUS
755.34 FEMUR NEC
755.37 FIBULA NEC
755.29 FINGER NEC
524.09 JAW
524.09 MANDIBLE
524.09 MAXILLA
752.69 PENIS
0 SEE ALSO BY ANATOMICAL SITE, 'ABSENCE CONGENITAL'

312.0# AGGRESSIVE CONDUCT DISORDER (OUTBURST)
5th Digit: 312.0
0. UNSPECIFIED
1. MILD
2. MODERATE
3. SEVERE

301.3 AGGRESSIVE PERSONALITY DISORDER
307.9 AGITATION
308.2 AGITATION STATE, ACUTE REACTION TO STRESS
750.11 AGLOSSIA CONGENITAL
784.69 AGNOSIA (AUDITORY) (VISUAL) (ORGANIC)
368.16 AGNOSIA VISUAL (PSYCHOPHYSICAL)
300.22 AGORAPHOBIA
300.21 AGORAPHOBIA WITH PANIC ATTACKS
288.0 AGRANULOCYTIC ANGINA
288.0 AGRANULOCYTOSIS
784.69 AGRAPHIA (AUDITORY) (VISUAL) (ORGANIC)
742.2 AGYRIA CONGENITAL
253.1 AHUMADA-DEL CASTILLO SYNDROME (NONPUERPERAL GALACTORRHEA AND AMENORRHEA)

AIDS, ARC AND SYMPTOMATIC HIV INFECTIONS ALL USE CODE 042. THIS CODE SHOULD BE SEQUENCED AS THE PRINCIPAL DIAGNOSIS WITH AN ADDITIONAL CODE FOR ANY MANIFESTATION. EXCEPTION: IF THE ENCOUNTER IS FOR AN UNRELATED CONDITION SUCH AS A TRAUMA, SEQUENCE THE TRAUMA AS THE PRINCIPAL DIAGNOSIS, FOLLOWED BY THE 042 CODE, AND THEN THE ADDITIONAL CODES FOR THE MANIFESTATIONS.

AIDS
042 NOS
042 NOS DUE TO HIV II [079.53]
V65.44 COUNSELING
V01.7 EXPOSURE
795.71 INCONCLUSIVE (NONSPECIFIC SEROLOGIC EVIDENCE)
042 LIKE SYNDROME
647.6# MATERNAL CURRENT (CO-EXISTENT) IN PREGNANCY [042]
5th Digit: 647.6
0. EPISODE OF CARE NOS OR N/A
1. DELIVERED
2. DELIVERED WITH POSTPARTUM COMPLICATION
3. ANTEPARTUM COMPLICATION
4. POSTPARTUM COMPLICATION
042 RELATED COMPLEX
042 RELATED COMPLEX DUE TO HIV II [079.53]

136.0 AINHUM
0 AIR BLAST CONCUSSION SYNDROME SEE ANATOMICAL SITE, INJURY

AIR EMBOLISM
999.1 FOLLOWING INFUSION PERFUSION OR TRANSFUSION
673.0# MATERNAL DUE TO PREGNANCY
5th Digit: 673.0
0. EPISODE OF CARE NOS OR N/A
1. DELIVERED
2. DELIVERED WITH POSTPARTUM COMPLICATION
3. ANTEPARTUM COMPLICATION
4. POSTPARTUM COMPLICATION
958.0 TRAUMATIC
908.6 TRAUMATIC LATE EFFECT

306.1 AIR HUNGER PSYCHOGENIC
993.9 AIR PRESSURE EFFECT
909.4 AIR PRESSURE LATE EFFECT
993.8 AIR PRESSURE OTHER SPECIFIED EFFECTS
994.6 AIR SICKNESS
909.4 AIR SICKNESS LATE EFFECT

AIRWAY
493.90 DISEASE REACTIVE (SEE ALSO 'ASTHMA')
519.8 OBSTRUCTION NEC
496 OBSTRUCTION CHRONIC
519.1 OBSTRUCTION DUE TO BRONCHOSPASM
934.9 OBSTRUCTION DUE TO FOREIGN BODY
506.9 OBSTRUCTION DUE TO INHALATION OF FUMES OR VAPORS
478.75 OBSTRUCTION DUE TO LARYNGOSPASM
495.9 OBSTRUCTION WITH ALLERGIC ALVEOLITIS NEC
0 OBSTRUCTION WITH ASTHMA SEE 'ASTHMA'
494 OBSTRUCTION WITH BRONCHIECTASIS
0 OBSTRUCTION WITH BRONCHITIS SEE 'BRONCHITIS', OBSTRUCTIVE
492.8 OBSTRUCTION WITH EMPHYSEMA NEC

081.2 AKAMUSHI DISEASE (SCRUB TYPHUS)
333.99 AKATHISIA DUE TO DRUGS
291.1 AKS (SEE ALSO 'PSYCHOSIS ALCOHOLIC')
049.8 AKUREYRI DISEASE

ALALIA
784.3 ACQUIRED
315.31 DEVELOPMENTAL - EXPRESSIVE
315.32 DEVELOPMENTAL - RECEPTIVE (EXPRESSIVE - RECEPTIVE) MIXED

270.8 ALANINE METABOLISM DISORDERS
270.8 ALANINEMIA
050.1 ALASTRIM
599.0 ALBARRAN'S (COLIBACILLURIA) DISEASE
756.52 ALBERS-SCHONBERG'S SYNDROME
726.71 ALBERT'S DISEASE
270.2 ALBINISM
270.2 ALBINISM AMINO ACID METABOLISM AROMATIC DISTURBANCES
270.2 ALBINISM OCULAR
275.49 ALBRIGHT-MARTIN (-BANTAM) SYNDROME (PSEUDOHYPOPARATHYROIDISM)
756.59 ALBRIGHT-MCCUNE-STERNBERG SYNDROME (OSTEITIS FIBROSA DISSEMINATA)
756.59 ALBRIGHT STERNBERG SYNDROME
273.8 ALBUMIN ABSENCE (BLOOD)
790.99 ALBUMIN GLOBULIN RATIO ABNORMAL
791.0 ALBUMINURIA ABNORMAL FINDINGS
646.2# ALBUMINURIA MATERNAL COMPLICATING PREGNANCY WITHOUT MENTION OF HYPERTENSION

5th Digit: 646.2

- **0. EPISODE OF CARE UNSPECIFIED OR N/A**
- **1. DELIVERED**
- **2. DELIVERED WITH POSTPARTUM COMPLICATION**
- **3. ANTEPARTUM COMPLICATION**
- **4. POSTPARTUM COMPLICATION**

> *SUBSTANCE ABUSE DESCRIBES THE PRACTICE OF USING DRUGS OR ALCOHOL TO EXCESS WITHOUT REACHING THE STATE OF PHYSICAL DEPENDENCE. **SUBSTANCE DEPENDENCE** IS ADDICTION. DEPENDENCE INVOLVES THE LOSS OF CONTROL AND JUDGMENT AND/OR THE INABILITY TO USE IN MODERATION. DEPENDENCE IS MARKED BY COMPULSIVE PHYSICAL DEMANDS WHICH ARE TRIGGERED BY FURTHER INGESTION.*

ALCOHOL

303.0# ABUSE DEPENDENT - ACUTE INTOXICATION
303.9# ABUSE DEPENDENT - IN CHRONIC ALCOHOLISM
305.0# ABUSE NONDEPENDENT

5th Digit: 303.0, 9, 305.0

- **0. NOS**
- **1. CONTINUOUS**
- **2. EPISODIC**
- **3. IN REMISSION**

790.3 BLOOD LEVEL EXCESSIVE (ELEVATED)
V70.4 BLOOD TEST FOR ALCOHOL
760.71 FETAL SYNDROME
760.71 TRANSMITTED VIA PLACENTA OR BREAST MILK AFFECTING FETUS OR NEWBORN

ALCOHOL INTOXICATION

303.0# ACUTE DEPENDENT
305.0# ACUTE NONDEPENDENT

5th Digit: 303.0, 305.0

- **0. NOS**
- **1. CONTINUOUS**
- **2. EPISODIC**
- **3. IN REMISSION**

291.4 ACUTE PATHOLOGIC (IDIOSYNCRATIC)

> *ALCOHOLIC (ALCOHOLISM INDUCED) CONDITIONS REQUIRE TWO CODES: ONE FOR THE ALCOHOLIC CONDITION, AND ONE FOR THE DEPENDENCE. SEE 'ALCOHOL ABUSE', (DEPENDENT). SEQUENCING DEPENDS ON THE REASON FOR ENCOUNTER. **ALCOHOLIC PSYCHOSES, 291.#(#),** HOWEVER, CODE FIRST WITH THE DEPENDENCE CODE SECOND.*

ALCOHOLIC (ALCOHOLISM INDUCED)

291.81 ABSTINENCE SYMPTOMS OR SYNDROME
291.1 AMNESTIC SYNDROME
291.89 ANXIETY
291.2 BRAIN SYNDROME (CHRONIC)
425.5 CARDIOMYOPATHY
303.9# CEREBELLAR ATAXIA [334.4]
303.9# CEREBRAL DEGENERATION DISEASE [331.7]

5th Digit: 303.9

- **0. UNSPECIFIED**
- **1. CONTINUOUS**
- **2. EPISODIC**
- **3. IN REMISSION**

571.2 CIRRHOSIS OF LIVER
291.5 DELUSIONS
291.2 DEMENTIA
291.81 DEPRIVATION SYMPTOMS OR SYNDROME
345.## EPILEPSY

4th Digit: 345

- **0. GENERALIZED NONCONVULSIVE**
- **1. GENERALIZED CONVULSIVE**
- **4. PARTIAL, WITH IMPAIRMENT OF CONSCIOUSNESS**
- **5. PARTIAL, WITHOUT IMPAIRMENT OF CONSCIOUSNESS**
- **6. INFANTILE SPASMS**
- **7. EPILEPSIA PARTIALIS CONTINUA**
- **8. OTHER FORMS**
- **9. UNSPECIFIED, NOS**

5th Digit: 345

- **0. WITHOUT MENTION OF INTRACTABLE EPILEPSY**
- **1. WITH INTRACTABLE EPILEPSY**

345.3 EPILEPSY GRAND MAL STATUS
345.2 EPILEPSY PETIT MAL STATUS
571.2 FATTY LIVER
535.3# GASTRITIS

5th Digit : 535.3

- **0. WITHOUT HEMORRHAGE**
- **1. WITH HEMORRHAGE**

571.1 HEPATITIS
303.0# INTOXICATION ACUTE

5th Digit: 303.0

- **0. NOS**
- **1. CONTINUOUS**
- **2. EPISODIC**
- **3. IN REMISSION**

291.4 INTOXICATION PATHOLOGICAL (IDIOSYNCRATIC)
291.5 JEALOUSY
291.1 KORSAKOFF SYNDROME (AKS)
571.3 LIVER DAMAGE
571.1 LIVER DISEASE ACUTE
571.3 LIVER DISEASE CHRONIC
291.9 MANIA NOS
0 MENTAL DISORDER SEE 'PSYCHOSIS ALCOHOLIC'
291.89 MOOD
357.5 NEUROPATHY
291.1 NEUROPATHY WITH PSYCHOSIS
291.2 ORGANIC BRAIN SYNDROME
291.5 PARANOIA (JEALOUSY)
0 PSYCHOSIS SEE 'PSYCHOSIS ALCOHOLIC'
V79.1 SCREENING
291.0 WITHDRAWAL - DELIRIUM (TREMENS)
291.3 WITHDRAWAL - HALLUCINOSIS (PSYCHOSIS)
291.81 WITHDRAWAL - SYMPTOMS OR SYNDROME
760.71 WITHDRAWAL - SYMPTOMS OR SYNDROME NEWBORN

ALCOHOLISM

303.0# ACUTE
303.9# CHRONIC
5th Digit: 303.0, 9
0. NOS
1. CONTINUOUS
2. EPISODIC
3. IN REMISSION

V61.41 FAMILY PROBLEMS (REASON FOR ENCOUNTER)
V11.3 HISTORY OF ALCOHOLISM
655.4# MATERNAL WITH SUSPECTED DAMAGE TO FETUS
5th Digit: 655.4
0. EPISODE OF CARE NOS OR N/A
1. DELIVERED
3. ANTEPARTUM COMPLICATION

V79.1 SCREENING

288.2 ALDER'S (REILLY) SYNDROME (LEUKOCYTE GRANULATION ANOMALY)
271.2 ALDOLASE (HEREDITARY) DEFICIENCY
255.1 ALDOSTERONISM (PRIMARY)
255.1 ALDOSTERONISM (SECONDARY)
237.2 ALDOSTERONOMA
279.12 ALDRICH (-WISKOTT) SYNDROME (ECZEMA-THROMBOCYTOPENIA)

085.1 ALEPPO BOIL
288.0 ALEUKIA CONGENITAL
284.# ALEUKIA HEMORRHAGICA (APLASTIC ANEMIA)
4th Digit: 284
0. CONGENITAL
8. ACQUIRED (SECONDARY)
9. UNSPECIFIED

315.01 ALEXIA DELAY IN DEVELOPMENT
784.61 ALEXIA WITH AGRAPHIA
733.7 ALGONEURODYSTROPHY

300.29 ALGOPHOBIA
202.1# ALIBERT-BAZIN SYNDROME (MYCOSIS FUNGOIDES) M9700/3
202.1# ALIBERT'S DISEASE (MYCOSIS FUNGOIDES) M9700/3
5th Digit: 202.1
0. UNSPECIFIED SITE, EXTRANODAL AND SOLID ORGAN SITES
1. LYMPH NODES OF HEAD FACE NECK
2. LYMPH NODES INTRATHORACIC
3. LYMPH NODES ABDOMINAL
4. LYMPH NODES AXILLA AND UPPER LIMB
5. LYMPH NODES INGUINAL REGION AND LOWER LIMB
6. LYMPH NODES INTRAPELVIC
7. SPLEEN
8. LYMPH NODES MULTIPLE SITES

293.89 ALICE IN WONDERLAND SYNDROME

560.9 ALIMENTARY CANAL OBSTRUCTION (SEE ALSO 'INTESTINE, INTESTINAL', OBSTRUCTION)

751.8 ALIMENTARY TRACT NOS - ABSENCE OR ATRESIA (COMPLETE) (PARTIAL) (CONGENITAL)
751.5 ALIMENTARY TRACT LOWER - ABSENCE (COMPLETE) (PARTIAL) (CONGENITAL)
751.2 ALIMENTARY TRACT LOWER - ATRESIA (CONGENITAL)
750.8 ALIMENTARY TRACT UPPER - ABSENCE OR ATRESIA (COMPLETE) (PARTIAL) (CONGENITAL)
750.9 ALIMENTARY TRACT UPPER - ANOMALY UNSPECIFIED CONGENITAL
750.8 ALIMENTARY TRACT UPPER - ANOMALY OTHER SPECIFIED CONGENITAL

790.5 ALKALINE PHOSPHATASE ABNORMAL BLOOD LEVEL
790.4 ALKALINE PHOSPHATASE ELEVATED

ALKALOSIS

276.3 NOS
276.3 METABOLIC
276.3 RESPIRATORY

270.2 ALKAPTONURIA AMINO ACID METABOLISM AROMATIC DISTURBANCES
270.2 ALKAPTONURIC OCHRONOSIS
620.6 ALLEN-MASTERS SYNDROME

ALLERGY, ALLERGIC

0 ANAPHYLACTIC SHOCK SEE 'ANAPHYLAXIS, ANAPHYLACTIC'
493.0# ASTHMA
5th Digit: 493.0
0. WITHOUT MENTION OF STATUS ASTHMATICUS
1. WITH STATUS ASTHMATICUS

518.6 BRONCHOPULMONARY ASPERGILLOSIS
558.9 COLITIS
372.14 CONJUNCTIVITIS (ECZEMATOUS)
0 DERMATITIS SEE ALSO 'DERMATITIS' AND 'DERMATITIS CONTACT'
V07.1 DESENSITIZATION
558.9 DIARRHEA
995.2 DRUG CORRECTLY ADMINISTERED
360.19 ENDOPHTHALMITIS
V19.6 FAMILY HISTORY OF ALLERGY DISORDERS
691.8 FOOD - ATOPIC DERMATITIS
692.5 FOOD - CONTACT WITH SKIN
V65.3 FOOD - COUNSELING AND SURVEILLANCE
693.1 FOOD - INGESTION DERMATITIS
535.4# GASTRITIS
5th Digit: 535.4
0. WITHOUT HEMORRHAGE
1. WITH HEMORRHAGE

558.9 GASTROENTERITIS
477.9 HAY FEVER
477.8 HAY FEVER - ANIMAL (DANDER) (HAIR) (FEATHERS)
477.8 HAY FEVER - DUST (HOUSE) (STOCK)
477.0 HAY FEVER - POLLENS (GRASS) (GRAINS) (RAGWEED) (TREES)
493.0# HAY FEVER - WITH ASTHMA
5th Digit: 493.0
0. WITHOUT MENTION OF STATUS ASTHMATICUS
1. WITH STATUS ASTHMATICUS

0 HISTORY SEE 'ALLERGY, ALLERGIC HISTORY'
995.3 HYPERSENSITIVITY
364.04 IRIDOCYCLITIS
995.2 MEDICINE CORRECTLY ADMINISTERED
287.0 PURPURA
995.3 REACTION
V15.0 REACTION HISTORY (SEE ALSO 'ALLERGY, ALLERGIC HISTORY')
909.9 REACTION LATE EFFECT
306.1 REACTION PSYCHOGENIC - RESPIRATORY
995.2 REACTION TO CORRECTLY ADMINISTERED SUBSTANCE
477.9 RHINITIS
477.8 RHINITIS - ANIMAL (DANDER) (HAIR) (DUST) (FEATHERS)
477.8 RHINITIS - DUST (HOUSE) (STOCK)
477.0 RHINITIS - POLLENS (GRASS) (GRAINS) (RAGWEED) (TREES)
493.0# RHINITIS - WITH ASTHMA
5th Digit: 493.0
0. WITHOUT MENTION OF STATUS ASTHMATICUS
1. WITH STATUS ASTHMATICUS

999.5 SERUM (PROPHYLACTIC) (THERAPEUTIC)
995.0 SHOCK
V07.1 SHOTS
692.9 SKIN REACTION
V72.7 TESTING
597.89 URETHRITIS
708.0 URTICARIA

	ALLERGY, ALLERGIC HISTORY
V15.0	UNSPECIFIED
V14.9	UNSPECIFIED MEDICATION
V14.6	ANALGESIC AGENT
V14.4	ANESTHETIC AGENT
V14.5	CODEINE
V14.5	NARCOTIC AGENT
V14.3	OTHER ANTI-INFECTIVE AGENT
V14.1	OTHER ANTIBIOTIC
V14.0	PENICILLIN
V14.2	SULFONAMIDES
V14.7	VACCINE
V14.8	OTHER SPECIFIED MEDICINAL AGENTS
V15.0	OTHER SPECIFIED NON-MEDICINAL AGENTS
117.6	ALLESCHERIA PETRIELLIDIUM BOYDII INFECTIONS
117.6	ALLESCHERIOSIS
757.1	ALLIGATOR BABY SYNDROME (ICHTHYOSIS CONGENITA)
701.1	ALLIGATOR SKIN DISEASE ACQUIRED
757.1	ALLIGATOR SKIN DISEASE CONGENITAL
116.1	ALMEIDA'S (BRAZILIAN BLASTOMYCOSIS)
	ALOPECIA
704.00	NOS
704.01	ANDROGENETIC
704.01	AREATA
757.4	CONGENITAL
316	PSYCHOGENIC [704.00]
091.82	SYPHILITIC
704.02	TELOGEN EFFLUVIUM
330.8	ALPERS' DISEASE OR GRAY-MATTER DEGENERATION
277.6	ALPHA 1 ANTITRYPSIN DEFICIENCY
277.6	ALPHA 1 TRYPSIN INHIBITOR DEFICIENCY
255.2	ALPHA (17) (20) HYDROXYLASE DEFICIENCY
792.3	ALPHA FETOPROTEIN ABNORMAL FINDING IN AMNIOTIC FLUID
790.99	ALPHA FETOPROTEIN ABNORMAL FINDING IN BLOOD
V28.1	ALPHA FETOPROTEIN SCREENING BY AMNIOCENTESIS
271.8	ALPHA FUCOSIDASE DEFICIENCY
272.5	ALPHA LIPOPROTEIN DEFICIENCY
271.8	ALPHA MANNOSIDASE DEFICIENCY
993.2	ALPINE SICKNESS
909.4	ALPINE SICKNESS LATE EFFECT
759.89	ALPORT'S SYNDROME (HEREDITARY HEMATURIA-NEPHROPATHY-DEAFNESS)
335.20	ALS MOTOR NEURON DISEASE (BULBAR) (MIXED TYPE)
0	ALTE (APPARENT LIFE-THREATENING EVENT) CODE INDIVIDUAL SYMPTOM(S)
780.0#	ALTERATION OF CONSCIOUSNESS
	5th Digit: 780.0
	1. COMA
	2. TRANSIENT AWARENESS
	3. PERSISTENT VEGETATIVE STATE
	9. OTHER (STUPOR, DROWSINESS, SOMNOLENCE, SEMICOMA, UNCONSCIOUSNESS)
780.9	ALTERED MENTAL STATUS
118	ALTERNARIA INFECTION TO COMPROMISED HOST ONLY
993.2	ALTITUDE SICKNESS
909.4	ALTITUDE SICKNESS LATE EFFECT
435.9	ALVAREZ SYNDROME (TRANSIENT CEREBRAL ISCHEMIA)
	ALVEOLAR
526.5	JAW ALVEOLITIS
516.3	CAPILLARY BLOCK SYNDROME
524.70	DENTAL - ANOMALY UNSPECIFIED
524.79	DENTAL - ANOMALY OTHER SPECIFIED
524.72	DENTAL - MANDIBULAR HYPERPLASIA
524.74	DENTAL - MANDIBULAR HYPOPLASIA
524.71	DENTAL - MAXILLARY HYPERPLASIA
524.73	DENTAL - MAXILLARY HYPOPLASIA
959.09	INJURY
525.8	PROCESS ABSENCE
750.26	PROCESS ABSENCE CONGENITAL
525.2	PROCESS ATROPHY
525.8	PROCESS IRREGULAR
525.8	RIDGE CLEFT
525.8	RIDGE ENLARGEMENT NOS
	ALVEOLITIS
495.9	ALLERGIC (EXTRINSIC)
495.7	ALLERGIC (EXTRINSIC) - VENTILATION
495.8	ALLERGIC (EXTRINSIC) - SPECIFIED TYPE NEC
495.4	DUE TO ASPERGILLUS CLAVATUS
495.6	DUE TO CRYPTOSTROMA CORTICALE
516.3	FIBROSING IDIOPATHIC (LUNG)
714.81	FIBROSING IDIOPATHIC (LUNG) - RHEUMATOID
526.5	JAW
526.5	SICCA DOLOROSA
	ALZHEIMERS
331.0	DEMENTIA [294.1]
331.0	DISEASE
331.0	DISEASE WITH DEMENTIA [294.1]
331.0	SCLEROSIS
331.0	SCLEROSIS WITH DEMENTIA [294.1]
V15.81	AMA DISCHARGE (AGAINST MEDICAL ADVICE)
330.1	AMAUROTIC FAMILIAL IDIOCY
	AMAUROSIS
369.00	NOS BOTH EYES
362.34	FUGAX
300.11	HYSTERICAL
362.76	LEBER'S CONGENITAL
377.34	TOBACCO
377.34	TOXIC
0	UREMIC SEE 'UREMIA'
	AMBLYOPIA
368.00	NOS
368.02	DEPRIVATION INDUCED
368.03	REFRACTIVE
368.01	STRABISMIC (SUPPRESSIVE)
377.34	TOXIC
	AMEBIC (AMEBIASIS)
006.0	ACUTE INFECTION
006.8	AMEBOMA
006.8	APPENDICITIS
006.8	BALANITIS
006.5	BRAIN ABSCESS (AND LIVER) (AND LUNG)
V02.2	CARRIER
006.1	CHRONIC
006.6	CUTANEOUS
007.8	DUE TO ORGANISMS OTHER THAN ENTAMOEBA HISTOLYTICA
006.0	DYSENTERY ACUTE
006.1	DYSENTERY CHRONIC
006.3	HEPATIC
006.9	INFECTION
136.2	INFECTION FREE-LIVING SPECIFIC
006.8	INFECTION OTHER SITES

AMEBIC (AMEBIASIS) (continued)
006.3 LIVER ABSCESS
006.4 LUNG ABSCESS (AND LIVER)
136.2 MENINGOENCEPHALITIS (NAEGLERIA)
006.2 NONDYSENTERIC COLITIS
006.6 SKIN ULCERATION
006.6 ULCERATION SKIN

755.4 AMELIA
755.31 AMELIA LOWER LIMB
755.21 AMELIA UPPER LIMB ABSENCE CONGENITAL
0 AMEBIASIS SEE 'AMEBIC (AMEBIASIS)'

AMELOBLASTOMA
213.# NOS (BY SITE) M9310/0
4th Digit: 213
0. SKULL FACE UPPER JAW
1. LOWER JAW NOS (OR IF UNSPECIFIED)
2. SPINE
3. RIB STERNUM CLAVICLE
4. UPPER LIMB LONG BONES SCAPULA
5. UPPER LIMB SHORT BONES
6. PELVIS SACRUM COCCYX
7. LOWER LIMB LONG BONE
8. LOWER LIMB SHORT BONE
9. SITE NOS

170.# MALIGNANT (BY SITE) M9310/3
4th Digit: 170
0. SKULL AND FACE
1. MANDIBLE (OR IF SITE UNSPECIFIED)
2. VERTEBRAL COLUMN
3. RIBS STERNUM CLAVICLE
4. SCAPULA LONG BONES UPPER LIMB
5. SHORT BONES UPPER LIMB
6. PELVIC BONES SACRUM COCCYX
7. LONG BONES LOWER LIMB
8. SHORT BONES LOWER LIMB
9. SITE NOS

520.5 AMELOGENESIS IMPERFECTA
626.0 AMENORRHEA PRIMARY OR SECONDARY
256.8 AMENORRHEA HYPERHORMONAL [626.0]
066.1 AMERICAN MOUNTAIN TICK BORNE FEVER
0 AMI (ACUTE MYOCARDIAL INFARCTION)) SEE 'MYOCARDIAL INFARCTION ACUTE'
270.9 AMINO ACID DEFICIENCY
270.9 AMINO ACID METABOLISM DISORDER
270.2 AMINO ACID METABOLISM DISORDER AROMATIC
775.8 AMINO ACID METABOLISM DISORDER NEONATAL TRANSITORY
270.8 AMINO ACID METABOLISM DISORDER OTHER
V09.4 AMINOGLYCOSIDES RESISTANT INFECTION (SEE DRUG RESISTANT MICROORGANISMS FOR COMPLETE LISTING)
270.6 AMMONIA METABOLISM DISORDER

AMNESIA
292.83 DRUG INDUCED
300.12 HYSTERICAL
300.12 PSYCHOGENIC
780.9 RETROGRADE
437.7 TRANSIENT GLOBAL

AMNESTIC SYNDROME
294.0 NOS
291.1 ALCOHOLIC (PSYCHOTIC)
294.0 CHRONIC (NONALCOHOLIC)
294.0 CONFABULATORY
292.83 DRUG INDUCED
291.1 KORSAKOFF'S
294.0 POSTTRAUMATIC

AMNIOCENTESIS
V28.0 CHROMOSOMAL SCREENING ANOMALY
762.1 DAMAGING PLACENTA AFFECTING FETUS OR NEWBORN
V28.1 FOR ALPHAFETOPROTEIN SCREENING
V28.2 FOR OTHER SCREENING

AMNION, AMNIOTIC
762.9 ABNORMALITY - NOS AFFECTING FETUS OR NEWBORN
762.8 ABNORMALITY - OTHER SPECIFIED AFFECTING FETUS OR NEWBORN
762.8 BAND AFFECTING FETUS OR NEWBORN
658.8# BAND COMPLICATING PREGNANCY
5th Digit: 658.8
0. EPISODE OF CARE NOS OR N/A
1. DELIVERED
3. ANTEPARTUM COMPLICATION

792.3 FLUID ABNORMAL
673.1# FLUID EMBOLISM MATERNAL DUE TO PREGNANCY
5th Digit: 673.1
0. EPISODE OF CARE NOS OR N/A
1. DELIVERED
2. DELIVERED WITH POSTPARTUM COMPLICATION
3. ANTEPARTUM COMPLICATION
4. POSTPARTUM COMPLICATION

658.8# FLUID LEAKAGE
0 INFECTION (CAVITY) SEE 'AMNIONITIS'
658.9# MEMBRANE OR CAVITY PROBLEM
658.8# NODOSUM
658.1# SAC RUPTURE PREMATURE
5th Digit: 658.1, 8-9
0. EPISODE OF CARE NOS OR N/A
1. DELIVERED
3. ANTEPARTUM COMPLICATION

658.4# AMNIONITIS
5th Digit: 658.4
0. EPISODE OF CARE NOS OR N/A
1. DELIVERED
3. ANTEPARTUM COMPLICATION

762.7 AMNIONITIS AFFECTING FETUS OR NEWBORN
301.7 AMORAL PERSONALITY
292.89 AMOTIVATIONAL SYNDROME
305.7# AMPHETAMINE ABUSE (NONDEPENDENT)
304.4# AMPHETAMINE ADDICTION (DEPENDENT)
5th Digit: 304.4, 305.7
0. NOS
1. CONTINUOUS
2. EPISODIC
3. IN REMISSION

530.89 AMPULLA ESOPHAGEAL
576.2 AMPULLA OF VATER OBSTRUCTION (OCCLUSION)
0 AMPULLA OF VATER OBSTRUCTION (OCCLUSION) WITH CALCULUS SEE 'CHOLEDOCHOLITHIASIS'
530.89 AMPULLA PHRENIC

A CURRENT COMPLICATED AMPUTATION IS A TRAUMATIC AMPUTATION WITH DELAYED HEALING OR TREATMENT, FOREIGN BODY, OR INFECTION.

AMPUTATION

0 AMPUTEE (BILATERAL) (OLD) ACQUIRED SEE 'AMPUTATION', STATUS, BY SITE

887.# ARM AND/OR HAND TRAUMATIC

4th Digit: 887

- **0. BELOW ELBOW UNILATERAL**
- **1. BELOW ELBOW UNILATERAL COMPLICATED ORIGINAL ADMISSION**
- **2. ABOVE ELBOW UNILATERAL**
- **3. ABOVE ELBOW UNILATERAL COMPLICATED ORIGINAL ADMISSION**
- **4. LEVEL NOS UNILATERAL**
- **5. LEVEL NOS UNILATERAL COMPLICATED ORIGINAL ADMISSION**
- **6. BILATERAL (ANY LEVEL)**
- **7. BILATERAL (ANY LEVEL) COMPLICATED ORIGINAL ADMISSION**

886.0 FINGER TRAUMATIC

886.1 FINGER TRAUMATIC - COMPLICATED ORIGINAL ADMISSION

896.0 FOOT TRAUMATIC UNILATERAL

896.1 FOOT TRAUMATIC UNILATERAL - COMPLICATED ORIGINAL ADMISSION

896.2 FOOT TRAUMATIC BILATERAL

896.3 FOOT TRAUMATIC BILATERAL - COMPLICATED ORIGINAL ADMISSION

997.62: INFECTION OF AN AMPUTATION STUMP, USE AN ADDITIONAL CODE TO IDENTIFY ORGANISM. SEE 'BACTERIAL INFECTION'.

997.62 INFECTION (LATE) (CHRONIC) STUMP

0 INFECTION CURRENT TRAUMATIC AMPUTATION SEE 'AMPUTATION' BY SITE, TRAUMATIC COMPLICATED

905.9 LATE EFFECT (SURGICAL) (TRAUMATIC)

997.6# LATE EFFECT STUMP

5th Digit: 997.6

- **0. NOS**
- **1. NEUROMA OF STUMP**
- **2. INFECTION (CHRONIC)**
- **9. OTHER**

897.# LEG

4th Digit: 897

- **0. UNILATERAL BELOW KNEE**
- **1. UNILATERAL BELOW KNEE COMPLICATED ORIGINAL ADMISSION**
- **2. UNILATERAL ABOVE KNEE**
- **3. UNILATERAL ABOVE KNEE COMPLICATED ORIGINAL ADMISSION**
- **4. UNILATERAL LEVEL NOS**
- **5. UNILATERAL LEVEL NOS COMPLICATED ORIGINAL ADMISSION**
- **6. BILATERAL ANY LEVEL**
- **7. BILATERAL ANY LEVEL COMPLICATED ORIGINAL ADMISSION**

878.0 PENIS TRAUMATIC

878.1 PENIS TRAUMATIC - COMPLICATED ORIGINAL ADMISSION

353.6 PHANTOM LIMB SYNDROME

878.2 SCROTUM AND TESTES TRAUMATIC

878.3 SCROTUM AND TESTES TRAUMATIC - COMPLICATED ORIGINAL ADMISSION

AMPUTATION (continued)

V49.7# STATUS - LOWER LIMB

5th Digit: V49.7

- **0. UNSPECIFIED LEVEL**
- **1. GREAT TOE**
- **2. OTHER TOE(S)**
- **3. FOOT**
- **4. ANKLE**
- **5. BELOW KNEE**
- **6. ABOVE KNEE**
- **7. HIP**

V49.6# STATUS - UPPER LIMB

5th Digit: V49.6

- **0. UNSPECIFIED LEVEL**
- **1. THUMB**
- **2. OTHER FINGER(S)**
- **3. HAND**
- **4. WRIST**
- **5. BELOW ELBOW**
- **6. ABOVE ELBOW**
- **7. SHOULDER**

997.6# STUMP COMPLICATION

5th Digit: 997.6

- **0. UNSPECIFIED**
- **1. NEUROMA**
- **2. INFECTION (CHRONIC)**
- **9. OTHER**

885.0 THUMB TRAUMATIC

885.1 THUMB TRAUMATIC - COMPLICATED ORIGINAL ADMISSION

895.0 TOE TRAUMATIC

895.1 TOE TRAUMATIC - COMPLICATED ORIGINAL ADMISSION

0 TRAUMATIC SEE 'OPEN WOUND', BY SITE

740.0 AMYELENCEPHALUS CONGENITAL

742.59 AMYELIA CONGENITAL

474.8 AMYGDALOLITH

790.5 AMYLASE ABNORMAL LEVEL

790.4 AMYLASE ELEVATED

277.3 AMYLOID DEGENERATION LIVER

AMYLOIDOSIS

277.3 NOS

277.3 CARDIOMYOPATHY [425.7]

277.3 HEREDITARY CARDIAC

277.3 INHERITED SYSTEMIC

277.3 NEPHROPATHIC

277.3 NEUROPATHIC (PORTUGUESE) (SWISS)

277.3 PERIPHERAL NERVE (AUTONOMIC) [337.1]

277.3 POLYNEUROPATHY [357.4]

277.3 RENAL DISEASE [583.81]

277.3 SECONDARY

277.3 WITH LUNG INVOLVEMENT [517.8]

277.3 WITH MYOPATHY [359.6]

271.0 AMYLOPECTINOSIS

275.1 AMYOSTATIC SYNDROME

728.2 AMYOTROPHIA

756.89 AMYOTROPHIA CONGENITA

353.5 AMYOTROPHIA NEURALGIC (NONDISCOGENIC)

335.20 AMYOTROPHIC LATERAL SCLEROSIS (SYNDROME)

AMYOTROPHY

005.1 BOTULISM [358.1]

250.6# DIABETIC [358.1]

5th Digit: 250.6

0. TYPE II, ADULT-ONSET, NON-INSULIN DEPENDENT (EVEN IF REQUIRING INSULIN), OR UNSPECIFIED; CONTROLLED

1. TYPE I, JUVENILE-ONSET OR INSULIN-DEPENDENT; CONTROLLED

2. TYPE II, ADULT-ONSET, NON-INSULIN DEPENDENT (EVEN IF REQUIRING INSULIN); UNCONTROLLED

3. TYPE I, JUVENILE-ONSET OR INSULIN-DEPENDENT; UNCONTROLLED

244.# HYPOTHYROID [358.1]

4th Digit: 244

0. POSTSURGICAL

1. POSTABLATIVE (IRRADIATION)

2. IODINE INGESTION

3. PAS, PHENYLBUT, RESORCINOL

8. SECONDARY NEC

9. NOS

281.0 PERNICIOUS ANEMIA [358.1]

335.21 SPINAL PROGRESSIVE

242.## THYROTOXIC [358.1]

4th Digit: 242

0. TOXIC DIFFUSE GOITER

1. TOXIC UNINODULAR GOITER

2. TOXIC MULTINODULAR GOITER

3. TOXIC NODULAR GOITER UNSPECIFIED

4. FROM ECTOPIC THYROID NODULE

8. OF OTHER SPECIFIED ORIGIN

9. WITHOUT GOITER OR OTHER CAUSE

5th Digit: 242

0. WITHOUT STORM

1. WITH STORM

795.79 ANA POSITIVE (ANTINUCLEAR ANTIBODIES)

008.46 ANAEROBIC ENTERITIS NOS

282.3 ANAEROBIC GLYCOLYSIS WITH ANEMIA

038.3 ANAEROBIC SEPSIS

0 ANAL SEE 'ANUS, ANAL'

763.5 ANALGESICS OF L&D AFFECTING FETUS OR NEWBORN

301.4 ANANCASTIC PERSONALITY DISORDER

ANAPHYLAXIS - ANAPHYLACTIC

995.0 NOS

909.9 NOS LATE EFFECT

995.0 ALLERGIC SHOCK

909.9 ALLERGIC SHOCK LATE EFFECT

995.0 DUE TO DRUG (MEDICINE) - CORRECTLY ADMINISTERED

909.9 DUE TO DRUG (MEDICINE) - CORRECTLY ADMINISTERED LATE EFFECT

977.9 DUE TO DRUG (MEDICINE) - IMPROPERLY ADMINISTERED

909.0 DUE TO DRUG (MEDICINE) - IMPROPERLY ADMINISTERED LATE EFFECT

995.0 DUE TO NONMEDICAL SUBSTANCE

909.9 DUE TO NONMEDICAL SUBSTANCE LATE EFFECT

977.9 DUE TO OVERDOSE

909.0 DUE TO OVERDOSE LATE EFFECT

999.4 DUE TO SERUM (IMMUNIZATION)

909.3 DUE TO SERUM (IMMUNIZATION) LATE EFFECT

287.0 PURPURA

995.0 REACTION

909.9 REACTION LATE EFFECT

995.0 SHOCK NOS

909.9 SHOCK NOS LATE EFFECT

ANAPHYLAXIS - ANAPHYLACTIC (continued)

995.6# SHOCK DUE TO FOOD NONPOISONOUS

5th Digit: 995.6

0. UNSPECIFIED FOOD

1. PEANUTS

2. CRUSTACEANS

3. FRUITS AND VEGETABLES

4. TREE NUTS AND SEEDS

5. FISH

6. FOOD ADDITIVES

7. MILK PRODUCTS

8. EGGS

9. OTHER SPECIFIED FOOD

909.9 SHOCK DUE TO FOOD LATE EFFECT

989.5 SHOCK DUE TO STING OR VENOM

909.1 SHOCK DUE TO STING OR VENOM LATE EFFECT

199.1 ANAPLASTIC CARCINOMA SITE NOS

0 ANAPLASTIC CARCINOMA SITE SPECIFIED SEE 'CANCER' BY SITE M8021/3

782.3 ANASARCA

752.62 ANASPADIAS CONGENITAL

747.60 ANASTOMOSIS ARTERIOVENOUS CONGENITAL NEC

997.4 ANASTOMOSIS COMPLICATION POSTSURGICAL - GASTROINTESTINAL

997.5 ANASTOMOSIS COMPLICATION POSTSURGICAL - URINARY

V45.3 ANASTOMOSIS GASTROINTESTINAL STATUS

534.## ANASTOMOTIC ULCER

4th Digit: 534

0. ACUTE WITH HEMORRHAGE

1. ACUTE WITH PERFORATION

2. ACUTE WITH HEMORRHAGE AND PERFORATION

3. ACUTE

4. CHRONIC OR UNSPECIFIED WITH HEMORRHAGE

5. CHRONIC OR UNSPECIFIED WITH PERFORATION

6. CHRONIC OR UNSPECIFIED WITH HEMORRHAGE AND PERFORATION

7. CHRONIC

9. UNSPECIFIED AS ACUTE OR CHRONIC

5th Digit: 534

0. WITHOUT OBSTRUCTION

1. OBSTRUCTED

ANCYLOSTOMA, ANCYLOSTOMIASIS

126.9 AND NECATORIASIS

126.2 BRAZILIENSE INFECTION

126.3 CEYLANICUM INFECTION

126.0 DUODENALE INFECTION

126.8 INFECTION OTHER SPECIFIED

126.1 NECATOR AMERICANUS

272.8 ANDERS (ADIPOSIS TUBEROSA SIMPLEX) DISEASE

271.0 ANDERSEN'S DISEASE (GLYCOGENOSIS IV)

272.7 ANDERSON'S DISEASE (ANGIOKERATOMA CORPORIS DIFFUSUM)

993.2 ANDES DISEASE

686.8 ANDREWS' DISEASE (PUSTULAR BACTERID)

CARCINOMAS AND NEOPLASMS SHOULD BE CODED BY SITE IF POSSIBLE. CODE BY CELL TYPE - "SITE NOS", IF AND ONLY IF A SITE IS NOT SPECIFIED IN THE DIAGNOSIS. OTHERWISE - REFER TO THE APPROPRIATE CATEGORY OF NEOPLASM FOR A MORE SPECIFIC CODE: SEE 'CANCER' 'CANCER METASTATIC', 'NEOPLASM UNCERTAIN BEHAVIOR', 'NEOPLASM UNSPECIFIED NATURE', OR 'BENIGN NEOPLASM'.

ANDROBLASTOMA

236.2 SITE NOS FEMALE
0 NOS FEMALE SITE SPECIFIED SEE 'NEOPLASM UNCERTAIN BEHAVIOR' BY SITE M8630/1
236.4 SITE NOS MALE
0 NOS MALE SITE SPECIFIED SEE 'NEOPLASM UNCERTAIN BEHAVIOR' BY SITE M8630/1

220 BENIGN FEMALE SITE NOS
0 BENIGN FEMALE SITE SPECIFIED SEE 'BENIGN NEOPLASM' BY SITE M8630/0
222.9 BENIGN MALE SITE NOS
0 BENIGN MALE SITE SPECIFIED SEE 'BENIGN NEOPLASM' BY SITE M8630/0

183.0 MALIGNANT FEMALE SITE NOS
0 MALIGNANT FEMALE SITE SPECIFIED SEE 'CANCER' BY SITE M9310/3
186.9 MALIGNANT MALE SITE NOS
0 MALIGNANT MALE SITE SPECIFIED SEE 'CANCER' BY SITE M9310/3

0 TUBULAR (WITH LIPID STORAGE) FEMALE SITE SPECIFIED SEE 'BENIGN NEOPLASM' BY SITE M8641/0
220 TUBULAR (WITH LIPID STORAGE) FEMALE SITE NOS
0 TUBULAR (WITH LIPID STORAGE) MALE SITE SPECIFIED SEE 'BENIGN NEOPLASM' BY SITE M8641/0
222.0 TUBULAR (WITH LIPID STORAGE) MALE SITE NOS M8641/0

256.1 ANDROGEN HYPERSECRETION OVARIAN
257.8 ANDROGEN INSENSITIVITY SYNDROME (TESTICULAR FEMINIZATION)

WHEN A PATIENT IS ADMITTED WITH, AND TREATED FOR ANEMIA, AND THE TREATMENT IS DIRECTED ONLY AT THAT CONDITION, THE ANEMIA WOULD BE THE PRINCIPAL DIAGNOSIS, REGARDLESS OF THE UNDERLYING CONDITION.

ANEMIA

285.9 NOS
282.2 6-PHOSPHOGLUCONIC DEHYDROGENASE DEFICIENCY
280.9 ACHLORHYDRIC
281.8 ACHRESTIC
281.0 ADDISON'S (PERNICIOUS)
281.0 ADDISON-BIERMER (PERNICIOUS)
288.0 AGRANULOCYTIC
281.4 AMINO ACID DEFICIENCY
282.3 ANAEROBIC GLYCOLYSIS DISORDER
284.# APLASTIC

4th Digit: 284

0. CONSTITUTIONAL (CONGENITAL) (FAMILIAL) (FANCONI'S) (INFANTILE) (PANCYTOPENIC) (PRIMARY) (RED CELL)

8. OTHER SPECIFIED (CHRONIC DISEASE) (DRUGS) (INFECTION) (PANCYTOPENIA) (RADIATION) (TOXIN)

9. NOS (APLASTIC) (AREGENERATIVE) (HYPOPLASTIC) (IDIOPATHIC) (NONREGENERATIVE) (REFRACTORY) (MEDULLARY HYPOPLASIA)

244.9 APLASTIC MYXEDEMA
284.8 APLASTIC RED CELL ACQUIRED (PURE) (WITH THYMOMA)
284.0 APLASTIC RED CELL CONGENITAL
284.9 AREGENERATIVE
284.0 AREGENERATIVE CONGENITAL
280.9 ASIDEROTIC
285.9 ATYPICAL (PRIMARY)
282.2 AUTOHEMOLYSIS OF SELWYN AND DACIE (TYPE I)
283.0 AUTOIMMUNE HEMOLYTIC

ANEMIA (continued)

282.2 BAGHDAD SPRING
007.0 BALANTIDIUM COLI
281.0 BIERMER'S (PERNICIOUS)
280.0 BLOOD LOSS NOS
285.1 BLOOD LOSS ACUTE ALL TYPES
<u>998.11</u> BLOOD LOSS ACUTE <u>RESULTING FROM A PROCEDURE</u> [285.1]
280.0 BLOOD LOSS CHRONIC ALL TYPES (IRON DEFICIENCY)
123.4 BOTHRIOCEPHALUS
126.9 BRICKMAKERS SEE ALSO 'ANCYLOSTOMIASIS'
437.8 CEREBRAL
285.9 CHILDHOOD
280.9 CHLOROTIC
284.8 CHRONIC SYSTEMIC DISEASE
281.9 CHRONIC SIMPLE
284.0 CHRONICA CONGENITA AREGENERATIVA
283.0 COLD TYPE (HEMOLYTIC) (SYMPTOMATIC) (SECONDARY)
281.0 <u>COMBINED SYSTEM DISEASE NEC</u> [<u>336.2</u>]
281.1 <u>COMBINED SYSTEM DISEASE DUE TO DIETARY DEFICIENCY</u> [<u>336.2</u>]

CONGENITAL

284.0 APLASTIC
776.5 DUE TO BLOOD LOSS (FETAL)
285.8 DYSHEMATOPOIETIC
285.8 DYSERYTHROPOIETIC
282.7 HEINZ-BODY (CASTLES)
282.9 HEREDITARY HEMOLYTIC
281.0 INTRINSIC FACTOR DEFICIENCY (CASTLE'S)
773.2 ISOIMMUNIZATION
282.2 NONSPHEROCYTIC TYPE I
282.3 NONSPHEROCYTIC TYPE II
281.0 PERNICIOUS
282.0 SPHEROCYTIC

ANEMIA (continued)

282.4 COOLEY'S
0 CRESCENT SEE 'SICKLE CELL'
281.0 CYTOGENIC
282.2 DACIE'S (NONSPHEROCYTIC) TYPE I
282.3 DACIE'S (NONSPHEROCYTIC) TYPE II
284.9 DAVIDSON'S (REFRACTORY)

DEFICIENCY

281.9 NOS
282.3 2, 3 DIPHOSPHOGLYCURATE MUTASE
282.3 2, 3 PG
282.2 6-PGD
282.2 6- PHOSPHOGLURONIC DEHYDROGENASE
281.4 AMINO ACID
281.3 B12 AND FOLATE
282.2 ENZYME, DRUG INDUCED (HEMOLYTIC)
282.3 ENZYME DEFICIENCY NEC
282.2 ERYTHROCYTIC GLUTATHIONE
281.2 FOLATE (DIETARY) (DRUG-INDUCED)
281.2 FOLIC ACID (DIETARY) (DRUG INDUCED)
282.2 G-6-PD (ERTHROCYTIC) (GLUTATHIONE)
282.2 GGS-R
282.2 GLUCOSE-6-PHOSPHATE DEHYDROGENASE (G-6-PD)
282.3 GLUCOSE-PHOSPHATE ISOMERASE
282.2 GLUTATHIONE PEROXIDASE
282.2 GLUTATHIONE-REDUCTASE
282.3 GLYCERALDEHYDE PHOSPHATE DEHYDROGENASE
282.3 GPI
282.2 G SH
285.9 HEMOGLOBIN
282.3 HEXOKINASE
280.9 IRON (FE)
280.8 IRON (FE) OTHER SPECIFIED

ANEMIA (continued)

DEFICIENCY (continued)

281.9 NUTRITIONAL NOS
280.9 NUTRITIONAL WITH POOR IRON ABSORPTION
281.8 NUTRITIONAL WITH SPECIFIED DEFICIENCY NEC
280.1 NUTRITIONAL DUE TO INADEQUATE DIETARY IRON INTAKE
281.8 NUTRITIONAL OTHER
281.8 OTHER SPECIFIED NUTRITIONAL
282.2 PENTOSE PHOSPHATE PATHWAY
282.3 PFK
282.3 PHOSPHOFRUCTO-ALDOLASE
282.3 PHOSPHOFRUCTOKINASE
282.3 PHOSPHOGLYCERATE KINASE
282.3 PK
281.4 PROTEIN
282.3 PYRUVATE KINASE (PK)
V78.1 SCREENING UNSPECIFIED
282.3 TPI
282.3 TRIOSEPHOSPHATE ISOMERASE
281.1 VITAMIN B12 NEC
281.1 VITAMIN B12 DIETARY
281.0 VITAMIN B12 PERNICIOUS

ANEMIA (continued)

284.0 DIAMOND-BLACKFAN (CONGENITAL HYPOPLASTIC)
123.4 DIBOTHRIOCEPHALUS
281.9 DIMORPHIC
281.8 DIPHASIC
032.89 DIPHTHERITIC
123.4 DIPHYLLOBOTHRIUM
282.60 DREPANOCYTIC SEE ALSO 'SICKLE CELL'
283.9 DYKE-YOUNG TYPE (SECONDARY) (SYMPTOMATIC)
285.8 DYSERYTHROPOIETIC (CONGENITAL) (TYPES I, II, III)
285.8 DYSHEMOPOIETIC (CONGENITAL)
126.9 EGYPT (SEE ALSO 'ANCYLOSTOMA')
282.3 EMBDEN MEYERHOF PATHWAY GLYCOLYSIS DEFECT
282.1 ELLIPTOCYTIC SEE ALSO ELLIPTOCYTOSIS'
0 ENZYME DEFICIENCY SEE 'ANEMIA', DEFICIENCY
126.9 EPIDEMIC SEE ALSO 'ANCYLOSTOMA'
282.4 ERYTHROBLASTIC FAMILIAL
773.5 ERYTHROBLASTIC LATE
285.9 ESSENTIAL
281.9 EVANS'
280.9 FABER'S (ACHLORHYDRIC ANEMIA)
280.0 FACTITIOUS (SELF-INDUCED BLOOD LETTING)
284.0 FANCONI'S (CONGENITAL PANCYTOPENIA)
284.0 FAMILIAL HYPOPLASTIC
282.4 FAMILIAL MICROCYTIC (ERYTHROBLASTIC)
V18.2 FAMILY HISTORY
282.2 FAVISM
0 FETUS SEE 'ANEMIA', NEWBORN OR FETUS
123.4 FISH TAPEWORM (D. LATUM) INFESTATION
282.2 GLUTATHIONE METABOLISM DISORDER
281.2 GOAT'S MILK
288.0 GRANULOCYTIC
282.7 HEINZ-BODY CONGENITAL
282.# HEMOGLOBINOPATHY (SICKLE CELL) (THALASSEMIA)

4th Digit: 282

0. SPHEROCYTIC
1. ELLIPTOCYTOTIC
2. G6PD (GLUTATHIONE REDUCTASE)
3. HEXOKINASE (PK) (TPI) DEFICIENCY NONSPHEROCYTOTIC TYPE II
4. THALASSEMIA (MEDITERRANEAN) (COOLEY'S)
5. SICKLE CELL TRAIT
7. HEMOGLOBINOPATHY (HB-C) (HB-D) (HB-E) (FETAL) OR NOS
8. OTHER SPECIFIED (STOMATOCYTOSIS)
9. NOS

280.0 HEMORRHAGE (CHRONIC)
285.1 HEMORRHAGE ACUTE

ANEMIA (continued)

HEMOLYTIC

283.9 ACQUIRED NOS
283.0 ACQUIRED AUTOIMMUNE (DRUG INDUCED) (WARM OR COLD TYPE)
283.1# ACQUIRED NONAUTOIMMUNE

4th Digit: 283.1

0. UNSPECIFIED
1. HEMOLYTIC-UREMIC SYNDROME
9. OTHER NON-AUTOIMMUNE

283.2 ACQUIRED WITH HEMOGLOBINURIA NEC
283.9 ACUTE
282.3 ACUTE DUE TO ENZYME DEFICIENCY
283.0 AUTOIMMUNE (ACQUIRED) (COLD TYPE) (IDIOPATHIC) (PRIMARY) (SECONDARY) (SYMPTOMATIC) (WARM TYPE)
282.4 CHILDHOOD
282.9 CHRONIC
283.9 CHRONIC IDIOPATHIC
283.0 COLD TYPE
282.0 CONGENITAL SPHEROCYTIC
282.3 CONGENITAL NONSPHEROCYTIC
283.0 DRUG-INDUCED
283.19 DUE TO CARDIAC CONDITION
283.19 DUE TO PROSTHESIS OR SHUNT
283.19 DUE TO TRAUMATIC CARDIAC CONDITION
283.19 FRAGMENTATION (ACQUIRED)
282.9 FAMILIAL
282.# HEREDITARY

4th Digit: 282

0. SPHEROCYTIC (ACHOLURIC JAUNDICE) (CONGENITAL) (MINKOWSKI CHAUFFARD SYNDROME) (SPHEROCYTOSIS)
1. ELLIPTOCYTOTIC (OVALOCYTOSIS) (CONGENITAL) (HEREDITARY)
2. G6PD (GLUTATHIONE REDUCTASE) (ENZYME DEFICIENCY) (DRUG INDUCED) (GLUTATHIONE-REDUCTASE) (FAVISM)
3. HEXOKINASE DEFICIENCY (PK) (TPI) (HEXOKINASE) (NONSPHEROCYTOTIC TYPE II)
4. THALASSEMIA (MEDITERRANEAN) (COOLEY'S) (HEREDITARY) (MICRODREPANOCYTOSIS) (SICKLE CELL) (THALASSEMIA HB-S DISEASE)
5. SICKLE CELL TRAIT
7. HEMOGLOBINOPATHY (HB-C) (HB-D) (HB- E) (FETAL) OR NOS
8. OTHER SPECIFIED (STOMATOCYTOSIS)
9. NOS

283.9 IDIOPATHIC (CHRONIC)
283.19 INFECTIOUS (ACQUIRED)
283.0 INFECTIOUS AUTOIMMUNE
283.19 LEDERER'S (ACQUIRED INFECTIOUS HEMOLYTIC))
283.19 MECHANICAL (ACQUIRED)
283.19 MICROANGIOPATHIC (ACQUIRED)
0 NEWBORN SEE 'ANEMIA', NEWBORN OR FETUS
283.10 NON-AUTOIMMUNE (ACQUIRED)
282.2 NONSPHEROCYTIC (HEREDITARY) TYPE I
282.3 NONSPHEROCYTIC (HEREDITARY) TYPE II
283.19 SECONDARY
283.0 SECONDARY AUTOIMMUNE
282.7 STRANSKY REGALA TYPE (HB-E)
283.19 SYMPTOMATIC
283.0 SYMPTOMATIC AUTOIMMUNE
446.6 THROMBOTIC THROMBOCYTOPENIC PURPURA
283.19 TOXIC (ACQUIRED)
283.19 TRAUMATIC CARDIAC
283.11 UREMIC (ADULT) (CHILD)
283.0 WARM TYPE

ANEMIA (continued)

280.0 HEMORRHAGIC (CHRONIC)
285.1 HEMORRHAGIC ACUTE
285.8 HEMPAS
282.61 HERRICK'S (HEMOGLOBIN S DISEASE)
282.2 HEXOSE MONOPHOSPHATE (HMP) SHUNT DEFICIENCY
282.4 HIGH A2
126.9 HOOKWORM SEE ALSO 'ANCYLOSTOMA'
280.9 HYPOCHROMIC (IDIOPATHIC) (MICROCYTIC) (NORMOBLASTIC)
285.0 HYPOCHROMIC FAMILIAL SEX LINKED
285.0 HYPOCHROMIC PYRIDOXINE-RESPONSIVE
285.0 HYPOCHROMIC WITH IRON LOADING
284.0 HYPOPLASIA CONGENITAL OR FAMILIAL
284.8 HYPOPLASIA RED BLOOD CELLS
284.9 HYPOPLASTIC (IDIOPATHIC)
284.0 HYPOPLASTIC CONGENITAL OR FAMILIAL
284.0 HYPOPLASTIC OF CHILDHOOD
285.9 IDIOPATHIC
280.9 IMPAIRED ABSORPTION
285.9 INFANTILE
285.9 INFECTIVE
126.9 INTERTROPICAL SEE ALSO 'ANCYLOSTOMA'
280.# IRON DEFICIENCY

4th Digit: 280

0. DUE TO CHRONIC BLOOD LOSS
1. DUE TO INADEQUATE IRON INTAKE
8. OTHER SPECIFIED (PATTERSON) (PLUMMER VINSON)
9. NOS (ACHLORHYDRIC) (CHLOROTIC)

285.1 IRON DEFICIENCY DUE TO ACUTE BLOOD LOSS
280.8 IRON DEFICIENCY WITH SIDEROPENIC DYSPHAGIA
285.8 JAKSCH'S (PSEUDOLEUKEMIA INFANTUM)
284.0 JOSEPH-DIAMOND-BLACKFAN (CONGENITAL HYPOPLASTIC)
280.9 KOILONYCHIA
386.50 LABYRINTH
283.19 LEDERER'S (ACQUIRED INFECTIOUS HEMOLYTIC ANEMIA)
282.4 LEPTOCYTOSIS (HEREDITARY)
285.8 LEUKOERYTHROBLASTIC
281.9 MACROCYTIC
281.2 MACROCYTIC NUTRITIONAL
281.2 MACROCYTIC TROPICAL
281.1 MALABSORPTION (FAMILIAL) SELECTIVE B12 WITH PROTEINURIA
084.6 MALARIAL SEE ALSO 'MALARIA'
281.0 MALIGNANT (PROGRESSIVE)
281.9 MALNUTRITION
084.6 MARSH SEE ALSO 'MALARIA'

CODE THE SPECIFIC MATERNAL ANEMIA IN ADDITION TO 648.2#. SEE 'ANEMIA'

648.2# MATERNAL CURRENT (CO-EXISTENT) IN PREGNANCY

5th Digit: 648.2

0. EPISODE OF CARE UNSPECIFIED OR N/A
1. DELIVERED
2. DELIVERED WITH POSTPARTUM COMPLICATION
3. ANTEPARTUM COMPLICATION
4. POSTPARTUM COMPLICATION

282.4 MEDITERRANEAN
281.# MEGALOBLASTIC

4th Digit: 281

2. FOLATE DEFICIENCY (CONGENITAL) (GOAT'S MILK) (NUTRITIONAL MEGALOBLASTIC)
3. OTHER (B12 WITH FOLATE DEFICIENCY) (REFRACTORY)
9. NOS

281.9 MEGALOBLASTIC
281.2 MEGALOBLASTIC NUTRITION (OF INFANCY)
281.3 MEGALOBLASTIC REFRACTORY
281.9 MEGALOCYTIC

ANEMIA (continued)

283.19 MICROANGIOPATHIC HEMOLYTIC
280.9 MICROCYTIC (HYPOCHROMIC)
282.4 MICROCYTIC FAMILIAL
282.4 MICRODREPANOCYTOSIS
126.9 MINERS'
285.8 MYELOPATHIC
285.8 MYELOPHTHISIC (NORMOCYTIC)
244.9 MYXEDEMA
126.1 NECATOR AMERICANUS

NEWBORN OR FETUS

773.2 UNSPECIFIED
773.1 ABO HEMOLYTIC DISEASE
773.1 ABO DUE TO MATERNAL/FETAL INCOMPATIBILITY
760.8 AFFECTED BY MATERNAL ANEMIA
776.5 DUE TO FETAL BLOOD LOSS
773.2 DUE TO ISOIMMUNIZATION - NOS
773.1 DUE TO ISOIMMUNIZATION - ABO
773.0 DUE TO ISOIMMUNIZATION - RH ANTIBODIES
773.0 DUE TO ISOIMMUNIZATION - RH (RHESUS), ANTI-D (RH)
773.2 DUE TO ISOIMMUNIZATION - OTHER SPECIFIED
773.2 ERYTHROBLASTIC
773.5 LATE DUE TO ISOIMMUNIZATION
776.5 POSTHEMORRHAGIC
776.6 PREMATURITY NEONATAL
773.0 RH DUE TO MATERNAL/FETAL INCOMPATIBILITY

ANEMIA (continued)

284.9 NONREGENERATIVE
285.9 NORMOCYTIC (NOT DUE TO BLOOD LOSS) (INFECTIONAL)
284.8 NORMOCYTIC MYELOPHTHISIC
281.2 NUTRITION OF (INFANCY)
281.9 NUTRITIONAL (DEFICIENCY)
281.2 NUTRITIONAL MEGALOBLASTIC (INFANCY)
280.9 NUTRITIONAL WITH POOR IRON ABSORPTION
280.1 NUTRITIONAL WITH INADEQUATE DIETARY IRON INTAKE
281.4 OROTIC ACIDURIC (CONGENITAL) (HEREDITARY)
289.8 OSTEOSCLEROTIC
282.1 OVALOCYTOSIS (HEREDITARY)
084.6 PALUDAL
281.0 PERNICIOUS (ADDISON'S) (BIERMER'S) (CASTLE'S DEFICIENCY) (CONGENITAL) (DORSOLATERAL SPINAL DEGENERATION) (JUVENILE) (INTRINSIC FACTOR) (MYELOPATHY) (NEUROPATHY) (PRIMARY) (PROGRESSIVE)
285.9 PLEOCHROMIC
281.8 PLEOCHROMIC OF SPRUE
285.8 PORTAL
280.0 POSTHEMORRHAGIC (CHRONIC)
285.1 POSTHEMORRHAGIC ACUTE
285.9 PRESSURE
285.9 PRIMARY
285.9 PROFOUND
285.9 PROGRESSIVE
281.0 PROGRESSIVE MALIGNANT
281.0 PROGRESSIVE PERNICIOUS
285.8 PSEUDOLEUKEMICA INFANTUM
285.0 PYRIDOXINE RESPONSIVE (HYPOCHROMIC)
284.8 RED CELL
284.0 RED CELL CONGENITAL
281.3 REFRACTORY MEGALOBLASTIC
285.0 REFRACTORIA SIDEROBLASTICA
284.9 REFRACTORY (PRIMARY)
285.0 REFRACTORY WITH HEMOCHROMATOSIS
285.0 REFRACTORY SIDEROBLASTIC
280.9 REFRACTORY SIDEROPENIC
282.4 RIETTI-GREPPI-MICHELI (THALASSEMIA MINOR)

ANEMIA (continued)

281.8 SCORBUTIC
285.9 SECONDARY
284.9 SEMIPLASTIC
285.9 SEPTIC
282.6# SICKLE CELL
5th Digit: 282.6
0. NOS
1. WITHOUT CRISIS
2. WITH CRISIS
3. HB-C
9. HB-S/HBD HB-S/HB-E

282.5 SICKLE CELL TRAIT
285.0 SIDEROACHRESTIC
285.0 SIDEROBLASTIC (ACQUIRED) (CONGENITAL) (DRUG-INDUCED) (DUE TO DISEASE) (HEREDITARY) (PRIMARY) (PYRIDOXINE-RESPONSIVE) (REFRACTORY) (SECONDARY) (SEX-LINKED HYPOCHROMIC) (VITAMIN B6 RESPONSIVE)
280.9 SIDEROPENIC (REFRACTORY)
281.9 SIMPLE CHRONIC
282.0 SPHEROCYTIC (HEREDITARY)
285.8 SPLENIC
272.7 SPLENIC FAMILIAL (GAUCHER'S)
285.8 SPLENOMEGALIC
282.8 STOMATOCYTOSIS
095.8 SYPHILITIC
282.4 TARGET CELL (OVAL)
282.4 THALASSEMIA
287.5 THROMBOCYTOPENIA
284.8 TOXIC
281.2 TROPICAL, MACROCYTIC
017.9# TUBERCULOSIS SEE ALSO 'TUBERCULOSIS'
5th Digit: 017.9
0. UNSPECIFIED
1. LAB NOT DONE
2. LABS PENDING
3. MICROSCOPY POSITIVE (IN SPUTUM)
4. CULTURE POSITIVE - MICROSCOPY NEGATIVE
5. CULTURE NEGATIVE - MICROSCOPY POSITIVE
6. CULTURE AND MICROSCOPY NEGATIVE CONFIRMED BY OTHER METHODS

281.1 VEGAN'S
285.0 VITAMIN B6 RESPONSIVE
281.1 VITAMIN B12 MALABSORPTION WITH PROTEINURIA
285.8 VON JAKSCH'S (PSEUDOLEUKEMIA INFANTUM)
283.0 WARM TYPE (HEMOLYTIC)
280.9 WITTS' (ACHLORHYDRIC)
281.2 ZUELZER (OGDEN) (NUTRITIONAL MEGALOBLASTIC)
285.8 OTHER SPECIFIED TYPE

740.# ANENCEPHALUS CONGENITAL
4th Digit: 740
0. ANENCEPHALUS
1. CRANIORACHISCHISIS
2. INIENCEPHALY

655.0# ANENCEPHALY FETALIS AFFECTING PREGNANCY MANAGEMENT
5th Digit: 655.0
0. EPISODE OF CARE NOS OR N/A
1. DELIVERED
3. ANTEPARTUM COMPLICATION

ANESTHESIA

371.81 EYE
782.0 SKIN
995.4 SHOCK (TO CORRECTLY ADMINISTERED SUBSTANCE)
909.9 SHOCK (TO CORRECTLY ADMINISTERED SUBSTANCE) LATE EFFECT

668.##: USE AN ADDITIONAL CODE TO FURTHER SPECIFY THE COMPLICATION OF ANESTHESIA OR OTHER SEDATION.

ANESTHESIA COMPLICATING L & D

763.5 AFFECTING FETUS OR NEWBORN
668.9# COMPLICATION NOS
668.1# CARDIAC COMPLICATIONS
668.2# CENTRAL NERVOUS SYSTEM COMPLICATIONS
668.0# PULMONARY COMPLICATIONS
668.8# OTHER SPECIFIED COMPLICATIONS
5th Digit: 668.0-2, 8-9
0. EPISODE OF CARE NOS OR N/A
1. DELIVERED
2. DELIVERED WITH POSTPARTUM COMPLICATION
3. ANTEPARTUM COMPLICATION
4. POSTPARTUM COMPLICATION

701.3 ANETODERMA

ANEURYSM AORTIC

441.9 NOS
441.4 ABDOMINAL
441.3 ABDOMINAL RUPTURED
747.29 CONGENITAL
441.0# DISSECTING (RUPTURED)
5th Digit: 441.0
0. UNSPECIFIED SITE
1. THORACIC
2. ABDOMINAL
3. THORACOABDOMINAL

647.0# MATERNAL - SYPHILITIC CURRENT (CO-EXISTENT) IN PREGNANCY [093.0]
5th Digit: 647.0
0. EPISODE OF NOS OR N/A
1. DELIVERED
2. DELIVERED WITH POSTPARTUM COMPLICATION
3. ANTEPARTUM COMPLICATION
4. POSTPARTUM COMPLICATION

648.9#: USE AN ADDITIONAL CODE TO IDENTIFY THE SPECIFIC AORTIC ANEURSYM.

648.9# MATERNAL - VASCULAR CURRENT (CO-EXISTENT) IN PREGNANCY
5th Digit: 648.9
0. EPISODE OF NOS OR N/A
1. DELIVERED
2. DELIVERED WITH POSTPARTUM COMPLICATION
3. ANTEPARTUM COMPLICATION
4. POSTPARTUM COMPLICATION

441.5 RUPTURED SITE NOS
093.0 SYPHILITIC
441.2 THORACIC
441.1 THORACIC RUPTURED
441.7 THORACOABDOMINAL
441.6 THORACOABDOMINAL RUPTURED
0 TRAUMATIC SEE 'AORTA, AORTIC', INJURY

ANEURYSM ARTERIAL (CIRSOID) (FALSE) (VARICOSE) (RUPTURED)

442.9 ARTERY NOS
447.0 ARTERIOVENOUS ACQUIRED
0 ARTERIOVENOUS CONGENITAL SEE 'ANEURYSM CONGENITAL'
442.81 CAROTID ARTERY INTERNAL EXTRACRANIAL PORTION
0 CAROTID ARTERY INTERNAL INTRACRANIAL PORTION SEE 'ANEURYSM CEREBRAL'
442.84 CELIAC ARTERY
372.74 CONJUNCTIVAL

A

ANEURYSM ARTERIAL (CIRSOID) (FALSE) (VARICOSE) (RUPTURED) (continued)

442.3 FEMORAL ARTERY
442.84 GASTRODUODENAL ARTERY
442.84 GASTROEPIPLOIC ARTERY
421.0 HEART VALVE (ANY) INFECTIVE
442.84 HEPATIC ARTERY
442.2 ILIAC ARTERY
442.89 INNOMINATE ARTERY
442.3 LOWER EXTREMITY

> *648.9#: USE AN ADDITIONAL CODE TO IDENTIFY THE SPECIFIC ARTERIAL ANEURSYM.*

648.9# MATERNAL CURRENT (CO-EXISTENT) IN PREGNANCY
5th Digit: 648.9
0. EPISODE OF NOS OR N/A
1. DELIVERED
2. DELIVERED WITH POSTPARTUM COMPLICATION
3. ANTEPARTUM COMPLICATION
4. POSTPARTUM COMPLICATION

442.89 MEDIASTINAL ARTERY
442.84 MESENTERIC ARTERY
442.84 PANCREATICODUODENAL ARTERY
442.3 POPLITEAL ARTERY
417.1 PULMONARY ARTERY
442.1 RENAL ARTERY
442.89 SPINAL ARTERY
442.83 SPLENIC ARTERY
442.82 SUBCLAVIAN ARTERY
442.84 SUPERIOR MESENTERIC ARTERY
0 TRAUMATIC SEE SPECIFIC ARTERY, INJURY
442.0 UPPER EXTREMITY ARTERY
442.84 VISCERAL ARTERY

ANEURYSM CEREBRAL

437.3 NONRUPTURED NOS
747.81 NONRUPTURED ARTERIOVENOUS CONGENITAL
437.3 NONRUPTURED CAROTID ARTERY INTERNAL INTRACRANIAL PORTION
0 RUPTURED SEE 'HEMORRHAGE' BY SITE
094.87 RUPTURED SYPHILITIC

ANEURYSM CONGENITAL

747.6# ARTERIOVENOUS (PERIPHERAL)
5th Digit: 747.6
0. PERIPHERAL VASCULAR UNSPECIFIED SITE
1. GASTROINTESTINAL VESSEL
2. RENAL VESSEL
3. UPPER LIMB VESSEL
4. LOWER LIMB VESSEL
9. OTHER SPECIFIED SITE PERIPHERAL VASCULAR

747.89 ARTERY SITE NEC
747.81 CEREBRAL ARTERIOVENOUS
747.89 CIRCULATORY NEC
746.85 CORONARY
746.85 CORONARY ARTERY
747.6# PERIPHERAL
747.6# PERIPHERAL ARTERY
5th Digit: 747.6
0. PERIPHERAL VASCULAR UNSPECIFIED SITE
1. GASTROINTESTINAL VESSEL
2. RENAL VESSEL
3. UPPER LIMB VESSEL
4. LOWER LIMB VESSEL
9. OTHER SPECIFIED SITE PERIPHERAL VASCULAR

747.3 PULMONARY
747.3 PULMONARY ARTERIOVENOUS
747.3 PULMONARY ARTERY
747.62 RENAL (PERIPHERAL VASCULAR)

ANEURYSM CONGENITAL (continued)

743.58 RETINAL
743.58 RETINAL ARTERY
747.29 SINUS OF VALSALVA
747.82 SPINAL

ANEURYSM HEART

414.11 CORONARY VESSELS
414.10 MURAL
414.10 VENTRICULAR
414.10 WALL
429.79 POSTINFARCTION <8 WKS. **[410.##]**
4th Digit: 410
0. ANTERIOR LATERAL
1. ANTERIOR
2. INFERIOR LATERAL
3. INFERIOR POSTERIOR
4. INFERIOR OTHER
5. LATERAL
6. POSTERIOR
7. SUBENDOCARDIAL
8. OTHER SITE
9. SITE NOS
5th Digit: 410
0. EPISODE OF CARE
1. INITIAL EPISODE OF CARE
2. SUBSEQUENT EPISODE OF CARE

429.79 POSTINFARCTION >8 WKS. [414.8]
414.19 OTHER

758.3 ANGELMAN SYNDROME
312.0# ANGER REACTION
5th Digit: 312.0
0. UNSPECIFIED
1. MILD
2. MODERATE
3. SEVERE

ANGIITIS

447.6 ANGIITIS
446.4 ALLERGIC GRANULOMATOSIS (LUNG)
446.20 HYPERSENSITIVITY
446.21 HYPERSENSITIVITY - GOODPASTURE'S SYNDROME
446.29 HYPERSENSITIVITY - OTHER SPECIFIED

> *648.9#: USE AN ADDITIONAL CODE TO IDENTIFY THE SPECIFIC ANGIITIS.*

648.9# MATERNAL CURRENT (CO-EXISTENT) IN PREGNANCY
5th Digit: 648.9
0. EPISODE OF NOS OR N/A
1. DELIVERED
2. DELIVERED WITH POSTPARTUM COMPLICATION
3. ANTEPARTUM COMPLICATION
4. POSTPARTUM COMPLICATION

446.0 NECROTIZING

> *ALL CARRIERS DO NOT REGARD CARDIAC ANGINA, 413.9, WITH THE SAME DEGREE OF MEDICAL URGENCY AS PREINFARCTION ANGINA, 411.1. CODE TO THE SPECIFICITY DOCUMENTED.*

ANGINA CARDIAC

413.9 NOS
411.1 CRESCENDO
413.0 DECUBITUS
413.9 EFFORT
413.9 EXERTIONAL
411.1 INITIAL
413.0 NOCTURNAL

ANGINA CARDIAC (continued)
413.9 PECTORIS
411.1 PREINFARCTION
413.1 PRINZMETAL'S
411.1 PROGRESSIVE
306.2 PSYCHOGENIC
413.9 STABLE
413.9 SYNDROME (HEBERDEN'S)
411.1 UNSTABLE
413.1 VARIANT

ANGINA CRURIS
443.9 NOS
440.2# EXTREMITIES DUE TO ATHEROSCLEROSIS
5th Digit: 440.2
0. UNSPECIFIED
1. WITH INTERMITTENT CLAUDICATION
2. WITH REST PAIN, OR REST PAIN AND (INTERMITTENT CLAUDICATION)
3. WITH ULCERATION, OR ULCERATION AND (INTERMITTENT CLAUDICATION) (REST PAIN)
4. WITH ISCHEMIC GANGRENE, OR ISCHEMIC GANGRENE AND (INTERMITTENT CLAUDICATION) (REST PAIN) (ULCERATION)
9. OTHER ATHEROSCLEROSIS EXTREMITIES

ANGINA INFECTIOUS
034.0 ERYSIPELATOUS
462 ERYTHEMATOUS
476.0 EXUDATIVE CHRONIC
478.29 FAUCIUM
462 GANGRENOUS
462 MALIGNANT
034.0 SEPTIC
034.0 STREPTOCOCCAL

ANGINA MESENTERIC
557.1 ABDOMINAL
557.1 INTESTINAL
557.1 MESENTERIC

0 ANGIOBLASTOMA SITE SPECIFIED SEE 'NEOPLASM UNCERTAIN BEHAVIOR' M9161/1
0 ANGIOCHOLECYSTITIS SEE 'CHOLECYSTITIS', ACUTE

ANGIODYSPLASIA
569.84 INTESTINE
569.85 INTESTINE WITH HEMORRHAGE
537.82 STOMACH AND DUODENUM
537.83 STOMACH AND DUODENUM WITH HEMORRHAGE

995.1 ANGIOEDEMA (ALLERGIC) (TO CORRECTLY ADMINISTERED SUBSTANCE)
909.9 ANGIOEDEMA (ALLERGIC) (TO CORRECTLY ADMINISTERED SUBSTANCE) LATE EFFECT
277.6 ANGIOEDEMA HEREDITARY
210.7 ANGIOFIBROMA SITE NOS
0 ANGIOFIBROMA SITE SPECIFIED SEE 'BENIGN NEOPLASM' BY SITE M9160/0
286.4 ANGIOHEMOPHILIA (A) (B)
363.43 ANGIOID STREAKS CHOROID
216.# ANGIOKERATOMA M9141/0
4th Digit: 216
0. LIP (SKIN OF)
1. EYELID INCLUDING CANTHUS
2. EAR (EXTERNAL) (AURICLE) (PINNA)
3. FACE (CHEEK) (NOSE)
4. SCALP NECK
5. TRUNK BACK CHEST
6. UPPER LIMB INCLUDING SHOULDER
7. LOWER LIMB INCLUDING HIP
8. OTHER SPECIFIED SITES
9. SKIN NOS

214.# ANGIOLIPOMA M8861/1
4th Digit: 214
0. FACE SKIN AND SUBCUTANEOUS TISSUE
1. SKIN AND SUBCUTANEOUS TISSUE OTHER
2. INTRATHORACIC ORGANS
3. INTRA ABDOMINAL ORGANS
4. SPERMATIC CORD
8. OTHER SPECIFIED SITES
9. UNSPECIFIED SITE

238.1 ANGIOLIPOMA INFILTRATING SITE NOS
0 ANGIOLIPOMA INFILTRATING SITE SPECIFIED SEE 'NEOPLASM UNCERTAIN BEHAVIOR' BY SITE M8861/1
0 ANGIOMA SEE 'HEMANGIOMA'
709.1 ANGIOMA SERPIGINOSUM
757.32 ANGIOMATOSIS
083.8 ANGIOMATOSIS BACILLARY
228.09 ANGIOMATOSIS SYSTEMIC
223.0 ANGIOMYOLIPOMA SITE NOS
0 ANGIOMYOLIPOMA SITE SPECIFIED SEE 'BENIGN NEOPLASM' BY SITE M8860/0
171.# ANGIOMYOLIPOSARCOMA M8860/3
215.# ANGIOMYOMA M8894/0
171.# ANGIOMYOSARCOMA M8894/3
4th Digit: 171, 215
0. HEAD FACE NECK
2. UPPER LIMB SHOULDER
3. LOWER LIMB HIP
4. THORAX
5. ABDOMINAL HYPOCHONDRIUM
6. PELVIS BUTTOCK GROIN INGUINAL REGION PERINEUM
7. TRUNK NOS BACK NOS FLANK NOS
8. OTHER SPECIFIED SITES
9. SITE NOS

ANGIONEUROTIC EDEMA
995.1 ANGIONEUROTIC EDEMA
909.9 ANGIONEUROTIC EDEMA LATE EFFECT
999.5 DUE TO SERUM
909.3 DUE TO SERUM LATE EFFECT
995.1 GIANT
909.9 GIANT LATE EFFECT
995.1 QUINCKE'S
909.9 QUINCKE'S LATE EFFECT
995.1 URTICARIA
909.9 URTICARIA LATE EFFECT

ANGIOPATHY
459.9 NOS
443.9 PERIPHERAL NOS
250.7# PERIPHERAL DIABETIC [443.81]
5th Digit: 250.7
0. TYPE II, ADULT-ONSET, NON-INSULIN DEPENDENT (EVEN IF REQUIRING INSULIN), OR UNSPECIFIED; CONTROLLED
1. TYPE I, JUVENILE-ONSET OR INSULIN-DEPENDENT; CONTROLLED
2. TYPE II, ADULT-ONSET, NON-INSULIN DEPENDENT (EVEN IF REQUIRING INSULIN); UNCONTROLLED
3. TYPE I, JUVENILE-ONSET OR INSULIN-DEPENDENT; UNCONTROLLED

443.89 PERIPHERAL OTHER SPECIFIED

ANGIOPATHY (continued)
362.18 RETINALIS (JUVENILIS)
362.10 RETINALIS (JUVENILIS) BACKGROUND
250.5# RETINALIS (JUVENILIS) DIABETIC [362.01]

5th Digit: 250.5

0. TYPE II, ADULT-ONSET, NON-INSULIN DEPENDENT (EVEN IF REQUIRING INSULIN), OR UNSPECIFIED; CONTROLLED
1. TYPE I, JUVENILE-ONSET OR INSULIN-DEPENDENT; CONTROLLED
2. TYPE II, ADULT-ONSET, NON-INSULIN DEPENDENT (EVEN IF REQUIRING INSULIN); UNCONTROLLED
3. TYPE I, JUVENILE-ONSET OR INSULIN-DEPENDENT; UNCONTROLLED

362.29 RETINALIS (JUVENILIS) PROLIFERATIVE
0 RETINALIS (JUVENILIS) TUBERCULOUS SEE 'TUBERCULOSIS', RETINALIS

443.9 ANGIOPLASTIC DISEASE
435.9 ANGIOPLASTIC DISEASE CEREBRAL
459.89 ANGIOPLASTIC DISEASE VEIN
V45.82 ANGIOPLASTY STATUS (PTCA)

128.8 ANGIOSTRONGYLUS CANTONENSIS INFECTION
159.1 ANGIOSARCOMA SPLEEN M9120/3
368.42 ANGIOSCOTOMA ENLARGED

705.0 ANHIDROSIS

0 ANIMAL BITE (SKIN SURFACE INTACT) SEE 'CONTUSION', BY SITE
0 ANIMAL BITE (SKIN SURFACE PENETRATED) SEE 'OPEN WOUND', BY SITE

743.45 ANIRIDIA CONGENITAL

127.1 ANISAKIASIS
127.1 ANISAKIS LARVA INFECTION

367.32 ANISEIKONIA

379.41 ANISOCORIA
743.46 ANISOCORIA CONGENITAL
790.0 ANISOCYTOSIS
367.31 ANISOMETROPIA

ANKLE
V49.74 AMPUTATION STATUS
736.70 DEFORMITY ACQUIRED
755.69 DEFORMITY CONGENITAL
726.70 ENTHESOPATHY
959.7 INJURY
916.8 INJURY OTHER AND NOS SUPERFICIAL
916.9 INJURY OTHER AND NOS SUPERFICIAL (INFECTED)
718.97 JOINT CALCIFICATION
718.97 JOINT LIGAMENT RELAXATION
0 JOINT LIGAMENT TEAR SEE 'SPRAIN'
0 JOINT SEE ALSO 'JOINT'
718.17 LOOSE BODY (JOINT)
V43.66 REPLACEMENT STATUS
845.00 SEPARATION (RUPTURE) (TEAR) (LACERATION)
845.00 STRAIN (AVULSION) (HEMATHROSIS)
726.70 TENDINITIS OR BURSITIS

374.46 ANKYLOBLEPHARON
750.0 ANKYLOGLOSSIA SUPERIOR SYNDROME
720.0 ANKYLOSING SPONDYLITIS
721.6 ANKYLOSING VERTEBRAL HYPEROSTOSIS

ANKYLOSIS
385.22 EAR OSSICLES
385.21 EAR OSSICLES MALLEUS
718.54 FINGER
718.57 FOOT
718.55 HIP

ANKYLOSIS (continued)
718.5# JOINT (FIBROUS) (OSSEUS)

5th Digit: 718.5

0. SITE NOS
1. SHOULDER REGION
2. UPPER ARM (ELBOW) (HUMERUS)
3. FOREARM (RADIUS) (WRIST) (ULNA)
4. HAND (CARPAL) (METACARPAL) (FINGERS)
5. PELVIC REGION AND THIGH (HIP) (BUTTOCK) (FEMUR)
6. LOWER LEG (FIBULA) (KNEE) (PATELLA) (TIBIA)
7. ANKLE AND/OR FOOT (METATARSALS) (TOES) (TARSALS)
8. OTHER
9. MULTIPLE

718.56 KNEE
724.6 LUMBOSACRAL (NONVERTEBRAL) (NONDISCOGENIC)
385.21 MALLEUS
718.58 NECK
718.58 RIB
724.6 SACROILIAC (NONVERTEBRAL) (NONDISCOGENIC)
724.6 SACRUM (NONVERTEBRAL) (NONDISCOGENIC)
724.9 SPINE (NONVERTEBRAL) (NONDISCOGENIC)
718.57 TOES
521.6 TOOTH

520.0 ANODONTIA

0 ANOMALY, ANOMALOUS SEE BY SPECIFIC ANOMALY OR BY ANATOMICAL SITE
759.9 ANOMALY NOS CONGENITAL
759.7 ANOMALY MULTIPLE NOS CONGENITAL

757.5 ANONYCHIA CONGENITAL
360.89 ANOPHTHALMOS ACQUIRED
743.00 ANOPHTHALMOS CONGENITAL

752.8 ANORCHISM ABSENCE CONGENITAL

783.0 ANOREXIA
307.1 ANOREXIA NERVOSA

ANOSMIA
781.1 NOS
478.9 POSTINFECTIONAL
306.7 PSYCHOGENIC
951.8 TRAUMATIC

780.9 ANOSOGNOSIA
756.50 ANOSTEOPLASIA
744.09 ANOTIA
628.0 ANOVULATORY CYCLE

799.0 ANOXEMIA
770.8 ANOXEMIA NEWBORN

ANOXIA, ANOXIC
799.0 NOS

BIRTH
768.9 UNSPECIFIED
768.6 MILD
768.6 MODERATE
768.5 SEVERE
768.5 SEVERE WITH NEUROLOGIC INVOLVEMENT

ANOXIA, ANOXIC (continued)

> *THE CODES FOR ANOXIA AND ANOXIC BRAIN DAMAGE DURING LABOR OR AT BIRTH CANNOT BE USED ALONE. YOU MUST ALSO CODE THE CAUSE OF THE ANOXIA OR ANOXIC BRAIN DAMAGE. SEQUENCE THE ANOXIA FIRST AND THE CAUSE SECOND. (POST-OP ANOXIC BRAIN DAMAGE DOES NOT REQUIRE AN ADDITIONAL CODE.*

BRAIN DAMAGE

348.1 NOS
768.0 CAUSING FETAL DEATH - NOS OR BEFORE ONSET OF LABOR
768.1 CAUSING FETAL DEATH - DURING LABOR
997.01 DUE TO ABORTION
772.1 DUE TO HEMORRHAGE INTRAVENTRICULAR (PERINATAL)
772.2 DUE TO SUBARACHNOID HEMORRHAGE PERINATAL CAUSE
767.0 DUE TO SUBDURAL OR CEREBRAL HEMORRHAGE
997.01 DURING OR RESULTING FROM A PROCEDURE
639.8 FOLLOWING ABORTION, ECTOPIC OR MOLAR PREGNANCY
997.01 POST OP

ANOXIA, ANOXIC (continued)

348.1 CEREBRAL
997.01 CEREBRAL DUE TO PROCEDURE
348.1 ENCEPHALOPATHY
997.01 ENCEPHALOPATHY DUE TO A PROCEDURE
770.8 FETAL AFFECTING NEWBORN
993.2 HIGH ALTITUDE
909.4 HIGH ALTITUDE LATE EFFECT

> *FETAL OR NEWBORN CODES (760-779), SOMETIMES REQUIRE AN ADDITIONAL CODE TO FURTHER SPECIFY THE CAUSE OF THE CONDITION, THE INFECTING ORGANISM, OR COMPLICATING DIAGNOSES. WHENEVER APPROPRIATE, DESCRIBE THE PATIENT'S MEDICAL SITUATION AS CLEARLY AND CONCISELY AS POSSIBLE USING MULTIPLE CODES.*

INTRAUTERINE

768.9 LIVEBORN - NOS
768.4 LIVEBORN - NOS ONSET
768.2 LIVEBORN - ONSET BEFORE LABOR
768.3 LIVEBORN - ONSET DURING LABOR OR DELIVERY
768.0 STILLBORN - DEATH BEFORE ONSET OF LABOR
768.1 STILLBORN - DEATH DURING LABOR

989.5 ANT (FIRE ANT) BITE
995.0 ANT (FIRE ANT) BITE WITH ANAPHYLAXIS [989.5]

451.82 ANTECUBITAL VEIN PHLEBITIS
796.5 ANTENATAL SCREENING FINDINGS ABNORMAL

ANTEPARTUM HEMORRHAGE

641.9# NOS
5th Digit: 641.9
0. EPISODE OF CARE NOS OR N/A
1. DELIVERED
3. ANTEPARTUM COMPLICATION

762.1 AFFECTING FETUS OR NEWBORN
641.3# ASSOCIATED WITH COAGULATION DEFECTS
641.8# OTHER
5th Digit: 641.3, 8
0. EPISODE OF CARE NOS OR N/A
1. DELIVERED
3. ANTEPARTUM COMPLICATION

ANTERIOR

360.34 CHAMBER FLAT (POSTINFLAMMATORY) (POST OP) (POSTTRAUMATIC)
786.52 CHEST WALL SYNDROME
958.8 COMPARTMENT SYNDROME (TIBIAL)
717.83 CRUCIATE LIGAMENT DISRUPTION (OLD)
717.9 CRUCIATE LIGAMENT RELAXATION
844.2 CRUCIATE LIGAMENT TEAR (STRAIN) (RUPTURE) - ACUTE
335.9 HORN CELL DISEASE
335.8 HORN CELL DISEASE OTHER
433.8# SPINAL ARTERY SYNDROME
5th Digit: 433.8
0. WITHOUT CEREBRAL INFARCTION
1. WITH CEREBRAL INFARCTION

721.1 SPINAL ARTERY COMPRESSION SYNDROME
904.51 TIBIAL ARTERY INJURY
908.3 TIBIAL ARTERY INJURY LATE EFFECT
958.8 TIBIAL (COMPARTMENT) SYNDROME
904.52 TIBIAL VEIN INJURY
908.3 TIBIAL VEIN INJURY LATE EFFECT

500 ANTHRACOSILICOSIS
500 ANTHRACOSIS

ANTHRAX

022.9 NOS
022.2 COLITIS
022.0 CUTANEOUS
022.2 GASTROINTESTINAL
022.1 PNEUMONIA [484.5]
022.1 PULMONARY
022.1 RESPIRATORY
022.3 SEPSIS
022.8 OTHER SPECIFIED MANIFESTATIONS

286.5 ANTI VIII A INCREASE
286.5 ANTI IX A INCREASE
286.5 ANTI X INCREASE
286.5 ANTI XI A INCREASE
611.0 ANTIBIOMA BREAST
V07.39 ANTIBIOTIC PROPHYLACTIC ADMINISTRATION
V58.62 ANTIBIOTICS FOLLOW UP EXAM - CURRENT THERAPY
V09.1 ANTIBIOTICS (B-LACTAM) RESISTANT INFECTION (SEE DRUG RESISTANT MICROORGANISMS FOR COMPLETE LISTING)
760.74 ANTIBIOTICS TRANSMITTED VIA PLACENTA OR BREAST MILK AFFECTING FETUS OR NEWBORN
279.00 ANTIBODY DEFICIENCY SYNDROME (AGAMMAGLOBULINEMIC) (HYPOGAMMAGLOBULINEMIC)

279.04 ANTIBODY DEFICIENCY SYNDROME CONGENITAL
795.79 ANTIBODY TITER RAISED
795.79 ANTICARDIOLIPIN ANTIBODY SYNDROME
V67.51 ANTICOAGULANT FOLLOW UP EXAM - COMPLETED THERAPY
V58.61 ANTICOAGULANT FOLLOW UP EXAM - CURRENT THERAPY

305.8# ANTIDEPRESSANT ABUSE (NONDEPENDENT)
5th Digit: 305.8
0. NOS
1. CONTINUOUS
2. EPISODIC
3. IN REMISSION

0 ANTIDIURETIC HORMONE SEE ALSO 'ADH'
259.3 ANTIDIURETIC HORMONE SECRETION (ADH) ECTOPIC SECRETION
795.79 ANTIGEN ANTIBODY REACTION ABNORMAL

286.0 ANTIHEMOPHILIC FACTOR A DEFICIENCY
286.1 ANTIHEMOPHILIC FACTOR B DEFICIENCY
286.2 ANTIHEMOPHILIC FACTOR C DEFICIENCY
286.0 ANTIHEMOPHILIC GLOBULIN (AHG) DEFICIENCY
758.3 ANTIMONGOLISM SYNDROME
0 ANTIMYCOBACTERIAL RESISTANT INFECTION SEE 'DRUG RESISTANCE'
795.79 ANTINUCLEAR ANTIBODIES RAISED (POSITIVE)
795.79 ANTIPHOSPHOLIPID ANTIBODY SYNDROME
301.7 ANTISOCIAL PERSONALITY DISORDER
286.5 ANTITHROMBINEMIA HEMORRHAGIC DISORDER DUE TO CIRCULATING ANTICOAGULANTS
286.5 ANTITHROMBOPLASTINEMIA HEMORRHAGIC DISORDER DUE TO CIRCULATING ANTICOAGULANTS
286.5 ANTITHROMBOPLASTINOGENEMIA HEMORRHAGIC DISORDER DUE TO CIRCULATING ANTICOAGULANTS
277.6 ANTITRYPSIN DEFICIENCY
V07.2 ANTIVENIN ADMINISTRATION (PROPHYLACTIC)
307.9 ANTON BABINSKI SYNDROME (HEMIASOMATOGNOSIA)
461.0 ANTRITIS ACUTE
473.0 ANTRITIS CHRONIC

ANURIA
788.5 NOS
997.5 POSTOPERATIVE
997.5 SPECIFIED AS DUE TO PROCEDURE
958.5 TRAUMATIC
908.6 TRAUMATIC LATE EFFECT
788.5 UNKNOWN ETIOLOGY

ANUS, ANAL
911.0 ABRASION
911.1 ABRASION INFECTED
751.2 ABSENCE (CANAL) (CONGENITAL)
569.49 ANUSITIS
751.2 ATRESIA CONGENITAL
911.2 BLISTER
911.3 BLISTER INFECTED
099.52 CHLAMYDIA TRACHOMATIS INFECTION
569.49 CRYPT
564.89 CONTRACTURE
787.99 DISCHARGE NEC
569.49 DISEASE NEC
751.5 DUPLICATION CONGENITAL
751.5 ECTOPIC CONGENITAL
565.0 FISSURE
863.89 FISSURE TRAUMATIC
863.99 FISSURE TRAUMATIC WITH OPEN WOUND
751.5 FISTULA CONGENITAL
565.1 FISTULA (TO SKIN)
911.6 FOREIGN BODY SUPERFICIAL
911.7 FOREIGN BODY SUPERFICIAL INFECTED
751.2 IMPERFORATE CONGENITAL
569.49 INFECTION
569.49 INFLAMMATION
959.1 INJURY
911.8 INJURY SUPERFICIAL OTHER AND UNSPECIFIED
911.9 INJURY SUPERFICIAL OTHER AND UNSPECIFIED INFECTED
911.4 INSECT BITE
911.5 INSECT BITE INFECTED
787.99 MASS
787.99 NEURALGIA
569.49 OCCLUSION
751.2 OCCLUSION CONGENITAL

ANUS, ANAL (continued)
569.42 PAIN
569.49 PAPILLAE HYPERTROPHY
211.4 POLYP - ADENOMATOUS
569.0 POLYP - NONADENOMATOUS
569.1 PROLAPSE (CANAL) (SPHINCTER)
751.5 PROLAPSE (CANAL) (SPHINCTER) CONGENITAL
751.2 SEPTUM CONGENITAL
564.6 SPASM
564.89 SPHINCTER DILATATION
569.3 SPHINCTER HEMORRHAGE
569.2 SPHINCTER STRICTURE
569.2 STENOSIS
751.2 STENOSIS CONGENITAL
569.2 STRICTURE
751.2 STRICTURE CONGENITAL
911.6 SUPERFICIAL FB
911.7 SUPERFICIAL FB INFECTED
787.99 SWELLING
565.0 TEAR NONTRAUMATIC, NONPUERPERAL
564.89 TIGHTNESS
569.41 ULCER

569.49 ANUSITIS

ANXIETY
291.89 ALCOHOL INDUCED (PSYCHOTIC)
300.4 DEPRESSION
300.00 DISORDER
300.02 DISORDER GENERALIZED
300.09 DISORDER OTHER SPECIFIED
292.89 DRUG INDUCED (PSYCHOTIC)
293.84 DUE TO OR ASSOCIATED WITH PHYSICAL CONDITION
313.0 FEARFULNESS OF CHILDHOOD AND ADOLESCENCE
300.20 HYSTERIA
300.00 NEUROSIS

ORGANIC ANXIETY SYNDROME, 293.84 IS A TRANSIENT ORGANIC PSYCHOSIS SECONDARY TO A MEDICAL CONDITION. CODE THE MEDICAL CONDITION FIRST, FOLLOWED BY 293.84.

293.84 ORGANIC SYNDROME
300.00 REACTION
309.24 REACTION ADJUSTMENT (TRANSIENT)
309.21 REACTION SEPARATION
308.0 REACTION STRESS (ACUTE)
309.21 SEPARATION DISORDER
300.00 STATE
300.00 STATE NONSITUATIONAL
300.00 SYNDROME
293.84 SYNDROME PSYCHOTIC (ORGANIC) (TRANSIENT)

AORTA, AORTIC
747.22 ABSENCE CONGENITAL
746.89 ABSENCE VALVE CONGENITAL
441.9 ANEURYSM - NOS
441.4 ANEURYSM - ABDOMINAL
441.3 ANEURYSM - ABDOMINAL RUPTURED
747.29 ANEURYSM - CONGENITAL
441.0# ANEURYSM - DISSECTING (RUPTURED)
5th Digit: 441.0
0. UNSPECIFIED SITE
1. THORACIC
2. ABDOMINAL
3. THORACOABDOMINAL

AORTA, AORTIC (continued)

> *648.9#: USE AN ADDITIONAL CODE TO IDENTIFY THE AORTIC ANEURYSM.*

648.9# ANEURYSM - MATERNAL CURRENT (CO-EXISTENT) IN PREGNANCY
5th Digit: 648.9
0. EPISODE OF NOS OR N/A
1. DELIVERED
2. DELIVERED WITH POSTPARTUM COMPLICATION
3. ANTEPARTUM COMPLICATION
4. POSTPARTUM COMPLICATION

441.5 ANEURYSM - RUPTURED SITE NOS
093.0 ANEURYSM - SYPHILITIC
441.2 ANEURYSM - THORACIC
441.1 ANEURYSM - THORACIC RUPTURED
441.7 ANEURYSM - THORACOABDOMINAL
441.6 ANEURYSM - THORACOABDOMINAL RUPTURED
0 ANEURYSM - TRAUMATIC SEE 'AORTA, AORTIC', INJURY
747.20 ANOMALY CONGENITAL
747.22 APLASIA CONGENITAL
747.21 ARCH ANOMALIES CONGENITAL
747.11 ARCH ATRESIA (CONGENITAL)
747.21 ARCH DOUBLE CONGENITAL
747.10 ARCH HYPOPLASIA CONGENITAL
747.11 ARCH INTERRUPTION CONGENITAL
747.21 ARCH PERSISTENT CONVOLUTIONS
747.21 ARCH PERSISTENT RIGHT
446.7 ARCH SYNDROME
440.0 ARTERIOSCLEROSIS (DEGENERATION) (DEFORMANS)
747.22 ATRESIA (CONGENITAL)
746.7 ATRESIA (CONGENITAL) WITH HYPOPLASIA OF ASCENDING AORTA AND DEFECTIVE DEVELOPMENT OF LEFT VENTRICLE (WITH MITRAL VALVE ATRESIA)
996.1 BALLOON COMPLICATION (MECHANICAL)
444.0 BIFURCATION (OCCLUSION) SYNDROME
237.3 BODY TUMOR SITE NOS
0 BODY TUMOR SITE SPECIFIED SEE 'NEOPLASM UNCERTAIN BEHAVIOR' BY SITE M8691/1
440.0 CALCIFICATION (ARTERITIS)
747.10 COARCTATION (PREDUCTAL) (POSTDUCTAL) CONGENITAL
747.21 DEXTRAPOSITION CONGENITAL
745.11 DEXTRATRANSPOSITION CONGENITAL
093.0 DILATATION SYPHILITIC
747.29 DILATION CONGENITAL
447.9 DISEASE
093.89 DISEASE SYPHILITIC
441.0# DISSECTING
5th Digit: 441.0
0. UNSPECIFIED SITE
1. THORACIC
2. ABDOMINAL
3. THORACOABDOMINAL

996.1 GRAFT COMPLICATION (MECHANICAL)
0 INCOMPETENCE SEE 'AORTIC INSUFFICIENCY'
902.0 INJURY ABDOMINAL
908.4 INJURY LATE EFFECT
901.0 INJURY THORACIC
0 INSUFFICIENCY SEE 'AORTIC INSUFFICIENCY'
902.0 LACERATION ABDOMINAL (RUPTURE) (HEMATOMA) (AVULSION) (ANEURYSM) TRAUMATIC
901.0 LACERATION THORACIC (RUPTURE) (HEMATOMA) (AVULSION) (ANEURYSM) TRAUMATIC
0 OBSTRUCTION OR OCCLUSION SEE 'AORTA, AORTIC (VALVE) STENOSIS'
0 REGURGITATION SEE 'AORTIC INSUFFICIENCY'
747.21 RING (ATRESIA) SYNDROME (CONGENITAL)
745.0 SEPTAL DEFECT CONGENITAL
747.22 STRICTURE CONGENITAL

AORTA, AORTIC (continued)

746.89 VALVE ATRESIA (CONGENITAL)
746.4 VALVE BICUSPID CONGENITAL
395.9 VALVE DISEASE RHEUMATIC
424.1 VALVE DISORDER
747.21 VASCULAR RING CONGENITAL

AORTA, AORTIC (VALVE) INSUFFICIENCY

746.4 CONGENITAL
424.1 INSUFFICIENCY
421.0 INSUFFICIENCY BACTERIAL (ACUTE) (CHRONIC)
395.1 RHEUMATIC
396.3 WITH MITRAL INSUFFICIENCY
396.3 WITH MITRAL INSUFFICIENCY RHEUMATIC
396.1 WITH MITRAL STENOSIS
396.1 WITH MITRAL STENOSIS RHEUMATIC
093.22 WITH MITRAL STENOSIS SYPHILITIC
396.8 WITH OTHER VALVE MULTIPLE INVOLVEMENT, STENOSIS/INSUFFICIENCY (RHEUMATIC)

AORTA, AORTIC (VALVE) STENOSIS

424.1 AORTIC STENOSIS
396.0 ATYPICAL
421.0 BACTERIAL ACUTE
421.0 BACTERIAL CHRONIC
746.3 CONGENITAL
746.7 CONGENITAL IN HYPOPLASTIC LEFT HEART
746.81 CONGENITAL SUBAORTIC
747.22 CONGENITAL SUPRAVALVULAR
425.1 HYPERTROPHIC SUBAORTIC - IDIOPATHIC
395.0 RHEUMATIC
395.2 RHEUMATIC WITH INSUFFICIENCY
093.22 SYPHILITIC
424.1 WITH INSUFFICIENCY
421.0 WITH INSUFFICIENCY BACTERIAL (ACUTE) (CHRONIC)
093.22 WITH INSUFFICIENCY SYPHILITIC
396.2 WITH MITRAL INSUFFICIENCY
396.2 WITH MITRAL INSUFFICIENCY RHEUMATIC
093.22 WITH MITRAL INSUFFICIENCY SYPHILITIC
396.0 WITH MITRAL STENOSIS
396.0 WITH MITRAL STENOSIS RHEUMATIC
093.22 WITH MITRAL STENOSIS SYPHILITIC
396.8 WITH OTHER VALVE MULTIPLE INVOLVEMENT, STENOSIS/INSUFFICIENCY (RHEUMATIC)

AORTITIS

447.6 NOS
447.6 CALCIFIC
093.1 LUETIC
391.1 RHEUMATIC ACUTE
093.1 SYPHILITIC
090.5 SYPHILITIC (CONGENITAL)

0 AORTOCORONARY BYPASS GRAFT COMPLICATION SEE COMPLICATION
V45.81 AORTOCORONARY BYPASS STATUS
444.0 AORTOILIAC OBSTRUCTION (OCCLUSION)
745.0 AORTOPULMONARY DEFECT (COMMON TRUNCUS) (COMMUNICATION ABNORMAL) CONGENITAL

APEPSIA

536.8 NOS
536.0 ACHLORHYDRIC
306.4 PSYCHOGENIC

255.2 APERT-GALLAIS SYNDROME (ADRENOGENITAL)
755.55 APERT'S SYNDROME (ACROCEPHALOSYNDACTYLY)
787.2 APHAGIA
307.1 APHAGIA PSYCHOGENIC

APHAKIA

379.31	APHAKIA
743.35	CONGENITAL
379.31	POSTSURGICAL
V45.61	STATUS POST CATARACT EXTRACTION

APHASIA

784.3	UNSPECIFIED
784.69	APRAXIA-ALEXIA SYNDROME
315.31	DEVELOPMENTAL EXPRESSIVE
315.32	DEVELOPMENTAL RECEPTIVE (EXPRESSIVE - RECEPTIVE) MIXED
438.11	LATE EFFECT CEREBROVASCULAR DISEASE
784.3	UNKNOWN ETIOLOGY

784.41 APHONIA
784.49 APHONIA CLERICORUM

APHTHAE, APHTHOUS

074.0	ANGINA
078.4	APHTHAE EPIZOOTIC
529.0	CACHECTIC
078.4	EPIZOOTIC
078.4	FEVER
528.2	ORAL
528.2	STOMATITIS

APNEA, APNEIC (SPELLS)

786.03	NOS
770.8	PERINATAL PERIOD
306.1	PSYCHOGENIC
780.57	SLEEP
780.53	SLEEP WITH HYPERSOMNIA
780.51	SLEEP WITH HYPOSOMNIA
780.51	SLEEP WITH INSOMNIA
780.57	SLEEP WITH SLEEP DISTURBANCE OTHER

077.4 APOLLO CONJUNCTIVITIS
726.90 APONEUROSIS DISEASE

APOPHYSITIS (SEE ALSO 'OSTEOCHONDROSIS')

732.9	NOS
732.6	JUVENILE
732.5	JUVENILE CALCANEAL

641.2# APOPLEXIA UTEROPLACENTAL

5th Digit: 641.2
- **0. EPISODE OF CARE NOS OR N/A**
- **1. DELIVERED**
- **3. ANTEPARTUM COMPLICATION**

436 APOPLEXY
0 APOPLEXY WITH RESIDUAL SEE 'LATE EFFECT', CEREBROVASCULAR DISEASE
V12.59 APOPLEXY HISTORY WITHOUT RESIDUAL
0 APPARENT LIFE-THREATENING EVENT (ALTE) CODE INDIVIDUAL SYMPTOM(S)

APPENDICITIS

540.9	ACUTE
540.1	ACUTE WITH PERITONEAL ABSCESS
540.0	ACUTE WITH PERITONITIS
540.0	ACUTE WITH RUPTURE
540.9	ACUTE WITHOUT PERITONITIS
006.8	AMEBIC
542	CHRONIC
540.9	GANGRENOUS
540.1	GANGRENOUS WITH PERITONEAL ABSCESS
540.0	GANGRENOUS WITH PERITONITIS OR RUPTURE
542	RECURRENT
542	RELAPSING
541	RETROCECAL
542	SUBACUTE
541	UNQUALIFIED

V44.52 APPENDICO-VESICOSTOMY STATUS

APPENDIX, APPENDICEAL

751.2	ABSENCE CONGENITAL
543.9	ADHESION
543.9	ATROPHY
543.9	CALCULUS
543.9	DIVERTICULUM
751.5	DUPLICATION CONGENITAL
543.9	FECALITH
543.0	HYPERPLASIA LYMPHOID
863.85	INJURY TRAUMATIC
863.95	INJURY TRAUMATIC WITH OPEN WOUND INTO CAVITY
908.1	INJURY TRAUMATIC LATE EFFECT
543.9	INTUSSUSCEPTION
751.5	MEGALOAPPENDIX CONGENITAL
543.9	MUCOCELE
540.0	RUPTURE (WITH PERITONITIS)
543.9	STERCOLITH
751.5	TRANSPOSITION CONGENITAL

783.0 APPETITE LOSS
307.59 APPETITE LOSS PSYCHOGENIC ORIGIN
307.52 APPETITE PERVERTED NONORGANIC ORIGIN
300.16 APPROXIMATE ANSWERS SYNDROME
784.69 APRAXIA (AUDITORY) (VISUAL) (ORGANIC)
438.81 APRAXIA (AUDITORY) (VISUAL) (ORGANIC) LATE EFFECT OF CEREBROVASCULAR DISEASE
742.3 AQUEDUCT OF SYLVIUS ATRESIA
0 AQUEDUCT OF SYLVIUS ATRESIA WITH SPINA BIFIDA SEE 'SPINA BIFIDA' WITH CEREBRAL DEGENERATION
331.4 AQUEDUCT OF SYLVIUS OBSTRUCTION (OCCLUSION)
742.3 AQUEDUCT OF SYLVIUS OBSTRUCTION (OCCLUSION) CONGENITAL
741.0# AQUEDUCT OF SYLVIUS OBSTRUCTION (OCCLUSION) CONGENITAL WITH SPINA BIFIDA

5th Digit: 741.0
- **0. REGION NOS**
- **1. CERVICAL REGION**
- **2. DORSAL (THORACIC REGION)**
- **3. LUMBAR REGION**

AQUEOUS

364.04	CELLS
364.04	FIBRIN
364.04	FLARE

0 ARACHNOIDITIS SEE ALSO 'MENINGITIS'
335.21 ARAN-DUCHENNE MUSCULAR ATROPHY
066.9 ARBOVIRUS INFECTION

> *AIDS, ARC AND SYMPTOMATIC HIV INFECTIONS ALL CODE TO 042. THIS CODE SHOULD BE SEQUENCED AS THE PRINCIPAL DIAGNOSIS WITH AN ADDITIONAL CODE FOR ANY MANIFESTATION. EXCEPTION: IF THE ENCOUNTER IS FOR AN UNRELATED CONDITION SUCH AS A TRAUMA, SEQUENCE THE TRAUMA AS THE PRINCIPAL DIAGNOSIS, FOLLOWED BY THE 042 CODE, AND THEN THE ADDITIONAL CODES FOR THE MANIFESTATIONS.*

042 ARC
042 ARC DUE TO HIV II [079.53]
503 ARC WELDER'S LUNG DISEASE
370.24 ARC WELDER'S SYNDROME (PHOTOKERATITIS)
734 ARCHES FALLEN
447.4 ARCUATE LIGAMENT (-CELIAC AXIS) SYNDROME
446.7 ARCUS AORTAE SYNDROME
743.43 ARCUS JUVENILIS
743.42 ARCUS JUVENILIS INTERFERING WITH VISION
371.41 ARCUS SENILIS

ARDS
507.0 ASSOCIATED WITH ASPIRATION PNEUMONIA
514 ASSOCIATED WITH HYPOSTATIC PNEUMONIA
518.81 ASSOCIATED WITH RESPIRATORY FAILURE - ACUTE IN OTHER CONDITIONS
518.84 ASSOCIATED WITH RESPIRATORY FAILURE - ACUTE AND CHRONIC IN OTHER CONDITIONS
518.83 ASSOCIATED WITH RESPIRATORY FAILURE - CHRONIC IN OTHER CONDITIONS
518.5 ASSOCIATED WITH SHOCK
518.82 ASSOCIATED WITH OTHER CONDITIONS
518.5 FOLLOWING TRAUMA AND SURGERY
518.5 TRAUMATIC OR POSTSURGICAL
518.82 OTHER CAUSES NEC

259.2 ARGENTAFFIN, ARGINTAFFINOMA SYNDROME
371.16 ARGENTOUS DEPOSITS CORNEA
270.6 ARGININE METABOLISM DISORDERS
270.6 ARGININOSUCCINATE SYNTHETASE OR LYASE DEFICIENCY
270.6 ARGININOSUCCINIC ACID METABOLISM DISORDERS
253.1 ARGONZ-DEL CASTILLO SYNDROME (NONPUERPERAL GALACTORRHEA AND AMENORRHEA
379.45 ARGYLL ROBERTSON PUPIL SYNDROME (ATYPICAL) (NONSYPHILITIC)
094.89 ARGYLL ROBERTSON PUPIL SYNDROME SYPHILITIC
371.16 ARGYRIA CORNEA
709.09 ARGYRIA SKIN FROM DRUG OR CORRECT SUBSTANCE PROPERLY ADMINISTERED
372.55 ARGYROSIS CONJUNCTIVAL
742.2 ARHINENCEPHALY CONGENITAL
315.1 ARITHMETICAL DISORDER SPECIFIC (DELAY IN DEVELOPMENT)
008.1 ARIZONA GROUP OF PARACOLON BACILLI GASTROENTERITIS

ARM
V49.60 ABSENCE (ACQUIRED) - NOS
V49.66 ABSENCE (ACQUIRED) - ABOVE ELBOW
V49.65 ABSENCE (ACQUIRED) - BELOW ELBOW
0 ABSENCE CONGENITAL - LOWER SEE 'FOREARM'
755.24 ABSENCE CONGENITAL - UPPER WITH INCOMPLETE ABSENCE OF DISTAL ELEMENTS
755.21 ABSENCE CONGENITAL - UPPER WITH COMPLETE ABSENCE OF DISTAL ELEMENTS
755.23 ABSENCE CONGENITAL - UPPER WITH FOREARM (INCOMPLETE)
0 AMPUTATION STATUS SEE 'AMPUTATION' STATUS UPPER LIMB
728.2 ATROPHY
903.9 BLOOD VESSEL INJURY NOS
903.8 BLOOD VESSEL INJURY MULTIPLE
903.8 BLOOD VESSEL INJURY SPECIFIED NEC
736.89 DEFORMITY (ACQUIRED) NEC
959.2 INJURY (PROXIMAL)
V52.0 PROSTHESIS (FITTING AND ADJUSTMENT) (REMOVAL)
840.9 SEPARATION (RUPTURE) (TEAR) (LACERATION)
755.20 SHORTENING CONGENITAL
337.9 SHOULDER SYNDROME SEE ALSO 'NEUROPATHY PERIPHERAL' AUTONOMIC
840.9 STRAIN (SPRAIN) (AVULSION) (HEMARTHROSIS)

277.3 ARMENIAN DISEASE

ARNOLD CHIARI SYNDROME
348.4 TYPE I
741.0# TYPE II
5th Digit: 741.0
0. REGION NOS
1. CERVICAL REGION
2. DORSAL (THORACIC REGION)
3. LUMBAR REGION

742.0 TYPE III
742.2 TYPE IV

ARRHYTHMIA
427.9 NOS
427.9 AURICULAR
427.89 BIGEMINY
426.9 BLOCK NOS (SEE ALSO 'HEART BLOCK')
427.89 BRADYCARDIA
427.9 CARDIAC
427.89 CORONARY SINUS
427.89 ECTOPIC
427.60 EXTRASYSTOLIC
427.9 JUVENILE
427.9 NODAL
997.1 POSTOPERATIVE (DURING OR RESULTING FROM A PROCEDURE)
306.2 PSYCHOGENIC
427.9 REFLEX
0 SEE ALSO 'DYSRHYTHMIA'
427.9 SINUS
427.9 SUPRAVENTRICULAR
427.9 TRANSITORY
780.2 VAGAL
427.9 VENTRICULAR

416.0 ARRILLAGA-AYERZA SYNDROME (PULMONARY ARTERY SCLEROSIS WITH PULMONARY HYPERTENSION)
709.09 ARSENICAL PIGMENTATION DUE TO DRUG OR CORRECT SUBSTANCE PROPERLY ADMINISTERED
0 ARTERIAL SEE 'ARTERY, ARTERIAL'
447.9 ARTERIOLE DISORDER NOS
447.8 ARTERIOLE DISORDER OTHER NEC
537.89 ARTERIOMESENTERIC DUODENUM OCCLUSION SYNDROME

DO NOT USE CODE 996.03, COMPLICATION OF A DEVICE, IMPLANT OR GRAFT MECHANICAL CARDIAC, WHEN THE PHYSICIAN DOCUMENTS THAT ARTERIOSCLEROSIS HAS CAUSED AN OCCLUSION OF A BYPASS GRAFT. IN CODING TERMS, THIS IS CONSIDERED TO BE A NORMAL PROGRESSION OF ARTERIOSCLEROSIS RATHER THAN A COMPLICATION OF A GRAFT. ASSIGN CODE 414.0#, ARTERIOSCLEROSIS BYPASS GRAFT, CORONARY.

ARTERIOSCLEROSIS, ARTERIOSCLEROTIC
440.9 GENERALIZED AND UNSPECIFIED
440.0 AORTA
424.1 AORTIC VALVE
433.0# BASILAR ARTERY
5th Digit: 433.0
0. WITHOUT CEREBRAL INFARCTION
1. WITH CEREBRAL INFARCTION

414.0# BYPASS GRAFT CORONARY
5th Digit: 414.0
2. AUTOLOGOUS VEIN BYPASS GRAFT
3. NONAUTOLOGOUS BIOLOGICAL BYPASS GRAFT
4. AUTOLOGOUS ARTERY BYPASS GRAFT (GASTROEPIPLOIC) (INTERNAL MAMMARY)
5. UNSPECIFIED TYPE OF BYPASS GRAFT

440.3# BYPASS GRAFT OF THE EXTREMITIES
5th Digit: 440.3
0. UNSPECIFIED GRAFT
1. AUTOLOGOUS VEIN BYPASS GRAFT
2. NONAUTOLOGOUS BIOLOGICAL BYPASS GRAFT

~~429.2~~ ~~CARDIOVASCULAR DISEASE~~ (NONHYPERTENSIVE) [440.9]
433.1# CAROTID ARTERY
5th Digit: 433.1
0. WITHOUT CEREBRAL INFARCTION
1. WITH CEREBRAL INFARCTION

437.0 CENTRAL NERVOUS SYSTEM
437.0 CEREBRAL

ARTERIOSCLEROSIS, ARTERIOSCLEROTIC (continued)

414.0# CORONARY
5th Digit: 414.0
0. UNSPECIFIED TYPE OF VESSEL, NATIVE OR GRAFT
1. NATIVE CORONARY VESSEL
2. AUTOLOGOUS VEIN BYPASS GRAFT
3. NONAUTOLOGOUS BIOLOGICAL BYPASS GRAFT
4. AUTOLOGOUS ARTERY BYPASS GRAFT (GASTROEPIPLOIC) (INTERNAL MAMMARY)
5. UNSPECIFIED TYPE OF BYPASS GRAFT

290.4# DEMENTIA [437.0]
5th Digit: 290.4
0. NOS
1. WITH DELIRIUM
2. DELUSIONAL
3. DEPRESSIVE

440.2# EXTREMITIES ARTERIES
5th Digit: 440.2
0. UNSPECIFIED
1. WITH INTERMITTENT CLAUDICATION
2. WITH REST PAIN, OR REST PAIN AND (INTERMITTENT CLAUDICATION)
3. WITH ULCERATION, OR ULCERATION AND (INTERMITTENT CLAUDICATION) (REST PAIN)
4. WITH ISCHEMIC GANGRENE, OR ISCHEMIC GANGRENE AND (INTERMITTENT CLAUDICATION) (REST PAIN) (ULCERATION)
9. OTHER ATHEROSCLEROSIS EXTREMITIES

440.3# EXTREMITIES ARTERIES - BYPASS GRAFT
5th Digit: 440.3
0. UNSPECIFIED GRAFT
1. AUTOLOGOUS VEIN BYPASS GRAFT
2. NONAUTOLOGOUS BIOLOGICAL BYPASS GRAFT

414.0# HEART DISEASE (ASHD)
5th Digit: 414.0
0. UNSPECIFIED TYPE OF VESSEL, NATIVE OR GRAFT
1. NATIVE CORONARY VESSEL
2. AUTOLOGOUS VEIN BYPASS GRAFT
3. NONAUTOLOGOUS BIOLOGICAL BYPASS GRAFT
4. AUTOLOGOUS ARTERY BYPASS GRAFT (GASTROEPIPLOIC) (INTERNAL MAMMARY)
5. UNSPECIFIED TYPE OF BYPASS GRAFT

424.99 HEART VALVE UNSPECIFIED

648.5#: USE AN ADDITIONAL CODE TO IDENTIFY THE SPECIFIC CARDIOVASCULAR ARTERIOSCLEROTIC CONDITION.

648.5# MATERNAL - CARDIOVASCULAR CURRENT (CO-EXISTENT) IN PREGNANCY
674.0# MATERNAL - CEREBROVASCULAR DUE TO PREGNANCY
5th Digit: 648.5, 674.0
0. EPISODE OF NOS OR N/A
1. DELIVERED
2. DELIVERED WITH POSTPARTUM COMPLICATION
3. ANTEPARTUM COMPLICATION
4. POSTPARTUM COMPLICATION

648.9#: USE AN ADDITIONAL CODE TO IDENTIFY THE SPECIFIC ARTERIOSCLEROTIC CONDITION.

648.9# MATERNAL - OTHER CURRENT (CO-EXISTENT) IN PREGNANCY
5th Digit: 648.9
0. EPISODE OF NOS OR N/A
1. DELIVERED
2. DELIVERED WITH POSTPARTUM COMPLICATION
3. ANTEPARTUM COMPLICATION
4. POSTPARTUM COMPLICATION

557.1 MESENTERIC
424.0 MITRAL VALVE

ARTERIOSCLEROSIS, ARTERIOSCLEROTIC (continued)

440.8 OTHER SPECIFIED ARTERIES
433.9# PRECEREBRAL ARTERY
433.8# PRECEREBRAL ARTERY OTHER SPECIFIED
5th Digit: 433.8-9
0. WITHOUT CEREBRAL INFARCTION
1. WITH CEREBRAL INFARCTION

416.0 PULMONARY IDIOPATHIC
416.0 PULMONARY CHRONIC
424.3 PULMONARY VALVE
0 RENAL ARTERIOLES SEE 'HYPERTENSIVE'
440.1 RENAL ARTERY
440.8 RETINAL VASCULAR CHANGES [362.13]
440.8 RETINOPATHY VASCULAR (CHANGES) [362.13]
424.2 TRICUSPID VALVE
433.2# VERTEBRAL ARTERY
5th Digit: 433.2
0. WITHOUT CEREBRAL INFARCTION
1. WITH CEREBRAL INFARCTION

0 ARTERIOSCLEROTIC SEE 'ARTERIOSCLEROSIS, ARTERIOSCLEROTIC'

747.60 ARTERIOVENOUS ARTERY NEC (ABERRANT) (ABSENCE) (AGENESIS) (ACCESSORY) (ANEURYSM) (DEFORMITY) (HYPOPLASIA) (MALPOSITION)

0 ARTERIOVENOUS COMPLICATION INTERNAL SHUNT OR FISTULA (SURGICALLY CREATED) SEE 'COMPLICATION' VASCULAR

ARTERIOVENOUS (A-V) MALFORMATION

437.3 BRAIN ACQUIRED
747.81 BRAIN CONGENITAL
430 BRAIN RUPTURED, SUBARACHNOID
747.81 CEREBROVASCULAR SYSTEM CONGENITAL
746.85 CORONARY ARTERY CONGENITAL
747.6# PERIPHERAL VASCULAR SYSTEM CONGENITAL (ABERRANT) (ABSENCE) (AGENESIS) (ACCESSORY) (ANEURYSM) (DEFORMITY) (HYPOPLASIA) (MALPOSITION)
5th Digit: 747.6
0. PERIPHERAL VASCULAR UNSPECIFIED SITE
1. GASTROINTESTINAL VESSEL
2. RENAL VESSEL
3. UPPER LIMB VESSEL
4. LOWER LIMB VESSEL
9. OTHER SPECIFIED SITE PERIPHERAL VASCULAR

747.3 PULMONARY
743.58 RETINA
747.82 SPINAL VESSEL CONGENITAL
747.89 OTHER SPECIFIED

996.73 ARTERIOVENOUS STEAL SYNDROME
747.60 ARTERIOVENOUS VEIN NEC (ABERRANT) (ABSENCE) (AGENESIS) (ACCESSORY) (ANEURYSM) (DEFORMITY) (HYPOPLASIA) (MALPOSITION)

ARTERITIS

447.6 NOS
446.20 ALLERGIC
447.6 AORTA
446.7 AORTIC ARCH
437.4 BRAIN
446.7 BRANCHIAL
446.7 BRANCHIOCEPHALICA
437.4 CEREBRAL
414.0# CORONARY ARTERIOSCLEROTIC
5th Digit: 414.0
0. UNSPECIFIED TYPE OF VESSEL, NATIVE OR GRAFT
1. NATIVE CORONARY VESSEL
2. AUTOLOGOUS VEIN BYPASS GRAFT
3. NONAUTOLOGOUS BIOLOGICAL BYPASS GRAFT
4. AUTOLOGOUS ARTERY BYPASS GRAFT (GASTROEPIPLOIC) (INTERNAL MAMMARY)
5. UNSPECIFIED TYPE OF BYPASS GRAFT

ARTERITIS (continued)

391.9 CORONARY RHEUMATIC
398.99 CORONARY RHEUMATIC (CHRONIC)
446.5 CRANIAL (LEFT) (RIGHT)
446.5 GIANT CELL
674.0# MATERNAL - CEREBROVASCULAR DUE TO PREGNANCY
5th Digit: 674.0
0. EPISODE OF NOS OR N/A
1. DELIVERED
2. DELIVERED WITH POSTPARTUM COMPLICATION
3. ANTEPARTUM COMPLICATION
4. POSTPARTUM COMPLICATION

648.5#: USE AN ADDITIONAL CODE TO IDENTIFY CORONARY ARTERITIS.

648.5# MATERNAL - CORONARY CURRENT (CO-EXISTENT) IN PREGNANCY
5th Digit: 648.5
0. EPISODE OF NOS OR N/A
1. DELIVERED
2. DELIVERED WITH POSTPARTUM COMPLICATION
3. ANTEPARTUM COMPLICATION
4. POSTPARTUM COMPLICATION

648.9#: USE AN ADDITIONAL CODE TO IDENTIFY THE SPECIFIC ARTERITIS.

648.9# MATERNAL - OTHER CURRENT (CO-EXISTENT) IN PREGNANCY
5th Digit: 648.9
0. EPISODE OF NOS OR N/A
1. DELIVERED
2. DELIVERED WITH POSTPARTUM COMPLICATION
3. ANTEPARTUM COMPLICATION
4. POSTPARTUM COMPLICATION

446.0 NECROTIZING
446.7 OBLITERANS
446.0 POLY
417.8 PULMONARY
362.18 RETINAL
447.2 SUPPURATIVE
446.5 TEMPORAL
446.7 YOUNG FEMALE SYNDROME (OBLITERATIVE BRACHIOCEPHALIC)

ARTERITIS SYPHILITIC

093.1 AORTA
093.1 AORTITIS
094.89 BRAIN
093.89 CORONARY ARTERY
093.89 GENERAL

ARTERY, ARTERIAL

747.81 ANOMALY - CEREBRAL (ABERRANT) (ABSENCE) (AGENESIS) (ACCESSORY) (ANEURYSM) (ATRESIA) (DEFORMITY) (HYPOPLASIA)
746.85 ANOMALY - CORONARY (ABSENCE) (AGENESIS) (ACCESSORY) (ANEURYSM) (ATRESIA) (DEFORMITY) (HYPOPLASIA) (MALPOSITION)
747.6# ANOMALY - PERIPHERAL VASCULAR NEC (ABERRANT) (ABSENCE) (AGENESIS) (ACCESSORY) (ANEURYSM) (DEFORMITY) (HYPOPLASIA) (MALPOSITION)
5th Digit: 747.6
0. UNSPECIFIED SITE
1. GASTROINTESTINAL VESSEL
2. RENAL VESSEL
3. UPPER LIMB VESSEL
4. LOWER LIMB VESSEL
9. OTHER SPECIFIED SITE PERIPHERAL VASCULAR

ARTERY, ARTERIAL (continued)

747.3 ANOMALY - PULMONARY (ABSENCE) (AGENESIS) (ANEURYSM) (HYPOPLASIA) (MALPOSITION)
743.58 ANOMALY - RETINAL (ANEURYSM) (ATRESIA) (DEFORMITY) (HYPOPLASIA)
747.82 ANOMALY - SPINAL (ABERRANT) (ANEURYSM) (DEFORMITY) (HYPOPLASIA)
747.5 ANOMALY - UMBILICAL (ABSENCE) (AGENESIS) (ATRESIA) (HYPOPLASIA)
440.2# ARTERIOSCLEROSIS EXTREMITIES (DEGENERATION) (DEFORMANS) (ARTERITIS)
440.2# ARTERIOSCLEROSIS EXTREMITIES WITH OCCLUSION (DEGENERATION) (DEFORMANS) (ARTERITIS)
5th Digit: 440.2
0. UNSPECIFIED
1. WITH INTERMITTENT CLAUDICATION
2. WITH REST PAIN, OR REST PAIN AND (INTERMITTENT CLAUDICATION)
3. WITH ULCERATION, OR ULCERATION AND (INTERMITTENT CLAUDICATION) (REST PAIN)
4. WITH ISCHEMIC GANGRENE, OR ISCHEMIC GANGRENE AND (INTERMITTENT CLAUDICATION) (REST PAIN) (ULCERATION)
9. OTHER ATHEROSCLEROSIS EXTREMITIES

440.3# ARTERIOSCLEROSIS EXTREMITIES BYPASS GRAFT
5th Digit: 440.3
0. UNSPECIFIED GRAFT
1. AUTOLOGOUS VEIN BYPASS GRAFT
2. NONAUTOLOGOUS BIOLOGICAL BYPASS GRAFT

747.60 ATRESIA (ANOMALY NEC) CONGENITAL
747.3 ATRESIA PULMONARY
790.91 BLOOD GAS ABNORMAL
447.9 DISORDERS

648.9#: USE AN ADDITIONAL CODE TO IDENTIFY THE SPECIFIC ARTERIAL DISORDER.

648.9# DISORDERS MATERNAL CURRENT (CO-EXISTENT) IN PREGNANCY
5th Digit: 648.9
0. EPISODE OF NOS OR N/A
1. DELIVERED
2. DELIVERED WITH POSTPARTUM COMPLICATION
3. ANTEPARTUM COMPLICATION
4. POSTPARTUM COMPLICATION

447.8 DISORDERS OTHER NEC
447.8 FIBROMUSCULAR HYPERPLASIA
447.3 FIBROMUSCULAR HYPERPLASIA RENAL
996.62 GRAFT COMPLICATION - INFECTION OR INFLAMMATION
996.1 GRAFT COMPLICATION - MECHANICAL
996.74 GRAFT COMPLICATION - OTHER
447.8 HYPERPLASIA FIBROMUSCULAR
447.3 HYPERPLASIA FIBROMUSCULAR RENAL
0 INJURY TRAUMATIC SEE SPECIFIED ARTERY, INJURY
443.9 INSUFFICIENCY (PERIPHERAL)
447.5 NECROSIS
444.9 OBSTRUCTION OR OCCLUSION NEC (EMBOLISM) (INFARCTION) (THROMBOSIS)
447.1 OCCLUSION DUE TO STRICTURE OR STENOSIS
444.22 OCCLUSION LOWER EXTREMITIES
0 OCCLUSION LOWER EXTREMITIES WITHOUT THROMBUS OR EMBOLUS SEE 'ARTERY, ARTERIAL', ARTERIOSCLEROSIS EXTREMITIES
444.21 OCCLUSION UPPER EXTREMITIES
0 OCCLUSION UPPER EXTREMITIES WITHOUT THROMBUS OR EMBOLUS SEE 'ARTERY, ARTERIAL', ARTERIOSCLEROSIS EXTREMITIES
447.2 RUPTURE DUE TO EROSION (ULCERATION)
443.9 SPASM (PERIPHERAL ARTERY)
744.04 STAPEDIA (PERSISTENT)
447.1 STRICTURE
442.0 UPPER EXTREMITY (ANEURYSM) (A-V FISTULA) (CIRSOID) (FALSE) (VARICOSE)
447.2 WALL ABSCESS

A

719.4# ARTHRALGIA

5th Digit: 719.4

0. SITE NOS
1. SHOULDER REGION
2. UPPER ARM (ELBOW) (HUMERUS)
3. FOREARM (RADIUS) (WRIST) (ULNA)
4. HAND (CARPAL) (METACARPAL) (FINGERS)
5. PELVIC REGION AND THIGH (HIP) (BUTTOCK) (FEMUR)
6. LOWER LEG (FIBULA) (KNEE) (PATELLA) (TIBIA)
7. ANKLE AND/OR FOOT (METATARSALS) (TOES) (TARSALS)
8. OTHER
9. MULTIPLE

ARTHRITIS

716.9# NOS
716.2# ALLERGIC
714.0 ATROPHIC
720.9 ATROPHIC SPINE
716.3# CLIMACTERIC
098.50 GONOCOCCAL
274.0 GOUT
0 HYPERTROPHIC SEE 'OSTEOARTHRITIS'
711.9# INFECTIVE
714.9 INFLAMMATORY
716.3# MENOPAUSAL
716.6# MONOARTICULAR
0 NODOSA SEE 'ARTHRITIS OSTEOARTHRITIS'
716.4# TRANSIENT
716.1# TRAUMATIC
716.8# OTHER SPECIFIED

5th Digit: 711.9, 716.1-4, 6, 8-9

0. SITE NOS
1. SHOULDER REGION
2. UPPER ARM (ELBOW) (HUMERUS)
3. FOREARM (RADIUS) (WRIST) (ULNA)
4. HAND (CARPAL) (METACARPAL) (FINGERS)
5. PELVIC REGION AND THIGH (HIP) (BUTTOCK) (FEMUR)
6. LOWER LEG (FIBULA) (KNEE) (PATELLA) (TIBIA)
7. ANKLE AND/OR FOOT (METATARSALS) (TOES) (TARSALS)
8. OTHER (HEAD) (NECK) (RIB) (SKULL) (TRUNK) (VERTEBRAE)
9. MULTIPLE

OSTEOARTHRITIS IS THE MOST COMMON TYPE OF ARTHRITIS, SOMETIMES REFERRED TO AS DEGENERATIVE JOINT DISEASE. CLASSIFICATION IS GENERALLY CODED TO LOCALIZED (PRIMARY OR SECONDARY), OR GENERALIZED.

ARTHRITIS OSTEOARTHRITIS (DEGENERATIVE)

715.9# NOS
715.9# DEGENERATIVE JOINT DISEASE
715.3# LOCALIZED
715.1# LOCALIZED PRIMARY (BY JOINT)
715.2# LOCALIZED SECONDARY (BY JOINT)

5th Digit: 715.1-3, 9

0. SITE UNSPECIFIED
1. SHOULDER REGION
2. UPPER ARM (ELBOW) (HUMERUS)
3. FOREARM (RADIUS) (WRIST) (ULNA)
4. HAND (CARPAL) (METACARPAL) (FINGERS)
5. PELVIC REGION AND THIGH (HIP) (BUTTOCK) (FEMUR)
6. LOWER LEG (FIBULA) (KNEE) (PATELLA) (TIBIA)
7. ANKLE AND/OR FOOT (METATARSALS) (TOES) (TARSALS)
8. OTHER SPECIFIED EXCEPT SPINE

ARTHRITIS OSTEOARTHRITIS (DEGENERATIVE) (continued)

715.0# GENERALIZED

5th Digit: 715.0

0. SITE UNSPECIFIED
4. HAND (CARPAL) (METACARPAL) (FINGERS)
9. MULTIPLE

715.8# MULTIPLE SITES (BY JOINT) (NOT SPECIFIED AS GENERALIZED)

5th Digit: 715.8

0. SITE UNSPECIFIED
9. MULTIPLE

ARTHRITIS OSTEOARTHRITIS (DEGENERATIVE) OF SPINE:

-WITH OSTEOPOROSIS [733.0#]

721.0 CERVICAL
721.1 CERVICAL WITH MYELOPATHY (CORD COMPRESSION)
721.3 LUMBAR
721.42 LUMBAR WITH MYELOPATHY (CORD COMPRESSION)
721.3 LUMBOSACRAL
721.42 LUMBOSACRAL WITH MYELOPATHY (CORD COMPRESSION)
721.90 SPINE
721.91 SPINE WITH MYELOPATHY (CORD COMPRESSION)
721.2 THORACIC
721.41 THORACIC WITH MYELOPATHY (CORD COMPRESSION)
721.7 TRAUMATIC

WITH OSTEOPOROSIS [733.0#]

5th Digit: 733.0

0. UNSPECIFIED
1. SENILE
2. IDIOPATHIC
3. DISUSE
9. DRUG INDUCED

ARTHRITIS RHEUMATOID

714.0 ADULT
714.30 JUVENILE CHRONIC OR UNSPECIFIED
714.33 JUVENILE MONOARTICULAR
714.32 JUVENILE PAUCIARTICULAR
714.31 JUVENILE POLYARTICULAR ACUTE
720.0 SPINE
714.0 WITH MYOPATHY [359.6]
714.0 WITH POLYNEUROPATHY [357.1]
714.2 WITH VISCERAL OR SYSTEMIC INVOLVEMENT

ARTHRITIS OTHER SPECIFIED

253.0 ACROMEGALIC [713.0]
039.8 ACTINOMYCOTIC **[711.4#]**
117.6 ALLESCHERIOSIS **[711.6#]**
277.3 AMYLOID [713.7]
088.9 ARTHROPOD BORNE DISEASE **[711.8#]**
088.89 ARTHROPOD BORNE DISEASE (OTHER) **[711.8#]**
117.3 ASPERGILLA **[711.6#]**
0 BACTERIAL SEE 'ARTHRITIS' PYOGENIC
088.0 BARTONELLA **[711.8#]**
136.1 BEHCET'S SYNDROME **[711.2#]**

5th Digit: 711.2, 4, 6, 8,

0. SITE NOS
1. SHOULDER REGION
2. UPPER ARM (ELBOW) (HUMERUS)
3. FOREARM (RADIUS) (WRIST) (ULNA)
4. HAND (CARPAL) (METACARPAL) (FINGERS)
5. PELVIC REGION AND THIGH (HIP) (BUTTOCK) (FEMUR)
6. LOWER LEG (FIBULA) (KNEE) (PATELLA) (TIBIA)
7. ANKLE AND/OR FOOT (METATARSALS) (TOES) (TARSALS)
8. OTHER (HEAD) (NECK) (RIB) (SKULL) (TRUNK) (VERTEBRAE)
9. MULTIPLE

ARTHRITIS OTHER SPECIFIED (continued)

116.# BLASTOMYCOTIC [711.6#]

4th Digit: 116
- 0. BLASTOMYCOSIS
- 1. PARACOCCIDIOIDOMYCOSIS
- 2. LOBOMYCOSIS

5th Digit: 711.6
- 0. SITE NOS
- 1. SHOULDER REGION
- 2. UPPER ARM (ELBOW) (HUMERUS)
- 3. FOREARM (RADIUS) (WRIST) (ULNA)
- 4. HAND (CARPAL) (METACARPAL) (FINGERS)
- 5. PELVIC REGION AND THIGH (HIP) (BUTTOCK) (FEMUR)
- 6. LOWER LEG (FIBULA) (KNEE) (PATELLA) (TIBIA)
- 7. ANKLE AND/OR FOOT (METATARSALS) (TOES) (TARSALS)
- 8. OTHER (HEAD) (NECK) (RIB) (SKULL) (TRUNK) (VERTEBRAE)
- 9. MULTIPLE

081.1 BRILL'S DISEASE [711.8#]

112.89 CANDIDAL [711.6#]

133.8 CHIGGERS (DUE TO) [711.8#]

134.1 CHIGOE (SANDFLEA) [711.8#]

117.2 CHROMOBLASTOMYCOTIC [711.6#]

114.3 COCCIDIOIDOMYCOTIC [711.6#]

5th Digit: 711.6, 8
- 0. SITE NOS
- 1. SHOULDER REGION
- 2. UPPER ARM (ELBOW) (HUMERUS)
- 3. FOREARM (RADIUS) (WRIST) (ULNA)
- 4. HAND (CARPAL) (METACARPAL) (FINGERS)
- 5. PELVIC REGION AND THIGH (HIP) (BUTTOCK) (FEMUR)
- 6. LOWER LEG (FIBULA) (KNEE) (PATELLA) (TIBIA)
- 7. ANKLE AND/OR FOOT (METATARSALS) (TOES) (TARSALS)
- 8. OTHER (HEAD) (NECK) (RIB) (SKULL) (TRUNK) (VERTEBRAE)
- 9. MULTIPLE

THE CODE IN THE LEFT MARGIN ALWAYS SEQUENCES FIRST. THE ADDITIONAL CODE IN BRACKETS TO THE RIGHT OF THE DESCRIPTION IS SEQUENCED SECONDARILY. UNDERLINING SHOWS THE CODE NUMBER THAT CORRESPONDS TO THE UNDERLINED VERBAL DESCRIPTION. UNDERLINING NEVER IMPLIES CORRECT SEQUENCING.

094.0 CHARCOT'S [713.5]

0 CHONDROCALCINOSIS SEE 'CHONDROCALCINOSIS'

556.# COLITIS ULCERATIVE (DUE TO) [713.1]

4th Digit: 556
- 0. ENTEROCOLITIS (CHRONIC)
- 1. ILEOCOLITIS (CHRONIC)
- 2. PROCTITIS (CHRONIC)
- 3. PROCTOSIGMOIDITIS (CHRONIC)
- 4. PSEUDOPOLYPOSIS OF COLON
- 5. LEFT-SIDED (CHRONIC)
- 6. UNIVERSAL (CHRONIC)
- 8. OTHER ULCERATIVE COLITIS
- 9. ULCERATIVE COLITIS (ENTERITIS) UNSPECIFIED

478.79 CRICOARYTENOID CARTILAGE

555.9 CROHN'S (DUE TO CROHN'S DISEASE) [713.1]

ARTHRITIS OTHER SPECIFIED (continued)

117.5 CRYPTOCOCCAL [711.6#]

275.49 CRYSTAL INDUCED - UNSPECIFIED [712.9#]

0 CRYSTAL INDUCED - CHONDROCALCINOSIS SEE 'CHONDROCALCINOSIS'

274.0 CRYSTAL INDUCED - GOUTY

275.49 CRYSTAL INDUCED - OTHER SPECIFIED [712.8#]

110.8 DERMATOPHYTOSIS [711.6#]

5th Digit: 711.6, 712.8-9
- 0. SITE NOS
- 1. SHOULDER REGION
- 2. UPPER ARM (ELBOW) (HUMERUS)
- 3. FOREARM (RADIUS) (WRIST) (ULNA)
- 4. HAND (CARPAL) (METACARPAL) (FINGERS)
- 5. PELVIC REGION AND THIGH (HIP) (BUTTOCK) (FEMUR)
- 6. LOWER LEG (FIBULA) (KNEE) (PATELLA) (TIBIA)
- 7. ANKLE AND/OR FOOT (METATARSALS) (TOES) (TARSALS)
- 8. OTHER (HEAD) (NECK) (RIB) (SKULL) (TRUNK) (VERTEBRAE)
- 9. MULTIPLE

279.0# DUE TO HYPOGAMMAGLOBULINEMIA [713.0]

5th Digit: 279.0
- 0. UNSPECIFIED
- 1. SELECTIVE IGA
- 2. SELECTIVE IGM
- 3. SELECTIVE IGG
- 5. INCREASED IGM
- 6. VARIABLE
- 9. OTHER

0 DYSENTERIC SEE 'ARTHRITIS', POSTDYSENTERIC

695.1 ERYTHEMA MULTIFORME (DUE TO) [713.3]

695.2 ERYTHEMA NODOSUM (DUE TO) [713.3]

125.# FILARIAL [711.7#]

711.7# HELMINTHIASIS

4th Digit: 125
- 0. BANCROFTIAN
- 1. MALAYAN
- 2. LOIASIS
- 3. ONCHOCERCIASIS
- 4. DIPETALONEMIASIS
- 5. MANSONELLA OZZARDI INFECTION
- 6. OTHER SPECIFIED
- 7. DRACONTIASIS
- 9. UNSPECIFIED

5th Digit: 711.7
- 0. SITE NOS
- 1. SHOULDER REGION
- 2. UPPER ARM (ELBOW) (HUMERUS)
- 3. FOREARM (RADIUS) (WRIST) (ULNA)
- 4. HAND (CARPAL) (METACARPAL) (FINGERS)
- 5. PELVIC REGION AND THIGH (HIP) (BUTTOCK) (FEMUR)
- 6. LOWER LEG (FIBULA) (KNEE) (PATELLA) (TIBIA)
- 7. ANKLE AND/OR FOOT (METATARSALS) (TOES) (TARSALS)
- 8. OTHER (HEAD) (NECK) (RIB) (SKULL) (TRUNK) (VERTEBRAE)
- 9. MULTIPLE

282.4 HEMAGLOBINOPATHY (DUE TO) [713.2]

275.0 HEMOCHROMATOSIS (DUE TO) [713.0]

286.0 HEMOPHILIA VIII ARTHRITIS [713.2]

286.1 HEMOPHILIA IX ARTHRITIS [713.2]

286.0 HEMOPHILIAC [713.2]

287.0 HENOCH SCHONLEIN PURPURA (DUE TO) [713.6]

ARTHRITIS OTHER SPECIFIED (continued)

134.2 HIRUDINIASIS [711.8#]

115.9# HISTOPLASMOSIS [711.6#]

5th Digit: 115.9
- 0. CAPSULATUM
- 1. DUBOISII
- 9. UNSPECIFIED

5th Digit: 711.6, 8
- 0. SITE NOS
- 1. SHOULDER REGION
- 2. UPPER ARM (ELBOW) (HUMERUS)
- 3. FOREARM (RADIUS) (WRIST) (ULNA)
- 4. HAND (CARPAL) (METACARPAL) (FINGERS)
- 5. PELVIC REGION AND THIGH (HIP) (BUTTOCK) (FEMUR)
- 6. LOWER LEG (FIBULA) (KNEE) (PATELLA) (TIBIA)
- 7. ANKLE AND/OR FOOT (METATARSALS) (TOES) (TARSALS)
- 8. OTHER (HEAD) (NECK) (RIB) (SKULL) (TRUNK) (VERTEBRAE)
- 9. MULTIPLE

252.0 HYPERPARATHYROID [713.0]

244.# HYPOTHYROID ACQUIRED [713.0]

4th Digit: 244
- 0. POSTSURGICAL
- 1. POSTABLATIVE (IRRADIATION)
- 2. IODINE INGESTION
- 3. PAS, PHENYLBUT, RESORCINOL
- 8. SECONDARY NEC
- 9. NOS

243 HYPOTHYROID CONGENITAL (DUE TO) [713.0]

085.9 LEISHMANIASIS [711.8#]

030.# LEPROMATOUS [711.4#]

4th Digit: 030
- 0. TYPE L
- 1. TYPE T
- 2. GROUP I
- 3. GROUP B
- 8. OTHER SPECIFIED LEPROSY
- 9. NOS

5th Digit: 711.4, 8
- 0. SITE NOS
- 1. SHOULDER REGION
- 2. UPPER ARM (ELBOW) (HUMERUS)
- 3. FOREARM (RADIUS) (WRIST) (ULNA)
- 4. HAND (CARPAL) (METACARPAL) (FINGERS)
- 5. PELVIC REGION AND THIGH (HIP) (BUTTOCK) (FEMUR)
- 6. LOWER LEG (FIBULA) (KNEE) (PATELLA) (TIBIA)
- 7. ANKLE AND/OR FOOT (METATARSALS) (TOES) (TARSALS)
- 8. OTHER (HEAD) (NECK) (RIB) (SKULL) (TRUNK) (VERTEBRAE)
- 9. MULTIPLE

100.# LEPTOSPIROSIS [711.8#]

4th Digit: 100
- 0. ICTEROHEMORRHAGICA
- 9. LEPTOSPIROSIS NOS

5th Digit: 711.8
- 0. SITE NOS
- 1. SHOULDER REGION
- 2. UPPER ARM (ELBOW) (HUMERUS)
- 3. FOREARM (RADIUS) (WRIST) (ULNA)
- 4. HAND (CARPAL) (METACARPAL) (FINGERS)
- 5. PELVIC REGION AND THIGH (HIP) (BUTTOCK) (FEMUR)
- 6. LOWER LEG (FIBULA) (KNEE) (PATELLA) (TIBIA)
- 7. ANKLE AND/OR FOOT (METATARSALS) (TOES) (TARSALS)
- 8. OTHER (HEAD) (NECK) (RIB) (SKULL) (TRUNK) (VERTEBRAE)
- 9. MULTIPLE

ARTHRITIS OTHER SPECIFIED (continued)

272.0 LIPOID DISORDER (DUE TO) [713.0]

088.81 LYME DISEASE [711.8#]

117.4 MADURA [711.6#]

084.9 MALARIAL [711.8#]

5th Digit: 711.6, 8
- 0. SITE NOS
- 1. SHOULDER REGION
- 2. UPPER ARM (ELBOW) (HUMERUS)
- 3. FOREARM (RADIUS) (WRIST) (ULNA)
- 4. HAND (CARPAL) (METACARPAL) (FINGERS)
- 5. PELVIC REGION AND THIGH (HIP) (BUTTOCK) (FEMUR)
- 6. LOWER LEG (FIBULA) (KNEE) (PATELLA) (TIBIA)
- 7. ANKLE AND/OR FOOT (METATARSALS) (TOES) (TARSALS)
- 8. OTHER (HEAD) (NECK) (RIB) (SKULL) (TRUNK) (VERTEBRAE)
- 9. MULTIPLE

THE CODE IN THE LEFT MARGIN ALWAYS SEQUENCES FIRST. THE ADDITIONAL CODE IN BRACKETS TO THE RIGHT OF THE DESCRIPTION IS SEQUENCED SECONDARILY. UNDERLINING SHOWS THE CODE NUMBER THAT CORRESPONDS TO THE UNDERLINED VERBAL DESCRIPTION. UNDERLINING NEVER IMPLIES CORRECT SEQUENCING.

202.3# MALIGNANT RETICULOSIS (DUE TO) [713.2]

5th Digit: 202.3
- 0. NOS
- 1. LYMPH NODES OF HEAD FACE NECK
- 2. LYMPH NODES INTRATHORACIC
- 3. LYMPH NODES ABDOMINAL
- 4. LYMPH NODES AXILLA AND UPPER LIMB
- 5. LYMPH NODES INGUINAL REGION AND LOWER LIMB
- 6. LYMPH NODES INTRAPELVIC
- 7. SPLEEN
- 8. LYMPH NODES MULTIPLE SITES

CODE THE SPECIFIC MATERNAL ARTHRITIS IN ADDITION TO 648.7#. SEE 'ARTHRITIS'.

648.7# MATERNAL CURRENT (CO-EXISTENT) IN PREGNANCY

5th Digit: 648.7
- 0. EPISODE OF CARE NOS OR N/A
- 1. DELIVERED
- 2. DELIVERED WITH POSTPARTUM COMPLICATION
- 3. ANTEPARTUM COMPLICATION
- 4. POSTPARTUM COMPLICATION

277.3 MEDITERRANEAN FEVER (DUE TO) [713.7]

036.82 MENINGOCOCCAL

133.9 MITES (DUE TO) [711.8#]

117.7 MUCORMYCOTIC [711.6#]

203.0 MULTIPLE MYELOMA (DUE TO) [713.2]

110.8 MYCOTIC (EPIDERMA) (ACTINA) (NOCARDIA) [711.6#]

118 MYCOTIC (OPPORTUNISTIC) [711.6#]

711.8# MYIASIS [134.0]

5th Digit: 711.6, 8
- 0. SITE NOS
- 1. SHOULDER REGION
- 2. UPPER ARM (ELBOW) (HUMERUS)
- 3. FOREARM (RADIUS) (WRIST) (ULNA)
- 4. HAND (CARPAL) (METACARPAL) (FINGERS)
- 5. PELVIC REGION AND THIGH (HIP) (BUTTOCK) (FEMUR)
- 6. LOWER LEG (FIBULA) (KNEE) (PATELLA) (TIBIA)
- 7. ANKLE AND/OR FOOT (METATARSALS) (TOES) (TARSALS)
- 8. OTHER (HEAD) (NECK) (RIB) (SKULL) (TRUNK) (VERTEBRAE)
- 9. MULTIPLE

094.0 NEUROPATHIC JOINT DISEASE [713.5]

ARTHRITIS OTHER SPECIFIED (continued)

711.4#	OTHER BACTERIAL
711.8#	PARASITIC OR INFECTIOUS
132.9	PEDICULOSIS **[711.8#]**
117.8	PHAEHYPHOMYCOSIS **[711.6#]**
103.9	PINTA **[711.8#]**
714.89	POLY (OTHER SPECIFIED)
009.0	POSTDYSENTERIC **[711.3#]**

5th Digit: 711.3-4, 6, 8

0. SITE NOS
1. SHOULDER REGION
2. UPPER ARM (ELBOW) (HUMERUS)
3. FOREARM (RADIUS) (WRIST) (ULNA)
4. HAND (CARPAL) (METACARPAL) (FINGERS)
5. PELVIC REGION AND THIGH (HIP) (BUTTOCK) (FEMUR)
6. LOWER LEG (FIBULA) (KNEE) (PATELLA) (TIBIA)
7. ANKLE AND/OR FOOT (METATARSALS) (TOES) (TARSALS)
8. OTHER (HEAD) (NECK) (RIB) (SKULL) (TRUNK) (VERTEBRAE)
9. MULTIPLE

714.4	POSTRHEUMATIC CHRONIC
696.0	PSORIATIC
711.0#	PYOGENIC **[041.#(#)]**
711.0#	SEPTIC-PYOGENIC **[041.#(#)]**

5th Digit: 711.0

0. SITE NOS
1. SHOULDER REGION
2. UPPER ARM (ELBOW) (HUMERUS)
3. FOREARM (RADIUS) (WRIST) (ULNA)
4. HAND (CARPAL) (METACARPAL) (FINGERS)
5. PELVIC REGION AND THIGH (HIP) (BUTTOCK) (FEMUR)
6. LOWER LEG (FIBULA) (KNEE) (PATELLA) (TIBIA)
7. ANKLE AND/OR FOOT (METATARSALS) (TOES) (TARSALS)
8. OTHER (HEAD) (NECK) (RIB) (SKULL) (TRUNK) (VERTEBRAE)
9. MULTIPLE

4th or 4th and 5th Digit Code for Organism: 041

.85	**AEROBACTER AEROGENES**
.82	**BACILLUS FRAGILIS**
.84	**BACTEROIDES (FRAGILIS)**
.83	**CLOSTRIDIUM PERFRINGENS**
.4	**E. COLI**
.81	**EATON'S AGENT**
.04	**ENTEROCOCCUS**
.3	**FRIEDLANDER'S BACILLUS,**
.84	**GRAM-NEGATIVE ANAEROBES**
.85	**GRAM-NEGATIVE BACTERIA NOS**
.5	**H. INFLUENZAE**
.86	**H. PYLORI**
.3	**KLEBSIELLA**
.85	**MIMA POLYMORPHA**
.81	**MYCOPLASMA**
.81	**PLEUROPNEUMONIA LIKE ORGANISMS**
.2	**PNEUMOCOCCUS**
.6	**PROTEUS (MIRABILIS) (MORGANII)**
.7	**PSEUDOMONAS**
.85	**SERRATIA**
.10	**STAPHYLOCOCCUS UNSPECIFIED**
.11	**STAPHYLOCOCCUS AUREUS**
.19	**STAPHYLOCOCCUS OTHER**
.00	**STREPTOCOCCUS**
.01	**STREPTOCOCCUS GROUP A**
.02	**STREPTOCOCCUS GROUP B**
.03	**STREPTOCOCCUS GROUP C**
.04	**STREPTOCOCCUS GROUP D**
.05	**STREPTOCOCCUS GROUP G**
.09	**STREPTOCOCCUS OTHER**
.84	**OTHER ANAEROBES**
.89	**OTHER SPECIFIED BACTERIA**

ARTHRITIS OTHER SPECIFIED (continued)

083.0	Q FEVER **[711.8#]**
099.3	REITER'S DISEASE **(711.1#)**
087.0	RELAPSING FEVER **[711.8#]**
519.9	RESPIRATORY DISORDER RELATED [713.4]
390	RHEUMATIC ACUTE
117.0	RHINOSPORIDIOSIS **[711.6#]**
082.8	RICKETTSIAL (LONE STAR FEVER) **[711.8#]**
083.8	RICKETTSIAL (OTHER SPECIFIED) **[711.8#]**
083.2	RICKETTSIALPOX **[711.8#]**
083.9	RICKETTSIOSIS **[711.8#]**
082.0	ROCKY MOUNTAIN SPOTTED FEVER **[711.8#]**

5th Digit: 711.1, 6, 8

0. SITE NOS
1. SHOULDER REGION
2. UPPER ARM (ELBOW) (HUMERUS)
3. FOREARM (RADIUS) (WRIST) (ULNA)
4. HAND (CARPAL) (METACARPAL) (FINGERS)
5. PELVIC REGION AND THIGH (HIP) (BUTTOCK) (FEMUR)
6. LOWER LEG (FIBULA) (KNEE) (PATELLA) (TIBIA)
7. ANKLE AND/OR FOOT (METATARSALS) (TOES) (TARSALS)
8. OTHER (HEAD) (NECK) (RIB) (SKULL) (TRUNK) (VERTEBRAE)
9. MULTIPLE

056.71	RUBELLA
003.23	SALMONELLA

THE CODE IN THE LEFT MARGIN ALWAYS SEQUENCES FIRST. THE ADDITIONAL CODE IN BRACKETS TO THE RIGHT OF THE DESCRIPTION IS SEQUENCED SECONDARILY . UNDERLINING SHOWS THE CODE NUMBER THAT CORRESPONDS TO THE UNDERLINED VERBAL DESCRIPTION. UNDERLINING NEVER IMPLIES CORRECT SEQUENCING.

135	SARCOID [713.7]
133.0	SCABIES (DUE TO) **[711.8#]**
999.5	SERUM SICKNESS (DUE TO) [713.6]
282.60	SICKLE CELL ANEMIA ARTHRITIS [713.2]
282.5	SICKLE CELL TRAIT ARTHRITIS [713.2]
134.9	SKIN PARASITES **[711.8#]**
104.0	SPIROCHETAL (BEJEL) NJOVERNA **[711.8#]**
104.8	SPIROCHETAL (OTHER SPECIFIED) **[711.8#]**
104.9	SPIROCHETAL **[711.8#]**
117.1	SPOROTRICHOSIS **[711.6#]**

5th Digit: 711.6, 8

0. SITE NOS
1. SHOULDER REGION
2. UPPER ARM (ELBOW) (HUMERUS)
3. FOREARM (RADIUS) (WRIST) (ULNA)
4. HAND (CARPAL) (METACARPAL) (FINGERS)
5. PELVIC REGION AND THIGH (HIP) (BUTTOCK) (FEMUR)
6. LOWER LEG (FIBULA) (KNEE) (PATELLA) (TIBIA)
7. ANKLE AND/OR FOOT (METATARSALS) (TOES) (TARSALS)
8. OTHER (HEAD) (NECK) (RIB) (SKULL) (TRUNK) (VERTEBRAE)
9. MULTIPLE

094.0	SYPHILITIC (TABES DORSALIS) [713.5]
336.0	SYRINGOMYELIC [713.5]
282.4	THALASSEMIA ARTHRITIS [713.2]

A

ARTHRITIS OTHER SPECIFIED (continued)

111.0 TINEA (DERMATOMYCOTIC) [711.6#]
130.7 TOXOPLASMOSIS [711.8#]
716.4# TRANSIENT
719.3# TRANSIENT PALINDROMIC
083.1 TRENCH MOUTH (QUINTAN WOLHYNIAN) FEVER [711.8#]
131.8 TRICHOMONAL [711.8#]
086.9 TRYPANOSOMA [711.8#]

5th Digit: 711.6, 8, 716.4, 719.3
0. SITE NOS
1. SHOULDER REGION
2. UPPER ARM (ELBOW) (HUMERUS)
3. FOREARM (RADIUS) (WRIST) (ULNA)
4. HAND (CARPAL) (METACARPAL) (FINGERS)
5. PELVIC REGION AND THIGH (HIP) (BUTTOCK) (FEMUR)
6. LOWER LEG (FIBULA) (KNEE) (PATELLA) (TIBIA)
7. ANKLE AND/OR FOOT (METATARSALS) (TOES) (TARSALS)
8. OTHER
9. MULTIPLE

015.0# TUBERCULOUS [711.4#]
002.0 TYPHOID [711.3#]

5th Digit: 015.0
0. NOS
1. LAB NOT DONE
2. LABS PENDING
3. MICROSCOPY POSITIVE (IN SPUTUM)
4. CULTURE POSITIVE - MICROSCOPY NEGATIVE
5. CULTURE NEGATIVE - MICROSCOPY POSITIVE
6. CULTURE AND MICROSCOPY NEGATIVE CONFIRMED BY OTHER METHODS

5th Digit: 711.3-4
0. SITE NOS
1. SHOULDER REGION
2. UPPER ARM (ELBOW) (HUMERUS)
3. FOREARM (RADIUS) (WRIST) (ULNA)
4. HAND (CARPAL) (METACARPAL) (FINGERS)
5. PELVIC REGION AND THIGH (HIP) (BUTTOCK) (FEMUR)
6. LOWER LEG (FIBULA) (KNEE) (PATELLA) (TIBIA)
7. ANKLE AND/OR FOOT (METATARSALS) (TOES) (TARSALS)
8. OTHER (HEAD) (NECK) (RIB) (SKULL) (TRUNK) (VERTEBRAE)
9. MULTIPLE

082.1 TYPHUS (AFRICAN) (INDIAN) (MEDITERRANEAN) [711.8#]
080 TYPHUS (LOUSE BORNE) (EPIDEMIC) [711.8#]
081.0 TYPHUS (MURINE) [711.8#]
082.3 TYPHUS (QUEENSLAND TICK) [711.8#]
081.2 TYPHUS (SCRUB) [711.8#]
082.2 TYPHUS (SIBERIAN) [711.8#]
082.9 TYPHUS (TICK BORNE) [711.8#]
081.9 TYPHUS [711.8#]

5th Digit: 711.8
0. SITE NOS
1. SHOULDER REGION
2. UPPER ARM (ELBOW) (HUMERUS)
3. FOREARM (RADIUS) (WRIST) (ULNA)
4. HAND (CARPAL) (METACARPAL) (FINGERS)
5. PELVIC REGION AND THIGH (HIP) (BUTTOCK) (FEMUR)
6. LOWER LEG (FIBULA) (KNEE) (PATELLA) (TIBIA)
7. ANKLE AND/OR FOOT (METATARSALS) (TOES) (TARSALS)
8. OTHER (HEAD) (NECK) (RIB) (SKULL) (TRUNK) (VERTEBRAE)
9. MULTIPLE

ARTHRITIS OTHER SPECIFIED (continued)

556.# ULCERATIVE COLITIS (DUE TO) [713.1]

4th Digit: 556
0. ENTEROCOLITIS (CHRONIC)
1. ILEOCOLITIS (CHRONIC)
2. PROCTITIS (CHRONIC)
3. PROCTOSIGMOIDITIS (CHRONIC)
4. PSEUDOPOLYPOSIS OF COLON
5. LEFT-SIDED (CHRONIC)
6. UNIVERSAL (CHRONIC)
8. OTHER ULCERATIVE COLITIS
9. ULCERATIVE COLITIS (ENTERITIS) UNSPECIFIED

101 VINCENT'S ANGINA [711.8#]
079.99 VIRAL NEC [711.5#]
056.71 VIRAL (RUBELLA)
102.0 YAWS [711.8#]
716.8# OTHER SPECIFIED

5th Digit: 711.5, 8, 716.8
0. SITE NOS
1. SHOULDER REGION
2. UPPER ARM (ELBOW) (HUMERUS)
3. FOREARM (RADIUS) (WRIST) (ULNA)
4. HAND (CARPAL) (METACARPAL) (FINGERS)
5. PELVIC REGION AND THIGH (HIP) (BUTTOCK) (FEMUR)
6. LOWER LEG (FIBULA) (KNEE) (PATELLA) (TIBIA)
7. ANKLE AND/OR FOOT (METATARSALS) (TOES) (TARSALS)
8. OTHER (HEAD) (NECK) (RIB) (SKULL) (TRUNK) (VERTEBRAE)
9. MULTIPLE

V45.4 ARTHRODESIS STATUS
0 ARTHROFIBROSIS SEE 'ANKYLOSIS'
728.3 ARTHROGRYPOSIS
754.89 ARTHROGRYPOSIS MULTIPLEX CONGENITA
0 ARTHROPATHY SEE 'ARTHRITIS'
0 ARTHROPATHY SEPTIC SEE 'ARTHRITIS OTHER SPECIFIED' PYOGENIC
088.9 ARTHROPOD BORNE DISEASE
088.89 ARTHROPOD BORNE DISEASES OTHER SPECIFIED
718.0# ARTICULAR CARTILAGE DERANGEMENT

5th Digit: 718.0
0. SITE NOS
1. SHOULDER REGION
2. UPPER ARM (ELBOW) (HUMERUS)
3. FOREARM (RADIUS) (WRIST) (ULNA)
4. HAND (CARPAL) (METACARPAL) (FINGERS)
5. PELVIC REGION AND THIGH (HIP) (BUTTOCK) (FEMUR)
7. ANKLE AND/OR FOOT (METATARSALS) (TOES) (TARSALS)
8. OTHER SPECIIFIED SITES
9. MULTIPLE

717.9 ARTICULAR CARTILAGE DERANGEMENT KNEE
270.2 ARTICULAR CARTILAGE DISORDER IN OCHRONOSIS
524.63 ARTICULAR DISC DISORDER (REDUCING OR NON REDUCING)
315.39 ARTICULATION DISORDER SPEECH DEVELOPMENTAL
V26.1 ARTIFICIAL INSEMINATION
V55.9 ARTIFICIAL OPENING UNSPECIFIED - CARE (CLOSURE) (TOILET) (ATTENTION)
V55.8 ARTIFICIAL OPENING OTHER SPECIFIED - CARE (CLOSURE) (TOILET) (ATTENTION)
V44.8 ARTIFICIAL OPENING OTHER STATUS
V15.84 ASBESTOS EXPOSURE HISTORY
501 ASBESTOSIS
501 ASBESTOSIS LUNG (OCCUPATIONAL)
757.33 ASBOE-HANSEN'S DISEASE (INCONTINENTIA PIGMENTI)

127.0 ASCARIASIS
127.0 ASCARIDIASIS
127.0 ASCARIS LUMBRICOIDES INFECTION

ASCITES
789.5 NOS
197.6 CANCEROUS (MALIGNANT) M8000/6
457.8 CHYLOUS
125.9 CHYLOUS - FILARIAL
778.0 CONGENITAL
653.7# FETAL CAUSING FETOPELVIC DISPROPORTION
660.1# FETAL CAUSING FETOPELVIC DISPROPORTION OBSTRUCTING LABOR [653.7#]
5th Digit: 653.7, 660.1
0. EPISODE OF CARE UNSPECIFIED OR N/A
1. DELIVERED
3. ANTEPARTUM COMPLICATION

719.0# JOINT
719.3# JOINT INTERMITTENT
5th Digit: 719.0, 3
0. SITE UNSPECIFIED
1. SHOULDER REGION
2. UPPER ARM (ELBOW) (HUMERUS)
3. FOREARM (RADIUS) (WRIST) (ULNA)
4. HAND (CARPAL) (METACARPAL) (FINGERS)
5. PELVIS THIGH (HIP) (BUTTOCK) (FEMUR)
6. LOWER LEG (FIBULA) (KNEE) (PATELLA) (TIBIA)
7. ANKLE AND/OR FOOT (METATARSALS) (TOES) (TARSALS)
8. OTHER
9. MULTIPLE

789.5 PSEUDOCHYLOUS
095.2 SYPHILITIC
014.0# TUBERCULOUS
5th Digit: 014.0
0. NOS
1. LAB NOT PENDING
2. LABS PENDING
3. MICROSCOPY POSITIVE (IN SPUTUM)
4. CULTURE POSITIVE - MICROSCOPY NEGATIVE
5. CULTURE NEGATIVE - MICROSCOPY POSITIVE
6. CULTURE AND MICROSCOPY NEGATIVE CONFIRMED BY OTHER METHODS

117.4 ASCOMYCETES INFECTION
267 ASCORBIC ACID DEFICIENCY
429.2 ASCVD (NONHYPERTENSIVE) WITH ARTERIOSCLEROSIS [440.9]
0 ASD (ATRIAL SEPTAL DEFECT) SEE 'ATRIAL', SEPTAL DEFECT
047.9 ASEPTIC MENINGITIS SYNDROME

ASEPTIC NECROSIS
733.40 BONE SITE UNSPECIFIED
733.42 FEMUR (HEAD AND NECK OF)
733.49 HAND
733.42 HIP
733.41 HUMERUS (HEAD OF)
733.43 MEDIAL FEMORAL CONDYLE
733.49 OF OTHER BONE
733.44 TALUS

414.0# ASHD (ARTERIOSCLEROTIC HEART DISEASE)
5th Digit: 414.0
0. UNSPECIFIED TYPE OF VESSEL, NATIVE OR GRAFT
1. NATIVE CORONARY VESSEL
2. AUTOLOGOUS VEIN BYPASS GRAFT
3. NONAUTOLOGOUS BIOLOGICAL BYPASS GRAFT
4. AUTOLOGOUS ARTERY BYPASS GRAFT (GASTROEPIPLOIC) (INTERNAL MAMMARY)
5. UNSPECIFIED TYPE OF BYPASS GRAFT

621.5 ASHERMAN'S SYNDROME
781.8 ASOMATOGNOSIA
299.8# ASPERGER'S DISORDER
5th Digit: 299.8
0. CURRENT OR ACTIVE STATE
1. RESIDUAL STATE
117.3 ASPERGILLOSIS
518.6 ASPERGILLOSIS ALLERGIC BRONCHOPULMONARY
117.3 ASPERGILLOSIS WITH EXTERNAL OTITIS [380.15]

300.00 ASPHYCTIC SYNDROME

THE CODES FOR ASPHYXIA FETUS OR NEWBORN CANNOT STAND ALONE. CODE THE UNDERLYING CAUSE OF THE ASPHYXIA IN ADDITION TO THE 768.#. SEQUENCE THE ASPHYXIA FIRST, WITH THE UNDERLYING CAUSE SECOND.

ASPHYXIA, ASPHYXIATION
799.0 NOS
BIRTH
768.9 UNSPECIFIED
768.6 MILD
768.6 MODERATE
768.5 SEVERE
768.5 SEVERE WITH NEUROLOGIC INVOLVEMENT

ASPHYXIA, ASPHYXIATION (continued)
770.8 FETAL AFFECTING NEWBORN
FOOD, MUCUS OR FOREIGN BODY INHALATION
933.1 NOS
934.8 BRONCHIOLES
934.1 BRONCHUS MAIN
933.1 INHALATION FOOD CHOKING, REGURGITATED, LARYNX
934.9 INHALATION LIQUID, LOWER RESPIRATORY TRACT
933.1 INHALATION PHLEGM CHOKING, LARYNX
934.9 INHALATION VOMITUS, LOWER RESPIRATORY TRACT
933.1 LARYNX
934.8 LUNG
932 NASAL PASSAGES
933.0 NASOPHARYNX
770.1 NEWBORN
933.0 PHARYNX
934.9 RESPIRATORY TRACT NOS
934.8 RESPIRATORY TRACT OTHER SPECIFIED PART
0 SUFFOCATION SEE 'SUFFOCATION'
933.0 THROAT NOS
934.0 TRACHEA
770.1 VAGINAL (FETUS OR NEWBORN)

GASES, FUMES, OR VAPORS
987.9 UNSPECIFIED GAS, FUME, OR VAPOR
987.5 BROMOBENZYL CYANIDE
987.0 BUTANE
986 CARBON MONOXIDE
987.6 CHLORINE GAS
987.5 CHLOROACETOPHENONE
987.4 DICHLOROMONOFLUOROMETHANE
987.5 ETHYLIODOACETATE
987.4 FREON
987.7 HYDROCYANIC ACID GAS
987.5 LACRIMOGENIC GAS
987.2 NITROGEN DIOXIDE
987.2 NITROGEN OXIDES
987.2 NITROUS FUMES
987.8 PHOSGENE
987.8 POLYESTER FUMES
987.0 PROPANE
0 SUFFOCATION SEE 'SUFFOCATION'
987.3 SULFUR DIOXIDE
987.0 OTHER HYDROCARBON GAS
987.8 OTHER SPECIFIED GAS, FUME OR VAPOR

A

ASPHYXIA, ASPHYXIATION (continued)

INTRAUTERINE
768.4 LIVE OUTCOME - NOS ONSET
768.2 LIVE OUTCOME - ONSET BEFORE LABOR
768.3 LIVE OUTCOME - ONSET DURING LABOR OR DELIVERY
768.0 WITH FETAL DEATH - BEFORE ONSET OF LABOR
768.1 WITH FETAL DEATH - DURING LABOR

MECHANICAL
994.7 NOS
770.8 DURING BIRTH SEE ALSO 'FETAL DISTRESS'
909.4 LATE EFFECT

ASPIRATION
997.3 ACID PULMONARY (SYNDROME) (DUE TO A PROCEDURE)
668.0# ACID PULMONARY (SYNDROME) OBSTETRICAL
5th Digit: 668.0
0. EPISODE OF CARE NOS OR N/A
1. DELIVERED
2. DELIVERED WITH POSTPARTUM COMPLICATION
3. ANTEPARTUM COMPLICATION
4. POSTPARTUM COMPLICATION

770.1 AMNIOTIC FLUID
507.0 BRONCHITIS
0 FOOD, FOREIGN BODY, OR GASOLINE WITH ASPHYXIATION SEE 'ASPHYXIATION FOOD, MUCUS, OR FOREIGN BODY INHALATION'
770.1 MECONIUM

MUCUS
933.1 NOS
934.9 INTO LOWER RESPIRATORY TRACT NOS
934.8 INTO BRONCHIOLES
934.1 INTO BRONCHUS MAIN
934.8 INTO LUNG
934.0 INTO TRACHEA
934.8 INTO OTHER SPECIFIED PARTS
770.1 NEWBORN
770.1 VAGINAL (FETUS OR NEWBORN)

PNEUMONIA / PNEUMONITIS
507.0 NOS
770.1 FETAL
507.0 FOOD REGURGITATED
506.0 FUMES OR VAPORS (CHEMICAL) (ACUTE)
507.0 GASTRIC SECRETIONS
516.8 LIPOID ENDOGENOUS
507.1 LIPOID EXOGENOUS
770.1 NEWBORN

> ***668.0#:*** *WHEN CODING A MATERNAL ASPIRATION PNEUMONIA/PNEUMONITIS USE AN ADDITIONAL CODE TO SHOW THE TYPE OF ASPIRATION.*

668.0# OBSTETRICAL MATERNAL (MOTHER'S RECORD)
5th Digit: 668.0
0. EPISODE OF CARE NOS OR N/A
1. DELIVERED
2. DELIVERED WITH POSTPARTUM COMPLICATION
3. ANTEPARTUM COMPLICATION
4. POSTPARTUM COMPLICATION

507.1 OILS OR ESSENCES
997.3 POSTOPERATIVE
507.0 VOMITUS
507.8 OTHER SOLIDS OR LIQUIDS

ASPIRATION (continued)
668.0# PULMONARY OBSTETRICAL (FOLLOWING ANESTHESIA OR OTHER SEDATION IN L AND D)
5th Digit: 668.0
0. EPISODE OF CARE NOS OR N/A
1. DELIVERED
2. DELIVERED WITH POSTPARTUM COMPLICATION
3. ANTEPARTUM COMPLICATION
4. POSTPARTUM COMPLICATION

997.3 RESULTING FROM A PROCEDURE
770.1 SYNDROME MASSIVE (OF INFANT DURING BIRTH)
770.1 VERNIX CASEOSA

V46.0 ASPIRATOR DEPENDENCE
307.9 ASTASIA
781.3 ASTASIA ATACTICA (CHOREIC) (PAROSXYSMAL TREPIDENT) (SPASTIC) (TREMBLING) (TREPIDAN)
300.11 ASTASIA HYSTERICAL
706.8 ASTEATOSIS (CUTIS)
379.22 ASTEROID HYALITIS
780.79 ASTHENIA
306.2 ASTHENIA NEUROCIRCULATORY
300.5 ASTHENIA PSYCHOGENIC
301.6 ASTHENIC PERSONALITY DISORDER
368.13 ASTHENOPIA

> *YOUR CHOICE OF A FOURTH OR FIFTH DIGIT MAY SIGNIFICANTLY ALTER THE MEANING OF YOUR DIAGNOSIS. NOTE UNDER ASTHMA THAT THE FOURTH DIGIT CLEARLY DEFINES THE TYPE OF ASTHMA FROM UNSPECIFIED TO CHRONIC OBSTRUCTIVE WITH COPD. THE FIFTH DIGIT INDICATES WITH OR WITHOUT STATUS.*

ASTHMA, ASTHMATIC
493.9# NOS
493.9# ALLERGIC
493.0# ALLERGIC RHINITIS
493.0# ALLERGIC WITH STATED CAUSE
493.0# ATOPIC
493.9# BRONCHOSPASM
493.0# CHILDHOOD
5th Digit: 493.0, 9
0. WITHOUT MENTION OF STATUS ASTHMATICUS
1. WITH STATUS ASTHMATICUS

491.20 CHRONIC BRONCHITIC (OBSTRUCTIVE)
491.21 CHRONIC BRONCHITIC (OBSTRUCTIVE) WITH EXACERBATION
493.2# CHRONIC OBSTRUCTIVE WITH COPD
5th Digit: 493.2
0. WITHOUT MENTION OF STATUS ASTHMATICUS
1. WITH STATUS ASTHMATICUS

507.8 DETERGENT
518.3 EOSINOPHILIA
493.0# EXTRINSIC
5th Digit: 493.0
0. WITHOUT MENTION OF STATUS ASTHMATICUS
1. WITH STATUS ASTHMATICUS

V17.5 FAMILY HISTORY
493.0# HAY
493.1# INFECTIVE
493.1# INTRINSIC
493.1# LATE-ONSET
5th Digit: 493.0, 1
0. WITHOUT MENTION OF STATUS ASTHMATICUS
1. WITH STATUS ASTHMATICUS

500 MINERS'
493.0# NEW ORLEANS (EPIDEMIC)
316 PSYCHOGENIC **[493.9#]**
5th Digit: 493.0, 9
0. WITHOUT MENTION OF STATUS ASTHMATICUS
1. WITH STATUS ASTHMATICUS

V71.8 SCREENING FOR SUSPECTED ASTHMA
495.8 WOOD

ASTIGMATISM

367.20 NOS
367.22 IRREGULAR
367.21 REGULAR

755.67 ASTRAGALOSCAPHOID SYNOSTOSIS
191.9 ASTROBLASTOMA SITE NOS
0 ASTROBLASTOMA SITE SPECIFIED SEE 'CANCER' BY SITE M9430/3

CARCINOMAS AND NEOPLASMS SHOULD BE CODED BY SITE IF POSSIBLE. CODE BY CELL TYPE - "SITE NOS", IF AND ONLY IF A SITE IS NOT SPECIFIED IN THE DIAGNOSIS. OTHERWISE - REFER TO THE APPROPRIATE CATEGORY OF NEOPLASM FOR A MORE SPECIFIC CODE: SEE 'CANCER' 'CANCER METASTATIC', 'NEOPLASM UNCERTAIN BEHAVIOR', 'NEOPLASM UNSPECIFIED NATURE', OR 'BENIGN NEOPLASM'.

ASTROCYTOMA

191.9 SITE NOS
0 SITE SPECIFIED SEE 'CANCER' BY SITE M9400/3
191.9 ANAPLASTIC TYPE SITE NOS
0 ANAPLASTIC TYPE SITE SPECIFIED SEE 'CANCER' BY SITE M9401/3
191.9 FIBRILLARY SITE NOS
0 FIBRILLARY SITE SPECIFIED SEE 'CANCER' BY SITE M9420/3
191.9 GEMISTOCYTIC SITE NOS
0 GEMISTOCYTIC SITE SPECIFIED SEE 'CANCER' BY SITE M9411/3
191.9 PILOCYTIC SITE NOS
0 PILOCYTIC SITE SPECIFIED SEE 'CANCER' BY SITE M9421/3
191.9 PROTOPLASMIC SITE NOS
0 PROTOPLASMIC SITE SPECIFIED SEE 'CANCER' BY SITE M9410/3
237.5 SUBEPENDYMAL GIANT CELL SITE NOS
0 SUBEPENDYMAL GIANT CELL SITE SPECIFIED SEE 'NEOPLASM UNCERTAIN BEHAVIOR' BY SITE M9383/1

ATAXIA, ATAXIC

781.3 NOS
303.## ALCOHOLIC CEREBELLAR [334.4]
4th Digit: 303
0. ACUTE
9. CHRONIC
5th Digit: 303
0. UNSPECIFIED
1. CONTINUOUS
2. EPISODIC
3. IN REMISSION

331.89 BRAIN
334.3 CEREBELLAR
244.# CEREBELLAR HYPOTHYROID [334.4]
4th Digit: 244
0. POSTSURGICAL
1. POSTABLATIVE (IRRADIATION)
2. IODINE INGESTION
3. PAS, PHENYLBUT, RESORCINOL
8. SECONDARY NEC
9. NOS

334.2 CEREBELLAR MARIE'S (SANGER BROWN) (MYOCLONICA)
244.# CEREBELLAR MYXEDEMA [334.4]
4th Digit: 244
0. POSTSURGICAL
1. POSTABLATIVE (IRRADIATION)
2. IODINE INGESTION
3. PAS, PHENYLBUT, RESORCINOL
8. SECONDARY NEC
9. NOS

ATAXIA, ATAXIC (continued)

239.# CEREBELLAR NEOPLASTIC DISEASE [334.4]
4th Digit: 239
0. DIGESTIVE SYSTEM, ANAL
1. RESPIRATORY SYSTEM
2. BONE, SOFT TISSUE, SKIN, (ANAL SKIN MARGIN)
3. BREAST
4. BLADDER
5. OTHER GENITOURINARY
6. BRAIN
7. ENDOCRINE GLANDS AND OTHER PARTS OF NERVOUS SYSTEM
8. OTHER SPECIFIED SITES
9. SITE UNSPECIFIED

334.3 CEREBELLAR OTHER
331.89 CEREBRAL
250.6# DIABETIC LOCOMOTOR (PROGRESSIVE) [337.1]
5th Digit: 250.6
0. TYPE II, ADULT-ONSET, NON-INSULIN DEPENDENT (EVEN IF REQUIRING INSULIN), OR UNSPECIFIED; CONTROLLED
1. TYPE I, JUVENILE-ONSET OR INSULIN-DEPENDENT; CONTROLLED
2. TYPE II, ADULT-ONSET, NON-INSULIN DEPENDENT (EVEN IF REQUIRING INSULIN); UNCONTROLLED
3. TYPE I, JUVENILE-ONSET OR INSULIN-DEPENDENT; UNCONTROLLED

334.0 FRIEDREICH'S
781.2 GAIT
300.11 HYSTERICAL
094.0 LOCOMOTOR (PROGRESSIVE)
334.2 MARIE'S
094.0 PROGRESSIVE LOCOMOTOR
334.2 SANGER-BROWN
334.0 SPINAL HEREDITARY
094.0 SPINAL PROGRESSIVE LOCOMOTOR
334.8 TELANGIECTASIA SYNDROME (LOUIS BAR SYNDROME)

ATELECTASIS

518.0 NOS
770.5 CONGENITAL PARTIAL
770.4 CONGENITAL PRIMARY
770.5 PERINATAL
997.3 POSTOPERATIVE (SYMPTOMATIC)
770.4 PRIMARY PERINATAL
770.5 SECONDARY PERINATAL
011.8# TUBERCULOUS
5th Digit: 011.8
0. NOS
1. LAB NOT DONE
2. LABS PENDING
3. MICROSCOPY POSITIVE (IN SPUTUM)
4. CULTURE POSITIVE - MICROSCOPY NEGATIVE
5. CULTURE NEGATIVE - MICROSCOPY POSITIVE
6. CULTURE AND MICROSCOPY NEGATIVE CONFIRMED BY OTHER METHODS

742.59 ATELOMYELIA CONGENITAL
437.0 ATHEROMA CEREBRAL ARTERIES
706.2 ATHEROMA SKIN

DO NOT USE CODE 996.03, COMPLICATION OF A DEVICE, IMPLANT OR GRAFT MECHANICAL CARDIAC, WHEN THE PHYSICIAN DOCUMENTS THAT ARTERIOSCLEROSIS HAS CAUSED AN OCCLUSION OF A BYPASS GRAFT. IN CODING TERMS, THIS IS CONSIDERED TO BE A NORMAL PROGRESSION OF ARTERIOSCLEROSIS RATHER THAN A COMPLICATION OF A GRAFT. ASSIGN CODE 414.0#, ARTERIOSCLEROSIS BYPASS GRAFT, CORONARY.

440.3# ATHEROSCLEROSIS EXTREMITIES BYPASS GRAFT
5th Digit: 440.3
0. UNSPECIFIED GRAFT
1. AUTOLOGOUS VEIN BYPASS GRAFT
2. NONAUTOLOGOUS BIOLOGICAL BYPASS GRAFT

440.2# ATHEROSCLEROSIS EXTREMITIES PERIPHERAL
5th Digit: 440.2
0. UNSPECIFIED
1. WITH INTERMITTENT CLAUDICATION
2. WITH REST PAIN, OR REST PAIN AND (INTERMITTENT CLAUDICATION)
3. WITH ULCERATION, OR ULCERATION AND (INTERMITTENT CLAUDICATION) (REST PAIN)
4. WITH ISCHEMIC GANGRENE, OR ISCHEMIC GANGRENE AND (INTERMITTENT CLAUDICATION) (REST PAIN) (ULCERATION)
9. OTHER ATHEROSCLEROSIS EXTREMITIES

0 ATHEROSCLEROSIS RENAL ARTERIOLES SEE 'HYPERTENSIVE', RENAL DISEASE
0 ATHEROSCLEROSIS SEE 'ARTERIOSCLEROSIS, ARTERIOSCLEROTIC'
414.0# ATHEROSCLEROTIC HEART DISEASE
5th Digit: 414.0
0. UNSPECIFIED TYPE OF VESSEL, NATIVE OR GRAFT
1. NATIVE CORONARY VESSEL
2. AUTOLOGOUS VEIN BYPASS GRAFT
3. NONAUTOLOGOUS BIOLOGICAL BYPASS GRAFT
4. AUTOLOGOUS ARTERY BYPASS GRAFT (GASTROEPIPLOIC) (INTERNAL MAMMARY)
5. UNSPECIFIED TYPE OF BYPASS GRAFT

110.4 ATHLETE'S FOOT
0 ATHYROIDISM SEE 'HYPOTHYROIDISM'
536.3 ATONIA DYSPEPSIA
666.1# ATONY UTERINE
5th Digit: 666.1
0. EPISODE OF NOS OR N/A
2. DELIVERED WITH POSTPARTUM COMPLICATION
4. POSTPARTUM COMPLICATION

691.8 ATOPIC DERMATITIS
0 ATRESIA SEE ANATOMICAL SITE
759.89 ATRESIA NEC (CONGENITAL)

ATRIAL
427.31 FIBRILLATION (PAROXYSMAL)
427.32 FLUTTER
0 INFARCTION SEE 'MYOCARDIAL INFARCTION ACUTE'
427.61 PREMATURE BEATS CONTRACTIONS OR SYSTOLES
429.71 SEPTAL DEFECT ACQUIRED FOLLOWING MYOCARDIAL INFARCTION (>8 WEEKS) [414.8]

ATRIAL (continued)
429.71 SEPTAL DEFECT ACQUIRED POST MI ACUTE (< 8 WEEKS) [410.##]
4th Digit: 410
0. ANTEROLATERAL
1. ANTERIOR (WALL) ANTEROAPICAL ANTEROSEPTAL OTHER ANTERIOR
2. INFEROLATERAL
3. INFEROPOSTERIOR
4. INFERIOR OTHER
5. LATERAL APICAL, BASOLATERAL, POSTEROLATERAL, LATERAL OTHER
6. POSTERIOR (POSTEROBASAL)
7. SUBENDOCARDIAL
8. ATRIUM PAPILLARY OR SEPTUM ALONE
9. UNSPECIFIED

5th Digit: 410
0. EPISODE UNSPECIFIED
1. INITIAL EPISODE
2. SUBSEQUENT EPISODE

745.5 SEPTAL DEFECT OSTIUM SECUNDUM TYPE CONGENITAL
745.8 SEPTAL DEFECT OSTIUM SECUNDUM TYPE CONGENITAL SINUS VENOSUS
745.69 SEPTUM ABSENCE CONGENITAL
745.7 VENTRICULAR SEPTAL ABSENCE

757.4 ATRICHOSIS CONGENITAL
0 ATRIOVENTRICULAR BLOCK SEE 'HEART BLOCK'
745.69 ATRIOVENTRICULAR CANAL DEFECT CONGENITAL
745.69 ATRIUM COMMON CONGENITAL
745.5 ATRIUM SECUNDUM DEFECT CONGENITAL
709.09 ATROPHIA ALBA
701.8 ATROPHIA CUTIS SENILIS

ATROPHODERMA
701.9 ATROPHODERMA
701.3 MACULATUM
701.8 NEURITICUM

ATROPHY
701.3 BLANCHE (OF MILIAN)
733.7 BONE (DISUSE)
372.8 CONJUNCTIVA (SENILE)
728.2 MUSCULAR (DISUSE)
797 OLD AGE
376.45 ORBIT
359.1 PSEUDOHYPERTROPHIC
527.0 SALIVARY GLAND

313.89 ATTACHMENT DISORDER REACTIVE (INFANCY OR CHILDHOOD)

ATTENTION DEFICIT DISORDER - (ADULT) (CHILD)
314.00 NOS
314.00 INATTENTIVE
314.01 WITH HYPERACTIVITY / IMPULSIVENESS
314.8 WITH OTHER SPECIFIED MANIFESTATIONS

382.2 ATTICOANTRAL DISEASE CHRONIC (WITH POSTERIOR/SUPERIOR MARGINAL PERFORATION OF EAR DRUM)
786.59 ATYPICAL CHEST PAIN
413.1 ATYPICAL CHEST PAIN - CARDIAC ANGINA
626.9 AUB (ABNORMAL UTERINE BLEEDING)

A

AUDITORY

433.8# ARTERY, INTERNAL OCCLUSION

5th Digit: 433.8

0. WITHOUT CEREBRAL INFARCTION

1. WITH CEREBRAL INFARCTION

744.01 CANAL ABSENCE (CONGENITAL)
744.02 CANAL ATRESIA (CONGENITAL)
380.9 CANAL DISORDER
959.09 CANAL INJURY (EXTERNAL) (MEATUS)
388.43 DISCRIMINATION IMPAIRMENT
794.15 FUNCTION STUDIES ABNORMAL
388.5 NERVE ATROPHY
388.5 NERVE DISORDER
951.5 NERVE INJURY
388.40 PERCEPTION ABNORMAL
388.44 RECRUITMENT ABNORMALITY
V53.09 SUBSTITUTION DEVICE FITTING AND ADJUSTMENT

757.39 AUDRY'S SYNDROME (ACROPACHYDERMA)
078.89 AUJESZKY'S DISEASE

AURICLE EAR

744.01 ABSENCE CONGENITAL
744.1 ACCESSORY CONGENITAL
380.89 CALCIFICATION
380.30 DISORDER
744.49 FISTULA CONGENITAL
959.09 INJURY
744.29 PROMINENCE CONGENITAL
0 SEE ALSO 'EAR', EXTERNAL

429.71 AURICULAR SEPTAL DEFECT
745.5 AURICULAR SEPTAL DEFECT CONGENITAL
350.8 AURICULOTEMPORAL NERVE DISORDER
350.8 AURICULOTEMPORAL SYNDROME
062.4 AUSTRALIAN ARBOENCEPHALITIS
062.4 AUSTRALIAN ENCEPHALITIS
062.4 AUSTRALIAN X DISEASE

AUTISM

299.00 INFANTILE (CHILDHOOD) ACTIVE STATE
299.01 INFANTILE (CHILDHOOD) RESIDUAL STATE

AUTOIMMUNE DISEASE

279.4 NOS
283.0 HEMOLYTIC (COLD/WARM TYPE)
252.1 PARATHYROID
245.2 THYROID

337.3 AUTONOMIC DYSREFLEXIA
337.3 AUTONOMIC DYSREFLEXIA WITH DECUBITUS ULCER [707.0]
337.3 AUTONOMIC DYSREFLEXIA WITH FECAL IMPACTION [560.39]

URINARY TRACT INFECTION: USE ADDITIONAL CODE FOR ORGANISM. SEE 'BACTERIAL INFECTION'.

337.3 AUTONOMIC DYSREFLEXIA WITH URINARY TRACT INFECTION [599.0]
337.9 AUTONOMIC NERVOUS SYSTEM DISORDER

AUTOSOME, AUTOSOMAL

758.5 ACCESSORY CONGENITAL
758.0 ACCESSORY - 21 OR 22
758.1 ACCESSORY - D1
758.2 ACCESSORY - E3
758.0 ACCESSORY - G
758.81 ACCESSORY - SEX
758.5 ANOMALIES OTHER CONDITIONS
758.3 DELETION SYNDROMES
758.4 TRANSLOCATION BALANCED IN NORMAL INDIVIDUAL

A-V (ARTERIOVENOUS) FISTULA

447.0 ACQUIRED

648.9#: USE AN ADDITIONAL CODE TO IDENTIFY THE AV FISTULA.

648.9# ACQUIRED MATERNAL CURRENT (CO-EXISTENT) IN PREGNANCY

5th Digit: 648.9

0. EPISODE OF NOS OR N/A

1. DELIVERED

2. DELIVERED WITH POSTPARTUM COMPLICATION

3. ANTEPARTUM COMPLICATION

4. POSTPARTUM COMPLICATION

900.01 CAROTID ARTERY COMMON TRAUMATIC
900.00 CAROTID ARTERY TRAUMATIC
908.3 CAROTID ARTERY TRAUMATIC LATE EFFECT
996.62 COMPLICATION (SHUNT) (SURGICALLY CREATED) - INFECTION OR INFLAMMATION
996.1 COMPLICATION (SHUNT) (SURGICALLY CREATED) - MECHANICAL
996.74 COMPLICATION (SHUNT) (SURGICALLY CREATED) - OTHER
414.19 HEART ACQUIRED
417.0 PULMONARY VESSELS
747.3 PULMONARY VESSELS CONGENITAL
996.62 SHUNT INFECTION OR INFLAMMATION

A-V (ARTERIOVENOUS) MALFORMATION

437.3 BRAIN ACQUIRED
747.81 BRAIN CONGENITAL
430 BRAIN RUPTURED, SUBARACHNOID
094.87 BRAIN RUPTURED, SYPHILITIC
747.81 CEREBROVASCULAR SYSTEM CONGENITAL
746.85 CORONARY ARTERY CONGENITAL
747.6# PERIPHERAL VASCULAR SYSTEM CONGENITAL (ABERRANT) (ABSENCE) (AGENESIS) (ACCESSORY) (ANEURYSM) (DEFORMITY) (HYPOPLASIA) (MALPOSITION)

5th Digit: 747.6

0. PERIPHERAL VASCULAR UNSPECIFIED SITE

1. GASTROINTESTINAL VESSEL

2. RENAL VESSEL

3. UPPER LIMB VESSEL

4. LOWER LIMB VESSEL

9. OTHER SPECIFIED SITE PERIPHERAL VASCULAR

747.3 PULMONARY
743.58 RETINA
747.82 SPINAL VESSEL CONGENITAL
747.89 OTHER SPECIFIED

0 AV BLOCK SEE 'HEART BLOCK'
426.89 AV DISSOCIATION
426.89 AV TACHYCARDIA NONPAROXYSMAL

AVASCULAR NECROSIS

733.40 BONE SITE UNSPECIFIED
733.42 FEMUR (HEAD AND NECK OF)
733.49 HAND
733.42 HIP
733.41 HUMERUS (HEAD OF)
733.43 MEDIAL FEMORAL CONDYLE
733.44 TALUS
733.49 OTHER BONE

344.89 AVELLIS' SYNDROME
993.2 AVIATOR'S DISEASE
268.9 AVITAMINOSIS D
301.82 AVOIDANT PERSONALITY

871.3 AVULSION EYE
871.3 AVULSION GLOBE
0 AVULSION INTERNAL ORGAN OR SITE SEE SPECIFIC ORGAN OR SITE, INJURY
0 AVULSION JOINT CAPSULE, LIGAMENT OR TENDON SEE 'SPRAIN', BY SITE
0 AVULSION OTHER SEE 'OPEN WOUND', BY SITE

A

780.02 AWARENESS TRANSIENT
502 AX GRINDER'S DISEASE
743.44 AXENFELD'S ANOMALY (SYNDROME)

AXILLA
959.2 INJURY
912.8 INJURY OTHER AND UNSPECIFIED SUPERFICIAL
912.9 INJURY OTHER AND UNSPECIFIED SUPERFICIAL INFECTED

AXILLARY
444.21 ARTERY (EMBOLISM) (THROMBOSIS) (OCCLUSION) (INFARCTION)
442.0 ARTERY ANEURYSM (RUPTURED) (CIRSOID) (VARIX) (FALSE)
440.2# ARTERY ARTERIOSCLEROSIS (DEGENERATION) (DEFORMANS) (ARTERITIS)

5th Digit: 440.2

0. UNSPECIFIED
1. WITH INTERMITTENT CLAUDICATION
2. WITH REST PAIN, OR REST PAIN AND (INTERMITTENT CLAUDICATION)
3. WITH ULCERATION, OR ULCERATION AND (INTERMITTENT CLAUDICATION) (REST PAIN)
4. WITH ISCHEMIC GANGRENE, OR ISCHEMIC GANGRENE AND (INTERMITTENT CLAUDICATION) (REST PAIN) (ULCERATION)
9. OTHER ATHEROSCLEROSIS EXTREMITIES

440.3# ARTERY BYPASS GRAFT ARTERIOSCLEROSIS (EXTREMITIES)

5th Digit: 440.3

0. UNSPECIFIED GRAFT
1. AUTOLOGOUS VEIN BYPASS GRAFT
2. NONAUTOLOGOUS BIOLOGICAL BYPASS GRAFT

903.01 ARTERY INJURY
908.3 ARTERY INJURY LATE EFFECT
903.01 ARTERY LACERATION (RUPTURE) (HEMATOMA) (AVULSION) (ANEURYSM) TRAUMATIC
908.3 ARTERY LACERATION LATE EFFECT

AXILLARY (continued)
353.0 NERVE DISORDER
955.0 NERVE INJURY
353.0 NERVE NEURITIS
903.02 VEIN INJURY
908.3 VEIN INJURY LATE EFFECT
903.02 VEIN LACERATION (RUPTURE) (HEMATOMA) (AVULSION) (ANEURYSM) TRAUMATIC
908.3 VEIN LACERATION LATE EFFECT
451.89 VEIN PHLEBITIS
903.00 VESSEL INJURY NOS
908.3 VESSEL INJURY LATE EFFECT
903.00 VESSEL LACERATION (RUPTURE) (HEMATOMA) (AVULSION) (ANEURYSM) UNSPECIFIED
908.3 VESSEL LACERATION LATE EFFECT

756.89 AYALA'S DISEASE
416.0 AYERZA'S DISEASE OR SYNDROME (PULMONARY ARTERY SCLEROSIS WITH PULMONARY HYPERTENSION)
606.0 AZOOSPERMIA
790.6 AZOTEMIA
788.9 AZOTEMIA PRERENAL
588.0 AZOTEMIC OSTEODYSTROPHY

AZYGOS
748.69 LOBE FISSURE CONGENITAL (OF LUNG)
901.89 VEIN INJURY
908.4 VEIN INJURY LATE EFFECT
901.89 VEIN LACERATION (RUPTURE) (HEMATOMA) (AVULSION) (ANEURYSM) TRAUMATIC
908.4 VEIN LACERATION LATE EFFECT

V09.1 B-LACTAM ANTIBIOTICS RESISTANT INFECTION (SEE 'DRUG RESISTANCE' FOR COMPLETE LISTING)
695.1 BAADER'S SYNDROME (ERYTHEMA MULTIFORME EXUDATIVUM)
721.5 BAASTRUP'S SYNDROME
088.82 BABESIASIS
088.82 BABESIOSIS
448.0 BABINGTON'S DISEASE

BABINSKI
253.8 FROHLICH SYNDROME (ADIPOSOGENITAL DYSTROPHY)
344.89 NAGEOTTE SYNDROME
093.89 VAQUEZ SYNDROME (CARDIOVASCULAR SYPHILIS)

0 BABY SEE 'INFANT'
791.9 BACILLURIA
005.89 BACILLUS CEREUS FOOD POISONING
041.82 BACILLUS FRAGILIS

BACK
307.89 ACHE PSYCHOGENIC
724.6 ACHE SACROILIAC
724.5 ACHE VERTEBROGENIC (POSTURAL)
724.9 DISORDER OTHER AND UNSPECIFIED
306.0 DISORDER PSYCHOGENIC (MUSCULOSKELETAL)
959.1 INJURY
911.8 INJURY SUPERFICIAL OTHER AND UNSPECIFIED
911.9 INJURY SUPERFICIAL OTHER AND UNSPECIFIED (INFECTED)
736.5 KNEE (GENU RECURVATUM)
724.2 PAIN LOW BACK
724.5 PAIN POSTURAL
307.89 PAIN PSYCHOGENIC
847.9 SEPARATION (RUPTURE) (TEAR) (LACERATION) UNSPECIFIED
724.8 STIFF
847.9 STRAIN (SPRAIN) (AVULSION) (HEMARTHROSIS) UNSPECIFIED
846.9 STRAIN (SPRAIN) LOW
724.8 OTHER SYMPTOMS REFERABLE TO BACK

307.89 BACKACHE PSYCHOGENIC
724.6 BACKACHE SACROILIAC
724.5 BACKACHE VERTEBROGENIC (POSTURAL)
362.10 BACKGROUND RETINOPATHY

BACTEREMIA: USE ADDITIONAL CODE FOR ORGANISM. SEE 'BACTERIAL INFECTION'.

BACTEREMIA
790.7 NOS
647.8# MATERNAL CURRENT (CO-EXISTENT) IN PREGNANCY
5th Digit: 647.8
0. EPISODE OF CARE NOS OR N/A
1. DELIVERED
2. DELIVERED WITH POSTPARTUM COMPLICATION
3. ANTEPARTUM COMPLICATION
4. POSTPARTUM COMPLICATION

659.3# MATERNAL DURING LABOR
5th Digit: 659.3
0. EPISODE OF CARE NOS OR N/A
1. DELIVERED
3. ANTEPARTUM COMPLICATION

031.2 MYCOBACTERIUM AVIUM-INTRACELLULARE COMPLEX (MAC)
0 WITH SEPSIS SEE 'SEPSIS', BY ORGANISM

BACTERIAL
040.89 DISEASE OTHER SPECIFIED
027.9 DISEASE ZOONOTIC
027.8 DISEASE ZOONOTIC OTHER SPECIFIED
008.5 GASTROENTERITIS
041.9 INFECTION
320.9 MENINGITIS

CODES FROM THIS CATEGORY ARE TO BE USED AS ADDITIONAL CODES TO IDENTIFY BACTERIAL AGENTS IN DISEASES THAT ARE CLASSIFIED ELSEWHERE.

BACTERIAL INFECTION
041.9 NOS
041.85 AEROBACTER AEROGENES
041.82 BACILLUS FRAGILIS
041.84 BACTEROIDES (FRAGILIS)
041.83 CLOSTRIDIUM PERFRINGENS
041.4 E. COLI
041.81 EATON'S AGENT
041.04 ENTEROCOCCUS
041.3 FRIEDLANDER'S BACILLUS,
041.84 GRAM-NEGATIVE ANAEROBES
041.85 GRAM-NEGATIVE BACTERIA NOS
041.5 H. INFLUENZAE
041.86 H. PYLORI (HELICOBACTER PYLORI)
041.3 KLEBSIELLA
041.85 MIMA POLYMORPHA
041.81 MYCOPLASMA
041.81 PLEUROPNEUMONIA LIKE ORGANISMS
041.2 PNEUMOCOCCUS
041.6 PROTEUS (MIRABILIS) (MORGANII)
041.7 PSEUDOMONAS
041.85 SERRATIA
041.10 STAPHYLOCOCCUS UNSPECIFIED
041.11 STAPHYLOCOCCUS AUREUS
041.19 STAPHYLOCOCCUS OTHER
041.00 STREPTOCOCCUS
041.01 STREPTOCOCCUS GROUP A
041.02 STREPTOCOCCUS GROUP B
041.03 STREPTOCOCCUS GROUP C
041.04 STREPTOCOCCUS GROUP D (ENTEROCOCCUS)
041.05 STREPTOCOCCUS GROUP G
041.09 STREPTOCOCCUS OTHER
041.84 OTHER ANAEROBES
041.89 OTHER SPECIFIED BACTERIA

686.8 BACTERID, BACTERIDE (ANDREWS' PUSTULAR)

BACTERIURIA: USE ADDITIONAL CODE FOR ORGANISM. SEE 'BACTERIAL INFECTION'.

BACTERIURIA
791.9 BACTERIURIA
599.0 BACTERIURIA WITH UTI
760.1 AFFECTING FETUS OR NEWBORN
791.9 ASYMPTOMATIC
V81.5 ASYMPTOMATIC (SCREENING FOR)
646.5# ASYMPTOMATIC COMPLICATING PREGNANCY [791.9]
5th Digit: 646.5
0. EPISODE OF CARE NOS OR N/A
1. DELIVERED
2. DELIVERED WITH POSTPARTUM COMPLICATION
3. ANTEPARTUM COMPLICATION
4. POSTPARTUM COMPLICATION

B

041.84 BACTEROIDES INFECTION (ORGANISM)
008.46 BACTEROIDES (FRAGILIS) INTESTINAL INFECTION
446.6 BAEHR-SCHIFFRIN DISEASE (THROMBOTIC THROMBOCYTOPENIC PURPURA)

528.5 BAELZ'S DISEASE
110.3 BAERENSPRUNG'S DISEASE (ECZEMA MARGINATUM)

495.1 BAGASSOSIS
085.1 BAGHDAD BOIL
446.5 BAGRATUNI'S SYNDROME (TEMPORAL ARTERITIS)

727.51 BAKER'S CYST (KNEE)
692.89 BAKER'S ITCH
756.89 BAKWIN KRIDA SYNDROME

BALANITIS
607.1 NOS
006.8 AMEBIC
112.2 CANDIDAL
099.53 CHLAMYDIAL
099.0 DUCREY'S BACILLUS
607.1 GANGRENOUS
098.0 GONOCOCCAL (ACUTE)
098.2 GONOCOCCAL (CHRONIC)
607.1 NONGONOCOCCAL
607.1 PHAGEDENIC
099.8 VENEREAL NEC
607.81 XEROTICA OBLITERANS

607.1 BALANOPOSTHITIS
099.53 BALANOPOSTHITIS CHLAMYDIAL
007.0 BALANTIDIASIS
007.0 BALANTIDIASIS INTESTINAL
007.0 BALANTIDIUM COLI INTESTINAL INFECTION
307.0 BALBUTIES BALBUTIO
704.00 BALDNESS
205.3# BALFOURS DISEASE (CHLOROMA)

5th Digit: 205.3
0. WITHOUT MENTION OF REMISSION
1. IN REMISSION

368.16 BALINT'S SYNDROME (PSYCHIC PARALYSIS OF VISUAL DISORIENTATION)
083.0 BALKAN GRIPPE
766.2 BALLANTYNE (-RUNGE) SYNDROME (POSTMATURITY)

V72.85 BALLISTOCARDIOGRAM
794.39 BALLISTOCARDIOGRAM ABNORMAL
V72.81 BALLISTOCARDIOGRAM PREOPERATIVE

993.2 BALLOON DISEASE
424.0 BALLOONING POSTERIOR LEAFLET SYNDROME
341.1 BALO'S CONCENTRIC SCLEROSIS
731.2 BAMBERGER MARIE DISEASE
661.4# BANDL'S RING COMPLICATING DELIVERY

5th Digit: 661.4
0. EPISODE OF CARE NOS OR N/A
1. DELIVERED
3. ANTEPARTUM COMPLICATION

023.1 BANGS DISEASE
995.1 BANNISTERS DISEASE
909.9 BANNISTERS LATE EFFECT
275.49 BANTAM ALBRIGHT MARTIN DISEASE (PSEUDOHYPOPARATHYROIDISM)
0 BANTI'S DISEASE OR SYNDROME SEE 'CIRRHOSIS'

780.9 BARAGNOSIS
266.2 BARASHEH
305.4# BARBITURATE ABUSE (NONDEPENDENT)
304.1# BARBITURATE ADDICTION (DEPENDENT)

5th Digit: 304.1, 305.4
0. NOS
1. CONTINUOUS
2. EPISODIC
3. IN REMISSION

707.9 BARCOO DISEASE (SEE ALSO 'ULCER, ULCERATION SKIN')
157.0 BARD-PIC SYNDROME (CARCINOMA HEAD OF PANCREAS)
157.0 BARD PIC CANCER
759.89 BARDET-BIEDL (OBESITY, POLYDACTYLY AND MENTAL RETARDATION)
503 BARITOSIS
503 BARIUM LUNG DISEASE
267 BARLOW (-MOLLER) SYNDROME (INFANTILE SCURVY)
424.0 BARLOW'S SYNDROME (MITRAL VALVE PROLAPSE)
993.2 BARODONTALGIA
909.4 BARODONTALGIA LATE EFFECT
985.0 BAROMETER MAKER'S DISEASE
301.51 BARON MUNCHAUSEN SYNDROME

BAROTRAUMA
909.4 LATE EFFECT
993.2 ODONTALGIA
993.0 OTITIC
993.1 SINUS

272.6 BARRAQUER SIMONS DISEASE (PROGRESSIVE LIPOSYSTROPHY)
357.0 BARRE-GUILLAIN SYNDROME
723.2 BARRE LIEOU SYNDROME
738.3 BARREL CHEST
530.2 BARRETTS SYNDROME (CHRONIC PEPTIC ULCER OF ESOPHAGUS)
530.5 BARSONY POLGAR SYNDROME (CORKSCREW ESOPHAGUS)
530.5 BARSONY TESCHENDORF SYNDROME (CORKSCREW ESOPHAGUS)

BARTHOLIN
616.3 ABSCESS MARSUPIALIZATION (NONOBSTETRICAL)
616.3 GLAND ABSCESS (NONOBSTETRICAL)
616.2 GLAND CYST (NONOBSTETRICAL)

BARTHOLINITIS
098.0 GONOCOCCAL ACUTE
098.2 GONOCOCCAL CHRONIC
616.8 SUPPURATING

088.0 BARTONELLOSIS
255.1 BARTTER'S SYNDROME (SECONDARY HYPERALDOSTERONISM WITH JUXTAGLOMERULAR HYPERPLASIA)

173.# BASAL CELL CARCINOMA M8090/3
173.# BASAL CELL CARCINOMA FIBROEPITHELIAL TYPE M8093/3

4th Digit: 173
0. SKIN OF LIP
1. EYELID INCLUDING CANTHUS
2. SKIN OF EAR AURICULAR CANAL (EXTERNAL) EXTERNAL MEATUS PINNA
3. SKIN OF UNSPECIFIED PARTS OF FACE CHEEK (EXTERNAL) CHIN EYEBROW FOREHEAD NOSE (EXT)
4. SCALP AND SKIN OF NECK
5. ALL SKIN TRUNK AXILLARY FOLD PERIANAL ABDOMINAL WALL ANUS BACK BREAST (OR MASTECTOMY SITE) BUTTOCK
6. ALL SKIN UPPER LIMB SHOULDER ARM FINGER FOREARM HAND
7. ALL SKIN LOWER LIMB HIP ANKLE FOOT HEEL KNEE LEG THIGH TOE POPLITEAL AREA
8. OTHER SPECIFIED SKIN SITES CONTIGUOUS OVERLAPPING SITES UNDETERMINED POINT OF ORIGIN
9. SITE NOS

THE CODING OF CANCERS IS COMPLEX AND CODING BY CELL TYPE IS USED ONLY IF THE SITE IS NOT SPECIFIED.

173.# BASAL CELL CARCINOMA MORPHEA TYPE M8092/3
173.# BASAL CELL CARCINOMA MULTICENTRIC M8091/3
4th Digit: 173
0. SKIN OF LIP
1. EYELID INCLUDING CANTHUS
2. SKIN OF EAR AURICULAR CANAL (EXTERNAL) EXTERNAL MEATUS PINNA
3. SKIN OF UNSPECIFIED PARTS OF FACE CHEEK (EXTERNAL) CHIN EYEBROW FOREHEAD NOSE (EXT)
4. SCALP AND SKIN OF NECK
5. ALL SKIN TRUNK AXILLARY FOLD PERIANAL ABDOMINAL WALL ANUS BACK BREAST (OR MASTECTOMY SITE) BUTTOCK
6. ALL SKIN UPPER LIMB SHOULDER ARM FINGER FOREARM HAND
7. ALL SKIN LOWER LIMB HIP ANKLE FOOT HEEL KNEE LEG THIGH TOE POPLITEAL AREA
8. OTHER SPECIFIED SKIN SITES CONTIGUOUS OVERLAPPING SITES UNDETERMINED POINT OF ORIGIN
9. SITE NOS

238.2 BASAL CELL TUMOR SITE NOS
0 BASAL CELL TUMOR SITE SPECIFIED SEE 'NEOPLASM UNCERTAIN BEHAVIOR' BY SITE M8090/1

333.90 BASAL GANGLION DISEASE
333.0 BASAL GANGLION DISEASE DEGENERATIVE
333.89 BASAL GANGLION DISEASE SPECIFIED NEC

794.7 BASAL METABOLIC RATE ABNORMAL
V72.6 BASAL METABOLIC RATE TESTING

199.1 BASALOID CARCINOMA SITE NOS
0 BASALOID CARCINOMA SITE SPECIFIED SEE 'CANCER' BY SITE M8123/3

757.31 BASAN'S DYSPLASIA
842.13 BASEBALL FINGER

242.00 BASEDOW'S DISEASE OR SYNDROME (EXOPHTHALMIC GOITER)
242.01 BASEDOW'S DISEASE WITH THYROTOXIC CRISIS OR STORM
583.89 BASEMENT MEMBRANE DISEASE NEC
446.21 BASEMENT MEMBRANE DISEASE NEC WITH PULMONARY HEMORRHAGE [583.81]

117.7 BASIDIOBOLUS INFECTION

BASILAR ARTERY
433.0# ARTERIOSCLEROSIS (DEGENERATION) (DEFORMANS) (ARTERITIS)
433.0# EMBOLISM THROMBOSIS OR OBSTRUCTION
5th Digit: 433.0
0. WITHOUT CEREBRAL INFARCTION
1. WITH CEREBRAL INFARCTION

431 HEMORRHAGE (RUPTURE)
433.0# OCCLUSION (THROMBOSIS) (OBSTRUCTION) (EMBOLISM) (NARROWING) (STENOSIS)
433.3# OCCLUSION BILATERAL OR WITH CAROTID AND/OR VERTEBRAL
5th Digit: 433.0, 3
0. WITHOUT CEREBRAL INFARCTION
1. WITH CEREBRAL INFARCTION

435.0 SYNDROME (INSUFFICIENCY)

903.1 BASILIC VEIN INJURY
451.82 BASILIC VEIN PHLEBITIS

377.04 BASOFRONTAL SYNDROME
288.0 BASOPENIA
194.3 BASOPHIL CARCINOMA SITE NOS
0 BASOPHIL CARCINOMA SITE SPECIFIED SEE 'CANCER' BY SITE M8300/3

288.8 BASOPHILIA
255.0 BASOPHILISM (CUSHING SYNDROME)
173.# BASOSQUAMOUS CARCINOMA (MULTICENTRIC) M8094/3
4th Digit: 173
0. SKIN OF LIP
1. EYELID INCLUDING CANTHUS
2. SKIN OF EAR AURICULAR CANAL (EXTERNAL) EXTERNAL MEATUS PINNA
3. SKIN OF UNSPECIFIED PARTS OF FACE CHEEK (EXTERNAL) CHIN EYEBROW FOREHEAD NOSE (EXT)
4. SCALP AND SKIN OF NECK
5. ALL SKIN TRUNK AXILLARY PERIANAL ABDOMINAL WALL ANUS BACK BREAST (OR MASTECTOMY SITE) BUTTOCK
6. ALL SKIN UPPER LIMB SHOULDER ARM FINGER FOREARM HAND
7. ALL SKIN LOWER LIMB HIP ANKLE FOOT HEEL KNEE LEG THIGH TOE POPLITEAL AREA
8. OTHER SPECIFIED SKIN SITES CONTIGUOUS OVERLAPPING SITES UNDETERMINED POINT OF ORIGIN
9. SITE NOS

272.5 BASSEN KORNZWEIG RETINAL DYSTROPHY [362.72]
272.5 BASSEN KORNZWEIG SYNDROME (ABETALIPOPROTEINEMIA)

744.29 BAT EAR CONGENITAL

078.0 BATEMAN'S DISEASE
287.2 BATEMAN'S PURPURA

994.1 BATHING CRAMP
909.4 BATHING CRAMP LATE EFFECT
300.23 BATHOPHOBIA

330.1 BATTEN DISEASE (CEREBRAL LIPIDOSES WITH CEREBRORETINAL DYSTROPHY)[362.71]

359.2 BATTEN-STEINERT DISEASE OR SYNDROME

WHEN THE CAUSE OF AN INJURY IS STATED TO BE ABUSE, MULTIPLE CODES SHOULD BE ASSIGNED, IF APPLICABLE, TO IDENTIFY ANY ASSOCIATED INJURIES. THEY ARE TO BE SEQUENCED IN THE FOLLOWING ORDER:

1. TYPE OF ABUSE - CHILD OR ADULT (995.5, 995.8)

2. TYPE OF INJURY

3. PERPETRATOR OF THE ABUSE - SEE E-CODE DIRECTORY 'ASSAULT' (E967)

4. NATURE OF THE ABUSE - SEE E-CODE DIRECTORY 'ASSAULT' (E904.0, E960-E966, E968)

995.81 BATTERED ADULT (SPOUSE) SYNDROME
995.54 BATTERED CHILD (BABY) SYNDROME
V15.41 BATTERED HISTORY
995.81 BATTERED WIFE (SPOUSE) (WOMAN)

031.0 BATTEY DISEASE
571.5 BAUMGARTEN-CRUVEILHIER DISEASE OR SYNDROME (CIRRHOSIS OF LIVER)
571.5 BAUMGARTEN-CRUVEILHIER DISEASE (CIRRHOSIS OF LIVER) WITH ESOPHAGEAL VARICES [**456.2#**]
5th Digit: 456.2
0. WITH BLEEDING
1. WITHOUT BLEEDING

503 BAUXITE-WORKERS DISEASE
094.1 BAYLE'S DISEASE (DEMENTIA PARALYTICA)

B

B

017.1# BAZIN'S DISEASE (PRIMARY) (SEE ALSO 'TUBERCULOSIS')

5th Digit: 017.1

0. NOS
1. LAB NOT DONE
2. LAB UNKNOWN AT PRESENT
3. MICROSCOPY POSITIVE - (IN SPUTUM)
4. CULTURE POSITIVE - MICROSCOPY NEGATIVE
5. CULTURE NEGATIVE - MICROSCOPY POSITIVE
6. CULTURE AND MICROSCOPY NEGATIVE - CONFIRMED BY OTHER METHODS

0 BBB (BUNDLE BRANCH BLOCK) SEE 'BUNDLE BRANCH BLOCK'
757.4 BEADED HAIR CONGENITAL
300.5 BEARD'S DISEASE (NEURASTHENIA)
571.49 BEARN-KUNKEL (-SLATER) SYNDROME (LUPOID HEPATITIS)
727.2 BEAT ELBOW (OCCUPATIONAL)
727.2 BEAT HAND (OCCUPATIONAL)
727.2 BEAT KNEE (OCCUPATIONAL)
429.1 BEAU'S MYOCARDIAL DEGENERATION
429.1 BEAU'S SYNDROME
720.0 BECHTEREW-STRUMPELL-MARIE SYNDROME (ANKYLOSING SPONDYLITIS)
720.0 BECHTEREW'S ANKYLOSING SPONDYLITIS
425.2 BECKER'S DISEASE

433.8# BECK'S SYNDROME (ANTERIOR SPINAL ARTERY OCCLUSION)

5th Digit: 433.8

0. WITHOUT CEREBRAL INFARCTION
1. WITH CEREBRAL INFARCTION

759.89 BECKWITH (-WIEDEMANN) SYNDROME
079.98 BEDSONIA
079.88 BEDSONIA SPECIFIED NEC
707.0 BED SORE
707.0 BED SORE WITH GANGRENE [785.4]
788.36 BEDWETTING
989.5 BEE STING
995.0 BEE STING WITH ANAPHYLAXIS [989.5]

242.0# BEGBIE'S EXOPHTHALMIC GOITER

5th Digit: 242.0

0. WITHOUT MENTION OF THYROTOXIC CRISIS OR STORM
1. WITH MENTION OF THYROTOXIC CRISIS OR STORM

V40.9 BEHAVIORAL PROBLEM
V40.3 BEHAVIORAL PROBLEM OTHER SPECIFIED
136.1 BEHCET'S DISEASE WITH VULVA ULCER [616.51]
136.1 BEHCET'S SYNDROME
0 BEHCET'S SYNDROME ARTHRITIS SEE 'ARTHRITIS OTHER SPECIFIED', BEHCET'S SYNDROME
362.50 BEHR'S DISEASE
111.2 BEIGEL'S WHITE PIEDRA
104.0 BEJEL
720.0 BEKHTEREV'S ANKYLOSING SPONDYLITIS
720.0 BEKHTEREV-STRUMPELL-MARIE SYNDROME (ANKYLOSING SPONDYLITIS)
0 BELCHING SEE 'ERUCTATION'

296.0# BELL'S AFFECTIVE PSYCHOSIS

5th Digit: 296.0

1. MILD
2. MODERATE
3. SEVERE WITHOUT MENTION OF PSYCHOTIC BEHAVIOR
4. SEVERE SPECIFIED AS WITH PSYCHOTIC BEHAVIOR
5. IN PARTIAL OR NOS REMISSION
6. IN FULL REMISSION

351.0 BELL'S PALSY

791.0 BENCE JONES PROTEINURIA ABNORMAL
993.3 BENDS
909.4 BENDS LATE EFFECT
344.89 BENEDIKT'S SYNDROME (PARALYSIS)
348.2 BENIGN INTRACRANIAL HYPERTENSION
0 BENIGN LESION SEE 'BENIGN NEOPLASM'

BENIGN NEOPLASM

215.5 ABDOMEN CONNECTIVE TISSUE
210.7 ADENOID TISSUE
227.0 ADRENAL GLAND
211.9 ALIMENTARY TRACT
211.5 AMPULLA OF VATER
211.4 ANAL CANAL OR SPHINCTER
216.5 ANUS (MARGIN) (SKIN) (PERIANAL)
211.4 ANUS
211.3 APPENDIX
212.1 ARYTENOID CARTILAGE
210.8 ARYTENOID FOLD
215.7 BACK CONNECTIVE TISSUE
221.2 BARTHOLIN'S GLAND
223.3 BLADDER

215.# BLOOD VESSEL

4th Digit: 215

0. HEAD FACE NECK
2. UPPER LIMB SHOULDER
3. LOWER LIMB HIP
4. THORAX
5. ABDOMINAL HYPOCHONDRIUM
6. PELVIS BUTTOCK GROIN INGUINAL REGION PERINEUM
7. TRUNK NOS BACK NOS FLANK NOS
8. OTHER SPECIFIED SITES
9. SITE NOS

213.# BONE AND ARTICULAR CARTILAGE

4th Digit: 213

0. SKULL FACE UPPER JAW
1. LOWER JAW NOS
2. SPINE
3. RIB STERNUM CLAVICLE
4. UPPER LIMB LONG BONES SCAPULA
5. UPPER LIMB SHORT BONES
6. PELVIS SACRUM COCCYX
7. LOWER LIMB LONG BONE
8. LOWER LIMB SHORT BONE
9. SITE NOS

225.0 BRAIN
210.6 BRANCHIAL CLEFT (VESTIGES)
610.0 BREAST CYST
610.2 BREAST FIBROADENOSIS
610.1 BREAST FIBROCYSTIC DISEASE
217 BREAST GLANDULAR
610.8 BREAST SEBACEOUS CYST
217 BREAST SOFT AND CONNECTIVE TISSUES
212.3 BRONCHUS
210.4 BUCCAL MUCOSA

215.# BURSA

4th Digit: 215

0. HEAD FACE NECK
2. UPPER LIMB SHOULDER
3. LOWER LIMB HIP
4. THORAX
5. ABDOMINAL HYPOCHONDRIUM
6. PELVIS BUTTOCK GROIN INGUINAL REGION PERINEUM
7. TRUNK NOS BACK NOS FLANK NOS
8. OTHER SPECIFIED SITES
9. SITE NOS

215.6 BUTTOCK CONNECTIVE TISSUE

BENIGN NEOPLASM (continued)

211.1 CARDIA OF STOMACH
211.1 CARDIAC ORIFICE
212.3 CARINA
227.5 CAROTID BODY
213.# CARTILAGE ARTICULAR
4th Digit: 213
0. SKULL FACE UPPER JAW
1. LOWER JAW NOS
2. SPINE
3. RIB STERNUM CLAVICLE
4. UPPER LIMB LONG BONES SCAPULA
5. UPPER LIMB SHORT BONES
6. PELVIS SACRUM COCCYX
7. LOWER LIMB LONG BONE
8. LOWER LIMB SHORT BONE
9. SITE NOS
225.3 CAUDA EQUINA
211.3 CECUM
225.0 CEREBELLOPONTINE ANGLE
225.2 CEREBRAL MENINGES
219.0 CERVIX STUMP
224.6 CHOROID
224.0 CILIARY BODY
221.2 CLITORIS
227.6 COCCYGEAL BODY
211.3 COLON
211.4 COLON RECTOSIGMOID
211.5 COMMON BILE DUCT
224.3 CONJUNCTIVA
215.# CONNECTIVE TISSUE (SOFT TISSUE)
4th Digit: 215
0. HEAD FACE NECK
2. UPPER LIMB SHOULDER
3. LOWER LIMB HIP
4. THORAX
5. ABDOMINAL HYPOCHONDRIUM
6. PELVIS BUTTOCK GROIN INGUINAL REGION PERINEUM
7. TRUNK NOS BACK NOS FLANK NOS
8. OTHER SPECIFIED SITES
9. SITE NOS
224.4 CORNEA
222.1 CORPUS CAVERNOSUM
225.1 CRANIAL NERVES
227.3 CRANIOBUCCAL POUCH
212.1 CRICOID CARTILAGE
212.1 CUNEIFORM CARTILAGE
211.5 CYSTIC DUCT
211.9 DIGESTIVE OTHER AND UNSPECIFIED PARTS
211.2 DUODENUM
212.0 EAR (MIDDLE)
227.9 ENDOCRINE
227.6 ENDOCRINE AORTIC BODY AND PARAGANGLIA
227.5 ENDOCRINE CAROTID BODY
220 ENDOCRINE OVARY
211.6 ENDOCRINE PANCREAS
222.0 ENDOCRINE TESTES
227.8 ENDOCRINE OTHER
219.1 ENDOMETRIUM
222.3 EPIDIDYMIS
212.1 EPIGLOTTIS (SUPRAHYOID) (UNSPECIFIED)
210.6 EPIGLOTTIS ANTERIOR ASPECT
211.0 ESOPHAGUS
212.0 ETHMOID SINUS
212.0 EUSTACHIAN TUBE

BENIGN NEOPLASM (continued)

224.9 EYE
224.6 EYE CHOROID
224.0 EYE CILIARY BODY
224.3 EYE CONJUNCTIVA
224.4 EYE CORNEA
224.0 EYE EYEBALL
215.0 EYE EYELID (CARTILAGE)
216.1 EYE EYELID (SKIN)
224.2 EYE IRIS
224.7 EYE LACRIMAL DUCT
224.2 EYE LACRIMAL GLAND
224.6 EYE NEVUS CHOROIDAL
225.1 EYE OPTIC NERVE
224.1 EYE ORBIT
213.0 EYE ORBITAL BONE
224.5 EYE RETINA
228.03 EYE RETINAL HEMANGIOMA
224.0 EYE SCLERA
224.0 EYE UVEAL TRACT
224.8 EYE OTHER SPECIFIED
215.0 EYELID CARTILAGE
216.1 EYELID SKIN
215.0 FACE CONNECTIVE TISSUE
213.0 FACIAL BONES
221.0 FALLOPIAN TUBE
210.6 FAUCES
215.7 FLANK CONNECTIVE TISSUE
210.0 FRENULUM LABII
212.0 FRONTAL SINUS
211.1 FUNDUS OF STOMACH
219.1 FUNDUS UTERINE
211.5 GALLBLADDER
211.9 GASTROINTESTINAL TRACT NOS
221.9 GENITAL FEMALE
221.2 GENITAL FEMALE EXTERNAL
221.8 GENITAL FEMALE OTHER
222.9 GENITAL MALE
222.8 GENITAL MALE OTHER
221.9 GENITOURINARY TRACT FEMALE NOS
222.9 GENITOURINARY TRACT MALE NOS
211.9 GI TRACT
210.4 GINGIVA
222.1 GLANS PENIS
227.6 GLOMUS JUGULARE
212.1 GLOTTIS
215.4 GREAT VESSELS (THORAX)
215.6 GROIN CONNECTIVE TISSUE
210.4 GUM
215.0 HEAD CONNECTIVE TISSUE
212.7 HEART
211.5 HEPATIC DUCT
212.3 HILUS LUNG
215.3 HIP CONNECTIVE TISSUE
216.7 HIP SKIN
215.5 HYPOCHONDRIUM
210.8 HYPOPHARYNX
227.3 HYPOPHYSIS
211.3 ILEOCECAL VALVE
211.2 ILEUM
215.6 INGUINAL REGION
211.9 INTESTINE
211.3 INTESTINE LARGE
211.2 INTESTINE SMALL
229.8 INTRATHORACIC
224.0 IRIS
211.7 ISLETS OF LANGERHANS (ISLET CELL TUMOR)

B

BENIGN NEOPLASM (continued)

213.1 JAW LOWER BONE
211.2 JEJUNUM

> *IF A LESION IS REMOVED AND YOU ARE UNSURE OF ITS MALIGNANCY AT THE TIME, OR YOU ARE UNSURE WHETHER IT IS UNDERGOING MALIGNANT TRANSFORMATION (REQUIRING MORE EXTENSIVE STUDY OR PROCEDURES), CODE A NEOPLASM OF UNCERTAIN BEHAVIOR.*

213.# JOINT CARTILAGE
4th Digit: 213
0. SKULL FACE UPPER JAW
1. LOWER JAW NOS
2. SPINE
3. RIB STERNUM CLAVICLE
4. UPPER LIMB LONG BONES SCAPULA
5. UPPER LIMB SHORT BONES
6. PELVIS SACRUM COCCYX
7. LOWER LIMB LONG BONE
8. LOWER LIMB SHORT BONE
9. SITE NOS

223.0 KIDNEY
223.1 KIDNEY RENAL PELVIS
221.2 LABIA
210.4 LABIAL COMMISSURE
224.7 LACRIMAL DUCT
224.2 LACRIMAL GLAND
210.8 LARYNGOPHARYNX
212.1 LARYNX
215.# LIGAMENT
4th Digit: 215
0. HEAD FACE NECK
2. UPPER LIMB SHOULDER
3. LOWER LIMB HIP
4. THORAX
5. ABDOMINAL HYPOCHONDRIUM
6. PELVIS BUTTOCK GROIN INGUINAL REGION PERINEUM
7. TRUNK NOS BACK NOS FLANK NOS
8. OTHER SPECIFIED SITES
9. SITE NOS

210.0 LIP
210.4 LIP (LABIAL COMMISSURE)
216.0 LIP SKIN
211.5 LIVER BILIARY PASSAGES
213.1 LOWER JAW BONE
215.3 LOWER LIMB AND HIP CONNECTIVE TISSUE
212.3 LUNG
229.0 LYMPH NODES
210.7 LYMPHADENOID TISSUE
210.2 MAJOR SALIVARY GLANDS
212.0 MAXILLARY SINUS
212.5 MEDIASTINUM
225.2 MENINGES CEREBRAL
225.4 MENINGES SPINAL
211.8 MESENTERY
211.8 MESOCOLON
210.6 MESOPHARYNX
210.3 MOUTH FLOOR
210.4 MOUTH OTHER AND UNSPECIFIED PARTS
215.# MUSCLE
4th Digit: 215
0. HEAD FACE NECK
2. UPPER LIMB SHOULDER
3. LOWER LIMB HIP
4. THORAX
5. ABDOMINAL HYPOCHONDRIUM
6. PELVIS BUTTOCK GROIN INGUINAL REGION PERINEUM
7. TRUNK NOS BACK NOS FLANK NOS
8. OTHER SPECIFIED SITES
9. SITE NOS

219.1 MYOMETRIUM
212.0 NARES
229.8 NASAL
212.0 NASAL CARTILAGE
212.0 NASAL CAVITIES
471.8 NASAL POLYP ACCESSORY SINUS
212.0 NASAL SEPTUM
210.7 NASAL SEPTUM POSTERIOR
212.0 NASAL SINUSES
216.3 NASAL SKIN
224.7 NASOLACRIMAL DUCT
210.7 NASOPHARYNX
215.0 NECK CONNECTIVE TISSUE
225.0 NERVOUS SYSTEM BRAIN
225.2 NERVOUS SYSTEM MENINGES UNSPECIFIED
225.8 NERVOUS SYSTEM OTHER SPECIFIED SITES
225.9 NERVOUS SYSTEM PART UNSPECIFIED
225.3 NERVOUS SYSTEM SPINAL CORD
225.4 NERVOUS SYSTEM SPINAL MENINGES
229.8 NOSE
216.3 NOSE SKIN
225.1 OLFACTORY NERVE OR BULB
211.8 OMENTUM
225.1 OPTIC NERVE
210.4 ORAL CAVITY NOS
210.4 ORAL MUCOSA
224.1 ORBIT
213.0 ORBITAL (BONE)
210.6 OROPHARYNX OTHER PARTS
229.8 OTHER
220 OVARY
620.0 OVARY CYST FOLLICULAR
221.0 OVIDUCT
210.4 PALATE (HARD) (SOFT)
211.6 PANCREAS
211.7 PANCREAS ISLETS OF LANGERHANS
227.6 PARA-AORTIC BODY
221.0 PARAMETRIUM
227.1 PARATHYROID GLAND
223.89 PARAURETHRAL GLANDS
210.2 PAROTID GLAND
215.6 PELVIS CONNECTIVE TISSUE
222.1 PENIS
212.7 PERICARDIUM
215.6 PERINEUM CONNECTIVE TISSUE
213.# PERIOSTEUM
4th Digit: 213
0. SKULL FACE UPPER JAW
1. LOWER JAW NOS
2. SPINE
3. RIB STERNUM CLAVICLE
4. UPPER LIMB LONG BONES SCAPULA
5. UPPER LIMB SHORT BONES
6. PELVIS SACRUM COCCYX
7. LOWER LIMB LONG BONE
8. LOWER LIMB SHORT BONE
9. SITE NOS

215.# PERIPHERAL NERVES AND GANGLIA
4th Digit: 215
0. HEAD FACE NECK
2. UPPER LIMB SHOULDER
3. LOWER LIMB HIP
4. THORAX
5. ABDOMINAL HYPOCHONDRIUM
6. PELVIS BUTTOCK GROIN INGUINAL REGION PERINEUM
7. TRUNK NOS BACK NOS FLANK NOS
8. OTHER SPECIFIED SITES
9. SITE NOS

BENIGN NEOPLASM (continued)

210.7 PHARYNGEAL TONSIL
210.9 PHARYNX
227.4 PINEAL GLAND
227.3 PITUITARY GLAND
212.4 PLEURA
210.8 POSTCRICOID REGION
222.1 PREPUCE
222.2 PROSTATE
600 PROSTATE ADENOMA
221.2 PUDENDUM
211.1 PYLORUS
210.8 PYRIFORM FOSSA
227.3 RATHKE'S POUCH
211.4 RECTOSIGMOID JUNCTION
211.4 RECTUM AND ANAL CANAL
223.1 RENAL PELVIS
223.1 RENAL PELVIS (CALYCES)
212.8 RESPIRATORY OTHER SPECIFIED SITE
212.9 RESPIRATORY SITE UNSPECIFIED
224.5 RETINA
228.03 RETINAL HEMANGIOMA
211.8 RETROPERITONEUM AND PERITONEUM
210.2 SALIVARY GLAND (MAJOR)
210.4 SALIVARY GLAND (MINOR) (UNSPECIFIED)
224.0 SCLERA
222.4 SCROTUM SKIN
227.3 SELLA TURCICA
222.8 SEMINAL VESICLE
215.2 SHOULDER CONNECTIVE TISSUE
216.6 SHOULDER SKIN
212.0 SINUS - ETHMOIDAL, FRONTAL, MAXILLARY, SPHENOIDAL
216.# SKIN

4th Digit: 216

0. LIP (SKIN OF)
1. EYELID INCLUDING CANTHUS
2. EAR (EXTERNAL) (AURICLE) (PINNA)
3. FACE (CHEEK) (NOSE) (EYEBROW)
4. SCALP NECK
5. TRUNK BACK CHEST
6. UPPER LIMB INCLUDING SHOULDER
7. LOWER LIMB INCLUDING HIP
8. OTHER SPECIFIED SITES
9. SKIN NOS

222.# SKIN OTHER MALE GENITAL

4th Digit: 222

0. TESTIS
1. PENIS
2. PROSTATE
3. EPIDIDYMIS
4. SCROTUM
8. OTHER SPECIFIED SITES
9. SITE UNSPECIFIED

213.0 SKULL, FACE AND UPPER JAW BONES
222.8 SPERMATIC CORD
212.0 SPHENOIDAL SINUS
211.5 SPHINCTER OF ODDI
225.3 SPINAL CORD
225.4 SPINAL MENINGES
211.9 SPLEEN NEC
211.1 STOMACH
210.2 SUBLINGUAL GLAND
210.2 SUBMANDIBULAR SALIVARY GLAND
227.0 SUPRARENAL GLAND

BENIGN NEOPLASM (continued)

215.# SYNOVIA
215.# TENDON (SHEATH)

4th Digit: 215

0. HEAD FACE NECK
2. UPPER LIMB SHOULDER
3. LOWER LIMB HIP
4. THORAX
5. ABDOMINAL HYPOCHONDRIUM
6. PELVIS BUTTOCK GROIN INGUINAL REGION PERINEUM
7. TRUNK NOS BACK NOS FLANK NOS
8. OTHER SPECIFIED SITES
9. SITE NOS

222.0 TESTIS
229.8 THORACIC
215.4 THORACIC CONNECTIVE TISSUE
215.4 THORACIC GREAT VESSELS
210.9 THROAT
212.6 THYMUS
226 THYROID
212.1 THYROID CARTILAGE
210.1 TONGUE
210.1 TONSIL LINGUAL
210.5 TONSIL PALATINE
210.7 TONSIL PHARYNGEAL
210.6 TONSIL FOSSA
210.6 TONSILLAR PILLARS
212.2 TRACHEA (TRACHEOBRONCHIAL)
215.7 TRUNK CONNECTIVE TISSUE
216.5 TRUNK SKIN
215.2 UPPER LIMB CONNECTIVE TISSUE
212.9 UPPER RESPIRATORY
223.2 URETER
223.3 URETER (ORIFICE OF BLADDER)
223.81 URETHRA
223.3 URETHRA (ORIFICE OF BLADDER)
223.89 URINARY ORGANS OTHER SPECIFIED
223.9 URINARY ORGANS
219.9 UTERUS
219.1 UTERUS BODY
219.0 UTERUS CERVIX UTERI
219.1 UTERUS ENDOMETRIUM
219.1 UTERUS FUNDUS
221.0 UTERUS LIGAMENTS
219.1 UTERUS MYOMETRIUM
221.0 UTERUS TUBE
219.8 UTERUS OTHER SPECIFIED PART
224.0 UVEAL TRACT
210.4 UVULA
221.1 VAGINA
210.6 VALLECULA
213.2 VERTEBRAL COLUMN
221.9 VESICOVAGINAL
221.2 VESTIBULAR (BARTHOLIN'S) GLAND
212.1 VOCAL CORDS (TRUE) (FALSE)
221.2 VULVA
210.2 WHARTON'S DUCT
227.6 ZUCKERKANDL'S ORGAN

694.5 BENIGN PEMPHIGUS
600 BENIGN PROSTATE HYPERTROPHY
333.93 BENIGN SHUDDERING ATTACKS
208.9# BENNET'S LEUKEMIA M9800/3

5th Digit: 208.9

0. WITHOUT MENTION OF REMISSION
1. IN REMISSION

379.22 BENSON'S DISEASE

B

B

305.4# BENZODIAZEPINE ABUSE (NONDEPENDENT)
304.1# BENZODIAZEPINE ADDICTION (DEPENDENT)

5th Digit: 304.1, 305.4

0. NOS
1. CONTINUOUS
2. EPISODIC
3. IN REMISSION

288.2 BEQUEZ CESAR (STEINBRINCK-CHEDIAK-HIGASHI) (CONGENITAL GIGANTISM OF PEROXIDASE GRANULES)
V62.82 BEREAVEMENT UNCOMPLICATED (REASON FOR ENCOUNTER)
300.11 BERGERON'S HYSTEROEPILEPSY
265.0 BERIBERI
265.0 BERIBERI CARDIOMYOPATHY [425.7]
265.0 BERIBERI CEREBRAL DEGENERATION DISEASE [331.7]
265.0 BERIBERI POLYNEUROPATHY [357.4]
921.3 BERLIN'S DISEASE
337.9 BERNARD-HORNER SYNDROME SEE ALSO 'NEUROPATHY PERIPHERAL' AUTONOMIC
255.4 BERNARD-SERGENT SYNDROME (ACUTE ADRENOCORTICAL INSUFFICIENCY)
287.1 BERNARD-SOULIER THROMBOPATHY DUE TO QUALITATIVE PLATELET DEFECTS
355.1 BERNHARDT - ROTH SYNDROME
428.0 BERNHEIM'S SYNDROME
430 BERRY ANEURYSM RUPTURED
123.8 BERTIELLIASIS
756.15 BERTOLOTTI'S SYNDROME (SACRALIZATION OF FIFTH LUMBAR VERTEBRA)
503 BERYLLIOSIS
503 BERYLLIOSIS (OCCUPATIONAL)
135 BESNIER-BOECK-SCHAUMANN DISEASE OR SYNDROME (SARCOIDOSIS)
362.76 BEST'S DISEASE
302.1 BESTIALITY
255.2 BETA 3 HYDROXYSTEROID DEHYDROGENASE DEFICIENCY
255.2 BETA 11 HYDROXYLASE DEFICIENCY
277.2 BETA-AMINO-ISOBUTYRICACIDURIA AMINO ACID DISTURBANCE (METABOLIC)
V69.3 BETTING AND GAMBLING PROBLEM
117.1 BEURMANN'S DISEASE (SPOROTRICHOSIS)
935.2 BEZOAR GASTRIC
936 BEZOAR INTESTINE
784.69 BIANCHI'S SYNDROME (APHASIA-APRAXIA-ALEXIA SYNDROME)
276.9 BICARBONATE ABNORMAL FINDINGS
891.2 BICEPS FEMORI TENDON LACERATION
880.23 BICEPS TENDON LACERATION
727.62 BICEPS TENDON RUPTURE (LONG HEAD) NONTRAUMATIC
726.12 BICIPITAL TENDONITIS
759.89 BIEDL-BARDET SYNDROME (OBESITY, POLYDACTYLY AND MENTAL RETARDATION)
330.1 BIELSCHOWSKY'S DISEASE
759.89 BIEMOND'S SYNDROME (OBESITY, POLYDACTYLY AND MENTAL RETARDATION)
281.0 BIERMER'S ANEMIA
695.4 BIETT'S DISEASE
755.66 BIFID DIGIT
289.4 BIG SPLEEN SYNDROME
427.89 BIGEMINY
256.4 BILATERAL POLYCYSTIC OVARIAN SYNDROME

BILE DUCT

751.61 ABSENCE (COMMON) (CONGENITAL)
576.8 ADHESIONS
751.60 ANOMALY NOS
751.69 ANOMALY OTHER SPECIFIED
576.2 ATRESIA
751.61 ATRESIA CONGENITAL
576.8 ATROPHY
576.8 CONTRACTION
576.8 CYST
576.9 DISORDERS
576.8 DISORDERS OTHER SPECIFIED
751.69 DUPLICATION CONGENITAL
576.4 FISTULA
576.8 HYPERTROPHY (STASIS) (CYST)
751.61 HYPOPLASIA CONGENITAL
868.02 INJURY TRAUMATIC
868.12 INJURY TRAUMATIC WITH OPEN WOUND INTO CAVITY
908.1 INJURY LATE EFFECT
751.61 OBSTRUCTION (OCCLUSION) CONGENITAL
751.61 OBSTRUCTION (OCCLUSION) CONGENITAL WITH JAUNDICE [774.5]
0 OBSTRUCTION (OCCLUSION) DUE TO GALLSTONE SEE 'CHOLEDOCHOLITHIASIS'
576.2 OBSTRUCTION (OCCLUSION) WITHOUT MENTION OF CALCULUS
576.3 PERFORATION
996.69 PROSTHESIS COMPLICATION - INFECTION OR INFLAMMATION
996.59 PROSTHESIS COMPLICATION - MECHANICAL
996.79 PROSTHESIS COMPLICATION - OTHER
576.3 RUPTURE (NON TRAUMATIC)
576.2 STENOSIS (STRICTURE) (OCCLUSION) WITHOUT CALCULUS
0 STENOSIS (STRICTURE) (OCCLUSION) WITH CALCULUS SEE 'CHOLEDOCHOLITHIASIS'
576.8 ULCER

791.4 BILE IN URINE
0 BILHARZIASIS SEE 'SCHISTOSOMA, SCHISTOSOMIASIS'

BILIARY

751.61 ATRESIA CONGENITAL
574.20 COLIC
574.21 COLIC WITH OBSTRUCTION
751.69 DUCT DUPLICATION OF CONGENITAL
575.8 DYSKINESIA
576.9 TRACT DISORDER
793.3 TRACT FILLING DEFECT

277.4 BILIRUBIN ABNORMAL FINDING
277.4 BILIRUBIN EXCRETION DISORDER
791.4 BILIURIA
741.9# BILLROTH'S MENINGOCELE

5th Digit: 741.9

0. REGION NOS
1. CERVICAL
2. DORSAL
3. LUMBAR

346.2# BING HORTON SYNDROME

5th Digit: 346.2

0. WITHOUT MENTION INTRACTABLE MIGRAINE
1. WITH INTRACTABLE MIGRAINE

BINOCULAR VISION

368.34 ABNORMAL RETINAL CORRESPONDENCE
368.30 DISORDER
368.33 FUSION WITH DEFECTIVE STEREOPSIS
368.31 SUPPRESSION
368.32 WITHOUT FUSION

290.12 BINSWANGERS DEMENTIA
259.2 BIORCK (-THORSON) SYNDROME (MALIGNANT CARCINOID)
277.6 BIOTINDTDASE DEFICIENCY

BIPOLAR DISORDER (PSYCHOSIS)

296.7 NOS
296.7 CIRCULAR TYPE I
296.7 CIRCULAR TYPE, NOT SPECIFIED AS MANIC OR DEPRESSIVE
296.4# CIRCULAR MANIC
296.5# CIRCULAR DEPRESSED
296.6# CIRCULAR TYPE MIXED
296.5# DEPRESSED
296.4# HYPOMANIC
296.4# MANIC

5th Digit: 296.4-6
0. NOS
1. MILD
2. MODERATE
3. SEVERE WITHOUT MENTION OF PSYCHOTIC BEHAVIOR
4. SEVERE SPECIFIED AS WITH PSYCHOTIC BEHAVIOR
5. IN PARTIAL OR NOS REMISSION
6. IN FULL REMISSION

296.7 TYPE I
296.89 TYPE II
296.8# OTHER MANIC DEPRESSIVE

5th Digit: 296.8
0. UNSPECIFIED
1. ATYPICAL MANIC
2. ATYPICAL DEPRESSIVE
9. OTHER (MIXED)

754.82 BIRD CHEST CONGENITAL
495.2 BIRD FANCIERS' LUNG
271.8 BIRD'S DISEASE (OXALURIA)
767.9 BIRTH INJURY
767.9 BIRTH TRAUMA
767.8 BIRTH TRAUMA SCALPEL WOUND
757.32 BIRTHMARKS CONGENITAL
0 BIRTHWEIGHT HIGH SEE 'LARGE BABY'
0 BIRTHWEIGHT LOW, NORMAL GESTATION SEE 'LIGHT FOR DATES'
0 BIRTHWEIGHT LOW, PREMATURE INFANT SEE 'PREMATURE INFANT'
273.8 BISALBUMINEMIA

ALL BITES AND STINGS ARE CODED AS TO VENOMOUS OR NONVENOMOUS. NONVENOMOUS BITES ARE CLASSIFIED BY TYPE OF INJURY. IF, WITH LACERATION OR PUNCTURE CODE TO 'OPEN WOUND'. IF SKIN IS INTACT, CODE TO 'CONTUSION'. NONVENOMOUS INSECTS, HOWEVER, ARE CONSIDERED SUPERFICIAL INJURIES AND ARE FOUND UNDER 'INSECT BITE' IN EASY CODER. VENOMOUS INSECT BITES CAN BE FOUND UNDER THE CATEGORY, 'STING VENOMOUS', OR 'BITES VENOMOUS'.

BITE NONVENOMOUS

0 ANIMAL (SKIN INTACT) SEE 'CONTUSION', BY SITE
0 ANIMAL (WITH LACERATION OR PUNCTURE) SEE 'OPEN WOUND', BY SITE
133.8 CHIGGER (RED BUG)
0 FLEA SEE 'INSECT BITE NONVENOMOUS', BY SITE
0 HUMAN (SKIN SURFACE INTACT) SEE 'CONTUSION', BY SITE
0 HUMAN (LACERATION OR PUNCTURE) SEE 'OPEN WOUND', BY SITE, COMPLICATED'
0 INSECT SEE 'INSECT BITE NONVENOMOUS', BY SITE OR 'INSECT BITE VENOMOUS'
0 TICK SEE 'INSECT BITE NONVENOMOUS', BY SITE

BITE VENOMOUS

989.5 ANT (FIRE ANT)
995.0 ANT (FIRE ANT) WITH ANAPHYLAXIS [989.5]
989.5 BLACK WIDOW SPIDER
995.0 BLACK WIDOW SPIDER WITH ANAPHYLAXIS [989.5]
989.5 BROWN SPIDER
995.0 BROWN SPIDER WITH ANAPHYLAXIS [989.5]
989.5 CENTIPEDE
995.0 CENTIPEDE WITH ANAPHYLAXIS [989.5]
989.5 COPPERHEAD SNAKE
995.0 COPPERHEAD SNAKE WITH ANAPHYLAXIS [989.5]
989.5 CORAL SNAKE
995.0 CORAL SNAKE WITH ANAPHYLAXIS [989.5]
989.5 FER DE LANCE
995.0 FER DE LANCE WITH ANAPHYLAXIS [989.5]
989.5 GILA MONSTER
995.0 GILA MONSTER WITH ANAPHYLAXIS [989.5]
909.1 LATE EFFECT
909.9 LATE EFFECT WITH ANAPHYLAXIS
989.5 LIZARD
995.0 LIZARD WITH ANAPHYLAXIS [989.5]
989.5 RATTLESNAKE
995.0 RATTLESNAKE WITH ANAPHYLAXIS [989.5]
989.5 SEA SNAKE
995.0 SEA SNAKE WITH ANAPHYLAXIS [989.5]
989.5 SNAKE VENOMOUS
995.0 SNAKE VENOMOUS WITH ANAPHYLAXIS [989.5]
989.5 TARANTULA
995.0 TARANTULA WITH ANAPHYLAXIS [989.5]
989.5 VENOMOUS
989.5 VIPER
995.0 VIPER WITH ANAPHYLAXIS [989.5]
989.5 WATER MOCCASIN
995.0 WATER MOCCASIN WITH ANAPHYLAXIS [989.5]

264.1 BITOT'S SPOT IN YOUNG CHILD
020.9 BLACK DEATH
921.0 BLACK EYE
500 BLACK LUNG DISEASE OR SYNDROME
111.3 BLACK PIEDRA
284.0 BLACKFAN DIAMOND ANEMIA
284.0 BLACKFAN-DIAMOND SYNDROME (CONGENITAL HYPOPLASTIC ANEMIA)
706.1 BLACKHEAD
780.2 BLACKOUT
084.8 BLACKWATER FEVER
989.5 BLACK WIDOW SPIDER BITE (SYNDROME)
995.0 BLACK WIDOW SPIDER BITE WITH ANAPHYLAXIS [989.5]

B

***BLADDER DISORDERS WITH INCONTINENCE (RETENTION):** WHEN CODING THE DISORDERS BELOW, CODE THE DISORDER FIRST, THEN ADD THE APPROPRIATE ADDITIONAL CODE FOR THE INCONTINENCE (RETENTION) - 788.2#, 788.3#, OR 625.6. **THE DISORDER SEQUENCES BEFORE THE INCONTINENCE (RETENTION).** FOR EXAMPLE,THE CODES FOR BLADDER WALL HEMORRHAGE WITH STRESS INCONTINENCE, FEMALE WOULD BE; 596.7 (BLADDER HEMORRHAGE) AND 625.6, (STRESS INCONTINENCE).*

BLADDER DISORDERS:

-WITH INCONTINENCE [788.3#]

-WITH STRESS INCONTINENCE, FEMALE [625.6]

-WITH URINARY RETENTION [788.2#]

596.8 ABSENCE
344.61 ACONTRACTILE
596.8 ADHESION (SPHINCTER)
596.4 ATONY OR INERTIA
344.61 ATONY OR INERTIA NEUROGENIC
596.8 ATROPHY
344.61 AUTONOMIC HYPERREFLEXIA
596.8 CALCIFICATION
594.1 CALCULUS
594.0 CALCULUS IN DIVERTICULUM
596.4 COMPLIANCE HIGH
596.52 COMPLIANCE LOW
596.8 CONTRACTED
596.0 CONTRACTURE ACQUIRED DISORDER
344.61 CORD
596.8 DEFORMITY
596.59 DETRUSOR INSTABILITY
596.55 DETRUSOR SPHINCTER DYSSYNERGIA
596.8 DILATATION
654.4# DILATATION MATERNAL COMPLICATING PREGNANCY
660.2# DILATATION MATERNAL COMPLICATING PREGNANCY OBSTRUCTING LABOR **[654.4#]**

5th Digit: 654.4
- **0. EPISODE OF CARE NOS OR N/A**
- **1. DELIVERED**
- **2. DELIVERED WITH POSTPARTUM COMPLICATION**
- **3. ANTEPARTUM COMPLICATION**
- **4. POSTPARTUM COMPLICATION**

5th Digit: 660.2
- **0. EPISODE OF CARE NOS OR N/A**
- **1. DELIVERED**
- **3. ANTEPARTUM COMPLICATION**

WITH INCONTINENCE [788.3#]

5th Digit: 788.3
- **0. UNSPECIFIED**
- **1. URGE INCONTINENCE**
- **2. STRESS, MALE**
- **3. MIXED URGE AND STRESS (MALE) (FEMALE)**
- **4. WITHOUT SENSORY AWARENESS**
- **5. POST-VOID DRIBBLING**
- **6. NOCTURNAL ENURESIS**
- **7. CONTINUOUS LEAKAGE**
- **8. OTHER**

WITH RETENTION [788.2#]

5th Digit: 788.2
- **0. UNSPECIFIED**
- **1. INCOMPLETE BLADDER EMPTYING**
- **9. OTHER SPECIFIED RETENTION**

***BLADDER DISORDERS WITH INCONTINENCE (RETENTION):** WHEN CODING THE DISORDERS BELOW, CODE THE DISORDER FIRST, THEN ADD THE APPROPRIATE ADDITIONAL CODE FOR THE INCONTINENCE (RETENTION) - 788.2#, 788.3#, OR 625.6. **THE DISORDER SEQUENCES BEFORE THE INCONTINENCE (RETENTION).** FOR EXAMPLE,THE CODES FOR BLADDER WALL HEMORRHAGE WITH STRESS INCONTINENCE, FEMALE WOULD BE; 596.7 (BLADDER HEMORRHAGE) AND 625.6, (STRESS INCONTINENCE).*

BLADDER DISORDERS: (continued)

-WITH INCONTINENCE [788.3#]

-WITH STRESS INCONTINENCE, FEMALE [625.6]

-WITH URINARY RETENTION [788.2#]

596.9 DISORDER
596.59 DISORDER DETRUSOR INSTABILITY
596.59 DISORDER FUNCTIONAL
0 DISORDER NEUROGENIC SEE UNDER SPECIFIC NEUROGENIC DISORDER
596.8 DISORDER SPECIFIED NEC
596.3 DIVERTICULITIS
596.3 DIVERTICULUM
594.0 DIVERTICULUM WITH CALCULUS
596.8 EVERSION
596.8 FIBROSIS
595.1 FIBROSIS INTERSTITIAL
595.1 FIBROSIS PANMURAL
793.5 FILLING DEFECT
596.2 FISTULA NOS
619.0 FISTULA FEMALE, BLADDER AND GENITAL TRACT
596.1 FISTULA INTESTINOVESICAL
596.2 FISTULA VESICAL NEC
794.9 FUNCTION ABNORMAL FINDING
596.59 FUNCTIONAL DISORDER OTHER
596.8 HEMORRHAGE
596.7 HEMORRHAGE BLADDER WALL
595.0 HEMORRHAGE DUE TO ACUTE CYSTITIS
618.0 HERNIA FEMALE
596.8 HERNIA MALE
596.51 HYPERACTIVE
596.7 HYPEREMIA
344.61 HYPERFLEXIA DETRUSOR
596.54 HYPERREFLEXIA (AUTONOMIC)
344.61 HYPERREFLEXIA (AUTONOMIC) WITH CAUDA EQUINA
596.51 HYPERTONICITY (OF SPHINCTER)
596.8 HYPERTROPHY
596.4 HYPOTONICITY
639.2 INJURY FOLLOWING ABORTION, ECTOPIC OR MOLAR PREGNANCY
665.5# INJURY - OBSTETRICAL

5th Digit: 665.5
- **0. EPISODE OF CARE NOS OR N/A**
- **1. DELIVERED**
- **4. POSTPARTUM COMPLICATION**

867.0 INJURY TRAUMATIC
867.1 INJURY TRAUMATIC WITH OPEN WOUND INTO CAVITY
908.2 INJURY TRAUMATIC LATE EFFECT

WITH INCONTINENCE [788.3#]

5th Digit: 788.3
- **0. UNSPECIFIED**
- **1. URGE INCONTINENCE**
- **2. STRESS, MALE**
- **3. MIXED URGE AND STRESS (MALE) (FEMALE)**
- **4. WITHOUT SENSORY AWARENESS**
- **5. POST-VOID DRIBBLING**
- **6. NOCTURNAL ENURESIS**
- **7. CONTINUOUS LEAKAGE**
- **8. OTHER**

WITH RETENTION [788.2#]

5th Digit: 788.2
- **0. UNSPECIFIED**
- **1. INCOMPLETE BLADDER EMPTYING**
- **9. OTHER SPECIFIED RETENTION**

BLADDER DISORDERS WITH INCONTINENCE (RETENTION): *WHEN CODING THE DISORDERS BELOW, CODE THE DISORDER FIRST, THEN ADD THE APPROPRIATE ADDITIONAL CODE FOR THE INCONTINENCE (RETENTION) - 788.2#, 788.3#, OR 625.6.* ***THE DISORDER SEQUENCES BEFORE THE INCONTINENCE (RETENTION).*** *FOR EXAMPLE,THE CODES FOR BLADDER WALL HEMORRHAGE WITH STRESS INCONTINENCE, FEMALE WOULD BE; 596.7 (BLADDER HEMORRHAGE) AND 625.6, (STRESS INCONTINENCE).*

BLADDER DISORDERS: (continued)

-WITH INCONTINENCE [788.3#]

-WITH STRESS INCONTINENCE, FEMALE [625.6]

-WITH URINARY RETENTION [788.2#]

596.59 INSTABILITY DETRUSOR
596.9 LESION
596.8 LEUKOPLAKIA VESICAL
596.52 LOW COMPLIANCE
596.8 MALACOPLAKIA
788.30 NECK SYNDROME
596.8 NECROSIS
596.54 NEUROGENIC NOS
344.61 NEUROGENIC WITH CAUDA EQUINA
596.0 OBSTRUCTION NECK
997.5 OBSTRUCTION NECK POSTOPERATIVE [596.0]
596.0 OBSTRUCTION VESICOURETHRAL ORIFICE
788.9 PAIN
596.53 PARALYSIS
596.54 PARALYSIS NEUROGENIC (SENSORY)
344.61 PARALYSIS NEUROGENIC (SENSORY) WITH CAUDA EQUINA
596.54 PARALYSIS SPASTIC (SENSORY)
344.61 PARALYSIS SPASTIC (SENSORY) WITH CAUDA EQUINA
596.53 PARALYSIS SPHINCTER
596.53 PARALYSIS VESICAL
618.0 PROLAPSE FEMALE
596.8 PROLAPSE MALE
794.9 RADIOISOTOPE STUDY ABNORMAL
596.59 RELAXATION
596.59 RELAXATION VESICAL
V43.5 REPLACEMENT (ARTIFICIAL) (PROSTHESIS)
788.20 RETENTION NEC
596.6 RUPTURE NONTRAUMATIC
867.0 RUPTURE TRAUMATIC
794.9 SCAN ABNORMAL
V76.3 SCREENING (CANCER) (MASS)
596.8 SPASM
596.0 STENOSIS
596.0 STENOSIS BLADDER NECK (ACQUIRED)
596.0 STRICTURE BLADDER NECK
788.9 TENESMUS

WITH INCONTINENCE [788.3#]

5th Digit: 788.3

0. UNSPECIFIED
1. URGE INCONTINENCE
2. STRESS, MALE
3. MIXED URGE AND STRESS (MALE) (FEMALE)
4. WITHOUT SENSORY AWARENESS
5. POST-VOID DRIBBLING
6. NOCTURNAL ENURESIS
7. CONTINUOUS LEAKAGE
8. OTHER

WITH RETENTION [788.2#]

5th Digit: 788.2

0. UNSPECIFIED
1. INCOMPLETE BLADDER EMPTYING
9. OTHER SPECIFIED RETENTION

BLADDER CONGENITAL

753.8 ABSENCE
753.8 ACCESSORY
753.9 ANOMALY NOS
753.8 ANOMALY OTHER SPECIFIED
753.6 ATRESIA (NECK)
753.9 DEFORMITY NOS
753.8 DILATATION
763.1 DILATATION WITH OBSTRUCTED LABOR AFFECTING FETUS OR NEWBORN
753.8 DIVERTICULUM
753.5 ECTOPIC
753.5 EXSTROPHY
753.5 EXTROVERSION
756.71 HERNIA CONGENITAL (FEMALE) (MALE)
753.6 OBSTRUCTION NECK
753.6 OBSTRUCTION VESICOURETHRAL ORIFICE
756.71 PROLAPSE (FEMALE) (MALE)
753.6 STENOSIS (NECK)

701.3 BLANCHE (OF MILIAN) ATROPHY

BLAST

921.3 BLINDNESS
0 CONCUSSION SEE 'BLAST', INJURY
869.0 INJURY NOS
869.1 INJURY NOS WITH OPEN WOUND
0 INJURY ABDOMEN OR THORAX SEE ANATOMICAL SITE, INJURY
850.9 INJURY BRAIN (SEE ALSO 'CONCUSSION')
0 INJURY BRAIN WITH SKULL FRACTURE SEE 'FRACTURE', SKULL
951.5 INJURY EAR (ACOUSTIC NERVE TRAUMA)
872.61 INJURY EAR (ACOUSTIC NERVE TRAUMA) WITH TYMPANIC MEMBRANE PERFORATION TRAUMATIC
872.71 INJURY EAR (ACOUSTIC NERVE TRAUMA) WITH TYMPANIC MEMBRANE PERFORATION TRAUMATIC COMPLICATED
0 INJURY INTERNAL ORGANS SEE SPECIFIC ORGAN, INJURY
861.20 INJURY LUNG
388.11 INJURY OTITIC (EXPLOSIVE)
0 SYNDROME SEE 'BLAST' INJURY

116.0 BLASTOMYCES (AJELLOMYCES) DERMATITIDIS INFECTION

116.2 BLASTOMYCES LOBOI INFECTIONS

BLASTOMYCOSIS

116.1 BRAZILIAN
116.0 CUTANEOUS
116.0 DERMATITIS
116.0 DISSEMINATED
116.2 KELOIDAL
116.2 LOBO'S
116.0 NORTH AMERICAN
116.1 PARACOCCIDIOID BLOCK
116.0 PULMONARY PRIMARY
116.1 SOUTH AMERICAN

709.8 BLEB
V45.69 BLEB FILTERING, EYE (POSTGLAUCOMA) (STATUS)
997.99 BLEB FILTERING, EYE (POSTGLAUCOMA) (STATUS) WITH COMPLICATION
997.99 BLEB FILTERING, EYE (POSTGLAUCOMA) (STATUS) POST CATARACT EXTRACTION
492.0 BLEB LUNG
770.5 BLEB LUNG CONGENITAL

B

B

BLEEDING

569.3	ANAL
628.0	ANOVULATORY CYCLE
448.9	CAPILLARY
0	COAGULATION DEFECT SEE 'COAGULATION DEFECT'
621.1	DUE TO SUBINVOLUTION UTERUS
666.2#	DUE TO SUBINVOLUTION UTERUS PUERPERAL
	5th Digit: 666.2
	0. EPISODE OF CARE NOS OR N/A
	2. DELIVERED
	4. POSTPARTUM COMPLICATION
388.69	EAR
627.0	EXCESSIVE MENOPAUSAL ONSET - MENORRHAGIA
626.3	EXCESSIVE MENSTRUAL ONSET - MENORRHAGIA PUBERTAL
286.9	FAMILIAL (SEE ALSO 'COAGULATION DEFECT')
626.7	FOLLOWING INTERCOURSE
578.9	GI CAUSE UNSPECIFIED
523.8	GUMS
455.8	HEMORRHOIDS NOS (SEE ALSO 'HEMORRHOIDS')
626.6	INTERMENSTRUAL IRREGULAR
626.5	INTERMENSTRUAL REGULAR
998.11	INTRAOPERATIVE COMPLICATING A PROCEDURE
626.4	IRREGULAR NEC
627.0	MENOPAUSAL
626.0	MENSTRUAL - ABSENCE
626.9	MENSTRUAL - DISORDER
306.52	MENSTRUAL - DISORDER PSYCHOGENIC
626.8	MENSTRUAL - DISORDER OTHER
626.2	MENSTRUAL - EXCESSIVE HEAVY PERIODS
627.0	MENSTRUAL - EXCESSIVE MENOPAUSAL
626.3	MENSTRUAL - EXCESSIVE ONSET OF PUBERTY
627.0	MENSTRUAL - EXCESSIVE PREMENOPAUSAL
V25.3	MENSTRUAL - EXTRACTION
626.1	MENSTRUAL - INFREQUENT
626.4	MENSTRUAL - IRREGULAR
627.1	MENSTRUAL - POSTMENOPAUSAL BLEEDING
626.5	MENSTRUAL - REGULAR
V25.3	MENSTRUAL - REGULATION
626.1	MENSTRUAL - SCANTY
626.8	MENSTRUAL - SUPPRESSION
626.8	MENSTRUAL - OTHER SPECIFIED
528.9	MOUTH
611.79	NIPPLE
784.7	NOSEBLEED
528.9	ORAL SOFT TISSUE
626.5	OVULATION
626.7	POSTCOITAL
627.1	POSTMENOPAUSAL
998.11	POSTOPERATIVE COMPLICATING A PROCEDURE
666.1#	POSTPARTUM (ATONIC)
666.2#	POSTPARTUM DELAYED OR SECONDARY
666.0#	POSTPARTUM THIRD STAGE
	5th Digit: 666.0-2
	0. EPISODE OF CARE NOS OR N/A
	2. DELIVERED
	4. POSTPARTUM COMPLICATION
626.3	PUBERTAL EXCESSIVE (MENSTRUAL ONSET)
569.3	RECTAL
784.8	THROAT
790.92	TIME ABNORMAL FINDING
286.9	TIME PROLONGED COAGULATION DEFECT - (SEE ALSO 'COAGULATION DEFECT')
789.9	UMBILICAL
772.3	UMBILICAL CORD STUMP AFTER BIRTH

BLEEDING (continued)

626.9	UTERINE NOS
627.0	UTERINE CLIMACTERIC
626.8	UTERINE DYSFUNCTIONAL (DUB)
621.1	UTERINE SUBINVOLUTION (DUE TO)
666.2#	UTERINE SUBINVOLUTION PUERPERAL (DUE TO)
	5th Digit: 666.2
	0. EPISODE OF CARE NOS OR N/A
	2. DELIVERED
	4. POSTPARTUM COMPLICATION
626.6	UTERINE UNRELATED TO MENSTRUAL CYCLE
623.8	VAGINAL NOS
641.9#	VAGINAL NOS IN PREGNANCY
641.2#	VAGINAL ABRUPTIO PLACENTAE IN PREGNANCY
641.1#	VAGINAL PLACENTA PREVIA IN PREGNANCY
	5th Digit: 641.1-2, 9
	0. EPISODE OF CARE NOS OR N/A
	1. DELIVERED
	3. ANTEPARTUM COMPLICATION
626.7	VAGINAL POSTCOITAL IRREGULAR
625.8	VICARIOUS MENSTRUATION

BLEPHARITIS

373.00	NOS
373.02	SQUAMOUS
373.01	ULCERATIVE
374.34	**BLEPHAROCHALASIS**

BLEPHAROCONJUNCTIVITIS

372.20	NOS
372.21	ANGULAR
372.22	CONTACT
374.46	BLEPHAROPHIMOSIS
374.89	BLEPHAROPLEGIA
0	BLEPHAROPTOSIS SEE 'PTOSIS OF THE EYE'
333.81	BLEPHAROSPASM
362.62	BLESSIG'S CYST
631	BLIGHTED OVUM
631	BLIGHTED OVUM WITH <u>COMPLICATION</u> DURING TREATMENT [<u>**639.#**</u>]
639.#	BLIGHTED OVUM WITH COMPLICATION FOLLOWING TREATMENT
	4th Digit: 639
	0. GENITAL TRACT AND PELVIC INFECTION
	1. DELAYED OR EXCESSIVE HEMORRHAGE
	2. DAMAGE TO PELVIC ORGANS AND TISSUE
	3. RENAL FAILURE
	4. METABOLIC DISORDERS
	5. SHOCK
	6. EMBOLISM
	8. OTHER SPECIFIED COMPLICATION
	9. UNSPECIFIED COMPLICATION

BLIND

0	COLOR SEE 'BLIND (COLOR BLINDNESS)'
377.75	CORTICAL
V19.0	FAMILY HISTORY (BLINDNESS)
360.42	HYPERTENSIVE EYE
360.41	HYPOTENSIVE EYE
300.11	HYSTERICAL
369.4	LEGAL (USA DEFINITION)
369.00	LEGAL (WHO DEFINITION)
579.2	LOOP SYNDROME (POSTOPERATIVE)
264.5	NIGHT VITAMIN A DEFICIENCY
369.60	ONE EYE
784.69	PSYCHIC
306.7	PSYCHOGENIC
363.31	SUN (SOLAR)
368.12	TEMPORARY (TRANSIENT)
369.01	TOTAL BOTH EYES
950.9	TRAUMATIC

BLIND (COLOR BLINDNESS)
368.54 ACHROMATOPSIA (TOTAL)
368.55 ACQUIRED
368.52 DEUTAN DEFECT (GREEN)
V19.0 FAMILY HISTORY
368.54 MONOCHROMATIC (CONE) (ROD)
368.51 PROTAN DEFECT (RED)
368.53 TRITAN DEFECT (BLUE)
368.54 TOTAL
368.59 OTHER

374.45 **BLINK REFLEX DEFICIENT**

BLISTER
919.2 SITE NOS
919.3 SITE NOS INFECTED
911.2 ABDOMINAL WALL
911.3 ABDOMINAL WALL INFECTED
916.2 ANKLE
916.3 ANKLE INFECTED
911.2 ANUS
911.3 ANUS INFECTED
912.2 ARM (UPPER)
912.3 ARM (UPPER) INFECTED
912.2 AXILLA
912.3 AXILLA INFECTED
911.2 BACK
911.3 BACK INFECTED
911.2 BREAST
911.3 BREAST INFECTED
911.2 BUTTOCK
911.3 BUTTOCK INFECTED
916.2 CALF
916.3 CALF INFECTED
910.2 CHEEK
910.3 CHEEK INFECTED
911.2 CHEST WALL
911.3 CHEST WALL INFECTED
910.2 EAR
910.3 EAR INFECTED
913.2 ELBOW
913.3 ELBOW INFECTED
910.2 FACE
910.3 FACE INFECTED
915.2 FINGER
915.3 FINGER INFECTED
911.2 FLANK
911.3 FLANK INFECTED
917.2 FOOT
917.3 FOOT INFECTED
913.2 FOREARM
913.3 FOREARM INFECTED
911.2 GROIN
911.3 GROIN INFECTED
910.2 GUM
910.3 GUM INFECTED
914.2 HAND
914.3 HAND INFECTED
917.2 HEEL
917.3 HEEL INFECTED
916.2 HIP
916.3 HIP INFECTED
911.2 INTERSCAPULAR REGION
911.3 INTERSCAPULAR REGION INFECTED
916.2 KNEE
916.3 KNEE INFECTED
911.2 LABIA
911.3 LABIA INFECTED
906.2 LATE EFFECT
916.2 LEG
916.3 LEG INFECTED
910.2 LIP
910.3 LIP INFECTED

BLISTER (continued)
919.2 MULTIPLE
919.3 MULTIPLE INFECTED
910.2 NECK
910.3 NECK INFECTED
910.2 NOSE
910.3 NOSE INFECTED
911.2 PENIS
911.3 PENIS INFECTED
911.2 PERINEUM
911.3 PERINEUM INFECTED
910.2 SCALP
910.3 SCALP INFECTED
912.2 SCAPULAR REGION
912.3 SCAPULAR REGION INFECTED
911.2 SCROTUM
911.3 SCROTUM INFECTED
912.2 SHOULDER
912.3 SHOULDER INFECTED
911.2 TESTIS
911.3 TESTIS INFECTED
916.2 THIGH
916.3 THIGH INFECTED
910.2 THROAT
910.3 THROAT INFECTED
915.2 THUMB
915.3 THUMB INFECTED
917.2 TOE
917.3 TOE INFECTED
911.2 TRUNK
911.3 TRUNK INFECTED
911.2 VAGINA
911.3 VAGINA INFECTED
911.2 VULVA
911.3 VULVA INFECTED
913.2 WRIST
913.3 WRIST INFECTED
919.2 OTHER SITES
919.3 OTHER SITES INFECTED

787.3 **BLOATING ABDOMINAL**

757.33 **BLOCH SIEMENS SYNDROME**
757.33 **BLOCH SULZBERGER INCONTINENTIA PIGMENTI**

307.9 **BLOCQ'S SYNDROME (ASTASIA-ABASIA)**

BLOOD
V70.4 ALCOHOL TEST
790.7 CULTURE POSITIVE (ABNORMAL FINDINGS)
289.9 DISORDER NOS
V18.3 DISORDER FAMILY HISTORY
V12.3 DISORDER PERSONAL HISTORY
306.8 DISORDER PSYCHOGENIC
V78.9 DISORDER SCREENING
V78.8 DISORDER SCREENING OTHER SPECIFIED
289.8 DISORDER SPECIFIED NEC
V59.0# DONOR NON-AUTOGENOUS
5th Digit: V59.0
1. WHOLE
2. STEM CELLS
9. OTHER

0 DONOR SELF DONATION - CODE UNDERLYING DISEASE
289.9 DYSCRASIA
776.9 DYSCRASIA FETUS OR NEWBORN NEC
289.9 FORMING ORGAN DISORDER NOS
V12.3 FORMING ORGAN DISORDER HISTORY
289.8 FORMING ORGAN DISORDER NEC
790.91 GAS LEVEL ABNORMAL
790.2 GLUCOSE ABNORMAL FINDINGS
790.2 GLUCOSE HIGH ABNORMAL FINDINGS
251.2 GLUCOSE LOW ABNORMAL FINDINGS
792.1 IN FECES (OCCULT)
599.7 IN URINE

B

BLOOD (continued)

772.0 LOSS FETAL
762.1 LOSS MATERNAL AFFECTING FETUS OR NEWBORN
790.6 NITROGEN DERIVATIVES ABNORMAL
796.2 PRESSURE ELEVATED WITHOUT CURRENT OR PAST DIAGNOSIS OF HYPERTENSION
796.4 PRESSURE FLUCTUATING
796.2 PRESSURE LABILE
796.3 PRESSURE LOW READING
371.12 STAINING CORNEA
790.2 SUGAR ABNORMAL FINDINGS
790.2 SUGAR HIGH ABNORMAL FINDINGS
251.2 SUGAR LOW ABNORMAL FINDINGS
V58.2 TRANSFUSION WITHOUT REPORTED DIAGNOSIS
656.2# TYPE INCOMPATIBILITY MATERNAL COMPLICATING PREGNANCY - ABO
656.1# TYPE INCOMPATIBILITY MATERNAL COMPLICATING PREGNANCY - ANTI-D ANTIBODIES (RH)
656.1# TYPE INCOMPATIBILITY MATERNAL COMPLICATING PREGNANCY - RHESUS (RH)
656.2# TYPE INCOMPATIBILITY MATERNAL COMPLICATING PREGNANCY - OTHER SPECIFIED

5th Digit: 656.1-2

0. EPISODE OF CARE UNSPECIFIED OR N/A
1. DELIVERED
3. ANTEPARTUM COMPLICATION

773.1 TYPE REACTION ABO HEMOLYTIC PERINATAL
773.2 TYPE REACTION HEMOLYTIC PERINATAL
773.0 TYPE REACTION RH HEMOLYTIC PERINATAL
747.60 VESSEL ATRESIA NEC (CONGENITAL)
459.9 VESSEL DISORDER
0 VESSEL INJURY SEE 'BLOOD VESSEL INJURY'
0 VESSEL GRAFT COMPLICATION SEE 'COMPLICATION' VASCULAR
459.9 VESSEL OCCLUSION NEC
V43.4 VESSEL REPLACEMENT (ARTIFICIAL) (PROSTHESIS) (VESSEL)
459.0 VESSEL RUPTURE SPONTANEOUS
V42.89 VESSEL TRANSPLANT STATUS

INJURY OF A BLOOD VESSEL CAN BE A LACERATION, A-V FISTULA, ANEURYSM, OR HEMATOMA. USE THE "INJURY" CODE FOUND BY ANATOMICAL SITE (THE NAME OF THE BLOOD VESSEL).

THE BLOOD VESSELS BELOW ARE THOSE VAGUELY DEFINED, POORLY SPECIFIED VESSELS IN GENERAL BODY AREAS. SPECIFIC ARTERY AND VEIN INJURIES CAN BE FOUND UNDER THEIR ANATOMICAL NAME. I.E., CAROTID ARTERY OR AORTA.

BLOOD VESSEL INJURY

902.9 ABDOMEN AND PELVIS
902.87 ABDOMEN AND PELVIS MULTIPLE
902.89 ABDOMEN AND PELVIS OTHER
902.87 ABDOMEN MULTIPLE
903.00 AXILLARY
903.1 BRACHIAL
904.6 DEEP PLANTAR
903.5 DIGITAL
900.9 HEAD AND NECK NOS
900.82 HEAD AND NECK MULTIPLE
900.89 HEAD AND NECK MULTIPLE OTHER
900.9 HEAD NOS
902.50 ILIAC
902.59 ILIAC OTHER

BLOOD VESSEL INJURY (continued)

908.4 LATE EFFECT - ABDOMEN AND PELVIS VESSELS
908.3 LATE EFFECT - HEAD AND NECK VESSELS
908.3 LATE EFFECT - LOWER EXTREMITY AND UNSPECIFIED VESSELS
908.4 LATE EFFECT - THORAX VESSELS
908.3 LATE EFFECT - UPPER EXTREMITY VESSELS
904.8 LOWER EXTREMITY UNSPECIFIED
904.7 LOWER EXTREMITY OTHER SPECIFIED
900.9 NECK NOS
902.9 PELVIS NOS
902.87 PELVIS AND ABDOMEN (MULTIPLE)
902.87 PELVIS MULTIPLE
904.40 POPLITEAL
901.40 PULMONARY
903.2 RADIAL
902.40 RENAL
901.9 THORAX
901.83 THORAX MULTIPLE
904.50 TIBIAL
903.3 ULNAR
903.9 UPPER EXTREMITY UNSPECIFIED
903.8 UPPER EXTREMITY OTHER SPECIFIED
904.9 SITE UNSPECIFIED

610.1 BLOODGOOD'S DISEASE
757.39 BLOOM (-MACHACEK) (-TORRE) SYNDROME
732.4 BLOUNT-BARBER SYNDROME (TIBIA VARA)
732.4 BLOUNT'S DISEASE (TIBIA VARA)
802.6 BLOW OUT FRACTURE ORBIT CLOSED
802.7 BLOW OUT FRACTURE ORBIT OPEN
491.20 BLUE BLOATER (SYNDROME)
491.21 BLUE BLOATER (SYNDROME) WITH ACUTE BRONCHITIS OR EXACERBATION
270.0 BLUE DIAPER SYNDROME
746.9 BLUE DISEASE (CONGENITAL HEART ANOMALY)
381.02 BLUE DRUM SYNDROME
216.# BLUE NEVUS M8780/0

4th Digit: 216

0. LIP (SKIN OF)
1. EYELID INCLUDING CANTHUS
2. EAR (EXTERNAL) (AURICLE) (PINNA)
3. FACE (CHEEK) (NOSE)
4. SCALP NECK
5. TRUNK BACK CHEST
6. UPPER LIMB INCLUDING SHOULDER
7. LOWER LIMB INCLUDING HIP
8. OTHER SPECIFIED SITES
9. SKIN NOS

173.# BLUE NEVUS MALIGNANT M8780/3

4th Digit: 173

0. SKIN OF LIP
1. EYELID INCLUDING CANTHUS
2. SKIN OF EAR AURICULAR CANAL (EXTERNAL) MEATUS PINNA
3. SKIN OF UNSPECIFIED PARTS OF FACE CHEEK CHIN EYEBROW FOREHEAD NOSE (EXTERNAL)
4. SCALP AND SKIN OF NECK
5. ALL SKIN TRUNK AXILLA PERIANAL ABDOMINAL WALL ANUS BACK BREAST (OR MASTECTOMY SITE) BUTTOCK
6. ALL SKIN UPPER LIMB SHOULDER ARM FINGER HAND
7. ALL SKIN LOWER LIMB HIP ANKLE FOOT KNEE LEG THIGH TOE POPLITEAL AREA
8. OTHER SPECIFIED SKIN SITES CONTIGUOUS SITES UNDETERMINED POINT OF ORIGIN
9. SITE NOS

756.51	BLUE SCLERA SYNDROME
0	BLUE TOE SYNDROME SEE 'ARTERIOSCLEROSIS, ARTERIOSCLEROTIC', EXTREMITIES
862.8	BLUNT CHEST TRAUMA
862.9	BLUNT CHEST TRAUMA WITH OPEN WOUND (INTRATHORACIC)
908.0	BLUNT CHEST TRAUMA LATE EFFECT
0	BLUNT TRAUMA INTERNAL ORGANS SEE SPECIFIC ORGAN, INJURY
368.8	BLURRED VISION
782.62	BLUSHING EXCESSIVE
794.7	BMR ABNORMAL
V65.0	BOARDER (SEEKING CONSULTATION) ACCOMPANYING SICK PERSON
704.8	BOCKHART'S IMPETIGO (SUPERFICIAL FOLLICULITIS)
046.2	BODECHTEL GUTTMANN DISEASE
334.8	BODER-SEDGWICK SYNDROME (ATAXIA-TELANGIECTASIA)
V15.85	BODY FLUID EXPOSURE HISTORY
132.1	BODY LICE
307.3	BODY ROCKING
135	BOECK'S DISEASE (SARCOIDOSIS)
530.4	BOERHAAVE'S SYNDROME (SPONTANEOUS ESOPHAGEAL RUPTURE)
0	BOIL SEE 'CARBUNCLE'
284.9	BOMFORD RHOADS ANEMIA

BONE

756.9	ABSENCE CONGENITAL
756.9	AGENESIS
733.99	ATROPHY - NOS
733.7	ATROPHY - DUE TO DISUSE
733.99	ATROPHY - DUE TO INFECTION
733.99	ATROPHY - POSTTRAUMATIC
733.2#	CYST

5th Digit: 733.2

0. UNSPECIFIED (LOCALIZED)
1. SOLITARY OR UNICAMERAL
2. ANEURYSMAL
9. OTHER

733.90	DISORDER (AND CARTILAGE)
648.7#	DISORDER BACK, PELVIS AND LOWER LIMBS MATERNAL CURRENT (CO-EXISTENT) IN PREGNANCY

5th Digit: 648.7

0. EPISODE OF CARE NOS OR N/A
1. DELIVERED
2. DELIVERED WITH POSTPARTUM COMPLICATION
3. ANTEPARTUM COMPLICATION
4. POSTPARTUM COMPLICATION

733.29	DISORDER (AND CARTILAGE) FIBROCYSTIC
733.99	DISORDER (AND CARTILAGE) OTHER SPECIFIED NEC
V59.2	DONOR NON-AUTOGENOUS
0	DONOR SELF-DONATION, CODE UNDERLYING DISEASE
756.59	FIBROSIS (DIFFUSE) CONGENITAL
756.54	FIBROUS DYSPLASIA POLYOSTOTIC CONGENITAL
794.9	FUNCTION STUDY ABNORMAL
996.67	GRAFT COMPLICATION - INFECTION OR INFLAMMATION
996.4	GRAFT COMPLICATION - MECHANICAL
996.78	GRAFT COMPLICATION - OTHER
996.67	GROWTH STIMULATOR COMPLICATION - INFECTION OR INFLAMMATION
996.4	GROWTH STIMULATOR COMPLICATION - MECHANICAL
996.78	GROWTH STIMULATOR COMPLICATION - OTHER
733.99	HYPERPLASIA
733.99	HYPERTROPHY

BONE (continued)

730.9#	INFECTION

5th Digit: 730.9

0. SITE NOS
1. SHOULDER REGION
2. UPPER ARM (ELBOW) (HUMERUS)
3. FOREARM (RADIUS) (WRIST) (ULNA)
4. HAND (CARPAL) (METACARPAL) (FINGERS)
5. PELVIC REGION (HIP) (BUTTOCK) (FEMUR)
6. LOWER LEG (FIBULA) (KNEE) (PATELLA) (TIBIA)
7. ANKLE AND FOOT (METATARSALS) (TOES) (TARSALS)
8. OTHER (HEAD) (NECK) (RIB) (SKULL) (TRUNK) (VERTEBRAE)
9. MULTIPLE

284.9	MARROW ABSENCE - NOS (IDIOPATHIC)
284.8	MARROW ABSENCE - ACQUIRED (SECONDARY)
284.0	MARROW ABSENCE - CONGENITAL
289.9	MARROW DISORDER
V59.3	MARROW DONOR NON-AUTOGENOUS
0	MARROW DONOR SELF-DONATION CODE UNDERLYING DISEASE
996.85	MARROW GRAFT-VERSUS-HOST DISEASE (ACUTE) (CHRONIC)
289.9	MARROW HYPERPLASIA
996.85	MARROW TRANSPLANT FAILURE
V42.81	MARROW TRANSPLANT STATUS
794.9	SCAN ABNORMAL
V59.2	TISSUE DONOR NON-AUTOGENOUS
0	TISSUE DONOR SELF-DONATION CODE UNDERLYING DISEASE
V42.4	TISSUE TRANSPLANT STATUS

BONE SPUR

726.91	NOS
726.73	CALCANEUS
726.39	ELBOW
726.73	FOOT
726.4	HAND
726.73	HEEL
726.5	HIP
726.5	ILIAC CREST
726.60	KNEE
726.91	NOSE
726.33	OLECRANON
726.69	PREPATELLAR OR SUBPATELLAR
726.4	WRIST
726.8	OTHER SPECIFIED SITE

0	BONIFIL'S DISEASE SEE 'HODGKIN'S' DISEASE
758.6	BONNEVIE ULLRICH SYNDROME
386.19	BONNIER'S SYNDROME
780.79	BONVALE DAM FEVER
0	BORDERLINE GLAUCOMA SEE 'GLAUCOMA', BORDERLINE
301.83	BORDERLINE PERSONALITY
062.9	BORNA DISEASE
074.1	BORNHOLM DISEASE (EPIDEMIC PLEURODYNIA)
477.9	BOSTOCK'S DISEASE (SEE ALSO 'HAY FEVER')
048	BOSTON EXANTHEM
005.1	BOTULISM
005.1	BOTULISM FOOD POISONING
005.1	BOTULISM WITH MYASTHENIA [358.1]

B

536.1 BOUCHARD'S DISEASE (MYOPATHIC GASTRIC DILATATION)
298.3 BOUFFEE DELIRANTE
391.9 BOUILLAUD'S SYNDROME (RHEUMATIC HEART DISEASE)
759.5 BOURNEVILLE (-PRINGLE) SYNDROME (TUBEROUS SCLEROSIS)
082.1 BOUTONNEUSE FEVER
736.21 BOUTONNIERE DEFORMITY FINGER (ACQUIRED)
427.2 BOUVERET-HOFFMANN SYNDROME (PAROXYSMAL TACHYCARDIA)

BOWEL
787.99 HABITS CHANGE
564.1 HYPERACTIVE SYNDROME
0 INFLAMMATORY SEE 'ENTERITIS'
639.2 INJURY POST ABORTIVE
564.1 IRRITABLE SYNDROME
557.# ISCHEMIC SYNDROME
4th Digit: 557
0. ACUTE
1. CHRONIC
9. UNSPECIFIED TRANSIENT

564.81 NEUROGENIC
560.9 OBSTRUCTION (STENOSIS) (STRICTURE) (OCCLUSION)
751.1 OBSTRUCTION CONGENITAL AND INFANTILE
560.81 OBSTRUCTION DUE TO ADHESIONS
560.89 OBSTRUCTION DUE TO MURAL THICKENING
560.31 OBSTRUCTION GALLSTONE
997.4 OBSTRUCTION POST OP
560.81 OBSTRUCTION POST OP DUE TO ADHESIONS
579.3 SHORT SYNDROME
787.5 SOUNDS ABNORMAL
787.5 SOUNDS ABSENT
787.5 SOUNDS HYPERACTIVE
560.2 VOLVULUS (TORSION) (STRANGULATION)

232.9 BOWEN'S DISEASE SITE UNSPECIFIED
0 BOWEN'S DISEASE SITE SPECIFIED SEE 'CA IN SITU' SKIN BY SITE M8081/2
736.42 BOWLEG ACQUIRED
754.44 BOWLEG CONGENITAL
268.1 BOWLEG RACHITIC
371.31 BOWMAN'S MEMBRANE FOLDS AND RUPTURE
0 BOXER'S FRACTURE SEE 'FRACTURE', METACARPAL
004.2 BOYD'S DYSENTERY - GROUP C SHIGELLA (SHIGELLA BOYDII)
203.0# BOZZOLO'S MULTIPLE MYELOMA M9730/3
5th Digit: 203.0
0. WITHOUT MENTION OF REMISSION
1. IN REMISSION

600 BPH
600 BPH WITH BLADDER NECK OBSTRUCTION [596.0]
V53.7 BRACE DEVICE (ORTHOPEDIC) FITTING AND ADJUSTMENT

BRACHIAL
442.0 ARTERY ANEURYSM (RUPTURED) (CIRSOID) (VARIX) (FALSE)
440.2# ARTERY ARTERIOSCLEROSIS (DEGENERATION)
5th Digit: 440.2
0. UNSPECIFIED
1. WITH INTERMITTENT CLAUDICATION
2. WITH REST PAIN, OR REST PAIN AND (INTERMITTENT CLAUDICATION)
3. WITH ULCERATION, OR ULCERATION AND (INTERMITTENT CLAUDICATION) (REST PAIN)
4. WITH ISCHEMIC GANGRENE, OR ISCHEMIC GANGRENE AND (INTERMITTENT CLAUDICATION) (REST PAIN) (ULCERATION)
9. OTHER ATHEROSCLEROSIS EXTREMITIES

BRACHIAL (continued)
440.3# ARTERY BYPASS GRAFT ARTERIOSCLEROSIS - EXTREMITIES
5th Digit: 440.3
0. UNSPECIFIED GRAFT
1. AUTOLOGOUS VEIN BYPASS GRAFT
2. NONAUTOLOGOUS BIOLOGICAL BYPASS GRAFT

444.21 ARTERY EMBOLISM (THROMBOSIS) (OCCLUSION) (INFARCTION)
903.1 ARTERY INJURY
908.3 ARTERY INJURY LATE EFFECT
903.1 BLOOD VESSELS INJURY
903.1 BLOOD VESSELS LACERATION (RUPTURE) (HEMATOMA) (AVULSION) (ANEURYSM) TRAUMATIC
908.3 BLOOD VESSELS LACERATION LATE EFFECT
723.4 NEURITIS
353.0 PLEXUS DISORDERS (NONDISCOGENIC)
742.8 PLEXUS DISPLACEMENT CONGENITAL
953.4 PLEXUS INJURY
767.6 PLEXUS INJURY (BIRTH TRAUMA)
353.0 PLEXUS SYNDROME
0 RADICULITIS (DISCOGENIC) SEE 'CERVICAL DISC DISORDER'
723.4 RADICULITIS (NONDISCOGENIC)
451.83 VEIN PHLEBITIS

INJURY TO NERVE INCLUDES LACERATION, TRAUMATIC NEUROMA, OR LESION IN CONTINUITY. USE THE ANATOMICAL SEARCH. (THE NAME OF THE NERVE).

759.89 BRACHMAN-DE LANGE SYNDROME (AMSTERDAM DWARF, MENTAL RETARDATION AND BRACHYCEPHALY)
756.0 BRACHYCEPHALY HEMIFACIAL
759.89 BRACHYMORPHISM ECTOPIA LENTIS
078.82 BRADLEY'S DISEASE (EPIDEMIC VOMITING)

BRADYCARDIA
427.89 UNSPECIFIED
427.81 CHRONIC
763.83 NEWBORN
427.89 NODAL
997.1 POSTOPERATIVE (DURING OR RESULTING FROM A PROCEDURE)
337.0 REFLEX
427.89 SINOATRIAL
427.89 SINUS
427.81 SINUS (PERSISTENT) (SEVERE)
427.81 TACHYCARDIA SYNDROME
427.89 VAGAL
427.81 WITH PAT

277.6 BRADYKINASE 1 DEFICIENCY
277.5 BRAILSFORD MORQUIO SYNDROME (MUCOPOLYSACCHARIDOSIS IV)
732.3 BRAILSFORD'S DISEASE (RADIAL HEAD)
732.5 BRAILSFORD'S DISEASE (TARSAL SCAPHOID)

BRAIN
794.01 ABNORMAL ECHOENCEPHALOGRAM
794.02 ABNORMAL ELECTROENCEPHALOGRAM (EEG)
794.00 ABNORMAL FUNCTION STUDY
794.09 ABNORMAL SCAN
740.0 ABSENCE - CONGENITAL
742.2 ABSENCE - SPECIFIED PART CONGENITAL
742.2 AGENESIS - SPECIFIED PART CONGENITAL
742.4 ANOMALIES (MULTIPLE) NOS CONGENITAL
742.2 APLASIA - SPECIFIED PART CONGENITAL

BRAIN (continued)

331.9 ATROPHY
290.10 ATROPHY - NOS WITH DEMENTIA
331.0 ATROPHY - ALZHEIMER'S
331.0 ATROPHY - ALZHEIMER'S WITH DEMENTIA [294.1]
331.1 ATROPHY - CIRCUMSCRIBED (PICK'S)
331.1 ATROPHY - CIRCUMSCRIBED (PICK'S) WITH DEMENTIA [294.1]
742.4 ATROPHY - CONGENITAL
331.2 ATROPHY - SENILE
348.4 COMPRESSION
767.0 COMPRESSION DUE TO HEMORRHAGIC INJURY AT BIRTH
348.9 CONDITION
348.8 CONDITION OTHER SPECIFIED
0 CONCUSSION SEE 'CEREBRAL CONCUSSION'
0 CONTUSION SEE 'CEREBRAL CONTUSION'
348.9 DAMAGE
348.1 DAMAGE - ANOXIC
0 DAMAGE - CHILD NEC SEE 'CEREBRAL PALSY'
767.0 DAMAGE - DUE TO BIRTH INJURY
997.01 DAMAGE - RESULTING FROM A PROCEDURE
348.8 DEATH
742.9 DEFORMITY CONGENITAL
742.2 DEFORMITY REDUCTION CONGENITAL
0 DEGENERATION SEE 'CEREBRAL DEGENERATION'
0 DISEASE INFLAMMATORY SEE 'ENCEPHALITIS'
348.9 DISEASE ORGANIC
437.0 DISEASE ORGANIC ARTERIOSCLEROTIC
331.2 DISEASE SENILE
996.63 ELECTRODE COMPLICATION - INFECTION OR INFLAMMATION
996.2 ELECTRODE COMPLICATION - MECHANICAL
996.75 ELECTRODE COMPLICATION - OTHER
794.00 FUNCTION STUDY ABNORMAL (SEE ALSO 'BRAIN', ABNORMAL)
674.0# HEMORRHAGE MATERNAL DUE TO PREGNANCY

5th Digit: 674.0
- **0. EPISODE OF CARE NOS OR N/A**
- **1. DELIVERED**
- **2. DELIVERED WITH POSTPARTUM COMPLICATION**
- **3. ANTEPARTUM COMPLICATION**
- **4. POSTPARTUM COMPLICATION**

742.2 HYPOPLASIA
854.## INJURY NOS

4th Digit: 854
- **0. WITHOUT MENTION OF OPEN INTRACRANIAL WOUND**
- **1. WITH MENTION OF OPEN INTRACRANIAL WOUND**

5th Digit: 854
- **0. LEVEL OF CONSCIOUSNESS NOS**
- **1. NO LOC**
- **2. LOC < 1 HR**
- **3. LOC 1 - 24 HRS**
- **4. LOC > 24 HRS WITH RETURN TO PRIOR LEVEL**
- **5. LOC > 24 HRS WITHOUT RETURN TO PRIOR LEVEL: OR DEATH BEFORE REGAINING CONSCIOUSNESS, REGARDLESS OF DURATION OF LOC**
- **6. LOC DURATION NOS**
- **9. WITH CONCUSSION NOS**

348.8 LESION
742.9 LESION CONGENITAL
437.9 LESION VASCULAR NOS
437.1 LESION VASCULAR DEGENERATIVE
437.2 LESION VASCULAR HYPERTENSIVE
V12.59 LESION VASCULAR OLD WITHOUT RESIDUAL
0 LESION VASCULAR WITH RESIDUAL SEE 'LATE EFFECT', CEREBROVASCULAR DISEASE
348.8 MASS
742.4 MULTIPLE CONGENITAL
V53.02 NEUROPACEMAKER FITTING AND ADJUSTMENT

BRAIN (continued)

0 OCCLUSION SEE 'BRAIN', INFARCT
0 PALSY SEE 'CEREBRAL PALSY'
794.09 SCAN ABNORMAL
341.9 SCLEROSIS (GENERAL) (LOBULAR)
331.0 SCLEROSIS LOBAR ATROPHIC
331.0 SCLEROSIS LOBAR ATROPHIC WITH DEMENTIA [294.1]

SOFTENING (NECROTIC) (PROGRESSIVE)

434.9# NOS

5th Digit: 434.9
- **0. WITHOUT CEREBRAL INFARCTION**
- **1. WITH CEREBRAL INFARCTION**

437.0 ARTERIOSCLEROTIC
742.4 CONGENITAL
434.1# EMBOLIC

5th Digit: 434.1
- **0. WITHOUT CEREBRAL INFARCTION**
- **1. WITH CEREBRAL INFARCTION**

431 HEMORRHAGIC
434.0# THROMBOTIC

5th Digit: 434.0
- **0. WITHOUT CEREBRAL INFARCTION**
- **1. WITH CEREBRAL INFARCTION**

SYNDROME

310.9 NOS
291.2 CHRONIC ALCOHOLIC
319 CONGENITAL
310.9 ORGANIC
310.2 POSTCONTUSIONAL
310.2 POSTTRAUMATIC
293.9 POSTTRAUMATIC PSYCHOTIC
293.0 POSTTRAUMATIC PSYCHOTIC - ACUTE
294.8 POSTTRAUMATIC PSYCHOTIC - CHRONIC
293.1 POSTTRAUMATIC PSYCHOTIC - SUBACUTE
310.9 PSYCHO-ORGANIC
294.9 PSYCHOTIC
290.0 SENILE
290.10 WITH PRESENILE BRAIN DISEASE
294.9 WITH PSYCHOSIS, PSYCHOTIC REACTION

BRAIN STEM

348.4 COMPRESSION
851.4# CONTUSION
851.5# CONTUSION WITH OPEN INTRACRANIAL WOUND

5th Digit: 851.4-5
- **0. LEVEL OF CONSCIOUSNESS NOS**
- **1. NO LOC**
- **2. LOC < 1 HR**
- **3. LOC 1 - 24 HRS**
- **4. LOC > 24 HRS WITH RETURN TO PRIOR LEVEL**
- **5. LOC > 24 HRS WITHOUT RETURN TO PRIOR LEVEL: OR DEATH BEFORE REGAINING CONSCIOUSNESS, REGARDLESS OF DURATION OF LOC**
- **6. LOC DURATION NOS**
- **9. WITH CONCUSSION NOS**

348.4 HERNIATION
434.91 INFARCTION
434.11 INFARCTION EMBOLIC
997.02 INFARCTION IATROGENIC
0 INFARCTION OLD WITH RESIDUAL SEE 'LATE EFFECT', CEREBROVASCULAR DISEASE
V12.59 INFARCTION OLD WITHOUT RESIDUAL
997.02 INFARCTION POSTOPERATIVE
434.01 INFARCTION THROMBOTIC

B

BRAIN STEM (continued)
851.6# LACERATION
851.7# LACERATION WITH OPEN INTRACRANIAL WOUND
5th Digit: 851.6-7
0. LEVEL OF CONSCIOUSNESS NOS
1. NO LOC
2. LOC < 1 HR
3. LOC 1 - 24 HRS
4. LOC > 24 HRS WITH RETURN TO PRIOR LEVEL
5. LOC > 24 HRS WITHOUT RETURN TO PRIOR LEVEL: OR DEATH BEFORE REGAINING CONSCIOUSNESS, REGARDLESS OF DURATION OF LOC
6. LOC DURATION NOS
9. WITH CONCUSSION NOS

744.41 BRANCHIAL ARCH SYNDROME

BRANCHIAL CLEFT
744.42 CYST CONGENITAL
744.41 FISTULA
744.41 SINUS OR FISTULA CONGENITAL
744.41 VESTIGE

686.8 BRANDT'S SYNDROME (ACRODERMATITIS ENTEROPATHICA)
644.1# BRAXTON HICKS CONTRACTIONS
5th Digit: 644.1
0. EPISODE OF CARE NOS OR N/A
3. ANTEPARTUM COMPLICATION

985.8 BRAZIERS DISEASE
116.1 BRAZILIAN BLASTOMYCOSIS
061 BREAKBONE FEVER

BREAST
793.8 ABNORMAL (X-RAY) (ULTRASOUND) (THERMOGRAPHY)
757.6 ABSENCE CONGENITAL (OR NIPPLE)
V45.71 ABSENCE POSTSURGICAL
757.6 ACCESSORY CONGENITAL (OR NIPPLE)
675.9# AND NIPPLE INFECTION MATERNAL DUE TO PREGNANCY
675.8# AND NIPPLE INFECTION OTHER SPECIFIED MATERNAL DUE TO PREGNANCY
5th Digit: 675.8-9
0. EPISODE OF CARE NOS OR N/A
1. DELIVERED
2. DELIVERED WITH POSTPARTUM COMPLICATION
3. ANTEPARTUM COMPLICATION
4. POSTPARTUM COMPLICATION

611.4 ATROPHY
676.3# ATROPHY PUERPERAL
5th Digit: 676.3
0. EPISODE OF CARE NOS OR N/A
1. DELIVERED
2. DELIVERED WITH POSTPARTUM COMPLICATION
3. ANTEPARTUM COMPLICATION
4. POSTPARTUM COMPLICATION

V50.1 AUGMENTATION (ELECTIVE) (FOR UNACCEPTABLE COSMETIC APPEARANCE)
259.1 BUDS (PREMATURE)
611.79 CALCIFICATION
V10.3 CANCER HISTORY
V76.10 CANCER SCREENING UNSPECIFIED
V76.11 CANCER SCREENING MAMMOGRAM FOR HIGH RISK PATIENT
V76.12 CANCER SCREENING MAMMOGRAM NEC
V76.19 CANCER SCREENING SPECIFIED TYPE NEC
610.1 DISEASE CYSTIC CHRONIC
610.1 DISEASE FIBROCYSTIC
611.0 DISEASE INFLAMMATORY

BREAST (continued)
676.9# DISORDER LACTATING NOS MATERNAL DUE TO PREGNANCY
676.8# DISORDER LACTATING OTHER MATERNAL DUE TO PREGNANCY
676.3# DISORDER OTHER AND UNSPECIFIED MATERNAL DUE TO PREGNANCY
5th Digit: 676.3, 8-9
0. EPISODE OF CARE NOS OR N/A
1. DELIVERED
2. DELIVERED WITH POSTPARTUM COMPLICATION
3. ANTEPARTUM COMPLICATION
4. POSTPARTUM COMPLICATION

611.9 DISORDER NONPUERPERAL NOS
611.8 DISORDER NONPUERPERAL OTHER SPECIFIED
611.8 DUCT OCCLUSION NONPUERPERAL
778.7 ENGORGEMENT NEWBORN
676.2# ENGORGEMENT MATERNAL DUE TO PREGNANCY
676.8# FEEDING DIFFICULTY MATERNAL DUE TO PREGNANCY
675.9# INFECTION NIPPLE MATERNAL DUE TO PREGNANCY
675.8# INFECTION NIPPLE MATERNAL OTHER DUE TO PREGNANCY
5th Digit: 675.8-9, 676.2, 8
0. EPISODE OF CARE NOS OR N/A
1. DELIVERED
2. DELIVERED WITH POSTPARTUM COMPLICATION
3. ANTEPARTUM COMPLICATION
4. POSTPARTUM COMPLICATION

610.2 FIBROADENOSIS
610.1 FIBROCYSTIC DISEASE
610.3 FIBROSCLEROSIS
611.8 HEMATOMA NONTRAUMATIC NONPUERPERAL
611.1 HYPERPLASIA NONPUERPERAL
611.1 HYPERTROPHY NONPUERPERAL
757.6 HYPOPLASIA CONGENITAL
V52.4 IMPLANT - FITTING AND ADJUSTMENT
V50.1 IMPLANT - INSERTION ADMISSION
V52.4 IMPLANT - REMOVAL ADMISSION
V45.83 IMPLANT - REMOVAL STATUS
V43.82 IMPLANT - STATUS
996.69 IMPLANT COMPLICATION - INFECTION OR INFLAMMATION
996.54 IMPLANT COMPLICATION - MECHANICAL
996.79 IMPLANT COMPLICATION - OTHER
611.79 INDURATION NONPUERPERAL
611.8 INFARCTION NONPUERPERAL
959.1 INJURY
911.8 INJURY OTHER AND UNSPECIFIED SUPERFICIAL
911.9 INJURY OTHER AND UNSPECIFIED SUPERFICIAL (INFECTED)
611.72 MASS OR LUMP NONPUERPERAL
611.8 PENDULOUS
V50.1 REDUCTION (ELECTIVE) (FOR UNACCEPTABLE COSMETIC APPEARANCE)
V50.41 REMOVAL PROPHYLACTIC
611.8 SUBINVOLUTION (POSTLACTATIONAL) (POSTPARTUM) NONPUERPERAL
757.6 SUPERNUMERARY CONGENITAL (OR NIPPLE)
611.79 SYMPTOMS OTHER
757.6 TISSUE ECTOPIC
611.0 ULCER

312.81 BREATH HOLDING CHILD
786.9 BREATH HOLDING SPELL
V57.0 BREATHING EXERCISES
786.09 BREATHING LABORED
102.9 BREDA'S DISEASE

BREECH

652.2# DELIVERY
763.0 DELIVERY AND EXTRACTION AFFECTING FETUS OR NEWBORN
660.0# DELIVERY OBSTRUCTING LABOR **[652.2#]**

5th Digit: 652.2, 660.0
0. EPISODE OF CARE NOS OR N/A
1. DELIVERED
3. ANTEPARTUM COMPLICATION

669.6# DELIVERY WITH BREECH EXTRACTION
669.6# EXTRACTION

5th Digit: 669.6
0. EPISODE OF CARE NOS OR N/A
1. DELIVERED

761.7 PRESENTATION AFFECTING FETUS OR NEWBORN BEFORE L&D
652.2# PRESENTATION BUTTOCKS, COMPLETE OR FRANK
660.0# PRESENTATION BUTTOCKS, COMPLETE OR FRANK OBSTRUCTING LABOR **[652.2#]**
652.8# PRESENTATION FOOTLING OR INCOMPLETE
660.0# PRESENTATION FOOTLING OR INCOMPLETE OBSTRUCTING LABOR **[652.8#]**
652.6# PRESENTATION WITH MULTIPLE GESTATION
660.0# PRESENTATION WITH MULTIPLE GESTATION OBSTRUCTING LABOR **[652.6#]**
652.1# PRESENTATION CONVERTED TO CEPHALIC PRESENTATION (OR OTHER MALPRESENTATION)
660.0# PRESENTATION CONVERTED TO CEPHALIC PRESENTATION (OR OTHER MALPRESENTATION) OBSTRUCTING LABOR **[652.1#]**

5th Digit: 652.1-2, 6, 8, 660.0
0. EPISODE OF CARE NOS OR N/A
1. DELIVERED
3. ANTEPARTUM COMPLICATION

624.0 BREISKY'S DISEASE (KRAUROSIS VULVAE)
289.2 BRENNEMANN'S SYNDROME

BRENNER TUMOR

220 SITE NOS
0 SITE SPECIFIED SEE 'BENIGN NEOPLASM' BY SITE M9000/0
236.2 BORDERLINE MALIGNANCY SITE NOS
0 BORDERLINE MALIGNANCY SITE SPECIFIED SEE 'NEOPLASM UNCERTAIN BEHAVIOR' BY SITE M9000/1
183.0 MALIGNANT SITE NOS
0 MALIGNANT SITE SPECIFIED SEE 'CANCER' BY SITE M9000/3

032.0 BRETONNEAU'S DISEASE (DIPHTHERITIC MALIGNANT ANGINA)
631 BREUS MOLE
631 BREUS MOLE WITH COMPLICATION DURING TREATMENT [639.#]
639.# BREUS MOLE WITH COMPLICATION FOLLOWING TREATMENT

4th Digit: 639
0. GENITAL TRACT AND PELVIC INFECTION
1. DELAYED OR EXCESSIVE HEMORRHAGE
2. DAMAGE TO PELVIC ORGANS AND TISSUE
3. RENAL FAILURE
4. METABOLIC DISORDERS
5. SHOCK
6. EMBOLISM
8. OTHER SPECIFIED COMPLICATION
9. UNSPECIFIED COMPLICATION

756.16 BREVIOCOLLIS
583.9 BRIGHT'S DISEASE (SEE ALSO 'NEPHRITIS')
0 BRIGHT'S DISEASE ARTERIOSCLEROTIC SEE 'HYPERTENSIVE', RENAL DISEASE

202.0# BRILL SYMMERS DISEASE

5th Digit: 202.0
0. NOS
1. LYMPH NODES OF HEAD FACE NECK
2. LYMPH NODES INTRATHORACIC
3. LYMPH NODES ABDOMINAL
4. LYMPH NODES AXILLA AND UPPER LIMB
5. LYMPH NODES INGUINAL REGION AND LOWER LIMB
6. LYMPH NODES INTRAPELVIC
7. SPLEEN
8. LYMPH NODES MULTIPLE SITES

081.1 BRILL ZINSSER DISEASE
081.0 BRILL'S RECRUDESCENT TYPHUS - FLEA BORNE
081.1 BRILL'S RECRUDESCENT TYPHUS - LOUSE BORNE
151.9 BRINTON'S DISEASE (LEATHER BOTTLE STOMACH)
002.9 BRION-KAYSER DISEASE
300.81 BRIQUET'S DISORDER OR SYNDROME

BRISSAUD'S

307.23 TIC (MOTOR VERBAL)
244.# INFANTILISM

4th Digit: 244
0. POSTSURGICAL
1. POSTABLATIVE (IRRADIATION)
2. IODINE INGESTION
3. PAS, PHENYLBUT, RESORCINOL
8. SECONDARY NEC
9. NOS

243 INFANTILISM CONGENITAL
244.9 MEIGE SYNDROME (INFANTILE MYXEDEMA)

272.2 BROAD-BETALIPOPROTEINEMIA

BROAD LIGAMENT

752.19 ABSENCE CONGENITAL
752.19 ACCESSORY CONGENITAL
752.10 ANOMALY CONGENITAL
752.19 ATRESIA CONGENITAL
620.8 CYST OR POLYP
620.9 DISORDER NONINFLAMMATORY
620.8 DISORDER SPECIFIED NEC
620.7 HEMATOMA (HEMATOCELE)
620.8 INFARCTION
867.6 INJURY (TRAUMATIC)
867.7 INJURY (TRAUMATIC) WITH OPEN WOUND
639.2 INJURY POST ABORTIVE
620.6 LACERATION SYNDROME
620.8 POLYP
620.8 RUPTURE

518.0 BROCK'S SYNDROME (ATELECTASIS DUE TO ENLARGED LYMPH NODES)

BROCQ'S DISEASE

694.0 HERPETIC DERMATITIS
698.3 LICHEN SIMPLEX CHRONICUS
691.8 NEURODERMATITIS (ATOPIC) (DIFFUSE)
696.2 PARAPSORIASIS
698.2 PRURIGO

730.1# BRODIE'S JOINT DISEASE

5th Digit: 730.1
0. SITE NOS
1. SHOULDER REGION
2. UPPER ARM (ELBOW) (HUMERUS)
3. FOREARM (RADIUS) (WRIST) (ULNA)
4. HAND (CARPAL) (METACARPAL) (FINGERS)
5. PELVIC REGION AND THIGH (HIP) (BUTTOCK) (FEMUR)
6. LOWER LEG (FIBULA) (KNEE) (PATELLA) (TIBIA)
7. ANKLE AND/OR FOOT (METATARSALS) (TOES)
8. OTHER (HEAD) (NECK) (RIB) (SKULL) (VERTEBRAE)
9. MULTIPLE

B

705.89 BROMHIDROSIS

349.82 BROMIDISM (BROMISM) ACUTE DUE TO CORRECT SUBSTANCE PROPERLY ADMINISTERED

0 BROMIDISM (BROMISM) ACUTE DUE TO OVERDOSE OR POISONING SEE 'TABLE OF DRUGS AND CHEMICALS'

304.1# BROMIDISM (BROMISM) CHRONIC

5th Digit: 304.1

0. NOS
1. CONTINUOUS
2. EPISODIC
3. IN REMISSION

0 BRONCHIAL SEE 'BRONCHUS, BRONCHIAL'

BRONCHIECTASIS

494 NOS
748.61 CONGENITAL
494 FUSIFORM
494 POSTINFECTIOUS
494 RECURRENT
011.5# TUBERCULOUS

5th Digit: 011.5

0. NOS
1. LAB NOT DONE
2. LABS PENDING
3. MICROSCOPY POSITIVE (IN SPUTUM)
4. CULTURE POSITIVE - MICROSCOPY NEGATIVE
5. CULTURE NEGATIVE - MICROSCOPY POSITIVE
6. CULTURE AND MICRO NEGATIVE CONFIRMED BY OTHER METHODS

WHEN CODING AN INFECTION, USE AN ADDITIONAL CODE, [041.#(#)], TO IDENTIFY THE ORGANISM. SEE 'BACTERIAL INFECTION'.

BRONCHIOLITIS

ACUTE (SUBACUTE) (INFECTIOUS)

466.19 NOS
466.19 CATARRHAL
466.11 DUE TO RSV (RESPIRATORY SYNCYTIAL VIRUS)
466.11 DUE TO RSV (RESPIRATORY SYNCYTIAL VIRUS) WITH BRONCHOSPASM OR OBSTRUCTION
487.1 INFLUENZAL
466.19 WITH BRONCHOSPASM OR OBSTRUCTION
466.19 DUE TO OTHER SPECIFIED ORGANISM

BRONCHIOLITIS (continued)

491.8 CHRONIC
491.8 OBLITERANS
996.84 OBLITERANS STATUS POST LUNG TRANSPLANT
516.8 OBLITERANS WITH ORGANIZING PNEUMONIA (BOOP)
506.4 OBLITERATIVE DUE TO FUMES AND VAPORS CHRONIC

BRONCHITIS QUICK REFERENCE

490 NOS
466.0 ACUTE
491.21 ACUTE WITH EMPHYSEMA
493.9# ALLERGIC NOS
493.0# ALLERGIC WITH STATED CAUSE

5th Digit: 493.0, 9

0. WITHOUT MENTION OF STATUS ASTHMATICUS
1. WITH STATUS ASTHMATICUS

BRONCHITIS QUICK REFERENCE (continued)

493.## ASTHMATIC ACUTE

4th Digit: 493

0. EXTRINSIC (OR ALLERGIC WITH STATED CAUSE)
1. INTRINSIC
2. CHRONIC OBSTRUCTIVE WITH COPD
9. NOS (OR ALLERGIC CAUSE NOT STATED)

5th Digit: 493

0. WITHOUT MENTION OF STATUS ASTHMATICUS
1. WITH STATUS ASTHMATICUS

491.2# ASTHMATIC CHRONIC
491.9 CHRONIC
491.2# CHRONIC OBSTRUCTIVE
491.2# CHRONIC WITH EMPHYSEMA
491.21 CHRONIC WITH EXACERBATION

5th Digit: 491.2

0. WITHOUT MENTION OF ACUTE EXACERBATION
1. WITH ACUTE EXACERBATION

490 WITH TRACHEITIS (TRACHEOBRONCHITIS)
466.0 WITH TRACHEITIS (TRACHEOBRONCHITIS) ACUTE
491.8 WITH TRACHEITIS (TRACHEOBRONCHITIS) CHRONIC

BRONCHITIS

934.1 ARACHIDIC
507.0 ASPIRATION FOOD OR VOMITUS
466.19 CAPILLARY ACUTE (WITH BRONCHOSPASM OR OBSTRUCTION)
491.8 CAPILLARY CHRONIC
011.3# CASEOUS (TUBERCULOUS)

5th Digit: 011.3

0. NOS
1. LAB NOT DONE
2. LABS PENDING
3. MICROSCOPY POSITIVE (IN SPUTUM)
4. CULTURE POSITIVE - MICROSCOPY NEGATIVE
5. CULTURE NEGATIVE - MICROSCOPY POSITIVE
6. CULTURE AND MICROSCOPY NEGATIVE CONFIRMED BY OTHER METHODS

104.8 CASTELLANI'S
490 CATARRHAL
466.0 CATARRHAL ACUTE
491.0 CATARRHAL CHRONIC
506.0 CHEMICAL (OR FUMES)(VAPOR) ACUTE
506.4 CHEMICAL (OR FUMES)(VAPOR) CHRONIC
466.0 CROUPOUS
466.0 EXUDATIVE (FIBRINOUS) (MEMBRANOUS) (PSEUDOMEMBRANOUS) ACUTE OR SUBACUTE
502 MOULDER'S
466.0 MUCOPURULENT (PURULENT) ACUTE
491.1 MUCOPURULENT (PURULENT) CHRONIC
491.8 OBLITERANS
491.2# OBSTRUCTIVE
491.2# OBSTRUCTIVE ASTHMATIC CHRONIC

5th Digit: 491.2

0. WITHOUT MENTION OF ACUTE EXACERBATION
1. WITH ACUTE EXACERBATION

491.21 OBSTRUCTIVE WITH ACUTE BRONCHITIS OR EXACERBATION
491.20 OBSTRUCTIVE WITH CHRONIC BRONCHITIS
491.1 PITUITIOUS
466.0 PNEUMOCOCCAL ACUTE OR SUBACUTE (WITH BONCHOSPASM OR OBSTRUCTION)
466.0 PSEUDOMEMBRANOUS
508.8 RADIATION
490 SIMPLE
491.8 ULCERATIVE
487.1 WITH INFLUENZA, FLU, GRIPPE

IF THE DIAGNOSIS IS NOT SPECIFIED AS ACUTE ON THE RECORD, SELECT THE CHRONIC OR NOS CODE. IF THE MEDICAL RECORD INDICATES THAT THE REASON THE PATIENT SOUGHT CARE WAS DUE TO AN EXACERBATION OF A CHRONIC CONDITION, CONSULT THE PHYSICIAN FOR FURTHER DOCUMENTATION.

BRONCHITIS ACUTE

466.0 NOS
507.0 ASPIRATION FOOD OR VOMITUS
493.## ASTHMATIC
4th Digit: 493
0. EXTRINSIC (OR ALLERGIC WITH STATED CAUSE)
1. INTRINSIC
2. CHRONIC OBSTRUCTIVE WITH COPD
9. NOS (OR ALLERGIC CAUSE NOT STATED)
5th Digit: 493
0. WITHOUT MENTION OF STATUS ASTHMATICUS
1. WITH STATUS ASTHMATICUS
466.19 CAPILLARY (WITH BRONCHOSPASM OR OBSTRUCTION)
466.0 CATARRHAL
506.0 CHEMICAL (OR FUMES)
466.0 CROUPOUS
466.0 EXUDATIVE (FIBRINOUS) (MEMBRANOUS) (PSEUDOMEMBRANOUS)(SEPTIC)
466.0 MUCOPURULENT (PURULENT)
466.0 PNEUMOCOCCAL (VIRAL)(PURULENT)
508.8 RADIATION
466.0 SIMPLE
466.0 SUBACUTE
466.0 WITH BRONCHOSPASM
491.21 WITH CHRONIC OBSTRUCTIVE PULMONARY DISEASE (COPD)
491.21 WITH EMPHYSEMA
466.0 WITH TRACHEITIS (TRACHEOBRONCHITIS)

IF THE DIAGNOSIS IS NOT SPECIFIED AS ACUTE ON THE RECORD, SELECT THE CHRONIC OR NOS CODE. IF THE MEDICAL RECORD INDICATES THAT THE REASON THE PATIENT SOUGHT CARE WAS DUE TO AN EXACERBATION OF A CHRONIC CONDITION, CONSULT THE PHYSICIAN FOR FURTHER DOCUMENTATION.

BRONCHITIS CHRONIC

491.9 NOS
491.2# ASTHMATIC
5th Digit: 491.2
0.WITHOUT MENTION OF ACUTE EXACERBATION
1.WITH ACUTE EXACERBATION
491.8 CAPILLARY
491.0 CATARRHAL
506.4 CHEMICAL (OR FUMES)
506.4 DUE TO FUMES AND VAPORS
491.1 FETID
502 MOULDER'S
491.1 MUCOPURULENT (PURULENT)
491.8 OBLITERANS
491.2# OBSTRUCTIVE
491.2# OBSTRUCTIVE ASTHMATIC CHRONIC
491.2# OBSTRUCTIVE WITH CHRONIC OBSTRUCTIVE PULMONARY DISEASE (COPD)
491.2# OBSTRUCTIVE WITH EMPHYSEMA
5th Digit: 491.2
0.WITHOUT MENTION OF ACUTE EXACERBATION
1.WITH ACUTE EXACERBATION
491.21 OBSTRUCTIVE WITH EXACERBATION
491.1 PITUITIOUS
508.8 RADIATION
V81.3 SCREENING
491.0 SIMPLE
491.0 SMOKERS'

BRONCHITIS CHRONIC (continued)

491.2# WITH ACUTE BRONCHITIS
5th Digit: 491.2
0.WITHOUT MENTION OF ACUTE EXACERBATION
1.WITH ACUTE EXACERBATION
487.1 WITH INFLUENZA, FLU, GRIPPE
491.8 WITH TRACHEOBRONCHITIS OR TRACHEITIS
491.8 OTHER SPECIFIED

485 BRONCHOALVEOLITIS
519.1 BRONCHOCELE
530.89 BRONCHOESOPHAGEAL FISTULA
117.9 BRONCHOHEMISPOROSIS
518.89 BRONCHOLITHIASIS
748.3 BRONCHOMALACIA
112.89 BRONCHOMONILIASIS

BRONCHOPNEUMONIA (SEE ALSO 'PNEUMONIA')

485 NOS
466.19 WITH ACUTE BRONCHIOLITIS
466.11 WITH ACUTE BRONCHIOLITIS DUE TO RSV (RESPIRATORY SYNCYTIAL VIRUS)

WHEN CODING AN INFECTION, USE AN ADDITIONAL CODE, [041.#(#)], TO IDENTIFY THE ORGANISM. SEE 'BACTERIAL INFECTION'.

466.19 WITH ACUTE BRONCHIOLITIS DUE TO OTHER INFECTIOUS ORGANISM
491.8 WITH CHRONIC BRONCHIOLITIS

518.6 BRONCHOPULMONARY ASPERGILLOSIS ALLERGIC
519.1 BRONCHOPULMONARY DISEASE
770.7 BRONCHOPULMONARY DYSPLASIA ARISING IN PERINATAL PERIOD

BRONCHOSPASM IS AN INTEGRAL PART OF ASTHMA AND SHOULD BE CODED ONLY AS A SIGN OR SYMPTOM AND ONLY IF THE UNDERLYING DISEASE IS NOT IDENTIFIED.

519.1 BRONCHOSPASM NOS
0 BRONCHOSPASM WITH ASTHMA SEE 'ASTHMA'
0 BRONCHOSPASM WITH BRONCHITIS SEE 'BRONCHITIS'
466.11 BRONCHOSPASM WITH BRONCHIOLITIS (ACUTE) DUE TO RSV (RESPIRATORY SYNCYTIAL VIRUS)

WHEN CODING AN INFECTION, USE AN ADDITIONAL CODE, [041.#(#)], TO IDENTIFY THE ORGANISM. SEE 'BACTERIAL INFECTION'.

466.19 BRONCHOSPASM WITH BRONCHIOLITIS (ACUTE) DUE TO OTHER INFECTIOUS ORGANISM
496 BRONCHOSPASM WITH CHRONIC OBSTRUCTIVE PULMONARY DISEASE (COPD)
0 BRONCHOSPASM WITH EMPHYSEMA SEE 'EMPHYSEMA'
519.1 BRONCHOSTENOSIS

BRONCHUS, BRONCHIAL

748.3 ABSENCE, AGENESIS OR ATRESIA (CONGENITAL)
901.89 BLOOD VESSEL INJURY
519.1 CALCIFICATION
519.1 DISEASE
494 DIVERTICULUM
748.3 DIVERTICULUM CONGENITAL
862.21 INJURY
862.31 INJURY WITH OPEN WOUND
908.0 INJURY LATE EFFECT
519.1 OBSTRUCTION
748.3 RUDIMENTARY TRACHEAL CONGENITAL
519.1 STENOSIS
748.3 STENOSIS CONGENITAL
519.1 ULCER

255.4 BRONZE DISEASE (ADDISON'S)
275.0 BRONZED DIABETES (IRON)
959.09 BROW INJURY

B

652.4# BROW PRESENTATION
660.0# BROW PRESENTATION OBSTRUCTING LABOR [652.4#]
652.6# BROW PRESENTATION WITH MULTIPLE GESTATION
660.0# BROW PRESENTATION WITH MULTIPLE GESTATION OBSTRUCTING LABOR [652.6#]

5th Digit: 652.4, 6, 660.0

0. EPISODE OF CARE NOS OR N/A
1. DELIVERED
3. ANTEPARTUM COMPLICATION

344.89 BROWN SEQUARD'S SYNDROME
989.5 BROWN SPIDER BITE
995.0 BROWN SPIDER BITE WITH ANAPHYLAXIS [989.5]
756.59 BROWN SPOT SYNDROME
378.61 BROWN'S (TENDON SHEATH) SYNDROME

BRUCELLA
023.1 ABORTUS INFECTION
023.3 CANIS INFECTION
023.9 INFECTION
023.8 INFECTION OTHER
023.0 MELITENSIS INFECTION
023.2 SUIS INFECTION
V74.8 SCREENING EXAM

759.89 BRUCK DE LANGE SYNDROME
733.99 BRUCK'S DISEASE
125.1 BRUG'S FILARIASIS
757.39 BRUGSCH'S SYNDROME (ACROPACHYDERMA)
285.8 BRUHL'S DISEASE
285.8 BRUHL'S SPLENIC ANEMIA WITH FEVER
0 BRUISE SEE 'CONTUSION'
772.6 BRUISING FETUS OR NEWBORN
785.9 BRUIT ARTERIAL
279.04 BRUTON'S X-LINKED AGAMMAGLOBULINEMIA
306.8 BRUXISM
770.7 BUBBLY LUNG SYNDROME

BUBO
289.3 NOS
099.0 CHANCROIDAL
099.1 CLIMATIC
098.89 GONOCOCCAL
099.0 HEMOPHILUS DUCREYI
099.8 INDOLENT
099.8 INGUINAL
099.8 PHAGEDENIC
099.1 TROPICAL
099.8 VENEREAL

0 BUBONOCELE SEE 'HERNIA', INGUINAL
020.0 BUBONIC PLAGUE
528.9 BUCCAL CAVITY DISEASE
732.1 BUCHANAN'S JUVENILE OSTEOCHONDROSIS
733.3 BUCHEM'S SYNDROME (HYPEROSTOSIS CORTICALIS)

BUCKET HANDLE TEAR
717.0 CARTILAGE (OLD)
717.0 KNEE (OLD)
836.0 MEDIAL MENISCUS ACUTE

453.0 BUDD - CHIARI SYNDROME (HEPATIC VEIN THROMBOSIS)
648.9# BUDD - CHIARI SYNDROME (HEPATIC VEIN THROMBOSIS) MATERNAL CURRENT (CO-EXISTENT) IN PREGNANCY [453.0]

5th Digit: 648.9

0. EPISODE OF NOS OR N/A
1. DELIVERED
2. DELIVERED WITH POSTPARTUM COMPLICATION
3. ANTEPARTUM COMPLICATION
4. POSTPARTUM COMPLICATION

495.2 BUDGERIGAR-FANCIERS' DISEASE
717.89 BUDINGER-LUDLOFF-LAWEN DISEASE OR SYNDROME
443.1 BUERGER'S DISEASE
431 BULBAR ARTERY HEMORRHAGE (RUPTURE)
335.22 BULBAR PALSY PROGRESSIVE
344.89 BULBAR PALSY SUPRANUCLEAR NEC
335.22 BULBAR SYNDROME
436 BULBAR SYNDROME LATERAL
756.0 BULGING FONTANELS
783.6 BULIMIA
307.51 BULIMIA NONORGANIC
787.7 BULKY STOOLS
709.8 BULLA(AE)
082.8 BULLIS FEVER SYNDROME

BULLOUS
694.9 DERMATOSES
646.8# DERMATOSES HERPES GESTATIONIS

5th Digit: 646.8

0. EPISODE OF CARE NOS OR N/A
1. DELIVERED
2. DELIVERED WITH POSTPARTUM COMPLICATION
3. ANTEPARTUM COMPLICATION
4. POSTPARTUM COMPLICATION

694.8 DERMATOSES OTHER SPECIFIED
684 IMPETIGO
371.23 KERATOPATHY CORNEAL
384.01 MYRINGITIS ACUTE WITHOUT OTITIS MEDIA
694.5 PEMPHIGOID

790.6 BUN AND CREATINE ELEVATED

BUNDLE BRANCH BLOCK
426.50 NOS
426.53 BIFASCICULAR NOS
426.53 BILATERAL NOS
426.3 LEFT NOS
426.2 LEFT ANTERIOR FASCICULAR
426.3 LEFT ANTERIOR WITH LEFT POSTERIOR
426.3 LEFT COMPLETE
426.2 LEFT HEMIBLOCK
426.2 LEFT POSTERIOR FASCICULAR
0 LEFT WITH RIGHT SEE 'BUNDLE BRANCH BLOCK', RIGHT
426.4 RIGHT NOS
426.53 RIGHT WITH LEFT NOS (INCOMPLETE) (MAIN STEM)
426.52 RIGHT WITH LEFT ANTERIOR FASCICULAR
426.54 RIGHT WITH LEFT ANTERIOR WITH LEFT POSTERIOR
426.51 RIGHT WITH LEFT POSTERIOR FASCICULAR
426.54 TRIFASCICULAR
426.4 WILSON'S TYPE

426.7 BUNDLE OF KENT SYNDROME (ANOMALOUS ATRIOVENTRICULAR EXCITATION)
040.81 BUNGPAGGA
727.1 BUNION
066.3 BUNYAMWERA FEVER (VIRAL)

BUPHTHALMOS
743.20 CONGENITAL
743.22 KERATOGLOBUS CONGENITAL
743.22 MEGALOCORNEA CONGENITAL
743.21 SIMPLE CONGENITAL
743.22 WITH OTHER OCULAR ANOMALIES CONGENITAL

272.3 BURGER-GRUTZ SYNDROME (ESSENTIAL FAMILIAL HYPERLIPEMIA)
577.8 BURKE'S SYNDROME (PANCREATIC INSUFFICIENCY AND CHRONIC NEUTROPENIA)

BURKITT'S

200.2# LYMPHOMA

200.2# TUMOR SITE M9750/3

5th Digit: 200.2

0. NOS, EXTRANODAL AND SOLID ORGAN SITES
1. LYMPH NODES OF HEAD FACE NECK
2. LYMPH NODES INTRATHORACIC
3. LYMPH NODES ABDOMINAL
4. LYMPH NODES AXILLA AND UPPER LIMB
5. LYMPH NODES INGUINAL REGION AND LOWER LIMB
6. LYMPH NODES INTRAPELVIC
7. SPLEEN
8. LYMPH NODES MULTIPLE SITES

> *"RULE OF NINES" : A GENERAL GUIDELINE TO ESTIMATE PERCENTAGE OF BODY SURFACE.*
>
> *EACH ARM =9%, EACH LEG = 18%, ANTERIOR TRUNK = 18%, POSTERIOR TRUNK = 18%, GENITALIA = 9%.*

BURN

949.# NOS SITE OR NOS PERCENTAGE OF BODY SURFACE

4th Digit: 949

0. UNSPECIFIED DEGREE
1. ERYTHEMA (FIRST DEGREE)
2. BLISTERS (SECOND DEGREE)
3. FULL THICKNESS SKIN (THIRD DEGREE NOS)
4. NECROSIS OF UNDERLYING TISSUES (DEEP THIRD DEGREE) WITHOUT LOSS OF A BODY PART
5. NECROSIS OF UNDERLYING TISSUES (DEEP THIRD DEGREE) WITH LOSS OF A BODY PART

> *CODE 948.## IS RECOMMENDED AS AN ADDITIONAL CODE TO SPECIFY THE PERCENTAGE OF BODY SURFACE INVOLVED.*

948.## CLASSIFIED ACCORDING TO % OF BODY SURFACE

4th Digit: 948

0. BURN {ANY DEGREE} INVOLVING LESS THAN 10%
1. BURN {ANY DEGREE} 10-19 %
2. BURN {ANY DEGREE} 20-29 %
3. BURN {ANY DEGREE} 30-39 %
4. BURN {ANY DEGREE} 40-49 %
5. BURN {ANY DEGREE} 50-59 %
6. BURN {ANY DEGREE} 60-69 %
7. BURN {ANY DEGREE} 70-79 %
8. BURN {ANY DEGREE} 80-89 %
9. BURN {ANY DEGREE} 90 % OR MORE

5th Digit: 948

0. WITH THIRD DEGREE LESS THAN 10% OR UNSPECIFIED
1. WITH THIRD DEGREE 10-19%
2. WITH THIRD DEGREE 20-29%
3. WITH THIRD DEGREE 30-39%
4. WITH THIRD DEGREE 40-49%
5. WITH THIRD DEGREE 50-59%
6. WITH THIRD DEGREE 60-69%
7. WITH THIRD DEGREE 70-79%
8. WITH THIRD DEGREE 80-89%
9. WITH THIRD DEGREE 90% OR MORE OF BODY SURFACE

940.# EYE AND ADNEXA

4th Digit: 940

0. CHEMICAL BURN OF EYELIDS AND PERIOCULAR AREA
1. OTHER BURNS OF EYELIDS AND PERIOCULAR AREA
2. ALKALINE CHEMICAL BURN CORNEA AND CONJUNCTIVA
3. ACID CHEMICAL BURN OF CORNEA AND CONJUNCTIVAL
4. OTHER BURN OF CORNEA AND CONJUNCTIVAL
5. BURN WITH RESULTING RUPTURE AND DESTRUCTION OF EYEBALL
9. UNSPECIFIED BURN OF EYE AND ADNEXA

> *THE MAJOR ELEMENTS IN DETERMINING BURN SEVERITY ARE: SIZE OF THE BURN AND DEPTH OF THE BURN. ANY SIGNIFICANT PRE-EXISTING ILLNESSES AND/OR ASSOCIATED INJURIES SHOULD BE NOTED.*

941.## HEAD NECK FACE

4th Digit: 941

0. UNSPECIFIED DEGREE
1. ERYTHEMA (FIRST DEGREE)
2. BLISTERS (SECOND DEGREE)
3. FULL THICKNESS SKIN (THIRD DEGREE NOS)
4. NECROSIS OF UNDERLYING TISSUES (DEEP THIRD DEGREE) WITHOUT LOSS OF A BODY PART
5. NECROSIS OF UNDERLYING TISSUES (DEEP THIRD DEGREE) WITH LOSS OF A BODY PART

5th Digit: 941

0. FACE AND HEAD UNSPECIFIED SITE
1. EAR (ANY PART)
2. EYE (WITH OTHER PARTS OF FACE HEAD AND NECK)
3. LIP (S)
4. CHIN
5. NOSE (SEPTUM)
6. SCALP (ANY PART)
7. FOREHEAD AND CHEEK
8. NECK
9. MULTIPLE SITES [EXCEPT WITH EYE] OF FACE HEAD NECK

958.3 INFECTED

947.# INTERNAL ORGANS (CHEMICAL)

4th Digit: 947

0. MOUTH AND PHARYNX; GUM TONGUE
1. LARYNX TRACHEA LUNG
2. ESOPHAGUS
3. GASTROINTESTINAL TRACT; COLON RECTUM SMALL INTESTINE STOMACH
4. VAGINA UTERUS
8. OTHER SPECIFIED SITES
9. UNSPECIFIED SITES

906.9 LATE EFFECT - UNSPECIFIED SITE

906.5 LATE EFFECT - EYE FACE HEAD NECK

906.6 LATE EFFECT - WRIST HAND

906.7 LATE EFFECT - OTHER EXTREMITIES

906.8 LATE EFFECT - OTHER SPECIFIED SITES

945.## LOWER LIMB THIGH KNEE ANKLE FOOT TOE

4th Digit: 945

0. UNSPECIFIED DEGREE
1. ERYTHEMA (FIRST DEGREE)
2. BLISTERS (SECOND DEGREE)
3. FULL THICKNESS SKIN (THIRD DEGREE NOS)
4. NECROSIS OF UNDERLYING TISSUES (DEEP THIRD DEGREE) WITHOUT LOSS OF A BODY PART
5. NECROSIS OF UNDERLYING TISSUES (DEEP THIRD DEGREE) WITH LOSS OF A BODY PART

5th Digit: 945

0. LOWER LIMB [LEG] UNSPECIFIED SITE
1. TOE (S) (NAIL)
2. FOOT
3. ANKLE
4. LOWER LEG
5. KNEE
6. THIGH (ANY PART)
9. MULTIPLE SITES OF LOWER LIMB (S)

946.# MULTIPLE SPECIFIED SITE

4th Digit: 946

0. UNSPECIFIED DEGREE
1. ERYTHEMA (FIRST DEGREE)
2. BLISTERS (SECOND DEGREE)
3. FULL THICKNESS SKIN (THIRD DEGREE NOS)
4. NECROSIS OF UNDERLYING TISSUES (DEEP THIRD DEGREE) WITHOUT LOSS OF A BODY PART
5. NECROSIS OF UNDERLYING TISSUES (DEEP THIRD DEGREE) WITH LOSS OF A BODY PART

B

BURN (continued)

692.71 SUNBURN

942.## TRUNK CHEST WALL ABDOMINAL WALL BACK GENITALIA

4th Digit: 942

- **0. UNSPECIFIED DEGREE**
- **1. ERYTHEMA (FIRST DEGREE)**
- **2. BLISTERS (SECOND DEGREE)**
- **3. FULL THICKNESS SKIN (THIRD DEGREE NOS)**
- **4. NECROSIS OF UNDERLYING TISSUES (DEEP THIRD DEGREE) WITHOUT LOSS OF A BODY PART**
- **5. NECROSIS OF UNDERLYING TISSUES (DEEP THIRD DEGREE) WITH LOSS OF A BODY PART**

5th Digit: 942

- **0. TRUNK UNSPECIFIED SITE**
- **1. BREAST**
- **2. CHEST WALL EXCLUDING BREAST AND NIPPLE**
- **3. ABDOMINAL WALL**
- **4. BACK (ANY PART)**
- **5. GENITALIA**
- **9. OTHER AND MULTIPLE SITES OF TRUNK**

943.## UPPER LIMB EXCEPT WRIST AND HAND

4th Digit: 943

- **0. UNSPECIFIED DEGREE**
- **1. ERYTHEMA (FIRST DEGREE)**
- **2. BLISTERS (SECOND DEGREE)**
- **3. FULL THICKNESS SKIN (THIRD DEGREE NOS)**
- **4. NECROSIS OF UNDERLYING TISSUES (DEEP THIRD DEGREE) WITHOUT LOSS OF A BODY PART**
- **5. NECROSIS OF UNDERLYING TISSUES (DEEP THIRD DEGREE) WITH LOSS OF A BODY PART**

5th Digit: 943

- **0. UPPER LIMB UNSPECIFIED SITE**
- **1. FOREARM**
- **2. ELBOW**
- **3. UPPER ARM**
- **4. AXILLA**
- **5. SHOULDER**
- **6. SCAPULAR REGION**
- **9. MULTIPLE EXCEPT WRIST AND HAND**

944.## WRIST AND HAND FINGERS THUMBS

4th Digit: 944

- **0. UNSPECIFIED DEGREE**
- **1. ERYTHEMA (FIRST DEGREE)**
- **2. BLISTERS (SECOND DEGREE)**
- **3. FULL THICKNESS SKIN (THIRD DEGREE NOS)**
- **4. NECROSIS OF UNDERLYING TISSUES (DEEP THIRD DEGREE) WITHOUT LOSS OF A BODY PART**
- **5. NECROSIS OF UNDERLYING TISSUES (DEEP THIRD DEGREE) WITH LOSS OF A BODY PART**

5th Digit: 944

- **0. HAND UNSPECIFIED SITE**
- **1. SINGLE DIGIT [FINGER (NAIL)] OTHER THAN THUMB**
- **2. THUMB (NAIL)**
- **3. TWO OR MORE DIGITS NOT INCLUDING THUMB**
- **4. TWO OR MORE DIGITS INCLUDING THUMB**
- **5. PALM**
- **6. BACK OF HAND**
- **7. WRIST**
- **8. MULTIPLE SITES OF WRIST (S) AND HAND(S)**

BURN LATE EFFECT

906.9 UNSPECIFIED SITE
906.5 EYE FACE HEAD NECK
906.6 WRIST HAND
906.7 OTHER EXTREMITIES
906.8 OTHER SPECIFIED SITES

732.3 BURN'S DISEASE (LOWER ULNA)
999.9 BURNETT'S SYNDROME (MILK-ALKALI)
253.3 BURNIER'S SYNDROME (HYPOPHYSEAL DWARFISM)
266.2 BURNING FEET SYNDROME
782.0 BURNING SENSATION SKIN
727.82 BURSA CALCIFICATION
727.9 BURSA DISORDER
727.89 BURSA OTHER DISORDER

BURSITIS

727.3 NOS
726.71 ACHILLES
726.90 ADHESIVE SITE UNSPECIFIED
726.79 ANKLE
726.5 BUTTOCK
726.79 CALCANEAL
727.82 CALCIFICATION
727.2 CARPENTER'S OCCUPATIONAL
726.63 COLLATERAL LIGAMENT - FIBULA
726.62 COLLATERAL LIGAMENT - TIBIA
726.19 DELTOID
726.2 DUPLAY'S
726.33 ELBOW
727.2 ELBOW OCCUPATIONAL
726.63 FIBULAR
726.63 FIBULAR COLLATERAL LIGAMENT
726.8 FINGER
726.79 FOOT
098.52 GONOCOCCAL
726.4 HAND
727.2 HAND OCCUPATIONAL
726.4 HAND OR WRIST
726.5 HIP
726.69 INFRAPATELLAR
726.5 ISCHIOGLUTEAL
726.60 KNEE
727.2 KNEE OCCUPATIONAL
727.2 OCCUPATIONAL ORIGIN (DUE TO)
726.33 OLECRANON
726.61 PES ANSERINUS
478.29 PHARYNGEAL
727.51 POPLITEAL
726.65 PREPATELLAR
727.3 RADIOHUMERAL
726.19 SCAPULOHUMERAL
726.0 SCAPULOHUMERAL (ADHESIVE)
726.10 SHOULDER
726.0 SHOULDER ADHESIVE
726.19 SUBACROMIAL
726.0 SUBACROMIAL (ADHESIVE)
726.19 SUBCORACOID
726.19 SUBDELTOID
726.0 SUBDELTOID ADHESIVE
726.69 SUBPATELLAR
095.7 SYPHILITIC
726.62 TIBIAL
726.62 TIBIAL COLLATERAL LIGAMENT
726.79 TOE
726.5 TROCHANTERIC
726.4 WRIST
0 SEE ALSO 'TENDINITIS'

031.1 BURULI ULCER
695.89 BURY'S DISEASE (ERYTHEMA ELEVATUM DIUTINUM)
710.1 BUSCHKE'S DISEASE (SCLERODERMA)
730.1# BUSQUET'S DISEASE

5th Digit: 730.1

0. SITE NOS
1. SHOULDER REGION
2. UPPER ARM (ELBOW) (HUMERUS)
3. FOREARM (RADIUS) (WRIST) (ULNA)
4. HAND (CARPAL) (METACARPAL) (FINGERS)
5. PELVIC REGION AND THIGH (HIP) (BUTTOCK) (FEMUR)
6. LOWER LEG (FIBULA) (KNEE) (PATELLA) (TIBIA)
7. ANKLE AND/OR FOOT (METATARSALS) (TOES)
8. OTHER (HEAD) (NECK) (RIB) (SKULL) (VERTEBRAE)
9. MULTIPLE

117.5 BUSSE BUSCHKE'S DISEASE (CRYPTOCOCCOSIS)
959.1 BUTTOCK INJURY
911.8 BUTTOCK INJURY OTHER AND UNSPECIFIED SUPERFICIAL
911.9 BUTTOCK INJURY OTHER AND UNSPECIFIED SUPERFICIAL (INFECTED)
085.1 BUTTON BISKRA DELHI ORIENTAL
736.21 BUTTONHOLE HAND
066.3 BWAMBA FEVER (VIRAL)

DO NOT USE CODE 996.03, COMPLICATION OF A DEVICE, IMPLANT OR GRAFT MECHANICAL CARDIAC, WHEN THE PHYSICIAN DOCUMENTS THAT ARTERIOSCLEROSIS HAS CAUSED AN OCCLUSION OF A BYPASS GRAFT. IN CODING TERMS, THIS IS CONSIDERED TO BE A NORMAL PROGRESSION OF ARTERIOSCLEROSIS RATHER THAN A COMPLICATION OF A GRAFT. ASSIGN CODE 414.0#, ARTERIOSCLEROSIS BYPASS GRAFT, CORONARY.

414.0# BYPASS GRAFT ARTERIOSCLEROSIS CORONARY

5th Digit: 414.0

2. AUTOLOGOUS VEIN BYPASS GRAFT
3. NONAUTOLOGOUS BIOLOGICAL BYPASS GRAFT
4. AUTOLOGOUS ARTERY BYPASS GRAFT (GASTROEPIPLOIC) (INTERNAL MAMMARY)
5. UNSPECIFIED TYPE OF BYPASS GRAFT

440.3# BYPASS GRAFT ARTERIOSCLEROSIS EXTREMITIES

5th Digit: 440.3

0. UNSPECIFIED GRAFT
1. AUTOLOGOUS VEIN BYPASS GRAFT
2. NONAUTOLOGOUS BIOLOGICAL BYPASS GRAFT

V45.81 BYPASS STATUS CORONARY
V45.3 BYPASS STATUS INTESTINAL
504 BYSSINOSIS
958.5 BYWATERS SYNDROME
908.6 BYWATERS SYNDROME LATE EFFECT

005.2 C. WELCHII FOOD POISONING

0 CA IN SITU SEE 'CARCINOMA IN SITU', BY SITE

0 CA METASTATIC SEE 'CANCER', BY SITE, METASTATIC OR 'CANCER METASTATIC'

0 CA SEE 'CANCER', BY SITE

799.4 CACHEXIA

414.0# CAD (CORONARY ARTERY DISEASE)

5th Digit: 414.0

- **0. UNSPECIFIED TYPE OF VESSEL, NATIVE OR GRAFT**
- **1. NATIVE CORONARY VESSEL**
- **2. AUTOLOGOUS VEIN BYPASS GRAFT**
- **3. NONAUTOLOGOUS BIOLOGICAL BYPASS GRAFT**
- **4. AUTOLOGOUS ARTERY BYPASS GRAFT (GASTROEPIPLOIC) (INTERNAL MAMMARY)**
- **5. UNSPECIFIED TYPE OF BYPASS GRAFT**

709.09 CAFE' AU LAIT SPOTS

305.9# CAFFEINE ABUSE NONDEPENDENT

5th Digit: 305.9

- **0. UNSPECIFIED**
- **1. CONTINUOUS**
- **2. EPISODIC**
- **3. IN REMISSION**

756.59 CAFFEY'S SYNDROME (INFANTILE CORTICAL HYPEROSTOSIS)

993.3 CAISSON DISEASE

909.4 CAISSON DISEASE LATE EFFECT

732.5 CALCANEAL APOPHYSITIS (JUVENILE)

726.73 CALCANEAL SPUR

845.02 CALCANEOFIBULAR SEPARATION (RUPTURE) (TEAR) (LACERATION)

845.02 CALCANEOFIBULAR STRAIN (SPRAIN) (AVULSION) (HEMARTHROSIS)

755.67 CALCANEONAVICULAR BAR

755.67 CALCANEUS COALITION

736.76 CALCANEUS DEFORMITY OTHER (ACQUIRED)

275.49 CALCAREOUS DEGENERATION NEC

502 CALCICOSIS LUNG (OCCUPATIONAL)

727.82 CALCIFIC TENDINITIS

726.11 CALCIFIC TENDINITIS SHOULDER

275.40 CALCIFICATION GENERAL

275.40 CALCIFICATION METASTATIC

0 CALCIFICATION SEE ANATOMICAL SITE

275.49 CALCINOSIS

709.3 CALCINOSIS CIRCUMSCRIPTA

709.3 CALCINOSIS CUTIS

275.49 CALCINOSIS INTERVERTEBRALIS **[722.9#]**

5th Digit: 722.9

- **0. UNSPECIFIED**
- **1. CERVICAL**
- **2. THORACIC**
- **3. LUMBAR**

246.0 CALCITONIN HYPERSECRETION

CALCIUM

275.41 DEFICIENCY
269.3 DEFICIENCY (DIETARY)
275.49 DEGENERATION NEC
275.42 EXCESS
275.49 INFILTRATE (MUSCLE)
275.40 METABOLISM DISORDER NOS
252.0 METABOLISM DISORDER (HYPERPARATHYROID)
252.1 METABOLISM DISORDER (HYPOPARATHYROID)
252.9 METABOLISM DISORDER (PARATHYROID GLAND DISORDER)
252.8 METABOLISM DISORDER (PARATHYROID GLAND DISORDER) (OTHER SPECIFIED)

CALCIUM (continued)

268.2 METABOLISM DISORDERS WITH OSTEOMALACIA
268.0 METABOLISM DISORDERS WITH RICKETS ACTIVE
268.1 METABOLISM DISORDERS WITH RICKETS LATE EFFECT
268.9 METABOLISM DISORDERS WITH VITAMIN D DEFICIENCY
275.40 THESAURISMOSIS

CALCULUS, CALCULOUS

543.9 APPENDIX
0 BILE DUCT (ANY) SEE 'CHOLEDOCHOLITHIASIS'
594.1 BLADDER
594.0 BLADDER DIVERTICULUM
518.89 BRONCHUS
0 CHOLESTEROL (PURE) (SOLITARY) SEE 'CHOLELITHIASIS'
372.54 CONJUNCTIVA
523.6 DENTAL (SUBGINGIVAL) (SUPRAGINGIVAL)
592.9 DISEASE
608.89 EPIDIDYMIS
0 GALLBLADDER SEE 'CHOLELITHIASIS'
751.69 GALLBLADDER CONGENITAL
0 HEPATIC (DUCT) SEE 'CHOLEDOCHOLITHIASIS'
560.39 INTESTINE (OBSTRUCTED)
592.0 KIDNEY
753.3 KIDNEY CONGENITAL
592.0 KIDNEY STAGHORN
274.11 KIDNEY URIC ACID
375.57 LACRIMAL PASSAGES
0 LIVER (IMPACTED) SEE 'CHOLEDOCHOLITHIASIS'
518.89 LUNG
478.1 NOSE
577.8 PANCREATIC (DUCT)
527.5 PAROTID GLAND
602.0 PROSTATE
592.0 RENAL
753.3 RENAL CONGENITAL
274.11 RENAL (URIC ACID)
527.5 SALIVARY SYSTEM
608.89 SEMINAL VESICLE
592.0 STAGHORN KIDNEY
527.5 STENSEN'S DUCT
527.5 SUBLINGUAL (DUCT) (GLAND)
750.26 SUBLINGUAL (DUCT) (GLAND) CONGENITAL
527.5 SUBMAXILLARY (DUCT) (GLAND)
594.8 SUBURETHRAL
474.8 TONSIL
523.6 TOOTH, TEETH
608.89 TUNICA VAGINALIS
592.1 URETER
594.2 URETHRAL
274.11 URIC ACID KIDNEY
592.9 URINARY
594.9 URINARY TRACT LOWER UNSPECIFIED
594.8 URINARY TRACT LOWER OTHER
623.8 VAGINA
594.1 VESICAL (IMPACTED)
527.5 WHARTON'S DUCT

916.8 CALF INJURY OTHER AND UNSPECIFIED SUPERFICIAL

916.9 CALF INJURY OTHER AND UNSPECIFIED SUPERFICIAL INFECTED

0 CALIFORNIA DISEASE SEE 'COCCIDIOIDOMYCOSIS'

062.5 CALIFORNIA VIRUS ENCEPHALITIS

371.03 CALIGO CORNEA

700 CALLUS

732.1 CALVE-LEGG-PERTHES SYNDROME (OSTEOCHONDROSIS FEMORAL CAPITAL)

732.1 CALVE (-PERTHES) OSTEOCHONDROSIS FEMORAL CAPITAL

755.59 CAMPTODACTYLY (CONGENITAL)

008.43 CAMPYLOBACTER INFECTION INTESTINE

756.59 CAMURATI-ENGELMANN DIAPHYSEAL SCLEROSIS

752.8 CANAL OF NUCK DEFORMITY

C

375.31 CANALICULITIS LACRIMAL ACUTE
375.41 CANALICULITIS LACRIMAL CHRONIC
743.65 CANALICULUS LACRIMALIS ABSENCE CONGENITAL
330.0 CANAVAN'S DISEASE

CANCER SITE UNSPECIFIED
199.1 OR BY MORPHOLOGY
199.1 METASTATIC

CANCER
195.2 ABDOMEN CAVITY, ORGAN VISCERA, ILL- DEFINED (NON GI)
198.89 ABDOMEN CAVITY, ORGAN VISCERA, ILL- DEFINED (NON GI) METASTATIC
173.5 ABDOMEN SKIN
198.2 ABDOMEN SKIN METASTATIC
173.5 ABDOMEN WALL ILL-DEFINED
198.2 ABDOMEN WALL ILL-DEFINED METASTATIC
171.5 ABDOMEN WALL SOFT TISSUE
198.89 ABDOMEN WALL SOFT TISSUE METASTATIC

195.8 ABDOMINOPELVIC
198.89 ABDOMINOPELVIC METASTATIC

160.9 ACCESSORY SINUS
197.3 ACCESSORY SINUS METASTATIC

170.4 ACROMION
198.5 ACROMION METASTATIC

147.1 ADENOID
198.89 ADENOID METASTATIC

183.9 ADNEXA (UTERINE) NEC
198.82 ADNEXA (UTERINE) NEC METASTATIC
183.8 ADNEXA (UTERINE) OTHER SPECIFIED SITES
183.8 ADNEXA (UTERINE) OVERLAPPING SITES

194.0 ADRENAL CORTEX
194.0 ADRENAL GLAND
194.0 ADRENAL MEDULLA
198.7 ADRENAL METASTATIC

159.9 ALIMENTRY CANAL ILL-DEFINED
197.8 ALIMENTRY TRACT ILL-DEFINED METASTATIC

143.9 ALVEOLAR (ALVEOLUS) NOS
198.89 ALVEOLAR (ALVEOLUS) NOS METASTATIC
143.9 ALVEOLAR (ALVEOLUS) MUCOSA NOS
143.1 ALVEOLAR (ALVEOLUS) MUCOSA LOWER
198.89 ALVEOLAR (ALVEOLUS) MUCOSA METASTATIC
143.0 ALVEOLAR (ALVEOLUS) MUCOSA UPPER
170.1 ALVEOLAR RIDGE OR PROCESS (UPPER OR LOWER) (ODONTOGENIC)
198.5 ALVEOLAR RIDGE OR PROCESS (UPPER OR LOWER) (ODONTOGENIC) METASTATIC

IF ENCOUNTER IS FOR CHEMOTHERAPY OR RADIOTHERAPY, SEQUENCE THE CHEMO OR RADIOTHERAPY FIRST, WITH THE CANCER AS AN ADDITIONAL CODE.

156.2 AMPULLA OF VATER
197.8 AMPULLA OF VATER METASTATIC

159.1 ANGIOSARCOMA OF SPLEEN

170.8 ANKLE BONE
198.5 ANKLE BONE METASTATIC
173.7 ANKLE SKIN
198.2 ANKLE SKIN METASTATIC

154.8 ANORECTUM
197.5 ANORECTUM METASTATIC

164.2 ANTERIOR MEDIASTINUM
197.1 ANTERIOR MEDIASTINUM METASTATIC

CANCER (continued)
160.2 ANTRUM MAXILLARY (HIGHMORE)
197.3 ANTRUM MAXILLARY (HIGHMORE) METASTATIC
151.2 ANTRUM PYLORIC
197.8 ANTRUM PYLORIC METASTATIC
160.1 ANTRUM TYMPANICUM
197.3 ANTRUM TYMPANICUM METASTATIC

154.3 ANUS NOS
197.5 ANUS NOS METASTATIC
154.2 ANUS CANAL
197.5 ANUS CANAL METASTATIC
173.5 ANUS CANAL SKIN
172.5 ANUS CANAL SKIN MELANOMA
198.2 ANUS CANAL SKIN METASTAIC
V10.06 ANUS HISTORY OF MALIGNANT NEOPLASM
172.5 ANUS MARGIN MELANOMA
173.5 ANUS SKIN
198.2 ANUS SKIN METASTATIC
154.2 ANUS SPHINCTER
197.5 ANUS SPHINCTER METASTATIC
173.5 ANUS SPHINCTER SKIN
172.5 ANUS SPHINCTER SKIN MELANOMA
198.2 ANUS SPHINCTER SKIN METASTATIC
154.8 ANUS UNDETERMINED ORIGIN OVERLAPPING

194.6 AORTIC BODY
198.89 AORTIC BODY METASTATIC

153.5 APPENDIX
197.5 APPENDIX METASTATIC

174.0 AREOLA FEMALE SOFT TISSUE
175.0 AREOLA MALE SOFT TISSUE
198.81 AREOLA METASTATIC

173.6 ARM SKIN
198.2 ARM SKIN METASTATIC
171.2 ARM SOFT TISSUE
198.89 ARM SOFT TISSUE METASTATIC

170.9 ARTICULAR CARTILAGE
198.5 ARTICULAR CARTILAGE METASTATIC

148.2 ARYEPIGLOTTIC FOLD NOS (HYPOPHARYNGEAL) (MARGINAL ZONE)
198.89 ARYEPIGLOTTIC FOLD NOS (HYPOPHARYNGEAL) (MARGINAL ZONE) METASTATIC
161.1 ARYEPIGLOTTIC FOLD LARYNGEAL ASPECT
197.3 ARYEPIGLOTTIC FOLD LARYNGEAL ASPECT METASTATIC

161.3 ARYTENOID CARTILAGE
197.3 ARYTENOID CARTILAGE METASTATIC

170.8 ASTRAGALUS
198.5 ASTRAGALUS METASTATIC

147.2 AUDITORY TUBE OPENING
198.89 AUDITORY TUBE OPENING METASTATIC

195.1 AXILLA ILL-DEFINED
198.89 AXILLA ILL-DEFINED METASTATIC
196.3 AXILLA NODES METASTATIC
171.4 AXILLA SOFT TISSUE
198.89 AXILLA SOFT TISSUE METASTATIC

195.8 BACK ILL-DEFINED
198.89 BACK ILL-DEFINED METASTATIC
173.5 BACK SKIN
198.2 BACK SKIN METASTATIC

WHEN ENCOUNTER IS FOR PLACEMENT OF RADIOACTIVE IMPLANTS, USE THE CODE FOR THE CANCER, RATHER THAN THE "ENCOUNTER FOR" V-CODES.

171.7 BACK SOFT TISSUE
198.89 BACK SOFT TISSUE METASTATIC

184.1 BARTHOLIN GLAND
198.82 BARTHOLIN GLAND METASTATIC

191.0 BASAL GANGLIA
198.3 BASAL GANGLIA METASTATIC

156.1 BILE DUCT COMMON
156.1 BILE DUCT CYSTIC
156.1 BILE DUCT EXTRAHEPATIC
156.1 BILE DUCT HEPATIC
155.1 BILE DUCT INTRAHEPATIC
156.9 BILE DUCT INTRAHEPATIC AND EXTRAHEPATIC
197.8 BILE DUCT METASTATIC

155.1 BILIARY CANALICULI INTRAHEPATIC
155.1 BILIARY CANALS INTERLOBULAR
155.1 BILIARY GALL DUCT INTRAHEPATIC
197.8 BILIARY METASTATIC
156.1 BILIARY PASSAGES NOS
155.1 BILIARY PASSAGES INTRAHEPATIC
156.9 BILARY TRACT

188.9 BLADDER
188.3 BLADDER ANTERIOR WALL
188.1 BLADDER DOME
V10.51 BLADDER HISTORY
188.2 BLADDER LATERAL WALL
198.1 BLADDER METASTATIC
188.5 BLADDER NECK
188.4 BLADDER POSTERIOR WALL
188.0 BLADDER TRIGONE
188.7 BLADDER URACHUS
188.5 BLADDER URETHRAL ORIFICE
188.9 BLADDER WALL NOS
188.8 BLADDER OTHER SPECIFIED SITES

171.# BLOOD VESSEL

4th Digit: 171

- **0. HEAD FACE NECK**
- **2. UPPER LIMB LIMB SHOULDER**
- **3. LOWER LIMB HIP**
- **4. THORAX**
- **5. ABDOMINAL HYPOCHONDRIUM**
- **6. PELVIS BUTTOCK GROIN INGUINAL REGION PERINEUM**
- **7. TRUNK NOS BACK NOS FLANK NOS**
- **8. OTHER SPECIFIED SITES**
- **9. SITE NOS**

198.89 BLOOD VESSEL METASTATIC

170.# BONE AND ARTICULAR CARTILAGE

4th Digit: 170

- **0. SKULL AND FACE**
- **1. MANDIBLE (OF IF SITE UNSPECIFIED)**
- **2. VERTEBRAL COLUMN**
- **3. RIBS STERNUM CLAVICLE**
- **4. SCAPULA LONG BONES UPPER LIMB**
- **5. SHORT BONES UPPER LIMB**
- **6. PELVIC BONES SACRUM COCCYX**
- **7. LONG BONES LOWER LIMB**
- **8. SHORT BONES LOWER LIMB**
- **9. SITE NOS**

198.5 BONE AND ARTICULAR CARTILAGE METASTATIC

170.9 BONE NOS
198.5 BONE NOS METASTATIC
170.8 BONE CUBOID
198.5 BONE CUBOID METASTATIC
170.5 BONE HANDS
198.5 BONE HANDS METASTATIC
V10.81 BONE HISTORY OF MALIGNANT NEOPLASM
170.9 BONE LIMB NOS
198.5 BONE LIMB NOS METASTATIC
170.7 BONE LOWER LIMB LONG BONES

CANCER (continued)

SYMPTOMS OF A MALIGNANCY SUCH AS PAIN OR NAUSEA, SHOULD NOT REPLACE THE CANCER CODE. SEQUENCE THE CANCER FIRST.

170.8 BONE LOWER LIMB SHORT BONES
198.5 BONE LOWER LIMB SHORT OR LONG METASTATIC
170.1 BONE MANDIBLE (ODONTOGENIC)
198.5 BONE MANDIBLE METASTATIC
202.90 BONE MARROW
198.5 BONE MARROW METASTATIC
170.0 BONE MAXILLA (ODONTOGENIC)
198.5 BONE MAXILLA (ODONTOGENIC) METASTATIC
198.5 BONE OR MARROW METASTATIC
170.8 BONE PATELLA
198.5 BONE PATELLA METASTATIC
170.3 BONE RIBS STERNUM
198.5 BONE RIBS STERNUM METASTATIC
170.0 BONE SKULL
198.5 BONE SKULL METASTATIC
170.2 BONE SPINE
198.5 BONE SPINE METASTATIC
170.4 BONE UPPER LIMB LONG BONES
170.5 BONE UPPER LIMB SHORT BONES
198.5 BONE UPPER LIMB SHORT OR LONG BONES METASTATIC
170.2 BONE VERTEBRA
198.5 BONE VERTEBRA METASTATIC

196.3 BRACHIAL NODES METASTATIC

191.9 BRAIN NOS
198.3 BRAIN NOS METASTATIC
191.6 BRAIN CEREBELLUM
198.3 BRAIN CEREBELLUM METASTATIC
191.0 BRAIN CEREBRUM (EXCEPT LOBES OR VENTRICLES)
198.3 BRAIN CEREBRUM (EXCEPT LOBES OR VENTRICLES) METASTATIC
191.1 BRAIN CEREBRUM FRONTAL LOBE
198.3 BRAIN CEREBRUM FRONTAL LOBE METASTATIC
191.4 BRAIN CEREBRUM OCCIPITAL LOBE
198.3 BRAIN CEREBRUM OCCIPITAL LOBE METASTATIC
191.3 BRAIN CEREBRUM PARIETAL LOBE
198.3 BRAIN CEREBRUM PARIETAL LOBE METASTATIC
191.2 BRAIN CEREBRUM TEMPORAL LOBE
198.3 BRAIN CEREBRUM TEMPORAL LOBE METASTATIC
V10.85 BRAIN HISTORY OF MALIGNANT NEOPLASM
191.8 BRAIN OVERLAPPING SITES
191.7 BRAIN STEM
198.3 BRAIN STEM METASTATIC
191.5 BRAIN VENTRICLES
198.3 BRAIN VENTRICLES METASTATIC
191.8 BRAIN OTHER PARTS
198.3 BRAIN OTHER PARTS METASTATIC

146.8 BRANCHIAL CLEFT
198.89 BRANCHIAL CLEFT METASTATIC

WHEN BOTH A PRIMARY AND SECONDARY SITE ARE PRESENT AND TREATED EQUALLY, SEQUENCE THE PRIMARY SITE FIRST.

174.# BREAST FEMALE CONNECTIVE SOFT TISSUE

4th Digit: 174

- **0. NIPPLE AND AREOLA**
- **1. CENTRAL PORTION**
- **2. UPPER INNER QUADRANT**
- **3. LOWER INNER QUADRANT**
- **4. UPPER OUTER QUADRANT**
- **5. LOWER OUTER QUADRANT**
- **6. AXILLARY TAIL**
- **8. MASTECTOMY SITE, INNER LOWER MIDLINE OUTER UPPER ECTOPIC SITES CONTIGUOUS OVERLAPPING SITES UNDETERMINED**
- **9. BREAST (FEMALE) SITE NOS**

198.81 BREAST FEMALE CONNECTIVE SOFT TISSUE METASTATIC
V16.3 BREAST HISTORY FAMILY OF MALIGNANT NEOPLASM
V10.3 BREAST HISTORY PERSONAL OF MALIGNANT NEOPLASM

C

CANCER (continued)

175.9 BREAST MALE NOS OR ECTOPIC TISSUE
198.81 BREAST MALE NOS OR ECTOPIC TISSUE METASTATIC
175.0 BREAST MALE AREOLA
198.81 BREAST MALE AREOLA METASTATIC
175.0 BREAST MALE NIPPLE
198.81 BREAST MALE NIPPLE METASTATIC
175.0 BREAST MALE SOFT TISSUE
198.81 BREAST MALE SOFT TISSUE METASTATIC
173.5 BREAST SKIN
173.5 BREAST SKIN MASTECTOMY SITE
198.2 BREAST SKIN METASTATIC
174.8 BREAST TISSUE MASTECTOMY SITE
198.81 BREAST TISSUE MASTECTOMY SITE, METASTATIC

183.3 BROAD LIGAMENT
198.82 BROAD LIGAMENT MESTASTATIC

196.1 BRONCHOPULMONARY NODES METASTATIC

162.9 BRONCHUS
V16.1 BRONCHUS HISTORY FAMILY OF MALIGNANT NEOPLASM
V10.11 BRONCHUS HISTORY PERSONAL OF MALIGNANT NEOPLASM
162.5 BRONCHUS LOWER LOBE
162.2 BRONCHUS MAIN BRONCHUS
197.0 BRONCHUS METASTATIC
162.4 BRONCHUS MIDDLE LOBE
162.8 BRONCHUS UNDETERMINED ORIGIN
162.3 BRONCHUS UPPER LOBE

145.9 BUCCAL CAVITY NOS
198.89 BUCCAL METASTATIC
145.0 BUCCAL MUCOSA
145.1 BUCCAL SULCUS (UPPER) (LOWER)

171.# BURSA

4th Digit: 171

- **0. HEAD FACE NECK**
- **2. UPPER LIMB SHOULDER**
- **3. LOWER LIMB HIP**
- **4. THORAX**
- **5. ABDOMINAL HYPOCHONDRIUM**
- **6. PELVIS BUTTOCK GROIN INGUINAL REGION PERINEUM**
- **7. TRUNK NOS BACK NOS FLANK NOS**
- **8. OTHER SPECIFIED SITES**
- **9. SITE NOS**

198.89 BURSA METASTATIC

173.5 BUTTOCKS SKIN
198.2 BUTTOCKS SKIN METASTATIC
171.6 BUTTOCKS SOFT TISSUE
198.89 BUTTOCKS SOFT TISSUE METASTATIC

170.8 CALCANEOUS
198.5 CALCANEOUS METASTATIC

155.1 CANALICULI BILIFERI
197.8 CANALICULI BILIFERI METASTATIC

173.1 CANTHUS SKIN
198.2 CANTHUS SKIN METASTATIC

IF TREATMENT IS DIRECTED TOWARDS THE METASTATIC SITE, THEN THAT SITE IS CODED FIRST, EVEN IF THE PRIMARY SITE IS KNOWN.

199.1 CARCINOMA
199.0 CARCINOMATOSIS

151.0 CARDIA (GASTRIC)
197.8 CARDIA (GASTRIC) METASTATIC

164.1 CARDIAC
198.89 CARDIAC METASTATIC

151.0 CARDIAC ORIFICE (STOMACH)
197.8 CARDIAC ORIFICE (STOMACH) METASTATIC

CANCER (continued)

151.0 CARDIO-ESOPHAGEAL JUNCTION
197.8 CARDIO-ESOPHAGEAL JUNCTION METASTATIC

162.2 CARINA
197.0 CARINA - BRONCHUS METASTATIC
197.3 CARINA - TRACHEA METASTATIC

194.5 CAROTID BODY
198.89 CAROTID BODY METASTATIC

170.5 CARPAL BONE
198.5 CARPAL BONE METASTATIC

192.2 CAUDA EQUINA
198.3 CAUDA EQUINA METASTATIC

192.9 CENTRAL NERVOUS SYSTEM
198.4 CENTRAL NERVOUS SYSTEM METASTATIC

191.6 CEREBELLOPONTINE ANGLE
198.3 CEREBELLOPONTINE ANGLE METASTATIC

191.6 CEREBELLUM
198.3 CEREBELLUM METASTATIC

191.0 CEREBRAL CORTEX
198.3 CEREBRAL CORTEX METASTATIC
192.1 CEREBRAL MENINGES
198.4 CEREBRAL MENINGES METASTATIC
191.7 CEREBRAL PEDUNCLE
198.3 CEREBRAL PEDUNCLE METASTATIC

191.1 CEREBRUM FRONTAL LOBE
198.3 CEREBRUM FRONTAL LOBE METASTATIC
191.4 CEREBRUM OCCIPITAL LOBE
198.3 CEREBRUM OCCIPITAL LOBE METASTATIC
191.3 CEREBRUM PARIETAL LOBE
198.3 CEREBRUM PARIETAL LOBE METASTATIC
191.2 CEREBRUM TEMPORAL LOBE
198.3 CEREBRUM TEMPORAL LOBE METASTATIC

196.0 CERVICAL NODES METASTATIC
196.0 CERVICOFACIAL NODES METASTATIC

180.9 CERVIX
180.0 CERVIX CANAL
180.0 CERVIX ENDOCERVIX
180.1 CERVIX EXOCERVIX
V10.41 CERVIX HISTORY OF MALIGNANT NEOPLASM
198.82 CERVIX METASTATIC
180.8 CERVIX SQUAMOCOLUMNAR JUNCTION
180.8 CERVIX STUMP
180.8 CERVIX OTHER SPECIFIED SITES

195.0 CHEEK ILL-DEFINED
145.0 CHEEK INNER ASPECT
198.89 CHEEK INNER ASPECT OR ILL-DEFINED METASTATIC
173.3 CHEEK SKIN (EXTERNAL)
198.2 CHEEK SKIN (EXTERNAL) METASTATIC

195.1 CHEST WALL ILL-DEFINED
198.89 CHEST WALL ILL-DEFINED METASTATIC
173.5 CHEST WALL SKIN
198.2 CHEST WALL SKIN METASTATIC

173.3 CHIN SKIN
198.2 CHIN SKIN METASTATIC

147.3 CHOANAE POSTERIOR MARGIN
198.89 CHOANAE POSTERIOR MARGIN METASTATIC

181 CHORIOCARCINOMA
186.9 CHORIOCARCINOMA MALE
181 CHORIOEPITHELIOMA

CANCER (continued)

190.6	CHOROID
198.4	CHOROID METASTATIC
191.5	CHOROID PLEXUS
198.3	CHOROID PLEXUS METASTATIC
190.0	CILIARY BODY
198.4	CILIARY BODY METASTATIC
170.3	CLAVICLE
198.5	CLAVICLE METASTATIC
184.3	CLITORIS
198.82	CLITORIS METASTATIC
154.8	CLOACOGENIC ZONE
197.5	CLOACOGENIC ZONE METASTATIC
192.9	CNS
198.4	CNS METASTATIC
194.6	COCCYGEAL BODY
198.89	COCCYGEAL BODY METASTATIC
170.6	COCCYX
198.5	COCCYX METASTATIC
153.9	COLON
153.5	COLON APPENDIX
153.6	COLON ASCENDING
153.4	COLON CECUM
153.2	COLON DESCENDING
V16.0	COLON FAMILY HISTORY OF MALIGNANT NEOPLASM
153.0	COLON HEPATIC FLEXURE
153.4	COLON ILEOCECAL VALVE
153.2	COLON LEFT
197.5	COLON METASTATIC
154.0	COLON RECTOSIGMOID
153.6	COLON RIGHT
153.3	COLON SIGMOID
153.7	COLON SPLENIC FLEXURE
153.1	COLON TRANSVERSE
153.8	COLON UNDETERMINED SITE
154.0	COLON WITH RECTUM
153.8	COLON OTHER SPECIFIED SITE
156.1	COMMON DUCT
197.8	COMMON DUCT METASTATIC
190.3	CONJUNCTIVA
198.4	CONJUNCTIVA METASTATIC
171.#	CONNECTIVE TISSUE

4th Digit: 171

0. HEAD FACE NECK
2. UPPER LIMB SHOULDER
3. LOWER LIMB HIP
4. THORAX
5. ABDOMINAL HYPOCHONDRIUM
6. PELVIS BUTTOCK GROIN INGUINAL REGION PERINEUM
7. TRUNK NOS BACK NOS FLANK NOS
8. OTHER SPECIFIED SITES
9. SITE NOS

198.89	CONNECTIVE TISSUE METASTATIC
190.4	CORNEA
198.4	CORNEA METASTATIC
182.0	CORNU
198.82	CORNU METASTATIC
191.8	CORPUS CALLOSUM
198.3	CORPUS CALLOSUM METASTATIC
187.3	CORPUS CAVERNOSUM
198.82	CORPUS CAVERNOSUM METASTATIC
191.0	CORPUS STRIATUM
198.3	CORPUS STRIATUM METASTATIC

IF ENCOUNTER IS FOR CHEMOTHERAPY OR RADIOTHERAPY AND A COMPLICATION OF THE THERAPY DEVELOPS, SEQUENCE THE THERAPY FIRST, THE COMPLICATION SECOND, THEN THE CANCER.

CANCER (continued)

170.3	COSTAL CARTILAGE
198.5	COSTAL CARTILAGE METASTATIC
170.3	COSTOVERTEBRAL JOINT
198.5	COSTOVERTEBRAL JOINT METASTATIC
191.9	CRANIAL FOSSA
198.3	CRANIAL FOSSA METASTATIC
192.0	CRANIAL NERVES
198.4	CRANIAL NERVES METASTATIC
194.3	CRANIOBUCCAL POUCH
198.89	CRANIOBUCCAL POUCH METASTATIC
194.3	CRANIOPHARYNGEAL TRACT
198.89	CRANIOPHARYNGEAL TRACT METASTATIC
161.3	CRICOID CARTILAGE
197.3	CRICOID CARTILAGE METASTATIC
190.0	CRYSTALLINE LENS
198.4	CRYSTALLINE LENS METASTATIC
170.8	CUBOID
198.5	CUBOID METASTATIC
158.8	CUL DE SAC (DOUGLAS)
197.6	CUL DE SAC (DOUGLAS) METASTATIC
170.8	CUNEIFORM ANKLE
198.5	CUNEIFORM ANKLE METASTATIC
161.3	CUNEIFORM CARTILAGE
197.3	CUNEIFORM CARTILAGE METASTATIC
170.5	CUNEIFORM WRIST
198.5	CUNEIFORM WRIST METASTATIC
156.1	CYSTIC DUCT
197.8	CYSTIC DUCT METASTATIC
171.4	DIAPHRAGM
198.89	DIAPHRAGM METASTATIC
159.8	DIGESTIVE ORGAN SITES NEC
197.8	DIGESTIVE ORGAN SITES NEC METASTATIC
199.0	DISSEMINATED
199.0	DISSEMINATED METASATIC
157.3	DUCT OF SANTORINI
197.8	DUCT OF SANTORINI METASTATIC
157.3	DUCT OF WIRSUNG
197.8	DUCT OF WIRSUNG METASTATIC
152.8	DUODENOJEJUNAL JUNCTION
197.4	DUODENOJEJUNAL JUNCTION METASTATIC
152.0	DUODENUM
197.4	DUODENUM METASTATIC
192.1	DURA (MATER)
198.4	DURA (MATER) METASTATIC
171.0	EAR CARTILAGE
198.89	EAR CARTILAGE METASTATIC
V10.22	EAR MIDDLE HISTORY OF MALIGNANT NEOPLASM
173.2	EAR SKIN
198.2	EAR SKIN METASTATIC
164.1	ENDOCARDIUM
198.89	ENDOCARDIUM METASTATIC
180.0	ENDOCERVICAL CANAL
180.0	ENDOCERVICAL GLAND
198.82	ENDOCERVICAL METASTATIC

CANCER (continued)

194.9	ENDOCRINE GLAND
198.89	ENDOCRINE GLAND METASTATIC
157.4	ENDOCRINE ISLETS LANGERHANS
197.8	ENDOCRINE ISLETS LANGERHANS METASTATIC
183.0	ENDOCRINE OVARY
198.6	ENDOCRINE OVARY METASTATIC

IF TREATMENT IS DIRECTED TOWARD THE METASTATIC SITE, THEN THAT SITE IS CODED FIRST, EVEN IF THE PRIMARY SITE IS KNOWN.

186.9	ENDOCRINE TESTIS DESCENDED
198.82	ENDOCRINE TESTIS METASTATIC
186.0	ENDOCRINE TESTIS UNDESCENDED
164.0	ENDOCRINE THYMUS
198.89	ENDOCRINE THYMUS METASTATIC
194.8	ENDOCRINE OTHER AND MULTIPLE GLANDS
198.89	ENDOCRINE OTHER AND MULTIPLE GLANDS METASTATIC
182.0	ENDOMETRIUM
198.82	ENDOMETRIUM METASTATIC
164.1	EPICARDIUM
198.89	EPICARDIUM METASTATIC
187.5	EPIDIDYMIS
V10.48	EPIDIDYMIS HISTORY OF MALIGNANT NEOPLASM
198.82	EPIDIDYMIS METASTATIC
161.1	EPIGLOTTIS NOS
197.3	EPIGLOTTIS NOS METASTATIC
146.4	EPIGLOTTIS ANTERIOR ONLY OROPHARYNX
198.89	EPIGLOTTIS ANTERIOR ONLY OROPHARYNX METASTATIC
146.4	EPIGLOTTIS FREE BORDER (MARGIN)
198.89	EPIGLOTTIS FREE BORDER (MARGIN) METASTATIC
161.1	EPIGLOTTIS POSTERIOR
197.3	EPIGLOTTIS POSTERIOR METASTATIC
161.1	EPIGLOTTIS SUPRAHYOID PORTION OR NOS
197.3	EPIGLOTTIS SUPRAHYOID PORTION OR NOS METASTATIC
196.3	EPITROCHLEAR NODES METASTATIC
150.9	ESOPHAGUS
150.2	ESOPHAGUS ABDOMINAL SEGMENT
151.0	ESOPHAGUS ABDOMINAL SEGMENT ADENOCARCINOMA
151.0	ESOPHAGUS CARDIOESOPHAGEAL
150.0	ESOPHAGUS CERVICAL SEGMENT
150.5	ESOPHAGUS DISTAL THIRD
V10.03	ESOPHAGUS HISTORY OF MALIGNANT NEOPLASM
150.5	ESOPHAGUS LOWER THIRD
151.0	ESOPHAGUS LOWER THIRD ADENOCARCINOMA
197.8	ESOPHAGUS METASTATIC
150.4	ESOPHAGUS MIDDLE THIRD
150.8	ESOPHAGUS OVERLAPPING SITES
150.3	ESOPHAGUS PROXIMAL THIRD
150.1	ESOPHAGUS THORACIC SEGMENT
150.3	ESOPHAGUS UPPER THIRD
150.8	ESOPHAGUS OTHER SPECIFIED
170.0	ETHMOID BONE (CARTILAGE) (JOINT) (PERIOSTEUM)
198.5	ETHMOID BONE (CARTILAGE) (JOINT) (PERIOSTEUM) METASTATIC
160.3	ETHMOID SINUS
197.3	ETHMOID SINUS METASTATIC
160.1	EUSTACHIAN TUBE
197.3	EUSTACHIAN TUBE METASTATIC
V71.1	EVALUATION NONE FOUND
173.2	EXTERNAL AUDITORY CANAL SKIN
198.2	EXTERNAL AUDITORY CANAL SKIN METASTATIC
156.1	EXTRAHEPATIC BILE DUCT
156.2	EXTRAHEPATIC BILE DUCT AMPULLA OF VATER
197.8	EXTRAHEPATIC BILE DUCT METASTATIC
190.1	EXTRAOCULAR MUSCLE
198.4	EXTRAOCULAR MUSCLE METASTATIC

CANCER (continued)

SYMPTOMS OF A MALIGNANCY SUCH AS PAIN OR NAUSEA, SHOULD NOT REPLACE THE CANCER CODE. SEQUENCE THE CANCER FIRST

190.# EYE

4th Digit: 190

0. EYEBALL
1. ORBIT SOFT TISSUE
2 LACRIMAL GLAND
3. CONJUNCTIVA
4. CORNEA
5. RETINA
6. CHOROID
7. LACRIMAL DUCT
8. OTHER SPECIFIED OR OVERLAPPING
9. NOS

V10.84	EYE HISTORY OF MALIGNANT NEOPLASM
190.0	EYE LENS
198.4	EYE METASTATIC
170.0	EYE ORBIT BONE
198.5	EYE ORBIT BONE METASTATIC
190.1	EYE ORBIT CONNECTIVE TISSUE
190.8	EYE UNDETERMINED SITE
190.8	EYE OTHER SPECIFIED SITES
190.0	EYEBALL (INTERNAL STRUCTURES)
190.0	EYEBALL CILIARY BODY
198.4	EYEBALL METASTATIC
173.3	EYEBROW SKIN
198.2	EYEBROW SKIN METASTATIC
171.0	EYELID CARTILAGE
198.89	EYELID CARTILAGE METASTATIC
173.1	EYELID SKIN
198.2	EYELID SKIN METASTATIC
195.0	FACE ILL-DEFINED
198.89	FACE ILL-DEFINED METASTATIC
173.3	FACE SKIN OTHER UNSPECIFIED PARTS
198.2	FACE SKIN OTHER UNSPECIFIED PARTS METASTATIC
170.0	FACIAL BONES
198.5	FACIAL BONES METASTATIC
183.2	FALLOPIAN TUBE
198.82	FALLOPIAN TUBE METASTATIC
161.1	FALSE CORDS
197.3	FALSE CORDS METASTATIC
192.1	FALX (CEREBELLI) (CEREBRI)
198.4	FALX (CEREBELLI) (CEREBRI) METASTATIC
0	FAMILY HISTORY SEE 'FAMILY' HISTORY
171.#	FASCIA
198.89	FASCIA METASTATIC
171.#	FAT

4th Digit: 171

0. HEAD FACE NECK
2. UPPER LIMB SHOULDER
3. LOWER LIMB HIP
4. THORAX
5. ABDOMINAL HYPOCHONDRIUM
6. PELVIS BUTTOCK GROIN INGUINAL REGION PERINEUM
7. TRUNK NOS BACK NOS FLANK NOS
8. OTHER SPECIFIED SITES
9. SITE NOS

198.89	FAT METASTATIC
196.5	FEMORAL LYMPH NODES METASTATIC
170.7	FEMUR
198.5	FEMUR METASTATIC

170.7 FIBULA
198.5 FIBULA METASTATIC

173.6 FINGER SKIN
198.2 FINGER SKIN METASTATIC
171.2 FINGER SOFT TISSUE
198.89 FINGER SOFT TISSUE METASTATIC

195.8 FLANK ILL-DEFINED
198.89 FLANK METASTATIC
171.7 FLANK SOFT TISSUE

170.8 FOOT BONE
198.5 FOOT BONE METASTATIC
173.7 FOOT SKIN
198.2 FOOT SKIN METASTATIC
171.3 FOOT SOFT TISSUE
198.89 FOOT SOFT TISSUE METASTATIC

173.6 FOREARM SKIN
198.2 FOREARM SKIN METASTATIC
171.2 FOREARM SOFT TISSUE
198.89 FOREARM SOFT TISSUE METASTATIC

173.3 FOREHEAD SKIN
198.2 FOREHEAD SKIN METASTATIC

187.1 FORESKIN
198.82 FORESKIN METASTATIC

147.2 FOSSA OF ROSENMULLER
198.89 FOSSA OF ROSENMULLER METASTATIC

170.0 FRONTAL BONE (CARTILAGE) (JOINT) (PERIOSTEUM)
198.5 FRONTAL BONE (CARTILAGE) (JOINT) (PERIOSTEUM) METASTATIC
191.1 FRONTAL LOBE
198.3 FRONTAL LOBE METASTATIC
160.4 FRONTAL SINUS
197.3 FRONTAL SINUS METASTATIC

182.0 FUNDUS UTERINE
198.82 FUNDUS UTERINE METASTATIC

156.0 GALLBLADDER
156.8 GALLBLADDER EXTRA HEPATIC DUCTS (OVERLAPPING)
197.8 GALLBLADDER METASTATIC

156.1 GALL DUCT EXTRAHEPATIC
155.1 GALL DUCT INTRAHEPATIC
197.8 GALL DUCT METASTATIC

171.# GANGLIA

4th Digit: 171

- **0. HEAD FACE NECK**
- **2. UPPER LIMB SHOULDER**
- **3. LOWER LIMB HIP**
- **4. THORAX**
- **5. ABDOMINAL HYPOCHONDRIUM**
- **6. PELVIS BUTTOCK GROIN INGUINAL REGION PERINEUM**
- **7. TRUNK NOS BACK NOS FLANK NOS**
- **8. OTHER SPECIFIED SITES**
- **9. SITE NOS**

198.89 GANGLIA METASTATIC

192.0 GANGLIA CRANIAL
198.4 GANGLIA CRANIAL METASTATIC

184.0 GARTNER'S DUCT
198.82 GARTNER'S DUCT METASTATIC

CANCER (continued)

> *IF TREATMENT IS DIRECTED TOWARD THE METASTATIC SITE, THEN THAT SITE IS CODED FIRST, EVEN IF THE PRIMARY SITE IS KNOWN.*

151.9 GASTRIC
151.4 GASTRIC BODY
151.0 GASTRIC CARDIAC ORIFICE
150.2 GASTRIC CARDIAC ORIFICE SQUAMOUS CELL
151.0 GASTRIC CARDIOESOPHAGEAL JUNCTION
150.5 GASTRIC CARDIOESOPHAGEAL JUNCTION SQUAMOUS CELL
151.3 GASTRIC FUNDUS
151.6 GASTRIC GREATER CURVATURE
151.5 GASTRIC LESSER CURVATURE
197.8 GASTRIC METASTATIC
151.8 GASTRIC OVERLAPPING UNDETERMINED
151.2 GASTRIC PYLORIC ANTRUM
151.1 GASTRIC PYLORUS

159.9 GASTROINTESTINAL TRACT
V16.0 GASTROINTESTINAL TRACT HISTORY FAMILY OF MALIGNANT NEOPLASM
V10.00 GASTROINTESTINAL TRACT HISTORY PERSONAL OF MALIGNANT NEOPLASM
197.8 GASTROINTESTINAL TRACT METASTATIC

199.0 GENERALIZED CANCER UNSPECIFIED SITE

V10.40 GENITAL ORGANS FEMALE HISTORY PERSONAL OF MALIGNANT NEOPLASM
184.8 GENITAL ORGANS FEMALE OTHER SPECIFIED SITE
184.9 GENITAL ORGANS FEMALE SITE NOS
V16.40 GENITAL ORGANS FAMILY HISTORY NOS
V16.49 GENITAL ORGANS FAMILY HISTORY OTHER SPECIFIED ORGAN
187.9 GENITAL ORGANS MALE
198.82 GENITAL ORGANS METASTATIC

184.4 GENITALIA FEMALE EXTERNAL
198.82 GENITALIA FEMALE EXTERNAL METASTATIC

184.9 GENITOURINARY TRACT FEMALE NOS
198.82 GENITOURINARY TRACT FEMALE NOS METASTATIC

V16.0 GI TRACT HISTORY FAMILY OF MALIGNANT NEOPLASM
V10.00 GI TRACT HISTORY PERSONAL OF MALIGNANT NEOPLASM

143.1 GINGIVA LOWER
198.89 GINGIVA METASTATIC
143.8 GINGIVA SITES OVERLAPPING
143.0 GINGIVA UPPER

187.2 GLANS PENIS
198.82 GLANS PENIS METASTATIC

191.0 GLOBUS PALLIDUS
198.3 GLOBUS PALLIDUS METASTATIC

194.6 GLOMUS JUGULARE
198.89 GLOMUS JUGULARE METASTATIC

146.4 GLOSSOEPIGLOTTIC FOLD
198.89 GLOSSOEPIGLOTTIC FOLD METASTATIC

146.2 GLOSSOPALATINE FOLD
198.89 GLOSSOPALATINE FOLD METASTATIC

161.0 GLOTTIS
161.0 GLOTTIS LARYNX
197.3 GLOTTIS METASTATIC

171.4 GREAT VESSELS
198.89 GREAT VESSELS METASTATIC

184.1 GREATER VESTIBULAR GLAND
198.82 GREATER VESTIBULAR GLAND METASTATIC

195.3 GROIN ILL-DEFINED
198.89 GROIN ILL-DEFINED METASTATIC
196.5 GROIN LYMPH NODES METASTATIC

CANCER (continued)

173.5	GROIN SKIN
198.2	GROIN SKIN METASTATIC
171.6	GROIN SOFT TISSUE
198.89	GROIN SOFT TISSUE METASTATIC
143.9	GUM
198.89	GUM METASTATIC
143.1	GUM LOWER
170.1	GUM LOWER JAW ODONTOGENIC
198.5	GUM LOWER JAW ODONTOGENIC METASTATIC
198.89	GUM LOWER METASTATIC
143.0	GUM UPPER
198.89	GUM UPPER METASTATIC
170.0	GUM UPPER JAW ODONTOGENIC
198.5	GUM UPPER JAW ODONTOGENESIS METASTATIC
143.8	GUM OTHER SITE
198.89	GUM OTHER SITE METASTATIC
170.5	HAND BONES
198.5	HAND BONES METASTATIC
173.6	HAND SKIN
198.2	HAND SKIN METASTATIC
171.2	HAND SOFT TISSUE
198.89	HAND SOFT TISSUE METASTATIC
145.2	HARD PALATE
198.89	HARD PALATE METASTATIC
195.0	HEAD ILL-DEFINED
198.89	HEAD ILL-DEFINED METASTATIC
164.1	HEART
198.89	HEART METASTATIC
156.1	HEPATIC DUCT
197.8	HEPATIC DUCT METASTATIC
153.0	HEPATIC FLEXURE
197.5	HEPATIC FLEXURE METASTATIC
155.0	HEPATOBLASTOMA PRIMARY
155.0	HEPATOCELLULAR PRIMARY
162.2	HILUS OF LUNG
197.0	HILUS OF LUNG METASTATIC
173.7	HIP SKIN
198.2	HIP SKIN METASTATIC
191.2	HIPPOCAMPUS
198.3	HIPPOCAMPUS METASTATIC
0	HISTORY SEE 'HISTORY'
170.4	HUMERUS
198.5	HUMERUS METASTATIC
171.5	HYPOCHONDRIUM SOFT TISSUE
198.89	HYPOCHONDRIUM SOFT TISSUE METASTATIC
196.6	HYPOGASTRIC NODES METASTATIC
148.9	HYPOPHARYNX
148.2	HYPOPHARYNX ARYEPIGLOTTIC FOLD
198.89	HYPOPHARYNX METASTATIC
148.0	HYPOPHARYNX POSTCRICOID REGION
148.3	HYPOPHARYNX POSTERIOR WALL
148.1	HYPOPHARYNX PYRIFORM SINUS
148.9	HYPOPHARYNX WALL NOS
148.8	HYPOPHARYNX OTHER SITES
194.3	HYPOPHYSIS
198.89	HYPOPHYSIS METASTATIC
191.0	HYPOTHALAMUS
198.3	HYPOTHALAMUS METASTATIC
152.2	ILEUM
153.4	ILEUM (ILEOCECAL VALVE)
197.4	ILEUM METASTATIC

CANCER (continued)

196.6	ILIAC NODES METASTATIC
170.6	ILIUM
198.5	ILIUM METASTATIC
203.8#	IMMUNOPROLIFERATIVE **5th Digit: 203.8** **0. WITHOUT MENTION OF REMISSION** **1. IN REMISSION**
196.3	INFRACLAVICULAR NODES METASTATIC
195.3	INGUINAL REGION ILL-DEFINED
198.89	INGUINAL REGION METASTATIC
171.6	INGUINAL REGION SOFT TISSUE
198.89	INGUINAL REGION SOFT TISSUE METASTATIC
196.1	INTERCOSTAL NODES METASTATIC
0	INTERDENTAL PAPILLAE SEE 'CANCER' GUM
196.2	INTESTINAL NODES METASTATIC
159.0	INTESTINAL TRACT
197.8	INTESTINAL TRACT METASTATIC
195.2	INTRA ABDOMINAL ILL-DEFINED (NON GI)
198.89	INTRA ABDOMINAL ILL-DEFINED (NON GI) METASTATIC
196.2	INTRA ABDOMINAL NODES METASTATIC
196.6	INTRAPELVIC NODES METASTATIC
195.1	INTRATHORACIC ILL-DEFINED
198.89	INTRATHORACIC ILL-DEFINED METASTATIC
196.1	INTRATHORACIC METASTATIC
163.9	INTRATHORACIC PLEURA
197.2	INTRATHORACIC PLEURA METASTATIC
163.0	INTRATHORACIC PLEURA PARIETAL
163.1	INTRATHORACIC PLEURA VISCERAL
163.8	INTRATHORACIC PLEURA UNDETERMINED
164.8	INTRATHORACIC THYMUS HEART MEDIASTINUM UNDETERMINED
190.0	IRIS
198.4	IRIS METASTATIC
170.6	ISCHIUM
198.5	ISCHIUM METASTATIC
170.1	JAW BONE
170.1	JAW BONE LOWER
198.5	JAW BONE METASTATIC
170.0	JAW BONE UPPER
195.0	JAW ILL-DEFINED
198.89	JAW ILL-DEFINED METASTATIC
152.1	JEJUNUM
197.4	JEJUNUM METASTATIC
189.0	KIDNEY
V16.51	KIDNEY HISTORY FAMILY OF MALIGNANT NEOPLASM
V10.52	KIDNEY HISTORY OF MALIGNANT NEOPLASM
198.0	KIDNEY METASTATIC
189.0	KIDNEY PARENCHYMA
189.9	KIDNEY URETER
173.7	KNEE (POPLITEAL) SKIN
198.2	KNEE (POPLITEAL) SKIN METASTATIC
184.1	LABIA MAJORA
198.82	LABIA METASTATIC
184.2	LABIA MINORA
140.6	LABIAL COMMISSURE
198.89	LABIAL COMMISSURE OR SULCUS METASTATIC
145.1	LABIAL SULCUS MOUTH (UPPER) (LOWER)
190.7	LACRIMAL DUCT
198.4	LACRIMAL DUCT METASTATIC
190.2	LACRIMAL GLAND
198.4	LACRIMAL GLAND METASTATIC
153.9	LARGE INTESTINE
V10.05	LARGE INTESTINE HISTORY OF MALIGNANT NEOPLASM
197.5	LARGE INTESTINE METASTATIC

CANCER (continued)

161.#	LARYNX
	4th Digit: 161
	0. GLOTTIC, COMMISSURE
	1. SUPRAGLOTTIC, AREYEPIGLOTTIC FOLD, FALSE CORDS
	2. SUBGLOTTIC
	3. CARTILAGE
	8. OTHER SPECIFIED SITES
	9. SITE UNSPECIFIED
V10.21	LARYNX HISTORY OF MALIGNANT NEOPLASM
197.3	LARYNX METASTATIC
173.7	LEG SKIN
198.2	LEG SKIN METASTATIC
171.3	LEG SOFT TISSUE
198.89	LEG SOFT TISSUE METASTATIC
182.0	LEIOMYOSARCOMA
190.0	LENS EYE
198.4	LENS EYE METASTATIC
171.#	LIGAMENT EXCEPT UTERINE
	4th Digit: 171
	0. HEAD FACE NECK
	2. UPPER LIMB SHOULDER
	3. LOWER LIMB HIP
	4. THORAX
	5. ABDOMINAL HYPOCHONDRIUM
	6. PELVIS BUTTOCK GROIN INGUINAL REGION PERINEUM
	7. TRUNK NOS BACK NOS FLANK NOS
	8. OTHER SPECIFIED SITES
	9. SITE NOS
198.89	LIGAMENT EXCEPT UTERINE METASTATIC
141.3	LINGUAE FRENULUM
198.89	LINGUAE FRENULUM METASTATIC
141.6	LINGUAL TONSIL
198.89	LINGUAL TONSIL METASTATIC
140.6	LIP COMMISSURE
198.89	LIP COMMISSURE METASTATIC
140.5	LIP FRENULUM
140.4	LIP FRENULUM LOWER
198.89	LIP FRENULUM METASTATIC
140.3	LIP FRENULUM UPPER
149.9	LIP ILL DEFINED
140.5	LIP INNER
140.5	LIP INNER BUCCAL MUCOSA
140.5	LIP INNER ORAL ASPECT
140.1	LIP LOWER
140.4	LIP LOWER BUCCAL MUCOSA
140.1	LIP LOWER EXTERNAL
140.4	LIP LOWER FRENULUM
140.4	LIP LOWER INNER ASPECT
140.1	LIP LOWER LIPSTICK AREA
140.4	LIP LOWER MUCOSA
140.4	LIP LOWER ORAL ASPECT
140.1	LIP LOWER VERMILION BORDER
198.89	LIP METASTATIC
173.0	LIP SKIN
198.2	LIP SKIN METASTATIC
140.0	LIP UPPER
140.3	LIP UPPER BUCCAL MUCOSA
140.0	LIP UPPER EXTERNAL
140.3	LIP UPPER FRENULUM

CANCER (continued)

IF TREATMENT IS DIRECTED TOWARDS THE PRIMARY SITE, SEQUENCE THAT SITE FIRST.

140.3	LIP UPPER INNER ASPECT
140.0	LIP UPPER LIPSTICK AREA
140.3	LIP UPPER MUCOSA
140.3	LIP UPPER ORAL ASPECT
140.0	LIP UPPER VERMILION BORDER
140.9	LIP VERMILION BORDER EXTERNAL
140.9	LIP VERMILION BORDER LIPSTICK AREA
140.8	LIP OTHER OVERLAPPING SITES
149.8	LIP OTHER OVERLAPPING SITES WITH ORAL CAVITY
V10.07	LIVER HISTORY OF MALIGNANT NEOPLASM
155.1	LIVER INTRAHEPTIC BILE DUCTS
197.7	LIVER METASTATIC
155.0	LIVER PRIMARY
155.2	LIVER UNDETERMINED PRIMARY OR SECONDARY
171.3	LOWER LIMB AND HIP SOFT TISSUE
198.89	LOWER LIMB AND HIP SOFT TISSUE METASTATIC
195.5	LOWER LIMB ILL-DEFINED
198.89	LOWER LIMB ILL-DEFINED METASTATIC
173.7	LOWER LIMB SKIN
198.2	LOWER LIMB SKIN METASTATIC
162.5	LOWER LOBE BRONCHUS
197.0	LOWER LOBE BRONCHUS METASTATIC
170.5	LUNATE
198.5	LUNATE METASTATIC
162.9	LUNG
162.9	LUNG BRONCHUS
162.8	LUNG BRONCHUS UNDETERMINED ORIGIN
V16.1	LUNG HISTORY FAMILY OF MALIGNANT NEOPLASM
V10.11	LUNG HISTORY PERSONAL OF MALIGNANT NEOPLASM
162.5	LUNG LOWER LOBE
197.0	LUNG METASTATIC
162.4	LUNG MIDDLE LOBE
162.3	LUNG UPPER LOBE
202.9#	LYMPH NODE (ANY SITE) PRIMARY
	5th Digit: 202.9
	0. NOS, EXTRANODAL AND SOLID ORGAN SITES
	1. LYMPH NODES OF HEAD FACE NECK
	2. LYMPH NODES INTRATHORACIC
	3. LYMPH NODES ABDOMINAL
	4. LYMPH NODES AXILLA AND UPPER LIMB
	5. LYMPH NODES INGUINAL REGION AND LOWER LIMB
	6. LYMPH NODES INTRAPELVIC
	7. SPLEEN
	8. LYMPH NODES MULTIPLE SITES
196.#	LYMPH NODE METASTATIC
	4th Digit: 196
	0. HEAD FACE NECK CERVICAL SUPRACLAVICULAR
	1. INTRATHORACIC BRONCHOPULMONARY MEDIASTINAL TRACHEOBRONCHIAL
	2. INTRA ABDOMINAL MESENTERIC RETROPERITONEAL
	3. AXILLA UPPER LIMB BRACHIAL INTRACLAVICULAR PECTORAL
	5. LOWER LIMB INGUINAL FEMORAL GROIN TIBIAL
	6. INTRAPELVIC HYPOGASTRIC ILIAC PARAMETRIAL
	8. MULTIPLE SITES
	9. LYMPH NODES NOS

CANCER (continued)

WHEN TREATMENT IS DIRECTED TOWARD A SECONDARY SITE, EVEN IF THE PRIMARY SITE IS KNOWN, SEQUENCE THE SECONDARY SITE FIRST.

202.9# LYMPHOID HISTIOCYTIC TISSUE
200.1# LYMPHOSARCOMA
5th Digit: 200.1, 202.9
- **0. NOS, EXTRANODAL AND SOLID ORGAN SITES**
- **1. LYMPH NODES OF HEAD FACE NECK**
- **2. LYMPH NODES INTRATHORACIC**
- **3. LYMPH NODES ABDOMINAL**
- **4. LYMPH NODES AXILLA AND UPPER LIMB**
- **5. LYMPH NODES INGUINAL REGION AND LOWER LIMB**
- **6. LYMPH NODES INTRAPELVIC**
- **7. SPLEEN**
- **8. LYMPH NODES MULTIPLE SITES**

170.0 MALAR BONE (CARTILAGE) (JOINT) (PERIOSTEUM)
198.5 MALAR BONE (CARTILAGE) (JOINT) (PERIOSTEUM) METASTATIC

187.8 MALE GENITAL OTHER
198.82 MALE GENITAL OTHER METASTATIC

199.1 MALIGNANCY NOS

170.1 MANDIBLE
198.5 MANDIBLE METASTATIC

202.90 MARROW BONE
198.5 MARROW BONE METASTATIC

173.5 MASTECTOMY SITE BREAST SKIN
198.2 MASTECTOMY SITE BREAST SKIN, METASTATIC
174.8 MASTECTOMY SITE BREAST TISSUE
198.81 MASTECTOMY SITE BREAST TISSUE, METASTATIC

160.1 MASTOID AIR CELLS
197.3 MASTOID AIR CELLS METASTATIC

170.1 MAXILLA INFERIOR
198.5 MAXILLA METASTATIC
170.0 MAXILLA SUPERIOR
160.2 MAXILLARY ANTRUM
197.3 MAXILLARY ANTRUM METASTATIC
160.2 MAXILLARY SINUS
197.3 MAXILLARY SINUS METASTATIC

152.3 MECKEL'S DIVERTICULUM
197.4 MECKEL'S DIVERTICULUM METASTATIC

196.1 MEDIASTINAL NODES METASTATIC

164.9 MEDIASTINUM
164.2 MEDIASTINUM ANTERIOR
197.1 MEDIASTINUM METASTATIC
164.3 MEDIASTINUM POSTERIOR

194.0 MEDULLA ADRENAL
198.7 MEDULLA ADRENAL METASTATIC

191.7 MEDULLA OBLONGATA
198.3 MEDULLA OBLONGATA METASTATIC

172.# MELANOMA SKIN
4th Digit: 172
- **0. LIP**
- **1. EYELID CANTHUS**
- **2. EAR (AURICLE) AURICULAR CANAL (EXTERNAL) (ACOUSTIC) MEATUS PINNA**
- **3. UNSPECIFIED PARTS OF FACE CHEEK CHIN EYEBROW FOREHEAD NOSE TEMPLE**
- **4. SCALP AND NECK**
- **5. TRUNK AXILLA BREAST GROIN PERIANAL SKIN PERINEUM UMBILICUS**
- **6. UPPER LIMB SHOULDER**
- **7. LOWER LIMB HIP**
- **8. OTHER SPECIFIED SKIN SITES CONTIGUOUS OR OVERLAPPING UNDETERMINED POINT OF ORIGIN**
- **9. SITE NOS**

CANCER (continued)

SYMPTOMS OF A MALIGNANCY SUCH AS PAIN OR NAUSEA, SHOULD NOT REPLACE THE CANCER CODE. SEQUENCE THE CANCER FIRST

192.1 MENINGES CEREBRAL
198.4 MENINGES CEREBRAL METASTATIC
192.3 MENINGES SPINAL CORD
198.4 MENINGES SPINAL CORD METASTATIC

196.2 MESENTERIC NODES METASTATIC

158.8 MESENTERY
197.6 MESENTERY METASTATIC

158.8 MESOCOLON
197.6 MESOCOLON METASTATIC

183.3 MESOVARIUM
198.82 MESOVARIUM METASTATIC

170.5 METACARPALS
198.5 METACARPALS METASTATIC

170.8 METATARSAL
198.5 METATARSAL METASTATIC

199.1 METASTATIC SITE NOS

191.7 MIDBRAIN
198.3 MIDBRAIN METASTATIC

162.4 MIDDLE LOBE BRONCHUS
197.0 MIDDLE LOBE BRONCHUS METASTATIC

145.9 MOUTH
144.0 MOUTH ANTERIOR TO PREMOLAR-CANINE JUNCTION
145.0 MOUTH CHEEK
144.9 MOUTH FLOOR
144.0 MOUTH FLOOR ANTERIOR
144.1 MOUTH FLOOR LATERAL
144.8 MOUTH FLOOR OTHER SITES
145.2 MOUTH HARD PALATE
198.89 MOUTH METASTATIC
145.6 MOUTH RETROMOLAR
145.5 MOUTH ROOF
145.3 MOUTH SOFT PALATE
147.3 MOUTH SOFT PALATE POSTERIOR PORTION
145.4 MOUTH UVULA
145.1 MOUTH VESTIBULE
145.8 MOUTH OTHER SPECIFIED AREA

199.0 MULTIPLE CANCERS
203.0# MULTIPLE MYELOMA
5th Digit: 203.0
- **0. WITHOUT MENTION OF REMISSION**
- **1. IN REMISSION**

171.# MUSCLE
4th Digit: 171
- **0. HEAD FACE NECK**
- **2. UPPER LIMB SHOULDER**
- **3. LOWER LIMB HIP**
- **4. THORAX**
- **5. ABDOMINAL HYPOCHONDRIUM**
- **6. PELVIS BUTTOCK GROIN INGUINAL REGION PERINEUM**
- **7. TRUNK NOS BACK NOS FLANK NOS**
- **8. OTHER SPECIFIED SITES**
- **9. SITE NOS**

198.89 MUSCLE METASTATIC

164.1 MYOCARDIUM
198.89 MYOCARDIUM METASTATIC

182.0 MYOMETRIUM
198.82 MYOMETRIUM METASTATIC

WHEN A PRIMARY SITE HAS BEEN RESECTED, AND THE CURRENT ENCOUNTER IS FOR RECURRENCE IN THE ORIGINAL SITE, SEQUENCE THE PRIMARY SITE FIRST.

170.0 NASAL BONE (CARTILAGE) (JOINT) (PERIOSTEUM)
198.5 NASAL BONE METASTATIC
160.0 NASAL CARTILAGE
197.3 NASAL CARTILAGE METASTATIC
160.0 NASAL CAVITY
160.9 NASAL CAVITY ACCESSORY SINUSES
160.3 NASAL CAVITY ETHMOIDAL SINUS
160.4 NASAL CAVITY FRONTAL SINUS
160.2 NASAL CAVITY MAXILLARY SINUS
197.3 NASAL CAVITY METASTATIC
160.8 NASAL CAVITY ORIGIN UNDETERMINED
160.5 NASAL CAVITY SPHENOIDAL SINUS
147.3 NASAL CHOANAE (POSTERIOR MARGIN)
198.89 NASAL CHOANAE (POSTERIOR MARGIN) METASTATIC
160.0 NASAL CONCHAE NASAL TURBINATES
197.3 NASAL CONCHAE NASAL TURBINATES METASTATIC
192.0 NASAL OLFACTORY BULB
198.4 NASAL OLFACTORY BULB METASTATIC
160.0 NASAL SEPTUM
197.3 NASAL SEPTUM METASTATIC
147.3 NASAL SEPTUM POSTERIOR MARGIN
198.89 NASAL SEPTUM POSTERIOR MARGIN METASTATIC
172.3 NASAL SKIN (MELANOMA)
198.2 NASAL SKIN (MELANOMA) METASTATIC
170.0 NASAL TURBINATE BONE
198.5 NASAL TURBINATE BONE METASTATIC
160.0 NASAL TURBINATE MUCOSA
197.3 NASAL TURBINATE MUCOSA METASTATIC
160.0 NASAL VESTIBULE
197.3 NASAL VESTIBULE METASTATIC

190.7 NASOLACRIMAL DUCT
198.4 NASOLACRIMAL DUCT METASTATIC

147.9 NASOPHARYNX
147.3 NASOPHARYNX ANTERIOR WALL
147.3 NASOPHARYNX FLOOR
147.2 NASOPHARYNX FOSSA OF ROSENMULLER
147.2 NASOPHARYNX LATERAL WALL
198.89 NASOPHARYNX METASTATIC
147.1 NASOPHARYNX POSTERIOR WALL
147.0 NASOPHARYNX SUPERIOR WALL (ROOF)
147.9 NASOPHARYNX WALL NOS
147.8 NASOPHARYNX OTHER SPECIFIED SITES

170.8 NAVICULAR ANKLE
198.5 NAVICULAR ANKLE OR HAND METASTATIC
170.5 NAVICULAR HAND

195.0 NECK ILL-DEFINED
198.89 NECK ILL-DEFINED METASTATIC
173.4 NECK SKIN
198.2 NECK SKIN METASTATIC

171.# NERVE (PERIPHERAL) (SYMPATHETIC) (PARASYMPATHETIC)

4th Digit: 171

0. HEAD FACE NECK
2. UPPER LIMB SHOULDER
3. LOWER LIMB HIP
4. THORAX
5. ABDOMINAL HYPOCHONDRIUM
6. PELVIS BUTTOCK GROIN INGUINAL REGION PERINEUM
7. TRUNK NOS BACK NOS FLANK NOS
8. OTHER SPECIFIED SITES
9. SITE NOS

198.89 NERVE (PERIPHERAL) (SYMPATHETIC) (PARASYMPATHETIC) METASTATIC

192.0 NERVE CRANIAL
198.4 NERVE CRANIAL METASTATIC

192.9 NERVOUS SYSTEM
198.4 NERVOUS SYSTEM METASTATIC
192.8 NERVOUS SYSTEM OTHER SPECIFIED SITES

174.0 NIPPLE FEMALE SOFT TISSUE
175.0 NIPPLE MALE SOFT TISSUE
198.81 NIPPLE SOFT TISSUE METASTATIC

195.0 NOSE ILL DEFINED
198.89 NOSE ILL DEFINED METASTATIC
160.0 NOSE INTERNAL
197.3 NOSE INTERNAL METASTATIC
173.3 NOSE SKIN (EXTERNAL)
198.2 NOSE SKIN METASTATIC

V71.1 OBSERVATION NONE FOUND

196.6 OBTURATOR NODES METASTATIC

170.0 OCCIPITAL BONE (CARTILAGE) (JOINT) (PERIOSTEUM)
198.5 OCCIPITAL BONE (CARTILAGE) (JOINT) (PERIOSTEUM) METASTATIC
191.4 OCCIPITAL LOBE
198.3 OCCIPITAL LOBE METASTATIC

192.0 OLFACTORY BULB
198.4 OLFACTORY BULB METASTATIC

158.8 OMENTUM
197.6 OMENTUM METASTATIC

192.0 OPTIC NERVE
198.4 OPTIC NERVE METASTATIC

145.9 ORAL CAVITY NOS
149.9 ORAL CAVITY ILL-DEFINED
198.89 ORAL CAVITY METASTATIC
V10.02 ORAL CAVITY AND PHARYNX HISTORY OF MALIGNANT NEOPLASM
V76.42 ORAL CAVITY SCREENING FOR MALIGNANT NEOPLASM
149.8 ORAL CAVITY OTHER SPECIFIED

170.0 ORBIT BONE (CARTILAGE) (JOINT) (PERIOSTEUM)
198.5 ORBIT BONE (CARTILAGE) (JOINT) (PERIOSTEUM) METASTATIC
190.1 ORBIT CONNECTIVE TISSUE
198.4 ORBIT CONNECTIVE TISSUE METASTATIC
190.1 ORBIT RETROBULBAR
198.4 ORBIT RETROBULBAR METASTATIC

146.9 OROPHARYNX
146.5 OROPHARYNX JUNCTIONAL REGION
146.6 OROPHARYNX LATERAL WALL
146.7 OROPHARYNX POSTERIOR WALL
198.89 OROPHARYNX METASTATIC
146.2 OROPHARYNX TONSILLAR PILLARS ANTERIOR
146.8 OROPHARYNX OTHER SPECIFIED SITES

183.0 OVARY
V10.43 OVARY HISTORY OF MALIGNANT NEOPLASM
198.6 OVARY METASTATIC

183.2 OVIDUCT
198.82 OVIDUCT METASTATIC

145.5 PALATE
145.2 PALATE HARD
145.5 PALATE JUNCTION OF HARD AND SOFT
198.89 PALATE METASTATIC
145.3 PALATE SOFT
147.3 PALATE SOFT POSTERIOR PORTION

146.2 PALATOGLOSSAL ARCH
198.89 PALATOGLOSSAL ARCH METASTATIC

146.2 PALATOPHARYNGEAL ARCH
198.89 PALATOPHARYNGEAL ARCH METASTATIC

CANCER (continued)

157.9	PANCREAS
157.1	PANCREAS BODY
157.3	PANCREAS DUCTS
157.8	PANCREAS ECTOPIC TISSUE
157.0	PANCREAS HEAD
157.4	PANCREAS ISLETS OF LANGERHANS
197.8	PANCREAS METASTATIC
157.3	PANCREAS SANTORINI DUCT
157.2	PANCREAS TAIL
157.8	PANCREAS UNDETERMINED SITE
157.3	PANCREAS WIRSUNG DUCT
194.6	PARA AORTIC BODY
198.89	PARA AORTIC BODY METASTATIC
194.6	PARAGANGLIA RELATED
198.89	PARAGANGLIA RELATED METASTATIC
196.6	PARAMETRIAL NODES METASTATIC
183.4	PARAMETRIUM
198.82	PARAMETRIUM METASTATIC
194.1	PARATHYROID GLAND
198.89	PARATHYROID GLAND METASTATIC
189.4	PARAURETHRAL GLANDS
198.1	PARAURETHRAL GLANDS METASTATIC
170.0	PARIETAL BONE (CARTILAGE) (JOINT) (PERIOSTEUM)
198.5	PARIETAL BONE (CARTILAGE) (JOINT) (PERIOSTEUM) METASTATIC
191.3	PARIETAL LOBE
198.3	PARIETAL LOBE METASTATIC
158.8	PARIETAL PERITONEUM
197.6	PARIETAL PERITONEUM METASTATIC
163.0	PARIETAL PLEURA
197.2	PARIETAL PLEURA METASTATIC
142.0	PAROTID GLAND
198.89	PAROTID GLAND METASTATIC

WHEN TWO PRIMARY SITES ARE FOUND, SEQUENCE THE SITE RECEIVING THE MOST TREATMENT FIRST

183.3	PAROVARIAN REGION
198.82	PAROVARIAN REGION METASTATIC
170.8	PATELLA
198.5	PATELLA METASTATIC
196.3	PECTORAL NODES METASTATIC
158.8	PELVIC PERITONEUM
197.6	PELVIC PERITONEUM METASTATIC
195.3	PELVIS ILL-DEFINED
198.89	PELVIS ILL-DEFINED METASTATIC
171.6	PELVIS SOFT TISSUE
198.89	PELVIS SOFT TISSUE METASTATIC
187.4	PENIS
187.3	PENIS BODY
187.2	PENIS GLANS
198.82	PENIS METASTATIC
187.4	PENIS SKIN
158.0	PERIADRENAL TISSUE
197.6	PERIADRENAL TISSUE METASTATIC
164.1	PERICARDIUM
198.89	PERICARDIUM METASTATIC
158.0	PERINEPHRIC TISSUE
197.6	PERINEPHRIC TISSUE METASTATIC
173.5	PERINEUM SKIN
198.2	PERINEUM SKIN METASTATIC
171.6	PERINEUM SOFT TISSUE
198.89	PERINEUM SOFT TISSUE METASTATIC

CANCER (continued)

158.0	PERIRENAL TISSUE
197.6	PERIRENAL TISSUE METASTATIC
158.9	PERITONEUM
158.8	PERITONEUM CUL-DE-SAC
158.8	PERITONEUM MESENTERY
197.6	PERITONEUM METASTATIC
158.8	PERITONEUM OMENTUM
158.8	PERITONEUM SPECIFIED PARTS
170.8	PHALANGES FOOT
198.5	PHALANGES FOOT METASTATIC
170.5	PHALANGES HAND
198.5	PHALANGES HAND METASTATIC
146.3	PHARYNGOEPIGLOTTIC FOLD ANTERIOR AND MEDIAL SURFACE
198.89	PHARYNGOEPIGLOTTIC FOLD ANTERIOR AND MEDIAL SURFACE METASTATIC
149.0	PHARYNX
V10.02	PHARYNX HISTORY OF MALIGNANT NEOPLASM
149.9	PHARYNX ILL DEFINED
198.89	PHARYNX METASTATIC
147.2	PHARYNX RECESS
149.1	PHARYNX WALDEYER'S RING
149.8	PHARYNX OTHER SPECIFIED
194.4	PINEAL GLAND
198.89	PINEAL GLAND METASTATIC
170.5	PISIFORM
198.5	PISIFORM METASTATIC
194.3	PITUITARY AND CRANIOPHARYNGEAL DUCT
198.89	PITUITARY METASTATIC
181	PLACENTA
198.82	PLACENTA METASTATIC
163.9	PLEURA
197.2	PLEURA METASTATIC
163.8	PLEURA OTHER SPECIFIED SITES
194.8	PLURIGLANDULAR INVOLVEMENT
198.89	PLURIGLANDULAR INVOLVEMENT METASTATIC
191.7	PONS
198.3	PONS METASTATIC
196.5	POPLITEAL LYMPH NODES METASTATIC
171.3	POPLITEAL SOFT TISSUE
198.89	POPLITEAL SOFT TISSUE METASTATIC
164.3	POSTERIOR MEDIASTINUM
197.1	POSTERIOR MEDIASTINUM METASTATIC
187.1	PREPUCE
198.82	PREPUCE METASTATIC
151.1	PREPYLORUS
197.8	PREPYLORUS METASTATIC
195.3	PRESACRAL REGION ILL DEFINED
198.89	PRESACRAL REGION ILL DEFINED METASTATIC

WHEN ENCOUNTER IS FOR A COMPLICATION OF A SURGICAL PROCEDURE TO RESECT A CANCER, SEQUENCE THE COMPLICATION FIRST AND THE CANCER AS AN ADDITIONAL CODE.

185	PROSTATE
V10.46	PROSTATE HISTORY OF MALIGNANT NEOPLASM
198.82	PROSTATE METASTATIC
V76.44	PROSTATE SCREENING
170.6	PUBIS
198.5	PUBIS METASTATIC
184.4	PUDENDUM
198.82	PUDENDUM METASTATIC

CANCER (continued)

151.1 PYLORUS (CANAL)
197.8 PYLORUS (CANAL) METASTATIC

148.1 PYRIFORM SINUS
198.89 PYRIFORM SINUS METASTATIC

170.4 RADIUS
198.5 RADIUS METASTATIC

194.3 RATHKE'S POUCH
198.89 RATHKE'S POUCH METASTATIC

154.0 RECTOSIGMOID JUNCTION
197.5 RECTOSIGMOID JUNCTION METASTATIC
154.8 RECTOSIGMOID UNDETERMINED

158.8 RECTOUTERINE POUCH
197.6 RECTOUTERINE POUCH METASTATIC

195.3 RECTOVAGINAL (SEPTUM) ILL-DEFINED
198.89 RECTOVAGINAL METASTATIC
195.3 RECTOVAGINAL RECTOVESICAL OVERLAPPING SITES

195.3 RECTOVESICAL (SEPTUM) ILL-DEFINED
198.89 RECTOVESICAL (SEPTUM) ILL-DEFINED METASTATIC

154.1 RECTUM
154.1 RECTUM AMPULLA
197.5 RECTUM METASTATIC
V10.06 RECTUM (RECTOSIGMOID JUNCTION) (ANUS) HISTORY
V76.41 RECTUM SCREENING FOR MALIGNANT NEOPLASM
154.8 RECTUM UNDETERMINED

189.1 RENAL PELVIS
198.0 RENAL PELVIS METASTATIC

165.8 RESPIRATORY AND INTRATHORACIC OTHER SPECIFIED SITES
197.3 RESPIRATORY AND INTRATHORACIC OTHER SPECIFIED SITES METASTATIC
V10.29 RESPIRATORY AND INTRATHORACIC ORGANS HISTORY OTHER
V10.20 RESPIRATORY ORGAN HISTORY OF MALIGNANT NEOPLASM
165.9 RESPIRATORY ORGAN OR SYSTEM ILL DEFINED
197.3 RESPIRATORY ORGAN OR SYSTEM ILL DEFINED METASTATIC
V76.0 RESPIRATORY ORGAN SCREENING FOR MALIGNANT NEOPLASM

165.9 RESPIRATORY TRACT
165.9 RESPIRATORY TRACT ILL-DEFINED SITES
197.3 RESPIRATORY TRACT METASTATIC
165.8 RESPIRATORY TRACT OTHER SPECIFIED SITES

190.5 RETINA
198.4 RETINA METASTATIC

190.5 RETINOBLASTOMA

190.1 RETROBULBAR
198.4 RETROBULBAR METASTATIC

158.0 RETROCECAL TISSUE
197.6 RETROCECAL TISSUE METASTATIC
196.2 RETROPERITONEAL NODES METASTATIC

158.0 RETROPERITONEUM
197.6 RETROPERITONEUM METASTATIC

170.3 RIBS
198.5 RIBS METASTATIC

183.5 ROUND LIGAMENT
198.82 ROUND LIGAMENT METASTATIC

195.3 SACROCOCCYGEAL REGION ILL-DEFINED
198.89 SACROCOCCYGEAL REGION ILL-DEFINED METASTATIC

170.6 SACRUM
198.5 SACRUM METASTATIC

CANCER (continued)

WHEN TREATMENT IS DIRECTED TOWARD A SECONDARY SITE, EVEN IF THE PRIMARY SITE IS KNOWN, SEQUENCE THE SECONDARY SITE FIRST.

142.9 SALIVARY GLAND
145.9 SALIVARY GLAND (MINOR GLAND)
198.89 SALIVARY GLAND METASTATIC
142.8 SALIVARY GLAND OTHER
142.2 SALIVARY GLAND SUBLINGUAL
142.1 SALIVARY GLAND SUBMANDIBULAR OR SUBMAXILLARY

196.0 SCALENE NODES METASTATIC

173.4 SCALP SKIN
198.2 SCALP SKIN METASTATIC

170.5 SCAPHOID OF HAND
198.5 SCAPHOID OF HAND METASTATIC

170.4 SCAPULA
198.5 SCAPULA METASTATIC

190.0 SCLERA
198.4 SCLERA METASTATIC

187.7 SCROTUM (SKIN)
198.82 SCROTUM (SKIN) METASTATIC

173.# SEBACEOUS GLANDS

4th Digit: 173

0. SKIN OF LIP
1. EYELID INCLUDING CANTHUS
2. SKIN OF EAR AURICULAR CANAL (EXTERNAL) MEATUS PINNA
3. SKIN OF UNSPECIFIED PARTS OF FACE CHEEK CHIN EYEBROW FOREHEAD NOSE (EXT)
4. SCALP AND SKIN OF NECK
5. ALL SKIN TRUNK AXILLAPERIANAL ABDOMINAL WALL ANUS BACK BREAST (OR MASTECTOMY SITE) BUTTOCK
6. ALL SKIN UPPER LIMB SHOULDER ARM FINGER HAND
7. ALL SKIN LOWER LIMB HIP ANKLE FOOT KNEE LEG THIGH TOE POPLITEAL AREA
8. OTHER SPECIFIED SKIN SITES CONTIGUOUS SITES UNDETERMINED POINT OF ORIGIN
9. SITE NOS

198.2 SEBACEOUS GLAND METASTATIC

194.3 SELLA TURCICA PITUITARY
198.89 SELLA TURCICA PITUITARY METASTATIC

170.5 SEMILUNAR
198.5 SEMILUNAR METASTATIC

187.8 SEMINAL VESICLE
198.82 SEMINAL VESICLE METASTATIC

173.6 SHOULDER SKIN
198.2 SHOULDER SKIN METASTATIC

154.0 SIGMOID (RECTOSIGMOID)
153.3 SIGMOID FLEXURE
197.5 SIGMOID METASTATIC

199.1 SIMPLEX SITE NOS

160.9 SINUS ACCESSORY
197.3 SINUS ACCESSORY METASTATIC
V10.22 SINUS HISTORY OF MALIGNANT NEOPLASM

193 SIPPLE'S SYNDROME

IF ENCOUNTER IS FOR CHEMOTHERAPY OR RADIOTHERAPY AND A COMPLICATION OF THE THERAPY DEVELOPS, SEQUENCE THE THERAPY FIRST, THE COMPLICATION SECOND, THEN THE CANCER.

C

CANCER (continued)

WHEN THE REASON FOR ENCOUNTER IS TO EVALUATE THE EXTENT OF A CANCER ALREADY DIAGNOSED, YOU MAY CODE THE CANCER AGAIN AS THE REASON FOR ENCOUNTER, RATHER THAN JUST THE SYMPTOMS.

173.# SKIN
4th Digit: 173
0. SKIN OF LIP
1. EYELID INCLUDING CANTHUS
2. SKIN OF EAR AURICULAR CANAL (EXTERNAL) MEATUS PINNA
3. SKIN OF UNSPECIFIED PARTS OF FACE CHEEK CHIN EYEBROW FOREHEAD NOSE (EXTERNAL)
4. SCALP AND SKIN OF NECK
5. ALL SKIN TRUNK AXILLA PERIANAL ABDOMINAL WALL ANUS BACK BREAST (OR MASTECTOMY SITE) BUTTOCK
6. ALL SKIN UPPER LIMB SHOULDER ARM FINGER HAND
7. ALL SKIN LOWER LIMB HIP ANKLE FOOT KNEE LEG THIGH TOE POPLITEAL AREA
8. OTHER SPECIFIED SKIN SITES CONTIGUOUS SITES UNDETERMINED POINT OF ORIGIN
9. SITE NOS
198.2 SKIN METASTATIC
V10.83 SKIN (OTHER) HISTORY OF MALIGNANT NEOPLASM

170.0 SKULL CALVARIUM
198.5 SKULL CALVARIUM METASTATIC

152.3 SMALL BOWEL MECKEL'S DIVERTICULUM
197.4 SMALL BOWEL METASTATIC
152.9 SMALL BOWEL OTHER OR UNDETERMINED
152.8 SMALL BOWEL OTHER UNDETERMINED SITES OVERLAPPING

145.3 SOFT PALATE
198.89 SOFT PALATE METASTATIC
147.3 SOFT PALATE POSTERIOR PORTION

187.6 SPERMATIC CORD
198.82 SPERMATIC CORD METASTATIC

170.0 SPHENOID BONE (CARTILAGE) (JOINT) (PERIOSTEUM)
198.5 SPHENOID BONE (CARTILAGE) (JOINT) (PERIOSTEUM) METASTATIC
160.5 SPHENOID SINUS
197.3 SPHENOID SINUS METASTATIC

156.1 SPHINCTER OF ODDI
197.8 SPHINCTER OF ODDI METASTATIC

192.2 SPINAL CORD
198.3 SPINAL CORD METASTATIC
192.3 SPINAL MENINGES
198.4 SPINAL MENINGES METASTATIC

170.6 SPINE - SACRUM, COCCYX
170.2 SPINE - SPINAL COLUMN, VERTEBRA
198.5 SPINE - METASTATIC

159.1 SPLEEN
159.1 SPLEEN ANGIOSARCOMA
159.1 SPLEEN FIBROSARCOMA
200.17 SPLEEN LYMPHOSARCOMA
197.8 SPLEEN METASTATIC
200.07 SPLEEN RETICULOSARCOMA (LYMPHOMA)

170.3 STERNUM
198.5 STERNUM METASTATIC

151.9 STOMACH
151.4 STOMACH BODY
151.0 STOMACH CARDIAC ORIFICE
150.2 STOMACH CARDIAC ORIFICE SQUAMOUS CELL
151.0 STOMACH CARDIOESOPHAGEAL JUNCTION

CANCER (continued)
150.5 STOMACH CARDIOESOPHAGEAL SQUAMOUS CELL
V16.0 STOMACH FAMILY HISTORY OF MALIGNANT NEOPLASM
151.6 STOMACH GREATER CURVATURE
V10.04 STOMACH HISTORY OF MALIGNANT NEOPLASM
151.5 STOMACH LESSER CURVATURE
197.8 STOMACH METASTATIC
151.8 STOMACH OTHER UNDETERMINED OVERLAPPING
151.2 STOMACH PYLORIC ANTRUM
151.1 STOMACH PYLORUS

161.2 SUBGLOTTIS LARYNX
197.3 SUBGLOTTIS LARYNX METASTATIC

142.2 SUBLINGUAL GLAND
198.89 SUBLINGUAL GLAND METASTATIC

142.1 SUBMANDIBULAR GLAND
198.89 SUBMANDIBULAR GLAND METASTATIC

142.1 SUBMAXILLARY GLAND
198.89 SUBMAXILLARY GLAND METASTATIC

173.# SUDORIFEROUS SUDORIPAROUS GLANDS
4th Digit: 173
0. SKIN OF LIP
1. EYELID INCLUDING CANTHUS
2. SKIN OF EAR AURICULAR CANAL (EXTERNAL) MEATUS PINNA
3. SKIN OF UNSPECIFIED PARTS OF FACE CHEEK CHIN EYEBROW FOREHEAD NOSE (EXT)
4. SCALP AND SKIN OF NECK
5. ALL SKIN TRUNK AXILLA PERIANAL ABDOMINAL WALL ANUS BACK BREAST (OR MASTECTOMY SITE) BUTTOCK
6. ALL SKIN UPPER LIMB SHOULDER ARM FINGER HAND
7. ALL SKIN LOWER LIMB HIP ANKLE FOOT KNEE LEG THIGH TOE POPLITEAL AREA
8. OTHER SPECIFIED SKIN SITES CONTIGUOUS SITES UNDETERMINED POINT OF ORIGIN
9. SITE NOS

198.2 SUDORIFEROUS SUDORIPAROUS GLANDS METASTATIC

145.1 SULCUS BUCCAL UPPER LOWER
145.1 SULCUS LABIAL UPPER LOWER
198.89 SULCUS METASTATIC

196.0 SUPRACLAVICULAR GLAND METASTATIC
195.0 SUPRACLAVICULAR REGION ILL-DEFINED
198.89 SUPRACLAVICULAR REGION ILL-DEFINED METASTATIC

161.1 SUPRAGLOTTIS
197.3 SUPRAGLOTTIS METASTATIC

194.0 SUPRARENAL GLAND
198.7 SUPRARENAL GLAND METASTATIC

173.# SWEAT GLAND
4th Digit: 173
0. SKIN OF LIP
1. EYELID INCLUDING CANTHUS
2. SKIN OF EAR AURICULAR CANAL (EXTERNAL) MEATUS PINNA
3. SKIN OF UNSPECIFIED PARTS OF FACE CHEEK CHIN EYEBROW FOREHEAD NOSE (EXT)
4. SCALP AND SKIN OF NECK
5. ALL SKIN TRUNK AXILLA PERIANAL ABDOMINAL WALL ANUS BACK BREAST (OR MASTECTOMY SITE) BUTTOCK
6. ALL SKIN UPPER LIMB SHOULDER ARM FINGER HAND
7. ALL SKIN LOWER LIMB HIP ANKLE FOOT KNEE LEG THIGH TOE POPLITEAL AREA
8. OTHER SPECIFIED SKIN SITES CONTIGUOUS SITES UNDETERMINED POINT OF ORIGIN
9. SITE NOS

198.2 SWEAT GLAND METASTATIC

C

CANCER (continued)

171.# SYNOVIA

4th Digit: 171

- **0. HEAD FACE NECK**
- **2. UPPER LIMB SHOULDER**
- **3. LOWER LIMB HIP**
- **4. THORAX**
- **5. ABDOMINAL HYPOCHONDRIUM**
- **6. PELVIS BUTTOCK GROIN INGUINAL REGION PERINEUM**
- **7. TRUNK NOS BACK NOS FLANK NOS**
- **8. OTHER SPECIFIED SITES**
- **9. SITE NOS**

198.89 SYNOVIA METASTATIC

170.8 TALUS
198.5 TALUS METASTATIC

191.8 TAPETUM
198.3 TAPETUM METASTATIC

170.8 TARSAL BONE
198.5 TARSAL BONE METASTATIC

173.3 TEMPLE SKIN
198.2 TEMPLE SKIN METASTATIC

170.0 TEMPORAL BONE (CARTILAGE) (JOINT) (PERIOSTEUM)
198.5 TEMPORAL BONE (CARTILAGE) (JOINT) (PERIOSTEUM) METASTATIC
191.2 TEMPORAL LOBE
198.3 TEMPORAL LOBE METASTATIC
191.2 TEMPORAL LOBE UNCUS
198.3 TEMPORAL LOBE UNCUS METASTATIC

171.# TENDON (SHEATH)

4th Digit: 171

- **0. HEAD FACE NECK**
- **2. UPPER LIMB SHOULDER**
- **3. LOWER LIMB HIP**
- **4. THORAX**
- **5. ABDOMINAL HYPOCHONDRIUM**
- **6. PELVIS BUTTOCK GROIN INGUINAL REGION PERINEUM**
- **7. TRUNK NOS BACK NOS FLANK NOS**
- **8. OTHER SPECIFIED SITES**
- **9. SITE NOS**

198.89 TENDON (SHEATH) METASTATIC

192.1 TENTORIUM
198.4 TENTORIUM METASTATIC

186.9 TESTIS NOS
186.9 TESTIS CHORIOCARCINOMA
186.0 TESTIS CHORIOCARCINOMA UNDESCENDED
186.9 TESTIS DESCENDED
186.0 TESTIS ECTOPIC UNDESCENDED
V10.47 TESTIS HISTORY OF MALIGNANT NEOPLASM
198.82 TESTIS METASTATIC
186.0 TESTIS RETAINED
V76.45 TESTIS SCREENING
186.9 TESTIS SCROTAL
186.0 TESTIS UNDESCENDED TESTIS
186.9 TESTIS OTHER AND UNSPECIFIED

191.0 THALAMUS
198.3 THALAMUS METASTATIC

195.5 THIGH ILL DEFINED
198.89 THIGH ILL DEFINED METASTATIC
173.7 THIGH SKIN
198.2 THIGH SKIN METASTATIC
171.3 THIGH SOFT TISSUE
198.89 THIGH SOFT TISSUE METASTATIC

195.1 THORAX ILL DEFINED
198.89 THORAX METASTATIC
171.4 THORAX SOFT TISSUE

CANCER (continued)

149.0 THROAT
198.89 THROAT METASTATIC

164.0 THYMUS
198.89 THYMUS METASTATIC
V10.29 THYMUS HISTORY OF MALIGNANT NEOPLASM

193 THYROGLOSSAL DUCT
198.89 THYROGLOSSAL DUCT METASTATIC

161.3 THYROID CARTILAGE
197.3 THYROID CARTILAGE METASTATIC
193 THYROID GLAND
198.89 THYROID GLAND METASTATIC
V10.87 THYROID HISTORY OF MALIGNANT NEOPLASM

170.7 TIBIA
198.5 TIBIA METASTATIC

196.5 TIBIAL LYMPH NODES METASTATIC

195.5 TOE ILL DEFINED
198.89 TOE ILL DEFINED METASTATIC
173.7 TOE SKIN
198.2 TOE SKIN METASTATIC
171.3 TOE SOFT TISSUE
198.89 TOE SOFT TISSUE METASTATIC

141.9 TONGUE
141.4 TONGUE ANTERIOR TWO-THIRDS
141.1 TONGUE ANTERIOR TWO THIRDS, DORSAL SURFACE
141.3 TONGUE ANTERIOR TWO THIRDS, VENTRAL SURFACE
141.0 TONGUE BASE
141.0 TONGUE BASE DORSAL
141.1 TONGUE DORSAL
141.1 TONGUE DORSAL MIDLINE
141.0 TONGUE DORSAL SURFACE OF BASE
141.0 TONGUE FIXED PART
V10.01 TONGUE HISTORY OF MALIGNANT NEOPLASM
141.5 TONGUE JUNCTIONAL ZONE
141.2 TONGUE LATERAL BORDER
141.6 TONGUE LINGUAL TONSIL
198.89 TONGUE METASTATIC
141.4 TONGUE MOBILE PART NOS
141.2 TONGUE TIP
141.3 TONGUE VENTRAL
141.8 TONGUE OTHER OVERLAPPING
141.8 TONGUE OVERLAPPING ORIGIN NOT DETERMINED

> *SYMPTOMS OF A MALIGNANCY SUCH AS PAIN OR NAUSEA, SHOULD NOT REPLACE THE CANCER CODE. SEQUENCE THE CANCER FIRST*

146.0 TONSIL
146.0 TONSIL FAUCIAL
141.6 TONSIL LINGUAL
198.89 TONSIL OR TONSILLAR METASTATIC
146.0 TONSIL OROPHARYNX FAUCIAL
146.0 TONSIL OROPHARYNX PALATINE
146.0 TONSIL PALATINE
147.1 TONSIL PHARYNGEAL
146.1 TONSILLAR FOSSA
146.1 TONSILLAR FOSSA OROPHARYNX
146.2 TONSILLAR PILLARS

195.8 TORSO OTHER SPECIFIED SITES ILL DEFINED
198.89 TORSO OTHER SPECIFIED SITES ILL DEFINED METASTATIC

162.0 TRACHEA
162.0 TRACHEA CARTILAGE
V16.1 TRACHEA FAMILY HISTORY OF MALIGNANT NEOPLASM
V10.12 TRACHEA HISTORY OF MALIGNANT NEOPLASM
197.3 TRACHEA METASTATIC
162.0 TRACHEA MUCOSA

162.8 TRACHEOBRONCHIAL NOS
197.3 TRACHEOBRONCHIAL NOS METASTATIC

196.1 TRACHEOBRONCHIAL NODES METASTATIC

CANCER (continued)

170.5	TRAPEZIUM, TRAPEZOID
198.5	TRAPEZIUM, TRAPEZOID METASTATIC
195.8	TRUNK ILL DEFINED
198.89	TRUNK ILL DEFINED METASTATIC
173.5	TRUNK SKIN
198.2	TRUNK SKIN METASTATIC
171.7	TRUNK SOFT TISSUE
198.89	TRUNK SOFT TISSUE METASTATIC
183.8	TUBO OVARIAN
198.82	TUBO OVARIAN METASTATIC
187.8	TUNICA VAGINALIS
198.82	TUNICA VAGINALIS METASTATIC
170.0	TURBINATE BONE (CARTILAGE) (JOINT) (PERIOSTEUM)
198.5	TURBINATE BONE (CARTILAGE) (JOINT) (PERIOSTEUM) METASTATIC
160.1	TYMPANIC CAVITY
197.3	TYMPANIC CAVITY METASTATIC
170.4	ULNA
198.5	ULNA METASTATIC
173.5	UMBILICUS SKIN
198.2	UMBILICUS SKIN METASTATIC
170.5	UNCIFORM
198.5	UNCIFORM METASTATIC
191.2	UNCUS
198.3	UNCUS METASTATIC
199.1	UNDIFFERENTIATED TYPE SITE UNSPECIFIED
165.0	UPPER AIRWAY
197.3	UPPER AIRWAY METASTATIC
195.4	UPPER LIMB ILL DEFINED
198.89	UPPER LIMB ILL DEFINED METASTATIC
171.2	UPPER LIMB SHOULDER SOFT TISSUE
198.89	UPPER LIMB SHOULDER SOFT TISSUE METASTATIC
173.6	UPPER LIMB SKIN
198.2	UPPER LIMB SKIN METASTATIC
165.0	UPPER RESPIRATORY TRACT
197.3	UPPER RESPIRATORY TRACT METASTATIC
189.2	URETER
198.1	URETER METASTATIC
188.6	URETERIC ORIFICE BLADDER
198.1	URETERIC ORIFICE BLADDER METASTATIC
189.1	URETEROPELVIC JUNCTION
198.0	URETEROPELVIC JUNCTION METASTATIC
189.3	URETHRA
198.1	URETHRA METASTATIC
188.5	URETHRA ORIFICE OF BLADDER
189.9	URINARY ORGANS
V16.59	URINARY ORGANS FAMILY HISTORY OF MALIGNANT NEOPLASM
198.1	URINARY ORGANS METASTATIC
189.8	URINARY ORGANS OVERLAPPING SITES
189.9	URINARY SYSTEM NOS
198.1	URINARY SYSTEM NOS METASTATIC
V10.50	URINARY TRACT HISTORY UNSPECIFIED ORGAN
V10.59	URINARY TRACT HISTORY OTHER SPECIFIED ORGAN
183.8	UTERO OVARIAN
198.82	UTERO OVARIAN METASTATIC
183.4	UTEROSACRAL LIGAMENT
198.82	UTEROSACRAL LIGAMENT METASTATIC

CANCER (continued)

WHEN BOTH A PRIMARY AND SECONDARY SITE ARE PRESENT AND TREATED EQUALLY, SEQUENCE THE PRIMARY SITE FIRST.

179	UTERUS
182.0	UTERUS BODY CORPUS
180.9	UTERUS CERVIX
182.0	UTERUS CORNU
182.0	UTERUS FUNDUS
V10.42	UTERUS HISTORY (EXCLUDING CERVIX) MALIGNANT NEOPLASM
182.1	UTERUS ISTHMUS
183.4	UTERUS LIGAMENT
182.1	UTERUS LOWER SEGMENT
198.82	UTERUS METASTATIC
183.2	UTERUS TUBE
182.8	UTERUS OTHER SPECIFIED SITE
190.0	UVEAL TRACT
198.4	UVEAL TRACT METASTATIC
145.4	UVULA
198.89	UVULA METASTATIC
184.0	VAGINA
198.82	VAGINA METASTATIC
184.9	VAGINA SEPTUM
184.0	VAGINA VAULT
146.3	VALLECULA
198.89	VALLECULA METASTATIC
187.6	VAS DEFERENS (SPERMATIC CORD)
198.82	VAS DEFERENS (SPERMATIC CORD) METASTATIC
191.5	VENTRICLES CHOROID PLEXUS
198.3	VENTRICLES CHOROID PLEXUS METASTATIC
191.5	VENTRICLES FLOOR OF VENTRICLE
198.3	VENTRICLES FLOOR OF VENTRICLE METASTATIC
161.1	VENTRICULAR BANDS, SUPRAGLOTTIS
197.3	VENTRICULAR BANDS, SUPRAGLOTTIS METASTATIC
140.9	VERMILION BORDER
140.1	VERMILION BORDER LIP LOWER
140.0	VERMILION BORDER LIP UPPER
198.89	VERMILION BORDER METASTATIC
170.2	VERTEBRA
198.5	VERTEBRA METASTATIC
170.6	VERTEBRA - SACRUM, COCCYX
198.5	VERTEBRA - SACRUM, COCCYX METASTATIC
184.9	VESICOVAGINAL
198.82	VESICOVAGINAL METASTATIC
184.9	VESICOVAGINAL SEPTUM
198.82	VESICOVAGINAL SEPTUM METASTATIC
163.1	VISCERAL PLEURAL
197.2	VISCERAL PLEURAL METASTATIC
161.0	VOCAL CORDS TRUE
161.1	VOCAL CORDS FALSE
197.3	VOCAL CORDS (TRUE) (FALSE) METASTATIC
170.0	VOMER (CARTILAGE) (JOINT) (PERIOSTEUM)
198.5	VOMER (CARTILAGE) (JOINT) (PERIOSTEUM) METASTATIC
184.4	VULVA
198.82	VULVA METASTATIC
149.1	WALDEYER'S RING
198.89	WALDEYER'S RING METASTATIC
142.1	WHARTON'S DUCT
198.89	WHARTON'S DUCT METASTATIC
170.3	XIPHOID
198.5	XIPHOID METASTATIC

CANCER (continued)

194.6 ZUCKERKANDL'S ORGAN
198.89 ZUCKERKANDL'S ORGAN METASTATIC

170.0 ZYGOMATIC BONE
198.5 ZYGOMATIC BONE METASTATIC

> *IF TREATMENT IS DIRECTED TOWARDS THE METASTATIC SITE, THEN THAT SITE IS CODED FIRST, EVEN IF THE PRIMARY SITE IS KNOWN.*
>
> *WHEN BOTH A PRIMARY AND SECONDARY SITE ARE PRESENT AND TREATED EQUALLY, SEQUENCE THE PRIMARY SITE FIRST.*

CANCER METASTATIC

199.1 SITE NOS
197.# DIGESTIVE
4th Digit: 197
4. SMALL INTESTINE, DUODENUM
5. LARGE INTESTINE, RECTUM
6. RETROPERITONEUM AND PERITONEUM
7. LIVER, SPECIFIED AS SECONDARY
8. OTHER DIGESTIVE ORGANS AND SPLEEN

196.# LYMPH NODE METASTATIC
4th Digit: 196
0. HEAD FACE NECK CERVICAL SUPRACLAVICULAR
1. INTRATHORACIC BRONCHOPULMONARY MEDIASTINAL TRACHEOBRONCHIAL
2. INTRA ABDOMINAL MESENTERIC RETROPERITONEAL
3. AXILLA UPPER LIMB BRACHIAL INTRACLAVICULAR PECTORAL
5. LOWER LIMB INGUINAL FEMORAL GROIN TIBIAL
6. INTRAPELVIC HYPOGASTRIC ILIAC PARAMETRIAL
8. MULTIPLE SITES
9. LYMPH NODES NOS

197.# RESPIRATORY
4th Digit: 197
0. LUNG, BRONCHUS
1. MEDIASTINUM
2. PLEURA
3. OTHER RESPIRATORY ORGANS, TRACHEA

198.#(#) OTHER SPECIFIED SITES
4th or 4th and 5th Digit: 198
0. KIDNEY
1. OTHER URINARY ORGANS
2. SKIN AND SKIN OF BREAST (OR MASTECTOMY SITE SKIN)
3. BRAIN AND SPINAL CORD
4. OTHER PARTS OF NERVOUS SYSTEM, MENINGES (CEREBRAL) (SPINAL)
5. BONE AND BONE MARROW
6. OVARY
7. ADRENAL GLAND
8#. OTHER SPECIFIED SITES
81. BREAST SOFT TISSUE
82. GENITAL ORGANS
89. OTHER

CANCER SCREENING

V76.9 NOS
V76.3 BLADDER
V76.10 BREAST UNSPECIFIED
V76.11 BREAST MAMMOGRAM FOR HIGH RISK PATIENT
V76.12 BREAST MAMMOGRAM NEC
V76.19 BREAST SPECIFIED TYPE NEC
V76.2 CERVIX
V76.42 ORAL CAVITY
V76.44 PROSTATE
V76.41 RECTAL CANCER
V76.0 RESPIRATORY ORGANS
V76.43 SKIN
V76.45 TESTIS
V76.49 OTHER SITES
V76.8 OTHER NEOPLASMS (BENIGN) (TUMORS)

528.1 CANCRUM ORIS
112.5 CANDIDEMIA

CANDIDIASIS

112.9 UNSPECIFIED SITE
112.2 BALANITIS
112.5 DISSEMINATED
112.81 ENDOCARDITIS
112.85 ENTERITIS
112.84 ESOPHAGITIS
771.7 INFECTION NEONATAL
112.3 INTERTRIGO
112.85 INTESTINE
112.4 LUNG
112.83 MENINGITIS
112.0 MOUTH
112.3 NAILS
112.3 ONYCHIA
112.0 ORAL
112.82 OTITIS EXTERNA
112.3 PERIONYXIS (PARONYCHIA)
112.4 PNEUMONIA
112.2 PYELONEPHRITIS
112.3 SKIN
112.5 SYSTEMIC
112.2 URINARY TRACT
112.2 UTI
112.1 VULVOVAGINITIS
112.89 OTHER SPECIFIED SITE NEC

136.8 CANDIRU INFESTATION
528.2 CANKER SORE
504 CANNABINOSIS
305.2# CANNABIS ABUSE NONDEPENDENT
304.3# CANNABIS ADDICTION DEPENDENT
5th Digit: 304.3, 305.2
0. NOS
1. CONTINUOUS
2. EPISODIC
3. IN REMISSION

128.8 CAPILLARIA HEPATICA INFECTION
127.5 CAPILLARIA PHILIPPINENSIS INFECTION
127.5 CAPILLARIASIS
128.8 CAPILLARIASIS HEPATICA

CAPILLARY

448.9 DISEASE

> *648.9#: USE AN ADDITIONAL CODE TO IDENTIFY THE CAPILLARY DISEASE.*

648.9# DISEASE MATERNAL CURRENT (CO-EXISTENT) IN PREGNANCY
5th Digit: 648.9
0. EPISODE OF NOS OR N/A
1. DELIVERED
2. DELIVERED WITH POSTPARTUM COMPLICATION
3. ANTEPARTUM COMPLICATION
4. POSTPARTUM COMPLICATION

287.8 FRAGILITY (HEREDITARY)
448.9 HEMORRHAGE (THROMBOSIS) HYPERPERMEABILITY

714.81 CAPLAN (-COLINET) SYNDROME
434.0# CAPSULAR THROMBOSIS SYNDROME
5th Digit: 434.0
0. WITHOUT CEREBRAL INFARCTION
1. WITH CEREBRAL INFARCTION

	CAPSULITIS
726.90	SITE UNSPECIFIED
387.8	LABYRINTHINE
726.0	SHOULDER (ADHESIVE)
0	SITE SPECIFIED SEE 'BURSITIS'
767.1	CAPUT SUCCEDANEUM
087.1	CARAPATA DISEASE
271.9	CARBOHYDRATE TRANSPORT AND METABOLISM DISORDER
271.8	CARBOHYDRATE TRANSPORT AND METABOLISM DISORDER - OTHER SPECIFIED
786.09	CARBON DIOXIDE NARCOSIS
276.2	CARBON DIOXIDE RETENTION
276.9	CARBONATE ABNORMAL FINDINGS
	CARBUNCLE
680.9	SITE UNSPECIFIED
680.2	ABDOMINAL WALL
680.6	ANKLE
680.5	ANUS
680.3	ARM (ANY PART EXCEPT HAND)
680.3	AXILLA
680.2	BACK (ANY PART EXCEPT BUTTOCKS)
680.2	BREAST
680.5	BUTTOCKS
680.2	CHEST WALL
607.2	CORPUS CAVERNOSUM
680.0	EAR (ANY PART)
680.0	EXTERNAL AUDITORY CANAL
373.13	EYELID
680.0	FACE
680.4	FINGER (ANY)
680.2	FLANK
680.7	FOOT
680.3	FOREARM
616.4	GENITALIA FEMALE (NONOBSTETRICAL)
608.4	GENITALIA MALE
680.5	GLUTEAL REGION
680.2	GROIN
680.4	HAND
680.8	HEAD (ANY PART EXCEPT FACE)
680.7	HEEL
680.6	HIP
680.6	KNEE
375.31	LACRIMAL SYSTEM
680.6	LEG (EXCEPT FOOT)
680.9	MULTIPLE SITE
680.1	NECK
680.0	NOSE
680.0	NOSE (SEPTUM)
376.01	ORBIT
680.2	PECTORAL REGION
607.2	PENIS
680.2	PERINEUM
680.0	PINNA
680.8	SCALP
608.4	SCROTUM
680.3	SHOULDER
680.0	TEMPLE REGION
608.4	TESTIS
680.6	THIGH
680.4	THUMB
680.7	TOE
680.2	TRUNK
680.2	UMBILICUS
608.4	VAS DEFERENS
616.4	VULVA (NONOBSTETRICAL)
680.4	WRIST
795.79	CARCINOEMBRYONIC ANTIGEN POSITIVE
453.1	CARCINOGENIC THROMBOPHLEBITIS SYNDROME
	CARCINOID
238.9	SITE NOS
0	SITE SPECIFIED SEE 'NEOPLASM UNCERTAIN BEHAVIOR', BY SITE
199.1	COMPOSITE SITE NOS
0	COMPOSITE SITE SPECIFIED SEE 'CANCER' BY SITE M8244/3
236.2	STRUMAL SITE NOS
0	STRUMAL SITE SPECIFIED SEE 'NEOPLASM UNCERTAIN BEHAVIOR' BY SITE M9091/1
259.2	SYNDROME
238.9	TUMOR SITE NOS
0	TUMOR SITE SPECIFIED SEE 'NEOPLASM UNCERTAIN BEHAVIOR' BY SITE M8240/1
199.1	TUMOR (MALIGNANT) SITE NOS
0	TUMOR (MALIGNANT) SITE SPECIFIED SEE 'CANCER' BY SITE M8240/3
199.1	TUMOR ARGENTAFFIN MALIGNANT SITE NOS
0	TUMOR ARGENTAFFIN MALIGNANT SITE SPECIFIED SEE 'CANCER' BY SITE M8241/1
238.9	TUMOR ARGENTAFFIN SITE NOS
0	TUMOR ARGENTAFFIN SITE SPECIFIED SEE 'NEOPLASM UNCERTAIN BEHAVIOR' BY SITE M8241/1
199.1	TUMOR NONARGENTAFFIN MALIGNANT SITE NOS
0	TUMOR NONARGENTAFFIN MALIGNANT SITE SPECIFIED SEE 'CANCER' BY SITE M8242/1
238.9	TUMOR NONARGENTAFFIN SITE NOS
0	TUMOR NONARGENTAFFIN SITE SPECIFIED SEE 'NEOPLASM UNCERTAIN BEHAVIOR' BY SITE M8242/1
0	CARCINOMA SITE SPECIFIED SEE 'CANCER', BY SITE M8010/3

CARCINOMA IN SITU QUICK REFERENCE

230.# DIGESTIVE ORGANS

4th Digit: 230

- **0. LIP, ORAL CAVITY, PHARYNX, MARGINAL ZONE**
- **1. ESOPHAGUS**
- **2. STOMACH**
- **3. COLON**
- **4. RECTUM**
- **5. ANAL CANAL**
- **6. ANUS, UNSPECIFIED**
- **7. OTHER AND UNSPECIFIED PARTS OF INTESTINE**
- **8. LIVER AND BILIARY SYSTEM**
- **9. OTHER AND UNSPECIFIED DIGESTIVE ORGANS**

233.# GENITOURINARY AND BREAST

4th Digit: 233

- **0. BREAST**
- **1. CERVIX UTERI**
- **2. OTHER AND UNSPECIFIED PARTS OF UTERUS**
- **3. OTHER AND UNSPECIFIED FEMALE GENITAL ORGANS**
- **4. PROSTATE**
- **5. PENIS**
- **6. OTHER AND UNSPECIFIED MALE GENITAL ORGANS**
- **7. BLADDER**
- **9. OTHER AND UNSPECIFIED URINARY ORGANS**

231.# RESPIRATORY

4th Digit: 231

- **0. LARYNX, ARYTENOID / CRICOID / CUNEIFORM / THYROID CARTILAGE, EPIGLOTTIS (SUPRAHYOID), VOCAL CORDS**
- **1. TRACHEA**
- **2. BRONCHUS AND LUNG, CARINA, HILUS OF LUNG**
- **8. OTHER SPECIFIED PARTS OF RESPIRATORY SYSTEM: NASAL CAVITIES, MIDDLE EAR, PLEURA, ACCESSORY SINUS**
- **9. RESPIRATORY SYSTEM (ORGAN) NOS**

CARCINOMA IN SITU QUICK REFERENCE (continued)

232.# SKIN

4th Digit: 232

0. LIP
1. EYELID, CANTHUS
2. EAR, EXTERNAL AUDITORY CANAL
3. SKIN OF OTHER AND UNSPECIFIED PARTS OF FACE
4. SCALP, SKIN OF NECK
5. SKIN OF TRUNK EXCEPT SCROTUM: ABDOMINAL WALL, ANUS, ANAL MARGIN, AXILLARY FOLD, BACK, BREAST, BUTTOCK, CHEST WALL, GROIN, PERINEUM
6. SKIN OF UPPER LIMB, SHOULDER
7. SKIN OF LOWER LIMB, HIP
8. OTHER SPECIFIED SKIN SITE: NOSE NOS
9. SKIN SITE NOS

234.# OTHER AND UNSPECIFIED PARTS

4th Digit: 234

0. EYE
8. OTHER SPECIFIED SITES: ENDOCRINE GLAND (ANY), EYELID CARTILAGE, OPTIC NERVE, ORBIT BONE
9. SITE NOS: CA IN SITU NOS

CARCINOMA IN SITU

234.9 NOS
230.8 AMPULLA OF VATER
230.5 ANAL CANAL
230.6 ANUS
232.5 ANUS (MARGIN) (SKIN) (PERINAL)
232.5 ANUS SKIN OF (MARGIN)
230.3 APPENDIX
230.0 ARYEPIGLOTTIC FOLD
231.0 ARYEPIGLOTTIC FOLD, LARYNGEAL ASPECT
230.0 ARYEPIGLOTTIC HYPOPHARYNGEAL
230.0 ARYEPIGLOTTIC MARGINAL
231.0 ARYTENOID CARTILAGE
232.5 AXILLARY FOLD SKIN
230.8 BILIARY SYSTEM
230.2 BODY OF STOMACH
233.0 BREAST
232.5 BREAST SKIN
231.2 BRONCHUS
232.5 BUTTOCK SKIN
230.2 CARDIA OF STOMACH
230.2 CARDIAC ORIFICE
231.2 CARINA
230.3 CECUM
233.1 CERVIX (STUMP)
232.5 CHEST WALL SKIN
230.3 COLON
230.4 COLON RECTOSIGMOID
230.8 COMMON BILE DUCT
234.0 CONJUNCTIVA
234.0 CORNEA
231.0 CRICOID CARTILAGE
231.0 CUNEIFORM CARTILAGE
230.8 CYSTIC DUCT
230.7 DIGESTIVE INTESTINE OTHER
230.9 DIGESTIVE ORGANS OTHER AND UNSPECIFIED
230.7 DUODENUM
232.2 EAR EXTERNAL AUDITORY CANAL SKIN
234.8 ENDOCRINE
231.0 EPIGLOTTIS
231.0 EPIGLOTTIS POSTERIOR
231.0 EPIGLOTTIS SUPRAHYOID
230.1 ESOPHAGUS
234.0 EYE
234.8 EYELID CARTILAGE
232.1 EYELID SKIN
232.1 EYELID SKIN CANTHUS
232.3 FACE SKIN OTHER AND UNSPECIFIED PARTS
230.2 FUNDUS OF STOMACH

CARCINOMA IN SITU (continued)

230.8 GALLBLADDER
230.9 GASTROINTESTINAL
233.7 GENITOURINARY BLADDER
233.1 GENITOURINARY CERVIX
233.5 GENITOURINARY PENIS
233.4 GENITOURINARY PROSTATE
233.2 GENITOURINARY UTERUS
233.3 GENITOURINARY OTHER AND UNSPECIFIED FEMALE GENITAL ORGANS
233.6 GENITOURINARY OTHER AND UNSPECIFIED MALE GENITAL
233.9 GENITOURINARY OTHER AND UNSPECIFIED URINARY ORGAN
230.0 GINGIVA
232.5 GROIN SKIN
230.8 HEPATIC DUCT
231.2 HILUS OF LUNG
232.7 HIP LOWER LIMB SKIN
230.0 HYPOPHARYNGEAL
230.0 HYPOPHARYNX
230.3 ILEOCECAL VALVE
230.7 ILEUM
230.7 INTESTINE SMALL NOS
230.7 JEJUNUM
230.3 LARGE INTESTINE
231.0 LARYNX
230.0 LIP
232.0 LIP SKIN
230.8 LIVER
231.2 LUNG
230.0 MARGINAL
231.8 MIDDLE EAR
230.0 MOUTH
230.0 MOUTH (FLOOR)
231.8 NASAL CAVITIES
230.0 NASOPHARYNX
232.4 NECK SKIN
234.8 OPTIC NERVE
234.8 ORBIT (BONE)
230.0 OROPHARYNX
234.8 OTHER SPECIFIED SITES
230.9 PANCREAS
230.0 PAROTID GLAND IN SITU
232.5 PERINEUM SKIN
231.8 PLEURA
233.4 PROSTATE
230.2 PYLORUS
230.4 RECTOSIGMOID JUNCTION
230.4 RECTUM
231.9 RESPIRATORY
231.8 RESPIRATORY OTHER
230.0 SALIVARY GLAND OR DUCT
232.4 SCALP
232.6 SHOULDER UPPER LIMB SKIN
231.8 SINUS (ACCESSORY)
232.9 SKIN
232.8 SKIN OTHER SPECIFIED SITES
230.7 SMALL INTESTINE
230.8 SPHINCTER OF ODDI
230.9 SPLEEN
230.2 STOMACH
231.0 THYROID
231.0 THYROID CARTILAGE
230.0 TONGUE
231.1 TRACHEA
231.1 TRACHEOBRONCHIAL
232.5 TRUNK SKIN
232.5 UMBILICUS (SKIN)
233.3 VAGINAL VESICOVAGINAL SEPTUM
231.0 VOCAL CORDS
230.0 WHARTON'S DUCT

0 CARCINOMA METASTATIC SITE SPECIFIED SEE 'CANCER' BY SITE, METASTATIC M8010/6
0 CARCINOMA SIMPLEX SITE SPECIFIED SEE 'CANCER' BY SITE M8231/3
0 CARCINOMA SKIN APPENDAGE SITE SPECIFIED SEE 'CANCER' SKIN BY SITE M8231/3
0 CARCINOMA UNDIFFERENTIATED TYPE SITE SPECIFIED SEE 'CANCER' BY SITE M8020/3
0 CARCINOMA VENTRICULI SEE 'CANCER', STOMACH
199.0 CARCINOMATOSIS SITE NOS M8010/6
0 CARCINOMATOSIS SITE SPECIFIED SEE 'CANCER' BY SITE M8010/3
199.1 CARCINOSARCOMA EMBRYONAL TYPE SITE NOS
0 CARCINOSARCOMA EMBRYONAL TYPE SITE SPECIFIED SEE 'CANCER' BY SITE M8981/3
199.1 CARCINOSARCOMA SITE NOS
0 CARCINOSARCOMA SITE SPECIFIED SEE 'CANCER' BY SITE M8980/3

CARDIAC
428.1 ASTHMA (SYNDROME)
429.1 ATROPHY (SEE ALSO 'MYOCARDIAL', DEGENERATION)
996.09 CATHETER COMPLICATION MECHANICAL
V58.82 CATHETER NONVASCULAR ADJUSTMENT
V58.81 CATHETER VASCULAR ADJUSTMENT
426.9 CONDUCTION DELAY (VENTRICULAR)
861.01 CONTUSION
861.11 CONTUSION WITH OPEN WOUND
908.0 CONTUSION LATE EFFECT
0 DEFIBRILLATOR SEE 'CARDIAC DEFIBRILLATOR'
V53.39 DEVICE OTHER SPECIFIED - FITTING AND ADJUSTMENT
V45.00 DEVICE UNSPECIFIED - IN SITU STATUS
V45.09 DEVICE OTHER SPECIFIED - IN SITU STATUS
785.3 DULLNESS (INCREASED) (DECREASED)
0 DYSRHYTHMIA SEE 'DYSRHYTHMIAS' OR BY SPECIFIED DYSRHYTHMIA
794.30 FUNCTION STUDY ABNORMAL
861.00 INJURY NOS
861.10 INJURY NOS WITH OPEN WOUND INTO THORAX
908.0 INJURY NOS LATE EFFECT
429.4 INSUFFICIENCY FOLLOWING CARDIAC SURGERY
861.02 LACERATION
861.12 LACERATION WITH OPEN WOUND INTO CHEST
908.0 LACERATION LATE EFFECT
306.2 NEUROSIS PSYCHOGENIC
0 PACEMAKER SEE 'CARDIAC PACEMAKER'
423.9 TAMPONADE
746.89 VALVE ATRESIA
746.89 VEIN ATRESIA
746.89 VEIN HYPOPLASIA

CARDIAC ARREST IS NOT AN ACCEPTABLE PRINCIPAL DIAGNOSIS BY MOST CARRIERS. AS A GENERAL RULE, CODE FIRST THE DISEASE OR CONDITION WHICH LED IMMEDIATELY TO THE ARREST. EXCEPTION: IF THE REASON THE PATIENT PRESENTED WAS THE ARREST.

CARDIAC ARREST
427.5 NOS
997.1 DURING OR RESULTING FROM A PROCEDURE
639.8 FOLLOWING ABORTION
668.1# FOLLOWING ANESTHESIA (OR FAILURE) L AND D
669.4# FOLLOWING OBSTETRICAL SURGERY OR PROCEDURE OR DELIVERY
5th Digit: 668.1, 669.4
0. EPISODE OF CARE NOS OR N/A
1. DELIVERED
2. DELIVERED WITH POSTPARTUM COMPLICATION
3. ANTEPARTUM COMPLICATION
4. POSTPARTUM COMPLICATION

CARDIAC DEFIBRILLATOR
996.61 COMPLICATION - INFECTION OR INFLAMMATION
996.04 COMPLICATION - MECHANICAL
996.72 COMPLICATION - OTHER
V53.32 FITTING AND ADJUSTMENT
V45.02 IN SITU (AUTOMATIC IMPLANTABLE)

CARDIAC PACEMAKER
V53.31 BATTERY REPLACEMENT
996.61 COMPLICATION - INFECTION OR INFLAMMATION
996.01 COMPLICATION - MECHANICAL (BREAKDOWN) (PERFORATION) (DISPLACED)
996.72 COMPLICATION - OTHER
V53.31 FITTING AND ADJUSTMENT
V45.01 IN SITU STATUS
996.01 MALFUNCTION (BREAKDOWN) (PERFORATION) (DISPLACED)
V53.31 REPROGRAMMING
429.4 SYNDROME

416.0 CARDIACOS NEGROS SYNDROME
747.49 CARDINAL VEIN LEFT POSTERIOR PERSISTENT CONGENITAL
530.89 CARDIO-ESOPHAGEAL RELAXATION
530.81 CARDIOCHALASIA

CARDIOMEGALY
429.3 NOS
746.89 CONGENITAL
271.0 GLYCOGEN
402.## HYPERTENSIVE
4th Digit: 402
0. MALIGNANT
1. BENIGN
9. NOS
5th Digit: 402
0. WITHOUT CONGESTIVE HEART FAILURE
1. WITH CONGESTIVE HEART FAILURE
429.3 IDIOPATHIC

CARDIOMYOPATHY
425.4 NOS
425.5 ALCOHOLIC
429.1 ARTERIOSCLEROTIC [440.9]
425.5 COBALT-BEER
425.3 CONGENITAL
425.4 CONGESTIVE
425.4 CONSTRICTIVE
425.4 FAMILIAL
274.82 GOUTY
402.## HYPERTENSIVE
4th Digit: 402
0. MALIGNANT
1. BENIGN
9. NOS
5th Digit: 402
0. WITHOUT CHF
1. WITH CHF
425.4 HYPERTROPHIC
425.1 HYPERTROPHIC OBSTRUCTIVE
746.84 HYPERTROPHIC OBSTRUCTIVE CONGENITAL
425.4 IDIOPATHIC
425.2 IDIOPATHIC MURAL
414.8 ISCHEMIC
425.4 NONOBSTRUCTIVE
425.2 OBSCURE OF AFRICA
425.4 OBSTRUCTIVE
425.4 PRIMARY
425.4 RESTRICTIVE
425.9 SECONDARY
425.9 TOXIC NEC

CARDIOMYOPATHY OTHER

277.3 AMYLOID [425.7]
265.0 BERI BERI [425.7]
086.0 CHAGAS' DISEASE
425.3 ELASTOMYOFIBROSIS
425.0 ENDOMYOCARDIAL FIBROSIS
334.0 FRIEDREICH'S (ATAXIA) [425.8]
271.0 GLYCOGENIC (CARDIAC) [425.7]
487.8 INFLUENZA [425.8]

WHEN CODING A MATERNAL CARDIOMYOPATHY COMPLICATING PREGNANCY, 648.6#, USE AN ADDITIONAL CODE TO IDENTIFY THE CARDIOMYOPATHY.

648.6# MATERNAL CURRENT (CO-EXISTENT) IN PREGNANCY [425.9]
5th Digit: 648.6
0. EPISODE OF CARE NOS OR N/A
1. DELIVERED
2. DELIVERED WITH POSTPARTUM COMPLICATION
3. ANTEPARTUM COMPLICATION
4. POSTPARTUM COMPLICATION

674.8# MATERNAL POSTPARTUM
5th Digit: 674.8
0. EPISODE OF CARE NOS OR N/A
2. DELIVERED WITH POSTPARTUM COMPLICATION
4. POSTPARTUM COMPLICATION

277.5 MUCOPOLYSACCHARIDOSIS (DUE TO) [425.7]
359.1 MUSCULAR DYSTROPHY (DUE TO) [425.8]
359.2 MYOTONIA ATROPHICA [425.8]
265.0 NUTRITIONAL (BERIBERI) [425.7]
269.9 NUTRITIONAL MALNUTRITION [425.7]
135 SARCOID [425.8]
242.## THYROTOXIC [425.7]
4th Digit: 242
0. DIFFUSE
1. UNINODULAR
2. MULTINODULAR
3. NODULAR UNSPECIFIED
4. ECTOPIC THYROID NODULAR
8. OTHER SPECIFIED
9. NOS
5th Digit: 242
0. WITHOUT MENTION OF THYROTOXIC CRISIS OR STORM
1. WITH MENTION OF THYROTOXIC CRISIS OR STORM

017.9# TUBERCULOUS [425.8]
5th Digit: 017.9
0. UNSPECIFIED
1. LAB NOT DONE
2. LABS PENDING
3. MICROSCOPY POSITIVE (IN SPUTUM)
4. CULTURE POSITIVE - MICROSCOPY NEGATIVE
5. CULTURE NEGATIVE - MICROSCOPY POSITIVE
6. CULTURE AND MICROSCOPY NEGATIVE CONFIRMED BY OTHER METHODS

427.5 CARDIOPULMONARY ARREST
416.9 CARDIOPULMONARY DISEASE, CHRONIC
278.8 CARDIOPULMONARY OBESITY SYNDROME
404.90 CARDIORENAL SYNDROME
769 CARDIORESPIRATORY DISTRESS SYNDROME (IDIOPATHIC) NEWBORN
799.1 CARDIORESPIRATORY FAILURE
530.0 CARDIOSPASM
750.7 CARDIOSPASM CONGENITAL

CARDIOVASCULAR

794.30 ABNORMAL FUNCTION STUDY
794.31 ABNORMAL ELECTROCARDIOGRAM (ECG) (EKG)
794.39 ABNORMAL OTHER STUDY
425.4 COLLAGENOSIS
V81.2 CONDITONS UNSPECIFIED SCREENING
429.2 DISEASE (ARTERIOSCLEROTIC) [440.9]
746.9 DISEASE (ARTERIOSCLEROTIC) CONGENITAL
402.## DISEASE (ARTERIOSCLEROTIC) HYPERTENSIVE
4th Digit: 402
0. MALIGNANT
1. BENIGN
9. NOS
5th Digit: 402
0. WITHOUT CHF
1. WITH CHF

V12.50 DISEASE HISTORY UNSPECIFIED
V12.59 DISEASE HISTORY OTHER SPECIFIED

WHEN CODING A MATERNAL CARDIOVASCULAR DISEASE COMPLICATING PREGNANCY, 648.6#, USE AN ADDITIONAL CODE TO IDENTIFY THE CONDITION.

648.6# DISEASE MATERNAL CURRENT (CO-EXISTENT) IN PREGNANCY
5th Digit: 648.6
0. EPISODE OF CARE NOS OR N/A
1. DELIVERED
2. DELIVERED WITH POSTPARTUM COMPLICATION
3. ANTEPARTUM COMPLICATION
4. POSTPARTUM COMPLICATION

V17.4 DISEASE FAMILY HISTORY
306.2 DISORDER (SYSTEM) PSYCHOGENIC
306.2 NEUROSIS PSYCHOGENIC
404.90 RENAL SYNDROME
785.9 SYMPTOM OTHER

272.7 CARDIOVASORENAL SYNDROME

CARDITIS

429.89 NOS
074.20 COXSACKIE
0 HYPERTENSIVE SEE 'CARDIOMYOPATHY'
036.40 MENINGOCOCCAL
429.89 OTHER (NONHYPERTENSIVE)
391.9 RHEUMATIC ACUTE
398.90 RHEUMATIC CHRONIC

V60.5 CARE HOLIDAY RELIEF
V62.2 CAREER CHOICE PROBLEM CAUSING ENCOUNTER
757.1 CARINI'S SYNDROME (ICHTHYOSIS CONGENITA)
631 CARNEOUS MOLE
631 CARNEOUS MOLE WITH COMPLICATION DURING TREATMENT [639.#]
639.# CARNEOUS MOLE WITH COMPLICATION FOLLOWING TREATMENT
4th Digit: 639
0. GENITAL TRACT AND PELVIC INFECTION
1. DELAYED OR EXCESSIVE HEMORRHAGE
2. DAMAGE TO PELVIC ORGANS AND TISSUE
3. RENAL FAILURE
4. METABOLIC DISORDERS
5. SHOCK
6. EMBOLISM
8. OTHER SPECIFIED COMPLICATION
9. UNSPECIFIED COMPLICATION

270.5 CARNOSINEMIA

CAROTID ARTERY

437.3 ANEURYSM - INTERNAL NOS (INTRACRANIAL PORTION)
442.81 ANEURYSM - INTERNAL EXTRACRANIAL PORTION

C

CAROTID ARTERY (continued)

433.1# ARTERIOSCLEROSIS
5th Digit: 433.1
0. WITHOUT CEREBRAL INFARCTION
1. WITH CEREBRAL INFARCTION

237.3 BODY TUMOR SITE NOS
0 BODY TUMOR SITE SPECIFIED SEE 'NEOPLASM UNCERTAIN BEHAVIOR' BY SITE M8980/3
996.62 BYPASS GRAFT COMPLICATION - INFECTION OR INFLAMMATION
996.1 BYPASS GRAFT COMPLICATION - MECHANICAL
996.74 BYPASS GRAFT COMPLICATION - OTHER
433.1# DISEASE (ULCERATIVE)
433.1# EMBOLISM THROMBOSIS
5th Digit: 433.1
0. WITHOUT CEREBRAL INFARCTION
1. WITH CEREBRAL INFARCTION

447.8 HYPERPLASIA
900.00 INJURY - NOS
900.01 INJURY - COMMON CAROTID
900.02 INJURY - EXTERNAL CAROTID
900.03 INJURY - INTERNAL CAROTID
908.3 INJURY - LATE EFFECT

433.1# OCCLUSION (OBSTRUCTION) (THROMBOSIS) (EMBOLISM) (STENOSIS)
433.3# OCCLUSION BILATERAL OR WITH BASILAR AND/OR VERTEBRAL ARTERY
5th Digit: 433.1, 3
0. WITHOUT CEREBRAL INFARCTION
1. WITH CEREBRAL INFARCTION

337.0 PAIN
337.0 SINUS SYNCOPE
435.8 SYNDROME (INTERNAL)

INJURY OF A BLOOD VESSEL CAN BE A LACERATION, A-V FISTULA, ANEURYSM, OR HEMATOMA. USE THE "INJURY" CODE FOUND BY ANATOMICAL SITE (THE NAME OF THE BLOOD VESSEL).

CAROTID ARTERY INJURY

900.00 NOS
900.01 COMMON CAROTID
900.02 EXTERNAL CAROTID
900.03 INTERNAL CAROTID
908.3 LATE EFFECT

337.0 CAROTID BODY OR SINUS SYNDROME
259.8 CAROTID GLAND DISEASE
V53.39 CAROTID SINUS PACEMAKER FITTING AND ADJUSTMENT
V45.09 CAROTID SINUS PACEMAKER IN SITU
337.0 CAROTIDYNIA
278.3 CAROTINEMIA

CARPAL

755.21 ABSENCE WITH COMPLETE ABSENCE OF DISTAL ELEMENTS
755.28 ABSENCE WITH INCOMPLETE ABSENCE OF DISTAL ELEMENTS
755.56 ACCESSORY BONE
755.28 AGENESIS
842.01 SEPARATION (RUPTURE) (TEAR) (LACERATION)
842.01 STRAIN (SPRAIN) (AVULSION) (HEMARTHROSIS)
354.0 TUNNEL SYNDROME
755.28 OR METACARPALS AGENESIS

759.89 CARPENTER'S SYNDROME

CARPOMETACARPAL JOINT DISLOCATION

833.04 CARPOMETACARPAL CLOSED
833.14 CARPOMETACARPAL OPEN

833.05 METACARPAL BONE PROXIMAL CLOSED
833.15 METACARPAL BONE PROXIMAL OPEN

833.03 MIDCARPAL CLOSED
833.13 MIDCARPAL OPEN

842.11 CARPOMETACARPAL STRAIN (SPRAIN)
781.7 CARPOPEDAL SPASM

CARRIER

V02.2 AMEBIASIS
V02.0 CHOLERA
V02.4 DIPHTHERIA
V02.2 ENDAMOEBA HISTOLYTICA
V02.3 GASTROINTESTINAL OTHER PATHOGENS
V02.7 GONORRHEA
V02.61 HAA (HEPATITIS AUSTRALIAN-ANTIGEN)
V02.60 HEPATITIS VIRAL NOS
V02.61 HEPATITIS VIRAL B (HAA) (SERUM)
V02.62 HEPATITIS VIRAL C
V02.69 HEPATITIS VIRAL OTHER
V02.59 MENINGOCOCCAL
V02.3 SALMONELLA
V02.61 SERUM HEPATITIS
V02.3 SHIGELLA
V02.59 STAPHYLOCOCCAL
V02.51 STREPTOCOCCUS GROUP B
V02.52 STREPTOCOCCUS OTHER
V02.1 TYPHOID
V02.60 VIRAL HEPATITIS NOS
V02.61 VIRAL HEPATITIS B (HAA) (SERUM)
V02.62 VIRAL HEPATITIS C
V02.69 VIRAL HEPATITIS OTHER
V02.59 OTHER SPECIFIED BACTERIAL DISEASE
V02.9 OTHER SPECIFIED INFECTIOUS ORGANISM
V02.8 OTHER VENEREAL DISEASE

088.0 CARRION'S DISEASE (BARTONELLOSIS)

CARTILAGE

756.9 AGENESIS
733.99 ATROPHY (INFECTIONAL) (JOINT)
733.99 CALCIFICATION (POSTINFECTIONAL)
748.3 CLEFT CONGENITAL
718.0# DERANGEMENT (ARTICULAR) OLD
5th Digit: 718.0
0. SITE NOS
1. SHOULDER REGION
2. UPPER ARM (ELBOW) (HUMERUS)
3. FOREARM (RADIUS) (WRIST) (ULNA)
4. HAND (CARPAL) (METACARPAL) (FINGERS)
5. PELVIC REGION AND THIGH (HIP) (BUTTOCK) (FEMUR)
7. ANKLE AND/OR FOOT (METATARSALS) (TOES)
8. OTHER
9. MULTIPLE

718.3# DERANGEMENT (ARTICULAR) - RECURRENT
5th Digit: 718.3
0. SITE UNSPECIFIED
1. SHOULDER REGION
2. UPPER ARM (ELBOW) (HUMERUS)
3. FOREARM (RADIUS) (WRIST) (ULNA)
4. HAND (CARPAL) (METACARPAL) (FINGERS)
5. PELVIC REGION (HIP) (BUTTOCK) (FEMUR)
6. LOWER LEG (FIBULA) (KNEE) (PATELLA) (TIBIA)
7. ANKLE AND/OR FOOT (METATARSALS) (TOES) (TARSALS)
8. OTHER
9. MULTIPLE

717.9 DERANGEMENT KNEE - NOS OLD
0 DERANGEMENT KNEE - MENISCUS SEE 'MENISCUS', KNEE TEAR
717.5 DERANGEMENT KNEE - SEMILUNAR OLD
733.90 DISEASE OR DISORDER
733.99 DISEASE OR DISORDER - SPECIFIED NEC

CARUNCLE
372.00 CONJUNCTIVA
373.00 EYELID
616.8 LABIUM
375.30 LACRIMAL
599.3 URETHRA
616.8 VAGINA

537.6 CASCADE STOMACH
259.2 CASSIDY (-SCHOLTE) SYNDROME (MALIGNANT CARCINOID)

CAST
V54.8 AFTERCARE (ORTHOPEDIC) (PLASTER)
0 APPLICATION SEE SPECIFIC INJURY
V54.8 CHANGE
V54.8 CHECKING
V53.7 FITTING AND ADJUSTMENT
V54.8 REMOVAL
557.1 SYNDROME (BODY CAST) (MESENTERIC ARTERY ISCHEMIA)

104.8 CASTELLANI'S DISEASE
281.0 CASTLE'S DEFICIENCY
266.2 CASTLE'S DEFICIENCY WITHOUT ANEMIA
266.2 CASTLE'S DEFICIENCY WITHOUT ANEMIA OR SPINAL CORD DEGENERATION
0 CAT BITE SEE 'OPEN WOUND' BY SITE
758.3 CAT CRY SYNDROME
V72.5 CAT SCAN
078.3 CAT SCRATCH FEVER
347 CATAPLEXY

CATARACT
366.9 NOS
V45.61 EXTRACTION STATUS WITH ARTIFICIAL LENS STATUS [V43.1]
998.82 FRAGMENTS IN EYE FOLLOWING SURGERY
V80.2 SCREENING

CATARACT NONSENILE (INFANTILE) (JUVENILE) (PRESENILE)
366.00 NOS
366.03 CORTICAL
998.82 FRAGMENTS IN EYE FOLLOWING SURGERY
366.03 LAMELLAR
366.04 NUCLEAR
366.01 SUBCAPSULAR POLAR ANTERIOR
366.02 SUBCAPSULAR POLAR POSTERIOR
366.03 ZONULAR
366.09 OTHER AND COMBINED FORMS

CATARACT SENILE
366.10 NOS
366.12 CORONARY
366.15 CORTICAL
V45.61 EXTRACTION STATUS WITH ARTIFICIAL LENS STATUS [V43.1]
998.82 FRAGMENTS IN EYE FOLLOWING SURGERY
366.18 HYPERMATURE
366.12 IMMATURE
366.12 INCIPIENT
366.17 MATURE
366.18 MORGAGNI
366.16 NUCLEAR
366.11 PSEUDOEXFOLIATION OF LENS CAPSULE
366.12 PUNCTATE
V80.2 SCREENING
366.13 SUBCAPSULAR POLAR ANTERIOR
366.14 SUBCAPSULAR POLAR POSTERIOR
366.17 TOTAL
366.12 WATER CLEFTS
366.19 OTHER AND COMBINED FORMS

CATARACT TRAUMATIC
366.20 NOS
V45.61 EXTRACTION STATUS WITH ARTIFICIAL LENS STATUS [V43.1]
998.82 FRAGMENTS IN EYE FOLLOWING SURGERY
366.21 LOCALIZED OPACITIES
366.23 PARTIALLY RESOLVED
V80.2 SCREENING
366.22 TOTAL

CATARACT OTHER ETIOLOGIES
366.46 ASSOCIATED WITH RADIATION AND OTHER PHYSICAL INFLUENCES
275.40 CALCINOSIS (DUE TO) [366.42]
743.31 CAPSULAR AND SUBCAPSULAR CONGENITAL
360.24 CHALCOSIS [366.34]
363.20 CHOROIDITIS (CHRONIC) [366.32]
366.30 COMPLICATA
743.30 CONGENITAL
743.32 CORTICAL AND ZONULAR CONGENITAL
756.0 CRANIOFASCIAL DYSOSTOSIS [366.44]
366.34 DEGENERATIVE (IN DEGENERATIVE DISORDER)
250.5# DIABETIC [366.41]

5th Digit: 250.5

0. TYPE II, ADULT-ONSET, NON-INSULIN DEPENDENT (EVEN IF REQUIRING INSULIN), OR UNSPECIFIED; CONTROLLED
1. TYPE I, JUVENILE-ONSET OR INSULIN-DEPENDENT; CONTROLLED
2. TYPE II, ADULT-ONSET, NON-INSULIN DEPENDENT (EVEN IF REQUIRING INSULIN); UNCONTROLLED
3. TYPE I, JUVENILE-ONSET OR INSULIN-DEPENDENT; UNCONTROLLED

366.45 DRUG INDUCED
998.82 FRAGMENTS IN EYE FOLLOWING SURGERY
271.1 GALACTOSEMIC [366.44]
365.9 GLAUCOMA [366.31]
366.31 GLAUCOMATOUS FLECKS (SUBCAPSULAR)
252.1 HYPOPARATHYROIDISM (DUE TO) [366.42]
363.0# INFLAMMATORY (CHOROIDITIS) (RETINITIS) [366.32]

5th Digit: 363.0

0. FOCAL NOS
1. FOCAL JUXTAPAPILLARY
3. FOCAL POSTERIOR POLE
4. FOCAL PERIPHERAL
5. FOCAL JUXTAPAPILLARY WITH RETINOCHOROIDITIS
6. FOCAL MACULAR
7. FOCAL POSTERIOR POLE WITH RETINOCHORIODITIS
8. FOCAL PERIPHERAL RETINOCHORIODITIS

366.32 INFLAMMATORY (DISORDER)
364.10 IRIDOCYCLITIS (DUE TO) [366.33]
366.8 LENS CALCIFICATION
360.21 MYOPIC (DEGENERATIVE) [366.34]
359.2 MYOTONIC [366.43]
743.33 NUCLEAR CONGENITAL
743.39 OTHER CONGENITAL
362.74 PIGMENTARY RETINAL DYSTROPHY [366.34]
366.46 RADIATION AND OTHER PHYSICAL INFLUENCES (ASSOCIATED)
366.50 SECONDARY
366.30 SECONDARY TO OCULAR DISORDERS

CATARACT OTHER ETIOLOGIES (continued)

250.5# SNOWFLAKE [366.41]

5th Digit: 250.5

0. TYPE II, ADULT-ONSET, NON-INSULIN DEPENDENT (EVEN IF REQUIRING INSULIN), OR UNSPECIFIED; CONTROLLED
1. TYPE I, JUVENILE-ONSET OR INSULIN-DEPENDENT; CONTROLLED
2. TYPE II, ADULT-ONSET, NON-INSULIN DEPENDENT (EVEN IF REQUIRING INSULIN); UNCONTROLLED
3. TYPE I, JUVENILE-ONSET OR INSULIN-DEPENDENT; UNCONTROLLED

360.24 SUNFLOWER [366.34]
275.49 TETANIC DUE TO CALCINOSIS [366.42]
252.1 TETANIC DUE TO HYPOTHYROIDISM [366.42]
743.34 TOTAL AND SUBTOTAL CONGENITAL
366.45 TOXIC
366.33 WITH NEOVASCULARIZATION
743.32 ZONULAR CONGENITAL
366.03 ZONULAR JUVENILE

366.16 CATARACTA BRUNESCENS
366.30 CATARACTA COMPLICATA
462 CATARRHAL ANGINA

781.9 CATATONIA
293.89 CATATONIA DUE TO OR ASSOCIATED WITH PHYSICAL CONDITION
0 CATATONIA WITH AFFECTIVE PSYCHOSIS SEE 'MANIC DEPRESSIVE PSYCHOSIS'
0 CATATONIA WITH SCHIZOPHRENIA SEE 'SCHIZOPHRENIA'

791.9 CATECHOLAMINES ABNORMAL
255.6 CATECHOLAMINE SECRETION BY PHEOCHROMOCYTOMA
791.9 CATECHOLAMINES URINARY ELEVATION

CATHETER

V56.1 AFTERCARE - DIALYSIS EXTRACORPOREAL
V56.2 AFTERCARE - DIALYSIS PERITONEAL
V58.82 AFTERCARE - NONVASCULAR NEC
V53.6 AFTERCARE - URINARY
V58.81 AFTERCARE - VASCULAR NEC

996.09 CARDIAC COMPLICATION MECHANICAL

COMPLICATION

998.2 ACCIDENTAL LACERATION OR PUNCTURE (DURING A PROCEDURE)
996.62 INFECTION OR INFLAMMATION -(ARTERIAL) (VASCULAR) (ARTERIOVENOUS DIALYSIS) (VENOUS)
996.68 INFECTION OR INFLAMMATION - PERITONEAL DIALYSIS
996.1 MECHANICAL - (ARTERIAL) (VASCULAR) (ARTERIOVENOUS DIALYSIS) (VENOUS)
996.09 MECHANICAL - CARDIAC CATHETER
996.56 MECHANICAL - PERITONEAL DIALYSIS
996.74 OTHER SPECIFIED COMPLICATION - (ARTERIAL) (VASCULAR) (VENOUS)
996.73 OTHER SPECIFIED COMPLICATION - HEMODIALYSIS (EXTRACORPOREAL)

DIALYSIS

V56.1 HEMODIALYSIS (EXTRACORPOREAL) CARE (FITTING) (ADJUSTMENT) (REMOVAL) (REPLACEMENT) (TOILET) (CLEANSING)
996.62 HEMODIALYSIS (EXTRACORPOREAL) COMPLICATION - INFECTION OR INFLAMMATION
996.1 HEMODIALYSIS (EXTRACORPOREAL) COMPLICATION - MECHANICAL
996.73 HEMODIALYSIS (EXTRACORPOREAL) COMPLICATION - OTHER SPECIFIED COMPLICATION

CATHETER (continued)

DIALYSIS (continued)

V56.2 PERITONEAL CARE - (FITTING) (ADJUSTMENT) (REMOVAL) (REPLACEMENT) (TOILET) (CLEANSING)
996.68 PERITONEAL COMPLICATION - INFECTION OR INFLAMMATION
996.56 PERITONEAL COMPLICATION - MECHANICAL
996.79 PERITONEAL COMPLICATION - OTHER SPECIFIED COMPLICATION

CATHETER (continued)

0 OSTOMY COMPLICATION SEE SPECIFIED OSTOMY

996.63 SPINAL COMPLICATION - INFECTION OR INFLAMMATION
996.2 SPINAL COMPLICATION - MECHANICAL
996.75 SPINAL COMPLICATION - OTHER SPECIFIED

V53.6 URINARY FITTING AND ADJUSTMENT (REMOVAL) (REPLACEMENT)
996.64 URINARY INDWELLING - INFECTION OR INFLAMMATION COMPLICATION
996.31 URINARY INDWELLING - MECHANICAL COMPLICATION
996.76 URINARY INDWELLING - OTHER SPECIFIED COMPLICATION

996.62 VASCULAR NEC COMPLICATION - INFECTION OR INFLAMMATION
996.1 VASCULAR NEC COMPLICATION - MECHANICAL
996.74 VASCULAR NEC COMPLICATION - OTHER SPECIFIED
V58.81 VASCULAR NEC FITTING AND ADJUSTMENT (REMOVAL) (REPLACEMENT)

996.63 VENTRICULAR SHUNT COMPLICATION - INFECTION OR INFLAMMATION
996.2 VENTRICULAR SHUNT COMPLICATION - MECHANICAL
996.75 VENTRICULAR SHUNT COMPLICATION - OTHER SPECIFIED

996.69 COMPLICATION OTHER SPECIFIED CATHETER - INFECTION OR INFLAMMATION
996.59 COMPLICATION OTHER SPECIFIED CATHETER - MECHANICAL
996.79 COMPLICATION OTHER SPECIFIED CATHETER - OTHER SPECIFIED

CAUDA EQUINA

742.59 DEVELOPMENT DEFECTIVE
806.6# SPINAL CORD INJURY WITH FRACTURE CLOSED
806.7# SPINAL CORD INJURY WITH FRACTURE OPEN

5th Digit: 806.6-7

0. CORD INJURY UNSPECIFIED
1. COMPLETE CAUDA EQUINA INJURY
2. OTHER CAUDA EQUINA INJURY
9. WITH OTHER SPINAL CORD INJURY

952.4 SPINAL CORD INJURY WITHOUT FRACTURE
344.60 SYNDROME (OLD) (CAUSE OTHER OR UNSPECIFIED)
344.61 SYNDROME (OLD) (CAUSE OTHER OR UNSPECIFIED) WITH NEUROGENIC BLADDER

738.7 CAULIFLOWER EAR

CAUSALGIA (SYNDROME)

355.9 NOS
355.71 LOWER LIMB
354.4 UPPER LIMB

359.3 CAVARE'S FAMILIAL PERIODIC PARALYSIS

228.0# CAVERNOUS NEVUS

5th Digit: 228.0

0. SITE NOS
1. SKIN AND SUBCUTANEOUS TISSUE
2. INTRACRANIAL STRUCTURES
3. RETINA
4. INTRA ABDOMINAL STRUCTURES
9. OTHER SITES

437.6 CAVERNOUS SINUS SYNDROME
325 CAVERNOUS SINUS THROMBOSIS
326 CAVERNOUS SINUS THROMBOSIS LATE EFFECT

736.75 CAVOVARUS FOOT DEFORMITY (ACQUIRED)
754.59 CAVOVARUS FOOT DEFORMITY CONGENITAL

736.73 CAVUS FOOT
754.71 CAVUS FOOT CONGENITAL
736.74 CAVUS FOOT WITH CLAW FOOT

694.4 CAZENAVE'S PEMPHIGUS
795.79 CEA (CARCINOEMBRYONIC ANTIGEN) POSITIVE
0 CECITIS SEE 'APPENDICITIS'

CECOSTOMY

V53.5 CARE - DEVICE
V55.4 CARE - STOMA
V55.4 CATHETER CARE
V55.4 CLOSURE
569.60 COMPLICATION - NOS
569.62 COMPLICATION - MECHANICAL
569.69 COMPLICATION - OTHER
569.69 FISTULA
569.69 HERNIA

WHEN CODING AN INFECTION OF AN OSTOMY, USE AN ADDITIONAL CODE TO SPECIFY THE ORGANISM. SEE 'BACTERIAL INFECTION'

569.61 INFECTION
569.61 INFECTION WITH CELLULITIS OF ABDOMEN [682.2]
569.61 INFECTION WITH SEPSIS [**038.#(#)**]

4th or 4th and 5th Digit Code for Organism: 038

- **.9 NOS**
- **.3 ANAEROBIC**
- **.3 BACTEROIDES**
- **.3 CLOSTRIDIUM**
- **.42 E COLI**
- **.49 ENTEROBACTER AEROGENES**
- **.40 GRAM NEGATIVE**
- **.49 GRAM NEGATIVE OTHER**
- **.41 HEMOPHILUS INFLUENZAE**
- **.2 PNEUMOCOCCAL**
- **.49 PROTEUS**
- **.43 PSEUDOMONAS**
- **.44 SERRATIA**
- **.10 STAPHYLOCOCCAL NOS**
- **.11 STAPHYLOCOCCAL AUREUS**
- **.19 STAPHYLOCOCCAL OTHER**
- **.0 STREPTOCOCCAL (ANAEROBIC)**
- **.49 YERSINIA ENTEROCOLITICA**
- **.8 OTHER SPECIFIED**

569.62 MALFUNCTION
569.69 PROLAPSE
V55.4 REMOVAL OR REPLACEMENT
V44.4 STATUS

CECUM

751.2 ABSENCE CONGENITAL
V45.72 ABSENCE POSTSURGICAL
564.89 ATONY
751.2 ATRESIA (CONGENITAL)
564.89 DILATATION
569.9 DISEASE
562.10 DIVERTICULUM
751.5 DIVERTICULUM CONGENITAL
751.5 DUPLICATION CONGENITAL
863.89 INJURY (TRAUMATIC)
863.99 INJURY (TRAUMATIC) WITH OPEN WOUND
560.9 OBSTRUCTION (SEE ALSO 'INTESTINE, INTESTINAL', OBSTRUCTION)
211.3 POLYP
751.4 ROTATION (FAILURE) (INCOMPLETE) (INSUFFICIENT) CONGENITAL
564.89 STASIS

CELIAC

442.84 ARTERY (ANEURYSM) (A-V FISTULA) (CIRSOID) (FALSE) (VARICOSE) (RUPTURED)
447.4 ARTERY COMPRESSION SYNDROME
648.9# ARTERY COMPRESSION SYNDROME MATERNAL CURRENT (CO-EXISTENT) IN PREGNANCY [447.4]

5th Digit: 648.9

- **0. EPISODE OF NOS OR N/A**
- **1. DELIVERED**
- **2. DELIVERED WITH POSTPARTUM COMPLICATION**
- **3. ANTEPARTUM COMPLICATION**
- **4. POSTPARTUM COMPLICATION**

902.20 ARTERY INJURY NOS
902.24 ARTERY INJURY OTHER NEC
908.4 ARTERY INJURY LATE EFFECT
902.24 AXIS INJURY OTHER SPECIFIED BRANCHES
908.4 AXIS INJURY LATE EFFECT
902.24 AXIS LACERATION (RUPTURE) (HEMATOMA) (AVULSION) (ANEURYSM) TRAUMATIC
908.4 AXIS LACERATION LATE EFFECT
447.4 AXIS SYNDROME
579.0 CRISIS
579.0 DISEASE (INFANTILISM) (RICKETS)
579.0 DISEASE SPRUE
954.1 GANGLION OR PLEXUS INJURY
579.0 SYNDROME

709.09 CELLULAR TISSUE DISEASE NEC

CELLULITIS, 681-682: CODING CELLULITIS ASSOCIATED WITH OR SECONDARY TO A SUPERFICIAL INJURY, OPEN WOUND, BURN, OR BITES REQUIRE TWO CODES: ONE FOR INJURY COMPLICATED AND ONE FOR THE CELLULITIS. SEQUENCING OF THE TWO CODES DEPEND ON THE CIRCUMSTANCES OF ADMISSION TO A DOCTOR'S OFFICE OR HOSPITAL.

CELLULITIS:

-WITH ORGANISM KNOWN [041.#(#)]

682.9 NOS
682.2 ABDOMINAL WALL
040.0 ANAEROBIC
566 ANAL
682.6 ANKLE
611.0 AREOLA
682.3 ARM
682.3 AXILLA
682.2 BACK
682.5 BACK BUTTOCK
611.0 BREAST
675.1# BREAST COMPLICATING PREGNANCY AND THE PUERPERIUM

5th Digit: 675.1

- **0. EPISODE OF CARE NOS OR N/A**
- **1. DELIVERED**
- **2. DELIVERED WITH POSTPARTUM COMPLICATION**
- **3. ANTEPARTUM COMPLICATION**
- **4. POSTPARTUM COMPLICATION**

611.0 BREAST NIPPLE
614.4 BROAD LIGAMENT
614.3 BROAD LIGAMENT ACUTE
614.4 BROAD LIGAMENT CHRONIC
682.5 BUTTOCK
569.61 CECOSTOMY WITH CELLULITIS OF ABDOMEN [682.2]
616.0 CERVIX
682.0 CHEEK EXTERNAL
528.3 CHEEK INTERNAL
682.2 CHEST WALL
682.0 CHIN
569.61 COLOSTOMY WITH CELLULITIS OF ABDOMEN [682.2]
607.2 CORPUS CAVERNOSUM

C

CELLULITIS: (continued)

-WITH ORGANISM KNOWN [041.#(#])

IN ORDER TO CORRECTLY CODE DIABETIC CELLULITIS, YOU MUST USE AN ADDITIONAL CODE TO IDENTIFY THE SPECIFIED SITE OF THE CELLULITIS. IE. STAPHYLOCOCCAL DIABETIC CELLULITIS FOOT 250.80, 682.7 AND 041.10.

250.8# DIABETIC

5th Digit: 250.8

0. TYPE II, ADULT-ONSET, NON-INSULIN DEPENDENT (EVEN IF REQUIRING INSULIN), OR UNSPECIFIED; CONTROLLED
1. TYPE I, JUVENILE-ONSET OR INSULIN-DEPENDENT; CONTROLLED
2. TYPE II, ADULT-ONSET, NON-INSULIN DEPENDENT (EVEN IF REQUIRING INSULIN); UNCONTROLLED
3. TYPE I, JUVENILE-ONSET OR INSULIN-DEPENDENT; UNCONTROLLED

WHEN CODING AN INFECTION, USE AN ADDITIONAL CODE, [041.#(#)], TO IDENTIFY THE ORGANISM.

681.9 DIGIT
614.4 DOUGLAS' CUL-DE-SAC NOS
614.3 DOUGLAS' CUL-DE-SAC ACUTE
614.4 DOUGLAS' CUL-DE-SAC CHRONIC
998.59 DRAINAGE SITE POSTOPERATIVE
380.10 EAR EXTERNAL AUDITORY CANAL
380.11 EAR PINNA
569.61 ENTEROSTOMY WITH CELLULITIS OF ABDOMEN [682.2]
035 ERYSIPELAS (SEE ALSO 'ERYSIPELAS')
373.13 EYELID
682.0 FACE
681.01 FELON
681.00 FINGER
681.02 FINGER ONYCHIA AND PARONYCHIA
682.2 FLANK
999.3 FOLLOWING VACCINATION
682.7 FOOT
681.10 FOOT - TOE
681.11 FOOT - TOE ONYCHIA AND PARONYCHIA
682.3 FOREARM
682.0 FOREHEAD
785.4 GANGRENOUS (SEE ALSO 'GANGRENE')
536.41 GASTROSTOMY WITH CELLULITIS OF ABDOMEN [682.2]
616.9 GENITAL ORGAN FEMALE (SEE ALSO 'ABSCESS', BY SITE)
608.4 GENITAL ORGAN MALE
478.71 GLOTTIS
682.5 GLUTEAL REGION
098.0 GONOCOCCAL NEC
682.2 GROIN
682.4 HAND
681.00 HAND - FINGER
681.02 HAND - FINGER ONYCHIA
681.00 HAND - THUMB
682.8 HEAD
682.0 HEAD (FACE)
682.7 HEEL
682.6 HIP
569.61 ILEOSTOMY WITH CELLULITIS OF ABDOMEN [682.2]
566 ISCHIORECTAL
682.0 JAW
569.61 JEJUNOSTOMY WITH CELLULITIS OF ABDOMEN [682.2]
682.6 KNEE
616.10 LABIUM MAJUS MINUS (SEE ALSO 'VAGINITIS')
478.71 LARYNX
682.6 LEG
528.5 LIP
611.0 MAMMARY GLAND
528.3 MOUTH (FLOOR)

CELLULITIS: (continued)

-WITH ORGANISM KNOWN [041.#(#])

681.9 NAIL NOS (FINGER) (TOE)
478.1 NASAL CAVITY
478.21 NASOPHARYNX
682.2 NAVEL
771.4 NAVEL CORD NEWBORN
682.1 NECK
611.0 NIPPLE
682.0 NOSE EXTERNAL
681.02 ONYCHIA FINGER
681.11 ONYCHIA TOE
376.01 ORBITAL
998.59 OSTOMY EXTERNAL
682.8 OTHER SPECIFIED SITE
528.3 PALATE (SOFT)
681.02 PARONYCHIA FINGER
681.11 PARONYCHIA TOE
682.2 PECTORAL REGION
614.4 PELVIS
614.4 PELVIS CHRONIC
614.4 PELVIS FEMALE
614.3 PELVIS FEMALE - ACUTE
614.4 PELVIS FEMALE - CHRONIC
016.7# PELVIS FEMALE - TUBERCULOUS

5th Digit: 016.7

0. UNSPECIFIED
1. LAB NOT DONE
2. LABS PENDING
3. MICROSCOPY POSITIVE (IN SPUTUM)
4. CULTURE POSITIVE - MICROSCOPY NEGATIVE
5. CULTURE NEGATIVE - MICROSCOPY POSITIVE
6. CULTURE AND MICROSCOPY NEGATIVE CONFIRMED BY OTHER METHODS

639.0 PELVIS FOLLOWING ABORTION ECTOPIC OR MOLAR PREGNANCY
567.2 PELVIS MALE
670.0# PELVIS MATERNAL DUE TO PREGNANCY

5th Digit: 670.0

0. EPISODE OF CARE NOS OR N/A
2. DELIVERED WITH POSTPARTUM COMPLICATION
4. POSTPARTUM COMPLICATION

0 PELVIS WITH ABORTION SEE 'ABORTION', BY TYPE, WITH INFECTION
0 PELVIS WITH ECTOPIC PREGNANCY SEE 'ECTOPIC PREGNANCY'
0 PELVIS WITH MOLAR PREGNANCY SEE 'MOLAR PREGNANCY'
607.2 PENIS
566 PERIANAL
682.2 PERINEUM
566 PERIRECTAL
475 PERITONSILLAR
597.0 PERIURETHRAL
0 PERIUTERINE SEE 'CELLULITIS', PELVIC
478.21 PHARYNX OR NASOPHARYNX
682.9 PHLEGMONOUS NEC
380.11 PINNA
614.4 POUCH OF DOUGLAS CHRONIC
566 RECTAL
611.0 RETROMAMMARY
0 RETROPERITONEAL SEE 'PERITONITIS'
614.4 ROUND LIGAMENT
614.3 ROUND LIGAMENT - ACUTE
614.4 ROUND LIGAMENT - CHRONIC
682.8 SCALP
704.8 SCALP DISSECTING
608.4 SCROTUM
608.0 SEMINAL VESICLE
682.3 SHOULDER

CELLULITIS: (continued)

-WITH ORGANISM KNOWN [041.#(#])

682.9 SKIN NEC
017.0# SKIN AND SUBCUTANEOUS CELLULAR TISSUE - TUBERCULOUS (PRIMARY)

5th Digit: 017.0

0. UNSPECIFIED
1. LAB NOT DONE
2. LABS PENDING
3. MICROSCOPY POSITIVE (IN SPUTUM)
4. CULTURE POSITIVE - MICROSCOPY NEGATIVE
5. CULTURE NEGATIVE - MICROSCOPY POSITIVE
6. CULTURE AND MICROSCOPY NEGATIVE CONFIRMED BY OTHER METHODS

608.4 SPERMATIC CORD
682.0 SUBMANDIBULAR REGION
527.3 SUBMANDIBULAR GLAND
528.3 SUBMAXILLARY
527.3 SUBMAXILLARY GLAND
682.0 SUBMENTAL
527.3 SUBMENTAL GLAND
682.0 TEMPLE (REGION)
608.4 TESTIS
682.6 THIGH
681.00 THUMB
681.10 TOE
681.11 TOE ONYCHIA AND PARONYCHIA
475 TONSIL
519.01 TRACHEOSTOMY WITH CELLULITIS OF NECK [682.1]
682.2 TRUNK
608.4 TUNICA VAGINALIS
771.4 UMBILICAL CORD - NEWBORN
682.2 UMBILICUS
0 VAGINA SEE 'VAGINITIS'
608.4 VAS DEFERENS
478.5 VOCAL CORD
616.10 VULVA (SEE ALSO 'VULVITIS')
682.4 WRIST
682.8 OTHER SPECIFIED SITE

4th or 4th and 5th Digit Code for Organism: 041

.85 AEROBACTER AEROGENES
.82 BACILLUS FRAGILIS
.84 BACTEROIDES (FRAGILIS)
.83 CLOSTRIDIUM PERFRINGENS
.4 E. COLI
.81 EATON'S AGENT
.04 ENTEROCOCCUS
.3 FRIEDLANDER'S BACILLUS,
.84 GRAM-NEGATIVE ANAEROBES
.85 GRAM-NEGATIVE BACTERIA NOS
.5 H. INFLUENZAE
.86 H. PYLORI
.3 KLEBSIELLA
.85 MIMA POLYMORPHA
.81 MYCOPLASMA
.81 PLEUROPNEUMONIA LIKE ORGANISMS
.2 PNEUMOCOCCUS
.6 PROTEUS (MIRABILIS) (MORGANII)
.7 PSEUDOMONAS
.85 SERRATIA
.10 STAPHYLOCOCCUS UNSPECIFIED
.11 STAPHYLOCOCCUS AUREUS
.19 STAPHYLOCOCCUS OTHER
.00 STREPTOCOCCUS
.01 STREPTOCOCCUS GROUP A
.02 STREPTOCOCCUS GROUP B
.03 STREPTOCOCCUS GROUP C
.04 STREPTOCOCCUS GROUP D
.05 STREPTOCOCCUS GROUP G
.09 STREPTOCOCCUS OTHER
.84 OTHER ANAEROBES
.89 OTHER SPECIFIED BACTERIA

213.# CEMENTOBLASTOMA BENIGN M9273/0
213.# CEMENTOMA NOS M9272/0
213.# CEMENTOMA GIGANTIFORM M9276/0

4th Digit: 213

0. SKULL FACE UPPER JAW
1. LOWER JAW (OR IF SITE UNSPECIFIED)

520.4 CEMENTUM APLASIA AND HYPOPLASIA
521.5 CEMENTUM HYPERPLASIA
989.5 CENTIPEDE BITE
995.0 CENTIPEDE BITE WITH ANAPHYLAXIS [989.5]
359.0 CENTRAL CORE DISEASE
341.8 CENTRAL DEMYELINATION OF CORPUS CALLOSUM
063.2 CENTRAL EUROPEAN ENCEPHALITIS
996.62 CENTRAL LINE COMPLICATION - INFECTION OR INFLAMMATION
996.1 CENTRAL LINE COMPLICATION - MECHANICAL
996.74 CENTRAL LINE COMPLICATION - OTHER
794.00 CENTRAL NERVOUS SYSTEM ABNORMAL FUNCTION STUDY
779.2 CENTRAL NERVOUS SYSTEM DYSFUNCTION NEWBORN NOS
341.8 CENTRAL PONTINE MYELINOSIS
362.31 CENTRAL RETINAL ARTERY OCCLUSION
362.35 CENTRAL RETINAL VEIN OCCLUSION
365.63 CENTRAL RETINAL VEIN OCCLUSION CAUSING GLAUCOMA [362.35]
362.41 CENTRAL SEROUS RETINOPATHY
359.0 CENTRONUCLEAR MYOPATHY
0 CEPHALGIA SEE 'HEADACHE'
920 CEPHALHEMATOMA (TRAUMATIC)
767.1 CEPHALHEMATOMA (BIRTH TRAUMA)
903.1 CEPHALIC VEIN (ARM) INJURY
451.82 CEPHALIC VEIN PHLEBITIS
652.1# CEPHALIC VERSION
660.0# CEPHALIC VERSION OBSTRUCTING LABOR **[652.1#]**

5th Digit: 652.1, 660.0

0. EPISODE OF CARE NOS OR N/A
1. DELIVERED
3. ANTEPARTUM COMPLICATION

653.4# CEPHALOPELVIC DISPROPORTION NOS
660.1# CEPHALOPELVIC DISPROPORTION OBSTRUCTING LABOR NOS **[653.4#]**

5th Digit: 653.4, 660.1

0. EPISODE OF CARE NOS OR N/A
1. DELIVERED
3. ANTEPARTUM COMPLICATION

V09.1 CEPHALOSPORINS RESISTANT INFECTION (SEE 'DRUG RESISTANCE' FOR COMPLETE LISTING)
120.3 CERCARIAE OF SCHISTOSOMA INFECTION

CEREBELLAR

742.2 ABSENCE (CONGENITAL)
433.8# ARTERY THROMBOSIS (EMBOLISM) (DEFORMANS)
433.8# ARTERY OCCLUSION

5th Digit: 433.8

0. WITHOUT CEREBRAL INFARCTION
1. WITH CEREBRAL INFARCTION

334.3 ATAXIA
334.0 ATAXIA FRIEDRICH'S
334.2 ATAXIA MARIE'S
334.3 ATAXIA OTHER

C

CEREBELLAR (continued)

331.9 ATROPHY
851.4# CONTUSION
851.5# CONTUSION WITH OPEN INTRACRANIAL WOUND
5th Digitt: 851.4-5
0. LEVEL OF CONSCIOUSNESS NOS
1. NO LOC
2. LOC < 1 HR
3. LOC 1 - 24 HRS
4. LOC > 24 HRS WITH RETURN TO PRIOR LEVEL
5. LOC > 24 HRS WITHOUT RETURN TO PRIOR LEVEL: OR DEATH BEFORE REGAINING CONSCIOUSNESS, REGARDLESS OF DURATION OF LOC
6. LOC DURATION NOS
9. WITH CONCUSSION NOS

334.2 DEGENERATION PRIMARY (HEREDITARY) (SPORADIC)
431 HEMORRHAGE (RUPTURE)
674.0# HEMORRHAGE MATERNAL COMPLICATING PREGNANCY
5th Digit: 674.0
0. EPISODE OF CARE NOS OR N/A
1. DELIVERED
2. DELIVERED WITH POSTPARTUM COMPLICATION
3. ANTEPARTUM COMPLICATION
4. POSTPARTUM COMPLICATION

434.91 INFARCTION
434.11 INFARCTION EMBOLIC
434.01 INFARCTION THROMBOTIC
851.6# LACERATION
851.7# LACERATION WITH OPEN INTRACRANIAL WOUND
5th Digit: 851.6-7
0. LEVEL OF CONSCIOUSNESS NOS
1. NO LOC
2. LOC < 1 HR
3. LOC 1 - 24 HRS
4. LOC > 24 HRS WITH RETURN TO PRIOR LEVEL
5. LOC > 24 HRS WITHOUT RETURN TO PRIOR LEVEL: OR DEATH BEFORE REGAINING CONSCIOUSNESS, REGARDLESS OF DURATION OF LOC
6. LOC DURATION NOS
9. WITH CONCUSSION NOS

433.8# OCCLUSION
5th Digit: 433.8
0. WITHOUT CEREBRAL INFARCTION
1. WITH CEREBRAL INFARCTION

741.0# CEREBELLOMEDULLARY MALFORMATION SYNDROME
5th Digit: 741.0
0. REGION NOS
1. CERVICAL REGION
2. DORSAL (THORACIC REGION)
3. LUMBAR REGION

CEREBRAL

437.3 ANEURYSM NOS
747.81 ANEURYSM (A-V) CONGENITAL
430 ANEURYSM (A-V) RUPTURED
094.87 ANEURYSM (A-V) RUPTURED (SYPHILITIC)
437.3 ANEURYSM-INTERNAL CAROTID ARTERY NOS OR INTRACRANIAL PORTION
348.1 ANOXIA
0 ANOXIA OBSTETRICAL SEE 'CEREBRAL ANOXIA OBSTETRICAL'
437.0 ARTERIOSCLEROSIS (DEGENERATION) (DEFORMANS) (ARTERITIS)
437.4 ARTERITIS

CEREBRAL (continued)

747.81 ARTERY ATRESIA (CONGENITAL)
435.8 ARTERY INSUFFICIENCY (SPASM) WITH TIA
434.9# ARTERY OCCLUSION
434.0# ARTERY THROMBOSIS
5th Digit: 434.0, 9
0. WITHOUT CEREBRAL INFARCTION
1. WITH CEREBRAL INFARCTION

331.89 ATAXIA
437.0 ATHEROSCLEROSIS
331.9 ATROPHY
290.10 ATROPHY WITH DEMENTIA
331.0 ATROPHY - ALZHEIMER'S
331.0 ATROPHY - ALZHEIMER'S WITH DEMENTIA [294.1]
331.1 ATROPHY - CIRCUMSCRIBED (PICK'S)
331.1 ATROPHY - CIRCUMSCRIBED (PICK'S) WITH DEMENTIA [294.1]
742.4 ATROPHY - CONGENITAL
331.2 ATROPHY - SENILE
436 ATTACK
780.39 ATTACK - TOXIC
348.8 CALCIFICATION (CORTEX)
437.0 CALCIFICATION ARTERY
853.0# COMPRESSION TRAUMATIC
853.1# COMPRESSION TRAUMATIC WITH OPEN INTRACRANIAL WOUND
5th Digit: 853.0-1
0. LEVEL OF CONSCIOUSNESS NOS
1. NO LOC
2. LOC < 1 HR
3. LOC 1 - 24 HRS
4. LOC > 24 HRS WITH RETURN TO PRIOR LEVEL
5. LOC > 24 HRS WITHOUT RETURN TO PRIOR LEVEL: OR DEATH BEFORE REGAINING CONSCIOUSNESS, REGARDLESS OF DURATION OF LOC
6. LOC DURATION NOS
9. WITH CONCUSSION NOS

0 CONCUSSION SEE 'CEREBRAL CONCUSSION'
0 CONTUSION SEE 'CEREBRAL CONTUSION'
0 CRISIS SEE 'CEREBROVASCULAR DISEASE'
742.4 CYST CONGENITAL
0 DEGENERATION SEE 'CEREBRAL DEGENERATION'
779.2 DEPRESSION NEONATAL
348.9 DISEASE
437.9 DISEASE ARTERIAL
348.5 EDEMA
348.5 EDEMA ANOXIC
434.1# EMBOLISM
5th Digit: 434.1
0. WITHOUT CEREBRAL INFARCTION
1. WITH CEREBRAL INFARCTION

348.8 FUNGUS
253.0 GIGANTISM SYNDROME
767.0 HEMORRHAGE (BIRTH TRAUMA) (OR SUBDURAL)
853.0# HEMORRHAGE TRAUMATIC
853.1# HEMORRHAGE TRAUMATIC WITH OPEN INTRACRANIAL WOUND
5th Digit: 853.0-1
0. LEVEL OF CONSCIOUSNESS NOS
1. NO LOC
2. LOC < 1 HR
3. LOC 1 - 24 HRS
4. LOC > 24 HRS WITH RETURN TO PRIOR LEVEL
5. LOC > 24 HRS WITHOUT RETURN TO PRIOR LEVEL: OR DEATH BEFORE REGAINING CONSCIOUSNESS, REGARDLESS OF DURATION OF LOC
6. LOC DURATION NOS
9. WITH CONCUSSION NOS

CEREBRAL (continued)

348.1 HYPOXIA
997.01 HYPOXIA DURING OR RESULTING FROM A PROCEDURE
434.91 INFARCTION
434.11 INFARCTION EMBOLIC
779.1 IRRITABILITY NEWBORN OTHER AND UNSPECIFIED

437.1 ISCHEMIA (CHRONIC)
435.9 ISCHEMIA INTERMITTENT (TRANSIENT)
435.8 ISCHEMIAS OTHER SPECIFIED TRANSIENT

851.2# LACERATION (CORTEX)
851.3# LACERATION (CORTEX) WITH OPEN INTRACRANIAL WOUND

5th Digit: 851.2-3

0. LEVEL OF CONSCIOUSNESS NOS
1. NO LOC
2. LOC < 1 HR
3. LOC 1 - 24 HRS
4. LOC > 24 HRS WITH RETURN TO PRIOR LEVEL
5. LOC > 24 HRS WITHOUT RETURN TO PRIOR LEVEL: OR DEATH BEFORE REGAINING CONSCIOUSNESS, REGARDLESS OF DURATION OF LOC
6. LOC DURATION NOS
9. WITH CONCUSSION NOS

348.8 LESION
330.1 LIPIDOSES
330.1 LIPIDOSES WITH DEMENTIA [294.1]
0 NERVE SEE 'CRANIAL', NERVE
434.9# OCCLUSION ARTERY

5th Digit: 434.9

0. WITHOUT CEREBRAL INFARCTION
1. WITH CEREBRAL INFARCTION

0 PALSY SEE 'CEREBRAL PALSY'
341.9 SCLEROSIS (GENERAL) (LOBULAR)
331.0 SCLEROSIS LOBAR ATROPHIC
331.0 SCLEROSIS LOBAR ATROPHIC WITH DEMENTIA [294.1]
436 SEIZURE
434.0# THROMBOSIS ARTERY

5th Digit: 434.0

0. WITHOUT CEREBRAL INFARCTION
1. WITH CEREBRAL INFARCTION

671.5# THROMBOSIS (VENOUS SINUS) MATERNAL DUE TO PREGNANCY

5th Digit: 671.5

0. EPISODE OF CARE NOS OR N/A
1. DELIVERED
2. DELIVERED WITH POSTPARTUM COMPLICATION
3. ANTEPARTUM COMPLICATION
4. POSTPARTUM COMPLICATION

436 VASCULAR ACCIDENT ACUTE
V53.01 VENTRICLE (COMMUNICATING) SHUNT FITTING AND ADJUSTMENT
V45.2 VENTRICLE (COMMUNICATING) SHUNT IN SITU
747.81 VESSELS ANOMALIES CONGENITAL

CEREBRAL ANOXIA OBSTETRICAL

668.2# FOLLOWING ANESTHESIA OR OTHER SEDATION IN L AND D
669.4# FOLLOWING OBSTETRICAL SURGERY

5th Digit: 668.2, 669.4

0. EPISODE OF CARE NOS OR N/A
1. DELIVERED
2. DELIVERED WITH POSTPARTUM COMPLICATION
3. ANTEPARTUM COMPLICATION
4. POSTPARTUM COMPLICATION

*CEREBRAL CONCUSSION RESULTS FROM A BLOW TO THE HEAD, AND MAY BE CODED AS A TRAUMA. CODE IT AS A TRAUMA UNTIL THE PHYSICIAN STATES THAT THE ACTIVE PHASE OF THE CONCUSSION HAS SUBSIDED AND THE SYMPTOMS ARE NO LONGER ORGANIC IN NATURE. AS LONG AS THE DOCUMENTATION STATES THAT THE PATIENT'S SYMPTOMS ARE DIRECTLY RESULTANT FROM A CONCUSSION, **USE A TRAUMA CODE.***

CEREBRAL CONCUSSION

850.9 NOS
850.0 NO LOSS OF CONSCIOUSNESS
850.5 LOC UNSPECIFIED DURATION
850.1 WITH BRIEF LOSS OF CONSCIOUSNESS
850.2 LOC 1-24 HOURS
850.3 LOC >24 HOURS WITH COMPLETE RECOVERY
850.4 LOC >24 HOURS WITHOUT RETURN TO PRE-EXISTING CONSCIOUS LEVEL

POST-CONCUSSION SYNDROME IS A NEUROLOGICAL CONDITION RESULTING FROM THE CONCUSSION TRAUMA, AND ICD 9 ASSIGNS IT TO A NON-PSYCHOTIC MENTAL DISORDER. POST-CONCUSSION SYNDROME CANNOT BE ASSIGNED A TRAUMA CODE.

CEREBRAL CONTUSION

851.8# NOS
851.9# NOS WITH OPEN INTRACRANIAL WOUND
851.4# BRAIN STEM
851.5# BRAIN STEM WITH OPEN INTRACRANIAL WOUND
851.4# CEREBELLAR
851.5# CEREBELLAR WITH OPEN INTRACRANIAL WOUND
851.0# CORTEX
851.1# CORTEX WITH OPEN INTRACRANIAL WOUND
851.4# OCCIPITAL LOBE
851.5# OCCIPITAL LOBE WITH OPEN INTRACRANIAL WOUND
851.8# OTHER
851.9# OTHER WITH OPEN INTRACRANIAL WOUND

5th Digit: 851.0-1, 4-5, 8-9

0. LEVEL OF CONSCIOUSNESS NOS
1. NO LOC
2. LOC < 1 HR
3. LOC 1 - 24 HRS
4. LOC > 24 HRS WITH RETURN TO PRIOR LEVEL
5. LOC > 24 HRS WITHOUT RETURN TO PRIOR LEVEL: OR DEATH BEFORE REGAINING CONSCIOUSNESS, REGARDLESS OF DURATION OF LOC
6. LOC DURATION NOS
9. WITH CONCUSSION NOS

CEREBRAL DEGENERATION

331.9 NOS
437.0 ARTERIOSCLEROTIC
330.9 CHILDHOOD
330.8 CHILDHOOD OTHER SPECIFIED
742.4 CONGENITAL
348.0 CYSTIC
330.2 LIPIDOSES GENERALIZED
046.1 JAKOB CREUTZFELDT
046.3 PROGRESSIVE (MULTIFOCAL) (ENCEPHALOPATHY)
331.2 SENILE
046.1 SPONGIFORM (SUBACUTE)
331.89 OTHER

C

C

CEREBRAL PALSY

333.7 ATHETOID [VOGT'S DISEASE]
343.9 CONGENITAL
343.0 DIPLEGIC
343.1 HEMIPLEGIC
343.# INFANTILE

4th Digit: 343

0. PARAPLEGIC (DIPLEGIC)
1. HEMIPLEGIC
2. QUADRIPLEGIC
3. MONOPLEGIC
4. HEMIPLEGIC (POSTNATAL) NOS
8. OTHER SPECIFIED
9. NOS

343.3 MONOPLEGIC
437.8 NONINFANTILE, NONCONGENITAL
343.0 PARAPLEGIC
343.2 QUADRIPLEGIC
343.9 SPASTIC
344.89 SPASTIC NONINFANTILE, NONCONGENITAL
094.89 SYPHILITIC
090.49 SYPHILITIC CONGENITAL
343.2 TETRAPLEGIC

759.89 CEREBROHEPATORENAL SYNDROME

CEREBROSPINAL FLUID

792.0 ABNORMAL
V45.2 DRAINAGE DEVICE (PRESENCE OF) STATUS
997.09 LEAKAGE AT LUMBAR PUNCTURE SITE
388.61 OTORRHEA
349.81 RHINORRHEA
V45.2 SHUNT STATUS

REMEMBER, CODE 436 FOR CVA IS A NON-SPECIFIC CODE. CODE INSTEAD THE INFARCTION, EMBOLUS, OR THROMBUS IF DOCUMENTED IN THE PATIENT'S RECORD.

CEREBROVASCULAR

436 ACCIDENT
V12.59 ACCIDENT - HISTORY WITHOUT RESIDUAL
435.9 ACCIDENT - IMPENDING (TRANSIENT ISCHEMIC ATTACK)
434.91 ACCIDENT - LACUNAR INFARCT
0 ACCIDENT - LATE EFFECT SEE 'LATE EFFECT', CEREBROVASCULAR DISEASE
0 ACCIDENT - OLD WITH RESIDUAL SEE 'LATE EFFECT', CEREBROVASCULAR DISEASE
V12.59 ACCIDENT - OLD WITHOUT RESIDUAL
435.9 ACCIDENT - TRANSIENT ISCHEMIC ATTACK (TIA)
437.7 AMNESIA TRANSIENT GLOBAL
0 CRISIS SEE 'CEREBROVASCULAR', DISEASE
437.9 DISEASE
437.0 DISEASE ARTERIOSCLEROTIC
437.1 DISEASE ISCHEMIC GENERALIZED NEC
0 DISEASE LATE EFFECT SEE 'LATE EFFECT', CEREBROVASCULAR DISEASE
437.1 DISEASE OCCLUSIVE
437.8 DISEASE OTHER
674.0# DISORDER (PUERPERIUM) MATERNAL DUE PREGNANCY

5th Digit: 674.0

0. EPISODE OF CARE NOS OR N/A
1. DELIVERED
2. DELIVERED WITH POSTPARTUM COMPLICATION
3. ANTEPARTUM COMPLICATION
4. POSTPARTUM COMPLICATION

437.1 INSUFFICIENCY ACUTE
435.9 INSUFFICIENCY ACUTE WITH TRANSIENT NEUROLOGICAL SIGNS
434.9# OCCLUSION

5th Digit: 434.9

0. WITHOUT CEREBRAL INFARCTION
1. WITH CEREBRAL INFARCTION

437.0 OCCLUSION DIFFUSE
747.81 SYSTEM ANOMALIES OF CONGENITAL

272.7 CEROID STORAGE DISEASE

CERTIFICATE ISSUE

V68.0 DEATH
V68.0 FITNESS
V68.0 INCAPACITY
V68.0 MEDICAL

380.4 CERUMEN IMPACTED

CERVICAL

744.43 AURICLE CONGENITAL
723.4 BRACHIAL RADICULAR SYNDROME
952.0# CORD INJURY
806.0# CORD INJURY WITH CLOSED FRACTURE
806.1# CORD INJURY WITH OPEN FRACTURE

5th Digit: 806.0-1, 952.0

0. C1-C4 WITH CORD INJURY NOS
1. C1-C4 WITH COMPLETE CORD LESION
2. C1-C4 WITH ANTERIOR CORD SYNDROME
3. C1-C4 WITH CENTRAL CORD LESION
4. C1-C4 WITH INCOMPLETE CORD LESION NOS OR POSTERIOR CORD SYNDROME
5. C5-C7 WITH CORD INJURY NOS
6. C5-C7 COMPLETE LESION OF CORD
7. C5-C7 WITH ANTERIOR CORD SYNDROME
8. C5-C7 WITH CENTRAL CORD SYNDROME
9. C5-C7 WITH INCOMPLETE CORD LESION NOS OR POSTERIOR

0 DISC DISORDER SEE 'CERVICAL DISC DISORDER'
722.0 DISC HERNIATION (HNP)
722.71 DISC HERNIATION (HNP) WITH MYELOPATHY
744.43 EAR CONGENITAL
722.0 NERVE COMPRESSION - DISCOGENIC
722.71 NERVE COMPRESSION - DISCOGENIC WITH MYELOPATHY
723.4 NERVE COMPRESSION - ROOT (BY SCAR TISSUE) NEC
722.81 NERVE COMPRESSION - ROOT POSTOPERATIVE
723.2 POSTERIOR, SYMPATHETIC SYNDROME
0 RADICULITIS (DISCOGENIC) SEE 'CERVICAL DISC' DISORDER
723.4 RADICULITIS (NONDISCOGENIC)
723.9 REGION DISORDER NEC
739.1 REGION SEGMENTAL OR SOMATIC DYSFUNCTION
756.2 RIB
353.0 RIB SYNDROME (NONDISCOGENIC)
953.0 ROOT INJURY (NERVE)
353.2 ROOT LESIONS NEC (NONDISCOGENIC)
723.9 SPINE DISORDER (NONDISCOGENIC)
337.0 SYMPATHETIC DYSTROPHY OR PARALYSIS SYNDROME
954.0 SYMPATHETIC NERVE INJURY
847.0 TRAUMATIC SYNDROME (ACUTE) NEC
0 UTERUS SEE 'CERVIX'
723.8 SYNDROME NEC

WHEN CODING BACK DISORDERS DUE TO DEGENERATION, DISPLACEMENT OR HNP OF THE INTERVERTEBRAL DISC, IT IS IMPORTANT TO DISTINGUISH WHETHER THESE CONDITIONS ARE WITH OR WITHOUT MYELOPATHY. MYELOPATHY REFERS TO FUNCTIONAL DISTURBANCES AND/OR PATHOLOGICAL CHANGES IN THE SPINAL CORD THAT RESULT FROM COMPRESSION.

CERVICAL DISC DISORDER

722.91 UNSPECIFIED
722.91 CALCIFICATION OR DISCITIS
722.4 DISEASE/DEGENERATION
722.71 DISEASE/DEGENERATION - WITH MYELOPATHY
722.0 DISPLACEMENT (HERNIATION) (HNP) (PROTRUSION) (RUPTURE)
722.71 DISPLACEMENT (HERNIATION) (HNP) (PROTRUSION) (RUPTURE) WITH MYELOPATHY
722.71 SYNDROME
722.91 OTHER SPECIFIED

723.1	CERVICALGIA (NECK PAIN) (NONDISCOGENIC)

CERVICITIS

616.0	NOS
760.8	AFFECTING NEWBORN OR FETUS
616.0	ATROPHIC OR SENILE (NONOBSTETRICAL)
616.0	ECTROPION CERVICAL
616.0	EVERSION CERVIX
098.15	GONORRHEA (ACUTE)
0	GRAVID SEE 'PREGNANCY COMPLICATIONS', MATERNAL CONDITIONS
616.8	INFLAMMATORY DISEASE (OTHER)
616.0	NONOBSTETRICAL
095.8	SYPHILITIC
131.09	TRICHOMONAL
016.7#	TUBERCULOUS

5th Digit: 016.7

0. NOS
1. LAB NOT DONE
2. LABS PENDING
3. MICROSCOPY POSITIVE (IN SPUTUM)
4. CULTURE POSITIVE - MICROSCOPY NEGATIVE
5. CULTURE NEGATIVE - MICROSCOPY POSITIVE
6. CULTURE AND MICRO NEGATIVE CONFIRMED BY OTHER METHODS

744.49	CERVICOAURAL FISTULA CONGENITAL
723.3	CERVICOBRACHIAL SYNDROME (DIFFUSE)
723.2	CERVICOCRANIAL SYNDROME
353.2	CERVICODORSAL OUTLET SYNDROME
739.1	CERVICOTHORACIC REGION SEGMENTAL OR SOMATIC DYSFUNCTION

CERVIX (UTERI)

622.8	ABSENCE
752.49	ABSENCE CONGENITAL
622.3	ADHESION (BAND)
752.49	AGENESIS CONGENITAL
622.1	ANAPLASIA
752.40	ANOMALY CONGENITAL
752.49	ANOMALY CONGENITAL OTHER SPECIFIED
622.4	ATRESIA
752.49	ATRESIA CONGENITAL
622.8	ATROPHY (SENILE)
622.8	CALCIFICATION (UTERI)
622.1	CERVICAL ATYPISM
622.3	CICATRIX (POSTPARTUM)
622.4	CONTRACTURE
752.49	CONTRACTURE CONGENITAL
622.8	CYST
616.9	DISORDER INFLAMMATORY
616.8	DISORDER INFLAMMATORY SPECIFIED NEC
622.9	DISORDER NONINFLAMMATORY
622.8	DISORDER NONINFLAMMATORY SPECIFIED NEC
622.1	DYSPLASIA
622.1	DYSPLASIA - CIN I
622.1	DYSPLASIA - CIN II
233.1	DYSPLASIA - CIN III (SEVERE)
622.0	ECTROPION
622.1	EPIDERMIDIZATION
622.0	EROSION
622.0	EROSION AND ECTROPION
622.0	EVERSION
622.8	FIBROSIS
622.8	HEMORRHAGE
0	HYPERPLASIA SEE 'CERVIX', DYSPLASIA
752.49	HYPERPLASIA CONGENITAL
622.6	HYPERTROPHIC ELONGATION
622.5	INCOMPETENCE (NONPREGNANT)
761.0	INCOMPETENT AFFECTING FETUS OR NEWBORN
639.2	INJURY POSTABORTIVE
867.4	INJURY (TRAUMATIC)
867.5	INJURY (TRAUMATIC) WITH OPEN WOUND

CERVIX (UTERI) (continued)

622.1	INTRAEPITHELIAL NEOPLASIA I
622.1	INTRAEPITHELIAL NEOPLASIA II
233.1	INTRAEPITHELIAL NEOPLASIA III (SEVERE)
622.2	LEUKOPLAKIA
622.4	OCCLUSION
084.0	OCCLUSION BY FALCIPARUM MALARIA
752.49	OCCLUSION CONGENITAL
622.3	OLD LACERATION
622.7	POLYP
219.0	POLYP ADENOMATOUS
622.7	POLYP MUCOUS OR UNSPECIFIED
622.1	SQUAMOUS METAPLASIA
622.4	STRICTURE AND STENOSIS
752.49	STRICTURE OR STENOSIS CONGENITAL
622.0	ULCER

CERVIX COMPLICATING PREGNANCY CHILDBIRTH OR PUERPERIUM

654.6#	ABNORMALITY OR ATRESIA
660.2#	ABNORMALITY OR ATRESIA OBSTRUCTING LABOR **[654.6#]**
654.6#	CICATRIX
660.2#	CICATRIX OBSTRUCTING LABOR **[654.6#]**
661.0#	DILATION FAILURE
654.5#	INCOMPETENCE
660.2#	INCOMPETENCE OBSTRUCTING LABOR **[654.5#]**
654.6#	RIGID
660.2#	RIGID OBSTRUCTING LABOR **[654.6#]**
654.6#	STENOSIS
660.2#	STENOSIS OBSTRUCTING LABOR **[654.6#]**
654.6#	SURGERY PREVIOUS
660.2#	SURGERY PREVIOUS OBSTRUCTING LABOR **[654.6#]**
654.6#	TUMOR
660.2#	TUMOR OBSTRUCTING LABOR **[654.6#]**
654.6#	POLYP
660.2#	POLYP OBSTRUCTING LABOR **[654.6#]**

5th Digit: 654.5-6

0. EPISODE OF CARE NOS OR N/A
1. DELIVERED
2. DELIVERED WITH POSTPARTUM COMPLICATION
3. ANTEPARTUM COMPLICATION
4. POSTPARTUM COMPLICATION

5th Digit: 660.2, 661.0

0. EPISODE OF CARE NOS OR N/A
1. DELIVERED
3. ANTEPARTUM COMPLICATION

> *WHEN CODING A CESAREAN SECTION, CODE THE REASON THAT THE CESAREAN WAS DONE. USE THE CODES BELOW ONLY IF THE CESAREAN ITSELF IS A COMPLICATING FACTOR.*

CESAREAN

763.4	DELIVERY AFFECTING FETUS OR NEWBORN
654.2#	SECTION (PREVIOUS) COMPLICATING CHILDBIRTH
660.2#	SECTION (PREVIOUS) OBSTRUCTING LABOR **[654.2#]**

5th Digit: 654.2, 660.2

0. EPISODE OF CARE NOS OR N/A
1. DELIVERED
3. ANTEPARTUM COMPLICATION

763.4	SECTION AFFECTING FETUS OR NEWBORN
762.1	SECTION DAMAGE TO PLACENTA AFFECTING FETUS OR NEWBORN
763.89	SECTION SCAR PREVIOUS AFFECTING FETUS OR NEWBORN
669.7#	SECTION WITHOUT MENTION OF INDICATION

5th Digit: 669.7

0. EPISODE OF CARE NOS OR N/A
1. DELIVERED

674.1#	SECTION WOUND DEHISCENCE

5th Digit: 674.1

0. NOS
2. DELIVERED WITH POSTPARTUM COMPLICATION
4. POSTPARTUM COMPLICATION

344.89 CESTAN (-CHENAIS) SYNDROME
433.8# CESTAN (-RAYMOND) SYNDROME
5th Digit: 433.8
0. WITHOUT CEREBRAL INFARCTION
1. WITH CEREBRAL INFARCTION

022.9 CHABERT'S DISEASE

CHAGAS' DISEASE
086.2 UNSPECIFIED
V75.3 SCREENING EXAM
086.0 WITH HEART INVOLVEMENT
086.1 WITH OTHER ORGAN INVOLVEMENT
086.2 WITHOUT MENTION OF ORGAN INVOLVEMENT

530.81 CHALASIA (CARDIAC SPHINCTER)
373.2 CHALAZION
373.2 CHALAZION (NOT INFECTED)

CHALCOSIS
360.24 NOS (GLOBE)
371.15 CORNEA
360.24 CRYSTALLINE LENS [366.34]
360.24 RETINA

502 CHALICOSIS LUNG (OCCUPATIONAL)
360.34 CHAMBER ANGLE FLAT
364.77 CHAMBER ANGLE RECESSION (IRIS AND CILIARY BODY)
091.2 CHANCRE CONJUNCTIVA (PRIMARY SYPHILITIC)
099.0 CHANCRE DUCREY'S
091.2 CHANCRE EYELID (PRIMARY SYPHILITIC)
091.0 CHANCRE GENITAL
099.0 CHANCRE SIMPLE
099.0 CHANCRE SOFT
114.1 CHANCRIFORM SYNDROME COCCIDIOIDOMYCOSIS
099.0 CHANCROID
647.2# CHANCROID MATERNAL CURRENT (CO-EXISTENT) IN PREGNANCY [099.0]
5th Digit: 647.2
0. EPISODE OF CARE NOS OR N/A
1. DELIVERED
2. DELIVERED WITH POSTPARTUM COMPLICATION
3. ANTEPARTUM COMPLICATION
4. POSTPARTUM COMPLICATION

655.4# CHANCROID MATERNAL (WITH KNOWN / SUSPECTED DAMAGE TO FETUS)
5th Digit: 655.4
0. EPISODE OF CARE NOS OR N/A
1. DELIVERED
3. ANTEPARTUM COMPLICATION

066.8 CHANDIPURA FEVER
732.7 CHANDLER'S OSTEOCHONDRITIS DISSECANS, HIP
787.99 CHANGE BOWEL HABITS
066.0 CHANGUINOLA FEVER
301.9 CHARACTER DISORDER NOS

CHARCOT('S)
094.0 ARTHRITIS TABES OR SYPHILITIC [713.5]
094.0 JOINT DISEASE [713.5]
250.6# JOINT DIABETIC [713.5]
5th Digit: 250.6
0. TYPE II, ADULT-ONSET, NON-INSULIN DEPENDENT (EVEN IF REQUIRING INSULIN), OR UNSPECIFIED; CONTROLLED
1. TYPE I, JUVENILE-ONSET OR INSULIN-DEPENDENT; CONTROLLED
2. TYPE II, ADULT-ONSET, NON-INSULIN DEPENDENT (EVEN IF REQUIRING INSULIN); UNCONTROLLED
3. TYPE I, JUVENILE-ONSET OR INSULIN-DEPENDENT; UNCONTROLLED

356.1 MARIE TOOTH (SCOLIOSIS) [737.43]

CHARCOT('S) (continued)
443.9 SYNDROME - ANGINA CRURIS
443.9 SYNDROME - INTERMITTENT CLAUDICATION
440.21 SYNDROME - INTERMITTENT CLAUDICATION DUE TO ATHEROSCLEROSIS
440.3# SYNDROME - INTERMITTENT CLAUDICATION DUE TO BYPASS GRAFT ATHEROSCLEROSIS
5th Digit: 440.3
0. UNSPECIFIED GRAFT
1. AUTOLOGOUS VEIN BYPASS GRAFT
2. NONAUTOLOGOUS BIOLOGICAL BYPASS GRAFT

648.9#: USE AN ADDITIONAL CODE TO IDENTIFY THE SPECIFIC TYPE OF CHARCOT'S SYNDROME.

648.9# SYNDROME - MATERNAL CURRENT (CO-EXISTENT) IN PREGNANCY
5th Digit: 648.9
0. EPISODE OF NOS OR N/A
1. DELIVERED
2. DELIVERED WITH POSTPARTUM COMPLICATION
3. ANTEPARTUM COMPLICATION
4. POSTPARTUM COMPLICATION

337.0 WEISS-BAKER SYNDROME

102.9 CHARLOUIS' DISEASE
267 CHEADLE (-MOLLER) (-BARLOW) SYNDROME (INFANTILE SCURVY)
288.2 CHEDIAK STEINBRINCK (HIGASHI) SYNDROME

CHEEK
528.9 BITING
738.19 DEFORMITY
744.9 DEFORMITY CONGENITAL
528.9 DISEASE (INNER)
959.09 INJURY
925.1 INJURY CRUSH
910.8 INJURY OTHER AND UNSPECIFIED (SUPERFICIAL)
910.9 INJURY OTHER AND UNSPECIFIED (SUPERFICIAL) INFECTED

495.8 CHEESE WASHERS' LUNG

CHEILITIS
528.5 NOS
692.72 ACTINIC ACUTE DUE TO SUN
692.74 ACTINIC CHRONIC DUE TO SUN
692.82 ACTINIC DUE TO RADIATION (EXCEPT SUN)
702.0 ACTINIC SOLAR KERATOSIS
528.5 ACUTE OR CHRONIC
528.5 ANGULAR
528.5 CATARRHAL
528.5 EXFOLIATIVE
528.5 GANGRENOUS
528.5 GLANDULARIS APOSTEMATOSA
351.8 GRANULOMATOSA
528.5 INFECTIONAL
528.5 MEMBRANOUS
351.8 MIESCHER'S
692.71 SUNBURN
528.5 SUPPURATIVE
528.5 ULCERATIVE
528.5 VESICULAR

749.2# CHEILOPALATOSCHISIS
5th Digit: 749.2
0. CLEFT PALATE WITH CLEFT LIP UNSPECIFIED
1. CLEFT PALATE UNILATERAL COMPLETE
2. CLEFT PALATE UNILATERAL INCOMPLETE
3. CLEFT PALATE BILATERAL COMPLETE
4. CLEFT PALATE BILATERAL INCOMPLETE
5. CLEFT PALATE OTHER COMBINATIONS

749.1# CHEILOSCHISIS

5th Digit: 749.1

0. CLEFT NOS
1. CLEFT UNILATERAL COMPLETE
2. CLEFT UNILATERAL INCOMPLETE
3. CLEFT BILATERAL COMPLETE
4. CLEFT BILATERAL INCOMPLETE

528.5 CHEILOSIS
705.81 CHEIROPOMPHOLYX
701.4 CHELOID
0 CHEMICAL BURN SEE 'BURN', BY SITE
0 CHEMICAL BURN INGESTED AGENT SEE 'BURN', INTERNAL ORGANS, BY SITE
V82.5 CHEMICAL POISONING AND OTHER CONTAMINATION SCREENING

IF A PATIENT IS ADMINISTERED CHEMOTHERAPY AT THE TIME OF PORT-O-CATH OR HICKMAN CATHETER INSERTION, ASSIGN CODE V58.1 AS THE PRINCIPAL DIAGNOSIS AND THE MALIGNANCY AS THE SECONDARY CODE.

IF CHEMOTHERAPY IS NOT ADMINISTERED AT THE SAME TIME AS THE CATHETER INSERTION CODE THE MALIGNANCY AS THE PRINCIPAL DIAGNOSIS.

CHEMOTHERAPY

V58.1 ADMISSION
V58.1 CHEMOEMBOLIZATION THERAPY
V66.2 CONVALESCENCE
V58.1 ENCOUNTER
V67.2 FOLLOWUP EXAM
V58.1 INTRA-ARTERIAL
V58.1 MAINTENANCE

V07.39 CHEMOTHERAPEUTIC AGENT ADMINISTRATION PROPHYLACTIC NEC

CHEST

786.7 ABNORMAL PERCUSSION
862.8 CRUSHED
908.0 CRUSHED LATE EFFECT
738.3 DEFORMITY ACQUIRED
786.59 DISCOMFORT
519.9 DISEASE (RESPIRATORY)
754.81 FUNNEL CONGENITAL
786.6 MASS OR SWELLING
786.9 SYMPTOMS NEC
862.8 TRAUMA (WITH INJURY TO INTRATHORACIC ORGANS)
862.9 TRAUMA WITH OPEN WOUND (WITH INJURY TO INTRATHORACIC ORGANS)
908.0 TRAUMA LATE EFFECT
754.89 WALL DEFORMITY CONGENITAL
959.1 WALL INJURY
911.8 WALL INJURY OTHER AND UNSPECIFIED SUPERFICIAL
911.9 WALL INJURY OTHER AND UNSPECIFIED SUPERFICIAL INFECTED
786.52 WALL PAIN ANTERIOR
786.52 WALL SYNDROME (ANTERIOR)
V71.2 X-RAY FOR SUSPECTED TUBERCULOSIS
V72.5 X-RAY ROUTINE
793.1 X-RAY LUNG SHADOW

CHEST PAIN

786.50 NOS
786.59 ATYPICAL
413.1 ATYPICAL - ANGINA
786.51 MIDSTERNAL
786.59 MUSCULOSKELETAL
786.59 NONCARDIAC
786.51 PRECORDIAL
786.52 PLEURITIC
786.59 PRESSURE
786.51 SUBSTERNAL
786.59 TIGHTNESS

786.04 CHEYNE STOKES RESPIRATION

FOR CODING PURPOSES, CHF AND RIGHT VENTRICULAR FAILURE ARE CONSIDERED TO BE SYNONYMOUS AND BOTH ARE ASSIGNED A 4TH DIGIT OF "0". LEFT VENTRICULAR FAILURE IS NOT THE SAME AS CHF. LEFT VENTRICULAR FAILURE IS ASSIGNED A 4TH DIGIT OF "1".

CHF (CONGESTIVE HEART FAILURE)

428.0 ACUTE
0 ACUTE LEFT VENTRICULAR SEE 'HEART FAILURE', LEFT
0 ACUTE LEFT VENTRICULAR WITH PULMONARY EDEMA SEE 'HEART FAILURE', LEFT
428.0 ACUTE WITH PULMONARY EDEMA
428.0 COMBINED LEFT-RIGHT SIDED
428.0 COMPENSATED
428.0 DECOMPENSATED (RIGHT CONGESTIVE)
997.1 DURING A PROCEDURE
779.8 FETUS OR NEWBORN
402.91 HYPERTENSIVE NOS
402.11 HYPERTENSIVE BENIGN
402.01 HYPERTENSIVE MALIGNANT
404.91 HYPERTENSIVE HEART AND RENAL NOS
404.11 HYPERTENSIVE HEART AND RENAL BENIGN
404.01 HYPERTENSIVE HEART AND RENAL MALIGNANT
404.93 HYPERTENSIVE HEART AND RENAL WITH RENAL FAILURE NOS
404.13 HYPERTENSIVE HEART AND RENAL WITH RENAL FAILURE BENIGN
404.03 HYPERTENSIVE HEART AND RENAL WITH RENAL FAILURE MALIGNANT
0 LEFT VENTRICULAR SEE 'HEART FAILURE'

CARDIAC COMPLICATIONS POST-OP ARE DIVIDED INTO TWO TYPES: IMMEDIATE POST-OP (SURGERY TO DISCHARGE), 997.1, AND LATE OR FOLLOWING DISCHARGE, 429.4.

997.1 POST OP (RESULTING FROM A PROCEDURE)
997.1 POST OP HEART SURGERY - IMMEDIATE
429.4 POST OP HEART SURGERY - LATE
398.91 RHEUMATIC
391.8 RHEUMATIC ACUTE OR ACTIVE
398.91 RHEUMATIC CHRONIC OR INACTIVE (WITH CHOREA)
428.0 RIGHT SECONDARY TO LEFT
392.0 SYDENHAM'S CHOREA WITH HEART INVOLVEMENT
402.91 WITH HYPERTENSIVE CARDIOMYOPATHY
402.11 WITH HYPERTENSIVE CARDIOMYOPATHY BENIGN
402.01 WITH HYPERTENSIVE CARDIOMYOPATHY MALIGNANT

CHF (CONGESTIVE HEART FAILURE) OBSTETRICAL

635.7# COMPLICATING ABORTION

5th Digit: 635.7

0. UNSPECIFIED
1. INCOMPLETE
2. COMPLETE

669.4# COMPLICATING LABOR AND DELIVERY

5th Digit: 669.4

0. EPISODE OF CARE NOS
1. DELIVERED W/ OR W/O MENTION ANTEPARTUM CONDITION
2. DELIVERED WITH MENTION OF POSTPARTUM COMPLICATION
3. ANTEPARTUM COMPLICATION
4. POSTPARTUM COMPLICATION

***648.6#**, USE AN ADDITIONAL CODE TO SPECIFY THE CONGESTIVE HEART FAILURE. SEE 'CHF'.*

648.6# CURRENT (CO-EXISTENT) IN PREGNANCY
668.1# DUE TO ANESTHESIA, OTHER SEDATION IN L & D

5th Digit: 648.6, 668.1

0. EPISODE OF CARE NOS
1. DELIVERED W/ OR W/O MENTION ANTEPARTUM CONDITION
2. DELIVERED WITH MENTION OF POSTPARTUM COMPLICATION
3. ANTEPARTUM COMPLICATION
4. POSTPARTUM COMPLICATION

639.8 FOLLOWING ABORTION

C

CHIARI

453.0 DISEASE (HEPATIC VEIN THROMBOSIS)

676.6# FROMMEL SYNDROME MATERNAL DUE TO PREGNANCY

5th Digit: 676.6

0. EPISODE OF CARE NOS
1. DELIVERED W/ OR W/O MENTION ANTEPARTUM CONDITION
2. DELIVERED WITH MENTION OF POSTPARTUM COMPLICATION
3. ANTEPARTUM COMPLICATION
4. POSTPARTUM COMPLICATION

348.4 MALFORMATION TYPE I

741.0# MALFORMATION TYPE II

5th Digit: 741.0

0. REGION NOS
1. CERVICAL REGION
2. DORSAL (THORACIC REGION)
3. LUMBAR REGION

742.0 MALFORMATION TYPE III
742.2 MALFORMATION TYPE IV
453.0 SYNDROME (HEPATIC VEIN THROMBOSIS)

368.41 CHIASMATIC SYNDROME
116.0 CHICAGO DISEASE (NORTH AMERICAN BLASTOMYCOSIS)
0 CHICKENPOX SEE 'VARICELLA'
085.4 CHICLERO ULCER
133.8 CHIGGERS
767.1 CHIGNON (DUE TO VACUUM EXTRACTION)
111.2 CHIGNON (WHITE PIEDRA)
134.1 CHIGOE INFESTATION
066.3 CHIKUNGUNYA FEVER (VIRAL)
751.4 CHILAIDITI'S SYNDROME (SUBPHRENIC DISPLACEMENT, COLON)
991.5 CHILBLAINS
909.4 CHILBLAINS LATE EFFECT

WHEN THE CAUSE OF AN INJURY IS STATED TO BE ABUSE, MULTIPLE CODES SHOULD BE ASSIGNED, IF APPLICABLE, TO IDENTIFY ANY ASSOCIATED INJURIES. THEY ARE TO BE SEQUENCED IN THE FOLLOWING ORDER:

1. TYPE OF ABUSE - CHILD OR ADULT (995.5, 995.8)

2. TYPE OF INJURY

3. PERPETRATOR OF THE ABUSE - SEE E-CODE DIRECTORY 'ASSAULT' (E967)

4. NATURE OF THE ABUSE - SEE E-CODE DIRECTORY 'ASSAULT' (E904.0, E960-E966, E968)

CHILD

995.5# ABUSE (VICTIM)

5th Digit: 995.5

0. UNSPECIFIED
1. EMOTIONAL / PSYCHOLOGICAL (DEPRIVATION)
2. NEGLECT (NUTRITIONAL), DESERTION
3. SEXUAL
4. PHYSICAL
5. SHAKEN INFANT SYNDROME
9. OTHER ABUSE AND NEGLECT, MULTIPLE FORMS

V61.22 ABUSE COUNSELING - PERPETRATOR PARENT
V62.83 ABUSE COUNSELING - OTHER PERPETRATOR OF PHYSICAL / SEXUAL ABUSE
V61.21 ABUSE COUNSELING - VICTIM
V71.6 ABUSE EVALUATION - BATTERY (ALLEGED)
V71.5 ABUSE EVALUATION - SEXUAL (ALLEGED)

V15.4# ABUSE HISTORY

5th Digit: V15.4

1. PHYSICAL ABUSE, RAPE
2. EMOTIONAL ABUSE, NEGLECT
9. OTHER PSYCHOLOGICAL TRAUMA

995.52 DESERTION

CHILD (continued)

995.5# MALTREATMENT SYNDROME

5th Digit: 995.5

0. UNSPECIFIED
1. EMOTIONAL / PSYCHOLOGICAL (DEPRIVATION)
2. NEGLECT (NUTRITIONAL), DESERTION
3. SEXUAL
4. PHYSICAL
5. SHAKEN INFANT SYNDROME
9. OTHER ABUSE AND NEGLECT, MULTIPLE FORMS

780.9 CHILLS
780.6 CHILLS WITH FEVER

CHIN

744.89 ABSENCE CONGENITAL
524.05 HYPERPLASIA
524.06 HYPOPLASIA
959.09 INJURY
996.69 PROSTHESIS COMPLICATION - INFECTION OR INFLAMMATION
996.59 PROSTHESIS COMPLICATION - MECHANICAL
996.79 PROSTHESIS COMPLICATION - OTHER

121.1 CHINESE LIVER FLUKE DISEASE

CHLAMYDIA

079.98 INFECTION (ORGANISM)
079.88 INFECTION OTHER SPECIFIED CHLAMYDIAL
483.1 PNEUMONIA
V73.98 SCREENING UNSPECIFIED CHLAMYDIAL DISEASE
V73.88 SCREENING OTHER SPECIFIED CHLAMYDIAL DISEASE
099.50 TRACHOMATIS INFECTION UNSPECIFIED
099.52 TRACHOMATIS ANUS
099.53 TRACHOMATIS BLADDER [595.4]
099.53 TRACHOMATIS CERVIX [616.0]
099.54 TRACHOMATIS EPIDIDYMIS [604.91]
099.54 TRACHOMATIS GENITOURINARY SPECIFIED NEC
099.53 TRACHOMATIS LOWER GENITOURINARY SITES
099.54 TRACHOMATIS PELVIC INFLAMMATORY DISEASE [614.9]
099.56 TRACHOMATIS PERIHEPATIC
099.56 TRACHOMATIS PERITONEUM
099.51 TRACHOMATIS PHARYNX
099.52 TRACHOMATIS RECTUM
099.54 TRACHOMATIS TESTIS [604.91]
099.53 TRACHOMATIS VAGINA [616.11]
099.53 TRACHOMATIS VULVITIS [616.11]
099.53 TRACHOMATIS VULVOVAGINITIS [616.11]
099.59 VENEREAL SPECIFIED SITE NEC

CHLOASMA

709.09 NOS
709.09 CACHECTICORUM
709.09 EPHELIDES
374.52 EYELID
709.09 IDIOPATHIC
709.09 SYMPTOMATIC
709.09 VAGINAL

276.9 CHLORIDE ABNORMAL FINDINGS

748.0 CHOANAL ATRESIA CONGENITAL
748.0 CHOANAL OCCLUSION

617.1 CHOCOLATE CYST OVARY

933.1 CHOKING (FOOD REGURGITATED) (PHLEGM)
784.9 CHOKING SENSATION

155.1 CHOLANGIOCARCINOMA SITE NOS
0 CHOLANGIOCARCINOMA SITE SPECIFIED SEE 'CANCER' BY SITE M8160/3

CHOLANGITIS

576.1 CHOLANGITIS
576.1 ACUTE
576.1 ASCENDING (SCLEROSING) (SECONDARY) (RECURRENT)
576.1 CHRONIC
571.6 CHRONIC NONSUPPURATIVE
571.6 CHRONIC NONSUPPURATIVE WITH ESOPHAGEAL VARICES [456.2#]
5th Digit: 456.2
0. WITH BLEEDING
1. WITHOUT BLEEDING

576.1 SUPPURATIVE

575.9 CHOLECYSTIC DISEASE

> *A COMBINATION CODE IS USED TO CLASSIFY TWO DIAGNOSES OR A DIAGNOSIS WITH ITS MANIFESTATION OR COMPLICATION. EX. 574.00: CHOLECYSTITIS ACUTE WITH CHOLELITHIASIS*

CHOLECYSTITIS

575.10 NOS
574.4# NOS - WITH CHOLEDOCHOLITHIASIS
574.1# NOS - WITH CHOLELITHIASIS
574.7# NOS - WITH CHOLELITHIASIS AND CHOLEDOCHOLITHIASIS
5th Digit: 574.1, 4, 7
0. WITHOUT OBSTRUCTION
1. WITH OBSTRUCTION

575.0 ACUTE
574.3# ACUTE - WITH CHOLEDOCHOLITHIASIS
574.0# ACUTE - WITH CHOLELITHIASIS
574.6# ACUTE - WITH CHOLELITHIASIS AND CHOLEDOCHOLITHIASIS
5th Digit: 574.0, 3, 6
0. WITHOUT OBSTRUCTION
1. WITH OBSTRUCTION

575.12 ACUTE AND CHRONIC
574.8# ACUTE AND CHRONIC - WITH CHOLELITHIASIS AND CHOLEDOCHOLITHIASIS
5th Digit: 574.8
0. WITHOUT OBSTRUCTION
1. WITH OBSTRUCTION

575.11 CHRONIC
574.4# CHRONIC - WITH CHOLEDOCHOLITHIASIS
574.1# CHRONIC - WITH CHOLELITHIASIS
574.7# CHRONIC - WITH CHOLELITHIASIS AND CHOLEDOCHOLITHIASIS
5th Digit: 574.1, 4, 7,
0. WITHOUT OBSTRUCTION
1. WITH OBSTRUCTION

575.12 CHRONIC AND ACUTE
574.8# CHRONIC AND ACUTE WITH CHOLELITHIASIS AND CHOLEDOCHOLITHIASIS
5th Digit: 574.8
0. WITHOUT OBSTRUCTION
1. WITH OBSTRUCTION

0 EMPHYSEMATOUS SEE 'CHOLECYSTITIS', ACUTE
0 GANGRENOUS SEE 'CHOLECYSTITIS', ACUTE
0 SUPPURATIVE SEE 'CHOLECYSTITIS', ACUTE

CHOLEDOCHAL CYST

576.8 CHOLEDOCHAL CYST
751.69 CHOLEDOCHAL CYST CONGENITAL

CHOLEDOCHOLITHIASIS

574.5# NOS
574.9# NOS WITH CHOLELITHIASIS
574.4# WITH CHOLECYSTITIS NOS
574.3# WITH CHOLECYSTITIS ACUTE
574.6# WITH CHOLECYSTITIS ACUTE - WITH CHOLELITHIASIS
574.8# WITH CHOLECYSTITIS ACUTE AND CHRONIC- WITH CHOLELITHIASIS
574.4# WITH CHOLECYSTITIS CHRONIC
574.7# WITH CHOLECYSTITIS CHRONIC - WITH CHOLELITHIASIS
5th Digit: 574.3-9
0. WITHOUT OBSTRUCTION
1. WITH OBSTRUCTION

CHOLELITHIASIS

574.2# NOS
574.9# NOS WITH CHOLEDOCHOLITHIASIS
574.1# WITH CHOLECYSTITIS NOS
574.0# WITH CHOLECYSTITIS ACUTE
574.6# WITH CHOLECYSTITIS ACUTE - WITH CHOLEDOCHOLITHIASIS
574.8# WITH CHOLECYSTITIS ACUTE AND CHRONIC- WITH CHOLEDOCHOLITHIASIS
574.1# WITH CHOLECYSTITIS CHRONIC
574.7# WITH CHOLECYSTITIS CHRONIC - WITH CHOLEDOCHOLITHIASIS
5th Digit: 574.0-2, 6-9
0. WITHOUT OBSTRUCTION
1. WITH OBSTRUCTION

782.4 CHOLEMIA

CHOLERA

001.9 NOS
985.4 ANTIMONIAL
V02.0 CARRIER
V01.0 EXPOSURE
V74.0 SCREENING EXAM
V06.0 TYPHOID PARATYPHOID VACCINATION
V03.0 VACCINATION
001.0 VIBRIO
001.1 VIBRIO EL TOR

CHOLESTEATOMA

385.30 CHOLESTATOMA
385.31 ATTIC
385.35 DIFFUSE (CHOLESTEATOSIS)
380.21 EXTERNA
385.32 MIDDLE EAR
385.33 MIDDLE EAR AND MASTOID
383.32 POSTMASTOIDECTOMY

385.35 CHOLESTEATOSIS DIFFUSE
385.82 CHOLESTERIN GRANULOMA MIDDLE EAR AND MASTOID
272.9 CHOLESTEROL ABNORMAL (SERUM LEVEL)
593.81 CHOLESTEROL EMBOLIZATION SYNDROME (EMBOLUS RENAL ARTERIOLE DUE TO AORTIC ARTERIOSCLEROSIS) [440.0]
V77.9 CHOLESTEROL SCREENING
575.6 CHOLESTEROLOSIS GALLBLADDER
0 CHOLESTEROLOSIS MIDDLE EAR SEE 'CHOLESTEATOMA'
733.99 CHONDRITIS
733.6 CHONDRITIS COSTAL

C

CHONDROBLASTOMA

213.# NOS M9230/0

170.# MALIGNANT M9230/3

4th Digit: 170, 213

0. SKULL FACE UPPER JAW
1. LOWER JAW NOS
2. SPINE
3. RIB STERNUM CLAVICLE
4. UPPER LIMB LONG BONES SCAPULA
5. UPPER LIMB SHORT BONES
6. PELVIS SACRUM COCCYX
7. LOWER LIMB LONG BONE
8. LOWER LIMB SHORT BONE
9. SITE NOS

CHONDROCALCINOSIS

275.49 CRYSTAL DEPOSITION - NOS [712.3#]

275.49 CRYSTAL DEPOSITION - DICALCIUM PHOSPHATE [712.1#]

275.49 CRYSTAL DEPOSITION - PYROPHOSPHATE CRYSTALS [712.2#]

5th Digit: 712.1-3

0. SITE NOS
1. SHOULDER REGION
2. UPPER ARM (ELBOW) (HUMERUS)
3. FOREARM (RADIUS) (WRIST) (ULNA)
4. HAND (CARPAL) (METACARPAL) (FINGERS)
5. PELVIC REGION AND THIGH (HIP) (BUTTOCK) (FEMUR)
6. LOWER LEG (FIBULA) (KNEE) (PATELLA) (TIBIA)
7. ANKLE AND/OR FOOT (METATARSALS) (TOES) (TARSALS)
8. OTHER (HEAD) (NECK) (RIB) (SKULL) (TRUNK) (VERTEBRAE)
9. MULTIPLE

380.00 CHONDRODERMATITIS NODULARIS HELICIS (SEE ALSO 'PERICHONDRITIS EAR')

756.4 CHONDRODYSTROPHIA (FETALIS) CONGENITAL

756.4 CHONDRODYSTROPHY CONGENITAL

756.55 CHONDROECTODERMAL DYSPLASIA SYNDROME

CHONDROMA

213.# NOS M9220/0

213.# JUXTACORTICAL M9221/0

4th Digit: 213

0. SKULL FACE UPPER JAW
1. LOWER JAW NOS
2. SPINE
3. RIB STERNUM CLAVICLE
4. UPPER LIMB LONG BONES SCAPULA
5. UPPER LIMB SHORT BONES
6. PELVIS SACRUM COCCYX
7. LOWER LIMB LONG BONE
8. LOWER LIMB SHORT BONE
9. SITE NOS

CHONDROMALACIA

733.92 NOS

733.92 LOCALIZED

717.7 LOCALIZED PATELLA

733.92 SYSTEMIC

733.92 TIBIAL PLATEAU

238.0 CHONDROMATOSIS SITE NOS

0 CHONDROMATOSIS SITE SPECIFIED SEE 'NEOPLASM UNCERTAIN BEHAVIOR' BY SITE M9220/1

CHONDROSARCOMA

170.# CHRONDROSARCOMA M9220/3

170.# JUXTACORTICAL M9221/3

170.# MESENCHYMAL M9240/3

4th Digit: 170

0. SKULL AND FACE
1. MANDIBLE
2. VERTEBRAL COLUMN
3. RIBS STERNUM CLAVICLE
4. SCAPULA LONG BONES UPPER LIMB
5. SHORT BONES UPPER LIMB
6. PELVIC BONES SACRUM COCCYX
7. LONG BONES LOWER LIMB
8. SHORT BONES LOWER LIMB
9. SITE NOS

848.42 CHONDROSTERNAL SEPARATION (RUPTURE) (TEAR) (LACERATION)

848.42 CHONDROSTERNAL STRAIN (SPRAIN) (AVULSION) (HEMARTHROSIS)

429.5 CHORDAE TENDINEAE RUPTURE

429.5 CHORDAE TENDINEAE RUPTURE (POST INFARCTION) [410.90]

752.63 CHORDEE CONGENITAL

607.89 CHORDEE (NONVENEREAL)

478.5 CHORDITIS

CHORDOMA

199.1 SITE NOS

0 SITE SPECIFIED SEE 'CANCER' BY SITE M9370/3

CHOREA

275.1 ATHETOSIS-AGITANS SYNDROME

333.5 HEMIBALLISM (US)

333.4 HUNTINGTON'S

333.5 OTHER

333.5 PAROXYSMAL CHOREO-ATHETOSIS

344.89 POSTHEMIPLEGIC

392.9 RHEUMATIC ACUTE

392.0 RHEUMATIC WITH HEART INVOLVEMENT ACUTE

333.5 CHOREOATHETOSIS PAROXYSMAL

236.1 CHORIOADENOMA (DESTRUENS) M9100/1

762.7 CHORIOAMNIONITIS AFFECTING FETUS OR NEWBORN

0 CHORIOAMNIONITIS SEE 'AMNIONITIS'

CARCINOMAS AND NEOPLASMS SHOULD BE CODED BY SITE IF POSSIBLE. CODE BY CELL TYPE - "SITE NOS", IF AND ONLY IF A SITE IS NOT SPECIFIED IN THE DIAGNOSIS. OTHERWISE - REFER TO THE APPROPRIATE CATEGORY OF NEOPLASM FOR A MORE SPECIFIC CODE: SEE 'CANCER' 'CANCER METASTATIC', 'NEOPLASM UNCERTAIN BEHAVIOR', 'NEOPLASM UNSPECIFIED NATURE', OR 'BENIGN NEOPLASM.'

CHORIOCARCINOMA

181 NOS M9100/3

199.1 COMBINED WITH TERATOMA SITE NOS

0 COMBINED WITH TERATOMA SITE SPECIFIED SEE 'CANCER' BY SITE M9101/3

181 FEMALE SITE NOS

0 FEMALE SITE SPECIFIED SEE 'CANCER' BY SITE M9101/3

186.9 MALE SITE NOS

0 MALE SITE SPECIFIED SEE 'CANCER' BY SITE M9101/3

181 CHORIOEPITHELIOMA NOS M9100/3

762.9 CHORION AND AMNION ABNORMALITY AFFECTING FETUS OR NEWBORN

762.8 CHORION AND AMNION ABNORMALITIES OTHER SPECIFIED AFFECTING FETUS OR NEWBORN

CHORIORETINAL SCAR

363.30 NOS

363.35 DISSEMINATED

743.53 DEGENERATION CONGENITAL

CHORIORETINAL SCAR (continued)
363.32 MACULAR
363.34 PERIPHERAL
363.33 POSTERIOR POLE

CHORIORETINITIS
363.20 NOS
363.10 DISSEMINATED
363.00 FOCAL
363.01 FOCAL JUXTAPAPILLARY (AND CHOROIDITIS)
363.03 FOCAL OTHER POSTERIOR POLE (AND CHOROIDITIS)
363.04 FOCAL PERIPHERAL (AND CHOROIDITIS)
0 HISTOPLASMA SEE 'HISTOPLASMA'
363.21 PARS PLANITIS
362.18 PERIVASCULITIS
0 SEE ALSO 'RETINITIS'
090.0 SYPHILITIC CONGENITAL EARLY [363.13]
095.8 SYPHILITIC CONGENITAL LATE [363.13]
091.51 SYPHILITIC SECONDARY
130.2 TOXOPLASMOSIS
017.3# TUBERCULOUS [363.13]
5th Digit: 017.3
0. NOS
1. LAB NOT DONE
2. LAB UNKNOWN AT PRESENT
3. MICROSCOPY POSITIVE - (IN SPUTUM)
4. CULTURE POSITIVE - MICROSCOPY NEGATIVE
5. CULTURE NEGATIVE - MICROSCOPY POSITIVE
6. CULTURE AND MICROSCOPY NEGATIVE - CONFIRMED BY OTHER METHODS

CHOROID, CHOROIDAL
363.43 ANGIOID STREAKS

433.8# ARTERY OBSTRUCTION OR OCCLUSION
433.8# ARTERY THROMBOSIS (EMBOLISM) (DEFORMANS)
5th Digit: 433.8
0. WITHOUT CEREBRAL INFARCTION
1. WITH CEREBRAL INFARCTION

363.40 ATROPHY
363.42 ATROPHY DIFFUSE SECONDARY
0 ATROPHY HEREDITARY SEE 'CHOROID, CHOROIDAL', DYSTROPHY HEREDITARY
363.41 ATROPHY SENILE

743.59 DEFECT CONGENITAL
363.40 DEGENERATION

363.70 DETACHMENT
363.72 DETACHMENT HEMORRHAGIC
363.71 DETACHMENT SEROUS

363.9 DISORDER
363.8 DISORDER OTHER SPECIFIED

DYSTROPHY HEREDITARY
363.50 NOS
363.57 ATROPHIC (GENERALIZED GYRATE)
363.54 CENTRAL GYRATE
363.53 CENTRAL PARTIAL
363.54 CENTRAL TOTAL
363.55 CHOROIDEREMIA
363.53 CIRCINATE
363.51 CIRCUMPAPILLARY PARTIAL
363.52 CIRCUMPAPILLARY TOTAL
363.56 DIFFUSE SCLEROSIS
363.57 GENERALIZED GYRATE ATROPHY
363.52 HELICOID
363.56 SCLEROSIS
363.54 SERPIGINOUS
363.56 OTHER DIFFUSE OR GENERALIZED PARTIAL
363.57 OTHER DIFFUSE OR GENERALIZED TOTAL

CHOROID, CHOROIDAL (continued)
362.16 NEOVASCULARIZATION
363.63 RUPTURE

363.30 SCAR
363.35 SCAR DISSEMINATED
363.33 SCAR OF POSTERIOR POLE
363.34 SCAR PERIPHERAL
363.31 SCAR SOLAR

363.40 SCLEROSIS
363.56 SCLEROSIS DIFFUSE HEREDITARY

349.2 CHOROID PLEXUS CALCIFICATION

CHOROIDITIS
363.20 NOS
363.00 FOCAL
363.10 DISSEMINATED
363.11 DISSEMINATED POSTERIOR POLE (AND CHORIORETINITIS)
363.12 DISSEMINATED PERIPHERAL (AND CHORIORETINITIS)
363.13 DISSEMINATED GENERALIZED (AND CHORIORETINITIS)
091.51 SYPHILITIC SECONDARY
017.3# TUBERCULOUS [363.13]
5th Digit: 017.3
0. NOS
1. LAB NOT DONE
2. LAB UNKNOWN AT PRESENT
3. MICROSCOPY POSITIVE - (IN SPUTUM)
4. CULTURE POSITIVE - MICROSCOPY NEGATIVE
5. CULTURE NEGATIVE - MICROSCOPY POSITIVE
6. CULTURE AND MICROSCOPY NEGATIVE - CONFIRMED BY OTHER METHODS

0 SEE ALSO 'RETINITIS' OR 'CHORIORETINITIS'

729.30 CHRISTIAN-WEBER NODULAR NONSUPPURATIVE PANNICULITIS
277.8 CHRISTIAN'S SYNDROME (CHRONIC HISTIOCYTOSIS X)
286.1 CHRISTMAS DISEASE
705.89 CHROMHIDROSIS
117.2 CHROMOBLASTOMYCOSIS
117.2 CHROMOMYCOSIS
194.3 CHROMOPHOBE CARCINOMA SITE NOS
0 CHROMOPHOBE CARCINOMA SITE SPECIFIED SEE 'CANCER' BY SITE M8270/3
758.3 CHROMOSOME 4 SHORT ARM DELETION SYNDROME
758.81 CHROMOSOME ACCESSORY - SEX CHROMOSOME
758.5 CHROMOSOME ACCESSORY - NEC
795.2 CHROMOSOME ANALYSIS ABNORMAL
758.9 CHROMOSOME ANOMALY - UNSPECIFIED CHROMOSOME
758.9 CHROMOSOME ANOMALY - MOSAICS
758.81 CHROMOSOME ANOMALY - MOSAICS SEX CHROMOSOME
758.81 CHROMOSOME ANOMALY - SEX CHROMOSOME
758.89 CHROMOSOME ANOMALY - OTHER
V82.4 CHROMOSOME ANOMALY SCREENING (MATERNAL POSTNATAL)

0 CHRONIC BRONCHITIS SEE 'BRONCHITIS CHRONIC'
416.9 CHRONIC COR PULMONALE

WHEN A PATIENT IS ADMITTED IN ACUTE RESPIRATORY FAILURE, DUE TO ACUTE EXACERBATION OF A CHRONIC RESPIRATORY CONDITION, SEQUENCE THE FAILURE BEFORE THE CHRONIC DISEASE.

C

WHEN A PATIENT IS ADMITTED IN RESPIRATORY FAILURE DUE TO A NON RESPIRATORY CONDITION, SEQUENCE THAT CONDITION BEFORE THE RESPIRATORY FAILURE..

CHRONIC OBSTRUCTIVE PULMONARY DISEASE

496 NOS
491.21 ACUTE EXACERBATION
491.21 ACUTE EXACERBATION - ACUTE BRONCHITIS
491.21 ACUTE EXACERBATION - CHRONIC BRONCHITIS
518.5 ACUTE EXACERBATION - ARDS [496]
415.0 ACUTE EXACERBATION - COR PULMONALE [496]
486 ACUTE EXACERBATION - PNEUMONIA [496]
512.8 ACUTE EXACERBATION - PNEUMOTHORAX [496]
415.19 ACUTE EXACERBATION - PULMONARY EMBOLUS [496]
415.11 ACUTE EXACERBATION - PULMONARY EMBOLUS POST OP OR IATROGENIC [496]
518.81 ACUTE EXACERBATION - RESPIRATORY FAILURE [496]
495.6 FUNGAL (THERMOPHILIC) (ACTINOMYCETE) (OTHER)
495.4 WITH ALLERGIC ALVEOLITIS (ASPERGILLUS CLAVATUS)
495.9 WITH ALLERGIC ALVEOLITIS AND PNEUMONITIS
493.2# WITH ASTHMA

5th Digit: 493.2

0. WITHOUT MENTION OF STATUS ASTHMATICUS
1. WITH STATUS ASTHMATICUS

494 WITH BRONCHIECTASIS
491.20 WITH BRONCHITIS CHRONIC
496 WITH BRONCHOSPASM
492.8 WITH EMPHYSEMA
492.0 WITH EMPHYSEMA BULLOUS
491.20 WITH EMPHYSEMA WITH BRONCHITIS
491.21 WITH EMPHYSEMA WITH BRONCHITIS WITH EXACERBATION
496 WITH UNKNOWN EXACERBATION

457.8 CHYLOCELE
0 CHYLOCELE FILARIAL SEE 'FILARIASIS
608.84 CHYLOCELE TUNICA VAGINALIS

791.1 CHYLURIA
125.1 CHYLURIA DUE TO BRUGIA (WUCHERERIA) MALAYI
125.0 CHYLURIA DUE TO WUCHERERIA BANCROFTI
791.1 CHYLURIA NONFILARIAL ABNORMAL

CICATRIX

709.2 NOS
474.8 ADENOID
525.8 ALVEOLAR PROCESS
569.49 ANUS
380.89 AURICLE
576.8 BILE DUCT
596.8 BLADDER
733.99 BONE
348.8 BRAIN
622.3 CERVIX POSTPARTUM
654.6# CERVIX PREGNANCY OR CHILDBIRTH
660.2# CERVIX PREGNANCY OR CHILDBIRTH OBSTRUCTING LABOR [654.6#]

5th Digit: 654.6

0. EPISODE OF CARE UNSPECIFIED OR N/A
1. DELIVERED
2. DELIVERED WITH POSTPARTUM COMPLICATION
3. ANTEPARTUM COMPLICATION
4. POSTPARTUM COMPLICATION

5th Digit: 660.2

0. EPISODE OF CARE UNSPECIFIED OR N/A
1. DELIVERED
3. ANTEPARTUM COMPLICATION

CICATRIX (continued)

363.30 CHORIORETINAL - NOS
363.35 CHORIORETINAL - DISSEMINATED
743.53 CHORIORETINAL - DEGENERATION CONGENITAL
363.32 CHORIORETINAL - MACULAR
363.34 CHORIORETINAL - PERIPHERAL
363.33 CHORIORETINAL - POSTERIOR POLE NEC
576.8 COMMON DUCT
757.39 CONGENITAL
372.64 CONJUNCTIVA
371.00 CORNEA
537.3 DUODENUM (BULB)
530.3 ESOPHAGUS
374.46 EYELID
478.29 HYPOPHARYNX
717.5 KNEE, SEMILUNAR CARTILAGE
375.53 LACRIMAL CANALICULI
375.56 LACRIMAL DUCT ACQUIRED
375.55 LACRIMAL DUCT NEONATAL
375.52 LACRIMAL PUNCTUM
375.54 LACRIMAL SAC
478.79 LARYNX
518.89 LUNG
363.32 MACULAR
363.35 MACULAR - DISSEMINATED
363.34 MACULAR - PERIPHERAL
385.89 MIDDLE EAR
528.9 MOUTH
728.89 MUSCLE
375.56 NASOLACRIMAL DUCT ACQUIRED
375.55 NASOLACRIMAL DUCT NEONATAL
478.29 NASOPHARYNX
528.9 PALATE (SOFT)
607.89 PENIS
602.8 PROSTATE
569.49 RECTUM
363.30 RETINA - NOS
363.35 RETINA - DISSEMINATED
743.53 RETINA - DEGENERATION CONGENITAL
363.32 RETINA - MACULAR
363.34 RETINA - PERIPHERAL
363.33 RETINA - POSTERIOR POLE NEC
608.89 SEMINAL VESICLE
709.2 SKIN
686.8 SKIN INFECTED
478.29 THROAT
529.8 TONGUE
474.8 TONSIL
478.9 TRACHEA
593.89 URETER
599.84 URETHRA
621.8 UTERUS
623.4 VAGINA
478.5 VOCAL CORD
709.2 WRIST CONSTRICTING (ANNULAR)

374.89 CILIA ABSENCE CONGENITAL
743.63 CILIA AGENESIS ABSENCE CONGENITAL

364.57 CILIARY BODY DEGENERATIVE CHANGES (ATROPHY)
364.9 CILIARY BODY DISEASE
364.41 CILIARY BODY HEMORRHAGE
362.16 CILIARY BODY NEOVASCULARIZATION

622.1 CIN I
622.1 CIN II
233.1 CIN III (SEVERE)

307.45 CIRCADIAN RHYTHM DISRUPTION
747.89 CIRCULATION FETAL PERSISTENT
794.39 CIRCULATION TIME ABNORMAL

CIRCULATORY

747.9 ANOMALY CONGENITAL
639.5 COLLAPSE POST (ABORTIVE) (ECTOPIC) (MOLAR) PREGNANCY
V12.50 DISEASE HISTORY UNSPECIFIED
V12.59 DISEASE HISTORY OTHER SPECIFIED
760.3 DISEASE MATERNAL, CHRONIC AFFECTING FETUS OR NEWBORN
093.9 DISEASE SYPHILITIC
090.5 DISEASE SYPHILITIC CONGENITAL
459.9 DISORDER

648.9#: USE AN ADDITIONAL CODE TO IDENTIFY CIRCULATORY DISORDERS.

648.9# DISORDER MATERNAL CURRENT (CO-EXISTENT) IN PREGNANCY

5th Digit: 648.9

- **0. EPISODE OF NOS OR N/A**
- **1. DELIVERED**
- **2. DELIVERED WITH POSTPARTUM COMPLICATION**
- **3. ANTEPARTUM COMPLICATION**
- **4. POSTPARTUM COMPLICATION**

459.89 DISORDER OTHER SPECIFIED
459.9 OBSTRUCTION
747.89 SYSTEM ABSENCE CONGENITAL
747.89 SYSTEM ANOMALY SPECIFIED SITE NEC

V50.2 CIRCUMCISION ROUTINE OR RITUAL (ELECTIVE)

CIRRHOSIS:

-WITH ESOPHAGEAL VARICES [456.2#]

571.2 ALCOHOLIC (LIVER)
571.5 BAUMGARTEN-CRUVEILHIER
571.6 BILIARY
121.1 BILIARY DUE TO CLONORCHIASIS
121.3 BILIARY DUE TO FLUKES
331.9 BRAIN
571.5 CARDIAC
571.2 CARDIAC ALCOHOLIC
571.6 CHARCOT'S
571.6 CHOLANGITIC (CHOLESTATIC)
624.2 CLITORIS (HYPERTROPHIC)
777.8 CONGENITAL (DUE TO FAILURE OF OBLITERATION OF UMBILICAL VEIN)
571.5 CONGESTIVE (LIVER)
571.2 CONGESTIVE ALCOHOLIC (LIVER)
571.5 CRYPTOGENIC (LIVER)
571.2 CRYPTOGENIC ALCOHOLIC (LIVER)
571.8 FATTY (LIVER)
571.0 FATTY ALCOHOLIC (LIVER)
571.2 FLORID
571.5 GLISSON'S (LIVER)
571.2 GLISSON'S ALCOHOLIC (LIVER)
571.6 HANOT'S
571.5 HOBNAIL (LIVER)
571.2 HOBNAIL ALCOHOLIC (LIVER)
571.6 INTRAHEPATIC
571.5 JUVENILE (LIVER)
571.2 JUVENILE ALCOHOLIC (LIVER)
587 KIDNEY
571.5 LAENNEC'S (LIVER)
571.2 LAENNEC'S ALCOHOLIC (LIVER)
571.5 LIVER NOS
515 LUNG
571.5 MACRONODULAR (LIVER)
571.2 MACRONODULAR ALCOHOLIC (LIVER)
084.9 MALARIAL
571.5 MICRONODULAR (LIVER)
571.2 MICRONODULAR ALCOHOLIC (LIVER)

-WITH ESOPHAGEAL VARICES [456.2#]

5th Digit: 456.2

- **0. WITH BLEEDING**
- **1. WITHOUT BLEEDING**

CIRRHOSIS: (continued)

-WITH ESOPHAGEAL VARICES [456.2#]

587 NEPHROTIC
571.6 OBSTRUCTIVE (BILIARY) (EXTRAHEPATIC) (INTRAHEPATIC)
620.8 OVARIAN
084.9 PALUDAL
577.8 PANCREAS (DUCT)
275.0 PIGMENTARY (IRON)
571.5 PORTAL (LIVER)
571.2 PORTAL ALCOHOLIC (LIVER)
571.5 POSTHEPATITIC
571.5 POSTNECROTIC (LIVER)
571.2 POSTNECROTIC ALCOHOLIC (LIVER)
571.6 PRIMARY (INTRAHEPATIC)
515 PULMONARY
587 RENAL
571.5 SEPTAL
289.51 SPLEEN
571.5 SPLENOMEGALIC (LIVER)
571.2 SPLENOMEGALIC ALCOHOLIC (LIVER)
535.4 STOMACH
571.6 TODD'S
571.5 WITHOUT MENTION OF ALCOHOL
571.6 XANTHOMATOUS (BILIARY)
272.2 XANTHOMATOUS (BILIARY) DUE TO XANTHOMATOSIS

-WITH ESOPHAGEAL VARICES [456.2#]

5th Digit: 456.2

- **0. WITH BLEEDING**
- **1. WITHOUT BLEEDING**

270.6 CITRULLINE METABOLISM DISORDERS
270.6 CITRULLINEMIA
709.09 CIVATTE'S POIKILODERMA

117.2 CLADOSPORIDIUM CARRIONII INFECTION
111.1 CLADOSPORIUM SPECIES INFECTION
117.8 CLADOSPORIUM TRICHOIDES INFECTION

577.8 CLARKE-HADFIELD SYNDROME (PANCREATIC INFANTILISM)
704.2 CLASTOTHRIX
337.9 CLAUDE BERNARD-HORNER SYNDROME SEE ALSO 'NEUROPATHY PERIPHERAL' AUTONOMIC
352.6 CLAUDE'S SYNDROME

CLAUDICATION

440.21 DUE TO ATHEROSCLEROSIS
440.3# DUE TO ATHEROSCLEROSIS OF A BYPASS GRAFT EXTREMITIES

5th Digit: 440.3

- **0. UNSPECIFIED GRAFT**
- **1. AUTOLOGOUS VEIN BYPASS GRAFT**
- **2. NONAUTOLOGOUS BIOLOGICAL BYPASS GRAFT**

443.9 INTERMITTENT NOS
453.8 INTERMITTENT VENOUS
443.9 PERIPHERAL VASCULAR DISEASE

300.29 CLAUSTROPHOBIA
738.8 CLAVICLE DEFORMITY ACQUIRED
755.51 CLAVICLE DEFORMITY CONGENITAL
700 CLAVUS
736.74 CLAW FOOT ACQUIRED
736.06 CLAW HAND ACQUIRED
735.5 CLAW TOE ACQUIRED
229.9 CLEAR CELL ADENOFIBROMA SITE NOS
0 CLEAR CELL ADENOFIBROMA SITE SPECIFIED SEE 'BENIGN NEOPLASM' BY SITE M8313/0

C

CLEFT
755.58 HAND CONGENITAL
749.1# LIP
749.0# PALATE
5th Digit: 749.0-1
0. NOS
1. UNILATERAL COMPLETE
2. UNILATERAL INCOMPLETE
3. BILATERAL COMPLETE
4. BILATERAL INCOMPLETE

749.2# PALATE WITH CLEFT LIP
5th Digit: 749.2
0. PALATE WITH CLEFT LIP UNSPECIFIED
1. PALATE UNILATERAL COMPLETE
2. PALATE UNILATERAL INCOMPLETE
3. PALATE BILATERAL COMPLETE
4. PALATE BILATERAL INCOMPLETE
5. PALATE OTHER COMBINATIONS

749.02 UVULA

755.59 CLEIDOCRANIAL DYSOSTOSIS
763.89 CLEIDOTOMY, FETAL
348.8 CLERAMBAULT'S AUTOMATISM SYNDROME
297.8 CLERAMBAULT'S EROTOMANIA SYNDROME
766.2 CLIFFORD'S SYNDROME (POSTMATURITY)
608.89 CLIMACTERIC MALE
627.2 CLIMACTERIC SYNDROME (FEMALE)
099.1 CLIMATIC BUBO
796.4 CLINICAL FINDINGS OTHER ABNORMAL

CLITORIS, CLITORAL
752.49 ABSENCE (AGENESIS) (STRICTURE) CONGENITAL
752.49 ANOMALY NEC
752.49 HOODED CONGENITAL
752.49 HYPERPLASIA CONGENITAL
255.2 HYPERTROPHY - ADRENOGENITAL
624.2 HYPERTROPHY - NONENDOCRINE
256.1 HYPERTROPHY- OVARIAN ANDROGEN SECRETION

751.5 CLOACAL ANOMALY
154.8 CLOACOGENIC CARCINOMA SITE NOS
0 CLOACOGENIC CARCINOMA SITE SPECIFIED SEE 'CANCER' BY SITE M8124/3

121.1 CLONORCHIOSIS
121.1 CLONORCHIOSIS BILIARY CIRRHOSIS DUE TO

CLOSTRIDIUM
008.45 DIFFICILE
040.0 HISTOLYTICUM
771.8 INTRA-AMNIOTIC INFECTION OF FETUS
040.0 OEDEMATIENS
005.3 OTHER SPECIFIED TYPE FOOD POISONING
041.83 PERFRINGENS
005.2 PERFRINGENS FOOD POISONING
771.8 PERINATAL INTRA-AMNIOTIC
040.0 SEPTICUM
004.0 SORDELLII
005.2 WELCHII FOOD POISONING
040.0 WELCHII INFECTION (PREFRINGENS)

286.3 CLOTTING FACTOR DEFICIENCY OTHER
757.31 CLOUSTON'S SYNDROME (HIDROTIC ECTODERMAL DYSPLASIA)
756.0 CLOVERLEAF SKULL

CLUB
736.29 FINGER ACQUIRED
754.89 FINGER CONGENITAL
736.71 FOOT ACQUIRED
754.70 FOOT CONGENITAL
754.51 FOOT EQUINOVARUS
736.07 HAND ACQUIRED
754.89 HAND CONGENITAL
703.8 NAIL ACQUIRED
757.5 NAIL CONGENITAL

781.5 CLUBBING FINGER
315.4 CLUMSINESS SYNDROME

CMV (CYTOMEGALOVIRUS INFECTIONS)
078.5 CMV
771.1 CONGENITAL OR PERINATAL
V01.7 EXPOSURE
078.5 HEPATITIS [573.1]
078.5 INCLUSION DISEASE (GENERALIZED)
078.5 PNEUMONIA [484.1]

794.00 CNS ABNORMAL FUNCTION STUDY
779.2 CNS DYSFUNCTION NEWBORN NOS
786.09 CO 2 (CARBON DIOXIDE) NARCOSIS

COAGULATION
790.92 DELAY NEC
286.9 DISORDER
286.7 FACTOR DEFICIENCY ACQUIRED
776.0 FACTOR DEFICIENCY ACQUIRED NEWBORN
286.9 FACTOR DEFICIENCY CONGENITAL
776.2 NEWBORN INTRAVASCULAR DISSEMINATED
790.92 STUDY ABNORMAL
790.92 TIME PROLONGED

COAGULATION DEFECT
286.9 NOS
0 ABORTION (IN) SEE 'ABORTION', BY TYPE WITH HEMORRHAGE
286.7 ACQUIRED (ANY)
641.3# ANTEPARTUM OR INTRAPARTUM
5th Digit: 641.3
0. EPISODE OF CARE NOS OR N/A
1. DELIVERED
3. ANTEPARTUM

762.1 ANTEPARTUM OR INTRAPARTUM AFFECTING FETUS OR NEWBORN
286.7 DUE TO LIVER DISEASE
286.7 DUE TO VITAMIN K DEFICIENCY
286.7 HYPOPROTHROMBINEMIA ACQUIRED
776.3 NEONATAL OTHER TRANSIENT
666.3# POSTPARTUM
5th Digit: 666.3
0. NOS
2. DELIVERED WITH POSTPARTUM COMPLICATION
4. POSTPARTUM COMPLICATION

286.6 COAGULOPATHY CONSUMPTION
500 COAL WORKERS' PNEUMOCONIOSIS
747.11 COARCTATION AORTA CONGENTAL
747.3 COARCTATION PULMONARY ARTERY CONGENITAL
362.12 COATS' SYNDROME
790.6 COBALT ABNORMAL BLOOD LEVEL

305.6# COCAINE ABUSE (NONDEPENDENT)
304.2# COCAINE ADDICTION (DEPENDENT)

5th Digit: 304.2, 305.6
- **0. NOS**
- **1. CONTINUOUS**
- **2. EPISODIC**
- **3. IN REMISSION**

760.75 COCAINE AFFECTING FETUS OR NEWBORN - ASYMPTOMATIC
779.5 COCAINE AFFECTING FETUS OR NEWBORN - WITH WITHDRAWAL SYMPTOMS
0 COCCIDIOIDAL DISEASE SEE 'COCCIDIOIDOMYCOSIS'

COCCIDIOIDOMYCOSIS
114.9 NOS
114.1 CUTANEOUS PRIMARY
114.3 DISSEMINATED
114.1 EXTRAPULMONARY PRIMARY
114.3 GRANULOMA
114.4 GRANULOMA LUNG
114.2 MENINGES
114.2 MENINGITIS
114.0 PNEUMONIAL
114.3 PROSTATE
114.3 OTHER FORMS PROGRESSIVE
114.5 PULMONARY
114.0 PULMONARY ACUTE PRIMARY
114.4 PULMONARY CHRONIC SECONDARY
114.4 PULMONARY RESIDUAL
114.3 SPECIFIED SITE NEC

0 COCCIDIOIDOSIS SEE 'COCCIDIOIDOMYCOSIS'
007.2 COCCIDIOSIS INTESTINAL
041.89 COCCUS INFECTION OR ORGANISM
724.79 COCCYGODYNIA

COCCYX, COCCYGEAL
724.70 DISORDER
724.71 HYPERMOBILITY
959.1 INJURY NOS
665.6# INJURY OBSTETRICAL

5th Digit: 665.6
- **0. EPISODE OF CARE NOS OR N/A**
- **1. DELIVERED**
- **4. POSTPARTUM COMPLICATION**

724.79 PAIN
724.79 SPECIFIED DISORDER NEC
847.4 SEPARATION (RUPTURE) (TEAR) (LACERATION)
847.4 STRAIN (SPRAIN) (AVULSION) (HEMARTHROSIS)

085.1 COCHIN-CHINA ULCER
759.89 COCKAYNE'S SYNDROME (MICROENCEPHALY AND DWARFISM)
757.39 COCKAYNE-WEBER SYNDROME (EPIDERMOLYSIS BULLOSA)
V14.5 CODEINE ALLERGY HISTORY
495.8 COFFEE WORKERS' LUNG
370.52 COGAN'S SYNDROME (NONSYPHILITIC INTERSTITIAL KERATITIS)
294.9 COGNITIVE DISORDER
438.0 COGNITIVE DISORDER LATE EFFECT OF CEREBROVASCULAR DISEASE
793.1 COIN LESION (LUNG)

COLD
460 NOS
283.0 AGGLUTININ DISEASE OR HEMOGLOBINURIA
283.2 AGGLUTININ HEMOGLOBINURIA PAROXYSMAL
477.9 ALLERGIC (SEE ALSO 'RHINITIS', ALLERGIC)
460 COMMON
460 COMMON DUE TO RSV (RESPIRATORY SYNCYTIAL VIRUS) [079.6]
487.1 GRIPPY

COLD (continued)
460 HEAD COMMON
283.0 HEMAGGLUTININ DISEASE CHRONIC
487.1 INFLUENZAL
991.9 INJURY EFFECT OF REDUCED TEMPERATURE
909.4 INJURY EFFECT OF REDUCED TEMPERATURE - LATE EFFECT
991.8 INJURY EFFECT OF REDUCED TEMPERATURE - OTHER SPECIFIED
778.2 INJURY SYNDROME OF NEWBORN
780.9 INTOLERANCE
782.0 SENSE ABSENCE
283.0 TYPE HEMOLYTIC ANEMIA (SECONDARY) (SYMPTOMATIC)
V04.7 VACCINATION

COLIC
789.0# NOS
789.0# ABDOMINAL
789.0# INFANTILE

5th Digit: 789.0
- **0. UNSPECIFIED SITE**
- **1. UPPER RIGHT QUADRANT**
- **2. UPPER LEFT QUADRANT**
- **3. LOWER RIGHT QUADRANT**
- **4. LOWER LEFT QUADRANT**
- **5. PERIUMBILIC**
- **6. EPIGASTRIC**
- **7. GENERALIZED**
- **9. OTHER SPECIFIED SITE (MULTIPLE)**

788.0 KIDNEY UNKNOWN ETIOLOGY
788.0 RENAL
788.0 URETER
599.84 URETHRAL

902.26 COLICA DEXTRA INJURY

COLITIS
558.9 UNSPECIFIED
558.9 ACUTE
558.9 ALLERGIC
006.2 AMEBIC NONDYSENTERIC
022.2 ANTHRAX
007.0 BALANTIDIAL
558.9 CHRONIC
007.2 COCCIDIAL
007.4 CRYPTOSPORIDIAL
558.9 DIETARY
V65.3 DIETARY COUNSELING AND SURVEILLANCE
558.1 DUE TO RADIATION
557.0 FULMINANT
558.9 FUNCTIONAL
009.0 GANGRENOUS
555.1 GRANULOMATOUS
0 INFECTIOUS SEE 'ENTERITIS' BY SPECIFIED ORGANISM
009.0 INFECTIOUS (SEPTIC)
009.1 INFECTIOUS ORIGIN PRESUMED
564.1 IRRITABLE
306.4 IRRITABLE BOWEL PSYCHOGENIC
564.1 IRRITABLE BOWEL SYNDROME
557.9 ISCHEMIC - NOS
557.0 ISCHEMIC - ACUTE
557.1 ISCHEMIC - CHRONIC
557.1 ISCHEMIC - DUE TO MESENTERIC ARTERY INSUFFICIENCY
564.1 MEMBRANOUS (MUCOUS) (ADAPTIVE) (SPASTIC)
316 MEMBRANOUS (MUCOUS) (SPASTIC) PSYCHOGENIC [564.1]
009.0 NECROTIC
006.2 NONDYSENTERIC AMEBIC
558.9 NONINFECTIOUS

C

COLITIS (continued)

007.8	PROTOZOAL OTHER SPECIFIED
007.9	PROTOZOAL UNSPECIFIED
008.45	PSEUDOMEMBRANOUS
306.4	PSYCHOGENIC
555.1	REGIONAL
555.1	SEGMENTAL
009.0	SEPTIC (SEE ALSO 'ENTERITIS' BY SPECIFIC ORGANISM)
564.1	SPASTIC COLON
316	SPASTIC PSYCHOGENIC [564.1]
008.41	STAPHYLOCOCCUS
005.0	STAPHYLOCOCCUS DUE TO FOOD
557.0	THROMBOULCERATIVE
558.2	TOXIC
555.1	TRANSMURAL
014.8#	TUBERCULOSIS (ULCERATIVE)

5th Digit: 014.8
- **0. NOS**
- **1. LAB NOT DONE**
- **2. LABS PENDING**
- **3. MICROSCOPY POSITIVE (IN SPUTUM)**
- **4. CULTURE POSITIVE - MICROSCOPY NEGATIVE**
- **5. CULTURE NEGATIVE - MICROSCOPY POSITIVE**
- **6. CULTURE AND MICROSCOPY NEGATIVE CONFIRMED BY OTHER METHODS**

556.# ULCERATIVE

4th Digit: 556
- **0. ENTEROCOLITIS (CHRONIC)**
- **1. ILEOCOLITIS (CHRONIC)**
- **2. PROCTITIS (CHRONIC)**
- **3. PROCTOSIGMOIDITIS (CHRONIC)**
- **4. PSEUDOPOLYPOSIS OF COLON**
- **5. LEFT-SIDED (CHRONIC)**
- **6. UNIVERSAL (CHRONIC)**
- **8. OTHER ULCERATIVE COLITIS**
- **9. ULCERATIVE COLITIS (ENTERITIS) UNSPECIFIED**

COLLAGEN

710.9	DISEASE
446.20	DISEASE VASCULAR
446.21	DISEASE VASCULAR - GOODPASTURE'S

> *648.9#: USE AN ADDITIONAL CODE TO IDENTIFY THE SPECIFIC COLLAGEN DISEASE.*

648.9# DISEASE VASCULAR - MATERNAL CURRENT (CO-EXISTENT) IN PREGNANCY

5th Digit: 648.9
- **0. EPISODE OF NOS OR N/A**
- **1. DELIVERED**
- **2. DELIVERED WITH POSTPARTUM COMPLICATION**
- **3. ANTEPARTUM COMPLICATION**
- **4. POSTPARTUM COMPLICATION**

446.29	DISEASE VASCULAR - SPECIFIED NEC
V50.1	INJECTION, COSMETIC

425.4	COLLAGENOSIS CARDIOVASCULAR
780.2	COLLAPSE
459.89	COLLATERAL CIRCULATION (VENOUS) ANY SITE
0	COLLATERAL LIGAMENT RUPTURE SEE 'SPRAIN'
352.6	COLLET SICARD SYNDROME
701.3	COLLOID ATROPHY DEGENERATIVE
709.3	COLLOID MILIUM

COLOBOMA

743.59	CHOROID CONGENITAL
743.52	FUNDUS CONGENITAL
743.46	IRIS CONGENITAL
743.36	LENS CONGENITAL
743.62	LIDS CONGENITAL
377.23	OPTIC (DISC)
743.56	RETINA CONGENITAL
773.47	SCLERA CONGENITAL

> *INJURY TO INTERNAL ORGANS - LUNG, SPLEEN, LIVER, KIDNEY, ETC. - CAN BE A CONTUSION, LACERATION, TEAR, OR RUPTURE. USE THE "INJURY" CODE FOUND UNDER THE ANATOMICAL SITE.*

COLON

751.2	ABSENCE CONGENITAL
V45.72	ABSENCE POSTSURGICAL
751.3	AGANGLIONOSIS CONGENITAL
564.89	ATONY FUNCTIONAL
751.2	ATRESIA CONGENITAL
564.7	DILATATION
751.3	DILATATION CONGENITAL
560.89	DILATATION MECHANICAL OBSTRUCTION
306.4	DILATATION PSYCHOGENIC
569.9	DISORDER
751.3	DISORDER CONGENITAL
564.9	DISORDER FUNCTIONAL
751.3	DISORDER FUNCTIONAL CONGENITAL
564.81	DISORDER FUNCTIONAL NEUROGENIC
564.89	DISORDER FUNCTIONAL OTHER SPECIFIED
306.4	DISORDER PSYCHOGENIC
562.10	DIVERTICULUM
751.5	DIVERTICULUM CONGENITAL
863.4#	INJURY
863.5#	INJURY WITH OPEN WOUND

5th Digit: 863.4-5
- **0. COLON UNSPECIFIED SITE**
- **1. ASCENDING [RIGHT] COLON**
- **2. TRANSVERSE COLON**
- **3. DESCENDING [LEFT] COLON**
- **4. SIGMOID COLON**
- **5. RECTUM**
- **6. MULTIPLE SITES IN COLON AND RECTUM**
- **9. OTHER**

908.1	INJURY LATE EFFECT
560.0	INVAGINATION
564.1	IRRITABLE (SPASTIC)
557.#	ISCHEMIA

4th Digit: 557
- **0. ACUTE**
- **1. CHRONIC**
- **9. UNSPECIFIED TRANSIENT**

569.89	LESION
751.4	MALROTATION CONGENITAL
560.9	OBSTRUCTION (OCCLUSION) DUE TO STENOSIS OR STRICTURE
560.89	OBSTRUCTION SYMPATHICOTONIC
211.3	POLYP ADENOMATOUS
569.89	POLYP NONADENOMATOUS
V12.72	POLYP HISTORY
211.4	POLYP RECTOSIGMOID JUNCTION, ADENOMATOUS
556.4	PSEUDOPOLYPOSIS
564.1	SPASTIC
564.89	STASIS
751.5	TRANSPOSITION CONGENITAL
560.2	VOLVULUS (TORSION) (STRANGULATION)

COLOR BLINDNESS

368.54	ACHROMATOPSIA (TOTAL)
368.55	ACQUIRED
368.52	DEUTAN DEFECT (GREEN)
368.54	MONOCHROMATIC (CONE) (ROD)
368.51	PROTAN DEFECT (RED)
368.53	TRITAN DEFECT (BLUE)
368.59	OTHER

COLOSTOMY

V53.5 BELT FITTING AND ADJUSTMENT
V55.3 CARE
V55.3 CATHETER ADJUSTMENT OR REPOSITIONING
V55.3 CATHETER REMOVAL OR REPLACEMENT
V55.3 CLOSURE
569.60 COMPLICATION - NOS
569.62 COMPLICATION - MECHANICAL
569.69 COMPLICATION - OTHER
569.69 FISTULA
569.69 HERNIA

WHEN CODING AN INFECTION OF AN OSTOMY, USE AN ADDITIONAL CODE TO SPECIFY THE ORGANISM. SEE 'BACTERIAL INFECTION'

569.61 INFECTION
<u>569.61</u> <u>INFECTION</u> WITH CELLULITIS OF ABDOMEN [682.2]
<u>569.61</u> <u>INFECTION</u> WITH SEPSIS [**038.#(#)**]

4th or 4th <u>and</u> 5th Digit Code for Organism: 038

.9 NOS
.3 ANAEROBIC
.3 BACTEROIDES
.3 CLOSTRIDIUM
.42 E COLI
.49 ENTEROBACTER AEROGENES
.40 GRAM NEGATIVE
.49 GRAM NEGATIVE OTHER
.41 HEMOPHILUS INFLUENZAE
.2 PNEUMOCOCCAL
.49 PROTEUS
.43 PSEUDOMONAS
.44 SERRATIA
.10 STAPHYLOCOCCAL NOS
.11 STAPHYLOCOCCAL AUREUS
.19 STAPHYLOCOCCAL OTHER
.0 STREPTOCOCCAL (ANAEROBIC)
.49 YERSINIA ENTEROCOLITICA
.8 OTHER SPECIFIED

569.62 MALFUNCTION
569.69 PROLAPSE
V44.3 STATUS
V55.3 TOILET STOMA

625.1 COLPOSPASM

COMA

780.01 COMA
250.2# DIABETIC HYPEROSMOLAR NON KETOTIC
250.3# DIABETIC HYPOGLYCEMIC
250.3# DIABETIC INSULIN
250.3# DIABETIC KETOACIDOTIC

5th Digit: 250.2-3

0. TYPE II, ADULT-ONSET, NON-INSULIN DEPENDENT (EVEN IF REQUIRING INSULIN), OR UNSPECIFIED; CONTROLLED
1. TYPE I, JUVENILE-ONSET OR INSULIN-DEPENDENT; CONTROLLED
2. TYPE II, ADULT-ONSET, NON-INSULIN DEPENDENT (EVEN IF REQUIRING INSULIN); UNCONTROLLED
3. TYPE I, JUVENILE-ONSET OR INSULIN-DEPENDENT; UNCONTROLLED

COMA (continued)

0 DUE TO HEPATITIS SEE 'HEPATITIS'
780.39 ECLAMPTIC
572.2 HEPATIC (CHRONIC LIVER DISEASE)
251.0 HYPERINSULINISM ORGANIC
251.0 HYPOGLYCEMIC NON-DIABETIC
251.0 HYPOGLYCEMIC NON-DIABETIC, IATROGENIC
251.0 INSULIN NON-DIABETIC
779.2 NEONATAL
780.09 OTHER ALTERATION OF CONSCIOUSNESS
780.02 TRANSIENT ALTERATION OF AWARENESS
0 UREMIC SEE 'UREMIA'
780.03 VEGETATIVE STATE PERSISTENT
0 SEE ALSO 'ALTERATION OF CONSCIOUSNESS'

0 COMATOSE SEE 'COMA'
0 COMBAT FATIGUE SEE 'STRESS REACTION'
279.2 COMBINED IMMUNITY DEFICIENCY SYNDROME
706.1 COMEDO

COMEDOCARCINOMA

174.9 SITE NOS
0 SITE SPECIFIED SEE 'CANCER' BY SITE M8501/3
174.# BREAST SOFT TISSUE

4th Digit: 174

0. NIPPLE AND AREOLA
1. CENTRAL PORTION
2. UPPER INNER QUADRANT
3. LOWER INNER QUADRANT
4. UPPER OUTER QUADRANT
5. LOWER OUTER QUADRANT
6. AXILLARY TAIL
8. MASTECTOMY SITE, INNER LOWER MIDLINE OUTER UPPER ECTOPIC SITES CONTIGUOUS OVERLAPPIING SITES UNDETERMINED
9. BREAST (FEMALE) SITE NOS

0 NONINFILTRATING SITE SPECIFIED SEE 'CA IN SITU' BY SITE M8501/2
233.2 NONINFILTRATING SITE NOS

610.4 COMEDOMASTITIS

745.69 COMMON ATRIUM CONGENITAL
868.02 COMMON DUCT INJURY (TRAUMATIC)
868.12 COMMON DUCT INJURY (TRAUMATIC) WITH OPEN WOUND
0 COMMON DUCT OBSTRUCTION SEE 'BILE DUCT', OBSTRUCTION
0 COMMON DUCT STONE SEE 'CHOLEDOCHOLITHIASIS'
V01.9 COMMUNICABLE DISEASES EXPOSURE UNSPECIFIED
V01.8 COMMUNICABLE DISEASES EXPOSURE OTHER
433.8# COMMUNICATING POSTERIOR ARTERY OCCLUSION

5th Digit: 433.8

0. WITHOUT CEREBRAL INFARCTION
1. WITH CEREBRAL INFARCTION

V40.1 COMMUNICATION PROBLEM
0 COMMOTIO CEREBRI SEE 'CONCUSSION'
958.8 COMPARTMENT SYNDROME (ANTERIOR) (DEEP) (POSTERIOR) (TIBIAL)
908.6 COMPARTMENT SYNDROME (ANTERIOR) (DEEP) (POSTERIOR) (TIBIAL) LATE EFFECT
V65.5 COMPLAINT UNFOUNDED (FEARED CONDITION)
279.8 COMPLEMENT C1-C9 DEFICIENCY

COMPLICATION OF A DEVICE, IMPLANT OR GRAFT - MECHANICAL

A MECHANICAL COMPLICATION MAY BE A BREAK DOWN (MECHANICAL) DISPLACEMENT, LEAKAGE, OBSTRUCTION, PERFORATION, OR PROTUSION OF AN IMPLANTED DEVICE.

996.0# CARDIAC

5th Digit: 996.0

0. UNSPECIFIED DEVICE, IMPLANT OR GRAFT
1. CARDIAC PACEMAKER (ELECTRODE)
2. HEART VALVE PROSTHESIS
3. CORONARY BYPASS GRAFT
AORTOCORONARY GRAFT
ARTERIAL OCCLUSION
4. CARDIAC DEFIBRILLATOR (AUTOMATIC IMPLANTABLE)
9. OTHER
CARDIAC CATHETER

996.2 CENTRAL NERVOUS SYSTEM
BRAIN ELECTRODE
DORSAL COLUMN STIMULATOR
INTRATHECAL INFUSION PUMP
PACEMAKER BRAIN
PACEMAKER PHRENIC NERVE
PERIPHERAL NERVE
SPINAL COLUMN ELECTRODE
VENTRICULAR SHUNT

996.3# GENITOURINARY

5th Digit: 996.3

0. UNSPECIFIED DEVICE, IMPLANT OR GRAFT
1. DUE TO URETHRAL (INDWELLING CATHETER)
2. DUE TO INTRAUTERINE CONTRACEPTIVE DEVICE
IUD
9. OTHER
CATHETER CYSTOSTOMY
GRAFT NEC
PENILE PROSTHESIS
URETERAL REPAIR (GRAFT)
VAS DEFERENS PROSTHESIS / RECONSTRUCTION

996.4 ORTHOPEDIC INTERNAL
BONE GRAFT
CARTILAGE GRAFT
EXTERNAL FIXATION WITH INTERNAL COMPONENTS
MUSCLE GRAFT
NAIL, ROD OR PLATE
TENDON GRAFT

C

COMPLICATION OF A DEVICE, IMPLANT OR GRAFT - MECHANICAL (continued)

0 OSTOMY SEE SPECIFIC OSTOMY

996.1 VASCULAR
A-V FISTULA OR SHUNT
AORTIC (BIFURCATION) GRAFT (REPLACEMENT)
ARTERIAL GRAFT
BLOOD VESSEL GRAFT
CAROTID ARTERY BYPASS
CENTRAL LINE
ARTERIOVENOUS DIALYSIS CATHETER
FEMORAL POPLITEAL BYPASS GRAFT
INFUSION PUMP
INTRAAORTIC BALLOON
UMBRELLA VENA CAVA

996.5# OTHER SPECIFIED

5th Digit: 996.5

1. DUE TO CORNEAL GRAFT (REJECTION/ REACTION)
2. DUE TO GRAFT OF OTHER TISSUE NOT ELSEWHERE CLASSIFIED
GRAFT NEC
SKIN GRAFT FAILURE OR REJECTION
TISSUE NEC
3. DUE TO OCULAR LENS PROSTHESIS
4. DUE TO BREAST PROSTHESIS
BREAST CAPSULE
MAMMARY IMPLANT
5. DUE TO ARTIFICIAL SKIN GRAFT AND DECELLULARIZED ALLODERMIS
6. DUE TO PERITONEAL DIALYSIS CATHETER
9. DUE TO OTHER IMPLANT (INTERNAL DEVICE) NOT ELSEWHERE CLASSIFIED
BILE DUCT PROSTHESIS
CATHETER NEC
CHIN PROSTHESIS
CONTRACEPTIVE DEVICE SUBDERMAL
ELECTRODE IMPLANT NEC
EYE (GLOBE) PROSTHESIS
GASTROINTESTINAL DEVICE
IMPLANT NEC
MECHANICAL DEVICE NEC
NON-ABSORBABLE SURGICAL MATERIAL
ORBITAL GLOBE IMPLANT
PACEMAKER NEC
PE TUBE
PROSTHETIC DEVICE NEC
REIMPLANTATION NEC
RESPIRATORY
SHUNT NEC
STENT NEC
TOOTH IMPLANT
TYMPANOSTOMY TUBE

DO NOT ASSUME THAT A CONDITION IS A POST-OP COMPLICATION. IT MUST BE PERFECTLY CLEAR THAT THE CONDITION DEVELOPED DIRECTLY AS A RESULT OF SURGERY OR MEDICAL CARE. THE DOCTOR MUST DOCUMENT IN THE RECORD THAT THE CONDITION WAS DUE TO A PROCEDURE.

COMPLICATION OF AN INTERNAL PROSTHESIS IMPLANT OR GRAFT - INFECTION OR INFLAMMATION

996.60 UNSPECIFIED INTERNAL PROSTHESIS IMPLANT OR GRAFT
996.61 CARDIAC
ARTERIAL
CORONARY ARTERY BYPASS GRAFT
DEFIBRILLATOR
ELECTRODE
HEART VALVE PROSTHESIS
PACEMAKER
PULSE GENERATOR
SUBCUTANEOUS POCKET
996.65 GENITOURINARY OTHER
IUD
PENILE PROSTHESIS
VAS DEFERENS PROSTHESIS
996.66 JOINT PROSTHESIS INTERNAL
996.63 NERVOUS SYSTEM
SPINAL CATHETER
CATHETER VENTRICULAR SHUNT
BRAIN ELECTRODE
PERIPHERAL NERVE GRAFT
VENTRICULAR SHUNT
996.67 ORTHOPEDIC OTHER INTERNAL
BONE GROWTH STIMULATOR
EXTERNAL FIXATION WITH INTERNAL COMPONENTS
ORTHOPEDIC NEC
NAIL, PINS, RODS, PLATE OR SCREWS
0 OSTOMY SEE SPECIFIC OSTOMY
996.68 PERITONEAL DIALYSIS CATHETER-EXIT SITE
996.64 URINARY CATHETER (INDWELLING)
URETHRAL CATHETER
996.62 VASCULAR
A-V FISTULA OR SHUNT
ARTERIAL NEC
ARTERIAL RENAL DIALYSIS
CAROTID ARTERY GRAFT
CATHETER VASCULAR NEC
CENTRAL LINE
ARTERIOVENOUS DIALYSIS CATHETER
INFUSION PUMP
INTRAAORTIC BALLOON
996.69 OTHER INTERNAL PROSTHESIS
BILE DUCT IMPLANT
BREAST IMPLANT
CATHETER NEC
CHIN IMPLANT
CONTRACEPTIVE DEVICE SUBDERMAL
CORNEAL IMPLANT NEC
EYE (ORBIT) IMPLANT
GASTROINTESTINAL NEC
OCULAR LENS IMPLANT
PE TUBE
RESPIRATORY
SKIN GRAFT
TOOTH IMPLANT
TYMPANOSTOMY TUBE

NON-MECHANCIAL COMPLICATIONS ARE ABNORMAL BODY REACTIONS DUE TO THE PRESENCE OF A PROPERLY FUNCTIONING DEVICE, IMPLANT OR GRAFT AND INCLUDE: EMBOLISM, FIBROSIS, INFECTION, INFLAMMATION, HEMORRHAGE, PAIN, STENOSIS, REJECTION, THROMBOSIS, OTHER.

COMPLICATION OF AN INTERNAL PROSTHETIC DEVICE, IMPLANT OR GRAFT - OTHER SPECIFIED (EMBOLUS) (FIBROSIS) (HEMORRHAGE) (PAIN) (STENOSIS) (THROMBUS)

996.70 UNSPECIFIED INTERNAL PROSTHESIS IMPLANT OR GRAFT, OTHER SPECIFIED COMPLICATION
996.72 CARDIAC
CORONARY ARTERY BYPASS GRAFT
DEFIBRILLATOR
ELECTRODES
PACEMAKER
PACEMAKER SUBCUTANEOUS POCKET
996.76 GENITOURINARY
IUD
PENILE PROSTHESIS
URETHRAL CATHETER
URINARY INDWELLING CATHETER
VAS DEFERENS PROSTHESIS
996.71 HEART VALVE PROSTHESIS
996.75 NERVOUS SYSTEM
BRAIN ELECTRODES
SPINAL CATHETER
VENTRICULAR SHUNT
996.77 ORTHOPEDIC JOINT PROSTHESIS INTERNAL
996.78 ORTHOPEDIC OTHER
BONE GROWTH STIMULATOR
EXTERNAL FIXATION WITH INTERNAL COMPONENTS
NAIL, ROD OR PLATE (INTERNAL)
0 OSTOMY SEE SPECIFIC OSTOMY
996.73 RENAL DIALYSIS
DIALYSIS CATHETER
VASCULAR CATHETER NEC
996.74 VASCULAR
ARTERIAL
A-V FISTULA OR SHUNT
BLOOD VESSEL GRAFT
CAROTID ARTERY GRAFT
CATHETER NEC
CENTRAL LINE
INFUSION PUMP
INTRAAORTIC BALLOON
996.79 OTHER
BILE DUCT IMPLANT
BREAST IMPLANT
CATHETER NEC
CATHETER PERITONEAL DIALYSIS
CHIN IMPLANT
CONTRACEPTIVE DEVICE SUBDERMAL
CORNEAL GRAFT
EYE PROSTHESIS IMPLANT
GASTROINTESTINAL NEC
OCULAR LENS
ORBITAL
PE TUBE
RESPIRATORY
SKIN GRAFT NEC
TOOTH IMPLANT
TYMPANOSTOMY TUBE

WHEN CODING A COMPLICATION OF AN ORGAN TRANSPLANT, USE AN ADDITIONAL CODE TO IDENTIFY THE NATURE OF THE COMPLICATION, SUCH AS CMV INFECTION [078.5]

COMPLICATION ORGAN TRANSPLANT

996.80 ORGAN UNSPECIFIED
996.85 BONE MARROW
996.83 HEART
996.89 INTESTINES
996.81 KIDNEY
996.82 LIVER
996.84 LUNG
996.86 PANCREAS
996.89 ORGAN OTHER SPECIFIED

COMPLICATION REATTACHED EXTREMITY OR BODY PART - INFECTION OR REJECTION

996.90 UNSPECIFIED REATTACHED EXTREMITY OR BODY PART EXTREMITY
996.93 FINGER (S)
996.95 FOOT AND TOE(S)
996.91 FOREARM
996.92 HAND
996.96 LOWER EXTREMITY OTHER AND UNSPECIFIED
996.94 UPPER EXTREMITY OTHER AND UNSPECIFIED
996.99 OTHER SPECIFIED BODY PART

DO NOT ASSUME THAT A CONDITION IS A POST-OP COMPLICATION. IT MUST BE PERFECTLY CLEAR THAT THE CONDITION DEVELOPED DIRECTLY AS A RESULT OF SURGERY OR MEDICAL CARE. THE DOCTOR MUST DOCUMENT IN THE RECORD THAT THE CONDITION WAS DUE TO A PROCEDURE.

COMPLICATIONS AFFECTING SPECIFIED BODY SYSTEMS NOT ELSEWHERE CLASSIFIED

997.6# AMPUTATION STUMP (LATE)
5th Digit: 997.6
0. UNSPECIFIED COMPLICATION
1. NEUROMA
2. INFECTION (CHRONIC)
9. OTHER

997.1 CARDIAC
CARDIAC ARREST / INSUFFICIENCY
CARDIORESPIRATORY FAILURE
HEART FAILURE

997.4 DIGESTIVE SYSTEM
ANASTOMOSIS INTESTINAL
HEPATIC FAILURE
INTESTINAL OBSTRUCTION
MESENTERIC ARTERY
POSTOPERATIVE NEC

997.0# NERVOUS SYSTEM
5th Digit: 997.0
0. NOS
1. CENTRAL NERVOUS SYSTEM
ANOXIC BRAIN DAMAGE
CEREBRAL HYPOXIA
2. CEREBROVASCULAR INFARCTION OR HEMORRHAGE
IATROGENIC STROKE
POSTOPERATIVE STROKE
9. OTHER

0 OSTOMY MALFUNCTION SEE SPECIFIC OSTOMY

997.2 PERIPHERAL VASCULAR
PHLEBITITS
POSTOPERATIVE NEC
THROMBOPHLEBITIS

997.3 RESPIRATORY
MENDELSON'S SYNDROME
PNEUMONIA (ASPIRATION)
POSTOPERATIVE NEC

997.5 URINARY
ANASTOMOSIS URINARY TRACT
ANURIA
CYSTOSTOMY MALFUNCTION
NEPHROSTOMY MALFUNCTION
OLIGURIA
POSTCYSTOSCOPIC
POSTOPERATIVE NEC
PYELOGRAM
RENAL ARTERY
RENAL FAILURE / INSUFFICIENCY
TUBULAR NECROSIS (ACUTE)
URETEROSTOMY MALFUNCTION
URETHROSTOMY MALFUNCTION

997.9# OTHER
5th Digit: 997.9
1. HYPERTENSION
9. OTHER
ELEPHANTIASIS OR LYMPHEDEMA
VITREOUS TOUCH SYNDROME
OTHER BODY SYSTEM NEC

C

WHEN CODING AN INFECTION, USE AN ADDITIONAL CODE, [041.#(#)], TO IDENTIFY THE ORGANISM. SEE 'BACTERIAL INFECTION'.

COMPLICATIONS OTHER OF PROCEDURES NOT ELSEWHERE CLASSIFIED

998.9 UNSPECIFIED COMPLICATION NOT ELSEWHERE CLASSIFIED
SURGICAL PROCEDURE
THERAPEUTIC MISADVENTURE OF SURGICAL TREATMENT

998.7 ACUTE REACTION TO FOREIGN SUBSTANCE ACCIDENTALLY LEFT DURING A PROCEDURE
TALC GRANULOMA

998.3 DISRUPTION OF OPERATION WOUND
BURST STITCHES / SUTURES
DISRUPTION OF INTERNAL SUTURE
WOUND DEHISCENCE

998.6 FISTULA PERSISTENT POSTOPERATIVE

998.4 FOREIGN BODY ACCIDENTALLY LEFT DURING A PROCEDURE

998.12 HEMATOMA

998.11 HEMORRHAGE

998.5# INFECTION POSTOPERATIVE
5th Digit: 998.5
1. SEROMA
9. OTHER

ABSCESS POSTOPERATIVE
SEPTICEMIA POSTOPERATIVE

998.2 LACERATION OR PUNCTURE ACCIDENTAL DURING A PROCEDURE
BY CATHETER OR OTHER INSTRUMENT DURING A PROCEDURE (BLOOD VESSEL) (NERVE) (ORGAN)

998.83 NON-HEALING SURGICAL WOUND

0 OSTOMY SEE SPECIFIC OSTOMY

998.13 SEROMA COMPLICATING PROCEDURE

998.51 SEROMA INFECTED POSTOPERATIVE

998.0 SHOCK POSTOPERATIVE
COLLAPSE NOS
SHOCK (ENDOTOXIC) (HYPOVOLEMIC)(SEPTIC)

998.83 SURGICAL WOUND NON-HEALING

998.8# OTHER SPECIFIED COMPLICATIONS OF PROCEDURES NOT ELSEWHERE CLASSIFIED
5th Digit: 998.8
1. EMPHYSEMA (SUBCUTANEOUS)
2. CATARACT FRAGMENTS
3. NON-HEALING SURGICAL WOUND
9. OTHER COMPLICATIONS OF PROCEDURE NEC

DO NOT ASSUME THAT A CONDITION IS A POST-OP COMPLICATION. IT MUST BE PERFECTLY CLEAR THAT THE CONDITION DEVELOPED DIRECTLY AS A RESULT OF SURGERY OR MEDICAL CARE. THE DOCTOR MUST DOCUMENT IN THE RECORD THAT THE CONDITION WAS DUE TO A PROCEDURE.

COMPLICATIONS OF MEDICAL CARE NOT ELSEWHERE CLASSIFIED

999.9 OTHER AND UNSPECIFIED COMPLICATIONS OF MEDICAL CARE NOT ELSEWHERE CLASSIFIED
UNSPECIFIED MISADVENTURE
DIALYSIS NEC
DURING DIALYSIS
ELECTROSHOCK THERAPY
EXTRACORPOREAL CIRCULATION
HYPERALIMENTATION THERAPY
INFUSION / PERFUSION PROCEDURE NEC
INHALATION THERAPY
INJECTION PROCEDURE
THERAPEUTIC MISADVENTURE
THERAPY NEC
ULTRASOUND THERAPY
VACCINATION NEC
VENTILATION THERAPY

999.6 ABO INCOMPATIBILITY IN INFUSION PERFUSION OR TRANSFUSION

999.1 AIR EMBOLISM
TO ANY SITE FOLLOWING INFUSION PERFUSION OR TRANSFUSION

999.4 ANAPHYLACTIC SHOCK DUE TO SERUM
ALLERGIC ANAPHYLACTIC SHOCK
VACCINATION ANAPHYLAXIS

999.0 GENERAL VACCINIA

999.7 RH INCOMPATIBILITY REACTION IN INFUSION PERFUSION OR TRANSFUSION

999.2 OTHER VASCULAR COMPLICATIONS FOLLOWING INFUSION, PERFUSION, OR TRANSFUSION
EMBOLISM / THROMBUS
PHLEBITIS THROMBOPHLEBITIS

999.3 OTHER INFECTION FOLLOWING INFUSION, INJECTION, TRANSFUSION, OR VACCINATION
GENERAL LOCALIZED INFECTION
INFECTION NEC
INFUSION INFECTION / SEPSIS
SEPSIS NEC
SEPTICEMIA
VACCINATION CELLULITIS
VACCINIA LOCALIZED

999.5 OTHER SERUM REACTION
ALLERGIC REACTION
PROTEIN SICKNESS
SERUM SICKNESS / RASH / INTOXICATION
URTICARIA DUE TO SERUM

999.8 OTHER TRANSFUSION REACTION
BLOOD (LYMPHOCYTES) (PLASMA)
SHOCK OR REACTION
TRANSFUSION REACTION NOS

0 COMPLICATION OF LABOR AND DELIVERY SEE SPECIFIED COMPLICATION, OR 'LABOR AND DELIVERY COMPLICATIONS'

909.3 COMPLICATION OF SURGICAL AND MEDICAL CARE LATE EFFECT

COMPOUND PRESENTATION

652.8# NOS
660.0# NOS OBSTRUCTING LABOR [652.8#]
652.6# WITH MULTIPLE GESTATION
660.0# WITH MULTIPLE GESTATION OBSTRUCTING LABOR [652.6#]

5th Digit: 652.6, 8, 660.0
0. EPISODE OF CARE UNSPECIFIED OR N/A
1. DELIVERED
3. ANTEPARTUM COMPLICATION

993.3 COMPRESSED AIR DISEASE
344.60 COMPRESSION CAUDA EQUINA SYNDROME
344.61 COMPRESSION CAUDA EQUINA SYNDROME WITH NEUROGENIC BLADDER
0 COMPRESSION NERVE SEE SPECIFIC NERVE, DISORDER
724.9 COMPRESSION OF SPINAL NERVE ROOT NEC (NONVERTEBRAL) (NONDISCOGENIC)
958.5 COMPRESSION SYNDROME
301.4 COMPULSIVE PERSONALITY
423.2 CONCATO'S PERICARDIAL POLYSEROSITIS
568.82 CONCATO'S DISEASE PERITONEAL
309.81 CONCENTRATION CAMP SYNDROME
368.12 CONCENTRIC FADING
560.39 CONCRETION INTESTINE

*CEREBRAL CONCUSSION RESULTS FROM A BLOW TO THE HEAD, AND SHOULD BE CODED AS A TRAUMA. CODE IT AS A TRAUMA UNTIL THE PHYSICIAN STATES THAT THE ACTIVE PHASE OF THE CONCUSSION HAS SUBSIDED AND THE SYMPTOMS ARE NO LONGER ORGANIC IN NATURE. AS LONG AS THE DOCUMENTATION STATES THAT THE PATIENT'S SYMPTOMS ARE DIRECTLY RESULTANT FROM A CONCUSSION, **USE A TRAUMA CODE.***

CONCUSSION

850.9 NOS
0 INJURY INTERNAL ORGANS (EXCEPT CEREBRAL) SEE SPECIFIC ORGAN, INJURY
850.0 NO LOSS OF CONSCIOUSNESS
850.1 LOC < 1 HOUR
850.2 LOC 1-24 HOURS
850.3 LOC >24 HOURS WITH COMPLETE RECOVERY
850.4 LOC >24 HOURS WITHOUT RETURN TO PRE-EXISTING CONSCIOUS LEVEL
850.5 LOC UNSPECIFIED DURATION
V71.8 OBSERVATION FOR SUSPECTED
310.2 SYNDROME

117.7 CONDIOBOLUS INFECTION
799.8 CONDITIONS OTHER ILL-DEFINED

CONDUCT DISORDER

312.9 NOS
312.82 NOS ADOLESCENT ONSET
312.81 NOS CHILDHOOD ONSET
309.3 ADJUSTMENT REACTION
312.0# AGGRESSIVE

5th Digit: 312.0
0. NOS
1. MILD
2. MODERATE
3. SEVERE

312.23 AGGRESSIVE SOCIALIZED
312.4 DELINQUENCY NEUROTIC

CONDUCT DISORDER (continued)

312.3# EXPLOSIVE DISORDER

5th Digit: 312.3
4. INTERMITTENT IMPULSE CONTROL
5. ISOLATED IMPULSE CONTROL

312.31 GAMBLING PATHOLOGICAL
312.30 IMPULSE CONTROL DISORDER
312.39 IMPULSE CONTROL DISORDER OTHER SPECIFIED
312.9 JUVENILE DELINQUENCY
312.32 KLEPTOMANIA
312.4 MIXED WITH EMOTION DISTURBANCE
312.33 PYROMANIA
312.2# SOCIALIZED
312.1# UNAGGRESSIVE

5th Digit: 312.1-2
0. NOS
1. MILD
2. MODERATE
3. SEVERE

312.21 UNAGGRESSIVE SOCIALIZED
312.8# OTHER SPECIFIED NEC

5th Digit: 312.8
1. CHILDHOOD ONSET
2. ADOLESCENT ONSET
9. OTHER SPECIFIED

426.9 CONDUCTION DELAY (CARDIAC) (VENTRICULAR)

CONDYLOMA

078.10 NOS
078.11 ACUMINATUM
098.0 GONORRHEAL
091.3 LATUM
091.3 SYPHILITIC (VENEREAL) (LATUM)
090.0 SYPHILITIC CONGENITAL

701.8 CONFLUENT AND RETICULATE PAPILLOMATOSIS

CONFUSION

298.9 NOS
293.0 ACUTE
290.3 ACUTE WITH SENILE DEMENTIA
291.0 ALCOHOLIC
292.81 DRUG-INDUCED
298.2 PSYCHOGENIC
298.2 REACTIVE
293.0 STATE (ACUTE)

CONGENITAL

286.3 AFIBRINOGENEMIA
776.5 ANEMIA DUE TO BLOOD LOSS
V19.5 ANOMALIES FAMILY HISTORY
759.9 ANOMALY
759.7 ANOMALY MULTIPLE NOS
759.89 ANOMALY OTHER SPECIFIED
779.9 DEBILITY
759.7 DEFORMITY MULTIPLE NOS
717.5 DISCOID MENISCUS (KNEE)
757.31 ECTODERMAL DYSPLASIA
352.6 FACIAL DIPLEGIA SYNDROME
282.0 HEMOLYTIC ANEMIA SPHEROCYTIC
243 HYPOTHYROIDISM
757.0 LYMPHEDEMA
759.89 MUSCULAR HYPERTROPHY-CEREBRAL SYNDROME
751.62 POLYCYSTIC DISEASE LIVER
759.7 SYNDROME AFFECTING MORE THAN ONE SYSTEM
759.89 SYNDROME AFFECTING MORE THAN ONE SYSTEM , SPECIFIED TYPE NEC

CONGENITAL CONDITIONS COMPLICATING PREGNANCY

WHEN CODING A MATERNAL CARDIOVASCULAR DISEASE COMPLICATING PREGNANCY, 648.5#, USE AN ADDITIONAL CODE TO IDENTIFY THE CONDITION.

648.5# CARDIOVASCULAR DISORDER MATERNAL
648.5# HEART DISEASE MATERNAL
654.0# UTERINE ABNORMALITY COMPLICATING PREGNANCY
660.2# UTERINE ABNORMALITY COMPLICATING PREGNANCY OBSTRUCTING LABOR [**654.0#**]

5th Digit: 648.5, 654.0
0. EPISODE OF CARE NOS OR N/A
1. DELIVERED
2. DELIVERED WITH POSTPARTUM COMPLICATION
3. ANTEPARTUM COMPLICATION
4. POSTPARTUM COMPLICATION

5th Digit: 660.2
0. EPISODE OF CARE NOS OR N/A
1. DELIVERED
3. ANTEPARTUM

372.71 CONGESTION CONJUNCTIVA
362.89 CONGESTION RETINA
625.5 CONGESTION-FIBROSIS SYNDROME (PELVIC)

FOR CODING PURPOSES, CHF AND RIGHT VENTRICULAR FAILURE ARE CONSIDERED TO BE SYNONYMOUS AND BOTH ARE ASSIGNED A 4TH DIGIT OF "0". LEFT VENTRICULAR FAILURE IS NOT THE SAME AS CHF. LEFT VENTRICULAR FAILURE IS ASSIGNED A 4TH DIGIT OF "1".

CONGESTIVE HEART FAILURE (CHF)

428.0 ACUTE
0 ACUTE LEFT VENTRICULAR SEE 'HEART FAILURE' LEFT
0 ACUTE LEFT VENTRICULAR WITH PULMONARY EDEMA SEE 'HEART FAILURE' LEFT
428.0 ACUTE WITH PULMONARY EDEMA
428.0 COMBINED LEFT-RIGHT SIDED
428.0 COMPENSATED
428.0 DECOMPENSATED (RIGHT CONGESTIVE)
997.1 DURING A PROCEDURE
779.8 FETUS OR NEWBORN
402.91 HYPERTENSIVE NOS
402.11 HYPERTENSIVE BENIGN
402.01 HYPERTENSIVE MALIGNANT
404.91 HYPERTENSIVE HEART AND RENAL NOS
404.11 HYPERTENSIVE HEART AND RENAL BENIGN
404.01 HYPERTENSIVE HEART AND RENAL MALIGNANT
404.93 HYPERTENSIVE HEART AND RENAL WITH RENAL FAILURE NOS
404.13 HYPERTENSIVE HEART AND RENAL WITH RENAL FAILURE BENIGN
404.03 HYPERTENSIVE HEART AND RENAL WITH RENAL FAILURE MALIGNANT
0 LEFT VENTRICULAR SEE 'HEART FAILURE'
997.1 POST OP (RESULTING FROM A PROCEDURE)
997.1 POST OP HEART SURGERY - IMMEDIATE
429.4 POST OP HEART SURGERY - LATE
398.91 RHEUMATIC
391.8 RHEUMATIC (ACUTE OR ACTIVE)
398.91 RHEUMATIC (CHRONIC) (INACTIVE) (WITH CHOREA)
428.0 RIGHT SECONDARY TO LEFT
392.0 SYDENHAM'S CHOREA WITH HEART INVOLVEMENT
402.91 WITH HYPERTENSIVE CARDIOMYOPATHY - NOS
402.11 WITH HYPERTENSIVE CARDIOMYOPATHY - BENIGN
402.01 WITH HYPERTENSIVE CARDIOMYOPATHY - MALIGNANT

CONGESTIVE HEART FAILURE (CHF) OBSTETRICAL

635.7# COMPLICATING ABORTION

5th Digit: 635.7
0. UNSPECIFIED
1. INCOMPLETE
2. COMPLETE

CONGESTIVE HEART FAILURE (CHF) OBSTETRICAL (continued)

669.4# COMPLICATING LABOR AND DELIVERY
668.1# DUE TO ANESTHESIA, OTHER SEDATION IN L&D

5th Digit: 668.1, 669.4
0. EPISODE OF CARE NOS OR N/A
1. DELIVERED
2. DELIVERED WITH POSTPARTUM COMPLICATION
3. ANTEPARTUM COMPLICATION
4. POSTPARTUM COMPLICATION

639.8 FOLLOWING ABORTION
648.6# MATERNAL CURRENT (CO-EXISTENT)

5th Digit: 648.6
0. EPISODE OF CARE NOS OR N/A
1. DELIVERED
2. DELIVERED WITH POSTPARTUM COMPLICATION
3. ANTEPARTUM COMPLICATION
4. POSTPARTUM COMPLICATION

759.4 CONJOINED TWINS

CONJUGATE GAZE

378.85 ANOMALIES OF DIVERGENCE
378.83 CONVERGENCE INSUFFICIENCY OR PALSY
378.84 EXCESS OR SPASM
378.81 PALSY
378.87 SKEW DEVIATION
378.82 SPASM

CONJUNCTIVA, CONJUNCTIVAL

918.2 ABRASION
372.63 ADHESIONS (EXTENSIVE)
372.62 ADHESIONS AND STRANDS (LOCALIZED)
372.74 ANEURYSM
372.55 ARGYROSIS
372.8 ATROPHY
372.54 CALCIFICATION
372.73 CHEMOSIS
372.54 CONCRETIONS
372.75 CYST
372.50 DEGENERATION
277.3 DEGENERATION AMYLOID [372.50]
372.56 DEPOSITS
372.9 DISEASE (SEE ALSO 'CONJUNCTIVITIS')
372.9 DISORDER
372.8 DISORDER OTHER
372.73 EDEMA
372.02 FOLLICULOSIS ACUTE
372.61 GRANULOMA
372.72 HEMORRHAGE
372.71 HYPEREMIA
372.73 HYPERTROPHY LYMPHOID
918.2 INJURY SUPERFICIAL
372.55 PIGMENTATIONS
379.93 REDNESS
372.64 SCARRING (POST ENUCLEATION)
372.62 STRANDS
372.74 VASCULAR ABNORMALITIES
372.53 XEROSIS
264.0 XEROSIS VITAMIN A
264.1 XEROSIS VITAMIN A DEFICIENCY WITH BITOT'S SPOT

CONJUNCTIVITIS

372.30 NOS
372.00 ACUTE
372.05 ACUTE ATOPIC
372.03 ACUTE CATARRHAL
372.02 ACUTE FOLLICULAR
077.3 ACUTE FOLLICULAR ADENOVIRAL
077.4 ACUTE FOLLICULAR EPIDEMIC HEMORRHAGIC
077.8 ACUTE FOLLICULAR NEWCASTLE
077.2 ACUTE FOLLICULAR PHARYNCONJUNCTIVAL
372.03 ACUTE MUCOPURULENT
372.04 ACUTE PSEUDOMEMBRANOUS
372.01 ACUTE SEROUS

C

CONJUNCTIVITIS (continued)

372.14 ALLERGIC
372.05 ANAPHYLACTIC
372.03 ANGULAR
077.4 APOLLO
372.30 BACTERIAL
372.05 CHEMICAL
077.98 CHLAMYDIAL
0 CHLAMYDIAL TRACHOMATIS SEE 'TRACHOMA'
372.10 CHRONIC
372.14 CHRONIC ALLERGIC OTHER
372.12 CHRONIC FOLLICULAR
372.11 CHRONIC SIMPLE
372.13 CHRONIC VERNAL
032.81 DIPHTHERITIC
372.05 DUST (DUE TO)
370.31 ECZEMATOUS
077.4 ENTEROVIRUS TYPE 70
077.4 EPIDEMIC HEMORRHAGIC
077.1 EPIDEMIC KERATOCONJUNCTIVITIS
695.1 ERYTHEMA MULTIFORME [372.33]
125.9 FILARIAL [372.15]
077.3 FOLLICULAR ADENOVIRAL
076.1 FOLLICULAR TRACHOMATOUS
370.34 GLARE
098.49 GONOCOCCAL
098.40 GONOCOCCAL NEONATAL
076.1 GRANULAR TRACHOMATOUS
077.4 HEMORRHAGIC (ACUTE) (EPIDEMIC)
054.43 HERPETIC SIMPLEX
053.21 HERPETIC ZOSTER
077.0 INCLUSION
771.6 INCLUSION NEONATAL
372.03 INFLUENZAL
372.03 KOCH WEEKS
085.5 LEISHMANIASIS [372.15]
372.05 LIGHT
372.05 MEDICAMENTOSA
372.04 MEMBRANOUS ACUTE
036.89 MENINGOCOCCAL
372.02 MORAX AXENFELD
771.6 NEONATAL
077.8 NEWCASTLE
360.14 NODOSA
077.3 OF BEAL
085.5 PARASITIC MUCOCUTANEOUS LEISHMANIASIS [372.15]
077.0 PARATRACHOMA
372.02 PARINAUD'S
694.61 PEMPHIGOID
372.39 PETRIFICANS
077.2 PHARYNGOCONJUNCTIVAL FEVER
370.31 PHLYCTENULAR
372.30 PNEUMOCOCCAL
099.3 REITER'S [372.33]
695.3 ROSACEA [372.31]
V74.4 SCREENING EXAM (BACTERIAL)
077.99 SEROUS VIRAL
372.30 STAPHYLOCOCCAL
372.30 STREPTOCCAL, STREPTOCOCCUS
372.04 SUN LAMP
077.0 SWIMMING POOL
095.8 SYPHILIS [372.10]
130.1 TOXOPLASMOSIS
372.39 TRAUMATIC NEC

CONJUNCTIVITIS (continued)

017.3# TUBERCULOUS [370.31]
5th Digit: 017.3
0. NOS
1. LAB NOT DONE
2. LABS PENDING
3. MICROSCOPY POSITIVE (IN SPUTUM)
4. CULTURE POSITIVE - MICROSCOPY NEGATIVE
5. CULTURE NEGATIVE - MICROSCOPY POSITIVE
6. CULTURE AND MICRO NEGATIVE CONFIRMED BY OTHER METHODS

021.3 TULAREMIC
372.13 VERNAL
370.32 VERNAL LIMBAR AND CORNEAL INVOLVEMENT [372.13]
077.99 VIRAL
077.4 VIRAL ACUTE HEMORRHAGIC
077.8 VIRAL OTHER
372.39 OTHER

099.3 CONJUNCTIVOURETHROSYNOVIAL SYNDROME
099.3 CONJUNCTIVOURETHROSYNOVIAL SYNDROME WITH ARTHROPATHY [711.1#]
5th Digit: 711.1
0. SITE NOS
1. SHOULDER REGION
2. UPPER ARM (ELBOW) (HUMERUS)
3. FOREARM (RADIUS) (WRIST) (ULNA)
4. HAND (CARPAL) (METACARPAL) (FINGERS)
5. PELVIC REGION AND THIGH (HIP) (BUTTOCK) (FEMUR)
6. LOWER LEG (FIBULA) (KNEE) (PATELLA) (TIBIA)
7. ANKLE AND/OR FOOT (METATARSALS) (TOES) (TARSALS)
8. OTHER (HEAD) (NECK) (RIB) (SKULL) (TRUNK) (VERTEBRAE)
9. MULTIPLE

099.3 CONJUNCTIVOURETHROSYNOVIAL SYNDROME WITH CONJUNCTIVITIS [372.33]
710.9 CONNECTIVE TISSUE DISEASE NEC (SEE ALSO 'COLLAGEN')
255.1 CONN-LOUIS SYNDROME (PRIMARY ALDOSTERONISM)
255.1 CONN'S SYNDROME (PRIMARY ALDOSTERONISM)
082.1 CONOR AND BRUCH'S BOUTONNEUSE FEVER
756.59 CONRADI (-HUNERMANN) DISEASE OR SYNDROME (CHONDRODYSPLASIA CALCIFICANS CONGENITA)
V19.7 CONSANGUINITY FAMILY HISTORY
564.0 CONSTIPATION
306.4 CONSTIPATION PSYCHOGENIC

CONSTITUTIONAL STATE

V21.2 ADOLESCENCE
V21.0 DEVELOPMENT RAPID GROWTH
V21.9 IN DEVELOPMENT
V21.8 IN DEVELOPMENT OTHER SPECIFIED
V21.1 PUBERTY

286.4 CONSTITUTIONAL THROMBOPATHY
0 CONSULTATION SEE 'COUNSELING'
0 CONTACT DERMATITIS SEE 'DERMATITIS CONTACT'
371.82 CONTACT LENS CAUSING CORNEAL DISORDER
V53.1 CONTACT LENSES FITTING AND ADJUSTMENT
0 CONTACT WITH COMMUNICABLE DISEASE SEE 'EXPOSURE'
051.2 CONTAGIOUS PUSTULAR DERMATITIS

CONTRACEPTION, CONTRACEPTIVE

ADVICE / COUNSELING

V25.09 FAMILY PLANNING
V25.02 PRESCRIPTION OR USE - FOAMS, CREAMS OR OTHER AGENTS
V25.01 PRESCRIPTION OR USE - ORAL CONTRACEPTIVE
V25.09 TUBOPLASTY (PROPOSED)
V25.09 VASECTOMY (PROPOSED)
V25.09 OTHER SPECIFIED NEC

MANAGEMENT

V25.9 UNSPECIFIED
V25.02 DIAPHRAGM FITTING
V15.7 HISTORY
V45.52 IMPLANTABLE SUBDERMAL - IN SITU
V25.5 IMPLANTABLE SUBDERMAL - INSERTION
V25.43 IMPLANTABLE SUBDERMAL - CHECKING, REINSERTION OR REMOVAL
V25.02 INJECTION
V25.49 INJECTION REPEAT
V25.42 IUD CHECKING, REINSERTION OR REMOVAL
V45.51 IUD IN SITU
V25.1 IUD INSERTION
V25.3 MENSTRUAL REGULATION
V25.01 ORAL PRESCRIPTION
V25.41 ORAL REPEAT PRESCRIPTION
V25.02 PRESCRIPTION FOAMS, CREAMS
V25.02 PRESCRIPTION OTHER SPECIFIED AGENT NEC
V25.49 PRESCRIPTION OTHER SPECIFIED AGENT NEC - REPEAT
V25.8 SPERM COUNT POST-VASECTOMY
V25.2 STERILIZATION
V25.40 SURVEILLANCE
V25.2 TUBOPLASTY ENCOUNTER
V25.2 VASECTOMY ENCOUNTER
V25.49 OTHER SPECIFIED CONTRACEPTIVE METHOD NEC
V45.59 OTHER SPECIFIED DEVICE IN SITU
V25.8 OTHER SPECIFIED MANAGEMENT NEC

CONTRACTION

564.89 ANUS
728.85 FLACCID PARALYTIC MUSCLE
728.89 HAMSTRING
564.89 RECTUM, RECTAL (SPHINCTER)
763.7 RING AFFECTING FETUS OR NEWBORN

CONTRACTURE

729.9 AXILLA
709.2 CICATRICIAL
728.89 FASCIA LATA (POSTURAL)
736.29 FINGER (NON ARTICULAR)
755.59 FINGER CONGENITAL
718.4# JOINT

5th Digit: 718.4

0. SITE NOS
1. SHOULDER REGION
2. UPPER ARM (ELBOW) (HUMERUS)
3. FOREARM (RADIUS) (WRIST) (ULNA)
4. HAND (CARPAL) (METACARPAL) (FINGERS)
5. PELVIC REGION AND THIGH (HIP) (BUTTOCK) (FEMUR)
6. LOWER LEG (FIBULA) (KNEE) (PATELLA) (TIBIA)
7. ANKLE AND/OR FOOT (METATARSALS) (TOES) (TARSALS)
8. OTHER
9. MULTIPLE

728.89 LIGAMENT
728.6 PALMAR FASCIA

V64.1 CONTRAINDICATION CAUSING CANCELLATION OF PROCEDURE

A CONTUSION IS A COLLECTION OF BLOOD UNDER THE SURFACE OF THE SKIN WITH THE SKIN SURFACE INTACT RESULTING FROM AN INJURY. DO NOT CODE CONTUSIONS WHEN THEY ACCOMPANY A FRACTURE, DISLOCATION, LACERATION, OR A CRUSH INJURY. RATHER, USE A CODE FROM THESE CATEGORIES SINCE CONTUSIONS ARE CONSIDERED TO BE INCIDENTAL TO THE GREATER INJURY. FOR CONTUSIONS OF NERVES OR INTERNAL ORGANS, USE THE "INJURY" CODE FOUND UNDER THE SPECIFIC ANATOMICAL SITES.

CONTUSION

924.9 NOS
922.2 ABDOMEN WALL OR MUSCLE
868.00 ABDOMINAL ORGAN UNSPECIFIED
868.10 ABDOMINAL ORGAN UNSPECIFIED WITH OPEN WOUND
868.09 ABDOMINAL ORGAN OTHER OR MULTIPLE
868.19 ABDOMINAL ORGAN OTHER OR MULTIPLE WITH OPEN WOUND
921.9 ADNEXA EYE
868.01 ADRENAL GLAND
868.11 ADRENAL GLAND WITH OPEN WOUND
924.21 ANKLE
924.20 ANKLE AND FOOT
923.9 ARM
923.10 ARM LOWER
923.09 ARM AND SHOULDER
923.8 ARM MULTIPLE SITES
923.03 ARM UPPER
920 AUDITORY CANAL (EXTERNAL) (MEATUS)
920 AURICLE EAR
923.02 AXILLARY REGION
923.09 AXILLARY REGION AND SHOULDER
923.09 AXILLARY REGION AND UPPER ARM
922.31 BACK
868.02 BILE DUCT
868.12 BILE DUCT WITH OPEN WOUND
924.9 BONE UNSPECIFIED
0 BRAIN SEE 'CEREBRAL CONTUSION'
922.0 BREAST
920 BROW
922.32 BUTTOCK
921.1 CANTHUS
861.01 CARDIAC
861.11 CARDIAC WITH OPEN WOUND INTO THORAX
952.4 CAUDA EQUINA (SPINE)
0 CEREBELLUM SEE 'BRAIN STEM', CONTUSION
0 CEREBRAL SEE 'CEREBRAL CONTUSION'
920 CHEEK
922.1 CHEST (WALL)
920 CHIN
922.4 CLITORIS
921.1 CONJUNCTIVA
952.4 CONUS MEDULLARIS (SPINE)
921.3 CORNEA
922.4 CORPUS CAVERNOSUM
0 CORTEX SEE 'CEREBRAL CONTUSION'
922.1 COSTAL REGION
920 EAR (AURICLE)
923.11 ELBOW
923.10 ELBOW WITH FOREARM
922.4 EPIDIDYMIS
922.2 EPIGASTRIC REGION
924.5 EXTREMITY LOWER
924.4 EXTREMITY LOWER MULTIPLE SITES
923.9 EXTREMITY UPPER
923.8 EXTREMITY UPPER MULTIPLE SITES
921.9 EYE
921.0 EYE AND ADNEXA (BLACK EYE)
921.3 EYEBALL
921.1 EYELID
920 FACE
922.2 FEMORAL TRIANGLE
772.6 FETUS OR NEWBORN
923.3 FINGER
923.3 FINGERNAIL

C

CONTUSION (continued)	
922.2	FLANK
924.20	FOOT OR FOOT AND ANKLE
923.10	FOREARM
923.10	FOREARM AND ELBOW
920	FOREHEAD
868.02	GALLBLADDER
868.12	GALLBLADDER WITH OPEN WOUND
922.4	GENITAL ORGANS EXTERNAL
921.3	GLOBE (EYE)
922.2	GROIN
920	GUM
923.20	HAND
920	HEAD
861.01	HEART
861.11	HEART WITH OPEN WOUND OF THORAX
924.20	HEEL
924.01	HIP
924.00	HIP WITH THIGH
922.2	ILIAC REGION
922.2	INGUINAL REGION
922.33	INTERSCAPULAR REGION
862.8	INTRATHORACIC ORGANS MULTIPLE
862.9	INTRATHORACIC ORGANS MULTIPLE, WITH OPEN WOUND INTO CAVITY
921.3	IRIS (EYE)
866.01	KIDNEY
866.11	KIDNEY WITH OPEN WOUND INTO CAVITY
924.11	KNEE
924.10	KNEE WITH LOWER LEG
922.4	LABIA
921.1	LACRIMAL APPARATUS, GLAND OR SAC
920	LARYNX
906.3	LATE EFFECT
924.5	LEG
924.10	LEG LOWER
924.4	LEG MULTIPLE SITES
921.3	LENS
920	LINGUAL
920	LIP
864.01	LIVER
864.11	LIVER WITH OPEN WOUND
922.31	LUMBAR REGION
861.21	LUNG
861.31	LUNG WITH OPEN WOUND
920	MALAR REGION
920	MANDIBULAR JOINT AREA
920	MASTOID REGION
0	MEMBRANE, BRAIN SEE 'CEREBRAL CONTUSION'
922.1	MIDTHORACIC REGION
920	MOUTH
862.8	MULTIPLE INTRATHORACIC ORGANS
862.9	MULTIPLE INTRATHORACIC ORGANS WITH OPEN WOUND INTO CAVITY
924.8	MULTIPLE SITES
924.4	MULTIPLE SITES LOWER LIMB
922.8	MULTIPLE SITES TRUNK
923.8	MULTIPLE SITES UPPER LIMB
924.9	MUSCLE SITE UNSPECIFIED
861.01	MYOCARDIAL
861.11	MYOCARDIAL WITH OPEN WOUND OF THORAX
920	NASAL (SEPTUM)
920	NECK
920	NOSE
920	OCCIPITAL REGION
0	OCCIPITAL LOBE SEE 'CEREBRAL CONTUSION'
921.2	ORBITAL AREA
920	PALATE
920	PARIETAL REGION
0	PARIETAL LOBE SEE 'CEREBRAL CONTUSION'

CONTUSION (continued)	
922.9	PELVIS
922.4	PENIS
861.01	PERICARDIUM
861.11	PERICARDIUM WITH OPEN WOUND OF THORAX
922.4	PERINEUM
921.1	PERIOCULAR
921.2	PERIORBITAL
868.03	PERITONEUM
868.13	PERITONEUM WITH OPEN WOUND
920	PHARYNX
924.11	POPLITEAL SPACE
922.4	PREPUCE
922.4	PUBIC REGION
922.4	PUDENDA
861.21	PULMONARY
861.31	PULMONARY WITH OPEN WOUND
924.00	QUADRICEPS FEMORALIS
866.01	RENAL
866.11	RENAL WITH OPEN WOUND INTO CAVITY
921.2	RETROBULBAR
868.04	RETROPERITONEUM
868.14	RETROPERITONEUM WITH OPEN WOUND
922.1	RIB
922.32	SACRAL REGION
920	SALIVARY DUCTS OR GLAND
920	SCALP
923.01	SCAPULA
923.09	SCAPULA AND SHOULDER
923.01	SCAPULAR REGION
921.3	SCLERA (EYE)
922.4	SCROTUM
923.00	SHOULDER
923.09	SHOULDER AND ARM MULTIPLE SITES
923.00	SHOULDER REGION
924.9	SKIN UNSPECIFIED SITE
920	SKULL
922.4	SPERMATIC CORD
952.4	SPINAL CORD CAUDA EQUINA
952.4	SPINAL CORD CONUS MEDULLARIS
865.01	SPLEEN
865.11	SPLEEN WITH OPEN WOUND INTO CAVITY
922.1	STERNAL REGION
921.1	SUBCONJUNCTIVAL
924.9	SUBCUTANEOUS UNSPECIFIED SITE
920	SUBMAXILLARY REGION
920	SUBMENTAL REGION
924.9	SUBPERIOSTEAL
923.3	SUBUNGUAL FINGERNAIL
923.3	SUBUNGUAL THUMBNAIL
924.3	SUBUNGUAL TOENAIL
920	SUPRACLAVICULAR FOSSA
920	SUPRAORBITAL
920	TEMPLE
922.4	TESTIS
924.00	THIGH
924.00	THIGH AND HIP
922.1	THORAX
920	THROAT
923.3	THUMB
923.3	THUMBNAIL
924.3	TOE
924.3	TOENAIL
920	TONGUE
922.9	TRUNK
922.8	TRUNK MULTIPLE SITES
922.4	TUNICA VAGINALIS
920	TYMPANUM
920	UVULA
922.4	VAGINA
920	VOCAL CORD
922.4	VULVA
923.21	WRIST
923.20	WRIST AND HAND

743.57 CONUS (CONGENITAL)
371.60 CONUS ACQUIRED
336.8 CONUS MEDULLARIS SYNDROME

CONVALESCENCE
V66.9 UNSPECIFIED
V66.2 FOLLOWING CHEMOTHERAPY
V66.4 FOLLOWING FRACTURE
V66.3 FOLLOWING MENTAL DISORDER
V66.5 FOLLOWING OTHER TREATMENT
V66.3 FOLLOWING PSYCHOTHERAPY
V66.1 FOLLOWING RADIOTHERAPY
V66.0 FOLLOWING SURGERY

WHEN USING CODE V66.7, CODE THE TERMINAL ILLNESS FIRST.

V66.7 FOR END-OF-LIFE, HOSPICE OR TERMINAL CARE
V66.7 FOR PALLIATIVE CARE
V66.6 TREATMENT COMBINED

378.84 CONVERGENCE EXCESS OR SPASM
378.83 CONVERGENCE INSUFFICIENCY OR PALSY
300.11 CONVERSION DISORDER
300.11 CONVERSION HYSTERIA OR REACTION

CONVULSIONS
780.39 NOS
780.39 BRAIN, CEREBRAL, CEREBROSPINAL
780.39 DISORDER OR STATE
780.39 DUE TO ETHER ANESTHETIC CORRECT SUBSTANCE CORRECTLY ADMINISTERED
780.39 ECLAMPTIC
0 EPILEPTIC SEE 'EPILEPSY, EPILEPTIC'
780.39 EPILEPTIFORM, EPILEPTOID
780.31 FEBRILE
780.39 GENERALIZED
780.39 INFANTILE
779.0 NEWBORN
780.39 NONEPILEPTIC UNKNOWN ETIOLOGY OR UNSPECIFIED
780.39 RECURRENT
780.39 REPETITIVE
780.39 SPASMODIC
780.39 UNCINATE

255.2 COOKE-APERT-GALLAIS SYNDROME (ADRENOGENITAL)
282.4 COOLEY'S ERYTHROBLASTIC ANEMIA
610.1 COOPER'S DISEASE

315.4 COORDINATION DISORDER
781.3 COORDINATION LACK OF

WHEN A PATIENT IS ADMITTED IN ACUTE RESPIRATORY FAILURE, DUE TO ACUTE EXACERBATION OF A CHRONIC RESPIRATORY CONDITION, SEQUENCE THE FAILURE BEFORE THE CHRONIC DISEASE.

WHEN A PATIENT IS ADMITTED IN RESPIRATORY FAILURE DUE TO A NON RESPIRATORY CONDITION, SEQUENCE THAT CONDITION BEFORE THE RESPIRATORY FAILURE..

COPD
496 NOS
491.21 ACUTE EXACERBATION
491.21 ACUTE EXACERBATION - ACUTE BRONCHITIS
491.21 ACUTE EXACERBATION - CHRONIC BRONCHITIS
518.5 ACUTE EXACERBATION - ARDS [496]
415.0 ACUTE EXACERBATION - COR PULMONALE [496]
483 ACUTE EXACERBATION - MYCOPLASMA PNEUMONIA [496]
486 ACUTE EXACERBATION - PNEUMONIA [496]
512.8 ACUTE EXACERBATION - PNEUMOTHORAX [496]
415.19 ACUTE EXACERBATION - PULMONARY EMBOLUS [496]
415.11 ACUTE EXACERBATION - PULMONARY EMBOLUS POST OP OR IATROGENIC [496]
518.81 ACUTE EXACERBATION - RESPIRATORY FAILURE [496]

COPD (continued)
495.6 FUNGAL (THERMOPHILIC) (ACTINOMYCETE) (OTHER)
495.4 WITH ALLERGIC ALVEOLITIS (ASPERGILLUS CLAVATUS)
495.9 WITH ALLERGIC ALVEOLITIS AND PNEUMONITIS
493.2# WITH ASTHMA
5th Digit: 493.2
0. WITHOUT MENTION OF STATUS ASTHMATICUS
1. WITH STATUS ASTHMATICUS

494 WITH BRONCHIECTASIS
491.20 WITH BRONCHITIS CHRONIC
491.21 WITH BRONCHITIS CHRONIC WITH ACUTE EXACERBATION
496 WITH BRONCHOSPASM
492.8 WITH EMPHYSEMA
492.0 WITH EMPHYSEMA BULLOUS
491.20 WITH EMPHYSEMA WITH BRONCHITIS
491.21 WITH EMPHYSEMA WITH BRONCHITIS WITH EXACERBATION
496 WITH UNKNOWN EXACERBATION

790.6 COPPER ABNORMAL BLOOD LEVEL
275.1 COPPER METABOLISM DISORDER
989.5 COPPERHEAD SNAKE BITE
995.0 COPPERHEAD SNAKE BITE WITH ANAPHYLAXIS [989.5]

560.39 COPROLITH
302.89 COPROPHILIA
277.1 COPROPORPHYRIA HEREDITARY

745.7 COR BILOCULARE ATRIAL AND VENTRICULAR SEPTUM ABSENCE
415.0 COR PULMONALE ACUTE
416.9 COR PULMONALE CHRONIC
416.9 COR PULMONALE SYNDROME
746.82 COR TRIATRIATUM CONGENITAL
745.3 COR TRILOCULARE BIATRIATUM
745.69 COR TRILOCULARE BIVENTRICULARE

INJURY OF A TENDON, JOINT CAPSULE, OR LIGAMENT CAN BE A SEPARATION, TEAR, LACERATION, AVULSION, STRAIN, SPRAIN, OR HEMARTHROSIS. YOU CAN FIND THIS UNDER SPRAIN ALSO.

840.1 CORACOCLAVICULAR SEPARATION (RUPTURE) (TEAR) (LACERATION)
840.1 CORACOCLAVICULAR STRAIN (SPRAIN) (AVULSION) (HEMARTHROSIS)
840.2 CORACOHUMERAL SEPARATION (RUPTURE) (TEAR) (LACERATION)
840.2 CORACOHUMERAL STRAIN (SPRAIN) (AVULSION) (HEMARTHROSIS)
989.5 CORAL SNAKE BITE
995.0 CORAL SNAKE BITE WITH ANAPHYLAXIS [989.5]
607.1 CORBUS' DISEASE
762.5 CORD COMPRESSION (AROUND NECK) (ENTANGLEMENT) (KNOT) (TORSION) AFFECTING FETUS OR NEWBORN
762.4 CORD PROLAPSED (PRESENTATION) AFFECTING FETUS OR NEWBORN
762.6 CORD CONDITION OTHER AFFECTING FETUS OR NEWBORN

743.46 CORECTOPIA CONGENITAL
495.3 CORKHANDLER'S LUNG
530.5 CORKSCREW ESOPHAGUS
700 CORN

CORNEA, CORNEAL
918.1 ABRASION
371.81 ANESTHESIA AND HYPOESTHESIA
743.9 ANOMALIES NOS
743.41 ANOMALIES OF SIZE AND SHAPE CONGENITAL
743.49 ANOMALIES SPECIFIED NEC
371.16 ARGENTOUS DEPOSITS

C

CORNEA, CORNEAL (continued)
371.03 CALIGO
371.30 CHANGES MEMBRANE
371.41 CHANGES SENILE

DEFORMITY
371.70 NOS
743.9 NOS CONGENITAL
371.71 ECTASIA
371.72 DESCEMETOCELE
371.73 STAPHYLOMA

DEGENERATION
371.40 NOS
371.44 CALCEROUS
371.41 DELLEN
371.41 HYALINE
371.46 NODULAR
371.48 PERIPHERAL
371.41 SENILE

CORNEA, CORNEAL (continued)
371.41 DELLEN

DEPOSIT
371.10 NOS
371.15 ASSOCIATED WITH METABOLIC DISORDERS
371.16 ARGENTOUS
270.0 IN CYSTINOSIS [371.15]
277.5 IN MUCOPOLYSACCHARIDOSIS [371.15]

CORNEA, CORNEAL (continued)
371.72 DESCEMETOCELE

DISORDER
371.9 NOS
371.82 DUE TO CONTACT LENS
371.89 OTHER SPECIFIED

CORNEA, CORNEAL (continued)
743.41 DISTORTION CONGENITAL
V59.5 DONOR NON-AUTOGENOUS

DYSTROPHY
371.50 NOS
371.57 COMBINED
371.56 CRYSTALLINE
371.57 ENDOTHELIAL (FUCH'S)
371.53 GRANULAR
371.51 JUVENILE EPITHELIAL
371.54 LATTICE
371.55 MACULAR
371.52 MICROSCOPIC CYSTIC
371.58 POLYMORPHOUS
371.58 POSTERIOR
371.52 RING LIKE
371.56 STROMAL

CORNEA, CORNEAL (continued)
371.71 ECTASIA

EDEMA
371.20 NOS
371.21 IDIOPATHIC
371.22 SECONDARY
371.23 BULLOUS KERATOPATHY
371.24 DUE TO WEARING CONTACT LENSES

CORNEA, CORNEAL (continued)
371.42 EROSION RECURRENT
371.44 FACET
996.69 GRAFT COMPLICATION - INFECTION OR INFLAMMATION
996.51 GRAFT COMPLICATION - MECHANICAL
996.79 GRAFT COMPLICATION - OTHER
371.57 GUTTATA

CORNEA, CORNEAL (continued)
054.43 HERPES DISCIFORM (SIMPLEX)
054.43 HERPES SIMPLEX
053.21 HERPES ZOSTER
371.89 HYPERTROPHY
371.81 HYPERESTHESIA
371.81 HYPOESTHESIA
371.20 INFILTRATE
370.9 INFLAMMATION
370.00 INFLAMMATION WITH ULCER
371.82 INJURY (SUPERFICIAL) DUE TO CONTACT LENS
918.1 LACERATION SUPERFICIAL
371.04 LEUCOMA CENTRAL
371.02 MACULA
371.03 MACULA INTERFERING WITH CENTRAL VISION
371.30 MEMBRANE CHANGE
371.01 NEBULA

NEOVASCULARIZATION
370.60 NOS
370.61 LOCALIZED
370.62 PANNUS
370.63 DEEP VASCULARIZATION
370.64 GHOST VESSELS

OPACITY
371.00 NOS
371.03 CENTRAL
743.43 CONGENITAL
743.42 CONGENITAL INTERFERING WITH VISION
371.01 MINOR
371.02 PERIPHERAL

CORNEA, CORNEAL (continued)
017.3# PHTHISICAL TUBERCULOUS [371.05]

5th Digit: 017.3
0. NOS
1. LAB NOT DONE
2. LABS PENDING
3. MICROSCOPY POSITIVE (IN SPUTUM)
4. CULTURE POSITIVE - MICROSCOPY NEGATIVE
5. CULTURE NEGATIVE - MICROSCOPY POSITIVE
6. CULTURE AND MICROSCOPY NEGATIVE CONFIRMED BY OTHER METHODS

PIGMENTATIONS
371.10 NOS
371.11 ANTERIOR
371.13 POSTERIOR
371.12 STROMAL

CORNEA, CORNEAL (continued)
743.41 PLANA
371.00 SCAR
264.6 SCAR DUE TO VITAMIN A DEFICIENCY
370.54 SCLEROSIS
371.73 STAPHYLOMA
V45.69 STATUS POSTSURGICAL
V42.5 TRANSPLANT (STATUS)

ULCER
370.00 NOS
370.03 CENTRAL
264.3 DUE TO VITAMIN A DEFICIENCY
370.04 HYPOPYON ULCER
370.01 MARGINAL
370.07 MOOREN'S ULCER
370.05 MYCOTIC
370.06 PERFORATED
370.02 RING
370.04 SERPIGINOUS

CORNEA, CORNEAL (continued)
371.40 XEROSIS

759.89 CORNELIA DE LANGE'S SYNDROME (AMSTERDAM DWARF, MENTAL RETARDATION, AND BRACHYCEPHALY)

700 CORNS

700 CORNS AND CLAVUS

CORONARY

V45.82 ANGIOPLASTY STATUS (PTCA)

746.85 ARTERY ABSENCE CONGENITAL

746.85 ARTERY ANOMALOUS ORIGIN OR COMMUNICATION

414.11 ARTERY ANEURYSM

414.0# ARTERY DISEASE (ARTERIOSCLEROSIS) (DEFORMANS) (ARTERITIS)

5th Digit: 414.0

0. UNSPECIFIED TYPE OF VESSEL, NATIVE OR GRAFT
1. NATIVE CORONARY VESSEL
2. AUTOLOGOUS VEIN BYPASS GRAFT
3. NONAUTOLOGOUS BIOLOGICAL BYPASS GRAFT
4. AUTOLOGOUS ARTERY BYPASS GRAFT (GASTROEPIPLOIC) (INTERNAL MAMMARY)
5. UNSPECIFIED TYPE OF BYPASS GRAFT

411.81 ARTERY EMBOLISM (THROMBOSIS) WITHOUT INFARCTION

0 ARTERY EMBOLISM (THROMBOSIS) WITH INFARCTION SEE 'MI (MYOCARDIAL INFARCTION) ACUTE'

414.0# ATHEROSCLEROSIS

5th Digit: 414.0

0. UNSPECIFIED TYPE OF VESSEL, NATIVE OR GRAFT
1. NATIVE CORONARY VESSEL
2. AUTOLOGOUS VEIN BYPASS GRAFT
3. NONAUTOLOGOUS BIOLOGICAL BYPASS GRAFT
4. AUTOLOGOUS ARTERY BYPASS GRAFT (GASTROEPIPLOIC) (INTERNAL MAMMARY)
5. UNSPECIFIED TYPE OF BYPASS GRAFT

414.0# BYPASS GRAFT ARTERIOSCLEROSIS

5th Digit: 414.0

2. AUTOLOGOUS VEIN BYPASS GRAFT
3. NONAUTOLOGOUS BIOLOGICAL BYPASS GRAFT
4. AUTOLOGOUS ARTERY BYPASS GRAFT (GASTROEPIPLOIC) (INTERNAL MAMMARY)
5. UNSPECIFIED TYPE OF BYPASS GRAFT

996.61 BYPASS GRAFT COMPLICATION - INFECTION OR INFLAMMATION

996.03 BYPASS GRAFT COMPLICATION - MECHANICAL (LEAKAGE) (OBSTRUCTION) (PERFORATION)

996.72 BYPASS GRAFT COMPLICATION - OTHER

V45.81 BYPASS STATUS

414.9 DISEASE ISCHEMIC

746.85 DISEASE ISCHEMIC CONGENITAL

093.20 DISEASE OSTIAL SYPHILITIC

411.89 INSUFFICIENCY ACUTE

414.8 INSUFFICIENCY CHRONIC

411.1 INSUFFICIENCY OR INTERMEDIATE SYNDROME

411.81 OBSTRUCTION (OCCLUSION) ACUTE WITHOUT INFARCTION

0 OBSTRUCTION (OCCLUSION) ACUTE WITH INFARCTION SEE 'MI (MYOCARDIAL INFARCTION) ACUTE'

0 OBSTRUCTION (OCCLUSION) CHRONIC WITHOUT INFARCTION DUE TO ATHEROSCLEROSIS SEE 'CORONARY', ARTERY DISEASE

746.89 VEIN ANOMALY

620.2 CORPUS ALBICANS CYST

742.2 CORPUS CALLOSUM ABSENCE CONGENITAL

341.8 CORPUS CALLOSUM CENTRAL DYMYELINATION

CORPUS CAVERNOSUM

607.89 ATROPHY (FIBROSIS) (ULCER) (HYPERTROPHY)

607.89 CALCIFICATION

607.2 CELLULITIS (ABSCESS) (BOIL) (CARBUNCLE)

607.89 FIBROSIS

607.82 HEMATOMA (HEMORRHAGE) NONTRAUMATIC

607.82 THROMBOSIS

620.1 CORPUS LUTEUM CYST OR HEMATOMA

620.1 CORPUS LUTEUM CYST RUPTURE

0 CORRIGAN'S DISEASE SEE 'AORTA, AORTIC (VALVE) INSUFFICIENCY'

V53.7 CORSET FITTING AND ADJUSTMENT ORTHOPEDIC

0 CORTICAL ATROPHY SEE 'BRAIN', ATROPHY

377.75 CORTICAL BLINDNESS

255.4 CORTICOADRENAL INSUFFICIENCY

255.2 CORTICOSEXUAL SYNDROME

255.2 CORTICOSTEROID METABOLISM DISORDER NEC

334.8 CORTICOSTRIATAL SPINAL DEGENERATION

255.8 CORTISOL BINDING GLOBULIN ABNORMALITY

255.0 CORTISOL OVERPRODUCTION

0 CORYNEBACTERIUM DIPHTHERIAE INFECTION SEE 'DIPHTHERIA'

460 CORYZA ACUTE

V50.9 COSMETIC SURGERY UNSPECIFIED (ELECTIVE)

V50.8 COSMETIC SURGERY OTHER (ELECTIVE)

524.60 COSTEN'S SYNDROME (COMPLEX)

733.6 COSTOCHONDRAL JUNCTION SYNDROME

786.52 COSTOCHONDRAL PAIN

739.8 COSTOCHONDRAL REGION SEGMENTAL OR SOMATIC DYSFUNCTION

733.6 COSTOCHONDRITIS

353.0 COSTOCLAVICULAR SYNDROME (NONDISCOGENIC)

739.8 COSTOVERTEBRAL REGION SEGMENTAL OR SOMATIC DYSFUNCTION

798.0 COT DEATH

297.1 COTARD'S SYNDROME (PARANOIA)

362.83 COTTON WOOL SPOTS RETINAL

724.3 COTUGNO'S SCIATICA

COUGH

786.2 COUGH

306.1 PSYCHOGENIC

491.0 SMOKERS'

786.3 WITH HEMORRHAGE

> *COUMADIN, DIGOXIN, CHEMOTHERAPY DRUGS, AND ANY OTHER DRUGS WITH A RISK OF ADVERSE REACTIONS ARE CONSIDERED TO BE HIGH-RISK MEDICATION. CODES V58.61 AND V58.69 ARE TO BE USED TO IDENTIFY PATIENTS THAT ARE CURRENTLY BEING MONITORED WHILE TAKING HIGH RISK MEDICATION. CODE V67.51 IS TO BE USED TO IDENTIFY PATIENTS THAT HAVE COMPLETED HIGH RISK MEDICATION THERAPY.*

V67.51 COUMADIN FOLLOW UP EXAM - COMPLETED THERAPY

V58.61 COUMADIN FOLLOW UP EXAM - CURRENT THERAPY

COUNSELING

V65.9 UNSPECIFIED REASON

V61.22 ABUSE CHILD - PERPETRATOR PARENTAL

V62.83 ABUSE CHILD - PERPETRATOR OTHER

V61.21 ABUSE CHILD - VICTIM

V61.12 ABUSE SPOUSE (PARTNER) - PERPETRATOR

V61.11 ABUSE SPOUSE (PARTNER) - VICTIM

V62.83 ABUSE - OTHER PERPETRATOR OF PHYSICAL / SEXUAL ABUSE

V62.89 ABUSE - OTHER VICTIM

V61.29 ADOPTED CHILD PROBLEM

V65.42 ALCOHOL ABUSE

V65.8 BREAST IMPLANT REMOVAL (ELECTIVE)

CONTRACEPTION

V25.09 FAMILY PLANNING

V25.01 PRESCRIPTION OR USE - ORAL CONTRACEPTIVE

V25.02 PRESCRIPTION OR USE - FOAMS, CREAMS OR OTHER AGENTS

V25.09 TUBOPLASTY (PROPOSED)

V25.09 VASECTOMY (PROPOSED)

V25.09 OTHER SPECIFIED NEC

C

COUNSELING (continued)

V65.40 COUNSELING OTHER NEC
V65.3 DIET
V65.42 DRUG ABUSE
V65.49 EDUCATION
V65.41 EXERCISE
V65.49 EXPLANATION OF INVESTIGATIVE FINDINGS
V65.8 FOR OTHER REASONS
V61.29 FOSTER CHILD PROBLEM
V65.45 GONORRHEA
V65.49 HEALTH
V65.44 HIV
V65.43 INJURY PREVENTION
V65.49 INSTRUCTION
V65.49 LAB OR RESULTS OF STUDIES
V65.2 MALINGERER
V61.10 MARITAL PROBLEMS NOS
V65.49 MEDICATION
V61.20 PARENT - CHILD PROBLEM, UNSPECIFIED
V65.5 PATIENT WITH FEARED COMPLAINT IN WHOM NO DIAGNOSIS MADE
V65.8 PATIENT/PERSON FOR OTHER REASONS
V65.0 PERSON ACCOMPANYING SICK PERSON
V65.1 PERSON CONSULTING ON BEHALF OF ANOTHER PERSON
V65.1 PERSON OTHER THAN PATIENT
V26.4 PROCREATIVE
V65.49 SEX NEC
V65.45 SEXUALLY TRANSMITTED DISEASE
V65.49 SMOKING CESSATION
V65.42 SUBSTANCE ABUSE
V65.45 SYPHILIS
V65.49 TREATMENT PLAN
V65.49 WITHOUT COMPLAINT OR SICKNESS
V65.49 OTHER SPECIFIED COUNSELING

597.89 COWPERITIS
131.02 COWPERITIS TRICHOMONAL

051.0 COWPOX
999.0 COWPOX FROM VACCINATION

732.1 COXA PLANA HIP AND PELVIS JUVENILE
736.31 COXA VALGA
755.61 COXA VALGA CONGENITAL
736.32 COXA VARA
755.62 COXA VARA CONGENITAL

COXSACKIE

074.20 CARDITIS
074.22 ENDOCARDITIS
047.0 MENINGITIS
074.23 MYOCARDITIS
074.21 PERICARDITIS
079.2 VIRUS INFECTION (INFECTING AGENT)
074.8 VIRUS OTHER SPECIFIED DISEASES

CPD

653.4# NOS
660.1# NOS OBSTRUCTING LABOR **[653.4#]**
655.0# DUE TO ANENCEPHALY, HYDROCEPHALY, SPINA BIFIDA (SUSPECTED/KNOWN AFFECTING MANAGEMENT OF MOTHER)

5th Digit: 653.4, 655.0, 660.1

0. EPISODE OF CARE NOS OR N/A
1. DELIVERED
3. ANTEPARTUM COMPLICATION

790.5 CPK ELEVATED

> *'CRACK BABY': CODE ON BABY'S RECORD ONLY. DO NOT CODE MOTHER'S ABUSE/DEPENDENCE WITH THESE CODES.*

760.75 CRACK AFFECTING FETUS OR NEWBORN VIA PLACENTA OR BREAST MILK (CRACK BABY) - ASYMPTOMATIC
779.5 CRACK AFFECTING FETUS OR NEWBORN VIA PLACENTA OR BREAST MILK (CRACK BABY) - WITH WITHDRAWAL SYMPTOMS

690.11 CRADLE CAP (SEBORRHEA CAPITIS)

CRAMP

729.82 NOS
789.0# ABDOMINAL

5th Digit: 789.0

0. UNSPECIFIED SITE
1. UPPER RIGHT QUADRANT
2. UPPER LEFT QUADRANT
3. LOWER RIGHT QUADRANT
4. LOWER LEFT QUADRANT
5. PERIUMBILIC
6. EPIGASTRIC
7. GENERALIZED
9. OTHER SPECIFIED SITE (MULTIPLE)

994.1 BATHING
992.2 HEAT
300.11 HYSTERICAL
0 INTESTINAL SEE 'CRAMP', ABDOMINAL
625.3 MENSTRUAL
729.82 MUSCLE
994.1 MUSCLE DUE TO IMMERSION
307.89 PSYCHOGENIC
276.1 SALT DEPLETION
789.06 STOMACH
300.89 TELEGRAPHERS'
625.8 UTERINE
625.3 UTERINE MENSTRUAL

CRANIAL

352.9 NERVE ATROPHY
352.9 NERVE DISORDER
951.9 NERVE INJURY
767.7 NERVE INJURY DUE TO BIRTH TRAUMA
907.1 NERVE INJURY LATE EFFECT
352.6 NERVE PALSIES MULTIPLE
756.0 SUTURES DELAYED CLOSURE
756.0 SUTURES PREMATURE CLOSURE

763.89 CRANIOCLASIS, FETAL
376.44 CRANIOFACIAL DEFORMITIES WITH ASSOCIATED ORBIT DEFORMITY
759.4 CRANIOPAGUS

237.0 CRANIOPHARYNGIOMA SITE NOS
0 CRANIOPHARYNGIOMA SITE SPECIFIED SEE 'NEOPLASM UNCERTAIN BEHAVIOR' BY SITE M9350/1
740.1 CRANIORACHISCHISIS CONGENITAL
756.0 CRANIOSYNOSTOSIS
763.89 CRANIOTOMY, FETAL
723.2 CRANIOVERTEBRAL SYNDROME
738.19 CRANIUM DEFORMITY
0 CRANIUM DEFORMITY CONGENITAL SEE SPECIFIC DEFORMITY
790.6 CREATINE AND BUN ELEVATED
126.9 CREEPING ERUPTION NOS

CREPITUS

719.6# JOINT

5th Digit: 719.6

0. SITE NOS
1. SHOULDER REGION
2. UPPER ARM (ELBOW) (HUMERUS)
3. FOREARM (RADIUS) (WRIST) (ULNA)
4. HAND (CARPAL) (METACARPAL) (FINGERS)
5. PELVIC REGION AND THIGH (HIP) (BUTTOCK) (FEMUR)
6. LOWER LEG (FIBULA) (KNEE) (PATELLA) (TIBIA)
7. ANKLE AND/OR FOOT (METATARSALS) (TOES) (TARSALS)
8. OTHER
9. MULTIPLE

518.1 SUBCUTANEOUS - NONTRAUMATIC
998.81 SUBCUTANEOUS - SURGICAL
958.7 SUBCUTANEOUS - TRAUMATIC

243 CRETINISM (ATHYROTIC) (ENDEMIC)
246.1 CRETINISM GOITROUS (SPORADIC)
046.1 CREUTZFELDT-JAKOB CEREBRAL DEGENERATION
046.1 CREUTZFELDT-JAKOB CEREBRAL DEGENERATION WITH DEMENTIA [294.1]
758.3 CRI DU CHAT SYNDROME
798.0 CRIB DEATH SYNDROME
199.1 CRIBRIFORM CARCINOMA SITE NOS
0 CRIBRIFORM CARCINOMA SITE SPECIFIED SEE 'CANCER' BY SITE M8201/3

CRICOID
748.3 CARTILAGE ANOMALY (ABSENCE) CONGENITAL
748.3 CARTILAGE POSTERIOR CLEFT CONGENITAL
748.3 CLEFT (POSTERIOR) CONGENITAL

787.2 CRICOPHARYNGEAL SYNDROME
277.4 CRIGLER NAJJAR SYNDROME (CONGENITAL HYPERBILIRUBINEMIA)
0 CRISIS ASTHMATIC SEE 'ASTHMA'
0 CRISIS HYPERTENSIVE SEE 'HYPERTENSION, HYPERTENSIVE'
351.8 CROCODILE TEARS SYNDROME
443.89 CROCQ'S ACROCYANOSIS

CROHN'S DISEASE
555.9 NOS
555.1 LARGE INTESTINE
555.0 SMALL INTESTINE
555.2 SMALL INTESTINE AND LARGE INTESTINE

211.3 CRONKHITE-CANADA SYNDROME
524.2 CROSSBITE (ANTERIOR) (POSTERIOR)
464.4 CROUP (SYNDROME)
464.4 CROUPOUS ANGINA
756.0 CROUZON'S CRANIOFACIAL DYSOSTOSIS
710.1 CRST SYNDROME (CUTANEOUS SYSTEMIC SCLEROSIS)
049.8 CRUCHET'S ENCEPHALITIS LETHARGICA

CRUCIATE LIGAMENT (KNEE)
717.83 ANTERIOR - DISRUPTION (OLD)
717.9 ANTERIOR - RELAXATION
844.2 ANTERIOR - SPRAIN (RUPTURE) (STRAIN) (TEAR) ACUTE
717.84 POSTERIOR - DISRUPTION (OLD)
717.9 POSTERIOR - RELAXATION
844.2 POSTERIOR - SPRAIN (RUPTURE) (STRAIN) (TEAR) ACUTE

443.9 CRURAL ANGINA

CRUSH INJURY
929.9 SITE UNSPECIFIED
928.21 ANKLE
927.9 ARM
927.03 ARM (UPPER)
927.8 ARM MULTIPLE SITES
927.02 AXILLARY REGION
926.11 BACK
926.19 BREAST
926.12 BUTTOCK
925.1 CHEEK
862.8 CHEST
925.1 EAR
927.11 ELBOW
926.0 EXTERNAL GENITALIA
925.1 FACE
927.3 FINGER
928.20 FOOT
927.10 FOREARM
927.20 HAND
928.20 HEEL
928.01 HIP
0 INTERNAL ORGANS SEE SPECIFIC ORGAN, INJURY
928.11 KNEE

CRUSH INJURY (continued)
926.0 LABIA
925.2 LARYNX
906.4 LATE EFFECT
928.9 LEG
928.10 LEG (LOWER)
928.8 LEG MULTIPLE SITES
929.0 MULTIPLE SITES NEC
925.2 NECK
926.0 PENIS
925.2 PHARYNX
925.1 SCALP
927.01 SCAPULAR REGION
926.0 SCROTUM
927.00 SHOULDER
927.09 SHOULDER AND ARM MULTIPLE SITES
958.5 SYNDROME
908.6 SYNDROME LATE EFFECT
926.0 TESTIS
928.00 THIGH
925.2 THROAT
928.3 TOE (S)
925.2 TONSIL
926.9 TRUNK
926.8 TRUNK MULTIPLE SITES
926.19 TRUNK OTHER SITES
926.0 VULVA
927.21 WRIST

861.20 CRUSHED LUNG SYNDROME
690.11 CRUSTA LACTEA
571.5 CRUVEILHIER-BAUMGARTEN SYNDROME (CIRRHOSIS OF LIVER)
335.21 CRUVEILHIER'S DISEASE
086.2 CRUZ-CHAGAS DISEASE (SEE ALSO 'CHAGAS' DISEASE')
273.2 CRYOGLOBULINEMIA MIXED
569.49 CRYPTITIS (ANAL) (RECTAL)

CRYPTOCOCCOSIS
117.5 NOS
117.5 EUROPEAN
117.5 NEOFORMANS INFECTION
117.5 PULMONARY
117.5 SYSTEMIC

743.06 CRYPTOPHTHALMOS CONGENITAL
752.51 CRYPTORCHISM CONGENITAL
007.4 CRYPTOSPORIDIA INFECTION
495.6 CRYPTOSTROMA CORTICALE ALVEOLITIS

CRYSTALLOPATHY
275.49 NOS [**712.9#**]
275.49 CHONDROCALCINOSIS - CALCIUM PYROPHOSPHATE CRYSTALS [**712.2#**]
275.49 CHONDROCALCINOSIS - DICALCIUM PHOSPHATE [**712.1#**]
275.49 CHONDROCALCINOSIS - UNSPECIFIED [**712.3#**]
274.0 GOUTY
274.0 URIC ACID
275.49 OTHER SPECIFIED [**712.8#**]

5th Digit: 712.1-3, 8-9
0. SITE NOS
1. SHOULDER REGION
2. UPPER ARM (ELBOW) (HUMERUS)
3. FOREARM (RADIUS) (WRIST) (ULNA)
4. HAND (CARPAL) (METACARPAL) (FINGERS)
5. PELVIC REGION AND THIGH (HIP) (BUTTOCK) (FEMUR)
6. LOWER LEG (FIBULA) (KNEE) (PATELLA) (TIBIA)
7. ANKLE AND/OR FOOT (METATARSALS) (TOES) (TARSALS)
8. OTHER (HEAD) (NECK) (RIB) (SKULL) (TRUNK) (VERTEBRAE)
9. MULTIPLE

791.9 CRYSTALLURIA
791.9 CRYSTALLURIA ELEVATED URINE LEVELS
791.9 CRYSTALS URINE ABNORMAL
388.61 CSF OTORRHEA
349.81 CSF RHINORRHEA
701.0 CSILLAG'S LICHEN SCLEROSUS ET ATROPHICUS
354.0 CTS (CARPAL TUNNEL SYNDROME)
354.2 CUBITAL TUNNEL SYNDROME
736.01 CUBITUS VALGUS
755.59 CUBITUS VALGUS CONGENITAL
736.02 CUBITUS VARUS
755.59 CUBITUS VARUS CONGENITAL
162.3 CUIFFINI-PANCOAST SYNDROME (CARCINOMA, PULMONARY APEX) M8010/3

CULTURE ABNORMAL FINDINGS

790.7 BLOOD
V08 HIV
795.3 NOSE
795.3 SKIN LESION NEC
792.0 SPINAL FLUID
795.3 SPUTUM
792.1 STOOL
795.3 THROAT
791.9 URINE
795.3 WOUND
795.3 NEC

309.29 CULTURE SHOCK
117.7 CUNNINGHAMELLA INFECTION
530.5 CURLING ESOPHAGUS
359.2 CURSCHMANN'S (-BATTEN) (-STEINERT) DISEASE OR SYNDROME

CUSHING'S SYNDROME

255.0 NOS
255.2 DUE TO ADRENAL HYPERPLASIA
255.0 IATROGENIC
255.0 IDIOPATHIC
962.0 OVERDOSE OR WRONG SUBSTANCE GIVEN OR TAKEN
255.0 PITUITARY DEPENDENT
255.0 WITH MYOPATHY [359.5]

0 CUT SEE 'LACERATION', BY SITE
702.8 CUTANEOUS HORN
126.9 CUTANEOUS LARVA MIGRANS
782.2 CUTANEOUS NODULE
956.4 CUTANEOUS SENSORY NERVE INJURY LOWER LIMB
955.5 CUTANEOUS SENSORY NERVE INJURY UPPER LIMB
V44.51 CUTANEOUS-VESICOSTOMY STATUS
701.8 CUTIS LAXA SENILIS

REMEMBER, CODE 436 FOR CVA IS A NON-SPECIFIC CODE. CODE INSTEAD, IF POSSIBLE, THE INFARCTION, EMBOLUS, OR THROMBUS IF DOCUMENTED IN THE PATIENT'S RECORD.

CVA (CEREBROVASCULAR ACCIDENT)

436 CVA
436 ACUTE
V17.1 FAMILY HISTORY
V12.59 HISTORY WITHOUT RESIDUAL
997.02 IATROGENIC
435.9 IMPENDING (TRANSIENT ISCHEMIC ATTACK)
434.91 LACUNAR INFARCT

CVA (CEREBROVASCULAR ACCIDENT) (continued)

LATE EFFECT

438.9 UNSPECIFIED
438.81 APRAXIA
438.0 COGNITIVE DEFECT
438.82 DYSPHAGIA
438.2# PARALYTIC - HEMIPLEGIA OR HEMIPARESIS
438.4# PARALYTIC - MONOPLEGIA LOWER LIMB
438.3# PARALYTIC - MONOPLEGIA UPPER LIMB

5th Digit: 438.2-4
0. UNSPECIFIED SIDE
1. DOMINANT SIDE
2. NONDOMINANT SIDE

438.5# PARALYTIC - OTHER SYNDROME

5th Digit: 438.5
0. UNSPECIFIED SIDE
1. DOMINANT SIDE
2. NONDOMINANT SIDE
3. BILATERAL

438.1# SPEECH AND LANGUAGE DEFICIT

5th Digit: 438.1
0. UNSPECIFIED
1. APHASIA
2. DYSPHASIA
9. OTHER

438.89 OTHER SPECIFIED

CVA (CEREBROVASCULAR ACCIDENT) (continued)

0 OLD WITH RESIDUAL SEE 'CVA', LATE EFFECT
V12.59 OLD WITHOUT RESIDUAL
997.02 POSTOPERATIVE
435.9 TRANSIENT ISCHEMIC ATTACK (TIA)

266.2 CYANOCOBALAMIN DEFICIENCY (NUTRITIONAL)

CYANOSIS, CYANOTIC

782.5 NOS
770.8 ATTACKS PERINATAL PERIOD
770.8 CONGENITAL
372.71 CONJUNCTIVA
289.7 ENTEROGENOUS
770.8 NEWBORN
362.10 RETINAL

CYCLITIS

364.00 ACUTE SUBACUTE
098.41 GONOCOCCAL
054.44 HERPES SIMPLEX
053.22 HERPES ZOSTER
363.21 POSTERIOR
364.01 PRIMARY
364.02 RECURRENT
364.03 SECONDARY INFECTIOUS
364.04 SECONDARY NONINFECTIOUS
0 SEE ALSO 'IRIDOCYCLITIS'

378.44 CYCLOPHORIA
367.51 CYCLOPLEGIA
301.13 CYCLOTHYMIC DISORDER
378.33 CYCLOTROPIA
733.99 CYRIAX'S (SLIPPING RIB) SYNDROME

CYST

474.8 ADENOID (INFECTED)
255.8 ADRENAL GLAND
518.89 AIR LUNG
526.2 ALVEOLAR PROCESS
762.8 AMNION AFFECTING FETUS OR NEWBORN
658.8# AMNIOTIC COMPLICATING CHILDBIRTH

5th Digit: 658.8
0. EPISODE OF CARE NOS OR N/A
1. DELIVERED
3. ANTEPARTUM COMPLICATION

CYST (continued)

364.62 ANTERIOR CHAMBER - EXUDATIVE
364.60 ANTERIOR CHAMBER - IDIOPATHIC
364.61 ANTERIOR CHAMBER - IMPLANTATION
478.1 ANTRUM
569.49 ANUS
522.8 APICAL (PERIODONTAL)
543.9 APPENDIX
348.0 ARACHNOID
478.79 ARYTENOID
706.2 AURICLE
727.51 BAKER'S KNEE
015.2# BAKER'S KNEE TUBERCULOUS [727.51]

5th Digit: 015.2

0. NOS
1. LAB NOT DONE
2 . LABS PENDING
3. MICROSCOPY POSITIVE (IN SPUTUM)
4. CULTURE POSITIVE - MICROSCOPY
5. CULTURE NEGATIVE - MICROSCOPY POSITIVE
6. CULTURE AND MICROSCOPY NEGATIVE CONFIRMED BY OTHER METHODS

616.2 BARTHOLIN'S GLAND (DUCT)
576.8 BILE DUCT
596.8 BLADDER
362.62 BLESSIG'S
733.2# BONE

5th Digit: 733.2

0. UNSPECIFIED (LOCALIZED)
1. SOLITARY OR UNICAMERAL
2. ANEURYSMAL
9. OTHER

0 BONE JAW SEE 'CYST', JAW, BY TYPE
348.0 BRAIN (SEE ALSO 'CYST CONGENITAL' AND 'CYST OF THE NERVOUS SYSTEM')
0 BRAIN HYDATID SEE 'ECHINOCOCCUS'
610.0 BREAST - BENIGN
610.0 BREAST - BLUE DOME
610.4 BREAST - INVOLUTION
610.0 BREAST - NIPPLE
610.0 BREAST - PEDUNCULATED
610.8 BREAST - SEBACEOUS
610.0 BREAST - SOLITARY
610.0 BREAST - TRAUMATIC
620.8 BROAD LIGAMENT (NONPREGNANT)
518.89 BRONCHOGENIC (MEDIASTINAL) (SEQUESTRATION)
528.4 BUCCAL
599.89 BULBOURETHRAL
727.49 BURSA
629.1 CANAL OF NUCK ACQUIRED
372.75 CANTHUS
336.8 CAUDA EQUINA
348.0 CAVUM SEPTI PELLUCIDI NEC
348.0 CEREBRAL
348.0 CEREBRAL MENINGES
622.8 CERVIX
617.1 CHOCOLATE (OVARY)
576.8 CHOLEDOCHAL
658.8# CHORION COMPLICATING PREGNANCY

5th Digit: 658.8

0. EPISODE OF CARE NOS OR N/A
1. DELIVERED
3. ANTEPARTUM COMPLICATION

348.0 CHOROID PLEXUS
457.8 CHYLE MESENTERY
364.62 CILIARY BODY - EXUDATIVE
364.60 CILIARY BODY - IDIOPATHIC
364.61 CILIARY BODY - IMPLANTATION
364.60 CILIARY BODY - IRIS
624.8 CLITORIS

CYST (continued)

733.20 COCCYX (SEE 'CYST', BONE)
0 COLLOID THYROID GLAND SEE 'GOITER'
0 COLLOID THIRD VENTRICLE BRAIN SEE 'CYST CONGENITAL', CEREBRAL
569.89 COLON
576.8 COMMON BILE DUCT
0 CONGENITAL SEE 'CYST CONGENITAL'
372.75 CONJUNCTIVAL
371.23 CORNEA
348.0 CORPORA QUADRIGEMINA
620.2 CORPUS ALBICANS (OVARY)
620.1 CORPUS LUTEUM OVARY (RUPTURED)
599.89 COWPER'S GLAND
253.8 CRANIOBUCCAL POUCH
253.8 CRANIOPHARYNGEAL POUCH
575.8 CYSTIC DUCT
123.1 CYSTICERCUS (ANY SITE)
526.0 DENTAL PRIMORDIAL (KERATOCYST)
522.8 DENTAL ROOT
526.0 DENTIGEROUS
526.0 DENTIGEROUS MANDIBLE
526.0 DENTIGEROUS MAXILLA
522.8 DENTOALVEOLAR
0 DERMOID SEE 'BENIGN NEOPLASM' BY SITE
0 DERMOID WITH MALIGNANT TRANSFORMATION SEE 'CANCER' BY SITE
709.8 DERMOID IMPLANTATION SKIN NEC
623.8 DERMOID IMPLANTATION VAGINA
624.8 DERMOID IMPLANTATION VULVA
528.4 DERMOID MOUTH
528.4 DERMOID ORAL SOFT TISSUE
685.1 DERMOID SACROCOCCYGEAL
685.0 DERMOID SACROCOCCYGEAL WITH ABSCESS
348.0 DURA CEREBRAL
349.2 DURA SPINAL
706.2 EAR (EXTERNAL)
122.9 ECHINOCOCCAL (SEE 'ECHINOCOCCUS INFECTION')
621.8 ENDOMETRIAL
617.9 ENDOMETRIAL ECTOPIC
706.2 EPIDERMAL (INCLUSION) (SEE ALSO 'CYST' SKIN)
706.2 EPIDERMOID (INCLUSION) (SEE ALSO 'CYST' SKIN)
528.4 EPIDERMOID (INCLUSION) MOUTH
528.4 EPIDERMOID MOUTH
0 EPIDERMOID OTHER THAN SKIN SEE 'CYST' BY SITE
608.89 EPIDIDYMIS
478.79 EPIGLOTTIS
259.8 EPIPHYSIS CEREBRI
706.2 EPITHELIAL INCLUSION (SKIN)
530.89 ESOPHAGUS
364.62 EYE - ANTERIOR CHAMBER EXUDATIVE
364.60 EYE - ANTERIOR CHAMBER IDIOPATHIC
364.61 EYE - ANTERIOR CHAMBER IMPLANTATION
372.75 EYE - CANTHUS
371.23 EYE - CORNEA
364.62 EYE - IRIS EXUDATIVE
364.60 EYE - IRIS IDIOPATHIC
364.61 EYE - IRIS IMPLANTATION
364.55 EYE - IRIS MIOTIC PUPILLARY MARGIN
360.13 EYE - IRIS PARASITIC
379.39 EYE - LENS
373.2 EYE - MEIBOMIAN GLAND
377.54 EYE - OPTIC CHIASM (SEE ALSO 'OPTIC CHIASM')
361.19 EYE - ORA SERRATA
379.8 EYE - RETENTION
361.19 EYE - RETINAL PSEUDOCYST
361.19 EYE - RETINAL OTHER
379.19 EYE - SCLERA
379.29 EYE - VITREOUS HUMOR
706.2 EYEBROW
374.84 EYELID
373.13 EYELID INFECTED
374.84 EYELID SWEAT GLAND OR DUCT

C

CYST (continued)

573.8 FALCIFORM LIGAMENT LIVER (INFLAMMATORY)
620.8 FALLOPIAN TUBE
526.1 FISSURAL OF JAW
526.0 FOLLICULAR DENTIGEROUS
620.0 FOLLICULAR OVARIAN
575.8 GALLBLADDER
0 GANGLION SEE 'GANGLION'
568.89 GAS MESENTERY
629.8 GENITAL ORGAN FEMALE NEC
523.8 GINGIVA
374.84 GLAND OF MOLL
526.1 GLOBULOMAXILLARY
620.0 GRAAFIAN FOLLICLE OVARY
620.2 GRANULOSAL LUTEIN
0 HEMANGIOMATOUS SEE 'HEMANGIOMA'
0 HYDATID FALLOPIAN TUBE SEE 'CYST CONGENITAL', HYDATID
0 HYDATID SEE 'ECHINOCOCCUS'
623.8 HYMEN
478.26 HYPOPHARYNX
253.8 HYPOPHYSIS, HYPOPHYSEAL (DUCT)
253.8 HYPOPHYSIS CEREBRI
526.1 INCISOR
526.1 INCISOR CANAL
0 INCLUSION - SEE 'BENIGN NEOPLASM' BY SITE
706.2 INCLUSION - SKIN
348.0 INTRAMEDULLARY
364.62 IRIS - EXUDATIVE
364.60 IRIS - IDIOPATHIC
364.61 IRIS - IMPLANTATION
364.55 IRIS - MIOTIC PUPILLARY MARGIN
360.13 IRIS - PARASITIC
526.# JAW (BONE)

4th Digit: 526

0. ODONTOGENIC
1. FISSURAL
2. ANEURYSMAL, HEMORRHAGIC, NOS, OTHER, AND TRAUMATIC

526.89 JAW (BONE) LATENT
706.2 KERATIN
593.2 KIDNEY ACQUIRED
727.51 KNEE (BAKER'S)
717.5 KNEE MENISCUS
624.8 LABIUM (MAJUS) (MINUS)
624.8 LABIUM SEBACEOUS
375.43 LACRIMAL APPARATUS
375.12 LACRIMAL GLAND AND CYSTIC DEGENERATION
478.79 LARYNX
379.39 LENS (EYE)
573.8 LIVER
122.8 LIVER ECHINOCOCCAL
122.0 LIVER ECHINOCOCCAL - GRANULOSIS
122.5 LIVER ECHINOCOCCAL - MULTILOCULARIS
518.89 LUNG
492.0 LUNG GIANT BULLOUS
620.1 LUTEIN
228.1 LYMPHANGIOMATOUS
528.4 LYMPHOEPITHELIAL MOUTH
362.54 MACULAR (DEGENERATION) (HOLE OR PSEUDOHOLE)
0 MALIGNANT SEE 'CANCER' BY SITE
610.0 MAMMARY GLAND
611.5 MAMMARY GLAND (MILK)
526.1 MEDIAN ANTERIOR MAXILLARY
526.1 MEDIAN PALATAL
373.2 MEIBOMIAN (GLAND)
717.5 MENISCUS KNEE
457.8 MESENTERY CHYLE
568.89 MESENTERY (MESENTERIC GAS)
568.89 MESOTHELIAL PERITONEUM
568.89 MESOTHELIAL PLEURA (PERITONEAL)

CYST (continued)

528.4 MOUTH
528.4 MOUTH - EPSTEIN'S PEARL
523.8 MOUTH - GINGIVAL
529.8 MOUTH - TONGUE
383.31 MUCOSAL MASTOIDECTOMY COMPLICATION
383.31 MUCOSAL POSTMASTOIDECTOMY CAVITY
239.5 MULTILOCULAR OVARY
621.8 MYOMETRIUM
616.0 NABOTHIAN (GLAND) (NONOBSTETRICAL)
478.1 NASAL ANTRUM
478.1 NASAL CAVITY
478.1 NASAL SEPTUM
478.1 NASAL SINUS
733.20 NASAL TURBINATE
528.4 NASOALVEOLAR MOUTH
528.4 NASOLABIAL
526.1 NASOPALATINE
478.26 NASOPHARYNX
0 NERVOUS SYSTEM SEE 'CYST OF THE NERVOUS SYSTEM'
706.2 NOSE (SKIN OF)
213.1 ODONTOGENIC CALCIFYING
213.0 ODONTOGENIC CALCIFYING UPPER JAW (BONE)
526.0 ODONTOGENIC DEVELOPMENTAL
568.89 OMENTUM (LESSER)
377.54 OPTIC CHIASM (SEE ALSO 'OPTIC CHIASM')
528.4 ORAL SOFT TISSUE (IMPLANTATION)
361.19 ORA SERRATA
376.81 ORBITAL
0 OROPHARYNGEAL SEE 'CYST OROPHARYNGEAL'
763.89 OVARIAN AFFECTING FETUS OR NEWBORN
654.4# OVARIAN COMPLICATING PREGNANCY OR CHILDBIRTH
660.2# OVARIAN COMPLICATING PREGNANCY AND CAUSING OBSTRUCTED LABOR **[654.4#]**

5th Digit: 654.4

0. EPISODE OF CARE NOS OR N/A
1. DELIVERED
2. DELIVERED WITH POSTPARTUM COMPLICATION
3. ANTEPARTUM COMPLICATION
4. POSTPARTUM COMPLICATION

5th Digit: 660.2

0. EPISODE OF CARE NOS OR N/A
1. DELIVERED
3. ANTEPARTUM COMPLICATION

763.1 OVARIAN WITH OBSTRUCTED LABOR AFFECTING FETUS OR NEWBORN
620.2 OVARY
617.1 OVARY - CHOCOLATE
620.2 OVARY - CORPUS ALBICANS
752.0 OVARY - CONGENITAL
620.1 OVARY - CORPUS LUTEUM (HEMORRHAGE) (RUPTURED)
220 OVARY - CYSTADENOMA
620.2 OVARY - CYSTOMA SIMPLE
220 OVARY - DERMOID
620.2 OVARY - DUE TO INVOLUTION FAILURE
617.1 OVARY - ENDOMETRIAL CYSTOMA
620.0 OVARY - GRAAFIAN FOLLICLE
620.0 OVARY - FOLLICULAR
620.2 OVARY - HEMORRHAGIC
620.1 OVARY - LUTEIN
239.5 OVARY - MULTILOCULAR
220 OVARY - NEOPLASTIC
620.8 OVARY - OVIDUCT
220 OVARY - PSEUDOMUCINOUS
256.4 OVARY - POLYCYSTIC (STEIN-LEVENTHAL SYNDROME)
620.2 OVARY - RETENTION
617.1 OVARY - SAMPSON'S
620.2 OVARY - SEROUS
256.4 OVARY - STEIN LEVENTHAL
620.2 OVARY - THECA-LUTEIN
620.2 OVARY - TWISTED
620.2 OVARY - OTHER
620.8 OVIDUCT

CYST (continued)

526.1	PALATINE OF JAW
526.1	PALATINE OF PAPILLA
577.2	PANCREAS
593.2	PARANEPHRIC
136.9	PARASITIC NEC
252.8	PARATHYROID GLAND
599.89	PARAURETHRAL DUCT
593.2	PERIRENAL
527.6	PAROTID GLAND
364.64	PARS PLANA (EXUDATIVE)
364.63	PARS PLANA (PRIMARY)
763.89	PELVIC AFFECTING FETUS OR NEWBORN
654.4#	PELVIC COMPLICATING PREGNANCY OR CHILDBIRTH
660.2#	PELVIC COMPLICATING PREGNANCY AND CAUSING OBSTRUCTED LABOR **[654.4#]**

5th Digit: 654.4

0. EPISODE OF CARE NOS OR N/A
1. DELIVERED
2. DELIVERED WITH POSTPARTUM COMPLICATION
3. ANTEPARTUM COMPLICATION
4. POSTPARTUM COMPLICATION

5th Digit: 660.2

0. EPISODE OF CARE NOS OR N/A
1. DELIVERED
3. ANTEPARTUM COMPLICATION

763.1	PELVIC WITH OBSTRUCTED LABOR AFFECTING FETUS OR NEWBORN
607.89	PENIS (SEBACEOUS)
522.8	PERIAPICAL
423.8	PERICARDIAL ACQUIRED (SECONDARY)
624.8	PERINEUM - FEMALE
355.9	PERINEURAL (TARLOV'S)
522.8	PERIODONTAL
577.2	PERIPANCREATIC
593.2	PERIPELVIC (LYMPHATIC)
568.89	PERITONEAL
457.8	PERITONEAL CHYLOUS
478.26	PHARYNGEAL BURSA
478.26	PHARYNX
478.26	PHARYNX WALL
685.1	PILONIDAL
173.5	PILONIDAL MALIGNANT
685.0	PILONIDAL WITH ABSCESS
253.8	PITUITARY (DUCT) (GLAND)
348.0	PORENCEPHALIC
685.1	POSTANAL INFECTED
685.0	POSTANAL WITH ABSCESS
383.31	POSTMASTOIDECTOMY CAVITY (MUCOSAL CYST)
607.89	PREPUCE
526.0	PRIMORDIAL (JAW)
600	PROSTATE
624.8	PUDENDA (SWEAT GLANDS)
522.8	RADICULAR
522.8	RADICULODENTAL
527.6	RANULA (MOUTH FLOOR)
253.8	RATHKE'S POUCH
569.49	RECTUM (EPITHELIUM) (MUCOUS)
593.2	RENAL ACQUIRED
591	RENAL CALYCEAL OR PYELOGENIC
522.8	RESIDUAL (RADICULAR)
620.2	RETENTION OVARY
706.2	RETENTION SKIN
360.13	RETINAL
362.54	RETINAL MACULAR
360.13	RETINAL PARASITIC
361.13	RETINAL PRIMARY
361.14	RETINAL SECONDARY
361.19	RETINAL PSEUDOCYST
361.19	RETINAL OTHER
568.89	RETROPERITONEAL

CYST (continued)

685.1	SACROCOCCYGEAL (DERMOID)
685.0	SACROCOCCYGEAL (DERMOID) WITH ABSCESS
527.6	SALIVARY GLAND OR DUCT
617.1	SAMPSON'S
379.19	SCLERA
706.2	SEBACEOUS
610.8	SEBACEOUS - BREAST
374.84	SEBACEOUS - EYELID
629.8	SEBACEOUS - GENITAL ORGAN FEMALE
608.89	SEBACEOUS - GENITAL ORGAN MALE
706.2	SEBACEOUS - GLAND (DUCT)
706.2	SEBACEOUS - SCROTUM
717.5	SEMILUNAR CARTILAGE (KNEE) OLD
608.89	SEMINAL VESICLE
620.2	SEROUS (OVARY)
478.1	SINUS (ANTRAL) (ETHMOIDAL) (FRONTAL) (MAXILLARY) (NASAL)
599.89	SKENE'S GLAND
706.2	SKIN
610.8	SKIN - BREAST
706.2	SKIN - EAR (EXTERNAL)
374.84	SKIN - EYELID
216.3	SKIN - FACE NEOPLASTIC
629.8	SKIN - GENITAL ORGAN FEMALE
608.89	SKIN - GENITAL ORGAN MALE
216.3	SKIN - NOSE NEOPLASTIC
706.2	SKIN - SCROTUM
705.89	SKIN - SWEAT GLAND OR DUCT
608.89	SPERMATIC CORD
478.1	SPHENOID SINUS
349.2	SPINAL MENINGES
733.20	SPINE (BONE)
289.59	SPLEEN
348.0	SUBARACHNOID
348.0	SUBDURAL CEREBRAL
349.2	SUBDURAL SPINAL CORD
527.6	SUBLINGUAL GLAND
527.6	SUBMAXILLARY GLAND
599.89	SUBURETHRAL
255.8	SUPRARENAL GLAND
348.0	SUPRASELLAR
705.89	SWEAT GLAND OR DUCT
337.9	SYMPATHETIC NERVOUS SYSTEM
727.40	SYNOVIAL
727.51	SYNOVIAL POPLITEAL SPACE
355.9	TARLOV'S
727.42	TENDON (SHEATH)
608.89	TESTIS
620.2	THECA LUTEIN OF OVARY
478.26	THORNWALDT'S
254.8	THYMUS
246.2	THYROID
0	THYROID ADENOMATOUS SEE 'GOITER' NODULAR
0	THYROID COLLOID SEE 'GOITER'
226	THYROID WITH CYSTADENOMA
529.8	TONGUE
474.8	TONSIL
522.8	TOOTH (DENTAL ROOT)
478.26	TORNWALDT'S
620.8	TUBO OVARIAN
614.1	TUBO OVARIAN INFLAMMATORY
608.89	TUNICA VAGINALIS
733.20	TURBINATE (NOSE)
607.89	TYSON'S GLAND
593.89	URETER
593.89	URETEROVESICAL ORIFICE
599.84	URETHRA
599.89	URETHRAL GLAND
620.8	UTERINE LIGAMENT
621.8	UTERUS

CYST (continued)

386.8	UTRICLE EAR
599.89	UTRICLE PROSTATE
599.89	UTRICULUS MASCULINUS
623.8	VAGINA
478.79	VALLECULA
348.0	VENTRICLE (NEUROEPITHELIAL)
599.89	VERUMONTANUM
596.8	VESICAL ORIFICE
379.29	VITREOUS HUMOR
624.8	VULVA
624.8	VULVOVAGINAL GLAND
706.2	WEN

CYST CONGENITAL

752.11	ACCESSORY FALLOPIAN TUBE
759.1	ADRENAL GLANDS
753.7	ALLANTOIC
751.69	BILE DUCT (CHOLEDOCHAL)
742.4	BRAIN COLLOID THIRD VENTRICLE
744.42	BRANCHIAL CLEFT
752.11	BROAD LIGAMENT (EMBRYONIC)
748.4	BRONCHOGENIC (MEDIASTINAL) (SEQUESTRATION)
752.41	CANAL OF NUCK
746.89	CELOMIC (PERICARDIUM)
742.4	CEREBRAL
751.69	CHOLEDOCHAL
742.4	COLLOID BRAIN THIRD VENTRICLE
742.3	DANDY-WALKER
0	DANDY-WALKER WITH SPINA BIFIDA SEE 'SPINA BIFIDA'
752.11	EMBRYONIC - BROAD LIGAMENT
752.41	EMBRYONIC - CERVIX
752.11	EMBRYONIC - FALLOPIAN TUBES
752.41	EMBRYONIC - HYMEN
752.41	EMBRYONIC - VAGINA
752.11	EMBRYONIC - UTERINE LIGAMENT
752.3	EMBRYONIC - UTERUS
751.5	ENTERIC
751.5	ENTEROGENOUS
748.3	EPIGLOTTIS
752.11	EPOOPHORON
750.4	ESOPHAGUS
743.39	EYE LENS
743.54	EYE POSTERIOR SEGMENT
743.03	EYE RETENTION
752.11	FALLOPIAN TUBE ACCESSORY
752.11	FIMBRIAL
752.11	GARTNER'S DUCT
752.41	GENITALIA FEMALE EMBRYONIC
752.8	HYDATID CYST OF MORGAGNI
752.11	HYDATID CYST OF MORGAGNI - FALLOPIAN TUBES
752.41	HYMEN EMBRYONAL
751.5	INTESTINE (SMALL)
753.11	KIDNEY
0	KIDNEY CYSTIC (DISEASE OF) SEE 'KIDNEY CONGENITAL', CYSTIC DISEASE
0	KIDNEY POLYCYSTIC (DISEASE OF) SEE 'KIDNEY CONGENITAL', POLYCYSTIC
748.3	LARYNX
743.39	LENS
751.62	LIVER
748.4	LUNG (CYSTIC) (POLYCYSTIC)
748.8	MEDIASTINUM
752.8	MESONEPHRIC DUCT
750.26	MOUTH (SUBLINGUAL) (SUBMAXILLARY GLAND)
752.8	MULLERIAN DUCT
742.59	NEUROENTERIC
751.8	OMENTUM
752.0	OVARY
752.11	OVIDUCT

CYST CONGENITAL (continued)

751.7	PANCREAS
752.11	PAROOPHORON
752.11	PAROVARIAN
752.69	PENIS (SEBACEOUS)
746.89	PERICARDIUM
753.8	PERIURETHRAL (TISSUE)
742.4	PORENCEPHALIC
744.47	PREAURICULAR
752.69	PREPUCE
753.11	RENAL SINGLE
759.0	SPLEEN
750.26	SUBLINGUAL
750.26	SUBMAXILLARY GLAND
759.2	THYMUS GLAND
759.2	THYROGLOSSAL DUCT
759.2	THYROLINGUAL DUCT
750.19	TONGUE
759.89	UMBILICUS
753.7	URACHUS
753.4	URETEROVESICAL ORIFICE
752.3	UTERUS EMBRYONAL
752.41	VAGINA EMBRYONAL
752.41	VULVA
752.8	WOLFFIAN

CYST OF THE EYE AND PERIORBITAL STRUCTURES

364.62	ANTERIOR CHAMBER EXUDATIVE
364.60	ANTERIOR CHAMBER IDIOPATHIC
364.61	ANTERIOR CHAMBER IMPLANTATION
372.75	CANTHUS
364.62	CILIARY BODY EXUDATIVE
364.60	CILIARY BODY IDIOPATHIC
364.61	CILIARY BODY IMPLANTATION
372.75	CONJUNCTIVAL
371.23	CORNEA
379.8	EYE RETENTION
374.84	EYELID
364.62	IRIS EXUDATIVE
364.60	IRIS IDIOPATHIC
364.61	IRIS IMPLANTATION
364.55	IRIS MIOTIC PUPILLARY MARGIN
360.13	IRIS PARASITIC
375.12	LACRIMAL GLAND AND CYSTIC DEGENERATION
379.39	LENS
362.54	MACULAR (DEGENERATION) (HOLE OR PSEUDOHOLE)
373.2	MEIBOMIAN GLAND
377.54	OPTIC CHIASM (SEE ALSO 'OPTIC CHIASM')
361.19	ORA SERRATA
376.81	ORBITAL
364.64	PARS PLANA (EXUDATIVE)
364.63	PARS PLANA (PRIMARY)
379.8	RETENTION
360.13	RETINAL
360.13	RETINAL PARASITIC
361.13	RETINAL PRIMARY
361.19	RETINAL PSEUDOCYST
361.14	RETINAL SECONDARY
361.19	RETINAL OTHER
379.19	SCLERA
379.29	VITREOUS HUMOR

CYST OF THE NERVOUS SYSTEM

348.0	ARACHNOID
336.8	CAUDA EQUINA
348.0	CAVUM SEPTI PELLUCIDI NEC
348.0	CEREBRAL MENINGES
348.0	CHOROID PLEXUS
348.0	CORPORA QUADRIGEMINA
348.0	DURA (CEREBRAL)
349.2	DURA (SPINAL)
348.0	PORENCEPHALIC

CYST OF THE NERVOUS SYSTEM (continued)

349.2 SPINAL MENINGES
348.0 SUBARACHNOID
793.0 SUBARACHNOID INTRASELLAR ABNORMAL RADIOLOGICAL STUDY
348.0 SUBDURAL CEREBRAL
349.2 SUBDURAL SPINAL CORD
348.0 VENTRICLE (NEUROEPITHELIAL)

CYST OROPHARYNGEAL

526.2 ALVEOLAR PROCESS (JAW BONE)
526.0 DENTIGEROUS (MANDIBLE) (MAXILLA)
526.1 FISSURAL OF JAW
526.1 GLOBULOMAXILLARY
478.26 HYPOPHARYNX
526.1 INCISOR
526.1 INCISOR CANAL
526.2 JAW
526.2 JAW ANEURYSMAL
526.1 JAW FISSURAL
526.2 JAW HEMORRHAGIC
526.2 JAW TRAUMATIC
526.1 MEDIAN ANTERIOR MAXILLARY
526.1 MEDIAN PALATAL
523.8 MOUTH GINGIVAL
478.1 NASAL (ANTRUM) (CAVITY) (SINUS) (SEPTUM)
526.1 NASOPALATINE
526.0 ODONTOGENIC DEVELOPMENTAL
526.1 PALATINE OF JAW
526.1 PALATINE OF PAPILLA
527.6 PAROTID GLAND
478.26 PHARYNGEAL BURSA
478.26 PHARYNX
526.0 PRIMORDIAL (JAW)
522.8 RADICULAR
522.8 RADICULODENTAL
522.8 RESIDUAL (RADICULAR)
478.1 SINUS (ANTRAL) (ETHMOIDAL) (FRONTAL) (MAXILLARY) (NASAL)
478.1 SPHENOID SINUS
478.26 THORNWALDT'S
474.8 TONSIL

CARCINOMAS AND NEOPLASMS SHOULD BE CODED BY SITE IF POSSIBLE. CODE BY CELL TYPE - "SITE NOS", IF AND ONLY IF A SITE IS NOT SPECIFIED IN THE DIAGNOSIS. OTHERWISE - REFER TO THE APPROPRIATE CATEGORY OF NEOPLASM FOR A MORE SPECIFIC CODE: SEE 'CANCER' 'CANCER METASTATIC', 'NEOPLASM UNCERTAIN BEHAVIOR', 'NEOPLASM UNSPECIFIED NATURE', OR 'BENIGN NEOPLASM'.

CYSTADENOCARCINOMA

199.1 SITE NOS
0 SITE SPECIFIED SEE 'CANCER' BY SITE M8440/3
155.1 BILE DUCT SITE NOS
0 BILE DUCT SITE SPECIFIED SEE 'CANCER' BY SITE M8161/3
183.0 MUCINOUS SITE NOS
0 MUCINOUS SITE SPECIFIED SEE 'CANCER' BY SITE M8470/3
183.0 PAPILLARY MUCINOUS SITE NOS
0 PAPILLARY MUCINOUS SITE SPECIFIED SEE 'CANCER' BY SITE M8471/3
0 PAPILLARY SITE SPECIFIED SEE 'CANCER' BY SITE M8450/3
183.0 PAPILLARY SEROUS SITE NOS
0 PAPILLARY SEROUS SITE SPECIFIED SEE 'CANCER' BY SITE M8460/3
174.9 SEROUS SITE NOS
0 SEROUS SITE SPECIFIED SEE 'CANCER' BY SITE M8441/3

CARCINOMAS AND NEOPLASMS SHOULD BE CODED BY SITE IF POSSIBLE. CODE BY CELL TYPE - "SITE NOS", IF AND ONLY IF A SITE IS NOT SPECIFIED IN THE DIAGNOSIS. OTHERWISE - REFER TO THE APPROPRIATE CATEGORY OF NEOPLASM FOR A MORE SPECIFIC CODE: SEE 'CANCER' 'CANCER METASTATIC', 'NEOPLASM UNCERTAIN BEHAVIOR', 'NEOPLASM UNSPECIFIED NATURE', OR 'BENIGN NEOPLASM'.

CYSTADENOMA

229.9 SITE NOS
0 SITE SPECIFIED SEE 'BENIGN NEOPLASM' BY SITE M8440/0
211.5 BILE DUCT SITE NOS
0 BILE DUCT SITE SPECIFIED SEE 'BENIGN NEOPLASM' BY SITE M8161/0
220 MUCINOUS SITE NOS
0 MUCINOUS (BORDERLINE MALIGNANCY) SITE SPECIFIED SEE 'NEOPLASM UNCERTAIN BEHAVIOR' M8470/1
236.2 MUCINOUS (BORDERLINE MALIGNANCY) SITE NOS
0 MUCINOUS SITE SPECIFIED SEE 'BENIGN NEOPLASM' BY SITE M8470/0
220 PAPILLARY SITE NOS
0 PAPILLARY SITE SPECIFIED SEE 'BENIGN NEOPLASM' BY SITE M8450/0
236.2 PAPILLARY (BORDERLINE MALIGNANCY) SITE NOS M8450/1
0 PAPILLARY (BORDERLINE MALIGNANCY) SITE SPECIFIED SEE 'NEOPLASM UNCERTAIN BEHAVIOR' BY SITE
236.2 PAPILLARY MUCINOUS (BORDERLINE MALIGNANCY) SITE NOS
0 PAPILLARY MUCINOUS (BORDERLINE MALIGNANCY) SITE SPECIFIED SEE 'NEOPLASM UNCERTAIN BEHAVIOR', BY SITE M8471/1
220 PAPILLARY MUCINOUS SITE NOS
0 PAPILLARY MUCINOUS SITE SPECIFIED SEE 'BENIGN NEOPLASM' BY SITE M8471/0
236.2 PAPILLARY SEROUS (BORDERLINE MALIGNANCY) SITE NOS
0 PAPILLARY SEROUS (BORDERLINE MALIGNANCY) SITE SPECIFIED SEE 'NEOPLASM UNCERTAIN BEHAVIOR', BY SITE M8460/1
220 PAPILLARY SEROUS SITE NOS
0 PAPILLARY SEROUS SITE SPECIFIED SITE SPECIFIED SEE 'BENIGN NEOPLASM' BY SITE M8460/0
236.2 SEROUS (BORDERLINE MALIGNANCY) SITE NOS
0 SEROUS (BORDERLINE MALIGNANCY) SITE SPECIFIED SEE 'NEOPLASM UNCERTAIN BEHAVIOR' BY SITE M8441/1
229.9 SEROUS SITE NOS
0 SEROUS SITE SPECIFIED SEE 'BENIGN NEOPLASM' BY SITE M8441/0

270.4 **CYSTATHIONINE METABOLISM DISTURBANCES**

270.4 **CYSTATHIONINEMIA, CYSTATHIONINURIA**

123.1 **CYSTICERCIASIS**

123.1 **CYSTICERCUS CELLULOSAE INFECTION**

CYSTIC

902.24 ARTERY INJURY
908.4 ARTERY INJURY LATE EFFECT
742.4 BRAIN DEGENERATION CONGENITAL
610.1 BREAST DISEASE
620.1 CORPORA LUTEA
575.8 DUCT ADHESION (ATROPHY) (CYST) (ULCER) (DYSKINESIA)
575.8 DUCT ATRESIA
751.61 DUCT ATRESIA CONGENITAL
576.8 DUCT ATROPHY
0 DUCT CALCULUS SEE 'CHOLELITHIASIS'
751.69 DUCT DUPLICATION CONGENITAL
751.61 DUCT OBSTRUCTION (OCCLUSION) CONGENITAL
575.2 DUCT OBSTRUCTION (OCCLUSION) (STENOSIS) (STRICTURE)
0 DUCT OBSTRUCTION (OCCLUSION) (STENOSIS) (STRICTURE) WITH CALCULUS SEE 'CHOLECYSTITIS'
575.8 DUCT DISORDERS OTHER SPECIFIED
575.4 DUCT PERFORATION
576.0 DUCT STUMP SYNDROME

C

CYSTIC (continued)

743.03 EYEBALL CONGENITAL
277.00 FIBROSIS NOS
277.01 FIBROSIS WITH MECONIUM ILEUS
V77.6 FIBROSIS SCREENING
228.1 HYGROMA
0 KIDNEY DISEASE CONGENITAL SEE 'KIDNEY CONGENITAL'
751.62 LIVER DISEASE CONGENITAL
518.89 LUNG ACQUIRED
748.4 LUNG CONGENITAL
0 MASS SEE 'CYST'
610.1 MASTITIS, CHRONIC
620.2 OVARY NOS
751.7 PANCREAS DISEASE CONGENITAL
717.5 SEMILUNAR CARTILAGE DISEASE
902.39 VEIN INJURY
908.4 VEIN INJURY LATE EFFECT
902.39 VEIN LACERATION (RUPTURE) (HEMATOMA) (AVULSION) (ANEURYSM) TRAUMATIC
908.4 VEIN LACERATION LATE EFFECT

123.1 CYSTICERCOSIS
270.0 CYSTINE STORAGE METABOLISM DISORDER
270.0 CYSTINOSIS
270.0 CYSTINURIA

C

CYSTITIS

595.9 NOS
595.0 ACUTE
595.0 ACUTE HEMORRHAGIC
595.89 ALLERGIC
595.2 CHRONIC
595.1 CHRONIC INTERSTITIAL
099.53 CHLAMYDIAL LOWER GENITOURINARY SITES
595.3 FOLLICULAR
595.89 GANGRENOUS
098.11 GONOCOCCAL ACUTE
098.31 GONOCOCCAL CHRONIC
112.2 MONILIAL
595.2 SUBACUTE
595.1 SUBMUCOUS
131.09 TRICHAMONAL
595.3 TRIGONITIS
595.1 ULCERATIVE
595.89 OTHER SPECIFIED

CYSTITIS (OTHER)

039.8 ACTINOMYCOTIC [595.4]
006.8 AMEBIC [595.4]
120.9 BILHARZIASIS (DUE TO) [595.4]
595.89 BULLOUS EMPHYSEMATOUS GLANDULARIS
595.81 CYSTICA
032.84 DIPHTHERITIC
122.3 ECHINOCOCCUS GRANULOSUS [595.4]
122.6 ECHINOCOCCUS MULTICULARIS [595.4]
595.89 EMPHYSEMATOUS
595.82 IRRADIATION

646.6#: SPECIFY THE MATERNAL CYSTITIS WITH AN ADDITIONAL CODE.

646.6# MATERNAL COMPLICATING PREGNANCY
5th Digit: 646.6
0. EPISODE OF CARE NOS OR N/A
1. DELIVERED
2. DELIVERED WITH POSTPARTUM COMPLICATION
3. ANTEPARTUM COMPLICATION
4. POSTPARTUM COMPLICATION

CYSTITIS (OTHER) (continued)

016.1# TUBERCULOUS [595.4]
5th Digit: 016.1
0. NOS
1. LAB NOT DONE
2. LABS PENDING
3. MICROSCOPY POSITIVE (IN SPUTUM)
4. CULTURE POSITIVE - MICROSCOPY NEGATIVE
5. CULTURE NEGATIVE - MICROSCOPY POSITIVE
6. CULTURE AND MICROSCOPY NEGATIVE CONFIRMED BY OTHER METHODS

CYSTOCELE

618.# FEMALE
618.# FEMALE WITH STRESS INCONTINENCE [625.6]
618.# FEMALE WITH OTHER URINARY INCONTINENCE **[788.3#]**
4th Digit: 618
0. WITHOUT UTERINE PROLAPSE
2. WITH INCOMPLETE UTERINE PROLAPSE
3. WITH COMPLETE UTERINE PROLAPSE
4. UTERINE PROLAPSE UNSPECIFIED

5th Digit: 788.3
0. UNSPECIFIED
1. URGE INCONTINENCE
3. MIXED URGE AND STRESS (MALE) (FEMALE)
4 WITHOUT SENSORY AWARENESS
5. POST-VOID DRIBBLING
6. NOCTURNAL ENURESIS
7. CONTINUOUS LEAKAGE
9. OTHER

596.8 MALE

CYSTOCELE OBSTETRICAL

763.89 AFFECTING FETUS OR NEWBORN
654.4# COMPLICATING PREGNANCY
660.2# OBSTRUCTING LABOR **[654.4#]**
5th Digit: 654.4
0. EPISODE OF CARE NOS OR N/A
1. DELIVERED
2. DELIVERED WITH POSTPARTUM COMPLICATION
3. ANTEPARTUM COMPLICATION
4. POSTPARTUM COMPLICATION

5th Digit: 660.2
0. EPISODE OF CARE NOS OR N/A
1. DELIVERED
3. ANTEPARTUM COMPLICATION

763.1 OBSTRUCTING LABOR AFFECTING FETUS OR NEWBORN

594.1 CYSTOLITHIASIS
596.53 CYSTOPLEGIA

CYSTOSARCOMA PHYLLODES

174.9 MALIGNANT SITE NOS
0 MALIGNANT SITE SPECIFIED SEE 'CANCER' BY SITE M9020/3
239.3 SITE NOS
0 SITE SPECIFIED SEE 'NEOPLASM UNCERTAIN BEHAVIOR' BY SITE M9020/1

WHEN CODING AN INFECTION OF AN OSTOMY, USE AN ADDITIONAL CODE TO SPECIFY THE ORGANISM. SEE 'BACTERIAL INFECTION'

CYSTOSTOMY

V55.5 CARE
V55.5 CATHETER ADJUSTMENT OR REPOSITIONING
996.39 CATHETER COMPLICATION (MECHANICAL)
V55.5 CATHETER REMOVAL OR REPLACEMENT
V55.5 CLOSURE
996.39 COMPLICATION CATHETER (MECHANICAL)
997.5 COMPLICATION STOMA
V53.6 DEVICE FITTING AND ADJUSTMENT

CYSTOSTOMY (continued)

997.5 MALFUNCTION
V55.5 REMOVAL OR CHANGE
V44.50 STATUS - NOS
V44.52 STATUS - APPENDICO-VESICOSTOMY
V44.51 STATUS - CUTANEOUS-VESICOSTOMY
V44.59 STATUS - OTHER
V55.5 TOILET STOMA

618.0 CYSTOURETHROCELE (FEMALE) (WITHOUT UTERINE PROLAPSE)

618.0 CYSTOURETHROCELE (FEMALE) (WITHOUT UTERINE PROLAPSE) WITH STRESS INCONTINENCE [625.6]

618.0 CYSTOURETHROCELE (FEMALE) (WITHOUT UTERINE PROLAPSE) WITH OTHER URINARY INCONTINENCE [788.3#]

5th Digit: 788.3

0. UNSPECIFIED
1. URGE INCONTINENCE
3. MIXED URGE AND STRESS (MALE) (FEMALE)
4 WITHOUT SENSORY AWARENESS
5. POST-VOID DRIBBLING
6. NOCTURNAL ENURESIS
7. CONTINUOUS LEAKAGE
9. OTHER

CYTOMEGALOVIRUS INFECTIONS

078.5 CMV
771.1 CONGENITAL OR PERINATAL
V01.7 EXPOSURE
078.5 HEPATITIS [573.1]
078.5 INCLUSION DISEASE (GENERALIZED)
078.5 PNEUMONIA [484.1]

719.06 CZERNY'S PERIODIC HYDRARTHROSIS OF THE KNEE

C

306.2 DA COSTA'S SYNDROME (NEUROCIRCULATORY ASTHENIA)

074.1 DAAE (-FINSEN) EPIDEMIC PLEURODYNIA

DACRYOADENITIS

375.00 DACRYOADENITIS

375.01 ACUTE

375.02 CHRONIC

DACRYOCYSTITIS

375.30 NOS

375.32 ACUTE

375.42 CHRONIC

771.6 NEONATAL

771.6 OPHTHALMIA NEONATORUM

375.33 PHLEGMONOUS

375.57 DACRYOLITH

375.11 DACRYOPS

375.56 DACRYOSTENOSIS

136.0 DACTYLOLYSIS SPONTANEA

282.4 DAMESHEK'S SYNDROME (ERYTHROBLASTIC ANEMIA)

281.0 DANA-PUTNAM SYNDROME (SCLEROSIS SUBACUTE WITH PERNICIOUS ANEMIA) [336.2]

686.8 DANBOLT (-CLOSS) SYNDROME (ACRODERMATITIS ENTEROPATHICA)

297.8 DANCING DISEASE

690.18 DANDRUFF

742.3 DANDY WALKER SYNDROME (ATRESIA, FORAMEN OF MAGENDIE)

741.0# DANDY WALKER SYNDROME (ATRESIA, FORAMEN OF MAGENDIE) WITH SPINA BIFIDA

5th Digit: 741.0

0. REGION NOS

1. CERVICAL REGION

2. DORSAL (THORACIC REGION)

3. LUMBAR REGION

030.1 DANIELSSEN'S ANESTHETIC LEPROSY

756.83 DANLOS' SYNDROME

695.0 DARIER'S ERYTHEMA ANNULARE CENTRIFUGUM

757.39 DARIER'S KERATOSIS FOLLICULARIS CONGENITAL

135 DARIER-ROUSSY SARCOID

264.8 DARIER'S VITAMIN A DEFICIENCY

368.63 DARK ADAPTATION CURVE ABNORMAL

0 DARLING'S DISEASE SEE 'HISTOPLASMOSIS'

744.29 DARWIN'S TUBERCLE CONGENITAL

425.0 DAVIES' ENDOMYOCARDIAL FIBROSIS

733.99 DAVIES-COLLEY SYNDROME (SLIPPING RIB)

046.2 DAWSON'S INCLUSION BODY ENCEPHALITIS

117.1 DE BEURMANN-GOUGEROT SPOROTRICHOSIS

789.2 DEBOVE'S SPLENOMEGALY

727.04 DE QUERVAIN'S TENDINITIS

245.1 DE QUERVAIN'S THYROIDITIS

641.3# DEAD FETUS SYNDROME

5th Digit: 641.3

0. EPISODE OF CARE NOS OR N/A

1. DELIVERED

3. ANTEPARTUM COMPLICATION

389.7 DEAF MUTISM (NONSPEAKING) NEC

DEAFNESS

389.9 NOS

744.03 CONGENITAL

V19.2 FAMILY HISTORY HEARING LOSS

300.11 HYSTERICAL

388.02 ISCHEMIC (TRANSIENT)

389.12 NEURAL

306.7 PSYCHOGENIC

951.5 TRAUMATIC

0 SEE ALSO 'HEARING LOSS'

DEATH

348.8 BRAIN

V68.0 CERTIFICATE ISSUE

768.0 FETAL DUE TO ASPHYXIA OR ANOXIA BEFORE ONSET OF LABOR AND/OR UNSPECIFIED TIME

768.1 FETAL DUE TO ASPHYXIA OR ANOXIA DURING LABOR

779.6 FETAL DUE TO INDUCED ABORTION

779.6 FETAL DUE TO TERMINATION OF PREGNANCY

798.2 IN 24 HOURS FROM ONSET OF SYMPTOMS UNEXPLAINED

798.1 INSTANTANEOUS CAUSE UNKNOWN

761.6 MATERNAL AFFECTING FETUS OR NEWBORN

674.9# MATERNAL SUDDEN (UNKNOWN CAUSE) DUE TO PREGNANCY

5th Digit: 674.9

0. NOS

2. DELIVERED WITH POSTPARTUM COMPLICATION

4. POSTPARTUM COMPLICATION

798.0 SUDDEN INFANT SYNDROME (SIDS)

0 SUDDEN INFANT SYNDROME (SIDS) NEAR MISS - CODE INDIVIDUAL SYMPTOM(S)

798.9 UNATTENDED

798.2 UNEXPLAINED < 24 HOURS FROM ONSET OF SYMPTOMS

DEBILITY

799.3 NOS

780.79 ASTHENIC

779.9 CONGENITAL

300.5 NERVOUS

797 SENILE

874.9 DECAPITATION

993.3 DECOMPRESSION SICKNESS

909.4 DECOMPRESSION SICKNESS LATE EFFECT

DECUBITUS (ULCER)

707.0 ANY SITE

707.0 WITH CELLULITIS [**682.#**]

4th Digit: 682

0. FACE

1. NECK

2. TRUNK

3. UPPER ARM AND FOREARM

4. HAND, EXCEPT FINGERS AND THUMB

5. BUTTOCK

6. LEG, EXCEPT FOOT

7. FOOT, EXCEPT TOES

8. OTHER SPECIFIED SITES

9. UNSPECIFIED SITE

707.0 WITH GANGRENE [785.4]

0 DEER FLY BITE, SEE 'INSECT BITE NONVENOMOUS', BY SITE

021.9 DEER FLY TULAREMIA (SEE ALSO 'TULAREMIA')

255.2 DEFEMINIZATION SYNDROME

639.1 DEFIBRINATION SYNDROME POST ABORTION OR ECTOPIC/MOLAR PREGNANCY

V48.0 DEFICIENCY HEAD

V47.0 DEFICIENCY INTERNAL ORGANS (OF)

V48.1 DEFICIENCY NECK

V48.1 DEFICIENCY TRUNK

738.9 DEFORMITY (ACQUIRED) SITE NOS

0 DEFORMITY SEE ALSO BY ANATOMICAL SITE

759.9 DEFORMITY NOS CONGENITAL

759.7 DEFORMITY MULTIPLE NOS CONGENITAL

738.8 DEFORMITY (ACQUIRED) OTHER SPECIFIED SITE

0 DEGENERATIVE ARTHRITIS SEE 'OSTEOARTHRITIS'

701.3 DEGENERATIVE COLLOID ATROPHY

D

DEGENERATIVE DISC DISEASE

722.6 SITE NOS
722.70 SITE NOS WITH MYELOPATHY
722.4 CERVICAL
722.71 CERVICAL WITH MYELOPATHY
722.52 LUMBAR (LUMBOSACRAL)
722.73 LUMBAR (LUMBOSACRAL)WITH MYELOPATHY
722.51 THORACIC (THORACOLUMBAR)
722.72 THORACIC (THORACOLUMBAR) WITH MYELOPATHY

DEGENERATIVE JOINT DISEASE (DJD)

715.90 SITE UNSPECIFIED
715.97 ANKLE AND/OR FOOT (METATARSALS) (TOES) (TARSALS)
715.93 FOREARM (RADIUS) (WRIST) (ULNA)
715.94 HAND (CARPAL) (METACARPAL) (FINGERS)
715.96 LOWER LEG (FIBULA) (KNEE) (PATELLA) (TIBIA)
715.95 PELVIC REGION AND THIGH (HIP) (BUTTOCK) (FEMUR)
715.91 SHOULDER REGION
721.90 SPINE - NOS
721.0 SPINE - CERVICAL
721.3 SPINE - LUMBAR OR LUMBOSACRAL
721.2 SPINE - THORACIC
715.92 UPPER ARM (ELBOW) (HUMERUS)
715.98 OTHER SPECIFIED

0 DEGLOVING INJURY SEE 'OPEN WOUND' BY SITE

447.8 DEGOS' DISEASE OR SYNDROME

DEHISCENCE OF WOUND POST OP

998.3 ABDOMINAL WOUND POST OP
998.3 WOUND POST OP
674.1.# ABDOMINAL WOUND POST OP C SECTION
674.2.# EPISIOTOMY
674.1.# UTERINE WOUND POST OP C SECTION OR OBSTETRICAL PROCEDURE
674.2.# WOUND POST OP PERINEAL OBSTETRICAL PROCEDURE
674.2.# WOUND POST OP PERINEAL FIRST DEGREE THROUGH FOURTH DEGREE REPAIR

5th Digit: 674.1-2
0. NOS
2. DELIVERED WITH POSTPARTUM COMPLICATION
4. POSTPARTUM COMPLICATION

WHEN A PATIENT IS ADMITTED AND TREATED FOR DEHYDRATION, AND THE TREATMENT IS DIRECTED ONLY AT THAT CONDITION, THE DEHYDRATION WOULD BE THE PRINCIPAL DIAGNOSIS, REGARDLESS OF THE UNDERLYING CONDITION.

778.4 DEHYDRATION FEVER NEWBORN
775.5 DEHYDRATION NEWBORN
276.5 DEHYDRATION VOLUME DEPLETION

386.19 DEITERS' NUCLEUS SYNDROME

348.8 DEJERINE-ROUSSY SYNDROME
356.0 DEJERINE SOTTAS DISEASE
333.0 DEJERINE THOMAS SYNDROME

759.89 DE LANGE'S SYNDROME (AMSTERDAM DWARF, MENTAL RETARDATION AND BRACHYCEPHALY) (CORNELIA)
756.0 DELAYED CLOSURE CRANIAL SUTURES
606.0 DEL CASTILLO SYNDROME (GERMINAL APLASIA)
359.8 DELEAGE'S DISEASE
758.3 DELETION CHROMOSOMES SYNDROME
085.1 DELHI BOIL

DELINQUENCY CONDUCT DISORDER

312.4 NEUROTIC
312.2 GROUP
312.9 JUVENILE

DELIRIUM

780.09 NOS
293.0 ACUTE (TRANSIENT) (ORGANIC) (PSYCHOSIS)
291.0 ALCOHOLIC
292.81 DRUG INDUCED [**304.##**]

4th Digit: 304
0. OPIOID
1. BARBITURATE, SEDATIVES, TRANQUILIZERS WITH SIMILAR EFFECT
2. COCAINE
3. CANNABIS
4. AMPHETAMINE TYPE
5. HALLUCINOGENIC
6. OTHER SPECIFIED
7. MIXED WITH OPIOID
8. MIXED
9. NOS

5th Digit: 304
0. NOS
1. CONTINUOUS
2. EPISODIC
3. IN REMISSION

780.39 ECLAMPTIC
293.1 SUBACUTE (TRANSIENT) (ORGANIC) (PSYCHOSIS)
293.81 TRANSIENT ORGANIC WITH DELUSIONS
293.82 TRANSIENT ORGANIC WITH HALLUCINATIONS
291.0 TREMENS DT'S (ALCOHOL WITHDRAWAL DELIRIUM)
0 SEE ALSO 'PSYCHOSIS'

*650, '**NORMAL DELIVERY**' REFERS TO THE DELIVERY EPISODE OF CARE ONLY. IF A COMPLICATION OF PREGNANCY IS NO LONGER PRESENT AT THE TIME OF DELIVERY, THE DELIVERY ITSELF IS STILL ASSIGNED 650 AS THE PRINCIPAL DIAGNOSIS.*

DELIVERY

650 NORMAL IN COMPLICATED OR UNCOMPLICATED PREGNANCY - SINGLE LIVEBORN (CODE ON MOTHER'S RECORD) [V27.0]
V39.1 NOS - BORN BEFORE ADMISSION TO HOSPITAL (CODE ON INFANT'S RECORD)
V39.0# NOS - BORN IN HOSPITAL (CODE ON INFANT'S RECORD)

5th Digit: V39.0
0. DELIVERED
1. DELIVERED BY CESAREAN SECTION

V39.2 NOS - BORN OUTSIDE HOSPITAL, NOT HOSPITALIZED (CODE ON INFANT'S RECORD)
763.0 AFFECTING FETUS OR NEWBORN - BREECH DELIVERY AND EXTRACTION
763.6 AFFECTING FETUS OR NEWBORN - RAPID SECOND STAGE
669.7# CESAREAN WITHOUT INDICATION

5th Digit: 669.7
0. EPISODE OF CARE NOS OR N/A
1. DELIVERED

669.5# FORCEPS OR VACUUM EXTRACTION

5th Digit: 669.5
0. EPISODE OF CARE NOS OR N/A
1. DELIVERED

V30.1 SINGLE LIVEBORN - BORN BEFORE ADMISSION TO HOSPITAL (CODE ON INFANT'S RECORD)
V30.0# SINGLE LIVEBORN - BORN IN HOSPITAL (CODE ON INFANT'S RECORD)

5th Digit: V30.0
0. DELIVERED
1. DELIVERED BY CESAREAN SECTION

V30.2 SINGLE LIVEBORN - BORN OUTSIDE HOSPITAL, NOT HOSPITALIZED (CODE ON INFANT'S RECORD)
V27.0 SINGLE LIVEBORN (CODE ON MOTHER'S RECORD)
V27.1 SINGLE STILLBORN (CODE ON MOTHER'S RECORD)

DELIVERY (continued)

V31.# TWIN MATE, LIVEBORN - NOT BORN IN HOSPITAL (CODE ON INFANT'S RECORD)
4th Digit: V31
1. BORN BEFORE ADMISSION TO HOSPITAL
2. BORN OUTSIDE HOSPITAL AND NOT HOSPITALIZED

V31.0# TWIN MATE, LIVEBORN - BORN IN HOSPITAL (CODE ON INFANT'S RECORD)
5th Digit: V31.0
0. DELIVERED
1. DELIVERED BY CESAREAN SECTION

V32.# TWIN MATE, STILLBORN - NOT BORN IN HOSPITAL (CODE ON INFANT'S RECORD)
4th Digit: V32
1. BORN BEFORE ADMISSION TO HOSPITAL
2. BORN OUTSIDE HOSPITAL AND NOT HOSPITALIZED

V32.0# TWIN MATE, STILLBORN - BORN IN HOSPITAL (CODE ON INFANT'S RECORD)
5th Digit: V32.0
0. DELIVERED
1. DELIVERED BY CESAREAN SECTION

V33.# TWIN UNSPECIFIED - NOT BORN IN HOSPITAL (CODE ON INFANT'S RECORD)
4th Digit: V33
1. BORN BEFORE ADMISSION TO HOSPITAL
2. BORN OUTSIDE HOSPITAL AND NOT HOSPITALIZED

V33.0# TWIN UNSPECIFIED - BORN IN HOSPITAL (CODE ON INFANT'S RECORD)
5th Digit: V33.0
0. DELIVERED
1. DELIVERED BY CESAREAN SECTION

V27.2 TWINS BOTH LIVEBORN (CODE ON MOTHER'S RECORD)
V27.3 TWINS ONE LIVEBORN AND ONE STILLBORN (CODE ON MOTHER'S RECORD)
V27.4 TWINS BOTH STILLBORN (OUTCOME CODE ON MOTHER'S RECORD)

V34.# OTHER MULTIPLE, MATES ALL LIVEBORN - NOT BORN IN HOSPITAL (CODE ON INFANT'S RECORD)
4th Digit: V34
1. BORN BEFORE ADMISSION TO HOSPITAL
2. BORN OUTSIDE HOSPITAL AND NOT HOSPITALIZED

V34.0# OTHER MULTIPLE, MATES ALL LIVEBORN - BORN IN HOSPITAL (CODE ON INFANT'S RECORD)
5th Digit: V34 .0
0. DELIVERED
1. DELIVERED BY CESAREAN SECTION

V35.# OTHER MULTIPLE, MATES ALL STILLBORN - NOT BORN IN HOSPITAL (CODE ON INFANT'S RECORD)
4th Digit: V35
1. BORN BEFORE ADMISSION TO HOSPITAL
2. BORN OUTSIDE HOSPITAL AND NOT HOSPITALIZED

V35.0# OTHER MULTIPLE, MATES ALL STILLBORN - BORN IN HOSPITAL (CODE ON INFANT'S RECORD)
5th Digit: V35.0
0. DELIVERED
1. DELIVERED BY CESAREAN SECTION

V36.# OTHER MULTIPLE, MATES LIVE AND STILLBORN - NOT BORN IN HOSPITAL (CODE ON INFANT'S RECORD)
4th Digit: V36
1. BORN BEFORE ADMISSION TO HOSPITAL
2. BORN OUTSIDE HOSPITAL AND NOT HOSPITALIZED

V36.0# OTHER MULTIPLE, MATES LIVE AND STILLBORN - BORN IN HOSPITAL (CODE ON INFANT'S RECORD)
5th Digit: V36.0
0. DELIVERED
1. DELIVERED BY CESAREAN SECTION

DELIVERY (continued)

V37.# OTHER MULTIPLE, UNSPECIFIED - NOT BORN IN HOSPITAL (CODE ON INFANT'S RECORD)
4th Digit: V37
1. BORN BEFORE ADMISSION TO HOSPITAL
2. BORN OUTSIDE HOSPITAL AND NOT HOSPITALIZED

V37.0# OTHER MULTIPLE, UNSPECIFIED - BORN IN HOSPITAL (CODE ON INFANT'S RECORD)
5th Digit: V37.0
0. DELIVERED
1. DELIVERED BY CESAREAN SECTION

V27.5 OTHER MULTIPLE BIRTH ALL LIVEBORN (OUTCOME CODE ON MOTHER'S RECORD)
V27.6 OTHER MULTIPLE BIRTH SOME LIVEBORN (CODE ON MOTHER'S RECORD)
V27.7 OTHER MULTIPLE BIRTH ALL STILLBORN (CODE ON MOTHER'S RECORD)
V27.9 OUTCOME OF DELIVERY UNSPECIFIED (CODE ON MOTHER'S RECORD)

644.2# PREMATURE
5th Digit: 644.2
0. EPISODE OF CARE NOS OR N/A
1. DELIVERED

763.6 RAPID SECOND STAGE AFFECTING FETUS OR NEWBORN
0 SEE ALSO 'PREGNANCY COMPLICATIONS', DELIVERY PROBLEMS
0 SEE ALSO 'LABOR AND DELIVERY COMPLICATIONS'

DELIVERY DELAYED

658.3# AFTER ARTIFICIAL RUPTURE OF MEMBRANES
658.2# AFTER SPONTANEOUS RUPTURE OF MEMBRANES
662.1# BIRTH NEC
5th Digit: 658.2-3, 662.1
0. EPISODE OF CARE NOS OR N/A
1. DELIVERED
3. ANTEPARTUM COMPLICATION

763.89 BIRTH NEC AFFECTING FETUS OR NEWBORN
662.3# BIRTH OF SECOND TWIN, TRIPLET, ETC.
5th Digit: 662.3
0. EPISODE OF CARE NOS OR N/A
1. DELIVERED
3. ANTEPARTUM COMPLICATION

763.89 BIRTH OF SECOND TWIN, TRIPLET, ETC. AFFECTING FETUS OR NEWBORN

DELUSIONAL DISORDER (PARANOID STATE)

297.9 NOS
297.2 PARAPHRENIA
300.29 PARASITOSIS
297.3 SHARED PARANOID DISORDER
297.0 SIMPLE PARANOID STATE
297.1 SYSTEMATIZED (GRANDIOSE)
297.8 OTHER SPECIFIED

DELUSIONAL SYNDROME

291.5 ALCOHOL INDUCED (SEE ALSO 'PSYCHOSIS ALCOHOLIC')
290.42 ARTERIOSCLEROTIC [437.0]
292.11 DRUG INDUCED (SEE ALSO 'PSYCHOSIS DRUG INDUCED')
293.81 ORGANIC (TRANSIENT)

117.8 DEMATIACIOUS FUNGI INFECTION

DEMENTIA

294.8 NOS
042 AIDS [294.1]
0 ALCOHOLIC SEE 'PSYCHOSIS ALCOHOLIC'
331.0 ALZHEIMER'S (SENILE) (PRESENILE) [294.1]
299.1# APHONIA SYNDROME OF CHILDHOOD
5th Digit: 299.1
0. ACTIVE STATE
1. RESIDUAL STATE

D

DEMENTIA (continued)

> *290.#(#) DEMENTIA: CODE FIRST ANY ASSOCIATED NEUROLOGICAL CONDITION.*

290.4# ARTERIOSCLEROTIC [437.0]
- **5th Digit: 290.4**
  - **0. NOS**
  - **1. WITH DELIRIUM**
  - **2. DELUSIONAL**
  - **3. DEPRESSIVE**

330.1 CEREBRAL LIPIDOSIS [294.1]
294.8 DIALYSIS [E879.1]
985.8 DIALYSIS DUE TO ALUMINUM OVERLOAD [294.8] [E879.1]
293.9 DIALYSIS TRANSIENT [E879.1]
0 DRUG INDUCED SEE 'PSYCHOSIS DRUG INDUCED'
345.## EPILEPTIC [294.1]
- **4th Digit: 345**
  - **0. GENERALIZED NONCONVULSIVE**
  - **1. GENERALIZED CONVULSIVE**
  - **4. PARTIAL, WITH IMPAIRMENT OF CONSCIOUSNESS**
  - **5. PARTIAL, WITHOUT IMPAIRMENT OF CONSCIOUSNESS**
  - **6. INFANTILE SPASMS**
  - **7. EPILEPSIA PARTIALIS CONTINUA**
  - **8. OTHER FORMS**
  - **9. UNSPECIFIED, NOS**
- **5th Digit: 345**
  - **0. WITHOUT MENTION OF INTRACTABLE EPILEPSY**
  - **1. WITH INTRACTABLE EPILEPSY**

345.3 EPILEPTIC GRAND MAL STATUS [294.1]
345.2 EPILEPTIC PETIT MAL STATUS [294.1]
275.1 HEPATOLENTICULAR DEGENERATION [294.1]
333.4 HUNTINGTON'S CHOREA [294.1]
046.1 JAKOB CREUTZFELDT (PRESENILE) [294.1]
0 MULTI-INFARCT SEE 'DEMENTIA', ARTERIOSCLEROTIC
340 MULTIPLE SCLEROSIS [294.1]
0 NEUROSYPHILIS SEE 'NEUROSYPHILIS'
090.40 PARALYTICA JUVENILIS
333.0 PELIZAEUS-MERZBACHER DISEASE [294.1]
331.1 PICK'S DISEASE [294.1]
446.0 POLYARTERITIS NODOSA [294.1]

> *290.#(#) DEMENTIA: CODE FIRST ANY ASSOCIATED NEUROLOGICAL CONDITION.*

PRESENILE
290.10 NOS
290.11 WITH DELIRIUM
290.12 WITH DELUSIONS
290.13 WITH DEPRESSION

> *290.#(#) DEMENTIA: CODE FIRST ANY ASSOCIATED NEUROLOGICAL CONDITION.*

SENILE
290.0 NOS
290.4# ARTERIOSCLEROTIC [437.0]
- **5th Digit: 290.4**
  - **0. NOS**
  - **1. WITH DELIRIUM**
  - **2. DELUSIONAL**
  - **3. DEPRESSIVE**

290.20 DELUSIONAL
290.21 DEPRESSIVE
090.40 PARALYTICA JUVENILIS
290.20 PARANOID TYPE
094.1 SYPHILITIC [294.1]
290.3 WITH ACUTE CONFUSIONAL STATE
290.3 WITH DELIRIUM

D

DEMENTIA (continued)
094.1 SYPHILITIC [294.1]
275.1 WILSON'S DISEASE [294.1]

133.8 DEMODEX FOLLICULORUM INFESTATION
341.9 DEMYELINATING DISEASE OR SYNDROME (CENTRAL NERVOUS SYSTEM)
341.8 DEMYELINATING DISEASE OR SYNDROME (CENTRAL NERVOUS SYSTEM) OTHER SPECIFIED NEC
357.8 DEMYELINATING POLYNEURITIS CHRONIC INFLAMMATORY

DENGUE
061 DENGUE
V73.5 FEVER SCREENING EXAM
065.4 HEMORRHAGIC FEVER

307.9 DENIAL VISUAL HALLUCINATION SYNDROME
520.2 DENS EVAGINATUS (INVAGINATUS)
520.2 DENS IN DENTE

DENTAL
524.7# ALVEOLAR ANOMALY
- **5th Digit: 524.7**
  - **0. UNSPECIFIED**
  - **1. MAXILLARY HYPERPLASIA**
  - **2. MANDIBULAR HYPERPLASIA**
  - **3. MAXILLARY HYPOPLASIA**
  - **4. MANDIBULAR HYPOPLASIA**
  - **9. OTHER SPECIFIED**

523.6 CALCULUS SUBGINGIVAL
523.6 CALCULUS SUPRAGINGIVAL
521.0 CARIES
V52.3 PROSTHETIC DEVICE (FITTING AND ADJUSTMENT) (REMOVAL)
522.2 PULP CALCIFICATION
525.3 ROOT RETAINED

520.6 DENTIA PRAECOX

DENTIN
522.3 IRREGULAR (PULP)
520.5 OPALESCENT
522.3 SECONDARY (PULP)
521.8 SENSITIVE

520.5 DENTINAL DYSPLASIA
521.5 DENTINAL HYPERPLASIA
520.4 DENTINAL PAPILLA CALCIFICATION
520.5 DENTINOGENESIS IMPERFECTA
213.# DENTINOMA M9271/0
- **4th Digit: 213**
  - **0. SKULL FACE UPPER JAW**
  - **1. LOWER JAW (OR IF SITE UNSPECIFIED)**

520.6 DENTITION DISORDER (OBSTRUCTED) (DELAYED) (NEONATAL) (PREMATURE) (DELAYED)
524.7# DENTOALVEOLAR ANOMALIES
- **5th Digit: 524.7**
  - **0. UNSPECIFIED ALVEOLAR ANOMALY**
  - **1. ALVEOLAR MAXILLARY HYPERPLASIA**
  - **2. ALVEOLAR MANDIBULAR HYPERPLASIA**
  - **3. ALVEOLAR MAXILLARY HYPOPLASIA**
  - **4. ALVEOLAR MANDIBULAR HYPOPLASIA**
  - **9. OTHER SPECIFIED ALVEOLAR ANOMALY**

524.5 DENTOFACIAL ABNORMALITIES FUNCTIONAL
524.9 DENTOFACIAL ANOMALIES
524.8 DENTOFACIAL ANOMALIES OTHER SPECIFIED
528.9 DENTURE SORE
V52.3 DENTURES FITTING AND ADJUSTMENT

DEPENDENCE

V46.0 ASPIRATOR (MECHANICAL)

V46.8 HYPERBARIC CHAMBER

V46.9 MACHINE

V46.8 POSSUM

V46.1 RESPIRATORY

0 SUBSTANCE SEE SUBSTANCE ABUSE OR SEE BY SUBSTANCE

301.59 DEPENDENT PERSONALITY

300.6 DEPERSONALIZATION SYNDROME

V25.02 DEPO-PROVERA INJECTION

V25.49 DEPO-PROVERA INJECTION REPEAT

DEPRESSION

311 NOS

296.82 DISORDER ATYPICAL (PSYCHOSIS)

296.3# DISORDER RECURRENT EPISODE (PSYCHOSIS)

296.2# DISORDER SINGLE EPISODE (PSYCHOSIS)

292.84 DRUG INDUCED

296.3# ENDOGENOUS (PSYCHOTIC) RECURRENT EPISODE (PSYCHOSIS)

296.2# ENDOGENOUS (PSYCHOTIC) SINGLE EPISODE

296.3# INVOLUTIONAL RECURRENT (PSYCHOSIS)

296.2# INVOLUTIONAL SINGLE EPISODE OR UNSPECIFIED

5th Digit: 296.2-3

0. UNSPECIFIED
1. MILD
2. MODERATE
3. SEVERE WITHOUT MENTION OF PSYCHOTIC BEHAVIOR
4. SEVERE SPECIFIED AS WITH PSYCHOTIC BEHAVIOR
5. IN PARTIAL OR UNSPECIFIED REMISSION
6. IN FULL REMISSION

648.4# MATERNAL CURRENT (CO-EXISTENT) IN PREGNANCY

5th Digit: 648.4

0. EPISODE OF CARE NOS
1. DELIVERED WITH OR WITHOUT MENTION OF ANTEPARTUM CONDITION
2. DELIVERED WITH MENTION OF POSTPARTUM COMPLICATION
3. ANTEPARTUM CONDITION
4. POSTPARTUM COMPLICATION

296.2# MONOPOLAR (SINGLE EPISODE OR UNSPECIFIED)

296.3# MONOPOLAR RECURRENT

5th Digit: 296.2-3

0. UNSPECIFIED
1. MILD
2. MODERATE
3. SEVERE WITHOUT MENTION OF PSYCHOTIC BEHAVIOR
4. SEVERE SPECIFIED AS WITH PSYCHOTIC BEHAVIOR
5. IN PARTIAL OR UNSPECIFIED REMISSION
6. IN FULL REMISSION

300.4 NEUROTIC

DEPRESSION (continued)

648.4# POSTPARTUM - (BLUES)

648.4# POSTPARTUM - DEPRESSION NOS [311]

648.4# POSTPARTUM PSYCHOTIC - RECURRENT [**296.3#**]

648.4# POSTPARTUM PSYCHOTIC - SINGLE EPISODE [**296.2#**]

5th Digit: 648.4

0. EPISODE OF CARE NOS
1. DELIVERED WITH OR WITHOUT MENTION OF ANTEPARTUM CONDITION
2. DELIVERED WITH MENTION OF POSTPARTUM COMPLICATION
3. ANTEPARTUM CONDITION
4. POSTPARTUM COMPLICATION

5th Digit: 296.2-3

0. UNSPECIFIED
1. MILD
2. MODERATE
3. SEVERE WITHOUT MENTION OF PSYCHOTIC BEHAVIOR
4. SEVERE SPECIFIED AS WITH PSYCHOTIC BEHAVIOR
5. IN PARTIAL OR UNSPECIFIED REMISSION

300.4 REACTIVE NEUROSIS

298.0 REACTIVE PSYCHOTIC

V79.0 SCREENING

293.83 TRANSIENT (ORGANIC) (PSYCHOSIS) (ALCOHOLIC) (DRUGS)

300.4 WITH ANXIETY (NEUROTIC)

DEPRESSIVE

311 DISORDER UNSPECIFIED

296.82 DISORDER ATYPICAL (PSYCHOSIS)

311 DISORDER NEC

300.4 NEUROSIS (REACTIVE)

301.12 PERSONALITY DISORDER CHRONIC

298.0 PSYCHOSIS REACTIVE

296.3# PSYCHOSIS RECURRENT (MAJOR) EPISODE

296.2# PSYCHOSIS SINGLE EPISODE OR UNSPECIFIED

5th Digit: 296.2-3

0. UNSPECIFIED
1. MILD
2. MODERATE
3. SEVERE WITHOUT MENTION OF PSYCHOTIC BEHAVIOR
4. SEVERE SPECIFIED AS WITH PSYCHOTIC BEHAVIOR
5. IN PARTIAL OR UNSPECIFIED REMISSION
6. IN FULL REMISSION

300.4 REACTION (NEUROSIS)

309.0 REACTION BRIEF

309.1 REACTION PROLONGED (ADJUSTMENT REACTION)

309.4 REACTION WITH CONDUCT DISTURBANCE

290.43 SYNDROME ARTERIOSCLEROTIC [437.0]

596.55 DETRUSOR SPHINCTER DYSSYNERGIA

727.04 DEQUERVAIN TENDONITIS

245.1 DEQUERVAIN THYROIDITIS

0 DERANGEMENT JOINT SEE 'JOINT', DERANGEMENT

272.8 DERCUM'S SYNDROME (ADIPOSIS DOLOROSA)

300.6 DEREALIZATION (NEUROTIC)

757.39 DERMAL HYPOPLASIA

DERMATITIS

692.9 UNSPECIFIED
692.82 AB IGNE
692.70 ACTINIC SOLAR
692.72 ACTINIC SOLAR - ACUTE
692.74 ACTINIC SOLAR - CHRONIC
692.89 ACTINIC OTHER
698.4 ARTEFACTA
316 ARTEFACTA PSYCHOGENIC [698.4]
691.8 ATOPIC
701.8 ATROPHICANS (DIFFUSA)
701.3 ATROPHICANS MACULOSA
694.9 BULLOUS
694.9 BULLOSA
692.6 BULLOSA STRIATA PRATENSIS
120.3 CERCARIAL CUTANEOUS
991.5 CONGELATIONIS
0 CONTACT SEE 'DERMATITIS CONTACT'
695.2 CONTUSIFORMIS
032.85 DIPHTHERITICA
692.82 DUE TO OTHER RADIATION
692.3 DUE TO DRUGS AND MEDICINES APPLIED TO SKIN
693.0 DUE TO DRUGS AND MEDICINES INGESTED
692.5 DUE TO FOOD IN CONTACT WITH SKIN
693.1 DUE TO FOOD INGESTED
693.9 DUE TO SUBSTANCES - UNSPECIFIED INGESTED
693.0 DUE TO SUBSTANCES - SPECIFIED INGESTED
693.8 DUE TO SUBSTANCES - OTHER INGESTED
625.8 DYSMENORRHEICA
690.8 ECZEMATOUS INFECTIOUS
692.9 ECZEMATOUS NEC
695.89 EPIDEMICA
695.81 ERYSIPELATOSA
695.89 EXFOLIATIVA
695.81 EXFOLIATIVA (INFANTUM) (NEONATORUM)
0 EYELID SEE 'DERMATITIS EYELID'
698.4 FACTITIA (ARTEFACTA)
704.8 FOLLICULARIS
646.8# GESTATIONIS

5th Digit: 646.8

0. EPISODE OF CARE NOS OR N/A
1. DELIVERED
2. DELIVERED WITH POSTPARTUM COMPLICATION
3. ANTEPARTUM COMPLICATION
4. POSTPARTUM COMPLICATION

694.0 HERPETIFORMIS
694.2 HERPETIFORMIS JUVENILE
694.5 HERPETIFORMIS SENILE
692.89 HIEMALIS
690.12 INFANTILE
690.8 INFECTIOSA ECZEMATOIDES
686.9 INFECTIOUS (STAPHYLOCOCCAL) (STREPTOCOCCAL)
690.8 INFECTIOUS (STAPHYLOCOCCAL) (STREPTOCOCCAL) ECZEMATOID
695.89 INTERTRIGINOUS SUPERFICIAL DUE TO (HEAT) (MOISTURE) (FRICTION)
709.1 LICHENOIDES PURPURICA PIGMENTOSA
692.3 MEDICAMENTOSA APPLIED TO SKIN
693.0 MEDICAMENTOSA INGESTED
694.0 MULTIFORMIS
694.2 MULTIFORMIS JUVENILE
694.5 MULTIFORMIS SENILE
691.8 NEUROGENIC
694.0 NEUROTICA
706.1 PAPILLARIS CAPILLITII
695.3 PERIORAL
694.0 POLYMORPHA DOLOROSA
694.0 PRURIGINOSA
694.2 PSORIASIFORM NODULARIS
316 PSYCHOGENIC [692.9]
686.00 PURULENT

DERMATITIS (continued)

686.00 PYOCOCCAL, PYOCOCCIDE
686.09 PYOCYANEUS
686.00 PYOGENICA
690.10 SEBORRHEIC
690.10 SEBORRHEIC EXTERNAL EAR [380.13]
690.11 SEBORRHEIC CAPITIS
690.11 SEBORRHEIC CAPITIS EXTERNAL EAR [380.13]
690.12 SEBORRHEIC INFANTILE
690.12 SEBORRHEIC INFANTILE EXTERNAL EAR [380.13]
690.18 SEBORRHEIC OTHER
690.18 SEBORRHEIC OTHER EXTERNAL EAR [380.13]
686.00 SEPTIC
0 SOLAR SEE 'DERMATITIS SOLAR'
459.81 STASIS
459.81 STASIS ULCERATED [**707.#**]

4th Digit: 707

1. LOWER LIMB EXCEPT DECUBITUS
8. CHRONIC OF OTHER SPECIFIED SITE
9. CHRONIC SITE NOS

454.1 STASIS VARICOSE
454.2 STASIS VARICOSE ULCERATED
459.1 STASIS VARICOSE DUE TO POSTPHLEBITIC SYNDROME
459.1 STASIS VARICOSE SECONDARY TO DEEP VEIN THROMBOSIS
709.8 TRAUMATIC NEC
694.0 TROPHONEUROTICA
686.8 VEGETANS
117.2 VERRUCOSA

DERMATITIS CONTACT QUICK REFERENCE

692.9 NOS
692.4 CHEMICAL PRODUCTS
692.0 DETERGENTS
692.3 DRUGS AND MEDICINES (IN CONTACT WITH SKIN)
692.5 FOOD (IN CONTACT WITH SKIN)
692.1 OILS AND GREASES
692.6 PLANTS (EXCEPT FOOD)
692.7# SOLAR RADIATION

5th Digit: 692.7

0. NOS
1. SUNBURN
2. ACUTE DUE TO SOLAR RADIATION
3. ACTINIC RETICULOID AND ACTINIC GRANULOMA
4. CHRONIC DUE TO SOLAR RADIATION
9. OTHER DUE TO SOLAR RADIATION

692.2 SOLVENTS
686.00 SUPPURATIVE
692.8# OTHER SPECIFIED

5th Digit: 692.8

1. DUE TO COSMETICS
2. DUE TO OTHER RADIATION
3. DUE TO METALS, JEWELRY
9. OTHER SUBSTANCES OR TRANSIENT TEMPERATURE

DERMATITIS CONTACT

692.9 NOS
692.2 ACETONE
692.4 ACIDS
692.4 ADHESIVE PLASTER (TAPE)
692.4 ALCOHOL (IN CONTACT WITH SKIN)
692.4 ALKALIS
692.9 ALLERGY
692.4 AMMONIA (HOUSEHOLD) (LIQUID)
692.3 ARNICA (IN CONTACT WITH SKIN)
692.4 ARSENIC
692.89 BLISTER BEETLE

DERMATITIS CONTACT (continued)

692.89 CATERPILLAR
692.4 CAUSTICS
692.5 CEREAL (IN CONTACT WITH SKIN)
692.2 CHLOROCOMPOUND
692.5 COFFEE (IN CONTACT WITH SKIN)
692.89 COLD WEATHER
692.81 COSMETICS
692.2 CYCLOHEXANE
692.81 DEODORANT
692.0 DETERGENTS
692.4 DICHROMATES
692.3 DRUGS AND MEDICINES (IN CONTACT WITH SKIN)
692.89 DYES
692.2 ESTER
373.32 EYELIDS
692.5 FISH (IN CONTACT WITH SKIN)
692.5 FLOUR (IN CONTACT WITH SKIN)
692.5 FRUIT (IN CONTACT WITH SKIN)
692.3 FUNGICIDES (IN CONTACT WITH SKIN)
692.89 FUR
692.2 GLYCOL
692.1 GREASE
692.89 HOT WEATHER OR PLACES
692.2 HYDROCARBONS
692.82 INFRARED RAYS
692.4 INSECTICIDES
692.3 IODINE (IN CONTACT WITH SKIN)
692.3 IODOFORM (IN CONTACT WITH SKIN)
692.83 JEWELRY
692.3 KERATOLYTICS (IN CONTACT WITH SKIN)
692.2 KETONE GROUP
692.6 LACQUER TREE [RHUS VERNICIFLUA]
692.82 LIGHT, EXCEPT SUN
692.5 MEAT (IN CONTACT WITH SKIN)
692.3 MERCURIALS (IN CONTACT WITH SKIN)
692.83 METALS
692.5 MILK (IN CONTACT WITH SKIN)
692.3 NEOMYCIN (IN CONTACT WITH SKIN)
692.4 NYLON
692.1 OIL
692.2 PAINT
692.3 PEDICULOCIDES (IN CONTACT WITH SKIN)
692.4 PETROLEUM
692.3 PHENOLS (IN CONTACT WITH SKIN)
692.6 PLANTS
692.3 PLASTERS MEDICATED (IN CONTACT WITH SKIN)
692.4 PLASTIC
692.6 POISON IVY [RHUS TOXICODENDRON]
692.6 POISON OAK [RHUS DIVERSILOBA]
692.6 POISON SUMAC [RHUS VENENATA]
692.6 POISON VINE [RHUS RADICANS]
692.89 PRESERVATIVES
692.6 PRIMROSE [PRIMULA]
692.82 RADIOACTIVE SUBSTANCES
692.6 RAGWEED [SENECIO JACOBAE]
692.4 RUBBER
692.3 SCABICIDES (IN CONTACT WITH SKIN)
0 SOLAR SEE 'DERMATITIS SOLAR'
692.3 TOPICAL MEDICATIONS (IN CONTACT WITH SKIN)
692.2 TURPENTINE
692.82 ULTRAVIOLET RAYS, EXCEPT SUN
692.82 X-RAY
692.4 OTHER CHEMICAL PRODUCTS
692.6 OTHER PLANTS IN CONTACT WITH THE SKIN
692.82 OTHER RADIATION
692.89 OTHER SUBSTANCES

DERMATITIS EYELID

039.3 ACTINOMYCOTIC [373.5]
373.31 ECZEMATOUS
373.32 CONTACT AND ALLERGIC
110.8 DERMATOPHYTIC [373.5]
054.41 HERPES SIMPLEX
053.20 HERPES ZOSTER
684 IMPETIGO [373.5]
030.0 LEPROMATOUS [373.4]
017.0# LUPUS VULGARIS (TUBERCULOUS) [373.4]
5th Digit: 017.0
0. UNSPECIFIED
1. LAB NOT DONE
2. LABS PENDING
3. MICROSCOPY POSITIVE (IN SPUTUM)
4. CULTURE POSITIVE - MICROSCOPY NEGATIVE
5. CULTURE NEGATIVE - MICROSCOPY POSITIVE
6. CULTURE AND MICROSCOPY NEGATIVE CONFIRMED BY OTHER METHODS
111.9 MYCOTIC [373.5]
373.5 OTHER INFECTIVE
999.0 POST VACCINATION [373.5]
017.0# TUBERCULOUS [373.4]
5th Digit: 017.0
0. UNSPECIFIED
1. LAB NOT DONE
2. LABS PENDING
3. MICROSCOPY POSITIVE (IN SPUTUM)
4. CULTURE POSITIVE - MICROSCOPY NEGATIVE
5. CULTURE NEGATIVE - MICROSCOPY POSITIVE
6. CULTURE AND MICROSCOPY NEGATIVE CONFIRMED BY OTHER METHODS
051.0 VACCINIA [373.5]
102.9 YAWS [373.4]

DERMATITIS SOLAR

692.70 NOS
692.73 ACTINIC RETICULOID AND ACTINIC GRANULOMA
692.72 ACUTE DUE TO SOLAR RADIATION
692.72 ACUTE SOLAR SKIN DAMAGE NOS
692.72 BERLOQUE
692.74 CHRONIC DUE TO SOLAR RADIATION
692.74 CHRONIC SOLAR SKIN DAMAGE NOS
692.74 ELASTOSIS
692.72 PHOTOALLERGIC RESPONSE
692.72 PHOTOTOXIC RESPONSE
692.72 POLYMORPHUS LIGHT ERUPTION
692.79 SKIN DAMAGE NOS
692.71 SUNBURN
692.79 OTHER

134.0 DERMATOBIA (HOMINIS) INFESTATION
374.87 DERMATOCHALASIS
216.# DERMATOFIBROMA NOS M8832/0
4th Digit: 216
0. LIP (SKIN OF)
1. EYELID INCLUDING CANTHUS
2. EAR (EXTERNAL) (AURICLE) (PINNA)
3. FACE (CHEEK) (NOSE)
4. SCALP NECK
5. TRUNK BACK CHEST
6. UPPER LIMB INCLUDING SHOULDER
7. LOWER LIMB INCLUDING HIP
8. OTHER SPECIFIED SITES
9. SKIN UNSPECIFIED

238.2 DERMATOFIBROMA PROTUBERANS SITE NOS
0 DERMATOFIBROMA PROTUBERANS SEE 'NEOPLASM UNCERTAIN BEHAVIOR', SKIN, BY SITE M8832/1

171.9 DERMATOFIBROSARCOMA SITE NOS
0 DERMATOFIBROSARCOMA SITE SPECIFIED SEE 'CANCER', SKIN, BY SITE M8832/3

757.2 DERMATOGLYPHIC ANOMALIES CONGENITAL
708.3 DERMATOGRAPHIA
111.9 DERMATOMYCOSIS
111.8 DERMATOMYCOSIS OTHER SPECIFIED
710.3 DERMATOMYOSITIS
110.1 DERMATOPHYTIC ONYCHIA
110.# DERMATOPHYTOSIS

4th Digit: 110

0. SCALP AND BEARD
1. NAIL (UNGUIUM)
2. HAND (MANUUM)
3. GROIN AND PERIANAL (CRURIS)
4. FOOT (PEDIS)
5. BODY (CORPORUS)
6. DEEP SEATED (GRANULOMA TRICHOPHYTICUM)
8. OTHER SPECIFIED SITE
9. UNSPECIFIED SITE

698.8 DERMATOPIELINOSIS
701.0 DERMATOSCLEROSIS LOCALIZED

DERMATOSIS

709.9 NOS
691.8 ATOPIC
694.9 BULLOUS
690.8 ERYTHEMATOSQUAMOUS
695.89 EXFOLIATIVA
698.4 FACTITIAL
098.89 GONOCOCCAL
694.0 HERPETIFORMIS
694.2 HERPETIFORMIS JUVENILE
694.5 HERPETIFORMIS SENILE
709.8 MENSTRUAL
695.89 NEUTROPHILIC, ACUTE FEBRILE
709.8 PAPULOSA NIGRA
709.00 PIGMENTARY NEC
0 PREGNANCY SEE 'PUPP'
709.09 PROGRESSIVE PIGMENTARY
316 PSYCHOGENIC [709.9]
709.3 SENILE NEC
690.10 UNNA'S (SEBORRHEIC DERMATITIS)

229.9 DERMOID CYST SITE UNSPECIFIED
0 DERMOID CYST SITE SPECIFIED SEE 'BENIGN NEOPLASM' BY SITE M9084/0
183.0 DERMOID CYST WITH MALIGNANT TRANSFORMATION SITE NOS
0 DERMOID CYST WITH MALIGNANT TRANSFORMATION SITE SPECIFIED SEE 'CANCER' BY SITE M9084/3

655.5# DES (KNOWN) (SUSPECTED) DAMAGE TO FETUS COMPLICATING PREGNANCY MANAGEMENT

5th Digit: 655.5

0. EPISODE OF CARE UNSPECIFIED OR N/A
1. DELIVERED
3. ANTEPARTUM COMPLICATION

760.76 DES TRANSMITTED VIA PLACENTA OR BREAST MILK AFFECTING FETUS OR NEWBORN
371.32 DESCEMET'S MEMBRANE FOLDS
371.33 DESCEMET'S MEMBRANE RUPTURE
371.72 DESCEMETOCELE
V07.1 DESENSITIZATION ALLERGY
0 DESERT RHEUMATISM SEE 'COCCIDIOIDOMYCOSIS'
995.84 DESERTION ADULT
995.52 DESERTION CHILD (NEWBORN)
238.1 DESMOID TUMOR SITE UNSPECIFIED
0 DESMOID TUMOR (ABDOMINAL) SITE SPECIFIED SEE 'NEOPLASM UNCERTAIN BEHAVIOR' OTHER AND UNSPECIFIED SITES CONNECTIVE AND OTHER TISSUE M8822/1
0 DESMOID TUMOR (EXTRA-ABDOMINAL) SITE SPECIFIED SEE 'NEOPLASM UNCERTAIN BEHAVIOR' OTHER AND UNSPECIFIED SITES CONNECTIVE AND OTHER TISSUE M8821/1

362.43 DETACHMENT RETINAL PIGMENT EPITHELIUM HEMORRHAGIC
977.3 DETERRENT ALCOHOL
270.0 DE TONI-FANCONI (-DEBRE) SYNDROME (CYSTINOSIS)
596.59 DETRUSOR INSTABILITY
368.52 DEUTAN DEFECT
368.52 DEUTERANOMALY
368.52 DEUTERANOPIA
117.4 DEUTEROMYCETES INFECTION
0 DEUTSCHLANDER'S SEE 'FRACTURE' FOOT

DEVELOPMENTAL DISORDER

315.9 NOS
314.1 ASSOCIATED WITH HYPERKINESIA
315.4 CLUMSINESS SYNDROME
315.4 COORDINATION
783.4 DELAY (PHYSIOLOGICAL)
V79.9 HANDICAPS SCREENING
V79.3 HANDICAPS IN EARLY CHILDHOOD SCREENING
V79.8 HANDICAPS OTHER SPECIFIED SCREENING
315.31 LANGUAGE EXPRESSIVE
315.32 LANGUAGE RECEPTIVE (RECEPTIVE-EXPRESSIVE) (MIXED)
315.2 LEARNING
315.1 MATHEMATICS
315.5 MIXED
315.39 PHONOLOGICAL (SPEECH) (READING)
783.9 PHYSIOLOGICAL DEVELOPMENTAL PROBLEM
315.00 READING
315.39 READING PHONOLOGICAL
315.39 SPEECH PHONOLOGICAL
315.09 SPELLING
V20.2 TESTING (CHILD) (INFANT)
315.31 WORD DEAFNESS (DELAY IN DEVELOPMENT)
315.2 WRITTEN EXPRESSION
315.2 OTHER SPECIFIED LEARNING DISORDER
315.09 OTHER SPECIFIED READING OR SPELLING DISORDER
315.39 OTHER SPECIFIED SPEECH OR LANGUAGE DISORDER
315.8 OTHER SPECIFIED DELAY IN DEVELOPMENT

696.4 DEVERGIE'S PITYRIASIS RUBRA PILARIS
470 DEVIATED NASAL SEPTUM (ACQUIRED)
V53.9 DEVICE OTHER AND UNSPECIFIED FITTING AND ADJUSTMENT
341.0 DEVIC'S NEUROMYELITIS OPTICA
074.1 DEVIL'S GRIP
746.87 DEXTROCARDIA
759.3 DEXTROCARDIA WITH VISCERA

> *CLASSIFICATION OF DIABETES IS BASED ON INSULIN DEPENDENCE RATHER THAN THE MEDICAL DEFINITION. ADULT ONSET IS CONSIDERED TO BE TYPE I IF THE PATIENT IS INSULIN DEPENDENT. SHORT TERM USE OF INSULIN DOES NOT CHANGE THE CLASSIFICATION TO TYPE I. TYPE I IS DETERMINED BY THE LONG-TERM, EVERYDAY DEPENDENCE ON INSULIN.*

DIABETES, DIABETIC

250.0# NOS
250.0# UNCOMPLICATED
250.9# DIABETES WITH UNSPECIFIED COMPLICATION
0 ACIDOSIS SEE 'DIABETES, DIABETIC' KETOACIDOSIS

5th Digit: 250

0. TYPE II, ADULT-ONSET, NON-INSULIN DEPENDENT (EVEN IF REQUIRING INSULIN), OR UNSPECIFIED; CONTROLLED
1. TYPE I, JUVENILE-ONSET OR INSULIN-DEPENDENT; CONTROLLED
2. TYPE II, ADULT-ONSET, NON-INSULIN DEPENDENT (EVEN IF REQUIRING INSULIN); UNCONTROLLED
3. TYPE I, JUVENILE-ONSET OR INSULIN-DEPENDENT; UNCONTROLLED

DIABETES, DIABETIC (continued)

250.4# ACUTE RENAL FAILURE [584.#]

4th Digit: 584

5. WITH TUBULAR NECROSIS
6. RENAL CORTICAL NECROSIS
7. MEDULLARY (PAPILLARY) NECROSIS
8. SPECIFIED PATHOLOGICAL LESION
9. RENAL FAILURE UNSPECIFIED

250.6# AMYOTROPHY [358.1]
250.7# ANGIOPATHY (PERIPHERAL) [443.81]
250.6# ARTHROPATHY (NEUROGENIC) [713.5]

5th Digit: 250

0. TYPE II, ADULT-ONSET, NON-INSULIN DEPENDENT (EVEN IF REQUIRING INSULIN), OR UNSPECIFIED; CONTROLLED
1. TYPE I, JUVENILE-ONSET OR INSULIN-DEPENDENT; CONTROLLED
2. TYPE II, ADULT-ONSET, NON-INSULIN DEPENDENT (EVEN IF REQUIRING INSULIN); UNCONTROLLED
3. TYPE I, JUVENILE-ONSET OR INSULIN-DEPENDENT; UNCONTROLLED

DIABETIC BLINDNESS REQUIRES A SECOND CODE FOR THE AMOUNT OF IMPAIRMENT. SEE "VISION IMPAIRMENT" FOR SECOND CODE.

250.5# BLINDNESS
250.5# CATARACT [366.41]
250.4# CHRONIC RENAL FAILURE [585]
250.7# CIRCULATORY DISORDER PERIPHERAL
250.2# COMA HYPEROSMOLAR (NON KETOTIC)
250.3# COMA HYPOGLYCEMIC
250.3# COMA INSULIN
250.3# COMA KETOACIDOTIC
250.6# DORSAL SCLEROSIS [340]

5th Digit: 250

0. TYPE II, ADULT-ONSET, NON-INSULIN DEPENDENT (EVEN IF REQUIRING INSULIN), OR UNSPECIFIED; CONTROLLED
1. TYPE I, JUVENILE-ONSET OR INSULIN-DEPENDENT; CONTROLLED
2. TYPE II, ADULT-ONSET, NON-INSULIN DEPENDENT (EVEN IF REQUIRING INSULIN); UNCONTROLLED
3. TYPE I, JUVENILE-ONSET OR INSULIN-DEPENDENT; UNCONTROLLED

258.1 DWARFISM OBESITY SYNDROME
V18.0 FAMILY HISTORY

DIABETIC GANGRENE [785.4] REQUIRES CODE 250.7# BEFORE CODE 785.4. REMEMBER, THE CODE TO THE LEFT OF THE DESCRIPTION ALWAYS SEQUENCES FIRST.

250.7# GANGRENE [785.4]
250.6# GASTROPARALYSIS [337.1]
250.6# GASTROPARESIS [536.3]

5th Digit: 250

0. TYPE II, ADULT-ONSET, NON-INSULIN DEPENDENT (EVEN IF REQUIRING INSULIN), OR UNSPECIFIED; CONTROLLED
1. TYPE I, JUVENILE-ONSET OR INSULIN-DEPENDENT; CONTROLLED
2. TYPE II, ADULT-ONSET, NON-INSULIN DEPENDENT (EVEN IF REQUIRING INSULIN); UNCONTROLLED
3. TYPE I, JUVENILE-ONSET OR INSULIN-DEPENDENT; UNCONTROLLED

648.8# GESTATIONAL

5th Digit: 648.8

0. EPISODE OF CARE UNSPECIFIED OR N/A
1. DELIVERED
2. DELIVERED WITH POSTPARTUM COMPLICATION
3. ANTEPARTUM COMPLICATION
4. POSTPARTUM COMPLICATION

DIABETES, DIABETIC (continued)

250.5# GLAUCOMA [365.44]
250.4# GLOMERULOSCLEROSIS (INTERCAPILLARY) [581.81]
250.8# GLYCOGENOSIS, SECONDARY [259.8]
250.3# HYPEROSMOLAR (KETOACIDOTIC) COMA
250.2# HYPEROSMOLAR (NON KETOTIC) COMA
250.2# HYPEROSMOLARITY
250.4# HYPERTENSION-NEPHROSIS SYNDROME [581.81]
250.8# HYPOGLYCEMIA
250.3# HYPOGLYCEMIC COMA
250.8# HYPOGLYCEMIC SHOCK
253.5 INSIPIDUS
588.1 INSIPIDUS NEPHROGENIC
250.3# INSULIN COMA
250.5# IRITIS [364.42]
250.1# KETOACIDOSIS
250.3# KETOACIDOSIS COMA
250.4# KIMMELSTIEL WILSON DISEASE [581.81]
250.8# LANCEREAUX'S [261]
250.8# LIPOIDOSIS [272.7]
250.5# MACULAR EDEMA [362.01]
250.5# MACULAR EDEMA CYSTOID [362.53]

5th Digit: 250

0. TYPE II, ADULT-ONSET, NON-INSULIN DEPENDENT (EVEN IF REQUIRING INSULIN), OR UNSPECIFIED; CONTROLLED
1. TYPE I, JUVENILE-ONSET OR INSULIN-DEPENDENT; CONTROLLED
2. TYPE II, ADULT-ONSET, NON-INSULIN DEPENDENT (EVEN IF REQUIRING INSULIN); UNCONTROLLED
3. TYPE I, JUVENILE-ONSET OR INSULIN-DEPENDENT; UNCONTROLLED

775.0 MATERNAL AFFECTING INFANT WITH HYPOGLYCEMIA

648.0#: SPECIFY THE MATERNAL DIABETES WITH AN ADDITIONAL CODE FOR THE SPECIFIC DIABETES. SEE 'DIABETES, DIABETIC'.

648.0# MATERNAL CURRENT (CO-EXISTENT) IN PREGNANCY
648.8# MATERNAL GESTATIONAL

5th Digit: 648.0, 648.8

0. EPISODE OF CARE UNSPECIFIED OR N/A
1. DELIVERED
2. DELIVERED WITH POSTPARTUM COMPLICATION
3. ANTEPARTUM COMPLICATION
4. POSTPARTUM COMPLICATION

250.6# MONONEURITIS NOS [355.9]
250.6# MONONEURITIS LOWER LIMB [355.8]
250.6# MONONEURITIS UPPER LIMB [354.9]
250.6# MYASTHENIA [358.1]
250.8# NECROBIOSIS LIPOIDICA DIABETICORUM [709.3]
775.1 NEONATAL
588.1 NEPHROGENIC
250.4# NEPHRITIS [583.81]
250.4# NEPHRITIS WITH NEPHROTIC SYNDROME [581.81]
250.4# NEPHROPATHY [583.81]
250.4# NEPHROSIS [581.81]
250.4# NEPHROTIC SYNDROME [581.81]

5th Digit: 250

0. TYPE II, ADULT-ONSET, NON-INSULIN DEPENDENT (EVEN IF REQUIRING INSULIN), OR UNSPECIFIED; CONTROLLED
1. TYPE I, JUVENILE-ONSET OR INSULIN-DEPENDENT; CONTROLLED
2. TYPE II, ADULT-ONSET, NON-INSULIN DEPENDENT (EVEN IF REQUIRING INSULIN); UNCONTROLLED
3. TYPE I, JUVENILE-ONSET OR INSULIN-DEPENDENT; UNCONTROLLED

D

DIABETES, DIABETIC (continued)

250.6# NEURALGIA [357.2]
250.6# NEUROLOGICAL MANIFESTATIONS
250.6# NEUROPATHY NOS [357.2]
250.6# NEUROPATHY MONONEURITIS SITE NOS (355.9)
250.6# NEUROPATHY MONONEURITIS LOWER LIMB [355.8]
250.6# NEUROPATHY MONONEURITIS UPPER LIMB [354.9]
250.6# NEUROPATHY PERIPHERAL AUTONOMIC [337.1]
250.6# NEUROPATHY POLYNEUROPATHY [357.2]

5th Digit: 250

0. **TYPE II, ADULT-ONSET, NON-INSULIN DEPENDENT (EVEN IF REQUIRING INSULIN), OR UNSPECIFIED; CONTROLLED**
1. **TYPE I, JUVENILE-ONSET OR INSULIN-DEPENDENT; CONTROLLED**
2. **TYPE II, ADULT-ONSET, NON-INSULIN DEPENDENT (EVEN IF REQUIRING INSULIN); UNCONTROLLED**
3. **TYPE I, JUVENILE-ONSET OR INSULIN-DEPENDENT; UNCONTROLLED**

775.1 NEWBORN INFANT SYNDROME
790.2 NONCLINICAL
250.8# OSTEOPATHY [731.8]
250.8# OSTEOMYELITIS [731.8] [**730.0#**]

5th Digit: 250

0. **TYPE II, ADULT-ONSET, NON-INSULIN DEPENDENT (EVEN IF REQUIRING INSULIN), OR UNSPECIFIED; CONTROLLED**
1. **TYPE I, JUVENILE-ONSET OR INSULIN-DEPENDENT; CONTROLLED**
2. **TYPE II, ADULT-ONSET, NON-INSULIN DEPENDENT (EVEN IF REQUIRING INSULIN); UNCONTROLLED**
3. **TYPE I, JUVENILE-ONSET OR INSULIN-DEPENDENT; UNCONTROLLED**

5th Digit: 730.0

0. **SITE NOS**
1. **SHOULDER REGION**
2. **UPPER ARM (ELBOW) (HUMERUS)**
3. **FOREARM (RADIUS) (WRIST) (ULNA)**
4. **HAND (CARPAL) (METACARPAL) (FINGERS)**
5. **PELVIC REGION (HIP) (BUTTOCK) (FEMUR) AND THIGH**
6. **LOWER LEG (FIBULA) (KNEE) (PATELLA) (TIBIA)**
7. **ANKLE AND OR FOOT (METATARSALS) (TOES) (TARSALS)**
8. **OTHER (HEAD) (NECK) (RIB) (SKULL) (TRUNK) (VERTEBRAE)**
9. **MULTIPLE**

250.7# PERIPHERAL VASCULAR DISEASE [443.81]
253.5 PITUITARY
250.6# POLYNEUROPATHY [357.2]
250.4# RENAL DISEASE [583.81]
271.4 RENAL GLYCOSURIA
250.5# RETINAL EDEMA [362.83]
250.5# RETINAL HEMORRHAGE (MICROANEURYSMS) [362.01]
250.5# RETINITIS [362.01]
250.5# RETINOPATHY [362.01]
250.5# RETINOPATHY PROLIFERATIVE [362.02]
V77.1 SCREENING
251.8 STEROID INDUCED

5th Digit: 250

0. **TYPE II, ADULT-ONSET, NON-INSULIN DEPENDENT (EVEN IF REQUIRING INSULIN), OR UNSPECIFIED; CONTROLLED**
1. **TYPE I, JUVENILE-ONSET OR INSULIN-DEPENDENT; CONTROLLED**
2. **TYPE II, ADULT-ONSET, NON-INSULIN DEPENDENT (EVEN IF REQUIRING INSULIN); UNCONTROLLED**
3. **TYPE I, JUVENILE-ONSET OR INSULIN-DEPENDENT; UNCONTROLLED**

DIABETES, DIABETIC (continued)

250.8# ULCER [**707.#**]
250.6# ULCER - NEUROPATHIC [**707.#**]
250.7# ULCER - PERIPHERAL VASCULAR [**707.#**]

5th Digit: 250

0. **TYPE II, ADULT-ONSET, NON-INSULIN DEPENDENT (EVEN IF REQUIRING INSULIN), OR UNSPECIFIED; CONTROLLED**
1. **TYPE I, JUVENILE-ONSET OR INSULIN-DEPENDENT; CONTROLLED**
2. **TYPE II, ADULT-ONSET, NON-INSULIN DEPENDENT (EVEN IF REQUIRING INSULIN); UNCONTROLLED**
3. **TYPE I, JUVENILE-ONSET OR INSULIN-DEPENDENT; UNCONTROLLED**

4th Digit: 707

1. **LOWER LIMB EXCEPT DECUBITUS**
8. **CHRONIC OF OTHER SPECIFIED SITE**
9. **CHRONIC SITE NOS**

588.1 VASO-PRESSIN RESISTANT
250.9# WITH COMPLICATIONS (UNSPECIFIED)
250.7# WITH CIRCULATORY (PERIPHERAL) MANIFESTATIONS
250.2# WITH COMA HYPEROSMOLAR
250.3# WITH COMA OTHER (HYPOGLYCEMIC) (INSULIN)
250.1# WITH KETOACIDOSIS
250.6# WITH NEUROLOGICAL MANIFESTATIONS
250.5# WITH OPHTHALMIC MANIFESTATIONS
250.4# WITH RENAL MANIFESTATIONS
250.8# WITH OTHER SPECIFIED MANIFESTATIONS
250.8# XANTHOMA [272.2]

5th Digit: 250

0. **TYPE II, ADULT-ONSET, NON-INSULIN DEPENDENT (EVEN IF REQUIRING INSULIN), OR UNSPECIFIED; CONTROLLED**
1. **TYPE I, JUVENILE-ONSET OR INSULIN-DEPENDENT; CONTROLLED**
2. **TYPE II, ADULT-ONSET, NON-INSULIN DEPENDENT (EVEN IF REQUIRING INSULIN); UNCONTROLLED**
3. **TYPE I, JUVENILE-ONSET OR INSULIN-DEPENDENT; UNCONTROLLED**

> *V56.#, 'ADMISSION FOR DIALYSIS', SHOULD BE ASSIGNED AS THE PRINCIPAL DIAGNOSIS WHEN THE ENCOUNTER IS FOR THE SOLE PURPOSE OF DIALYSIS. USE AN ADDITIONAL CODE FOR THE CONDITION FOR WHICH DIALYSIS IS PERFORMED.*

DIALYSIS

V56.0 ADMISSION / ENCOUNTER FOR - EXTRACORPOREAL TREATMENT
V56.8 ADMISSION / ENCOUNTER FOR - PERITONEAL TREATMENT
996.62 A-V FISTULA OR SHUNT COMPLICATION - INFECTION OR INFLAMMATION
996.1 A-V FISTULA OR SHUNT COMPLICATION - MECHANICAL
996.74 A-V FISTULA OR SHUNT COMPLICATION - OTHER
999.9 COMPLICATION NOS MEDICAL (HEMODIALYSIS) (RENAL)
294.8 DEMENTIA [E879.1]
985.8 DEMENTIA DUE TO ALUMINUM OVERLOAD [294.8] [E879.1]
293.9 DEMENTIA TRANSIENT [E879.1]
276.9 DISEQUILIBRIUM [E879.1]
V56.1 EXTRACORPOREAL CATHETER CARE (REMOVAL) (REPLACEMENT) (TOILET) (CLEANSING)
996.62 EXTRACORPOREAL CATHETER COMPLICATION - INFECTION OR INFLAMMATION
996.1 EXTRACORPOREAL CATHETER COMPLICATION - MECHANICAL
996.73 EXTRACORPOREAL CATHETER COMPLICATION - OTHER
V45.1 EXTRACORPOREAL STATUS
V56.0 EXTRACORPOREAL TREATMENT ENCOUNTER (INTERMITTENT)

DIALYSIS (continued)

V56.2 PERITONEAL CATHETER CARE (REMOVAL) (REPLACEMENT) (TOILET) (CLEANSING)
996.68 PERITONEAL CATHETER COMPLICATION - INFECTION OR INFLAMMATION, EXIT SITE
996.56 PERITONEAL CATHETER COMPLICATION - MECHANICAL
996.79 PERITONEAL CATHETER COMPLICATION - OTHER
V56.8 PERITONEAL TREATMENT ENCOUNTER (INTERMITTENT)
0 PREPARATION - CODE UNDERLYING CONDITION
V56.1 RENAL CATHETER CARE (REMOVAL) (REPLACEMENT) (TOILET) (CLEANSING)
996.62 RENAL CATHETER COMPLICATION - INFECTION OR INFLAMMATION
996.1 RENAL CATHETER COMPLICATION - MECHANICAL
996.73 RENAL CATHETER COMPLICATION - OTHER
V45.1 RENAL STATUS
V56.0 RENAL TREATMENT ENCOUNTER (INTERMITTENT)

284.0 DIAMOND BLACKFAN ANEMIA (SYNDROME)
287.2 DIAMOND-GARDENER SYNDROME (AUTOERYTHROCYTE SENSITIZATION)

691.0 DIAPER DERMATITIS
691.0 DIAPER RASH
289.7 DIAPHORASE DEFICIENCY
780.8 DIAPHORESIS

DIAPHRAGM

756.6 ABSENCE (CONGENITAL)
756.6 DEFECT CONGENITAL
551.3 DEFECT HERNIA WITH GANGRENE
519.4 DISORDER
756.6 EVENTRATION CONGENITAL
V25.02 FITTING FOR CONTRACEPTION
756.6 HERNIA CONGENITAL
862.0 INJURY
862.1 INJURY WITH OPEN WOUND INTO CAVITY
908.0 INJURY LATE EFFECT
519.4 PARALYSIS
519.4 RELAXATION

519.4 DIAPHRAGMITIS
733.99 DIAPHYSITIS

DIARRHEA

787.91 NOS
787.91 ACUTE
558.9 ALLERGIC
007.0 BALANTIDIAL
787.91 CHRONIC
007.2 COCCIDIAL
007.4 CRYPTOSPORIDIAL
008.2 DUE TO ENTEROBACTER AEROGENES
009.2 DYSENTERIC
009.3 ENDEMIIC
009.3 EPIDEMIC
007.9 FLAGELLATE
564.5 FUNCTIONAL
007.1 GIARDIAL
009.2 INFECTIOUS
009.3 INFECTIOUS ORIGIN PRESUMED
558.9 INFLAMMATORY
787.91 NONINFECTIOUS
558.9 NONINFECTIOUS DUE TO GASTROENTERITIS OR COLITIS
564.4 POST GASTRECTOMY OR POST VAGOTOMY
564.4 POST OP GI SURGERY
007.# PROTOZOAL

4th Digit: 007

0. BALANTIDIASIS
1. GIARDIASIS
2. COCCIDIOSIS
3. TRICHOMONIASIS
4. CRYPTOSPORIDIOSIS
8. OTHER SPECIFIED
9. UNSPECIFIED

DIARRHEA (continued)

306.4 PSYCHOGENIC (CYCLICAL)
009.2 TRAVELERS
007.3 TRICHOMONAL
008.8 VIRAL

DIASTASIS

733.99 CRANIAL BONES
756.0 CRANIAL BONES (CONGENITAL)
728.84 MUSCLE
728.84 RECTUS ABDOMINIS
665.8# RECTUS ABDOMINIS COMPLICATING PREGNANCY

5th Digit: 665.8

0. EPISODE OF CARE NOS OR N/A
1. DELIVERED
2. DELIVERED WITH POSTPARTUM COMPLICATION
3. ANTEPARTUM COMPLICATION
4. POSTPARTUM COMPLICATION

756.79 RECTUS ABDOMINIS CONGENITAL

742.51 DIASTEMATOMYELIA SPINAL CORD CONGENITAL
502 DIATOMACEOUS EARTH DISEASE (OCCUPATIONAL)
732.5 DIAZ'S OSTEOCHONDROSIS ASTRAGALUS

963.1 DIBROMOMANNITOL

286.6 DIC (SYNDROME)
776.2 DIC NEWBORN
759.4 DICEPHALUS
V74.8 DICK SCREENING EXAM
121.8 DICROCOELIUM DENDRITICUM INFECTION

253.8 DIENCEPHALOHYPOPHYSEAL SYNDROME
V69.1 DIET AND EATING HABITS PROBLEM
V65.3 DIET COUNSELING
760.76 DIETHYLSTILBESTROL (DES) TRANSMITTED VIA PLACENTA OR BREAST MILK AFFECTING FETUS OR NEWBORN

0 DIEULAFOY'S ULCER SEE 'ULCER', PYLORIC

151.9 DIFFUSE CARCINOMA SITE NOS
0 DIFFUSE CARCINOMA SITE SPECIFIED SEE 'CANCER' BY SITE M8145/3
723.3 DIFFUSE CERVICOBRACHIAL SYNDROME
496 DIFFUSE OBSTRUCTIVE PULMONARY SYNDROME
286.6 DIFFUSE OR DISSEMINATED DIC SYNDROME

279.11 DIGEORGE'S SYNDROME (THYMIC HYPOPLASIA)

DIGESTIVE

751.8 ABSENCE ORGAN OR TRACT CONGENITAL
751.2 ABSENCE ORGAN OR TRACT CONGENITAL- LOWER
750.8 ABSENCE ORGAN OR TRACT CONGENITAL - UPPER
536.9 DISORDER
306.4 DISORDER PSYCHOGENIC
V12.70 HISTORY OF DISEASE
V12.79 HISTORY OF DISEASE OTHER SPECIFIED
751.8 ORGANS NOS DUPLICATION (MALPOSITION) CONGENITAL
V47.3 PROBLEM OTHER
751.9 SYSTEM ANOMALY NOS - CONGENITAL
751.8 SYSTEM ANOMALIES OTHER SPECIFIED- CONGENITAL
751.8 SYSTEM ATRESIA
777.9 SYSTEM DISORDER PERINATAL
777.8 SYSTEM DISORDER PERINATAL OTHER SPECIFIED
787.99 SYSTEM SYMPTOMS
V55.4 TRACT ARTIFICIAL OPENING CARE (OTHER)

756.51 DIGHTON'S SYNDROME
0 DIGIT SEE 'FINGER' OR 'THUMB' OR 'TOE'

903.5 DIGITAL ARTERY INJURY
908.3 DIGITAL ARTERY OR BLOOD VESSEL INJURY OR LACERATION LATE EFFECT
903.5 DIGITAL BLOOD VESSELS INJURY
903.5 DIGITAL BLOOD VESSELS LACERATION (RUPTURE) (HEMATOMA) (AVULSION) (ANEURYSM) TRAUMATIC
955.6 DIGITAL NERVE INJURY
907.4 DIGITAL NERVE INJURY LATE EFFECT
207.0# DI GUGLIELMO'S DISEASE OR SYNDROME (ERYTHREMIC MYELOSIS) M9841/3

5th Digit: 207.0
0. WITHOUT MENTION OF REMISSION
1. WITH MENTION OF REMISSION

796.0 DILANTIN TOXICITY - ASYMPTOMATIC
0 DILANTIN TOXICITY - SYMPTOMATIC SEE DRUGS AND CHEMICALS (APPENDIX B) OR 'POISONING MEDICINAL'
305.3# DIMETHYLTRYPTAMINE (DMT) ABUSE (NONDEPENDENT)
304.5# DIMETHYLTRYPTAMINE (DMT) ADDICTION (DEPENDENT)

5th Digit: 304.5, 305.3
0. UNSPECIFIED
1. CONTINUOUS
2. EPISODIC
3. IN REMISSION

759.6 DIMITRI-STURGE-WEBER ENCEPHALOCUTANEOUS ANGIOMATOSIS
125.4 DIPETALONEMA PERSTANS INFECTION
125.6 DIPETALONEMA STREPTOCERCA INFECTION
125.4 DIPETALONEMIASIS
752.69 DIPHALLUS

DIPHTHERIA
032.2 ANTERIOR NASAL
V02.4 CARRIER
032.81 CONJUNCTIVAL
032.85 CUTANEOUS
032.84 CYSTITIS
032.0 FAUCIAL
032.9 INFECTION
032.3 LARYNGEAL
032.82 MYOCARDITIS
032.1 NASOPHARYNGEAL
032.83 PERITONITIS
032.89 POLYNEUROPATHY [357.4]
032.3 TRACHEITIS
032.89 OTHER
V74.3 SCREENING EXAM
V06.5 VACCINATION (TETANUS - DIPTHERIA)
V03.5 VACCINATION (SINGLE)

DIPHTHERITIC
032.0 ANGINA GANGRENOUS
032.0 ANGINA MALIGNANT
032.0 ANGINA MEMBRANOUS
032.0 ANGINA PHLEGMONOUS

123.4 DIPHYLLOBOTHRIASIS INTESTINAL
123.4 DIPHYLLOBOTHRIUM INFECTION (ADULT)
123.5 DIPHYLLOBOTHRIUM LARVAE INFECTION
388.41 DIPLACUSIS
344.1 DIPLEGIA ACQUIRED LOWER LIMB (OLD)
438.53 DIPLEGIA ACQUIRED LOWER LIMB (OLD) - LATE EFFECT OF CEREBROVASCULAR DISEASE [344.1]
344.2 DIPLEGIA ACQUIRED UPPER LIMB (OLD)
438.53 DIPLEGIA ACQUIRED UPPER LIMB (OLD) - LATE EFFECT OF CEREBROVASCULAR DISEASE [344.2]
343.0 DIPLEGIA CONGENITAL
123.8 DIPLOGONOPORUS INFECTION (GRANDIS)
368.2 DIPLOPIA
368.15 DIPLOPIA REFRACTIVE
303.9# DIPSOMANIA

5th Digit: 303.9
0. NOS
1. CONTINUOUS
2. EPISODIC
3. IN REMISSION

123.8 DIPYLIDIUM INFECTION (CANINUM)
125.6 DIROFILARIA INFECTION
307.52 DIRT EATING CHILD
V68.0 DISABILITY CERTIFICATE ISSUE
0 DISARTICULATION SEE 'AMPUTATION'

WHEN CODING BACK DISORDERS DUE TO DEGENERATION, DISPLACEMENT OR HNP OF THE INTERVERTEBRAL DISC, IT IS IMPORTANT TO DISTINGUISH WHETHER THESE CONDITIONS ARE WITH OR WITHOUT MYELOPATHY. MYELOPATHY REFERS TO FUNCTIONAL DISTURBANCES AND/OR PATHOLOGICAL CHANGES IN THE SPINAL CORD THAT RESULT FROM COMPRESSION.

722.10 LUMBAR DISC HERNIATION (HNP)

722.73 LUMBAR DISC HERNIATION (HNP) WITH MYELOPATHY

DISC (INTERVERTEBRAL)

CALCIFICATION OR DISCITIS
722.90 NOS
722.91 CERVICAL
722.93 LUMBAR (LUMBOSACRAL)
722.92 THORACIC (THORACOLUMBAR)

DEGENERATIVE DISEASE (DEGENERATION)
722.6 SITE NOS
722.70 SITE NOS WITH MYELOPATHY
722.4 CERVICAL
722.71 CERVICAL WITH MYELOPATHY
722.52 LUMBAR (LUMBOSACRAL)
722.73 LUMBAR (LUMBOSACRAL)WITH MYELOPATHY
722.51 THORACIC (THORACOLUMBAR)
722.72 THORACIC (THORACOLUMBAR) WITH MYELOPATHY

DISORDER
722.90 UNSPECIFIED
722.70 UNSPECIFIED WITH MYELOPATHY

DISPLACEMENT (RUPTURE)
722.2 SITE NOS
722.70 SITE NOS WITH MYELOPATHY
722.0 CERVICAL
722.71 CERVICAL WITH MYELOPATHY
722.10 LUMBAR
722.73 LUMBAR WITH MYELOPATHY
722.11 THORACIC
722.72 THORACIC WITH MYELOPATHY

HERNIATION
722.2 SITE NOS
722.70 SITE NOS WITH MYELOPATHY
722.0 CERVICAL
722.71 CERVICAL WITH MYELOPATHY
722.10 LUMBAR
722.73 LUMBAR WITH MYELOPATHY
722.11 THORACIC
722.72 THORACIC WITH MYELOPATHY

0 DISC SYNDROME SEE 'INTERVERTEBRAL DISC'
0 DISCHARGE SEE BY ANATOMICAL SITE
722.9# DISCITIS (INTERVERTEBRAL)

5th Digit: 722.9
0. UNSPECIFIED
1. CERVICAL
2. THORACIC
3. LUMBAR

D

722.90 DISCOGENIC DISEASE OR SYNDROME (SEE ALSO 'INTERVERTEBRAL DISC')
373.34 DISCOID LUPUS ERYTHEMATOSUS EYELID
717.5 DISCOID MENISCUS - OLD
0 DISEASE SEE BY ANATOMICAL SITE OR SPECIFIED DISORDER
799.9 DISEASE UNDIAGNOSED CAUSE OF MORBIDITY AND MORTALITY
276.9 DISEQUILIBRIUM (ELECTROLYTES) SYNDROME
276.9 DISEQUILIBRIUM DUE TO DIALYSIS [E879.1]
V48.6 DISFIGUREMENT HEAD
V48.7 DISFIGUREMENT NECK
V48.7 DISFIGUREMENT TRUNK
299.1# DISINTEGRATIVE DISORDER (CHILDHOOD)

5th Digit: 299.1

0. CURRENT OR ACTIVE STATE
1. RESIDUAL STATE

IN CODING MULTIPLE INJURIES, SEQUENCE THE MOST SEVERE INJURY FIRST. OPEN DISLOCATIONS SEQUENCE BEFORE CLOSED DISLOCATIONS.

FOR PATHOLOGICAL DISLOCATIONS, LOOK UNDER "DISLOCATION PATHOLOGICAL".

DISLOCATION

839.8 NOS CLOSED
839.9 NOS OPEN

831.04 ACROMIOCLAVICULAR CLOSED
831.14 ACROMIOCLAVICULAR OPEN

837.0 ANKLE CLOSED
837.1 ANKLE OPEN

839.8 ARM CLOSED
839.9 ARM OPEN
839.8 ARM MULTIPLE AND ILL-DEFINED CLOSED
839.9 ARM MULTIPLE AND ILL-DEFINED OPEN

837.0 ASTRAGALUS CLOSED
837.1 ASTRAGALUS OPEN

839.01 ATLANTO AXIAL CLOSED
839.11 ATLANTO AXIAL OPEN
839.01 ATLAS CLOSED
839.11 ATLAS OPEN
839.02 AXIS CLOSED
839.12 AXIS OPEN

839.8 BACK CLOSED
839.9 BACK OPEN
839.8 BACK MULTIPLE AND ILL-DEFINED CLOSED
839.9 BACK MULTIPLE AND ILL-DEFINED OPEN

723.8 BELL-DALY

839.61 BREAST BONE CLOSED
839.71 BREAST BONE OPEN

833.00 CARPAL (BONE) CLOSED
833.10 CARPAL (BONE) OPEN

833.04 CARPOMETACARPAL CLOSED
833.14 CARPOMETACARPAL OPEN

DISLOCATION (continued)

839.0# CERVICAL SPINE (VERTEBRA) CLOSED
839.1# CERVICAL SPINE (VERTEBRA) OPEN

5th Digit: 839.0-1

0. CERVICAL VERTEBRA UNSPECIFIED
1. FIRST CERVICAL VERTEBRA
2. SECOND CERVICAL VERTEBRA
3. THIRD CERVICAL VERTEBRA
4. FOURTH CERVICAL VERTEBRA
5. FIFTH CERVICAL VERTEBRA
6. SIXTH CERVICAL VERTEBRA
7. SEVENTH CERVICAL VERTEBRA
8. MULTIPLE CERVICAL VERTEBRA

756.19 CERVICAL SPINE (VERTEBRA) CONGENITAL
723.8 CERVICAL SPINE (VERTEBRA) PATHOLOGIC OR RECURRENT

0 CHIROPRACTIC SEE 'LESION', NONALLOPATHIC

831.04 CLAVICLE CLOSED
831.14 CLAVICLE OPEN

839.41 COCCYX CLOSED
839.51 COCCYX OPEN
724.79 COCCYX PATHOLOGIC OR RECURRENT

831.04 COLLAR BONE CLOSED
831.14 COLLAR BONE OPEN

831.09 CORACOID CLOSED
831.19 CORACOID OPEN

839.69 COSTAL CARTILAGE CLOSED
839.79 COSTAL CARTILAGE OPEN

839.69 COSTOCHONDRAL CLOSED
839.79 COSTOCHONDRAL OPEN

839.69 CRICOARYTENOID ARTICULATION CLOSED
839.79 CRICOARYTENOID ARTICULATION OPEN

839.69 CRICOTHYROID (CARTILAGE) ARTICULATION CLOSED
839.79 CRICOTHYROID (CARTILAGE) ARTICULATION OPEN

385.23 EAR OSSICLES

832.0# ELBOW CLOSED
832.1# ELBOW OPEN

5th Digit: 832.0-1

0. UNSPECIFIED
1. ANTERIOR
2. POSTERIOR
3. MEDIAL
4. LATERAL
9. OTHER

754.89 ELBOW CONGENITAL
832.01 ELBOW NURSEMAID'S
718.22 ELBOW PATHOLOGICAL
718.32 ELBOW RECURRENT OLD

360.81 EYE OR EYEBALL
376.36 EYE OR EYEBALL LATERAL

0 FEMUR DISTAL END SEE 'DISLOCATION', KNEE
0 FEMUR PROXIMAL END SEE 'DISLOCATION', HIP

837.0 FIBULA DISTAL END CLOSED
837.1 FIBULA DISTAL END OPEN
0 FIBULA PROXIMAL END SEE 'DISLOCATION', KNEE

834.00 FINGER CLOSED
834.02 FINGER CLOSED INTERPHALANGEAL
834.01 FINGER CLOSED METACARPOPHALANGEAL
834.10 FINGER OPEN
834.12 FINGER OPEN INTERPHALANGEAL
834.11 FINGER OPEN METACARPOPHALANGEAL
718.24 FINGER PATHOLOGICAL
718.34 FINGER RECURRENT OLD

D

DISLOCATION (continued)

838.## FOOT
4th Digit: 838
0. CLOSED
1. OPEN
5th Digit: 838
0. FOOT UNSPECIFIED
1. TARSAL (BONE) JOINT UNSPECIFIED
2. MIDTARSAL (JOINT)
3. TARSOMETATARSAL (BONE)
4. METATARSAL (BONE) JOINT UNSPECIFIED
5. METATARSOPHALANGEAL (JOINT)
6. INTERPHALANGEAL (JOINT) FOOT
9. OTHER

718.27 FOOT PATHOLOGICAL
718.37 FOOT RECURRENT

831.09 GLENOID CLOSED
831.19 GLENOID OPEN

839.8 HAND CLOSED
839.9 HAND OPEN
839.8 HAND MULTIPLE AND ILL-DEFINED CLOSED
839.9 HAND MULTIPLE AND ILL-DEFINED OPEN

835.## HIP
4th Digit: 835
0. CLOSED
1. OPEN
5th Digit: 835
0. UNSPECIFIED
1. POSTERIOR
2. OBTURATOR
3. ANTERIOR

V82.3 HIP (CONGENITAL) SCREENING
754.30 HIP CONGENITAL
754.31 HIP CONGENITAL BILATERAL
754.35 HIP CONGENITAL WITH SUBLUXATION OF OTHER HIP
718.25 HIP PATHOLOGICAL
996.4 HIP PROSTHESIS
718.35 HIP RECURRENT OLD

0 HUMERUS DISTAL SEE 'DISLOCATION', ELBOW
831.0# HUMERUS PROXIMAL CLOSED
831.1# HUMERUS PROXIMAL OPEN
5th Digit: 831.0-1
0. UNSPECIFIED
1. ANTERIOR
2. POSTERIOR
3. INFERIOR

385.23 INCUS

831.01 INFRACORACOID CLOSED
831.11 INFRACORACOID OPEN

839.69 INNOMINATE (PUBIC JUNCTION) (SACRAL JUNCTION) CLOSED
839.79 INNOMINATE (PUBIC JUNCTION) (SACRAL JUNCTION) OPEN

0 INTERCARPAL SEE 'DISLOCATION', WRIST

834.02 INTERPHALANGEAL FINGER OR HAND CLOSED
834.12 INTERPHALANGEAL FINGER OR HAND OPEN

838.06 INTERPHALANGEAL FOOT OR TOE CLOSED
838.16 INTERPHALANGEAL FOOT OR TOE OPEN

830.0 JAW (CARTILAGE) (MENISCUS) CLOSED (TMJ)
830.1 JAW (CARTILAGE) (MENISCUS) OPEN (TMJ)
524.69 JAW RECURRENT

DISLOCATION (continued)

836.5# KNEE CLOSED
836.6# KNEE OPEN
5th Digit: 836.5-6
0. UNSPECIFIED
1. ANTERIOR
2. POSTERIOR
3. MEDIAL
4. LATERAL END
9. OTHER OR ROTATORY

754.41 KNEE CONGENITAL WITH GENU RECURVATUM
718.26 KNEE PATHOLOGICAL
836.59 KNEE ROTATORY CLOSED
836.69 KNEE ROTATORY OPEN
718.36 KNEE RECURRENT OLD

375.16 LACRIMAL GLAND
905.6 LATE EFFECT

839.8 LEG CLOSED
839.9 LEG OPEN

379.32 LENS (CRYSTALLINE) (COMPLETE) (PARTIAL)
379.33 LENS ANTERIOR
743.37 LENS CONGENITAL
379.34 LENS POSTERIOR
921.3 LENS TRAUMATIC

839.20 LUMBAR VERTEBRA CLOSED
839.30 LUMBAR VERTEBRA OPEN

839.20 LUMBOSACRAL CLOSED
839.30 LUMBOSACRAL OPEN
756.19 LUMBOSACRAL CONGENITAL
724.6 LUMBOSACRAL PATHOLOGIC OR RECURRENT

0 LUNATE SEE 'DISLOCATION', WRIST

830.0 MANDIBLE CLOSED (TMJ)
830.1 MANDIBLE OPEN (TMJ)

830.0 MAXILLA (INFERIOR) CLOSED
830.1 MAXILLA (INFERIOR) OPEN

834.01 METACARPAL (BONE) DISTAL END CLOSED
834.11 METACARPAL (BONE) DISTAL END OPEN
833.05 METACARPAL (BONE) PROXIMAL END CLOSED
833.15 METACARPAL (BONE) PROXIMAL END OPEN

834.01 METACARPOPHALANGEAL CLOSED
834.11 METACARPOPHALANGEAL OPEN

838.04 METATARSAL (BONE) CLOSED
838.14 METATARSAL (BONE) OPEN

838.05 METATARSOPHALANGEAL CLOSED
838.15 METATARSOPHALANGEAL OPEN

833.03 MIDCARPAL CLOSED
833.13 MIDCARPAL OPEN

838.02 MIDTARSAL CLOSED
838.12 MIDTARSAL OPEN

0 MONTEGGIA'S SEE 'DISLOCATION', HIP

839.8 MULTIPLE AND ILL-DEFINED CLOSED
839.9 MULTIPLE AND ILL-DEFINED OPEN

837.0 NAVICULAR FOOT CLOSED
837.1 NAVICULAR FOOT OPEN

0 NECK SEE 'DISLOCATION', CERVICAL SPINE

0 NELATON'S SEE 'DISLOCATION', ANKLE

D

DISLOCATION (continued)

832.01 NURSEMAID'S ELBOW
831.0# NURSEMAID'S SHOULDER
5th Digit: 831.0
0. UNSPECIFIED
1. ANTERIOR
2. POSTERIOR
3. INFERIOR
4. ACROMIOCLAVICULAR
9. SCAPULA

839.69 NOSE CLOSED
839.79 NOSE OPEN

839.01 OCCIPUT FROM ATLAS CLOSED
839.11 OCCIPUT FROM ATLAS OPEN

996.53 OCULAR IMPLANT

836.3 PATELLA CLOSED
836.4 PATELLA OPEN
755.64 PATELLA CONGENITAL
718.26 PATELLA PATHOLOGIC
718.36 PATELLA RECURRENT OLD

718.2# PATHOLOGICAL
5th Digit: 718.2
0. SITE UNSPECIFIED
1. SHOULDER REGION
2. UPPER ARM (ELBOW) (HUMERUS)
3. FOREARM (RADIUS) (WRIST) (ULNA)
4. HAND (CARPAL) (METACARPAL) (FINGERS)
5. PELVIC REGION (HIP) (BUTTOCK) (FEMUR)
6. LOWER LEG (FIBULA) (KNEE) (PATELLA) (TIBIA)
7. ANKLE AND OR FOOT (METATARSALS) (TOES) (TARSALS)
8. OTHER
9. MULTIPLE

724.8 PATHOLOGICAL SPINE - NOS
724.6 PATHOLOGICAL SPINE - LUMBOSACRAL JOINT
724.6 PATHOLOGICAL SPINE - SACROILIAC JOINT

839.69 PELVIS CLOSED
839.79 PELVIS OPEN

0 PHALANX OF FOOT OR TOE SEE 'DISLOCATION', TOE
0 PHALANX OF HAND SEE 'DISLOCATION', FINGER

832.01 RADIAL HEAD CLOSED
832.11 RADIAL HEAD OPEN

833.02 RADIOCARPAL CLOSED
833.12 RADIOCARPAL OPEN

833.01 RADIOULNAR DISTAL END CLOSED
833.11 RADIOULNAR DISTAL END OPEN
0 RADIOULNAR PROXIMAL END SEE 'DISLOCATION', ELBOW

833.00 RADIUS DISTAL END CLOSED
833.10 RADIUS DISTAL END OPEN
0 RADIUS PROXIMAL END SEE 'DISLOCATION', ELBOW

718.3# RECURRENT
5th Digit: 718.3
0. SITE UNSPECIFIED
1. SHOULDER REGION
2. UPPER ARM (ELBOW) (HUMERUS)
3. FOREARM (RADIUS) (WRIST) (ULNA)
4. HAND (CARPAL) (METACARPAL) (FINGERS)
5. PELVIC REGION (HIP) (BUTTOCK) (FEMUR)
6. LOWER LEG (FIBULA) (KNEE) (PATELLA) (TIBIA)
7. ANKLE AND OR FOOT (METATARSALS) (TOES) (TARSALS)
8. OTHER
9. MULTIPLE

724.9 RECURRENT SPINE - NOS
724.6 RECURRENT SPINE - LUMBOSACRAL JOINT
724.6 RECURRENT SPINE - SACROILIAC JOINT

839.69 RIB CLOSED
839.79 RIB OPEN
756.3 RIB CONGENITAL
718.28 RIB PATHOLOGICAL
718.38 RIB RECURRENT OLD

836.59 ROTATORY (KNEE) CLOSED
836.69 ROTATORY (KNEE) OPEN

839.42 SACROILIAC CLOSED
839.52 SACROILIAC OPEN
755.69 SACROILIAC CONGENITAL
724.6 SACROILIAC PATHOLOGIC OR RECURRENT

839.42 SACRUM CLOSED
839.52 SACRUM OPEN

837.0 SCAPHOID FOOT CLOSED
837.1 SCAPHOID FOOT OPEN
833.00 SCAPHOID WRIST CLOSED
833.10 SCAPHOID WRIST OPEN

831.09 SCAPULA CLOSED
831.19 SCAPULA OPEN

839.69 SEPTAL CARTILAGE (NOSE) CLOSED
839.79 SEPTAL CARTILAGE (NOSE) OPEN
470 SEPTUM (NASAL) (OLD)

831.0# SHOULDER CLOSED
831.1# SHOULDER OPEN
831.0# SHOULDER NURSEMAID'S
5th Digit: 831.0-1
0. UNSPECIFIED
1. ANTERIOR
2. POSTERIOR
3. INFERIOR
4. ACROMIOCLAVICULAR
9. SCAPULA

718.21 SHOULDER PATHOLOGIC
718.31 SHOULDER RECURRENT

838.00 SMITH'S EPIPHYSEAL CLOSED
838.10 SMITH'S EPIPHYSEAL OPEN

839.40 SPINE NOS CLOSED
839.50 SPINE NOS OPEN
756.19 SPINE NOS CONGENITAL
724.8 SPINE NOS PATHOLOGIC
724.9 SPINE NOS RECURRENT
767.4 SPINE OR SPINAL CORD BIRTH TRAUMA

0 SPONTANEOUS SEE 'DISLOCATION', PATHOLOGICAL

839.61 STERNOCLAVICULAR CLOSED
839.71 STERNOCLAVICULAR OPEN

839.61 STERNUM CLOSED
839.71 STERNUM OPEN

831.01 SUBGLENOID CLOSED
831.11 SUBGLENOID OPEN

838.## SUBTALAR
838.## TARSAL
4th Digit: 838
0. CLOSED
1. OPEN
5th Digit: 838
0. FOOT UNSPECIFIED
1. TARSAL (BONE) JOINT UNSPECIFIED
2. MIDTARSAL (JOINT)
3. TARSOMETATARSAL (BONE) JOINT UNSPECIFIED
4. METATARSAL (BONE) JOINT UNSPECIFIED
5. METATARSOPHALANGEAL (JOINT)
6. INTERPHALANGEAL (JOINT) FOOT
9. OTHER

DISLOCATION (continued)

718.27 TARSAL PATHOLOGIC
718.37 TARSAL RECURRENT

837.0 TARSONAVICULAR CLOSED
837.1 TARSONAVICULAR OPEN

830.0 TEMPOROMANDIBULAR CLOSED
830.1 TEMPOROMANDIBULAR OPEN
524.69 TEMPOROMANDIBULAR RECURRENT

839.21 THORACIC VERTEBRA CLOSED
839.31 THORACIC VERTEBRA OPEN
724.8 THORACIC PATHOLOGIC
724.9 THORACIC RECURRENT

839.69 THYROID CARTILAGE CLOSED
839.79 THYROID CARTILAGE OPEN

837.0 TIBIA DISTAL END CLOSED
837.1 TIBIA DISTAL END OPEN
0 TIBIA PROXIMAL END SEE 'DISLOCATION', KNEE

838.06 TOE INTERPHALANGEAL CLOSED
838.16 TOE INTERPHALANGEAL OPEN
838.09 TOE(S) OTHER CLOSED
838.19 TOE(S) OTHER OPEN
718.27 TOE(S) PATHOLOGICAL
718.37 TOE(S) RECURRENT OLD

839.69 TRACHEA CLOSED
839.79 TRACHEA OPEN

833.09 ULNA DISTAL END CLOSED
833.19 ULNA DISTAL END OPEN
0 ULNA PROXIMAL END SEE 'DISLOCATION', ELBOW

839.40 VERTEBRA NOS CLOSED
839.50 VERTEBRA NOS OPEN
756.19 VERTEBRA NOS OR OTHER CONGENITAL
724.8 VERTEBRA NOS OR OTHER PATHOLOGICAL
724.9 VERTEBRA NOS OR OTHER RECURRENT OLD
839.49 VERTEBRA OTHER CLOSED
839.59 VERTEBRA OTHER OPEN

833.## WRIST

4th Digit: 833
0. CLOSED
1. OPEN

5th Digit: 833
0. UNSPECIFIED PART
1. RADIOULNAR
2. RADIOCARPAL
3. MIDCARPAL
4. CARPOMETACARPAL
5. METACARPAL
9. OTHER

718.23 WRIST PATHOLOGICAL
718.33 WRIST RECURRENT OLD

839.61 XIPHOID CARTILAGE CLOSED
839.71 XIPHOID CARTILAGE OPEN

839.69 OTHER SPECIFIED BONE CLOSED
839.79 OTHER SPECIFIED BONE OPEN

0 DISORDER SEE BY ANATOMICAL SITE OR SPECIFIED DISORDER

0 DISPROPORTIONS INDICATING CARE IN PREGNANCY SEE 'PREGNANCY COMPLICATIONS', DISPROPORTIONS

286.6 DISSEMINATED INTRAVASCULAR COAGULATION

776.2 DISSEMINATED INTRAVASCULAR COAGULATION IN NEWBORN

031.2 DISSEMINATED MYCOBACTERIUM AVIUM-INTRACELLULARE COMPLEX (DMAC)

446.6 DISSEMINATED PLATELET THROMBOSIS SYNDROME

300.15 DISSOCIATIVE DISORDER OR REACTION
300.14 DISSOCIATIVE IDENTITY DISORDER

524.2 DISTO OCCLUSION

DISTOMIASIS

121.9 DISTOMIASIS
120.9 HEMIC
121.1 HEPATIC DUE TO CLONORCHIS SINENSIS
121.4 INTESTINAL
121.2 PULMONARY

782.0 DISTURBANCE OF SKIN SENSATION

733.7 DISUSE ATROPHY BONE
728.2 DISUSE ATROPHY MUSCLE
307.81 DITTHOMSKA SYNDROME
788.42 DIURESIS
993.3 DIVERS' PALSY OR PARALYSIS
909.4 DIVERS' PALSY OR PARALYSIS LATE EFFECT
378.85 DIVERGENCE ANOMALIES (EYE MOVEMENT)

0 DIVERTICULA SEE ANATOMICAL SITE

DIVERTICULITIS

596.3 BLADDER
562.1# COLON (LARGE INTESTINE)
562.1# COLON WITH ABSCESS [567.2]
562.1# COLON WITH PERITONITIS [567.9]
562.1# COLON WITH PERITONITIS (OTHER TYPE) [567.8]
562.1# COLON WITH PERITONITIS (PNEUMOCOCCAL) [567.1]
562.0# DUODENUM
562.0# ILEUM
562.0# JEJUNUM
562.0# SMALL INTESTINE
562.0# SMALL INTESTINE PERITONITIS [567.9]
562.0# SMALL INTESTINE WITH ABSCESS [567.2]
562.0# SMALL INTESTINE WITH PERITONITIS (OTHER TYPE) [567.8]

5th Digit: 562.0, 1
1. WITHOUT HEMORRHAGE
3. WITH HEMORRHAGE

DIVERTICULOSIS

562.1# COLON
562.1# COLON (LARGE BOWEL) (INTESTINE)
562.1# COLON WITH ABSCESS [567.2]
562.1# COLON WITH PERITONITIS [567.9]
562.1# COLON WITH PERITONITIS (OTHER TYPE) [567.8]
562.1# COLON WITH PERITONITIS (PNEUMOCOCCAL) [567.1]
562.0# DUODENUM
562.0# ILEUM
562.0# JEJUNUM
562.0# SMALL INTESTINE
562.0# SMALL INTESTINE WITH ABSCESS [567.2]
562.0# SMALL INTESTINE WITH PERITONITIS [567.9]

5th Digit: 562.0, 1
0. WITHOUT HEMORRHAGE
2. WITH HEMORRHAGE

0 DIVERTICULUM SEE ANATOMICAL SITE
V61.0 DIVORCE (REASON FOR ENCOUNTER)
386.12 DIX-HALLPIKE NEUROLABYRINTHITIS

DIZZINESS

780.4 NOS
300.11 HYSTERICAL
306.9 PSYCHOGENIC [780.4]

DJD (DEGENERATIVE JOINT DISEASE)
715.90 SITE UNSPECIFIED
715.97 ANKLE AND/OR FOOT (METATARSALS) (TOES) (TARSALS)
715.93 FOREARM (RADIUS) (WRIST) (ULNA)
715.94 HAND (CARPAL) (METACARPAL) (FINGERS)
715.96 LOWER LEG (FIBULA) (KNEE) (PATELLA) (TIBIA)
715.95 PELVIC REGION AND THIGH (HIP) (BUTTOCK) (FEMUR)
715.91 SHOULDER REGION
721.90 SPINE - NOS
721.0 SPINE - CERVICAL
721.3 SPINE- LUMBAR OR LUMBOSACRAL
721.2 SPINE - THORACIC
715.92 UPPER ARM (ELBOW) (HUMERUS)
715.98 OTHER SPECIFIED

250.1# DKA (DIABETIC KETOACIDOSIS)
250.3# DKA (DIABETIC KETOACIDOSIS) COMA
5th Digit: 250.1, 3
0. TYPE II, ADULT-ONSET, NON-INSULIN DEPENDENT (EVEN IF REQUIRING INSULIN), OR UNSPECIFIED; CONTROLLED
1. TYPE I, JUVENILE-ONSET OR INSULIN-DEPENDENT; CONTROLLED
2. TYPE II, ADULT-ONSET, NON-INSULIN DEPENDENT (EVEN IF REQUIRING INSULIN); UNCONTROLLED
3. TYPE I, JUVENILE-ONSET OR INSULIN-DEPENDENT; UNCONTROLLED

031.2 DMAC (DISSEMINATED MYCOBACTERIUM AVIUM INTRACELLULARE COMPLEX)
288.0 DOAN-WISEMAN SYNDROME (PRIMARY SPLENIC NEUTROPENIA)
0 DOG BITE SEE 'OPEN WOUND', BY SITE
123.8 DOG TAPEWORM (INFECTION)
093.1 DOHLE-HELLER AORTITIS
288.2 DOHLE BODY-PANMYELOPATHIC SYNDROME
754.0 DOLICHOCEPHALY
751.5 DOLICHOCOLON DIVERTICULUM CONGENITAL
759.82 DOLICHOSTENOMELIA
259.8 DONOHUE'S SYNDROME (LEPRECHAUNISM)

> ***TISSUE OR ORGAN DONOR:** DO NOT USE V59 FOR SELF-DONATION (AUTOGENOUS DONATION). RATHER, CODE THE UNDERLYING CONDITION.*

DONOR NON-AUTOGENOUS
V59.9 ORGAN OR TISSUE
V59.0# BLOOD
5th Digit: V59.0
1. WHOLE
2. STEM CELLS
9. OTHER

V59.2 BONE
V59.3 BONE MARROW
V59.5 CORNEA
V70.8 EXAM - POTENTIAL DONOR ORGAN OR TISSUE
V59.4 KIDNEY
V59.6 LIVER
V59.8 LUNG
V59.8 LYMPHOCYTE
V59.1 SKIN
V59.8 OTHER SPECIFIED ORGAN OR TISSUE

099.2 DONOVANOSIS
496 DOPS - DIFFUSE OBSTRUCTIVE PULMONARY SYNDROME

DORSAL COLUMN STIMULATOR
996.63 COMPLICATION - INFECTION OR INFLAMMATION
996.2 COMPLICATION - MECHANICAL (DISPLACED) (FAILED)
996.75 COMPLICATION - OTHER
V53.02 FITTING OR ADJUSTMENT

722.11 DORSAL DISC DISPLACEMENT
722.72 DORSAL DISC DISPLACEMENT WITH MYELOPATHY
953.1 DORSAL ROOT INJURY (NERVE)
0 DORSAL SEE ALSO THORACIC
436 DORSOLATERAL MEDULLARY SYNDROME
333.7 DOUBLE ATHETOSIS SYNDROME
759.4 DOUBLE MONSTER
368.2 DOUBLE VISION
360.81 DOUBLE WHAMMY SYNDROME
758.0 DOWN'S SYNDROME (MONGOLISM)
V19.5 DOWN'S SYNDROME (MONGOLISM) FAMILY HISTORY
V06.1 DPT VACCINATION
V06.3 DPT WITH POLIO VACCINATION
V06.2 DPT WITH TAB VACCINATION
125.7 DRACONTIASIS
125.7 DRACUNCULUS MEDINENSIS INFECTION
282.1 DRESBACH'S SYNDROME (ELLIPTOCYTOSIS)
117.8 DRESCHLERA HAWAIIENSIS INFECTION
118 DRESCHLERA INFECTION TO COMPROMISED HOST ONLY
V58.3 DRESSING CHANGE (SURGICAL AFTERCARE)
283.2 DRESSLER'S HEMOGLOBINURIA SYNDROME
411.0 DRESSLER'S SYNDROME (POSTMYOCARDIAL INFARCTION)

DROP
736.29 FINGER
736.79 FOOT
735.8 TOE
736.05 WRIST

782.3 DROPSY
994.1 DROWNING AND NONFATAL SUBMERSION
909.4 DROWNING AND NONFATAL SUBMERSION LATE EFFECT
780.09 DROWSINESS

> *ABUSE VERSUS DEPENDENCE IS THE MAJOR DISTINCTION TO MAKE WHEN CODING FOR A PATIENT WITH AN ALCOHOL OR DRUG PROBLEM. ADDICTION IS DEPENDENCE.*

DRUG
796.0 ABNORMAL LEVELS (BLOOD) (URINE) (OTHER TISSUE)
0 ABUSE SEE 'DRUG ABUSE'
995.2 HYPERSENSITIVITY NOS (PROPERLY ADMINISTERED)
292.2 INTOXICATION (PATHOLOGICAL) WITH BRIEF PSYCHOSIS
977.9 OVERDOSE UNSPECIFIED
995.2 REACTION NOS (PROPERLY ADMINISTERED)
V70.3 SCREEN ADMINISTRATIVE
V70.4 SCREEN MEDICOLEGAL
796.0 TEST ABNORMAL (BLOOD) (URINE) (OTHER TISSUE)
V70.3 TEST ADMINISTRATIVE
V70.4 TEST MEDICOLEGAL
V58.62 THERAPY LONG-TERM ANTIBIOTICS CURRENT
V58.61 THERAPY LONG-TERM ANTICOAGULANT CURRENT
V58.69 THERAPY LONG-TERM OTHER CURRENT
V58.1 THERAPY STATUS

SUBSTANCE ABUSE DESCRIBES THE PRACTICE OF USING DRUGS OR ALCOHOL TO EXCESS WITHOUT REACHING THE STATE OF PHYSICAL DEPENDENCE.

SUBSTANCE DEPENDENCE IS ADDICTION. DEPENDENCE INVOLVES THE LOSS OF CONTROL AND JUDGMENT AND/OR THE INABILITY TO USE IN MODERATION. DEPENDENCE IS MARKED BY COMPULSIVE PHYSICAL DEMANDS WHICH ARE TRIGGERED BY FURTHER INGESTION.

DRUG ABUSE

304.## DEPENDENT (ADDICTION)
4th Digit: 304
0. OPIOID
1. BARBITURATE, SEDATIVES, AND TRANQUILIZERS WITH A SIMILAR EFFECT
2. COCAINE
3. CANNABIS
4. AMPHETAMINE TYPE
5. HALLUCINOGENIC
6. OTHER SPECIFIED
7. MIXED WITH OPIOID
8. MIXED
9. NOS
5th Digit: 304
0. NOS
1. CONTINUOUS
2. EPISODIC
3. IN REMISSION

304.8# DEPENDENT POLYSUBSTANCE (ADDICTION)
5th Digit: 304.8
0. NOS
1. CONTINUOUS
2. EPISODIC
3. IN REMISSION

V11.8 HISTORY
305.## NONDEPENDENT (ABUSE)
4th Digit: 305
0. ALCOHOL
2. CANNABIS
3. HALLUCINOGEN
4. BARBITURATE, SEDATIVE, OR HYPNOTIC WITH A SIMILAR EFFECT
5. OPIOID
6. COCAINE
7. AMPHETAMINE TYPE
8. ANTIDEPRESSANT TYPE
9. MIXED OR OTHER SPECIFIED
5th Digit: 305
0. NOS
1. CONTINUOUS
2. EPISODIC
3. IN REMISSION

305.9# NONDEPENDENT POLYSUBSTANCE (ABUSE)
5th Digit: 305.9
0. NOS
1. CONTINUOUS
2. EPISODIC
3. IN REMISSION

648.3# : CODE THE SPECIFIC MATERNAL DRUG ABUSE OR DEPENDENCE WITH AN ADDITIONAL CODE. SEE 'ABUSE' DRUG.

DRUG ABUSE COMPLICATING PREGNANCY

648.3# MATERNAL CURRENT (CO-EXISTENT)
5th Digit: 648.3
0. EPISODE OF CARE UNSPECIFIED OR N/A
1. DELIVERED
2. DELIVERED WITH POSTPARTUM COMPLICATION
3. ANTEPARTUM COMPLICATION
4. POSTPARTUM COMPLICATION

DRUG ABUSE COMPLICATING PREGNANCY (continued)

655.5# MATERNAL WITH SUSPECTED DAMAGE TO FETUS
5th Digit: 655.5
0. EPISODE OF CARE UNSPECIFIED OR N/A
1. DELIVERED
3. ANTEPARTUM COMPLICATION

DRUG INDUCED MENTAL DISORDERS (WITH ASSOCIATED DRUG DEPENDENCE)

292.9 NOS [304.##]
292.84 AFFECTIVE SYNDROME ORGANIC [304.##]
292.83 AMNESIA [304.##]
292.89 ANXIETY [304.##]
4th Digit: 304
0. OPIOID
1. BARBITURATE, SEDATIVES, AND TRANQUILIZERS WITH A SIMILAR EFFECT
2. COCAINE
3. CANNABIS
4. AMPHETAMINE TYPE
5. HALLUCINOGENIC
6. OTHER SPECIFIED
7. MIXED WITH OPIOID
8. MIXED
9. NOS
5th Digit: 304
0. UNSPECIFIED
1. CONTINUOUS
2. EPISODIC
3. IN REMISSION

305.3 BAD TRIP (LSD) (HALLUCINOGENIC)
292.81 DELIRIUM [304.##]
292.11 DELUSIONAL PSYCHOSIS [304.##]
292.82 DEMENTIA OR PSYCHOSIS [304.##]
292.84 DEPRESSION [304.##]
292.12 HALLUCINATORY PSYCHOSIS [304.##]
292.2 INTOXICATION PATHOLOGICAL (RESULTING IN BRIEF PSYCHOTIC STATE) [304.##]
292.9 MENTAL DISORDER [304.##]
292.11 PARANOID STATE [304.##]
292.89 PERSONALITY [304.##]
292.9 PSYCHOSIS NOS [304.##]
292.0 WITHDRAWAL SYNDROME [304.##]
292.89 OTHER SPECIFIED MENTAL DISORDER [304.##]
4th Digit: 304
0. OPIOID
1. BARBITURATE, SEDATIVES, AND TRANQUILIZERS WITH A SIMILAR EFFECT
2. COCAINE
3. CANNABIS
4. AMPHETAMINE TYPE
5. HALLUCINOGENIC
6. OTHER SPECIFIED
7. MIXED WITH OPIOID
8. MIXED
9. NOS
5th Digit: 304
0. UNSPECIFIED
1. CONTINUOUS
2. EPISODIC
3. IN REMISSION

DRUG REACTION

292.2 UNSPECIFIED WITH BRIEF PSYCHOSIS (UNEXPECTED)
292.2 IDIOSYNCRATIC RESULTING IN BRIEF PSYCHOTIC STATE
763.5 MATERNAL AFFECTING FETUS OR NEWBORN
779.4 NEWBORN SPECIFIC TO NEWBORN
292.2 PATHOLOGIC RESULTING IN BRIEF PSYCHOTIC STATE

NEVER USE A CODE FOR DRUG RESISTANCE AS A PRINCIPAL DIAGNOSIS. THESE SHOULD BE USED AS ADDITIONAL CODES ONLY.

DO NOT ASSIGN THESE CODES SOLELY ON THE BASIS OF LAB REPORTS. ONLY THE PHYSICIAN CAN DIAGNOSE AN INFECTION WITH A DRUG RESISTANT ORGANISM.

SEQUENCING OF DRUG RESISTANT ORGANISMS: THE DISEASE OR COMPLICATION CODE IS FIRST, FOLLOWED BY THE ORGANISM CODE (IF KNOWN), FOLLOWED BY THE V09. CODE.

DRUG RESISTANCE

V09.90 DRUGS NOS
V09.91 DRUGS MULTIPLE NOS
V09.4 AMIKACIN
V09.4 AMINOGLYCOSIDES NEC
V09.5# AMODIAQUINE
V09.8# AMODIQUIN
5th Digit: V09.5, 8
0. WITHOUT RESISTANCE TO MULTIPLE DRUGS OF THIS CLASS
1. WITH RESISTANCE TO MULTIPLE DRUGS OF THIS CLASS

V09.0 AMOXICILLIN
V09.0 AMPICILLIN
V09.7# ANTIMYCOBACTERIAL AGENTS NEC
5th Digit: V09.7
0. WITHOUT RESISTANCE TO MULTIPLE DRUGS OF THIS CLASS
1. WITH RESISTANCE TO MULTIPLE DRUGS OF THIS CLASS

V09.2 AZITHROMYCIN
V09.0 AZLOCILLIN
V09.1 AZTREONAM
V09.1 B-LACTAM ANTIBIOTICS NEC
V09.0 BACAMPICILLIN
V09.8# BACITRACIN
V09.8# BENZNIDAZOLE
V09.7# CAPREOMYCIN
5th Digit: V09.7-8
0. WITHOUT RESISTANCE TO MULTIPLE DRUGS OF THIS CLASS
1. WITH RESISTANCE TO MULTIPLE DRUGS OF THIS CLASS

V09.0 CARBENICILLIN
V09.1 CEFACLOR
V09.1 CEFADROXIL
V09.1 CEFAMANDOLE
V09.1 CEFATETAN
V09.1 CEFAZOLIN
V09.1 CEFONICID
V09.1 CEFOPERAZONE
V09.1 CEFORANIDE
V09.1 CEFOTAXIME
V09.1 CEFOXITIN
V09.1 CEFTAZIDINE
V09.1 CEFTIZOXIME
V09.1 CEFTRIAXONE
V09.1 CEFUROXIME
V09.1 CEPHALOGLYCIN
V09.1 CEPHALORIDINE
V09.1 CEPHALOSPORINS NEC
V09.1 CEPHALOTHIN
V09.1 CEPHAPIRIN
V09.1 CEPHRADINE

DRUG RESISTANCE (continued)

V09.8# CHLORAMPHENICOL
V09.5# CHLORAQUINE
V09.8# CHLORGUANIDE
V09.8# CHLOROQUINE
V09.8# CHLORPROGUANIL
5th Digit: V09.5, 8
0. WITHOUT RESISTANCE TO MULTIPLE DRUGS OF THIS CLASS
1. WITH RESISTANCE TO MULTIPLE DRUGS OF THIS CLASS

V09.3 CHLORTETRACYCLINE
V09.5# CINOXACIN
V09.5# CIPROFLOXACIN
5th Digit: V09.5
0. WITHOUT RESISTANCE TO MULTIPLE DRUGS OF THIS CLASS
1. WITH RESISTANCE TO MULTIPLE DRUGS OF THIS CLASS

V09.2 CLARITHROMYCIN
V09.8# CLINDAMYCIN
V09.5# CLIOQUINOL
V09.7# CLOFAZIMINE
5th Digit: V09.5, 7-8
0. WITHOUT RESISTANCE TO MULTIPLE DRUGS OF THIS CLASS
1. WITH RESISTANCE TO MULTIPLE DRUGS OF THIS CLASS

V09.0 CLOXACILLIN
V09.0 CYCLACILLIN
V09.7# CYCLOSERINE
V09.7# DAPSONE (DZ)
5th Digit: V09.7
0. WITHOUT RESISTANCE TO MULTIPLE DRUGS OF THIS CLASS
1. WITH RESISTANCE TO MULTIPLE DRUGS OF THIS CLASS

V09.3 DEMECLOCYCLINE
V09.0 DICLOXACILLIN
V09.3 DOXYCYCLINE
V09.1 ECPHALEXIN
V09.5# ENOXACIN
5th Digit: V09.5
0. WITHOUT RESISTANCE TO MULTIPLE DRUGS OF THIS CLASS
1. WITH RESISTANCE TO MULTIPLE DRUGS OF THIS CLASS

V09.2 ERYTHROMYCIN
V09.7# ETHAMBUTOL (EMB)
V09.7# ETHIONAMIDE (ETA)
V09.5# FLUOROQUINOLONES
5th Digit: V09.5, 7
0. WITHOUT RESISTANCE TO MULTIPLE DRUGS OF THIS CLASS
1. WITH RESISTANCE TO MULTIPLE DRUGS OF THIS CLASS

V09.4 GENTAMICIN
V09.8# HALOFANTRINE
5th Digit: V09.8
0. WITHOUT RESISTANCE TO MULTIPLE DRUGS OF THIS CLASS
1. WITH RESISTANCE TO MULTIPLE DRUGS OF THIS CLASS

V09.1 IMIPENEM
V09.5# IODOQUINOL
V09.7# ISONIAZID (INH)
5th Digit: V09.5, 7
0. WITHOUT RESISTANCE TO MULTIPLE DRUGS OF THIS CLASS
1. WITH RESISTANCE TO MULTIPLE DRUGS OF THIS CLASS

DRUG RESISTANCE (continued)

V09.4 KANAMYCIN
V09.2 MACROLIDES NEC
V09.6 MAFENIDE
V09.8# MEFLOQUINE
V09.8# MELASSOPROL
5th Digit: V09.8
0. WITHOUT RESISTANCE TO MULTIPLE DRUGS OF THIS CLASS
1. WITH RESISTANCE TO MULTIPLE DRUGS OF THIS CLASS

V09.0 METHACILLIN
V09.3 METHACYCLINE
V09.8# METHENAMINE
V09.8# METRONIDAZOLE
5th Digit: V09.8
0. WITHOUT RESISTANCE TO MULTIPLE DRUGS OF THIS CLASS
1. WITH RESISTANCE TO MULTIPLE DRUGS OF THIS CLASS

V09.0 MEXLOCILLIN
V09.3 MINOCYCLINE
V09.0 NAFCILLIN
V09.5# NALIDIXIC ACID
5th Digit: V09.5
0. WITHOUT RESISTANCE TO MULTIPLE DRUGS OF THIS CLASS
1. WITH RESISTANCE TO MULTIPLE DRUGS OF THIS CLASS

V09.2 NATAMYCIN
V09.4 NEOMYCIN
V09.4 NETILMICIN
V09.8# NIMORAZOLE
V09.8# NITROFURANTOIN
V09.8# NITROFURTIMOX
V09.5# NORFLOXACIN
5th Digit: V09.5, 8
0. WITHOUT RESISTANCE TO MULTIPLE DRUGS OF THIS CLASS
1. WITH RESISTANCE TO MULTIPLE DRUGS OF THIS CLASS

V09.2 NYSTATIN
V09.5# OFLOXACIN
5th Digit: V09.5
0. WITHOUT RESISTANCE TO MULTIPLE DRUGS OF THIS CLASS
1. WITH RESISTANCE TO MULTIPLE DRUGS OF THIS CLASS

V09.2 OLEANDOMYCIN
V09.8# OTHER SPECIFIED DRUGS NEC
5th Digit: V09.8
0. WITHOUT RESISTANCE TO MULTIPLE DRUGS OF THIS CLASS
1. WITH RESISTANCE TO MULTIPLE DRUGS OF THIS CLASS

V09.0 OXACILLIN
V09.3 OXYTETRACYCLINE
V09.7# PARA-AMINO SALICYLIC ACID (PAS)
5th Digit: V09.7
0. WITHOUT RESISTANCE TO MULTIPLE DRUGS OF THIS CLASS
1. WITH RESISTANCE TO MULTIPLE DRUGS OF THIS CLASS

V09.4 PAROMOMYCIN
V09.0 PENICILLIN (G) (V) (VK)
V09.8# PENTAMIDINE
5th Digit: V09.8
0. WITHOUT RESISTANCE TO MULTIPLE DRUGS OF THIS CLASS
1. WITH RESISTANCE TO MULTIPLE DRUGS OF THIS CLASS

V09.0 PIPERACILLIN

V09.5# PRIMAQUINE
V09.8# PROGUANIL
V09.7# PYRAZINAMIDE (PZA)
V09.8# PYRIMETHAMINE/SULFALENE
V09.8# PYRIMETHAMINE/SULFODOXINE
V09.5# QUINACRINE
V09.8# QUINIDINE
V09.8# QUININE
V09.5# QUINOLONES NEC
V09.7# RIFABUTIN
V09.7# RIFAMPIN (RIF)
V09.7# RIFAMYCIN
5th Digit: V09.5, 7-8
0. WITHOUT RESISTANCE TO MULTIPLE DRUGS OF THIS CLASS
1. WITH RESISTANCE TO MULTIPLE DRUGS OF THIS CLASS

V09.3 ROLITETRACYCLINE
V09.8# SPECTINOMYCIN
5th Digit: V09.8
0. WITHOUT RESISTANCE TO MULTIPLE DRUGS OF THIS CLASS
1. WITH RESISTANCE TO MULTIPLE DRUGS OF THIS CLASS

V09.2 SPIRAMYCIN
V09.4 STREPTOMYCIN (SM)
V09.6 SULFACETAMIDE
V09.6 SULFACYTINE
V09.6 SULFADIAZINE
V09.6 SULFADOXINE
V09.6 SULFAMETHOXAZOLE
V09.6 SULFAPYRIDINE
V09.6 SULFASALIZINE
V09.6 SULFISOXAZOLE
V09.6 SULFONAMIDES
V09.7# SULFOXONE
5th Digit: V09.7
0. WITHOUT RESISTANCE TO MULTIPLE DRUGS OF THIS CLASS
1. WITH RESISTANCE TO MULTIPLE DRUGS OF THIS CLASS

V09.3 TETRACYCLINE
V09.3 TETRACYCLINES NEC
V09.8# THIAMPHENICOL
5th Digit: V09.8
0. WITHOUT RESISTANCE TO MULTIPLE DRUGS OF THIS CLASS
1. WITH RESISTANCE TO MULTIPLE DRUGS OF THIS CLASS

V09.0 TICARCILLIN
V09.8# TINIDAZOLE
5th Digit: V09.8
0. WITHOUT RESISTANCE TO MULTIPLE DRUGS OF THIS CLASS
1. WITH RESISTANCE TO MULTIPLE DRUGS OF THIS CLASS

V09.4 TOBRAMYCIN
V09.8# TRIAMPHENICOL
V09.8# TRIMETHOPRIM
V09.8# VANCOMYCIN
5th Digit: V09.8
0. WITHOUT RESISTANCE TO MULTIPLE DRUGS OF THIS CLASS
1. WITH RESISTANCE TO MULTIPLE DRUGS OF THIS CLASS

DRUG WITHDRAWAL

292.0 SYMPTOMS OR SYNDROME
779.5 SYMPTOMS OR SYNDROME NEWBORN OR INFANT OF DEPENDENT MOTHER

303.0# DRUNKENNESS ACUTE IN ALCOHOLISM
305.0# DRUNKENNESS NONDEPENDENT
5th Digit: 303.0, 305.0
0. UNSPECIFIED
1. CONTINUOUS
2. EPISODIC
3. IN REMISSION

291.4 DRUNKENNESS PATHOLOGIC

DRUSEN
362.57 DEGENERATIVE
362.77 HEREDITARY
377.21 OPTIC DISC

375.15 DRY EYE SYNDROME
701.1 DRY SKIN SYNDROME
526.5 DRY SOCKET
291.0 DT'S
300.14 DUAL PERSONALITY DISORDER
378.71 DUANE'S SYNDROME (DUANE-STILLING-TURK SYNDROME) (OCULAR RETRACTION)
626.8 DUB
277.4 DUBIN-JOHNSON SYNDROME (CONSTITUTIONAL HYPERBILIRUBINEMIA)
277.4 DUBIN-SPRINZ SYNDROME (CONSTITUTIONAL HYPERBILIRUBINEMIA)
049.8 DUBINI'S ELECTRIC CHOREA
090.5 DUBOIS' THYMUS GLAND (ABSCESS)

DUCHENNE'S
335.21 ARAN MUSCULAR ATROPHY
094.0 DISEASE
094.0 LOCOMOTOR ATAXIA
359.1 MUSCULAR DYSTROPHY
335.22 PARALYSIS
359.1 PSEUDOHYPERTROPHY MUSCLES
335.22 SYNDROME

747.89 DUCTUS ARTERIOSUS ABSENCE CONGENITAL
795.79 DUFFY ANTIGEN POSITIVE
694.0 DUHRING'S DISEASE (DERMATITIS HERPETIFORMIS)
057.8 DUKES FILATOW DISEASE
085.0 DUMDUM FEVER
564.2 DUMPING SYNDROME
536.8 DUMPING SYNDROME NONSURGICAL
0 DUODENAL SEE 'DUODENUM, DUODENAL'

DUODENUM, DUODENAL
V45.72 ABSENCE (ACQUIRED) (POSTOPERATIVE)
751.1 ATRESIA (ABSENCE) CONGENITAL
568.0 BAND DUE TO ADHESION
564.89 DILATATION
537.9 DISORDER
537.89 DISORDER OTHER SPECIFIED NEC
562.00 DIVERTICULA
751.5 DIVERTICULA CONGENITAL
535.6# DUODENITIS
5th Digit : 535.6
0. WITHOUT HEMORRHAGE
1. WITH HEMORRHAGE

793.4 FILLING DEFECT
537.4 FISTULA
537.2 ILEUS CHRONIC
863.21 INJURY TRAUMATIC
863.31 INJURY TRAUMATIC WITH OPEN WOUND
908.1 INJURY TRAUMATIC LATE EFFECT
564.89 IRRITABILITY
537.3 OBSTRUCTION
751.1 OBSTRUCTION CONGENITAL
0 OBSTRUCTION DUE TO ULCER SEE 'ULCER', DUODENAL
537.89 PROLAPSE

DUODENUM, DUODENAL (continued)
537.89 REFLUX
537.89 RUPTURE
564.89 SPASM
751.1 STENOSIS (CICATRIX) (STRUCTURE) CONGENITAL
537.3 STENOSIS (STRICTURE) (VOLVULUS) (CICATRIX)
532.## ULCER
532.## ULCER DUE TO HELICOBACTER PYLORI [041.86]
316 ULCER PSYCHOGENIC [532.##]
4th Digit: 532
0. ACUTE WITH HEMORRHAGE
1. ACUTE WITH PERFORATION
2. ACUTE WITH HEMORRHAGE AND PERFORATION
3. ACUTE
4. CHRONIC OR UNSPECIFIED WITH HEMORRHAGE
5. CHRONIC OR UNSPECIFIED WITH PERFORATION
6. CHRONIC OR UNSPECIFIED WITH HEMORRHAGE AND PERFORATION
7. CHRONIC
9. UNSPECIFIED AS ACUTE OR CHRONIC
5th Digit: 532
0. WITHOUT OBSTRUCTION
1. OBSTRUCTED

537.3 VOLVULUS

726.2 DUPLAY'S DISEASE OR SYNDROME
781.6 DUPRE'S SYNDROME (MENINGISM)
728.6 DUPUYTREN'S CONTRACTURE OF PALMAR FASCIA
099.1 DURAND-NICOLAS-FAVRE CLIMATIC BUBO
746.5 DUROZIEZ'S CONGENITAL MITRAL STENOSIS
086.9 DUTTON'S TRYPANOSOMIASIS
0 DVT (DEEP VEIN THROMBOSIS) SEE 'THROMBOSIS', SPECIFIED VEIN

DWARFISM
259.4 UNSPECIFIED
756.4 ACHONDROPLASIA
759.7 INTRAUTERINE
253.3 LORAIN LEVI
263.2 NUTRITIONAL
253.3 PITUITARY
259.8 PROGERIA
316 PSYCHOSOCIAL FACTORS [259.4]
588.0 RENAL

283.9 DYKE YOUNG SYNDROME (ACQUIRED MACROCYTIC HEMOLYTIC ANEMIA)
784.5 DYSARTHRIA
440.21 DYSBASIA ANGIOSCLEROTICA DUE TO ATHEROSCLEROSIS
315.1 DYSCALCULIA (DELAY IN DEVELOPMENT)
756.4 DYSCHONDROPLASIA CONGENITAL
756.4 DYSCHONDROPLASIA WITH HEMANGIOMATA
709.0# DYSCHROMIA
5th Digit: 709.0
0. UNSPECIFIED
1. VITILIGO
9. OTHER DYSCHROMIA

289.9 DYSCRASIA BLOOD
004.0 DYSENTERIAE SHIGELLA
009.2 DYSENTERIC DIARRHEA

DYSENTERY
009.2 UNSPECIFIED
006.0 AMEBIC ACUTE
006.1 AMEBIC CHRONIC
0 BACILLARY SEE 'DYSENTERY', SHIGELLA
009.0 CATARRHAL
007.4 CRYPTOSPORIDIAL
009.0 HEMORRHAGIC
009.0 INFECTIOUS
009.0 INFECTIOUS (HEMORRHAGIC)

D

DYSENTERY (continued)

007.# PROTOZOAL

4th Digit: 007

0. BALANTIDIASIS
1. GIARDIASIS
2. COCCIDIOSIS
3. TRICHOMONIASIS
4. CRYPTOSPORIDIOSIS
8. OTHER SPECIFIED
9. UNSPECIFIED

004.9 SHIGELLA
004.2 SHIGELLA BOYDII (GROUP C)
004.0 SHIGELLA DYSENTERIAE (GROUP A) (SCHMITZ) (SHIGA)
004.1 SHIGELLA FLEXNERI (GROUP B)
004.3 SHIGELLA SONNEI (GROUP D)
004.8 SHIGELLA OTHER SPECIFIED

780.4 DYSEQUILIBRIUM
286.3 DYSFIBRINOGENEMIA
626.8 DYSFUNCTIONAL UTERINE BLEEDING (HEMORRHAGE)
279.06 DYSGAMMAGLOBULINEMIA (ACQUIRED) (CONGENITAL) (PRIMARY)

DYSGERMINOMA

183.0 FEMALE SITE NOS
0 FEMALE SITE SPECIFIED SEE 'CANCER' BY SITE M9060/3
186.9 MALE SITE NOS
0 MALE SITE SPECIFIED SEE 'CANCER' BY SITE M9060/3

705.81 DYSHIDROSIS
795.0 DYSKARYOTIC CERVICAL SMEAR (PAP)

DYSKINESIA

781.3 DYSKINESIA
530.5 ESOPHAGUS
300.11 HYSTERICAL
564.89 INTESTINAL
333.82 OROFACIAL
307.9 PSYCHOGENIC
333.82 TARDIVE

784.5 DYSLALIA
315.39 DYSLALIA DEVELOPMENT

784.61 DYSLEXIA
315.02 DYSLEXIA DEVELOPMENTAL (DELAY IN DEVELOPMENT)

625.3 DYSMENORRHEA
306.52 DYSMENORRHEA PSYCHOGENIC
300.7 DYSMORPHIC BODY DISORDER

625.0 DYSPAREUNIA
608.89 DYSPAREUNIA MALE
302.76 DYSPAREUNIA PSYCHOGENIC
536.3 DYSPEPSIA ATONIC
536.8 DYSPEPSIA DISORDERS OTHER SPECIFIED FUNCTION OF STOMACH
564.89 DYSPEPSIA INTESTINAL
306.4 DYSPEPSIA PSYCHOGENIC (CYCLICAL)

787.2 DYSPHAGIA
438.82 DYSPHAGIA LATE EFFECT OF CEREBROVASCULAR DISEASE
288.1 DYSPHAGOCYTOSIS CONGENITAL

784.5 DYSPHASIA
438.12 DYSPHASIA LATE EFFECT CEREBROVASCULAR DISEASE

784.49 DYSPHONIA
374.52 DYSPIGMENTATION EYELID
253.9 DYSPITUITARISM

770.7 DYSPLASIA BRONCHOPULMONARY PERINATAL
622.1 DYSPLASIA CERVIX - CIN I
622.1 DYSPLASIA CERVIX - CIN II
233.1 DYSPLASIA CERVIX - CIN III (SEVERE)
623.0 DYSPLASIA VAGINA
624.8 DYSPLASIA VULVA
233.3 DYSPLASIA VULVA VIN III
786.09 DYSPNEA (PAROXYSMAL) (NOCTURNAL)
306.1 DYSPNEIC DISORDER PSYCHOGENIC
781.3 DYSPRAXIA
315.4 DYSPRAXIA SYNDROME
286.3 DYSPROTHROMBINEMIA
337.3 DYSREFLEXIA AUTONOMIC
337.3 DYSREFLEXIA AUTONOMIC WITH DECUBITUS ULCER [707.0]
337.3 DYSREFLEXIA AUTONOMIC WITH FECAL IMPACTION [560.39]

> *URINARY TRACT INFECTION: USE ADDITIONAL CODE FOR ORGANISM. SEE 'BACTERIAL INFECTION'.*

337.3 DYSREFLEXIA AUTONOMIC WITH URINARY TRACT INFECTION [599.0]

> *CARDIAC DYSRHYTHMIA , 427.9, IS A NON-SPECIFIC DIAGNOSIS. ALWAYS CODE THE SPECIFIC TYPE OF DYSRHYTHMIA WHEN POSSIBLE.*

DYSRHYTHMIAS

427.9 CARDIAC DYSRHYTHMIA
427.31 ATRIAL FIBRILLATION (PAROXYSMAL)
427.32 ATRIAL FLUTTER
427.61 ATRIAL PREMATURE BEATS CONTRACTIONS OR SYSTOLES
427.89 BIGEMINY
427.2 BOUVERET-HOFFMANN SYNDROME
427.81 BRADYCARDIA CHRONIC
337.0 BRADYCARDIA REFLEX
427.89 BRADYCARDIA SINUS
427.81 BRADYCARDIA SINUS (PERSISTENT) (SEVERE)
427.89 BRADYCARDIA VAGAL
427.81 BRADYCARDIA WITH PAT
427.5 CARDIAC ARREST NOS
337.0 CAROTID SINUS SYNCOPE
427.89 CORONARY SINUS ARRHYTHMIA
427.89 ECTOPIC ARRHYTHMIA
427.61 ECTOPIC AURICULAR BEATS
427.60 ECTOPIC BEATS
427.69 ECTOPIC VENTRICULAR BEATS
427.60 EXTRASYSTOLES
427.31 FIBRILLATION ATRIAL
427.41 FIBRILLATION VENTRICULAR
427.32 FLUTTER ATRIAL
427.42 FLUTTER VENTRICULAR
0 FOLLOWING ABORTION SEE 'ABORTION'
0 FOLLOWING ECTOPIC OR MOLAR PREGNANCY SEE 'ECTOPIC PREGNANCY' OR 'MOLAR PREGNANCY'
427.60 JUNCTIONAL PREMATURE CONTRACTION
429.4 LATE EFFECT OF CARDIAC SURGERY
427.60 NODAL PREMATURE CONTRACTION
427.61 PAC'S (PREMATURE ATRIAL CONTRACTIONS)
429.4 PACEMAKER SYNDROME
427.2 PAROXYSMAL TACHYCARDIA
427.0 PAROXYSMAL TACHYCARDIA ATRIAL
427.0 PAROXYSMAL TACHYCARDIA SUPRAVENTRICULAR
427.1 PAROXYSMAL TACHYCARDIA VENTRICULAR
427.0 PAT PAROXYSMAL ATRIAL TACHYCARDIA
316 PAT PSYCHOGENIC [427.0]
429.4 POSTCARDIOTOMY SYNDROME
997.1 POSTOPERATIVE (DURING OR RESULTING FROM A PROCEDURE)
429.4 POSTVALVULOTOMY SYNDROME

DYSRHYTHMIAS (continued)

427.61 PREMATURE ATRIAL CONTRACTIONS
427.60 PREMATURE JUNCTIONAL CONTRACTIONS
427.60 PREMATURE NODAL CONTRACTION
427.69 PREMATURE VENTRICULAR CONTRACTIONS
427.69 OTHER PREMATURE BEATS
427.69 PVC'S
427.81 SICK SINUS SYNDROME
427.81 SINOATRIAL NODE DYSFUNCTION
427.89 SINUS BRADYCARDIA
427.81 SINUS BRADYCARDIA PERSISTENT
427.81 SINUS BRADYCARDIA SEVERE
427.61 SUPRAVENTRICULAR PREMATURE BEATS
427.89 SUPRAVENTRICULAR TACHYCARDIA
427.0 SUPRAVENTRICULAR TACHYCARDIA PAROXYSMAL
427.81 TACHYBRADY SYNDROME
785.0 TACHYCARDIA
427.89 TACHYCARDIA ATRIAL
427.0 TACHYCARDIA ATRIAL PAROXYSMAL
427.0 TACHYCARDIA AV PAROXYSMAL
427.81 TACHYCARDIA BRADYCARDIA SYNDROME
427.0 TACHYCARDIA JUNCTIONAL PAROXYSMAL
427.2 TACHYCARDIA PAROXYSMAL
427.89 TACHYCARDIA SUPRAVENTRICULAR
427.0 TACHYCARDIA SUPRAVENTRICULAR PAROXYSMAL
427.1 TACHYCARDIA VENTRICULAR
427.41 TACHYCARDIA VENTRICULAR FIBRILLATION
427.42 TACHYCARDIA VENTRICULAR FLUTTER
427.1 TACHYCARDIA VENTRICULAR PAROXYSMAL
427.1 V TACH
427.1 V TACH PAROXYSMAL
427.69 VENTRICULAR ESCAPE BEATS
427.41 VENTRICULAR FIBRILLATION
427.42 VENTRICULAR FLUTTER
427.69 VENTRICULAR PREMATURE BEATS (CONTRACTIONS)
427.69 VENTRICULAR PREMATURE CONTRACTIONS
427.5 VENTRICULAR STANDSTILL
427.1 VENTRICULAR TACHYCARDIA
427.1 VENTRICULAR TACHYCARDIA PAROXYSMAL
427.89 WANDERING (ATRIAL) PACEMAKER
427.89 OTHER SPECIFIED

289.4 DYSSPLENISM
334.2 DYSSYNERGIA CEREBELLARIS MYOCLONICA
300.4 DYSTHYMIC DISORDER
660.9# DYSTOCIA WITH OBSTRUCTED LABOR
660.4# DYSTOCIA SHOULDER OBSTRUCTING LABOR

5th Digit: 660.4, 9

0. EPISODE OF CARE UNSPECIFIED OR N/A
1. DELIVERED
3. ANTEPARTUM COMPLICATION

654.9# DYSTOCIA SYNDROME (DYSTROPHIA)

5th Digit: 654.9

0. EPISODE OF CARE UNSPECIFIED OR N/A
1. DELIVERED
2. DELIVERED WITH POSTPARTUM COMPLICATION
3. ANTEPARTUM COMPLICATION
4. POSTPARTUM COMPLICATION

333.6 DYSTONIA DEFORMANS PROGRESSIVA
333.7 DYSTONIA DUE TO DRUGS
333.6 DYSTONIA IDIOPATHIC TORSION
333.6 DYSTONIA MUSCULORUM DEFORMANS
333.7 DYSTONIA SYMPTOMATIC TORSION

359.2 DYSTROPHIA MYOTONICA
703.8 DYSTROPHIA UNGUIUM

337.0 DYSTROPHY CERVICAL SYMPATHETIC (CAUSALGIA)
270.8 DYSTROPHY OCULOCEREBRORENAL
337.2# DYSTROPHY REFLEX/POSTTRAUMATIC SYMPATHETIC

5th Digit: 337.2

0. UNSPECIFIED
1. UPPER LIMB
2. LOWER LIMB
9. OTHER SPECIFIED SITE

788.1 DYSURIA
306.53 DYSURIA PSYCHOGENIC

041.4 E COLI INFECTION OR ORGANISM
771.8 E COLI INFECTION INTRA-AMNIOTIC (FETUS OR NEWBORN)
756.71 EAGLE-BARRETT SYNDROME
362.18 EALES' DISEASE OR SYNDROME

EAR

388.8 ABSENCE
0 ABSENCE CONGENITAL SEE 'EAR ANOMALY'
388.70 ACHE
0 ANOMALY SEE 'EAR ANOMALY'
388.9 ATROPHY
380.50 CANAL OBSTRUCTION
388.60 DISCHARGE
388.69 DISCHARGE BLOOD
388.61 DISCHARGE CEREBROSPINAL FLUID
384.20 DRUM PERFORATION (SEE ALSO 'TYMPANIC MEMBRANE PERFORATION')
V72.1 EXAM
0 EXTERNAL EAR SEE ALSO 'PINNA'
380.31 HEMATOMA AURICLE
388.69 HEMORRHAGE
380.10 INFECTION EXTERNAL NOS (SEE ALSO 'OTITIS EXTERNA')
386.30 INFECTION INNER NOS (SEE ALSO 'LABYRINTHITIS')
382.9 INFECTION MIDDLE (SEE ALSO 'OTITIS MEDIA')
380.11 INFECTION PINNA ACUTE
698.9 ITCHING
388.8 MASS
388.10 NOISE EFFECTS (TO INNER EAR)
388.70 PAIN
388.71 PAIN OTOGENIC
388.72 PAIN REFERRED
V50.3 PIERCING (ELECTIVE)
381.81 PRESSURE (EUSTACHIAN)
V41.3 PROBLEM OTHER SPECIFIED
380.12 SWIMMER'S
380.4 WAX
V80.3 DISEASES SCREENING

EAR ANOMALY

744.3 NOS
744.00 NOS WITH IMPAIRMENT OF HEARING
744.09 ABSENCE
744.01 ABSENCE EXTERNAL EAR
744.21 ABSENCE LOBE
744.04 ABSENCE OSSICLES
744.02 CANAL ATRESIA
744.3 DEFORMITY NOS
744.02 EXTERNAL EAR OTHER WITH IMPAIRMENT OF HEARING
744.05 INNER EAR
744.03 MIDDLE EAR EXCEPT OSSICLES
744.1 SUPERNUMERARY (EAR) (LOBULE)
744.09 OTHER SPECIFIED CAUSING IMPAIRMENT OF HEARING

EAR DISORDER

388.9 UNSPECIFIED
388.00 DEGENERATIVE
380.9 EXTERNAL
380.89 EXTERNAL OTHER
388.9 INNER CHRONIC NEC
385.9 MIDDLE (AND MASTOID)
385.10 MIDDLE (AND MASTOID) ADHESIVE
385.89 MIDDLE (AND MASTOID) OTHER
388.00 VASCULAR
388.8 OTHER SPECIFIED NEC

EAR INFECTION

380.10 EXTERNAL NOS (SEE ALSO 'OTITIS EXTERNA')
035 EXTERNAL (ACUTE) ERYSIPELAS [380.13]
684 EXTERNAL (ACUTE) IMPETIGINOUS [380.13]
690.10 EXTERNAL SEBORRHEIC DERMATITIS NOS [380.13]
690.11 EXTERNAL SEBORRHEIC DERMATITIS CAPITIS [380.13]
690.12 EXTERNAL SEBORRHEIC DERMATITIS INFANTILE [380.13]
690.18 EXTERNAL SEBORRHEIC DERMATITIS OTHER [380.13]
386.30 INNER NOS (SEE ALSO 'LABYRINTHITIS')
382.9 MIDDLE SEE 'OTITIS MEDIA'

EAR INJURY

959.09 UNSPECIFIED
388.11 BLAST TRAUMA (INNER EAR)
925.1 CRUSHING
910.8 OTHER AND UNSPECIFIED (SUPERFICIAL)
910.9 OTHER AND UNSPECIFIED (SUPERFICIAL) INFECTED

EAR OSSICLES

744.04 ANOMALIES CONGENITAL
385.23 DISCONTINUITY
385.23 DISLOCATION
385.22 IMPAIRED MOBILITY
385.21 IMPAIRED MOBILITY - MALLEUS
385.22 IMPAIRED MOBILITY - OTHER
385.24 PARTIAL LOSS OR NECROSIS

388.70 EARACHE
062.2 EASTERN EQUINE ENCEPHALITIS

EATING DISORDER

307.50 UNSPECIFIED
307.1 ANOREXIA NERVOSA
307.59 APPETITE LOSS PSYCHOGENIC
307.51 BULIMIA
783.3 DIFFICULTIES MISMANAGEMENT
783.6 EXCESSIVE
307.59 INFANTILE NONORGANIC
307.59 LOSS OF APPETITE NONORGANIC
307.52 PICA
V69.1 PROBLEM
307.50 PSYCHOGENIC NEC
307.53 RUMINATION PSYCHOGENIC
307.54 VOMITING PSYCHOGENIC
307.59 OTHER

EATON LAMBERT SYNDROME

005.1 BOTULISM [358.1]
250.6# DIABETIC [358.1]

5th Digit: 250.6

0. TYPE II, ADULT-ONSET, NON-INSULIN DEPENDENT (EVEN IF REQUIRING INSULIN), OR UNSPECIFIED; CONTROLLED
1. TYPE I, JUVENILE-ONSET OR INSULIN-DEPENDENT; CONTROLLED
2. TYPE II, ADULT-ONSET, NON-INSULIN DEPENDENT (EVEN IF REQUIRING INSULIN); UNCONTROLLED
3. TYPE I, JUVENILE-ONSET OR INSULIN-DEPENDENT; UNCONTROLLED

244.# HYPOTHYROID [358.1]

4th Digit: 244

0. POSTSURGICAL
1. POSTABLATIVE (IRRADIATION)
2. IODINE INGESTION
3. PAS, PHENYLBUT, RESORCINOL
8. SECONDARY NEC
9. NOS

281.0 PERNICIOUS ANEMIA [358.1]

E

EATON LAMBERT SYNDROME (continued)

242.## THYROTOXIC [358.1]

4th Digit: 242

0. TOXIC DIFFUSE GOITER
1. TOXIC UNINODULAR GOITER
2. TOXIC MULTINODULAR GOITER
3. TOXIC NODULAR GOITER UNSPECIFIED
4. FROM ECTOPIC THYROID NODULE
8. OF OTHER SPECIFIED ORIGIN
9. WITHOUT GOITER OR OTHER CAUSE

5th Digit: 242

0. WITHOUT STORM
1. WITH STORM

041.81 EATON'S AGENT INFECTION OR ORGANISM
002.2 EBERTH'S TYPHOID FEVER
065.8 EBOLA HEMORRHAGIC FEVER
065.8 EBOLA INFECTION (VIRUS)
746.2 EBSTEIN'S ANOMALY (HEART)
250.4# EBSTEIN'S NEPHROTIC SYNDROME (DIABETIC) [581.81]

5th Digit: 250.4

0. TYPE II, ADULT-ONSET, NON-INSULIN DEPENDENT (EVEN IF REQUIRING INSULIN), OR UNSPECIFIED; CONTROLLED
1. TYPE I, JUVENILE-ONSET OR INSULIN-DEPENDENT; CONTROLLED
2. TYPE II, ADULT-ONSET, NON-INSULIN DEPENDENT (EVEN IF REQUIRING INSULIN); UNCONTROLLED
3. TYPE I, JUVENILE-ONSET OR INSULIN-DEPENDENT; UNCONTROLLED

746.2 EBSTEIN'S SYNDROME (DOWNWARD DISPLACEMENT, TRICUSPID VALVE INTO RIGHT VENTRICLE)

ECCHYMOSES

459.89 NOS
372.72 CONJUNCTIVA
921.0 EYE (TRAUMATIC)
921.1 EYELID (TRAUMATIC)
772.6 FETUS OR NEWBORN
459.89 MULTIPLE
772.6 NEWBORN
782.7 SPONTANEOUS
0 TRAUMATIC SEE 'CONTUSION', BY SITE

216.# ECCRINE ACROSPIROMA M8402/0
216.# ECCRINE DERMAL CYLINDROMA M8200/0
216.# ECCRINE SPIRADENOMA M8403/0

4th Digit: 216

0. LIP (SKIN OF)
1. EYELID INCLUDING CANTHUS
2. EAR (EXTERNAL) (AURICLE) (PINNA)
3. FACE (CHEEK) (NOSE)
4. SCALP NECK
5. TRUNK BACK CHEST
6. UPPER LIMB INCLUDING SHOULDER
7. LOWER LIMB INCLUDING HIP
8. OTHER SPECIFIED SITES
9. SKIN UNSPECIFIED

794.31 ECG ABNORMAL
0 ECHINOCOCCIASIS SEE 'ECHINOCOCCUS'

ECHINOCOCCUS GRANULOSUS INFECTION

122.4 UNSPECIFIED
122.0 LIVER
122.1 LUNG
122.2 THYROID
122.3 OTHER

ECHINOCOCCUS INFECTION

122.9 UNSPECIFIED
122.8 LIVER
122.9 LUNG
122.9 THYROID
122.9 OTHER

ECHINOCOCCUS INFECTION OF ORBIT (EYE)

122.9 UNSPECIFIED [376.13]
122.3 GRANULOSUS [376.13]
122.6 MULTILOCULARIS [376.13]

ECHINOCOCCUS MULTILOCULARIS INFECTION

122.7 UNSPECIFIED
122.5 LIVER
122.6 LUNG
122.6 THYROID
122.6 OTHER

121.8 ECHINOSTOMA ILOCANUM INFECTION
078.89 ECHO VIRUS DISEASE NEC
079.1 ECHO VIRUS IN DISEASES CLASSIFIED ELSEWHERE
047.1 ECHO VIRUS MENINGITIS
793.2 ECHOCARDIOGRAM ABNORMAL
V72.81 ECHOCARDIOGRAM PREOPERATIVE
V72.85 ECHOCARDIOGRAM SCREENING
794.01 ECHOENCEPHALOGRAM ABNORMAL
793.# ECHOGRAM ABNORMAL FINDINGS (NONSPECIFIC) NEC

4th Digit: 793

0. SKULL AND HEAD
1. LUNG FIELD
2. OTHER INTRATHORACIC ORGAN
3. BILIARY TRACT
4. GASTROINTESTINAL TRACT
5. GENITOURINARY ORGANS
6. ABDOMINAL AREA INCLUDING RETROPERITONEUM
7. MUSCULOSKELETAL SYSTEM
8. BREAST
9. OTHER

780.39 ECLAMPSIA (COMA) (CONVULSIONS) (DELIRIUM) (NOT ASSOCIATED WITH CHILDBIRTH)
780.39 ECLAMPSIA MALE
642.6# ECLAMPSIA MATERNAL
642.7# ECLAMPSIA MATERNAL WITH PRE-EXISTING HYPERTENSION

5th Digit: 642.6-7

0. EPISODE OF CARE NOS OR N/A
1. DELIVERED
2. DELIVERED WITH POSTPARTUM COMPLICATIONS
3. ANTEPARTUM COMPLICATION
4. POSTPARTUM COMPLICATIONS

V60.9 ECONOMIC CIRCUMSTANCE (REASON FOR ENCOUNTER)
V60.8 ECONOMIC CIRCUMSTANCE OTHER SPECIFIED
049.8 ECONOMO'S ENCEPHALITIS LETHARGICA

ECTASIA

448.9 CAPILLARY
593.89 KIDNEY
448.9 PAPILLARY
527.8 SALIVARY GLAND (DUCT)

ECTHYMA

686.8 UNSPECIFIED
051.2 CONTAGIOSUM
686.09 GANGRENOSUM
051.2 INFECTIOSUM

757.31 ECTODERMAL DYSPLASIA CONGENITAL

ECTOPIC

255.0 ACTH SYNDROME
427.61 AURICULAR BEATS
427.60 BEATS
259.3 HORMONE SECRETION NEC
427.69 VENTRICULAR BEATS

ECTOPIC KIDNEY

753.3 UNSPECIFIED
654.4# PREGNANCY (CHILDBIRTH)
660.2# PREGNANCY (CHILDBIRTH) OBSTRUCTING LABOR [**654.4#**]

5th Digit: 654.4

0. EPISODE OF CARE UNSPECIFIED OR N/A
1. DELIVERED
2. DELIVERED WITH POSTPARTUM COMPLICATION
3. ANTEPARTUM COMPLICATION
4. POSTPARTUM COMPLICATION

5th Digit: 660.2

0. EPISODE OF CARE UNSPECIFIED OR N/A
1. DELIVERED
3. ANTEPARTUM COMPLICATION

ECTOPIC ORGANS CONGENITAL

751.8 ABDOMINAL VISCERA
756.79 ABDOMINAL VISCERA DUE TO DEFECT IN ANTERIOR ABDOMINAL WALL
759.1 ADRENAL GLAND
753.5 BLADDER
748.69 BONE AND CARTILAGE IN LUNG
742.4 BRAIN
757.6 BREAST TISSUE
746.87 CARDIUM
742.4 CEREBRUM
746.87 CORDIS
617.9 ENDOMETRIUM
751.69 GALLBLADDER
750.7 GASTRIC MUCOSA
743.37 LENTIS
752.0 OVARY CONGENITAL
751.7 PANCREAS
750.26 SEBACEOUS GLANDS MOUTH
752.51 TESTIS
759.2 THYROID
753.5 VESICAE

ECTOPIC PREGNANCY (RUPTURED) (UNRUPTURED)

633.9 UNSPECIFIED
633.9 UNSPECIFIED WITH COMPLICATION DURING TREATMENT [**639.#**]
639.# UNSPECIFIED WITH COMPLICATION FOLLOWING TREATMENT

4th Digit: 639

0. GENITAL TRACT AND PELVIC INFECTION
1. DELAYED OR EXCESSIVE HEMORRHAGE
2. DAMAGE TO PELVIC ORGANS AND TISSUE
3. RENAL FAILURE
4. METABOLIC DISORDERS
5. SHOCK
6. EMBOLISM
8. OTHER SPECIFIED COMPLICATION
9. UNSPECIFIED COMPLICATION

633.0 ABDOMINAL
761.4 ABDOMINAL AFFECTING FETUS OR NEWBORN
633.0 ABDOMINAL WITH COMPLICATION DURING TREATMENT [**639.#**]
639.# ABDOMINAL WITH COMPLICATION FOLLOWING TREATMENT

4th Digit: 639

0. GENITAL TRACT AND PELVIC INFECTION
1. DELAYED OR EXCESSIVE HEMORRHAGE
2. DAMAGE TO PELVIC ORGANS AND TISSUE
3. RENAL FAILURE
4. METABOLIC DISORDERS
5. SHOCK
6. EMBOLISM
8. OTHER SPECIFIED COMPLICATION
9. UNSPECIFIED COMPLICATION

761.4 AFFECTING FETUS OR NEWBORN

ECTOPIC PREGNANCY (RUPTURED) (UNRUPTURED) (continued)

639.# COMPLICATION FOLLOWING TREATMENT

4th Digit: 639

0. GENITAL TRACT AND PELVIC INFECTION
1. DELAYED OR EXCESSIVE HEMORRHAGE
2. DAMAGE TO PELVIC ORGANS AND TISSUE
3. RENAL FAILURE
4. METABOLIC DISORDERS
5. SHOCK
6. EMBOLISM
8. OTHER SPECIFIED COMPLICATION
9. UNSPECIFIED COMPLICATION

633.2 OVARIAN
633.2 OVARIAN WITH COMPLICATION DURING TREATMENT [**639.#**]
639.# OVARIAN WITH COMPLICATION FOLLOWING TREATMENT

4th Digit: 639

0. GENITAL TRACT AND PELVIC INFECTION
1. DELAYED OR EXCESSIVE HEMORRHAGE
2. DAMAGE TO PELVIC ORGANS AND TISSUE
3. RENAL FAILURE
4. METABOLIC DISORDERS
5. SHOCK
6. EMBOLISM
8. OTHER SPECIFIED COMPLICATION
9. UNSPECIFIED COMPLICATION

633.1 TUBAL
761.4 TUBAL AFFECTING FETUS OR NEWBORN
633.1 TUBAL WITH COMPLICATION DURING TREATMENT [**639.#**]
639.# TUBAL WITH COMPLICATION FOLLOWING TREATMENT

4th Digit: 639

0. GENITAL TRACT AND PELVIC INFECTION
1. DELAYED OR EXCESSIVE HEMORRHAGE
2. DAMAGE TO PELVIC ORGANS AND TISSUE
3. RENAL FAILURE
4. METABOLIC DISORDERS
5. SHOCK
6. EMBOLISM
8. OTHER SPECIFIED COMPLICATION
9. UNSPECIFIED COMPLICATION

633.8 OTHER
761.4 OTHER AFFECTING FETUS OR NEWBORN
633.8 OTHER WITH COMPLICATION DURING TREATMENT [**639.#**]
639.# OTHER WITH COMPLICATION FOLLOWING TREATMENT

4th Digit: 639

0. GENITAL TRACT AND PELVIC INFECTION
1. DELAYED OR EXCESSIVE HEMORRHAGE
2. DAMAGE TO PELVIC ORGANS AND TISSUE
3. RENAL FAILURE
4. METABOLIC DISORDERS
5. SHOCK
6. EMBOLISM
8. OTHER SPECIFIED COMPLICATION
9. UNSPECIFIED COMPLICATION

ECTOPIC SECRETION

259.3 ADH
259.3 ADRENALIN
255.0 ADRENCORTICOTROPIN
259.3 EPINEPHRINE
259.3 NOREPINEPHRINE
259.3 PITUITARY (POSTERIOR)

ECTROMELIA

755.4 UNSPECIFIED
755.30 LOWER LIMB
755.20 UPPER LIMB

ECTROPION

569.49	ANAL
622.0	CERVICAL
616.0	CERVICAL WITH CERVICITIS
374.10	EYELID
374.14	EYELID - CICATRICIAL
743.62	EYELID - CONGENITAL
374.12	EYELID - MECHANICAL
374.11	EYELID - SENILE
374.13	EYELID - SPASTIC
364.54	EYELID - UVEA
528.5	LIP
750.26	LIP CONGENITAL
569.49	RECTAL
599.84	URETHRAL

ECZEMA

692.9	NOS
692.9	ALLERGIC
706.8	ASTEATOTIC
691.8	ATOPIC
692.9	CONTACT NEC
692.9	DERMATITIS NEC
705.81	DYSHYDROTIC
380.22	EAR (EXTERNAL)
691.8	FLEXURAL
274.89	GOUTY
054.0	HERPETICUM HERPES SIMPLEX
701.8	HYPERTROPHICUM
684	IMPETIGINOUS
690.12	INFANTILE (SEBORRHEIC) (INTERTRIGINOUS)
692.9	INTERTRIGINOUS NEC
690.12	INTERTRIGINOUS INFANTILE (SEBORRHEIC)
691.8	INTRINSIC
692.9	LICHENIFIED NEC
110.3	MARGINATUM
692.9	NUMMULAR
316	PSYCHOGENIC [692.9]
316	PSYCHOGENIC (ATOPIC) [691.8]
686.8	PUSTULAR
690.18	SEBORRHEIC
690.12	SEBORRHEIC INFANTILE
692.79	SOLAR
454.1	STASIS (LOWER EXTREMITY)
454.2	STASIS (LOWER EXTREMITY) WITH ULCER
279.12	THROMBOCYTOPENIA SYNDROME
999.0	VACCINATUM
698.3	VERRUCOSUM CALLOSUM

756.51	**EDDOWES' SYNDROME (BRITTLE BONES AND BLUE SCLERA)**

EDEMA

782.3	NOS
995.1	ALLERGIC
909.9	ALLERGIC LATE EFFECT
372.73	CONJUNCTIVA
374.82	EYELID
782.3	EXTREMITIES LOWER
459.2	EXTREMITIES LOWER DUE TO VENOUS OBSTRUCTION
629.8	GENITALIA FEMALE
478.6	GLOTTIC
478.6	LARYNGEAL
782.3	LEG
459.2	LEGS DUE TO VENOUS OBSTRUCTION
757.0	LEGS HEREDITARY
782.3	LOCALIZED NOS
782.3	LOWER EXTREMITIES
459.2	LOWER EXTREMITIES DUE TO VENOUS OBSTRUCTION
362.83	MACULAR
362.53	MACULAR CYSTOID

EDEMA (continued)

250.5#	MACULAR DIABETIC [362.01]
250.5#	MACULAR DIABETIC CYSTOID [362.53]

5th Digit: 250.5

0. TYPE II, ADULT-ONSET, NON-INSULIN DEPENDENT (EVEN IF REQUIRING INSULIN), OR UNSPECIFIED; CONTROLLED

1. TYPE I, JUVENILE-ONSET OR INSULIN-DEPENDENT; CONTROLLED

2. TYPE II, ADULT-ONSET, NON-INSULIN DEPENDENT (EVEN IF REQUIRING INSULIN); UNCONTROLLED

3. TYPE I, JUVENILE-ONSET OR INSULIN-DEPENDENT; UNCONTROLLED

608.86	MALE GENITAL ORGANS
040.0	MALIGNANT
778.5	NEONATORUM
778.5	NEWBORN OTHER AND UNSPECIFIED
262	NUTRITIONAL WITHOUT MENTION OF DYSPIGMENTATION OF SKIN AND HAIR
376.33	ORBITAL
577.8	PANCREATIC
782.3	PEDAL
607.83	PENILE
478.25	PHARYNX OR NASOPHARYNX

PULMONARY

514	NOS
518.4	ACUTE
507.0	ACUTE ASPIRATION
428.1	ACUTE CARDIOGENIC
506.1	ACUTE CHEMICAL OR FUMES
518.4	ACUTE DUE TO PNEUMONIA
518.4	ACUTE POSTOPERATIVE
428.0	ACUTE WITH CHF (RIGHT HEART FAILURE)
402.91	ACUTE WITH HYPERTENSIVE HEART FAILURE - NOS
402.11	ACUTE WITH HYPERTENSIVE HEART FAILURE - BENIGN
402.01	ACUTE WITH HYPERTENSIVE HEART FAILURE - MALIGNANT
428.1	ACUTE WITH LEFT HEART FAILURE
518.5	ADULT RESPIRATORY DISTRESS SYNDROME ASSOCIATED WITH SHOCK
507.0	ASSOCIATED WITH ASPIRATION PNEUMONIA [518.82]
514	ASSOCIATED WITH HYPOSTATIC PNEUMONIA
518.81	ASSOCIATED WITH RESPIRATORY FAILURE - ACUTE IN OTHER CONDITIONS
518.84	ASSOCIATED WITH RESPIRATORY FAILURE - ACUTE AND CHRONIC IN OTHER CONDITIONS
518.83	ASSOCIATED WITH RESPIRATORY FAILURE - CHRONIC IN OTHER CONDITIONS
518.82	ASSOCIATED WITH OTHER CONDITIONS
514	CHRONIC
518.4	DUE TO ARDS [518.82]
518.4	DUE TO ARDS (DRUG OVERDOSE)
518.5	DUE TO ARDS (POST OP WITH SHOCK)
518.5	DUE TO ARDS (TRAUMATIC) [518.4]
508.1	DUE TO RADIATION CHRONIC
508.0	DUE TO RADIATION PNEUMONITIS
508.8	DUE TO OTHER EXTERNAL AGENTS
508.9	DUE TO UNSPECIFIED EXTERNAL AGENTS
518.4	DUE TO RENAL FAILURE [585]
518.4	DUE TO SEPSIS [038.39]
518.4	DUE TO SEPSIS (GRAM NEGATIVE) [785.59]
518.5	DUE TO SHOCK LUNG
518.5	DUE TO SHOCK TRAUMATIC
518.5	FOLLOWING TRAUMA AND SURGERY
518.4	POSTOPERATIVE ACUTE
518.4	POSTOPERATIVE ACUTE DUE TO FLUID OVERLOAD [276.6]
391.8	RHEUMATIC ACUTE
398.91	RHEUMATIC CHRONIC
392.0	RHEUMATIC WITH CHOREA
428.1	WITH HEART DISEASE OR FAILURE - LEFT
428.0	WITH HEART DISEASE OR FAILURE - RIGHT
428.0	WITH HEART DISEASE OR FAILURE - COMBINED

EDEMA (continued)
782.3 PITTING
581.9 RENAL
362.83 RETINAL (LOCALIZED) (MACULAR) (PERIPHERAL)
362.53 RETINAL (LOCALIZED) (MACULAR) (PERIPHERAL) CYSTOID
250.5# RETINAL DIABETIC [362.83]
5th Digit: 250.5
0. TYPE II, ADULT-ONSET, NON-INSULIN DEPENDENT (EVEN IF REQUIRING INSULIN), OR UNSPECIFIED; CONTROLLED
1. TYPE I, JUVENILE-ONSET OR INSULIN-DEPENDENT; CONTROLLED
2. TYPE II, ADULT-ONSET, NON-INSULIN DEPENDENT (EVEN IF REQUIRING INSULIN); UNCONTROLLED
3. TYPE I, JUVENILE-ONSET OR INSULIN-DEPENDENT; UNCONTROLLED
608.86 SCROTAL
336.1 SPINAL CORD ARTERIAL
478.6 SUBGLOTTIC
478.6 SUPRAGLOTTIC
782.3 TOXIC
782.3 UNKNOWN ETIOLOGY
624.8 VULVA (ACUTE)

992.2 EDSALL'S DISEASE
V62.3 EDUCATIONAL CIRCUMSTANCE (HANDICAP) CAUSING ENCOUNTER
758.2 EDWARD'S SYNDROME

EEG
794.02 ABNORMAL
V72.83 PREOPERATIVE
V72.85 SCREENING

537.89 EFFERENT LOOP SYNDROME
704.02 EFFLUVIUM TELOGEN
306.2 EFFORT SYNDROME (AVIATORS') (PSYCHOGENIC)

EFFUSION
490 BRONCHIAL (SEE ALSO 'BRONCHITIS')
348.5 CEREBRAL
719.0# JOINT
719.3# JOINT INTERMITTENT
5th Digit: 719.0, 3
0. SITE UNSPECIFIED
1. SHOULDER REGION
2. UPPER ARM (ELBOW) (HUMERUS)
3. FOREARM (RADIUS) (WRIST) (ULNA)
4. HAND (CARPAL) (METACARPAL) (FINGERS)
5. PELVIS THIGH (HIP) (BUTTOCK) (FEMUR)
6. LOWER LEG (FIBULA) (KNEE) (PATELLA) (TIBIA)
7. ANKLE AND/OR FOOT (METATARSALS) (TOES) (TARSALS)
8. OTHER
9. MULTIPLE
423.9 PERICARDIAL
420.90 PERICARDIAL ACUTE
568.82 PERITONEAL CHRONIC
789.5 PERITONEAL CHRONIC ASCITES
511.9 PLEURAL - UNSPECIFIED
511.9 PLEURAL - FETUS OR NEWBORN
197.2 PLEURAL - MALIGNANT
511.9 PLEURAL - PLEURISY NOS
997.3 PLEURAL - POST OP
511.1 PLEURAL - PNEUMOCOCCAL [041.2]
511.1 PLEURAL - STAPHYLOCOCCAL **[041.1#]**
5th Digit: 041.1
0. UNSPECIFIED
1. AUREUS
9. OTHER

EFFUSION (continued)
511.1 PLEURAL - STREPTOCOCCAL **[041.0#]**
5th Digit: 041.0
0. NOS
1. GROUP A
2. GROUP B
3. GROUP C
4. GROUP D (ENTEROCOCCUS)
5. GROUP G
9. OTHER STREP
862.29 PLEURAL - TRAUMATIC WITHOUT OPEN WOUND
862.39 PLEURAL - TRAUMATIC WITH OPEN WOUND
012.0# PLEURAL - TUBERCULOUS
010.1# PLEURAL - TUBERCULOUS PRIMARY PROGRESSIVE
5th Digit: 010.1, 012.0
0. UNSPECIFIED
1. LAB NOT DONE
2. LABS PENDING
3. MICROSCOPY POSITIVE (IN SPUTUM)
4. CULTURE POSITIVE - MICROSCOPY NEGATIVE
5. CULTURE NEGATIVE - MICROSCOPY POSITIVE
6. CULTURE AND MICROSCOPY NEGATIVE CONFIRMED BY OTHER METHODS
0 PULMONARY SEE 'EFFUSION', PLEURAL
322.9 SPINAL (SEE ALSO 'MENINGITIS')

756.83 EHLERS DANLOS SYNDROME
082.8 EHRLICHIA INFECTION
111.0 EICHSTEDT'S PITYRIASIS VERSICOLOR

EIGHTH
388.5 CRANIAL NERVE DISORDER (ATROPHY) (DEGENERATION)
951.5 CRANIAL NERVE INJURY
094.86 NERVE NEURITIS (SYPHILITIC)

745.4 EISENMENGER'S DEFECT, SYNDROME OR COMPLEX (VENTRICULAR SEPTAL DEFECT)

EJACULATE
792.2 BLOODY (PERSISTENT)
608.89 PAINFUL
306.59 PSYCHOGENIC

752.8 EJACULATORY DUCT ATRESIA (ABSENCE) (CONGENITAL)
608.89 EJACULATORY DUCT OBSTRUCTION
333.99 EKBOM'S SYNDROME (RESTLESS LEG)

EKG
794.31 ABNORMAL
412 M.I. DIAGNOSED, BUT PRESENTING NO SYMPTOMS
V71.7 NORMAL (EVALUATION FOR SUSPECTED HEART DISEASE)
V72.81 PREOPERATIVE EXAM

756.51 EKMAN'S SYNDROME (BRITTLE BONES AND BLUE SCLERA)
215.# ELASTOFIBROMA M8820/0
4th Digit: 215
0. HEAD FACE NECK
2. UPPER LIMB SHOULDER
3. LOWER LIMB HIP
4. THORAX
5. ABDOMINAL HYPOCHONDRIUM
6. PELVIS BUTTOCK GROIN INGUINAL REGION PERINEUM
7. TRUNK UNSPECIFIED BACK NOS FLANK NOS
8. OTHER SPECIFIED SITES
9. SITE UNSPECIFIED

701.8 ELASTOIDOSIS CUTANEA NODULARIS
757.39 ELASTOMA JUVENILE
701.8 ELASTOSIS
701.1 ELASTOSIS PERFORANS SERPIGINOSA
701.8 ELASTOSIS SENILIS
692.74 ELASTOSIS SOLAR

ELBOW

736.00 DEFORMITY ACQUIRED
726.30 INFLAMMATION (ENTHESOPATHY)
959.3 INJURY
913.8 INJURY OTHER AND UNSPECIFIED SUPERFICIAL
913.9 INJURY OTHER AND UNSPECIFIED SUPERFICIAL (INFECTED)
719.82 JOINT CALCIFICATION
718.92 JOINT LIGAMENT RELAXATION
0 JOINT LIGAMENT TEAR SEE 'SPRAIN'
0 JOINT SEE ALSO 'JOINT'
718.12 LOOSE BODY
726.39 OTHER SPECIFIED INFLAMMATION
V43.62 REPLACEMENT STATUS
841.9 SEPARATION (RUPTURE) (TEAR) (LACERATION)
841.8 SEPARATION (RUPTURE) (TEAR) (LACERATION) OTHER SPECIFIED SITES
841.9 STRAIN (SPRAIN) (AVULSION) (HEMARTHROSIS)
841.8 STRAIN (SPRAIN) (AVULSION) (HEMARTHROSIS) OTHER SPECIFIED SITES

INJURY OF A TENDON JOINT CAPSULE, OR LIGAMENT CAN BE A SEPARATION, TEAR, LACERATION, AVULSION, STRAIN, SPRAIN, OR HEMARTHROSIS. YOU CAN FIND THIS UNDER SPRAIN ALSO.

ELECTIVE SURGERY

V50.9 PROCEDURE UNSPECIFIED
V50.8 OTHER SPECIFIED SURGERY

266.2 ELECTRIC FEET SYNDROME
0 ELECTRICAL BURN SEE 'BURN', BY SITE
994.8 ELECTRICAL SHOCK NONFATAL
909.4 ELECTRICAL SHOCK LATE EFFECT
794.31 ELECTROCARDIOGRAM ABNORMAL
994.8 ELECTROCUTION
909.4 ELECTROCUTION LATE EFFECT
794.02 ELECTROENCEPHALOGRAM (EEG) ABNORMAL

ELECTROLYTE

791.9 ABNORMAL LEVEL - URINARY
276.9 DISORDER (IMBALANCE) NEC
276.9 DISORDER (IMBALANCE) UREMIC
276.2 IMBALANCE ACIDOSIS
276.3 IMBALANCE ALKALOSIS
643.1# IMBALANCE ASSOCIATED WITH HYPEREMESIS IN PREGNANCY

5th Digit: 643.1
0. EPISODE OF CARE UNSPECIFIED OR N/A
1. DELIVERED
3. ANTEPARTUM COMPLICATION

669.0# IMBALANCE COMPLICATING L AND D

5th Digit: 669.0
0. EPISODE OF CARE UNSPECIFIED OR N/A
1. DELIVERED
2. DELIVERED WITH POSTPARTUM COMPLICATION
3. ANTEPARTUM COMPLICATION
4. POSTPARTUM COMPLICATION

639.4 IMBALANCE FOLLOWING ABORTION / ECTOPIC / MOLAR PREGNANCY
791.9 LEVEL ABNORMAL - URINARY
775.5 NEONATAL TRANSITORY DISTURBANCE NEC

794.17 ELECTROMYOGRAM ABNORMAL EXCLUDES EYE
794.12 ELECTRO-OCULOGRAM ABNORMAL (EOG)
794.11 ELECTRORETINOGRAM (ERG) ABNORMAL
237.71 ELEPHANT MAN SYNDROME

ELEPHANTIASIS

457.1 NOS
125.1 DUE TO BRUGIA (WUCHERERIA) MALAYI
125.0 DUE TO WUCHERERIA BANCROFTI
125.9 FILARIAL

ELEPHANTIASIS (continued)

457.1 NONFILARIAL
757.0 NONFILARIAL CONGENITAL
374.83 NONFILARIAL EYELID
624.8 NONFILARIAL VULVA
457.0 POST MASTECTOMY
997.99 SURGICAL

352.4 ELEVENTH CRANIAL NERVE DISORDERS (ATROPHY)
951.6 ELEVENTH CRANIAL NERVE INJURY

ELLIPTOCYTOSIS

282.1 NOS (CONGENITAL) (HEREDITARY)
282.7 HB-C (DISEASE)
282.7 HEMOGLOBIN DISEASE
282.60 SICKLE-CELL (DISEASE)
282.5 SICKLE-CELL TRAIT

756.55 ELLIS-VAN CREVELD SYNDROME (CHONDROECTODERMAL DYSPLASIA)
251.5 ELLISON-ZOLLINGER (GASTRIC HYPERSECTION WITH PANCREATIC ISLET CELL TUMOR)
309.22 EMANCIPATION ADJUSTMENT REACTION (ADOLESCENT) (EARLY ADULT)

EMBOLISM

958.0 AIR (ANY SITE)
999.1 AIR FOLLOWING INFUSION, PERFUSION OR TRANSFUSION
908.6 AIR FOLLOWING TRAUMA LATE EFFECT
444.1 AORTA
444.0 AORTA ABDOMINAL
444.0 AORTA BIFURCATION
444.0 AORTA SADDLE
444.1 AORTA THORACIC
444.0 AORTOILIAC
444.9 ARTERY NOS
444.22 ARTERY LOWER EXTREMITY
444.21 ARTERY UPPER EXTREMITY
444.89 ARTERY SPECIFIED SITE NEC
433.8# AUDITORY ARTERY INTERNAL
433.0# BASILAR ARTERY
433.3# BASILAR ARTERY BILATERAL OR MULTIPLE

5th Digit: 433.0, 3, 8
0. WITHOUT CEREBRAL INFARCTION
1. WITH CEREBRAL INFARCTION

444.89 BLADDER ARTERY
444.21 BRACHIAL ARTERY
434.1# BRAIN

5th Digit: 434.1
0. WITHOUT CEREBRAL INFARCTION
1. WITH CEREBRAL INFARCTION

448.9 CAPILLARY
0 CARDIAC ACUTE WITH INFARCTION SEE 'MYOCARDIAL INFARCTION ACUTE'
433.1# CAROTID ARTERY
433.3# CAROTID ARTERY BILATERAL OR MULTIPLE
433.8# CEREBELLAR ARTERY
434.1# CEREBRAL ARTERY OR VEIN

5th Digit: 433.1, 3, 8, 434.1
0. WITHOUT CEREBRAL INFARCTION
1. WITH CEREBRAL INFARCTION

997.02 CEREBRAL ARTERY POSTOPERATIVE NEC
433.8# CHOROIDAL ARTERY
433.8# COMMUNICATING POSTERIOR ARTERY

5th Digit: 433.8
0. WITHOUT CEREBRAL INFARCTION
1. WITH CEREBRAL INFARCTION

0 COMPLICATING ABORTION SEE 'ABORTION', BY TYPE, WITH EMBOLISM
0 COMPLICATING ECTOPIC PREGNANCY SEE 'ECTOPIC PREGNANCY', BY SITE WITH COMPLICATION
0 COMPLICATING MOLAR PREGNANCY SEE 'MOLAR PREGNANCY', BY TYPE WITH COMPLICATION
0 CORONARY ARTERY OR VEIN ACUTE WITH INFARCTION SEE 'MYOCARDIAL INFARCTION ACUTE'
411.81 CORONARY ARTERY OR VEIN ACUTE WITHOUT MI

EMBOLISM (continued)

0	DUE TO A DEVICE SEE 'COMPLICATION OF A DEVICE, IMPLANT OR GRAFT - OTHER SPECIFIED'
434.1#	ENCEPHALOMALACIA
	5th Digit: 434.1
	0. WITHOUT CEREBRAL INFARCTION
	1. WITH CEREBRAL INFARCTION
444.22	EXTREMITY ARTERY NOS
444.22	EXTREMITY ARTERY LOWER
444.21	EXTREMITY ARTERY UPPER
0	EYE SEE 'RETINAL ARTERY OCCLUSION'
958.1	FAT (CEREBRAL) (PULMONARY) (SYSTEMIC)
958.1	FAT FOLLOWING TRAUMA
908.6	FAT FOLLOWING TRAUMA LATE EFFECT
444.22	FEMORAL ARTERY
453.8	FEMORAL VEIN
639.6	FOLLOWING ABORTION
639.6	FOLLOWING ECTOPIC OR MOLAR PREGNANCY
0	HEART ACUTE WITH INFARCTION SEE 'MYOCARDIAL INFARCTION ACUTE'
453.0	HEPATIC (VEIN)
433.8#	HYPOPHYSEAL ARTERY
	5th Digit: 433.8
	0. WITHOUT CEREBRAL INFARCTION
	1. WITH CEREBRAL INFARCTION
444.81	ILIAC (ARTERY)
444.81	ILIOFEMORAL
557.0	INTESTINE (ARTERY) (VEIN) (WITH GANGRENE)
434.1#	INTRACRANIAL
	5th Digit: 434.1
	0. WITHOUT CEREBRAL INFARCTION
	1. WITH CEREBRAL INFARCTION
326	INTRACRANIAL SINUS (SEPTIC) LATE EFFECT
325	INTRACRANIAL VENOUS SINUS (ANY)
437.6	INTRACRANIAL VENOUS SINUS NONPYOGENIC
593.81	KIDNEY (ARTERY)
434.1#	MENINGES
	5th Digit: 434.1
	0. WITHOUT CEREBRAL INFARCTION
	1. WITH CEREBRAL INFARCTION
557.0	MESENTERIC (ARTERY) (VEIN) (WITH GANGRENE)
444.9	MULTIPLE NEC
0	OPHTHALMIC ARTERY SEE 'RETINAL ARTERY OCCLUSION'
444.9	PARADOXICAL NEC
607.82	PENIS
444.22	PERIPHERAL ARTERY NEC
997.2	PERIPHERAL VASCULAR POSTOPERATIVE NEC
253.8	PITUITARY
433.8#	PONTINE ARTERY
	5th Digit: 433.8
	0. WITHOUT CEREBRAL INFARCTION
	1. WITH CEREBRAL INFARCTION
444.22	POPLITEAL (ARTERY)
452	PORTAL (VEIN)
433.8#	POSTERIOR COMMUNICATING ARTERY
	5th Digit: 433.8
	0. WITHOUT CEREBRAL INFARCTION
	1. WITH CEREBRAL INFARCTION
997.2	POSTOPERATIVE NEC
997.02	POSTOPERATIVE CEREBRAL ARTERY NEC
415.11	POSTOPERATIVE PULMONARY
433.9#	PRECEREBRAL ARTERY NOS
433.3#	PRECEREBRAL ARTERY BILATERAL OR MULTIPLE
433.8#	PRECEREBRAL ARTERY NEC
	5th Digit: 433.3, 8-9
	0. WITHOUT CEREBRAL INFARCTION
	1. WITH CEREBRAL INFARCTION

EMBOLISM (continued)

415.11	PULMONARY (ARTERY) (VEIN) IATROGENIC
415.19	PULMONARY (ARTERY) (VEIN) OTHER AND NOS
415.11	PULMONARY (ARTERY) (VEIN) POSTOPERATIVE
0	PYEMIC SEE 'SEPSIS'
593.81	RENAL ARTERY
453.3	RENAL VEIN
0	RETINAL ARTERY SEE 'RETINAL ARTERY OCCLUSION'
444.0	SADDLE AORTA
0	SOAP WITH ABORTION SEE 'ABORTION', BY TYPE WITH EMBOLISM
0	SOAP WITH ECTOPIC OR MOLAR PREGNANCY SEE 'ECTOPIC PREGNANCY' OR 'MOLAR PREGNANCY', BY SITE OR TYPE WITH COMPLICATION
444.89	SPINAL ARTERY
336.1	SPINAL CORD
324.1	SPINAL CORD SEPTIC OR PYOGENIC
444.89	SPLEEN (ARTERY)
999.2	THROMBUS FOLLOWING INFUSION, PERFUSION OR TRANSFUSION
444.21	ULNAR ARTERY
453.9	VEIN NOS
453.8	VEIN OTHER SPECIFIED SITE
0	VEIN WITH INFLAMMATION OR PHLEBITIS SEE 'THROMBOPHLEBITIS'
453.2	VENA CAVA
433.2#	VERTEBRAL ARTERY
433.3#	VERTEBRAL ARTERY BILATERAL OR MULTIPLE
	5th Digit: 433.2-3
	0. WITHOUT CEREBRAL INFARCTION
	1. WITH CEREBRAL INFARCTION

EMBOLISM COMPLICATING PREGNANCY

673.0#	AIR DUE TO PREGNANCY
673.1#	AMNIOTIC FLUID DUE TO PREGNANCY
673.2#	BLOOD-CLOT DUE TO PREGNANCY
674.0#	BRAIN DUE TO PREGNANCY
	5th Digit: 673.0-2, 674.0
	0. EPISODE OF CARE UNSPECIFIED OR N/A
	1. DELIVERED
	2. DELIVERED WITH POSTPARTUM COMPLICATION
	3. ANTEPARTUM COMPLICATION
	4. POSTPARTUM COMPLICATION

WHEN CODING A MATERNAL CARDIOVASCULAR DISEASE COMPLICATING PREGNANCY, 648.6#, USE AN ADDITIONAL CODE TO IDENTIFY THE CONDITION.

648.6#	CARDIAC CURRENT (CO-EXISTENT)
674.0#	CEREBRAL DUE TO PREGNANCY
673.8#	FAT DUE TO PREGNANCY
671.5#	INTRACRANIAL VENOUS SINUS NONPYOGENIC DUE TO PREGNANCY
673.2#	PULMONARY PUERPERAL NOS DUE TO PREGNANCY
673.8#	PULMONARY OTHER DUE TO PREGNANCY
673.3#	SEPTIC (PYEMIC) DUE TO PREGNANCY
671.5#	SPINAL DUE TO PREGNANCY
	5th Digit: 648.6, 671.5, 673.2-3, 8, 674.0
	0. EPISODE OF CARE UNSPECIFIED OR N/A
	1. DELIVERED
	2. DELIVERED WITH POSTPARTUM COMPLICATION
	3. ANTEPARTUM COMPLICATION
	4. POSTPARTUM COMPLICATION

EMBOLISM COMPLICATING PREGNANCY (continued)

> *648.9#: USE AN ADDITIONAL CODE TO IDENTIFY THE SPECIFIC VASCULAR OR LYMPHATIC EMBOLUS.*

648.9# VASCULAR AND LYMPHATIC MATERNAL CURRENT (CO-EXISTENT) IN PREGNANCY
5th Digit: 648.9
0. EPISODE OF CARE UNSPECIFIED OR N/A
1. DELIVERED
2. DELIVERED WITH POSTPARTUM COMPLICATION
3. ANTEPARTUM COMPLICATION
4. POSTPARTUM COMPLICATION

> *WHEN CODING A MATERNAL CARDIOVASCULAR DISEASE COMPLICATING PREGNANCY, 648.6#, USE AN ADDITIONAL CODE TO IDENTIFY THE CONDITION.*

648.6# OTHER SPECIFIED CARDIOVASCULAR DISEASE CURRENT (CO-EXISTENT) IN PREGNANCY
5th Digit: 648.6
0. EPISODE OF CARE NOS OR N/A
1. DELIVERED
2. DELIVERED WITH POSTPARTUM COMPLICATION
3. ANTEPARTUM COMPLICATION
4. POSTPARTUM COMPLICATION

186.9 EMBRYONAL CARCINOMA SITE NOS
0 EMBRYONAL CARCINOMA SITE SPECIFIED SEE 'CANCER' BY SITE M9070/3
752.41 EMBRYONIC CYST CERVIX VAGINA AND EXTERNAL FEMALE GENITALIA
270.2 EMBRYONIC FIXATION SYNDROME
787.03 EMESIS
787.01 EMESIS WITH NAUSEA

EMG
794.17 ABNORMAL
794.14 EYE ABNORMAL
V72.83 PREOPERATIVE
V72.85 SCREENING

EMOTIONAL, EMOTIONALLY
309.29 CRISIS NEC (SEE ALSO 'STRESS', 'ADJUSTMENT REACTION')
308.0 CRISIS, ACUTE REACTION TO STRESS
313.9 DISTURBANCE OF CHILDHOOD OR ADOLESCENCE - UNSPECIFIED
313.89 DISTURBANCE OF CHILDHOOD OR ADOLESCENCE - OTHER
301.3 INSTABILITY (EXCESSIVE)
301.3 PATHOLOGICAL
V40.9 PROBLEM
301.59 UNSTABLE

EMPHYSEMA NONPULMONARY
958.7 CELLULAR TISSUE
908.6 CELLULAR TISSUE LATE EFFECT
595.89 EMPHYSEMATOUS CYSTITIS
376.89 EYE
374.85 EYELID
416.9 HEART
958.7 MEDIASTINAL TRAUMATIC
908.6 MEDIASTINAL TRAUMATIC LATE EFFECT
376.89 ORBIT
958.7 SUBCUTANEOUS TRAUMATIC
908.6 SUBCUTANEOUS TRAUMATIC LATE EFFECT
998.81 SURGICAL RESULTING FROM A PROCEDURE
254.8 THYMUS (CONGENITAL)

EMPHYSEMA PULMONARY
492.8 UNSPECIFIED
492.8 ATROPHIC
492.0 BULLOUS
492.8 CENTRIACINAR
492.8 CENTRILOBULAR
518.2 COMPENSATORY
770.2 CONGENITAL
506.4 DUE TO FUMES AND VAPORS
492.0 EMPHYSEMATOUS BLEB
492.0 EMPHYSEMATOUS BLEB RUPTURED
518.1 INTERSTITIAL
770.2 INTERSTITIAL NEWBORN
518.1 MEDIASTINAL
770.2 MEDIASTINAL IN FETUS OR NEWBORN
492.8 OBSTRUCTIVE
492.8 PANACINAR
492.8 PANLOBULAR
492.0 RUPTURED EMPHYSEMATOUS BLEB
V81.3 SCREENING
492.8 VESICULAR
491.21 WITH ACUTE BRONCHITIS
491.20 WITH BRONCHITIS
491.21 WITH BRONCHITIS WITH EXACERBATION

492.0 EMPHYSEMATOUS BLEB
595.89 EMPHYSEMATOUS CYSTITIS
V62.1 EMPLOYMENT ADVERSE EFFECT OF ENVIRONMENT CAUSING ENCOUNTER
V62.2 EMPLOYMENT DISSATISFACTION CAUSING ENCOUNTER
253.8 EMPTY SELLA (TURCICA) SYNDROME

EMPYEMA NONPULMONARY
473.9 ACCESSORY SINUS
324.0 BRAIN
473.2 ETHMOID SINUS
473.1 FRONTAL SINUS
575.0 GALLBLADDER (SEE ALSO 'CHOLECYSTITIS', ACUTE)
383.00 MASTOID
526.4 MAXILLARY JAW
473.0 MAXILLARY SINUS
473.9 NASAL SINUS ACCESSORY
473.9 NASAL SINUS (CHRONIC)
473.3 SPHENOIDAL SINUS
324.9 SUBDURAL
593.89 URETERAL

EMPYEMA PULMONARY
510.9 UNSPECIFIED
510.9 LUNG
513.0 LUNG WITH ABSCESS
510.0 LUNG WITH FISTULA

ENAMEL HYPOPLASIA (TEETH)
520.4 NEONATAL
520.4 POSTNATAL
520.4 PRENATAL

ENCEPHALITIS
323.9 NOS
049.8 ACUTE INCLUSION BODY NECROTIZING
049.8 ACUTE NECROTIZING
136.2 AMEBIC (NAEGLERIA)
062.4 AUSTRALIAN
062.5 CALIFORNIA VIRUS
982.1 CARBON TETRACHLORIDE (SOLVENT) [323.7]
078.3 CAT SCRATCH DISEASE [323.0]
063.2 CENTRAL EUROPEAN
046.2 DAWSON'S INCLUSION BODY
062.2 EASTERN EQUINE
049.8 EPIDEMIC
323.5 FOLLOWING IMMUNIZATION PROCEDURES

E

ENCEPHALITIS (continued)

054.3 HERPES SIMPLEX
961.3 HYDROXYQUINOLINE DERIVATIVES TOXICITY [323.7]
062.8 ILHEUS VIRUS
487.8 INFLUENZA [323.4]
046.1 JAKOB CREUTZFELDT WITH PRESENILE DEMENTIA
062.0 JAPANESE
062.0 JAPANESE B
046.0 KURU
062.5 LA CROSSE
063.8 LANGAT
326 LATE EFFECT
139.8 LATE EFFECT - DUE TO INFECTIOUS DISEASES
326 LATE EFFECT - DUE TO NERVOUS SYSTEM DISEASES
139.0 LATE EFFECT - DUE TO VIRAL DISEASES
984.# LEAD TOXICITY [323.7]

4th Digit: 984
0. INORGANIC COMPOUNDS
1. ORGANIC COMPOUNDS
2. OTHER COMPOUNDS
9. UNSPECIFIED

049.8 LETHARGICA
046.3 LEUKOENCEPHALOPATHY (MULTIFOCAL)
046.3 LEUKOENCEPHALOPATHY (MULTIFOCAL) (PROGRESSIVE)
063.1 LOUPING ILL
710.0 LUPUS [323.8]
084.6 MALARIAL [323.2]
036.1 MENINGOCOCCAL
985.0 MERCURY TOXICITY [323.7]
075 MONONUCLEOSIS [323.0]
062.9 MOSQUITO BORNE VIRAL
V73.5 MOSQUITO BORNE VIRAL SCREENING EXAM
072.2 MUMPS
062.4 MURRAY VALLEY
064 NEGISHI VIRUS
073.7 ORNITHOSIS [323.0]
323.8 OTHER CAUSES
341.1 PERIAXIALIS (CONCENTRICA) (DIFFUSA)
052.0 POST CHICKENPOX
323.5 POSTIMMUNIZATION
136.9 POSTINFECTIOUS [323.6]
055.0 POSTMEASLES
052.0 POSTVARICELLA
049.8 POSTVIRAL NEC [326]
063.8 POWASSAN
083.9 RICKETTSIAL [323.1]
049.8 RIO BRAVO
056.01 RUBELLA
063.0 RUSSIAN SPRING SUMMER [TAIGA]
062.3 ST LOUIS
046.2 SUBACUTE SCLEROSING
094.81 SYPHILITIC
090.41 SYPHILITIC CONGENITAL
985.8 THALLIUM TOXICITY [323.7]
V73.5 TICK BORNE SCREENING EXAM
063.9 TICK BORNE VIRAL
063.2 TICK BORNE VIRAL CENTRAL EUROPEAN
063.1 TICK BORNE VIRAL LOUPING ILL
063.0 TICK BORNE VIRAL RUSSIAN SPRING-SUMMER
063.8 TICK BORNE VIRAL OTHER SPECIFIED
323.7 TOXIC
130.0 TOXOPLASMOSIS [323.4]
086.0 TRYPANOSOMAL [323.2]
013.6# TUBERCULOUS

5th Digit: 013.6
0. UNSPECIFIED
1. LAB NOT DONE
2. LABS PENDING
3. MICROSCOPY POSITIVE (IN SPUTUM)
4. CULTURE POSITIVE - MICROSCOPY NEGATIVE
5. CULTURE NEGATIVE - MICROSCOPY POSITIVE
6. CULTURE AND MICROSCOPY NEGATIVE CONFIRMED BY OTHER METHODS

ENCEPHALITIS (continued)

081.9 TYPHUS (FEVER) [323.1]
V05.0 VACCINATION (VIRAL ARTHROPOD BORNE)
046.2 VAN BOGAERT'S
066.2 VENEZUELAN EQUINE
049.9 VIRAL
064 VIRAL ARTHROPOD BORNE VECTOR UNKNOWN
139.0 VIRAL LATE EFFECTS
062.8 VIRAL OTHER SPECIFIED MOSQUITO BORNE
063.8 VIRAL OTHER SPECIFIED TICK BORNE
V73.5 VIRAL SCREENING EXAM
063.9 VIRAL TICK BORNE
062.1 WESTERN EQUINE
323.8 OTHER SPECIFIED CAUSE

742.0 ENCEPHALOCELE CONGENITAL
376.81 ENCEPHALOCELE ORBITAL
759.6 ENCEPHALOCUTANEOUS ANGIOMATOSIS
742.0 ENCEPHALOCYSTOCELE CONGENITAL

ENCEPHALOMALACIA

434.9# NOS

5th Digit: 434.9
0. WITHOUT CEREBRAL INFARCTION
1. WITH CEREBRAL INFARCTION

431 DUE TO HEMORRHAGE
435.9 DUE TO RECURRENT SPASM OF ARTERY
434.1# EMBOLIC

5th Digit: 434.1
0. WITHOUT CEREBRAL INFARCTION
1. WITH CEREBRAL INFARCTION

290.12 SUBCORTICALIS CHRONICUS ARTERIOSCLEROTICA
434.0# THROMBOTIC

5th Digit: 434.0
0. WITHOUT CEREBRAL INFARCTION
1. WITH CEREBRAL INFARCTION

0 ENCEPHALOMYELITIS ABACTERIAL SEE 'ENCEPHALITIS'
323.5 ENCEPHALOMYELITIS POSTIMMUNIZATION OR POSTVACCINAL
326 ENCEPHALOMYELITIS POSTIMMUNIZATION OR POSTVACCINAL LATE EFFECT
0 ENCEPHALOMYELITIS SEE 'ENCEPHALITIS'

742.0 ENCEPHALOMYELOCELE CONGENITAL

ENCEPHALOPATHY

348.3 UNSPECIFIED
348.3 ACUTE
291.2 ALCOHOLIC
348.1 ANOXIC
437.0 ARTERIOSCLEROTIC
572.2 HEPATIC
437.2 HYPERTENSIVE
251.2 HYPOGLYCEMIC

METABOLIC (TOXIC)

293.0 ACUTE BRAIN SYNDROME WITH TRANSIENT DELIRIUM
293.0 ACUTE DELIRIUM
291.0 ALCOHOL WITHDRAWAL WITH DELIRIUM TREMENS
293.0 DELIRIUM ASSOCIATED WITH SYSTEMIC INFECTION
292.81 DRUG INDUCED DELIRIUM
586 UREMIA

ENCEPHALOPATHY (continued)

349.82 TOXIC

ENCEPHALOPATHY DUE TO OTHER CAUSES
774.7 BILIRUBIN PERINATAL
742.9 CONGENITAL
294.8 DUE TO DIALYSIS
293.9 DUE TO DIALYSIS (TRANSIENT)
265.2 DUE TO NICOTINE ACID DEFICIENCY
310.2 DUE TO TRAUMA (POSTCONCUSSIONAL)
251.2 HYPOGLYCEMIC
487.8 INFLUENZA (DUE TO)
984.9 LEAD [323.7]
046.1 SPONGIFORM SUBACUTE
094.81 SYPHILITIC
349.82 TOXIC
086.9 TRYPANOSOMAL [323.2]
266.9 VITAMIN B DEFICIENCY
265.1 WERNICKE'S (POLIOENCEPHALITIS)

0 ENCEPHALORRHAGIA SEE 'HEMORRHAGE' BRAIN
756.4 ENCHONDROMATOSIS CONGENITAL
787.6 ENCOPRESIS
307.7 ENCOPRESIS PSYCHOGENIC

WHEN USING CODE V66.7, CODE THE TERMINAL ILLNESS FIRST.

V66.7 END-OF-LIFE CARE ENCOUNTER

ENDARTERITIS
447.6 UNSPECIFIED
414.0# CORONARY ARTERIOSCLEROTIC
5th Digit: 414.0
0. UNSPECIFIED TYPE OF VESSEL, NATIVE OR GRAFT
1. NATIVE CORONARY VESSEL
2. AUTOLOGOUS VEIN BYPASS GRAFT
3. NONAUTOLOGOUS BIOLOGICAL BYPASS GRAFT
4. AUTOLOGOUS ARTERY BYPASS GRAFT (GASTROEPIPLOIC) (INTERNAL MAMMARY)
5. UNSPECIFIED TYPE OF BYPASS GRAFT
391.9 CORONARY RHEUMATIC
398.99 CORONARY RHEUMATIC (CHRONIC)
417.8 PULMONARY
362.18 RETINAL
0 SEE ALSO 'ARTERITIS'

0 ENDEMIC POLYARTHRITIS SEE 'KASCHIN-BECK DISEASE'
745.60 ENDOCARDIAL CUSHION DEFECT CONGENITAL
425.3 ENDOCARDIAL FIBROELASTOSIS
424.90 ENDOCARDIAL OBSTRUCTION
424.99 ENDOCARDIAL OBSTRUCTION ARTERIOSCLEROTIC
424.99 ENDOCARDIAL OBSTRUCTION SPECIFIED CAUSE, NONRHEUMATIC

ENDOCARDITIS
424.90 NOS
397.9 NOS - RHEUMATIC INACTIVE OR QUIESCENT (WITH CHOREA)
421.9 ACUTE (SUBACUTE)
391.1 ACUTE (SUBACUTE) - RHEUMATIC
392.0 ACUTE (SUBACUTE) - RHEUMATIC WITH CHOREA

AORTIC
424.1 NOS (ARTERIOSCLEROTIC) (HYPERTENSIVE)
421.9 NOS ACUTE (SUBACUTE)
746.89 CONGENITAL
391.1 RHEUMATIC ACTIVE (ACUTE)
392.0 RHEUMATIC ACTIVE (ACUTE) - WITH CHOREA
396.9 RHEUMATIC ACTIVE (ACUTE) - WITH MITRAL DISEASE
395.9 RHEUMATIC INACTIVE (QUIESCENT) (WITH CHOREA)
396.9 RHEUMATIC INACTIVE (QUIESCENT) WITH MITRAL DISEASE (WITH CHOREA)
424.1 OTHER SPECIFIED CAUSE NONRHEUMATIC

ENDOCARDITIS (continued)
424.90 ASEPTIC
421.0 BACTERIAL
424.90 CHRONIC VALVULAR NOS
397.9 CHRONIC VALVULAR NOS - RHEUMATIC INACTIVE OR QUIESCENT
425.3 CONGENITAL
421.0 CONSTRICTIVE
425.3 FETAL
996.61 HEART VALVE PROSTHESIS COMPLICATION - INFECTION OR INFLAMMATION
424.99 HYPERTENSIVE
421.0 INFECTIOUS OR INFECTIVE
421.0 LENTA
421.0 LOEFFLER'S
421.0 MALIGNANT

MITRAL
394.9 NOS (RHEUMATIC)
391.1 ACUTE (ACTIVE)
421.0 ACUTE (ACTIVE) - BACTERIAL
396.9 ACUTE (ACTIVE) - WITH AORTIC DISEASE
392.0 ACUTE (ACTIVE) - WITH CHOREA
424.0 ARTERIOSCLEROTIC
746.89 CONGENITAL
424.0 HYPERTENSIVE
391.1 RHEUMATIC - ACUTE (ACTIVE)
392.0 RHEUMATIC - ACUTE (ACTIVE) WITH CHOREA
394.9 RHEUMATIC - INACTIVE (QUIESCENT) (WITH CHOREA)
396.9 RHEUMATIC - INACTIVE (QUIESCENT) WITH AORTIC VALVE DISEASE (WITH CHOREA)

PULMONARY
424.3 NOS (ARTERIOSCLEROTIC)
421.9 ACUTE OR SUBACUTE
391.1 ACUTE OR SUBACUTE - RHEUMATIC (ACTIVE)
392.0 ACUTE OR SUBACUTE - RHEUMATIC (ACTIVE) WITH CHOREA
746.09 CONGENITAL
424.3 HYPERTENSIVE
391.1 RHEUMATIC ACUTE (ACTIVE) (SUBACUTE)
392.0 RHEUMATIC ACUTE (ACTIVE) (SUBACUTE) WITH CHOREA
397.1 RHEUMATIC CHRONIC (INACTIVE)

ENDOCARDITIS (continued)
421.0 PURULENT
391.1 RHEUMATIC ACTIVE OR ACUTE VALVE NOS
392.0 RHEUMATIC ACTIVE OR ACUTE VALVE NOS WITH CHOREA
397.9 RHEUMATIC CHRONIC VALVE NOS
421.0 SEPTIC
0 SUBACUTE SEE 'ENDOCARDITIS', BY SITE, ACUTE
421.0 SUPPURATIVE
0 TOXIC SEE 'ENDOCARDITIS', BY SITE, ACUTE

TRICUSPID
397.0 NOS
391.1 ACTIVE OR ACUTE
392.0 ACTIVE OR ACUTE WITH CHOREA
397.0 CHRONIC, INACTIVE OR QUIESCENT
746.89 CONGENITAL
424.2 NONRHEUMATIC (ARTERIOSCLEROTIC) (HYPERTENSIVE)
421.9 NONRHEUMATIC ACUTE OR SUBACUTE
397.0 RHEUMATIC
391.1 RHEUMATIC ACTIVE (ACUTE)
392.0 RHEUMATIC ACTIVE (ACUTE) WITH CHOREA
397.0 RHEUMATIC INACTIVE (CHRONIC) (QUIESCENT)

ENDOCARDITIS (continued)
421.0 ULCERATIVE
421.0 VEGETATIVE

THE CODE IN THE LEFT MARGIN ALWAYS SEQUENCES FIRST. THE ADDITIONAL CODE IN BRACKETS TO THE RIGHT OF THE DESCRIPTION IS SEQUENCED SECONDARILY. UNDERLINING SHOWS THE CODE NUMBER THAT CORRESPONDS TO THE UNDERLINED VERBAL DESCRIPTION. UNDERLINING NEVER IMPLIES CORRECT SEQUENCING.

ENDOCARDITIS OTHER CAUSES

421.0 ACUTE BACTERIAL DUE TO STREPTOCOCCAL **[041.0#]**

5th Digit: 041.0
- **0. NOS**
- **1. GROUP A**
- **2. GROUP B**
- **3. GROUP C**
- **4. GROUP D (ENTEROCOCCUS)**
- **5. GROUP G**
- **9. OTHER STREP**

424.99 ARTERIOSCLEROTIC
116.0 BLASTOMYCOTIC [421.1]
112.81 CANDIDAL
996.61 CARDIAC VALVE PROSTHESIS
074.22 COXSACKIE
098.84 GONOCOCCAL
115.94 HISTOPLASMA
115.04 HISTOPLASMA CAPSULATUM
115.14 HISTOPLASMA DUBOISII
425.3 IN ENDOCARDIAL FIBROELASTOSIS
710.0 LIBMAN SACHS [424.91]
710.0 LUPUS [424.91]
036.42 MENINGOCOCCAL
112.81 MONILIASIS
421.0 MYCOTIC
421.0 PNEUMOCOCCIC [041.2]
083.0 Q FEVER (DUE TO) [421.1]
421.0 SERRATIA MARCESCENS
421.0 SUBACUTE BACTERIAL DUE TO STAPHYLOCOCCAL **[041.1#]**

5th Digit: 041.1
- **0. UNSPECIFIED**
- **1. AUREUS**
- **9. OTHER**

093.20 SYPHILITIC NEC
093.22 SYPHILITIC AORTIC VALVE
093.21 SYPHILITIC MITRAL VALVE
093.24 SYPHILITIC PULMONIC VALVE
093.23 SYPHILITIC TRICUSPID VALVE
017.9# TUBERCULOUS [424.91]

5th Digit: 017.9
- **0. UNSPECIFIED**
- **1. LAB NOT DONE**
- **2. LABS PENDING**
- **3. MICROSCOPY POSITIVE (IN SPUTUM)**
- **4. CULTURE POSITIVE - MICROSCOPY NEGATIVE**
- **5. CULTURE NEGATIVE - MICROSCOPY POSITIVE**
- **6. CULTURE AND MICROSCOPY NEGATIVE CONFIRMED BY OTHER METHODS**

002.0 TYPHOID [421.1]
424.90 VALVE UNSPECIFIED CAUSE UNSPECIFIED
397.9 VALVE UNSPECIFIED CAUSE RHEUMATIC
424.99 VALVE UNSPECIFIED CAUSE SPECIFIED
710.0 VERRUCOUS ATYPICAL [424.91]
425.3 WITH ENDOCARDIAL FIBROELASTOSIS
424.99 OTHER SPECIFIED CAUSE EXCEPT RHEUMATIC

616.0 ENDOCERVICITIS (NONOBSTETRICAL)

ENDOCRINE

258.0 ADENOMATOSIS MULTIPLE POLYGLANDULAR ACTIVITY
259.9 DISORDER
306.6 DISORDER PSYCHOGENIC
259.9 DISTURBANCE
775.9 DISTURBANCE FETUS AND NEWBORN
775.8 DISTURBANCE NEONATAL OTHER TRANSITORY
794.6 FUNCTION STUDY OTHER ABNORMAL
759.2 GLAND NEC ABSENCE (CONGENITAL)
255.3 HYPERTENSIVE SYNDROME
306.6 MALFUNCTION PSYCHOGENIC
V77.9 SCREENING FOR DISORDER
259.8 OTHER SPECIFIED DISORDER NEC

ENDODERMAL SINUS TUMOR

183.0 FEMALE SITE UNSPECIFIED
0 FEMALE SITE SPECIFIED SEE 'CANCER' BY SITE M9071/3
186.9 MALE SITE UNSPECIFIED
0 SITE SPECIFIED SEE 'CANCER' BY SITE M8931/1

236.0 ENDOLYMPHATIC STROMAL MYOSIS SITE NOS
0 ENDOLYMPHATIC STROMAL MYOSIS SITE SPECIFIED SEE 'NEOPLASM UNCERTAIN BEHAVIOR' BY SITE M8931/1
0 ENDOMETRIAL SEE 'ENDOMETRIUM, ENDOMETRIAL'
199.1 ENDOMETRIOID CARCINOMA SITE UNSPECIFIED
0 ENDOMETRIOID CARCINOMA SITE SPECIFIED SEE 'CANCER' BY SITE M8380/3

ENDOMETRIOSIS

617.9 ENDOMETRIOSIS
617.5 APPENDIX
617.8 BLADDER
617.3 BROAD LIGAMENT
617.0 CERVIX
617.5 COLON
617.3 DOUGLAS CUL DE SAC
617.2 FALLOPIAN TUBE
617.8 GALLBLADDER
617.8 GENITAL ORGAN NEC (FEMALE)
617.6 IN SCAR OF SKIN
617.0 INTERNAL
617.5 INTESTINE
617.8 LUNG
617.0 MYOMETRIUM
617.1 OVARY
617.3 PELVIC PERITONEUM
617.3 PERITONEAL PARAMETRIUM
617.4 RECTOVAGINAL SEPTUM AND VAGINA
617.5 RECTUM
617.3 ROUND LIGAMENT
617.6 SKIN
236.0 STROMAL
617.8 UMBILICUS
617.0 UTERUS
617.4 VAGINA
617.8 VULVA
617.8 OTHER SPECIFIED SITE NEC

ENDOMETRITIS

615.9 NOS
615.0 ACUTE
760.8 AFFECTING FETUS OR NEWBORN
616.0 CERVICAL (HYPERPLASTIC)
615.1 CHRONIC
098.16 GONOCOCCAL ACUTE
098.36 GONOCOCCAL CHRONIC
098.16 BLENNORRHAGIC ACUTE
098.36 BLENNORRHAGIC CHRONIC
639.0 FOLLOWING ECTOPIC MOLAR OR ABORTED PREGNANCY
621.3 HYPERPLASTIC
616.0 HYPERPLASTIC CERVIX

E

ENDOMETRITIS (continued)
615.9 SENILE (ATROPHIC)
016.7# TUBERCULOUS
5th Digit: 016.7
0. UNSPECIFIED
1. LAB NOT DONE
2. LABS PENDING
3. MICROSCOPY POSITIVE (IN SPUTUM)
4. CULTURE POSITIVE - MICROSCOPY NEGATIVE
5. CULTURE NEGATIVE - MICROSCOPY POSITIVE
6. CULTURE AND MICROSCOPY NEGATIVE CONFIRMED BY OTHER METHODS

ENDOMETRITIS OBSTETRICAL
760.8 AFFECTING FETUS
0 ASSOCIATED WITH PREGNANCY SEE SPECIFIC CONDITION
670.0# MATERNAL DUE TO PREGNANCY
5th Digit: 670.0
0. UNSPECIFIED
2. DELIVERED WITH POSTPARTUM COMPLICATION
4. POSTPARTUM COMPLICATION
639.0 POST ABORTION OR ECTOPIC/MOLAR PREGNANCY

ENDOMETRIUM, ENDOMETRIAL
621.8 ATROPHY (SENILE)
622.8 ATROPHY (SENILE) CERVIX
621.3 CYSTIC HYPERPLASIA
617.1 CYSTOMA (OVARIAN)
621.3 HYPERPLASIA
622.1 HYPERPLASIA CERVIX
621.8 METAPLASIA SQUAMOUS
621.0 POLYP

425.2 ENDOMYOCARDIAL DISEASE, IDIOPATHIC MURAL
425.0 ENDOMYOCARDIAL FIBROSIS
425.2 ENDOMYOCARDIOPATHY SOUTH AFRICAN
0 ENDOMYOMETRITIS SEE 'ENDOMETRITIS'
362.18 ENDOPHLEBITIS RETINA
0 ENDOPHLEBITIS SEE 'THROMBOPHLEBITIS'
0 ENDOPHTHALMIA SEE 'ENDOPHTHALMITIS'

ENDOPHTHALMITIS
360.01 ACUTE
360.03 CHRONIC
098.42 GONORRHEAL
360.13 PARASITIC
360.19 PHACOANAPHYLACTIC
360.00 PURULENT
360.19 SPECIFIED TYPE NEC
360.11 SYMPATHETIC

236.2 ENDOSALPINGIOMA SITE UNSPECIFIED
0 ENDOSALPINGIOMA SITE SPECIFIED SEE 'NEOPLASM UNCERTAIN BEHAVIOR' BY SITE M9111/1
287.8 ENDOTHELIOSIS
287.8 ENDOTHELIOSIS HEMORRHAGIC INFECTIONAL
585 END STAGE RENAL DISEASE (ESRD)
756.59 ENGELMANN'S DIAPHYSEAL SCLEROSIS
252.0 ENGEL-VON RECKLINGHAUSEN SYNDROME (OSTEITIS FIBROSA CYSTICA)
268.0 ENGLISH RICKETS
690.8 ENGMAN'S INFECTIOUS ECZEMATOID DERMATITIS
611.79 ENGORGEMENT BREAST NEC
778.7 ENGORGEMENT BREAST NEWBORN
362.37 ENGORGEMENT RETINAL VEIN
789.1 ENLARGEMENT OF LIVER UNSPECIFIED

ENOPHTHALMOS
376.50 NOS
376.51 ATROPHIC (OF ORBITAL TISSUE)
376.52 TRAUMATIC OR SURGERY

526.89 ENOSTOSIS
0 ENTAMOEBA HISTOLYTICA INFECTION SEE 'AMEBIC (AMEBIASIS)'
762.5 ENTANGLEMENT OF CORD AFFECTING FETUS OR NEWBORN

ENTERITIS COMMON TYPES
558.9 NOS
008.62 ADENOVIRUS
558.9 ALLERGIC NONINFECTIOUS
006.9 AMEBIC NOS
006.0 AMEBIC ACUTE
006.1 AMEBIC CHRONIC
004.9 BACILLARY NEC
001.1 CHOLERA EL TOR
001.1 CHOLERIFORMIS
007.4 CRYPTOSPORIDIAL
558.9 DIETARY NONINFECTIOUS
564.1 DUE TO IRRITABLE BOWEL SYNDROME
564.1 DUE TO MEMBRANOUS COLITIS
564.1 DUE TO MUCOUS COLITIS
564.1 DUE TO MYXOMEMBRANOUS COLITIS
564.1 DUE TO NEUROGENIC COLITIS
564.1 DUE TO SPASMODIC COLITIS
564.1 DUE TO SPASTIC COLON
008.0# E. COLI
5th Digit: 008.0
0. E. COLI
1. ENTEROPATHOGENIC
2. ENTEROTOXIGENIC
3. ENTEROINVASIVE
4. ENTEROHEMORRHAGIC
9. SPECIFIED TYPE NEC
008.67 ENTEROVIRUS NEC
009.0 EPIDEMIC
009.0 GANGRENOUS
007.1 GIARDIAL
009.0 INFECTIOUS NEC
009.0 INFECTIOUS (SEPTIC)
009.1 INFECTIOUS ORIGIN PRESUMED
487.8 INFLUENZAL
009.0 NECROTIC
558.9 NONINFECTIOUS (ALLERGIC) (DIETARY)
558.9 NONINFECTIOUS (OTHER AND UNSPECIFIED)
008.63 NORWALK-LIKE VIRUS
008.63 NORWALK VIRUS
007.# PROTOZOAL
4th Digit: 007
0. BALANTIDIASIS
1. GIARDIASIS
2. COCCIDIOSIS
3. TRICHOMONIASIS
4. CRYPTOSPORIDIOSIS
8. OTHER SPECIFIED
9. UNSPECIFIED
003.0 SALMONELLA INFECTION
003.0 SALMONELLOSIS
009.0 SEPTIC
004.9 SHIGELLA
008.41 STAPHYLOCOCCUS
007.3 TRICHOMONAL
556.9 ULCERATIVE (CHRONIC)
008.69 VIRUS SPECIFIED NEC
008.8 VIRUS
009.0 ZYMOTIC

ENTERITIS COMPLETE LISTING
008.62 ADENOVIRUS
008.2 AEROBACTER AEROGENES
558.9 ALLERGIC NONINFECTIOUS
006.0 AMEBIC ACUTE
006.1 AMEBIC CHRONIC
006.9 AMEBIC NOS

ENTERITIS COMPLETE LISTING (continued)

008.46 ANAEROBIC (COCCI) (GRAM-NEGATIVE) (GRAM-POSITIVE) (MIXED) NEC
008.1 ARIZONA BACILLUS
008.66 ASTROVIRUS
004.9 BACILLARY NEC
008.5 BACTERIA NEC
008.49 BACTERIA NEC SPECIFIED NEC
008.46 BACTEROIDES (FRAGILIS) (MELAN IN OGENISCUS) (ORALIS)
007.0 BALANTIDIAL
008.46 BUTYRIVIBRIO (FIBRIOSOLVENS)
008.65 CALCIVIRUS
008.43 CAMPLYOBACTER
112.85 CANDIDAL
007.8 CHILOMASTIX
001.1 CHOLERIFORMIS
008.45 CLOSTRIDIUM DIFFICILE
008.46 CLOSTRIDIUM HAEMOLYTICUM
008.46 CLOSTRIDIUM NOVYI
008.43 CLOSTRIDIUM SPECIFIED TYPE NEC
007.2 COCCIDIAL
557.0 COCKLE AGENT
008.67 COXSACKIE (VIRUS)
007.4 CRYPTOSPORIDIAL
558.9 DIETARY
008.64 DITCHLING AGENT
564.1 DUE TO IRRITABLE BOWEL SYNDROME
564.1 DUE TO MEMBRANOUS COLITIS
564.1 DUE TO MUCOUS COLITIS
564.1 DUE TO MYXOMEMBRANOUS COLITIS
564.1 DUE TO NEUROGENIC COLITIS
564.1 DUE TO SPASMODIC COLITIS
564.1 DUE TO SPASTIC COLON
008.0# E. COLI

5th Digit: 008.0

0. E. COLI
1. ENTEROPATHOGENIC
2. ENTEROTOXIGENIC
3. ENTEROINVASIVE
4. ENTEROHEMORRHAGIC
9. SPECIFIED TYPE NEC

008.67 ECHO VIRUS
001.1 EL TOR
007.8 EMBADOMONIAL
008.2 ENTEROBACTER AEROGENES
008.49 ENTEROCOCCI
008.67 ENTEROVIRUS NEC
009.0 EPIDEMIC
008.46 EUBACTERIUM
558.9 FERMENTATIVE
008.46 FUSOBACTERIUM (NUCLEATUM)
009.0 GANGRENOUS
007.1 GIARDIAL
008.47 GRAM-NEGATIVE BACTERIA NEC
008.46 GRAM-NEGATIVE BACTERIA NEC ANAEROBIC NEC
0 GRANULOMATOUS SEE 'CROHN'S DISEASE'
008.63 HAWAII AGENT
009.0 INFECTIOUS NEC
009.1 INFECTIOUS ORIGIN PRESUMED
009.0 INFECTIOUS (SEPTIC)
487.8 INFLUENZAL
558.9 IRRITATING FOODS (DUE TO)
557.9 ISCHEMIC NOS
557.0 ISCHEMIC ACUTE
557.1 ISCHEMIC CHRONIC
557.1 ISCHEMIC DUE TO MESENTERIC ARTERY INSUFFICIENCY
008.47 KLEBSIELLA AEROGENES
555.1 LARGE BOWEL NONINFECTIOUS
555.2 LARGE BOWEL WITH SMALL INTESTINE NONINFECTIOUS
008.66 MARIN COUNTY AGENT
008.63 MONTGOMERY COUNTY AGENT

ENTERITIS COMPLETE LISTING (continued)

009.0 NECROTIC
005.2 NECROTICANS
555.9 NONINFECTIOUS SITE NOS
558.9 NONINFECTIOUS (ALLERGIC) (DIETARY)
558.9 NONINFECTIOUS (OTHER AND UNSPECIFIED)
008.63 NORWALK VIRUS
008.63 NORWALK-LIKE VIRUS
008.63 OTOFUKE AGENT
008.1 PARACOLOBACTRUM ARIZONAE
008.47 PARACOLON BACILLUS NEC
008.64 PARAMATTA AGENT
002.9 PARATYPHOID (FEVER)
008.46 PEPTOCOCCUS
008.46 PEPTOSTREPTOCOCCUS
008.46 PROPRIONIBACTERIUM
007.# PROTOZOAL

4th Digit: 007

0. BALANTIDIASIS
1. GIARDIASIS
2. COCCIDIOSIS
3. TRICHOMONIASIS
4. CRYPTOSPORIDIOSIS
8. OTHER SPECIFIED
9. UNSPECIFIED

008.42 PSEUDOMONAS AERUGINOSA
008.61 ROTAVIRUS
003.0 SALMONELLA INFECTION
003.0 SALMONELLOSIS
008.63 SAPPORO AGENT
555.9 SEGMENTAL
009.0 SEPTIC
558.9 SIMPLE
004.9 SHIGELLA
555.0 SMALL INTESTINE
008.64 SMALL ROUND VIRUS (SRV) NEC
008.63 SMALL ROUND VIRUS (SRV) NEC FEATURELESS NEC
008.63 SMALL ROUND VIRUS (SRV) NEC STRUCTURED NEC
008.63 SNOW MOUNTAIN (SM) AGENT
008.49 SPECIFIED BACTERIA NEC
008.8 SPECIFIED ORGANISM, NONBACTERIAL NEC
008.41 STAPHYLOCOCCUS
008.49 STREPTOCOCCUS
008.46 STREPTOCOCCUS ANAEROBIC
008.63 TAUNTON AGENT
008.69 TOROVIRUS
558.2 TOXIC NONINFECTIOUS
008.46 TREPONEMA (DENTICOLA) (MACRODENTIUM)
007.3 TRICHOMONAL
002.0 TYPHOSA
556.9 ULCERATIVE (CHRONIC)
008.46 VEILLONELLA
008.8 VIRUS
008.69 VIRUS SPECIFIED NEC
008.64 WOLLAN (W) AGENT
008.44 YERSINIA ENTEROCOLITICA
009.0 ZYMOTIC
0 SEE 'AMEBIC, AMEBIASIS'
0 SEE ALSO 'GASTROENTERITIS'

099.3 ENTEROARTICULAR SYNDROME
099.3 ENTEROARTICULAR SYNDROME WITH ARTHROPATHY [711.1#]

5th Digit: 711.1

0. SITE NOS
1. SHOULDER REGION
2. UPPER ARM (ELBOW) (HUMERUS)
3. FOREARM (RADIUS) (WRIST) (ULNA)
4. HAND (CARPAL) (METACARPAL) (FINGERS)
5. PELVIC REGION AND THIGH (HIP) (BUTTOCK) (FEMUR)
6. LOWER LEG (FIBULA) (KNEE) (PATELLA) (TIBIA)
7. ANKLE AND/OR FOOT (METATARSALS) (TOES) (TARSALS)
8. OTHER (HEAD) (NECK) (RIB) (SKULL) (TRUNK) (VERTEBRAE)
9. MULTIPLE

099.3 ENTEROARTICULAR SYNDROME WITH CONJUNCTIVITIS [372.33]
127.4 ENTEROBIASIS INFECTION
127.4 ENTEROBIUS VERMICULARIS INFECTION
618.6 ENTEROCELE VAGINAL (CONGENITAL OR ACQUIRED)
618.6 ENTEROCELE VAGINAL (CONGENITAL OR ACQUIRED) WITH STRESS INCONTINENCE [625.6]
618.6 ENTEROCELE VAGINAL (CONGENITAL OR ACQUIRED)WITH OTHER URINARY INCONTINENCE [788.3#]

5th Digit: 788.3

0. UNSPECIFIED
1. URGE INCONTINENCE
3. MIXED URGE AND STRESS
4 WITHOUT SENSORY AWARENESS
5. POST-VOID DRIBBLING
6. NOCTURNAL ENURESIS
7. CONTINUOUS LEAKAGE
9. OTHER

041.04 ENTEROCOCCUS INFECTION NEC

ENTEROCOLITIS

558.1 DUE TO RADIATION
777.5 DUE TO RADIATION IN NEWBORN
777.8 FETUS OR NEWBORN
777.5 FETUS OR NEWBORN NECROTIZING
557.0 FULMINANT
555.2 GRANULOMATOSIS
557.0 HEMORRHAGIC (ACUTE)
557.1 HEMORRHAGIC (CHRONIC)
557.0 NECROTIZING (ACUTE MEMBRANOUS)
777.5 NECROTIZING IN FETUS OR NEWBORN
008.45 PSEUDOMEMBRANOUS
777.5 PSEUDOMEMBRANOUS IN NEWBORN
008.41 STAPHYLOCOCCAL
556.0 ULCERATIVE

560.39 ENTEROLITH

ENTEROPATHY

569.9 NOS
579.8 EXUDATIVE
579.0 GLUTEN
557.0 HEMORRHAGIC TERMINAL
579.8 PROTEIN LOSING

569.89 ENTEROPTOSIS INTESTINE
564.1 ENTEROSPASM

ENTEROSTOMY

V53.5 BELT FITTING AND ADJUSTMENT
V55.3 CARE
V55.3 CATHETER ADJUSTMENT OR REPOSITIONING
V55.3 CATHETER REMOVAL OR REPLACEMENT
V55.3 CLOSURE
569.60 COMPLICATION - NOS
569.62 COMPLICATION - MECHANICAL
569.69 COMPLICATION - OTHER
569.69 FISTULA
569.69 HERNIA

WHEN CODING AN INFECTION OF AN OSTOMY, USE AN ADDITIONAL CODE TO SPECIFY THE ORGANISM. SEE 'BACTERIAL INFECTION'

569.61 INFECTION
569.61 INFECTION WITH CELLULITIS OF ABDOMEN [682.2]
569.61 INFECTION WITH SEPSIS [038.#(#)]

4th or 4th and 5th Digit Code for Organism: 038

.9 NOS
.3 ANAEROBIC
.3 BACTEROIDES
.3 CLOSTRIDIUM
.42 E COLI
.49 ENTEROBACTER AEROGENES
.40 GRAM NEGATIVE
.49 GRAM NEGATIVE OTHER
.41 HEMOPHILUS INFLUENZAE
.2 PNEUMOCOCCAL
.49 PROTEUS
.43 PSEUDOMONAS
.44 SERRATIA
.10 STAPHYLOCOCCAL NOS
.11 STAPHYLOCOCCAL AUREUS
.19 STAPHYLOCOCCAL OTHER
.0 STREPTOCOCCAL (ANAEROBIC)
.49 YERSINIA ENTEROCOLITICA
.8 OTHER SPECIFIED

569.62 MALFUNCTION
569.69 PROLAPSE
V44.3 STATUS
V55.3 TOILET STOMA

078.89 ENTEROVIRUS DISEASE NEC
048 ENTEROVIRUS DISEASE CENTRAL NERVOUS SYSTEM NEC
008.67 ENTEROVIRUS GASTROENTERITIS
079.89 ENTEROVIRUS INFECTION IN DISEASES CLASSIFIED ELSEWHERE
077.4 ENTEROVIRUS TYPE 70 CONJUNCTIVITIS
117.7 ENTOMOPHTHORA INFECTION
368.15 ENTOPTIC PHENOMENA
0 ENTRAPMENT SYNDROME SEE 'NEUROPATHY' ENTRAPMENT

ENTROPION (EYELID)

374.00 NOS
374.04 CICATRICIAL
743.62 CONGENITAL
374.02 MECHANICAL
374.02 PARALYTIC
374.01 SENILE
374.03 SPASTIC
139.1 TRACHOMA (LATE EFFECT)

871.3 ENUCLEATION TRAUMATIC

ENURESIS

788.30 NOS
788.36 NOCTURNAL
307.6 PSYCHOGENIC

E

277.6 ENZYMES DEFICIENCY
790.5 ENZYMES SERUM NEC ABNORMAL
277.9 ENZYMOPATHY
794.12 EOG ABNORMAL
288.0 EOSINOPENIA

EOSINOPHILIA
288.3 ALLERGIC
288.3 HEREDITARY
288.3 IDIOPATHIC
710.5 MYALGIA SYNDROME
518.3 PULMONARY
288.3 SECONDARY
518.3 TROPICAL

277.8 EOSINOPHILIC GRANULOMA (BONE)

> *CARCINOMAS AND NEOPLASMS SHOULD BE CODED BY SITE IF POSSIBLE. CODE BY CELL TYPE - "SITE NOS", IF AND ONLY IF A SITE IS NOT SPECIFIED IN THE DIAGNOSIS. OTHERWISE - REFER TO THE APPROPRIATE CATEGORY OF NEOPLASM FOR A MORE SPECIFIC CODE: SEE 'CANCER' 'CANCER METASTATIC', 'NEOPLASM UNCERTAIN BEHAVIOR', 'NEOPLASM UNSPECIFIED NATURE', OR 'BENIGN NEOPLASM'.*

EPENDYMOMA
191.9 SITE UNSPECIFIED
0 SITE SPECIFIED SEE 'CANCER' BY SITE M9391/3
191.9 ANAPLASTIC TYPE SITE UNSPECIFIED
0 ANAPLASTIC TYPE SITE SPECIFIED SEE 'CANCER' BY SITE M9392/3
237.5 MYXOPAPILLARY SITE NOS
0 MYXOPAPILLARY SITE SPECIFIED SEE 'NEOPLASM UNCERTAIN BEHAVIOR' BY SITE M9394/1
237.5 PAPILLARY SITE NOS
0 PAPILLARY SITE SPECIFIED SEE 'NEOPLASM UNCERTAIN BEHAVIOR' BY SITE M9393/1

709.09 EPHELIDES
780.6 EPHEMERAL FEVER
743.62 EPIBLEPHARON CONGENITAL
743.63 EPICANTHUS (FOLD) (CONGENITAL)
726.32 EPICONDYLITIS LATERAL
726.31 EPICONDYLITIS MEDIAL

EPIDEMIC
078.89 CERVICAL MYALGIA
136.9 DISEASE NEC
077.4 HEMORRHAGIC CONJUNCTIVITIS
078.6 HEMORRHAGIC FEVER
077.1 KERATOCONJUNCTIVITIS
078.82 VOMITING SYNDROME

078.19 EPIDERMODYSPLASIA VERRUCIFORMIS
706.2 EPIDERMOID CYST

EPIDERMOLYSIS
757.39 BULLOSA CONGENITAL
695.1 COMBUSTIFORMIS (TOXICA)
977.9 DRUG INDUCED

110.# EPIDERMOPHYTON INFECTIONS
4th Digit: 110
0. SCALP AND BEARD
1. NAIL (UNGUIUM)
2. HAND (MANUUM)
3. GROIN AND PERIANAL (CRURIS)
4. FOOT (PEDIS)
5. BODY (CORPORUS)
6. DEEP SEATED (GRANULOMA TRICHOPHYTICUM)
8. OTHER SPECIFIED SITE
9. UNSPECIFIED SITE

385.30 EPIDERMOSIS EAR (MIDDLE)

EPIDIDYMIS
608.89 ABSENCE
752.8 ABSENCE CONGENITAL
608.3 ATROPHY
608.9 DISORDER
608.2 TORSION

EPIDIDYMITIS
604.90 NOS
604.0 AND ORCHITIS WITH ABSCESS
604.90 AND ORCHITIS WITHOUT ABSCESS
032.89 DIPHTHERITIC [604.91]
125.9 FILARIAL [604.91]
098.13 GONOCOCCAL ACUTE
098.33 GONOCOCCAL CHRONIC
604.0 WITH ABSCESS
604.0 WITH ORCHITIS AND ABSCESS
604.99 OTHER
095.8 SYPHILITIC [604.91]
016.4# TUBERCULOSIS
5th Digit: 016.4
0. UNSPECIFIED
1. LAB NOT DONE
2. LABS PENDING
3. MICROSCOPY POSITIVE (IN SPUTUM)
4. CULTURE POSITIVE - MICROSCOPY NEGATIVE
5. CULTURE NEGATIVE - MICROSCOPY POSITIVE
6. CULTURE AND MICROSCOPY NEGATIVE CONFIRMED BY OTHER METHODS

432.0 EPIDURAL HEMATOMA (HEMORRHAGE) NONTRAUMATIC
852.4# EPIDURAL HEMATOMA (HEMORRHAGE) TRAUMATIC
852.5# EPIDURAL HEMATOMA (HEMORRHAGE) TRAUMATIC WITH OPEN INTRACRANIAL WOUND
5th Digit: 852.4-5
0. LEVEL OF CONSCIOUSNESS UNSPECIFIED
1. NO LOC
2. LOC < 1 HR
3. LOC 1 - 24 HRS
4. LOC > 24 HRS WITH RETURN TO PRIOR LEVEL
5. LOC > 24 HRS WITHOUT RETURN TO PRIOR LEVEL: OR DEATH BEFORE REGAINING CONSCIOUSNESS, REGARDLESS OF DURATION OF LOC
6. LOC DURATION UNSPECIFIED
9. WITH CONCUSSION UNSPECIFIED

536.9 EPIGASTRIC DISORDER FUNCTIONAL
306.4 EPIGASTRIC DISORDER FUNCTIONAL - PSYCHOGENIC
789.36 EPIGASTRIC MASS
789.06 EPIGASTRIC PAIN
553.29 EPIGASTROCELE

EPIGLOTTIS
748.3 ANOMALY CONGENITAL
748.3 ATRESIA CONGENITAL
748.3 FISSURE CONGENITAL
959.09 INJURY

EPIGLOTTITIS
464.30 ACUTE
464.31 ACUTE WITH OBSTRUCTION
464.30 ACUTE VIRAL
464.31 ACUTE VIRAL WITH OBSTRUCTION
476.1 CHRONIC

759.4 EPIGNATHUS

DO NOT CODE EPILEPSY AS INTRACTABLE UNLESS THE PHYSICIAN STATES IT IS INTRACTABLE. RECURRENT SEIZURES ARE NOT ENOUGH TO INDICATE INTRACTABLE EPILEPSY.

EPILEPSY, EPILEPTIC

345.9# NOS
345.0# ABSENCE ATONIC
345.0# ABSENCE TYPICAL
5th Digit: 345.0, 9
0. WITHOUT MENTION OF INTRACTABLE EPILEPSY
1. WITH INTRACTABLE EPILEPSY

345.2 ABSENCE STATUS (PETIT MAL STATUS)
345.4# AUTOMATISM
345.5# BRAVAIS-JACKSONIAN NOS
345.1# CLONIC
5th Digit: 345.1, 4-5
0. WITHOUT MENTION OF INTRACTABLE EPILEPSY
1. WITH INTRACTABLE EPILEPSY

293.0 CONFUSIONAL STATE
345.9# CONVULSION NOS
345.8# CURSIVE (RUNNING) (GELASTIC)
5th Digit: 345.8-9
0. WITHOUT MENTION OF INTRACTABLE EPILEPSY
1. WITH INTRACTABLE EPILEPSY

345.## DEMENTIA [294.1]
345.## DETERIORATION [294.1]
4th Digit: 345
0. GENERALIZED NONCONVULSIVE
1. GENERALIZED CONVULSIVE
4. PARTIAL, WITH IMPAIRMENT OF CONSCIOUSNESS
5. PARTIAL, WITHOUT IMPAIRMENT OF CONSCIOUSNESS
6. INFANTILE SPASMS
7. EPILEPSIA PARTIALIS CONTINUA
8. OTHER FORMS
9. UNSPECIFIED, NOS

5th Digit: 345
0. WITHOUT MENTION OF INTRACTABLE EPILEPSY
1. WITH INTRACTABLE EPILEPSY

V17.2 FAMILY HISTORY
345.9# FIT NOS
345.5# FOCAL (MOTOR)
345.7# FOCAL (MOTOR) STATUS
345.1# GENERALIZED CONVULSIVE
345.0# GENERALIZED NONCONVULSIVE
345.1# GRAND MAL
5th Digit: 345.0-1, 5, 7, 9
0. WITHOUT MENTION OF INTRACTABLE EPILEPSY
1. WITH INTRACTABLE EPILEPSY

345.3 GRAND MAL STATUS
345.6# HYPSARRHYTHMIA
345.6# INFANTILE (SPASMS) (SALAAM) (LIGHTNING)
345.5# JACKSONIAN
345.4# LIMBIC SYSTEM
345.1# MAJOR (MOTOR)
5th Digit: 345.1, 4-6
0. WITHOUT MENTION OF INTRACTABLE EPILEPSY
1. WITH INTRACTABLE EPILEPSY

E

USE AN ADDITIONAL CODE TO IDENTIFY THE SPECIFIC MATERNAL EPILEPSY. SEE 'EPILEPSY, EPILEPTIC'.

648.9# MATERNAL CURRENT (CO-EXISTENT) IN PREGNANCY
5th Digit: 648.9
0. EPISODE OF CARE UNSPECIFIED OR N/A
1. DELIVERED
2. DELIVERED WITH POSTPARTUM COMPLICATION
3. ANTEPARTUM COMPLICATION
4. POSTPARTUM COMPLICATION

345.0# MINOR
345.1# MYOCLONIC
5th Digit: 345.0-1
0. WITHOUT MENTION OF INTRACTABLE EPILEPSY
1. WITH INTRACTABLE EPILEPSY

333.2 MYOCLONIC PROGRESSIVE
779.0 NEWBORN
345.5# PARTIAL NOS
345.5# PARTIAL MOTOR
345.4# PARTIAL PSYCHOSENSORY
345.4# PARTIAL SECONDARILY GENERALIZED
345.4# PARTIAL WITH IMPAIRMENT OF CONSCIOUSNESS
345.7# PARTIALIS CONTINUA (KOJEVNIKOV)
345.0# PETIT MAL
5th Digit: 345.0, 4-5, 7
0. WITHOUT MENTION OF INTRACTABLE EPILEPSY
1. WITH INTRACTABLE EPILEPSY

345.2 PETIT MAL STATUS
345.4# PSYCHOMOTOR
345.7# PSYCHOMOTOR STATUS
5th Digit: 345.4, 7
0. WITHOUT MENTION OF INTRACTABLE EPILEPSY
1. WITH INTRACTABLE EPILEPSY

294.8 PSYCHOSIS **[345.##]**
4th Digit: 345
0. GENERALIZED NONCONVULSIVE
1. GENERALIZED CONVULSIVE
4. PARTIAL, WITH IMPAIRMENT OF CONSCIOUSNESS
5. PARTIAL, WITHOUT IMPAIRMENT OF CONSCIOUSNESS
6. INFANTILE SPASMS
7. EPILEPSIA PARTIALIS CONTINUA
8. OTHER FORMS
9. UNSPECIFIED, NOS

5th Digit: 345
0. WITHOUT MENTION OF INTRACTABLE EPILEPSY
1. WITH INTRACTABLE EPILEPSY

345.0# PYKNO-EPILEPSY
345.9# SEIZURE NOS
345.0# SEIZURE AKINETIC
345.0# SEIZURE ATONIC
345.5# SENSORY-INDUCED
345.5# SOMATOMOTOR (SOMATOSENSORY)
5th Digit: 345.0, 5, 9
0. WITHOUT MENTION OF INTRACTABLE EPILEPSY
1. WITH INTRACTABLE EPILEPSY

345.3 STATUS EPILEPTICUS (GRAND MAL)

EPILEPSY, EPILEPTIC (continued)
345.4# TEMPORAL LOBE (PSYCHOMOTOR)
345.7# TEMPORAL LOBE (PSYCHOMOTOR) STATUS
345.1# TONIC (TONIC-CLONIC)
5th Digit: 345.1, 4, 7
0. WITHOUT MENTION OF INTRACTABLE EPILEPSY
1. WITH INTRACTABLE EPILEPSY

293.0 TWILIGHT STATE
345.5# VISCERAL
345.5# VISUAL
345.8# OTHER SPECIFIED
5th Digit: 345.5, 8
0. WITHOUT MENTION OF INTRACTABLE EPILEPSY
1. WITH INTRACTABLE EPILEPSY

780.39 EPILEPTIFORM ATTACK (CONVULSIONS) (SEIZURE)
301.3 EPILEPTOID PERSONALITY DISORDER
759.5 EPILOIA
259.3 EPINEPHRINE ECTOPIC SECRETION

EPIPHORA
375.21 DUE TO EXCESS LACRIMATION
375.22 DUE TO INSUFFICIENT DRAINAGE
375.20 UNSPECIFIED AS TO CAUSE

733.91 EPIPHYSEAL ARREST
732.2 EPIPHYSEAL ARREST FEMORAL HEAD
756.56 EPIPHYSEAL DYSPLASIA MULTIPLE CONGENITAL

732.2 EPIPHYSIS CAPITAL FEMORAL SLIPPED NONTRAUMATIC

EPIPHYSITIS
732.9 NOS
732.6 JUVENILE
732.6 JUVENILE OTHER SITE
732.5 OS CALCIS (JUVENILE)
732.0 VERTEBRAL (JUVENILE)

EPISCLERITIS
379.00 NOS
274.89 GOUTY [379.09]
379.09 NEC
379.02 NODULAR
379.01 PERIODICA FUGAX
379.00 STAPHYLOCOCCAL
379.00 SUPPURATIVE
095.0 SYPHILITIC
017.3# TUBERCULOSIS [379.09]
5th Digit: 017.3
0. UNSPECIFIED
1. LAB NOT DONE
2. LABS PENDING
3. MICROSCOPY POSITIVE (IN SPUTUM)
4. CULTURE POSITIVE - MICROSCOPY NEGATIVE
5. CULTURE NEGATIVE - MICROSCOPY POSITIVE
6. CULTURE AND MICROSCOPY NEGATIVE CONFIRMEDBY OTHER METHODS

674.3# EPISIOTOMY COMPLICATION (INFECTION) (OTHER)
674.2# EPISIOTOMY DISRUPTION (OF WOUND)
5th Digit: 674.2-3
0. UNSPECIFIED
2. DELIVERED WITH POSTPARTUM COMPLICATION
4. POSTPARTUM COMPLICATION

753.8 EPISPADIAS CONGENITAL - FEMALE
752.62 EPISPADIAS CONGENITAL - MALE

EPISTAXIS
784.7 NOS
448.0 HEREDITARY
784.7 RECURRENT (CHRONIC) (UNSPECIFIED) (SEVERE)
625.8 VICARIOUS MENSTRUATION

EPITHELIAL
364.61 DOWN GROWTH EYE (ANTERIOR CHAMBER)
709.8 HYPERPLASIA
611.8 HYPERPLASIA - NIPPLE
528.7 HYPERPLASIA - ORAL INCLUDING TONGUE
709.8 HYPERPLASIA - SKIN
623.0 HYPERPLASIA - VAGINAL WALL
229.9 TUMOR BENIGN SITE UNSPECIFIED
0 TUMOR BENIGN SITE SPECIFIED SEE 'BENIGN NEOPLASM' BY SITE M8010/0

CARCINOMAS AND NEOPLASMS SHOULD BE CODED BY SITE IF POSSIBLE. CODE BY CELL TYPE - "SITE NOS", IF AND ONLY IF A SITE IS NOT SPECIFIED IN THE DIAGNOSIS. OTHERWISE - REFER TO THE APPROPRIATE CATEGORY OF NEOPLASM FOR A MORE SPECIFIC CODE: SEE 'CANCER' 'CANCER METASTATIC', 'NEOPLASM UNCERTAIN BEHAVIOR', 'NEOPLASM UNSPECIFIED NATURE', OR 'BENIGN NEOPLASM.'

EPITHELIOMA
229.9 BENIGN SITE UNSPECIFIED
0 BENIGN SITE SPECIFIED SEE 'BENIGN NEOPLASM' BY SITE M8011/0
216.# INTRADERMAL
4th Digit: 216
0. LIP (SKIN OF)
1. EYELID INCLUDING CANTHUS
2. EAR (EXTERNAL) (AURICLE) (PINNA)
3. FACE (CHEEK) (NOSE)
4. SCALP NECK
5. TRUNK BACK CHEST
6. UPPER LIMB INCLUDING SHOULDER
7. LOWER LIMB INCLUDING HIP
8. OTHER SPECIFIED SITES
9. SKIN UNSPECIFIED

199.1 MALIGNANT SITE UNSPECIFIED
0 MALIGNANT SITE SPECIFIED SEE 'CANCER' BY SITE M8011/3

363.15 EPITHELIOPATHY
757.5 EPONYCHIA
752.11 EPOOPHORON CYST CONGENITAL
332.1 EPS (EXTRAPYRAMIDAL SYNDROME)

075 EPSTEIN BARRE INFECTION (VIRAL)
528.4 EPSTEIN'S PEARL (CYST MOUTH)
581.9 EPSTEIN'S SYNDROME
780.4 EQUILIBRIUM DISTURBANCE
024 EQUINIA
754.69 EQUINOVALGUS DEFORMITY CONGENITAL
754.51 EQUINOVARUS CONGENITAL
736.71 EQUINOVARUS DEFORMITY ACQUIRED
736.72 EQUINUS DEFORMITY OF FOOT ACQUIRED

767.6 ERB DUCHENNE PALSY OR PARALYSIS (BIRTH TRAUMA)
358.0 ERB (-OPPENHEIM) -GOLDFLAM SYNDROME
094.89 ERB'S DISEASE (SYPHILITIC)
359.1 ERB'S (-LANDOUZY) MUSCULAR DYSTROPHY
253.0 ERDHEIM'S SYNDROME (ACROMEGALIC MACROSPONDYLITIS)

607.84 ERECTILE DISORDER MALE - ORGANIC
302.72 ERECTILE DISORDER MALE - PSYCHOSEXUAL

607.3 ERECTION PAINFUL (PERSISTENT)
794.11 ERG ABNORMAL

349.82 ERGOTISM CORRECT SUBSTANCE (PROPERLY ADMINISTERED)
988.2 ERGOTISM DRUG THERAPY (MIGRAINE)
975.0 ERGOTISM OVERDOSE (WRONG SUBSTANCE)

300.16 ERICHSEN'S RAILWAY SPINE
732.4 ERLACHER BLOUNT SYNDROME (TIBIA VARA)

EROSION

447.2 ARTERY WITHOUT RUPTURE
535.4# GASTRIC
535.4# PYLORUS
535.4# STOMACH
5th Digit: 535.4
0. WITHOUT HEMORRHAGE
1. WITH HEMORRHAGE

302.89 EROTOMANIA

787.3 ERUCTATION
306.4 ERUCTATION NERVOUS OR PSYCHOGENIC

ERYSIPELAS

035 ERYSIPELAS
035 ERYSIPELAS EAR (EXTERNAL) [380.13]
035 ERYSIPELAS PINNA [380.13]

027.1 ERYSIPELOID OF ROSENBACH
027.1 ERYSIPELOTHRIX INFECTION

ERYTHEMA

695.9 NOS
695.0 ANNULARE (CENTRIFUGUM) (RHEUMATICUM)
695.1 BULLOSUM (GYRATUM)
088.81 CHRONICUM MIGRANS
695.1 CONJUNCTIVA
026.1 EPIDEMIC ARTHRITIC
017.1# INDURATUM
5th Digit: 017.1
0. NOS
1. LAB NOT DONE
2. LABS PENDING
3. MICROSCOPY POSITIVE (IN SPUTUM)
4. CULTURE POSITIVE - MICROSCOPY NEGATIVE
5. CULTURE NEGATIVE - MICROSCOPY POSITIVE
6. CULTURE AND MICROSCOPY NEGATIVE CONFIRMED BY OTHER METHODS

057.0 INFECTIOSUM
695.89 INTERTRIGO
695.1 IRIS
695.1 MULTIFORME
695.2 NODOSUM
017.1# NODOSUM, TUBERCULOUS
5th Digit: 017.1
0. NOS
1. LAB NOT DONE
2. LABS PENDING
3. MICROSCOPY POSITIVE (IN SPUTUM)
4. CULTURE POSITIVE - MICROSCOPY NEGATIVE
5. CULTURE NEGATIVE - MICROSCOPY POSITIVE
6. CULTURE AND MICROSCOPY NEGATIVE CONFIRMED BY OTHER METHODS

991.5 PERNIO
909.4 PERNIO LATE EFFECT
695.0 SCARLATINIFORM
695.0 TOXIC
695.0 VENENATUM

039.0 ERYTHRASMA

985.0 ERYTHREDEMA
985.0 ERYTHREDEMA POLYNEURITICA
985.0 ERYTHREDEMA POLYNEUROPATHY

ERYTHREMIA

207.0# ACUTE SITE UNSPECIFIED M9841/3
207.1# CHRONIC M9842/3
207.0# MYELOSIS M9841/3
5th Digit: 207.0, 1
0. WITHOUT MENTION OF REMISSION
1. WITH MENTION OF REMISSION

284.0 ERYTHROBLASTOPENIA CONGENITAL
284.8 ERYTHROBLASTOPENIA (SECONDARY)

773.2 ERYTHROBLASTOSIS FETALIS
773.1 ERYTHROBLASTOSIS FETALIS DUE TO ABO ANITIBODIES
773.0 ERYTHROBLASTOSIS FETALIS DUE TO RH ANTIBODIES

443.89 ERYTHROCYANOSIS
284.9 ERYTHROCYTE ABSENCE
283.19 ERYTHROCYTE FRAGMENTATION SYNDROME

ERYTHRODERMA

695.89 DESQUAMATIVA (INFANTS)
695.89 EXFOLIATIVE
757.1 ICTHYOSIFORM (CONGENITAL)
695.89 INFANTUM
696.2 MACULOPAPULAR
778.8 NEONATORUM
696.1 PSORIATORUM
695.9 SECONDARY

284.0 ERYTHROGENESIS IMPERFECTA
289.9 ERYTHROID HYPERPLASIA
207.0# ERYTHROLEUKEMIA M9840/3
5th Digit: 207.0
0. WITHOUT MENTION OF REMISSION
1. WITH MENTION OF REMISSION

443.89 ERYTHROMELALGIA
701.8 ERYTHROMELIA
289.9 ERYTHROPHAGOCYTOSIS
300.23 ERYTHROPHOBIA
528.7 ERYTHROPLAKIA ORAL (MOUTH) (TONGUE)
233.5 ERYTHROPLASIA SITE UNSPECIFIED
0 ERYTHROPLASIA SITE SPECIFIED SEE 'CARCINOMA IN SITU', BY SITE
284.9 ERYTHROPOIESIS ABSENCE
284.0 ERYTHROPOIESIS ABSENCE CONGENITAL

041.4 ESCHERICHIA COLI INFECTION OR ORGANISM
771.8 ESCHERICHIA COLI INFECTION INTRA-AMNIOTIC (FETUS OR NEWBORN)
530.89 ESOPHAGALGIA
0 ESOPHAGEAL SEE 'ESOPHAGUS, ESOPHAGEAL'

530.89 ESOPHAGECTASIS
530.0 ESOPHAGECTASIS CARDIOSPASM INDUCED

530.5 ESOPHAGISMUS

ESOPHAGITIS

530.10 ESOPHAGITIS
112.84 CANDIDAL
530.19 CHEMICAL PEPTIC
530.19 POSTOPERATIVE
530.11 REFLUX
530.19 SPECIFIED NEC
017.8# TUBERCULOUS
5th Digit: 017.8
0. UNSPECIFIED
1. LAB NOT DONE
2. LABS PENDING
3. MICROSCOPY POSITIVE (IN SPUTUM)
4. CULTURE POSITIVE - MICROSCOPY NEGATIVE
5. CULTURE NEGATIVE - MICROSCOPY POSITIVE
6. CULTURE AND MICROSCOPY NEGATIVE CONFIRMED BY OTHER METHODS

530.89 ESOPHAGOBRONCHIAL FISTULA
750.3 ESOPHAGOBRONCHIAL FISTULA CONGENITAL

530.89 ESOPHAGOCUTANEOUS FISTULA
530.6 ESOPHAGOCELE ACQUIRED
530.89 ESOPHAGODYNIA
530.89 ESOPHAGOMALACIA
530.89 ESOPHAGOPLEUROCUTANEOUS FISTULA
530.89 ESOPHAGOPTOSIS
530.5 ESOPHAGOSPASM

530.84 ESOPHAGOTRACHEAL FISTULA
750.3 ESOPHAGOTRACHEAL FISTULA CONGENITAL

ESOPHAGUS, ESOPHAGEAL

530.19 ABSCESS
750.3 ABSENCE (CONGENITAL)
530.89 AMPULLA
530.0 APERISTALSIS
530.3 COMPRESSION
530.5 CORKSCREW
530.5 CURLING
530.89 CYST
530.89 DEFORMITY (ACQUIRED)
530.89 DEVIATION (ACQUIRED)
530.89 DILATATION (ACQUIRED)
530.89 DISPLACEMENT (ACQUIRED)
530.9 DISORDER
530.5 DISORDER FUNCTIONAL
306.4 DISORDER FUNCTIONAL - PSYCHOGENIC
530.6 DIVERTICULUM ACQUIRED
530.5 DYSKINESIA
530.89 EROSION
530.89 ESOPHAGALGIA
530.89 FISTULA
530.82 HEMORRHAGE
530.89 HYPERSENSITIVE
530.10 INFLAMMATION
874.4 INJURY CERVICAL - TRAUMATIC
874.5 INJURY CERVICAL - TRAUMATIC WITH OPEN WOUND
908.0 INJURY LATE EFFECT
862.22 INJURY - TRAUMATIC
862.32 INJURY - TRAUMATIC WITH OPEN WOUND
530.89 LACERATION
530.83 LEUKOPLAKIA
530.7 MALLORY WEISS TEAR
530.89 NECROSIS
530.3 OBSTRUCTION
530.4 PERFORATION NONTRAUMATIC
530.6 POUCH ACQUIRED
530.81 REFLUX
530.4 RUPTURE NONTRAUMATIC
530.5 SPASM
530.3 STRICTURE AND STENOSIS
530.84 TRACHEOESOPHAGEAL FISTULA
530.2 ULCER
456.1 ULCER - VARICOSE
456.0 ULCER - VARICOSE WITH BLEEDING
530.89 DISORDERS OTHER SPECIFIED

ESOPHAGUS, ESOPHAGEAL CONGENITAL ANOMALIES

750.3 ABSENCE
750.3 ATRESIA
750.4 DILATATION
750.4 DISPLACEMENT
750.4 DIVERTICULUM
750.4 DUPLICATION
750.4 FISTULA
750.3 FISTULA TRACHEOESOPHAGEAL
750.4 GIANT
750.6 HERNIA (HIATAL)
750.3 IMPERFORATE
750.4 POUCH
750.3 RING
750.3 STENOSIS
750.3 STRICTURE
750.3 WEBBED

ESOPHAGUS, ESOPHAGEAL VARICES

456.1 NOS
571.5 DUE TO CIRRHOSIS (NON ALCOHOLIC)[456.21]
572.3 DUE TO PORTAL HYPERTENSION [456.21]
571.2 IN ALCOHOLIC CIRRHOSIS [456.21]
571.2 IN ALCOHOLIC CIRRHOSIS WITH BLEEDING [456.20]
571.6 IN BILIARY CIRRHOSIS [456.21]
571.6 IN BILIARY CIRRHOSIS WITH BLEEDING [456.20]
456.0 WITH BLEEDING
571.0 WITH BLEEDING DUE TO CIRRHOSIS [456.20]
572.3 WITH BLEEDING DUE TO PORTAL HYPERTENSION [456.20]

ESOPHORIA

378.84 CONVERGENCE EXCESS
378.85 DIVERGENCE INSUFFICIENCY
378.41 UNSPECIFIED

ESOTROPIA

378.0# NOS
378.0# CONVERGENT CONCOMITANT STRABISMUS

5th Digit: 378.0

0. UNSPECIFIED
1. MONOCULAR UNSPECIFIED
2. MONOCULAR WITH A PATTERN
3. MONOCULAR WITH V PATTERN
4. MONOCULAR WITH OTHER NONCOMITANCIES (X OR Y PATTERN)
5. ALTERNATING UNSPECIFIED
6. ALTERNATING WITH A PATTERN
7. ALTERNATING WITH V PATTERN
8. ALTERNATING WITH OTHER NONCOMITANCIES (X OR Y PATTERN)

378.20 INTERMITTENT
378.22 INTERMITTENT (ALTERNATING)
378.21 INTERMITTENT (MONOCULAR)
378.35 ACCOMMODATIVE COMPONENT
378.00 NONACCOMMODATIVE

085.5 ESPUNDIA
790.1 ESR ABNORMAL
585 ESRD (END STAGE RENAL DISEASE)

CARCINOMAS AND NEOPLASMS SHOULD BE CODED BY SITE IF POSSIBLE. CODE BY CELL TYPE - "SITE NOS", IF AND ONLY IF A SITE IS NOT SPECIFIED IN THE DIAGNOSIS. OTHERWISE - REFER TO THE APPROPRIATE CATEGORY OF NEOPLASM FOR A MORE SPECIFIC CODE: SEE 'CANCER' 'CANCER METASTATIC', 'NEOPLASM UNCERTAIN BEHAVIOR', 'NEOPLASM UNSPECIFIED NATURE', OR 'BENIGN NEOPLASM.'

160.0 ESTHESIONEUROBLASTOMA SITE UNSPECIFIED
0 ESTHESIONEUROBLASTOMA SITE SPECIFIED SEE 'CANCER' BY SITE M9522/3
160.0 ESTHESIONEUROCYTOMA SITE UNSPECIFIED
0 ESTHESIONEUROCYTOMA SITE SPECIFIED SEE 'CANCER' BY SITE M9521/3
160.0 ESTHESIONEUROEPITHELIOMA SITE UNSPECIFIED
0 ESTHESIONEUROEPITHELIOMA SITE SPECIFIED SEE 'CANCER' BY SITE M9523/3
099.1 ESTHIOMENE
V61.0 ESTRANGEMENT (REASON FOR ENCOUNTER)
256.0 ESTROGEN HYPERSECRETION
0 ETHANOL SEE 'ALCOHOL'
270.8 ETHANOLAMINE METABOLISM DISORDERS
270.8 ETHANOLAMINURIA
0 ETHANOLISM SEE 'ALCOHOLISM'
461.2 ETHMOIDAL SINUS (ABSCESS) (INFECTION) (INFLAMMATION) ACUTE
478.1 ETHMOIDITIS INFLUENZAL
359.2 EULENBURG'S CONGENITAL MYOTONIA
257.2 EUNUCHOIDISM

EUSTACHIAN

744.24 ABSENCE OR ATRESIA (CONGENITAL)
744.24 ANOMALIES SPECIFIED CONGENITAL
744.24 DILATATION CONGENITAL
381.9 DISORDER TUBE
381.89 DISORDER OTHER
381.81 DYSFUNCTION
381.50 INFECTION
381.51 INFECTION - ACUTE
381.52 INFECTION - CHRONIC
959.09 INJURY
381.60 OBSTRUCTION
381.63 OBSTRUCTION (EXTRINSIC) (CARTILAGENOUS) (COMPRESSION)
381.62 OBSTRUCTION (INTRINSIC) (CARTILAGENOUS)
381.61 OBSTRUCTION (OSSEOUS) (CHOLESTEATOMA) (POLYP) (OTHER LESION)
381.7 PATULOUS
381.81 PRESSURE
381.50 SALPINGITIS
381.51 SALPINGITIS ACUTE
381.52 SALPINGITIS CHRONIC
381.60 STENOSIS (TUBE)
381.60 STRICTURE (TUBE)

790.94 EUTHYROID SICK SYNDROME

> *V71 - V71.9 ARE ALWAYS SEQUENCED FIRST--THEY DESCRIBE THE EVALUATION AND OBSERVATION FOR SUSPECTED INJURY OR ILLNESS. EXAMPLE: EVALUATION OF A PATIENT IN A MOTOR VEHICLE ACCIDENT WITH NO APPARENT INJURY.*

EVALUATION FOR SUSPECTED CONDITION (UNDIAGNOSED) (UNPROVEN) NOT FOUND

V71.9 UNSPECIFIED
V71.6 ABUSE - CHILD OR ADULT
V71.3 ACCIDENT AT WORK
V71.4 ACCIDENT NEC
V71.8 ACUTE ABDOMEN
V71.01 ANTISOCIAL BEHAVIOR - ADULT
V71.02 ANTISOCIAL BEHAVIOR - CHILD OR ADOLESCENT
V71.6 ASSAULT WITH NO NEED FOR MEDICAL TREATMENT
V71.1 CANCER
V71.7 CARDIOVASCULAR DISEASE
V71.4 CONCUSSION - ACCIDENTAL
V71.6 CONCUSSION - INFLICTED
V71.3 CONCUSSION - WORK RELATED
V71.8 CVA (CEREBROVASCULAR ACCIDENT)
V71.8 FOREIGN BODY INGESTION
V71.01 GANG ACTIVITY ADULT WITH NO MANIFEST PSYCHIATRIC DISORDER
V71.02 GANG ACTIVITY CHILD WITH NO MANIFEST PSYCHIATRIC DISORDER
V71.8 HEMORRHAGE (NON TRAUMATIC) (POST OP)
V71.09 MENTAL CONDITION
V71.4 MVA (MOTOR VEHICLE ACCIDENT) WITH NO APPARENT INJURY
V71.7 MYOCARDIAL INFARCTION

NEWBORN (28 DAYS OR LESS)

V29.9 UNSPECIFIED
V29.8 CARDIOVASCULAR DISEASE
V29.8 CONGENITAL ABNORMALITY
V29.3 GENETIC CONDITION
V29.8 INGESTION FOREIGN OBJECT
V29.0 INFECTIOUS DISEASE
V29.8 INJURY
V29.3 METABOLIC CONDITION
V29.8 NEOPLASM
V29.1 NEUROLOGICAL DISEASE
V29.8 POISONING
V29.2 RESPIRATORY CONDITION
V29.8 SPECIFIED NEC

EVALUATION FOR SUSPECTED CONDITION (UNDIAGNOSED) (UNPROVEN) NOT FOUND (continued)

V71.02 PSYCHIATRIC DISORDER - ADOLESCENT OR CHILD WITH ANTISOCIAL BEHAVIOR (GANG ACTIVITY)
V71.01 PSYCHIATRIC DISORDER - ADULT WITH ANTISOCIAL BEHAVIOR (GANG ACTIVITY)
V71.09 PSYCHIATRIC DISORDER OTHER
V71.5 RAPE (ALLEGED)
V71.8 RUPTURE OF MEMBRANES PREMATURE
V71.5 SEDUCTION (ALLEGED)
V71.8 SEPSIS
V71.8 STROKE
V71.8 SUICIDE ATTEMPT (ALLEGED)
V71.2 TUBERCULOSIS
V71.4 OTHER ACCIDENT
V71.6 OTHER INFLICTED INJURY
V71.8 OTHER SPECIFIED SUSPECTED CONDITIONS

287.3 EVAN'S SYNDROME (THROMBOCYTOPENIC PURPURA)

EVERSION

596.8 BLADDER
616.0 CERVIX WITH CERVICITIS
622.0 CERVIX UTERI
755.67 FOOT CONGENITAL
736.79 FOOT NEC
375.51 LACRIMAL PUNCTUM
593.89 URETER (MEATUS)
599.84 URETHRA (MEATUS)
618.1 UTERUS SEE ALSO 'UTERUS, UTERINE PROLAPSE'

EVISCERATION

767.8 BIRTH TRAUMA
553.29 CONGENITAL
998.3 OPERATIVE WOUND
869.1 TRAUMATIC
871.3 TRAUMATIC - EYE (GLOBE)
908.2 TRAUMATIC - LATE EFFECT

> *V CODES ARE GENERALLY SEQUENCED SECONDARILY--EXCEPTION: IF THEY ARE THE "REASON" FOR THE ENCOUNTER. (REASON RULE)*

EXAM

V72.9 NOS
V70.3 ADMINISTRATIVE PURPOSES (GENERAL) (ADMINISTRATIVE)
V70.3 ADMISSION TO OLD AGE HOME (GENERAL) (ADMINISTRATIVE)
V70.3 ADOPTION (GENERAL) (ADMINISTRATIVE)
V72.7 ALLERGY
V70.0 ANNUAL ROUTINE (HEALTH CHECK-UP)
V20.2 ANNUAL ROUTINE (HEALTH CHECK-UP) INFANT OR CHILD
V70.3 CAMP (GENERAL) (ADMINISTRATIVE)
V72.5 CHEST X-RAY (ROUTINE)
V72.2 DENTAL
V70.8 DONOR POTENTIAL - ORGAN OR TISSUE
V70.3 DRIVING LICENSE (GENERAL) (ADMINISTRATIVE)
V70.3 DRUG SCREENING (GENERAL) (ADMINISTRATIVE)
V70.4 DRUG TEST MEDICOLEGAL
V72.1 EARS AND/OR HEARING
V72.0 EYE

EXAM (continued)

> *DO NOT CONFUSE FOLLOWUP OR ROUTINE AFTERCARE WITH "COMPLICATIONS." FOLLOWUP EXAMS AND ROUTINE AFTERCARE ARE PLANNED VISITS THAT ARE PART OF THE NORMAL COURSE OF TREATMENT. COMPLICATIONS ARE UNEXPECTED DEVELOPMENTS THAT REQUIRE SUBSEQUENT TREATMENT.*

FOLLOW-UP

V67.9	UNSPECIFIED
V67.2	CHEMOTHERAPY
V67.6	COMBINED TREATMENT
V67.4	FRACTURE TREATMENT - HEALED
0	FRACTURE TREATMENT - HEALING OR CURRENT SEE 'AFTERCARE', ORTHOPEDIC

> *ANTIBIOTICS, COUMADIN, DIGOXIN, CHEMOTHERAPY DRUGS, AND ANY OTHER DRUGS WITH A RISK OF ADVERSE REACTIONS ARE CONSIDERED TO BE HIGH-RISK MEDICATION.*

V67.51	HIGH RISK MEDICATION THERAPY - COMPLETED
V58.62	HIGH RISK MEDICATION ANTIBIOTIC - CURRENT THERAPY
V58.61	HIGH RISK MEDICATION ANTICOAGULANT - CURRENT THERAPY
V58.69	HIGH RISK MEDICATION OTHER - CURRENT THERAPY
V67.3	PSYCHOTHERAPY AND OTHER TREATMENT
V67.1	RADIOTHERAPY
V67.0	SURGERY
V67.59	OTHER TREATMENT NEC

EXAM (continued)

V70.9	GENERAL (MEDICAL)
V72.3	GYNECOLOGICAL (ROUTINE)
V70.3	IMMIGRATION AND NATURALIZATION (GENERAL) (ADMINISTRATIVE)
V70.6	IN POPULATION SURVEYS (HEALTH)
V20.2	INFANT / NEWBORN / CHILD ANNUAL ROUTINE (HEALTH CHECK-UP)
0	INFANT / NEWBORN SUSPECTED CONDITION (UNDIAGNOSED) (UNPROVEN) SEE 'EVALUATION NEWBORN / INFANT'
V70.3	INSURANCE CERTIFICATION (GENERAL) (ADMINISTRATIVE)
V72.6	LABORATORY (ROUTINE)
V70.3	MARRIAGE (GENERAL) (ADMINISTRATIVE)
V70.0	MEDICAL (ROUTINE) (GENERAL)
V20.2	NEWBORN / INFANT / CHILD ANNUAL ROUTINE (HEALTH CHECK-UP)
0	NEWBORN / INFANT SUSPECTED CONDITION (UNDIAGNOSED) (UNPROVEN) SEE 'EVALUATION NEWBORN / INFANT'
V70.7	NORMAL COMPARISON IN CLINICAL RESEARCH
V70.5	OCCUPATION (HEALTH)
V25.41	ORAL CONTRACEPTION (ROUTINE)
V70.8	OTHER GENERAL MEDICAL
V72.85	OTHER SPECIFIED SPECIAL EXAMINATION (SPECIFIED TYPE OR REASON NEC)
0	PAP SMEAR SEE 'EXAM' ROUTINE, PAP SMEAR
V70.4	PATERNITY TESTING
V72.3	PELVIC (ROUTINE)
V70.5	PREEMPLOYMENT (HEALTH)

PREGNANCY

V25.41	FOR ORAL CONTRACEPTION (ROUTINE)
V72.4	POSSIBLE UNCONFIRMED
V24.0	POSTPARTUM (IMMEDIATE)
V24.2	POSTPARTUM ROUTINE FOLLOWUP
V22.0	PRENATAL FIRST PREGNANCY
V22.1	PRENATAL SUBSEQUENT PREGNANCY
0	PRENATAL SEE 'SUPERVISION OF PREGNANCY'

EXAM (continued)

V70.3	PREMARITAL (GENERAL) (ADMINISTRATIVE)

> *V72.#, 'PREOPERATIVE EXAMINATION' IDENTIFIES THE TYPE OF EXAM DONE RATHER THAN THE TYPE OF SURGERY TO BE PERFORMED. THE PREOPERATIVE EXAMINATION CODE SHOULD BE LISTED FIRST FOLLOWED BY THE CODE FOR THE CONDITION NECESSITATING THE SURGERY.*

V72.8# PREOPERATIVE

5th Digit: V72.8

1. **CARDIOVASCULAR**
2. **RESPIRATORY**
3. **OTHER SPECIFIED PREOPERATIVE EXAM**
4. **PREOPERATIVE EXAM UNSPECIFIED**

V70.3	PRISON (GENERAL) (ADMINISTRATIVE)
V70.1	PSYCHIATRIC (GENERAL EXAM REQUESTED BY AUTHORITY)
V70.2	PSYCHIATRIC (GENERAL) OTHER OR UNSPECIFIED
V72.5	RADIOLOGICAL NEC

ROUTINE

V72.9	NOS
V72.7	ALLERGY
V72.2	DENTAL
V72.1	EARS AND/OR HEARING
V72.0	EYE
V72.3	GYNECOLOGICAL (ROUTINE)
V20.2	HEALTH CHECK INFANT OR CHILD
V72.6	LABORATORY (ROUTINE)
0	PAP SMEAR FOLLOWUP TO PREVIOUS TREATMENT WITH NO RECURRENCE SEE 'EXAM' FOLLOWUP
V71.1	PAP SMEAR SUSPECTED NEOPLASM (UNPROVEN) (UNDIAGNOSED)
V72.3	PAP SMEAR WITH GYN EXAM
V76.2	PAP SMEAR WITHOUT GYN EXAM
V72.3	PELVIC (ROUTINE)
0	PREGNANCY SEE 'EXAM' PREGNANCY
V72.5	RADIOLOGICAL NEC
V72.2	TEETH
V20.2	WELL BABY
V65.5	WELL-WORRIED
V65.5	WORRIED-WELL
V72.0	VISION
V72.85	OTHER SPECIFIED (SPECIFIED TYPE OR REASON NEC)

EXAM (continued)

V70.5	SCHOOL (HEALTH)
V70.3	SCHOOL ADMISSION (GENERAL) (ADMINISTRATIVE)
0	SCREENING SEE 'SCREENING'
V72.7	SKIN HYPERSENSITIVITY
V72.85	SPECIAL EXAMINATION OTHER (SPECIFIED TYPE OR REASON NEC)
V70.3	SPORTS COMPETITION (GENERAL) (ADMINISTRATIVE)
0	SUSPECTED CONDITION (UNDIAGNOSED) (UNPROVEN) SEE 'EVALUATION'
0	SUSPECTED CONDITION INFANT / NEWBORN (UNDIAGNOSED) (UNPROVEN) SEE 'EVALUATION NEWBORN / INFANT'
V72.2	TEETH
V72.0	VISION
0	WITH NO ILLNESS OR INJURY SEE 'OBSERVATION'
V65.5	WORRIED-WELL

782.1	EXANTHEM
057.9	EXANTHEM VIRAL
057.8	EXANTHEMA SUBITUM (SIXTH DISEASE)
255.0	EXCESS CORTISOL, IATROGENIC SYNDROME

EXCESSIVE

783.6 EATING
527.7 SALIVATION
786.4 SPUTUM
780.8 SWEATING
783.5 THIRST
701.5 TISSUE GRANULATION

298.1 EXCITATION REACTIVE (PSYCHOTIC)
698.4 EXCORIATION NEUROTIC
0 EXCORIATION (TRAUMATIC) SEE ANATOMICAL SITE, INJURY SUPERFICIAL
V65.41 EXERCISE COUNSELING
V47.2 EXERCISE INTOLERANCE CARDIOVASCULAR (RESPIRATORY) AT REST OR ORDINARY ACTIVITY
V69.0 EXERCISE PROBLEM (LACK OF)

EXHAUSTION

991.8 COLD
994.5 EXERTION EXCESSIVE
909.4 EXERTION EXCESSIVE LATE EFFECT
994.4 EXPOSURE
909.4 EXPOSURE LATE EFFECT
779.8 FETUS OR NEWBORN
992.5 HEAT
992.4 HEAT - SALT DEPLETION
992.3 HEAT - WATER DEPLETION
763.89 MATERNAL AFFECTING FETUS OR NEWBORN
669.8# MATERNAL COMPLICATING DELIVERY

5th Digit: 669.8

0. EPISODE OF CARE NOS OR N/A
1. DELIVERED
2. WITH POSTPARTUM COMPLICATION
3. ANTEPARTUM COMPLICATION
4. POSTPARTUM COMPLICATION

300.5 MENTAL
300.5 NERVOUS (PSYCHOGENIC)
797 OLD AGE (SENILE)
780.79 PHYSICAL NEC
780.79 POSTINFECTIONAL
300.5 SYNDROME

302.4 EXHIBITIONISM
756.79 EXOMPHALOS CONGENITAL

EXOPHORIA

378.42 EXOPHORIA
378.83 CONVERGENCE INSUFFICIENCY
378.85 DIVERGENCE EXCESS

EXOPHTHALMOS

376.30 NOS
743.66 CONGENITAL
376.31 CONSTANT
376.34 INTERMITTENT
376.22 OPHTHALMOPLEGIA
376.35 PULSATING
242.## THYROTOXIC [376.21]
242.## THYROTOXIC WITH OPHTHALMOPLEGIA [376.22]

4th Digit: 242

0 DIFFUSE
1. UNINODULAR
2. MULTINODULAR
3. NODULAR UNSPECIFIED
4. ECTOPIC THYROID NODULAR
8. OTHER SPECIFIED
9 UNSPECIFIED

5th Digit: 242

0. WITHOUT MENTION OF THYROTOXIC CRISIS OR STORM
1. WITH MENTION OF THYROTOXIC CRISIS OR STORM

EXOSTOSIS

726.91 SITE NOS
756.4 NOS CONGENITAL
380.81 EAR CANAL (EXTERNAL)
098.89 GONOCOCCAL
726.5 HIP
733.3 INTRACRANIAL
526.81 JAW
728.11 LUXURIANS
726.91 NASAL BONES
376.42 ORBIT
721.8 SPINE
095.5 SYPHILITIC
726.4 WRIST

EXOTROPIA

378.1# EXOTROPIA
378.1# DIVERGENT NONCOMITANT STRABISMUS

5th Digit: 378.1

0. UNSPECIFIED
1. MONOCULAR UNSPECIFIED
2. MONOCULAR WITH A PATTERN
3. MONOCULAR WITH V PATTERN
4. MONOCULAR WITH OTHER NONCOMITANCIES (X OR Y PATTERN)
5. ALTERNATING UNSPECIFIED
6. ALTERNATING WITH A PATTERN
7. ALTERNATING WITH V PATTERN
8. ALTERNATING WITH OTHER NONCOMITANCIES (X OR Y PATTERN)

378.20 INTERMITTENT
378.24 INTERMITTENT ALTERNATING
378.23 INTERMITTENT MONOCULAR

V68.2 EXPERT EVIDENCE REQUEST
993.4 EXPLOSION EFFECTS OF AIR PRESSURE
909.4 EXPLOSION EFFECTS OF AIR PRESSURE LATE EFFECT
312.3# EXPLOSIVE DISORDER

5th Digit: 312.3

4. INTERMITTENT IMPULSE CONTROL
5. ISOLATED IMPULSE CONTROL

EXPOSURE

994.9 NOS
V01.9 NOS COMMUNICABLE DISEASES
V01.7 AIDS
V15.84 ASBESTOS HISTORY
V15.85 BODY FLUIDS - POTENTIALLY HAZARDOUS HISTORY
V01.7 CHICKENPOX
V01.0 CHOLERA
V01.8 COCCIDIOIDOMYCOSIS
V01.7 COXSACKIE (CMV) (ADENOVIRUS)
V01.7 ECHO (VACINNIA) (HERPES SIMPLEX)
994.4 EXHAUSTION
909.4 EXHAUSTION LATE EFFECT
V01.6 GONORRHEA
V01.8 H. INFLUENZA
V15.85 HAZARDOUS BODY FLUIDS HISTORY
V01.7 HEPATITIS VIRAL A B OR OTHER
V01.6 HERPES GENITALIA
V01.8 HISTOPLASMOSIS
V01.7 HIV
V01.7 INFLUENZA
V15.86 LEAD HISTORY
V01.8 LICE
V01.7 MEASLES (RUBEOLA)
V01.8 MENINGOCOCCUS
V01.7 MONONUCLEOSIS
V01.7 MUMPS
V01.8 OTHER COMMUNICABLE DISEASES
V01.7 OTHER VIRAL DISEASES

EXPOSURE (continued)

V01.8 PEDICULOSIS
V01.8 PERTUSSIS
V01.8 PNEUMOCOCCUS
V01.2 POLIOMYELITIS
V15.85 POTENTIALLY HAZARDOUS - BODY FLUIDS HISTORY
V01.5 RABIES
V01.4 RUBELLA
V01.3 SMALLPOX
V01.8 STREPTOCOCCUS
V01.6 SYPHILIS
V01.1 TB
V01.8 TRICHOMONAS
V01.8 TULAREMIA
V01.6 VD
V01.6 VENEREAL DISEASE
V01.7 VIRAL HEPATITIS A B OR OTHER
0 SEE SPECIFIED AGENT I.E. RUBELLA

772.0 EXSANGUINATION FETAL

EXTENSOR

883.2 DIGITI MINIMI TENDON LACERATION FINGER
882.2 DIGITI MINIMI TENDON LACERATION HAND

891.2 HALLUCIS TENDON LACERATION ANKLE
892.2 HALLUCIS TENDON LACERATION FOOT
893.2 HALLUCIS TENDON LACERATION TOE

883.2 INDICUS PROPRIUS LACERATION FINGER
882.2 INDICUS PROPRIUS LACERATION HAND

881.20 POLLICIS LONGUS LACERATION FOREARM
882.2 POLLICIS LONGUS LACERATION HAND
883.2 POLLICIS LONGUS LACERATION THUMB
881.22 POLLICIS LONGUS LACERATION WRIST

883.2 POLLICIS BREVIS LACERATION FINGER
882.2 POLLICIS BREVIS LACERATION HAND

727.63 TENDON HAND AND WRIST RUPTURE NONTRAUMATIC

891.2 TENDON TOE LACERATION ANKLE
892.2 TENDON TOE LACERATION FOOT
893.2 TENDON TOE LACERATION TOE

900.81 EXTERNAL JUGULAR VEIN INJURY
908.3 EXTERNAL JUGULAR VEIN INJURY LATE EFFECT
763.89 EXTRACTION FETAL MANUAL OR WITH HOOK AFFECTING FETUS OR NEWBORN
660.7# EXTRACTION FORCEPS OR VACUUM (FAILED)

5th Digit: 660.7
0. EPISODE OF CARE UNSPECIFIED OR N/A
1. DELIVERED
3. ANTEPARTUM COMPLICATION

432.0 EXTRADURAL HEMATOMA
852.4# EXTRADURAL HEMATOMA TRAUMATIC
852.5# EXTRADURAL HEMATOMA TRAUMATIC - WITH OPEN INTRACRANIAL WOUND

5th Digit: 852.4-5
0. LEVEL OF CONSCIOUSNESS UNSPECIFIED
1. NO LOC
2. LOC < 1 HR
3. LOC 1 - 24 HRS
4. LOC > 24 HRS WITH RETURN TO PRIOR LEVEL
5. LOC > 24 HRS WITHOUT RETURN TO PRIOR LEVEL: OR DEATH BEFORE REGAINING CONSCIOUSNESS, REGARDLESS OF DURATION OF LOC
6. LOC DURATION UNSPECIFIED
9. WITH CONCUSSION UNSPECIFIED

333.90 EXTRAPYRAMIDAL DISEASE OR SYNDROME
781.0 EXTRAPYRAMIDAL SYMPTOMS
427.60 EXTRASYSTOLES
997.1 EXTRASYSTOLES POSTOPERATIVE (DURING OR RESULTING FROM A PROCEDURE)

EXTRAVASATION

459.0 BLOOD
457.8 CHYLE INTO MESENTERY
788.8 URINE

EYE

379.90 DISORDER UNSPECIFIED
360.89 ABSENCE
743.69 ABSENCE - ADNEXA
743.69 ABSENCE - MUSCLE EXTRINSIC
364.9 ANTERIOR CHAMBER
360.42 BLIND HYPERTENSIVE
360.41 BLIND HYPOTENSIVE
374.43 BLINKING
368.8 BLURRED VISION
379.93 CONJUNCTIVAL REDNESS
360.40 DEGENERATED
379.93 DISCHARGE
743.10 DYSPLASIA (CONGENITAL) - NOS
743.11 DYSPLASIA (CONGENITAL) - SIMPLE
743.12 DYSPLASIA (CONGENITAL) - WITH OTHER ANOMALIES OF EYE AND ADNEXA
364.61 EPITHELIAL DOWN GROWTH
360.41 EYEBALL ATROPHY
360.9 EYEBALL DISORDER
379.24 FLOATERS
360.9 GLOBE DISODERS NOS
360.81 GLOBE LUXATION
743.10 HYPOPLASIA (CONGENITAL) - NOS
743.11 HYPOPLASIA (CONGENITAL) - SIMPLE
743.12 HYPOPLASIA (CONGENITAL) - WITH OTHER ANOMALIES OF EYE AND ADNEXA
364.3 INFLAMMATORY
379.99 ITCHING
379.92 MASS
379.58 MOVEMENT IRREGULAR DEFICIENCIES OF SMOOTH PURSUIT (SEE ALSO BY SPECIFIC IRREGULARITY)
379.59 MOVEMENT OTHER IRREGULARITIES
378.9 MUSCLE
379.8 MUSCLES DEFORMITY ACQUIRED
379.91 PAIN (IN OR AROUND)
V41.1 PROBLEMS NEC
306.7 PSYCHOGENIC
379.93 REDNESS (CONJUNCTIVA)
378.71 RETRACTION SYNDROME
366.16 SCLEROSIS NUCLEAR (SENILE)
368.13 STRAIN
379.92 SWELLING
360.89 OTHER (GLOBE) DISORDERS
379.99 OTHER ILL-DEFINED EYE DISORDER
379.8 OTHER SPECIFIED EYE AND ADNEXA DISORDER

EYE ANOMALIES CONGENITAL

743.00 ABSENCE
743.69 ABSENCE - ADNEXA
743.69 ABSENCE - MUSCLE
743.48 ANOMALIES ANTERIOR SEGMENT MULTIPLE AND COMBINED
743.49 ANOMALIES ANTERIOR SEGMENT OTHER CONGENITAL
743.9 ANOMALY CONGENITAL
743.8 ANOMALY OTHER SPECIFIED CONGENITAL
743.9 DEFORMITY CONGENITAL
743.69 DEFORMITY ACCESSORY MUSCLES CONGENITAL
743.10 DYSPLASIA (CONGENITAL) - NOS
743.11 DYSPLASIA (CONGENITAL) - SIMPLE
743.12 DYSPLASIA (CONGENITAL) - WITH OTHER ANOMALIES OF EYE AND ADNEXA
743.10 HYPOPLASIA (CONGENITAL) - NOS
743.11 HYPOPLASIA (CONGENITAL) - SIMPLE
743.12 HYPOPLASIA (CONGENITAL) - WITH OTHER ANOMALIES OF EYE AND ADNEXA
743.69 MUSCLES DEFORMITY CONGENITAL
V80.2 SCREENING

EYE EXAM

V53.1 CONTACT LENS FITTING
V53.1 EYEGLASSES FITTING AND ADJUSTMENT
V72.0 ROUTINE
V80.2 SCREENING FOR CONGENITAL ANOMALY
V80.2 SCREENING FOR OTHER CONDITIONS

EYE INJURIES

921.9 NOS
918.9 NOS SUPERFICIAL
871.3 AVULSION
767.8 BIRTH TRAUMA DAMAGE
871.3 ENUCLEATION TRAUMATIC
921.3 EYEBALL
871.9 EYEBALL OPEN WOUND
871.5 EYEBALL PENETRATION WITH MAGNETIC FOREIGN BODY
871.6 EYEBALL PENETRATION WITH NONMAGNETIC FOREIGN BODY
918.9 EYEBALL SUPERFICIAL
918.1 EYEBALL SUPERFICIAL LACERATION
871.4 LACERATION UNSPECIFIED
871.0 LACERATION OCULAR
871.1 LACERATION OCULAR WITH PARTIAL LOSS OF INTRAOCULAR TISSUE
996.59 ORBITAL IMPLANT PROLAPSE
871.2 RUPTURE WITH PARTIAL LOSS OF INTRAOCULAR TISSUE

EYE PROSTHESIS

V45.69 AND ADNEXA SURGERY STATUS
996.69 COMPLICATION - INFECTION OR INFLAMMATION
996.59 COMPLICATION - MECHANICAL
996.79 COMPLICATION - OTHER
V52.2 FITTING AND ADJUSTMENT (REMOVAL)
V43.0 GLOBE REPLACEMENT (ARTIFICIAL) (PROSTHESIS)

959.09 EYEBROW INJURY

EYELID

374.89 ABSENCE ACQUIRED
743.62 ABSENCE CONGENITAL
743.62 ACCESSORY CONGENITAL
374.50 ATROPHY (SENILE)
374.84 CYST
743.62 DEFORMITIES CONGENITAL
743.63 DEFORMITY OTHER SPECIFIED CONGENITAL
0 DERMATITIS SEE 'DERMATITIS EYELID'
373.34 DISCOID LUPUS ERYTHEMATOSUS
374.9 DISORDER
374.43 DISORDER ABNORMAL INNERVATION SYNDROME
374.50 DISORDER DEGENERATIVE
374.56 DISORDER DEGENERATIVE OTHER
374.44 DISORDER SENSORY
374.89 DISORDER OTHER
374.45 DISORDER OTHER SENSORIMOTOR
374.52 DYSPIGMENTATION
374.82 EDEMA
373.13 FURUNCLE
374.82 HYPEREMIA
374.52 HYPERPIGMENTATION
374.54 HYPERTRICHOSIS
374.53 HYPOPIGMENTATION
374.55 HYPOTRICHOSIS
373.9 INFECTION UNSPECIFIED
373.9 INFILTRATE
373.9 INFLAMMATION
373.8 INFLAMMATION OTHER
921.1 INJURY
918.0 INJURY SUPERFICIAL
374.41 LAG OR RETRACTION (NERVOUS)
374.55 MADAROSIS
756.0 MALAR-MANDIBLE SYNDROME
373.11 STYE
374.85 VASCULAR ANCMALIES
374.56 OTHER DEGENERATIVE DISORDERS OF SKIN AFFECTING EYELID
374.89 OTHER DISORDERS

125.2 EYEWORM OF AFRICA

E

280.9 FABER'S ANEMIA (SYNDROME)
272.7 FABRY'S DISEASE OR SYNDROME (ANGIOKERATOMA CORPORIS DIFFUSUM)
272.7 FABRY'S DISEASE CEREBRAL DEGENERATION [330.2]

FACE, FACIAL
756.0 ABSENCE - BONES NEC CONGENITAL
744.89 ABSENCE - SPECIFIED PART NEC CONGENITAL
744.9 ANOMALY CONGENITAL
744.89 ANOMALY SPECIFIED NEC CONGENITAL
754.0 ASYMMETRY CONGENITAL
701.9 ATROPHY (SKIN)
754.0 COMPRESSION CONGENITAL
738.19 DEFORMITY
744.9 DEFORMITY NOS CONGENITAL
959.09 INJURY
925.1 INJURY CRUSH
910.8 INJURY OTHER AND UNSPECIFIED (SUPERFICIAL)
910.9 INJURY OTHER AND UNSPECIFIED (SUPERFICIAL) INFECTED
V50.1 LIFT (ELECTIVE) (FOR UNACCEPTABLE COSMETIC APPEARANCE)
351.8 MYOKYMIA
351.8 NERVE (7TH) ATROPHY
351.9 NERVE (7TH) DISORDER
951.4 NERVE (7TH) INJURY
767.5 NERVE (7TH) INJURY NEWBORN (BIRTH TRAUMA)
351.8 NERVE (7TH) NEURITIS
351.8 NERVE (7TH) PAIN
351.0 NERVE (7TH) PALSY
767.5 NERVE (7TH) PALSY NEWBORN (BIRTH TRAUMA)
997.09 NERVE (7TH) PALSY POSTOPERATIVE
351.0 NERVE (7TH) PARALYSIS
351.8 NERVE (7TH) DISORDER OTHER SPECIFIED NEC
784.0 PAIN
350.2 PAIN ATYPICAL
351.8 PAIN NERVE
374.43 PARADOXICAL MOVEMENT
652.4# PRESENTATION
660.0# PRESENTATION OBSTRUCTING LABOR **[652.4#]**
652.6# PRESENTATION WITH MULTIPLE GESTATION
660.0# PRESENTATION WITH MULTIPLE GESTATION OBSTRUCTING LABOR **[652.6#]**
652.1# PRESENTATION WITH VERSION
660.0# PRESENTATION WITH VERSION OBSTRUCTING LABOR **[652.1#]**

5th Digit: 652.1, 4, 6, 660.0
0. EPISODE OF CARE UNSPECIFIED OR N/A
1. DELIVERED
3. ANTEPARTUM COMPLICATION

724.8 FACET SYNDROME
0 FACIAL SEE 'FACE, FACIAL'
300.19 FACTITIOUS ILLNESS NOS
301.51 FACTITIOUS ILLNESS CHRONIC WITH PHYSICAL SYMPTOMS
300.19 FACTITIOUS ILLNESS WITH COMBINED PHYSICAL AND PSYCHOLOGICAL SYMPTOMS
300.19 FACTITIOUS ILLNESS WITH PHYSICAL SYMPTOMS
300.16 FACTITIOUS ILLNESS WITH PSYCHOLOGICAL SYMPTOMS

FACTOR
286.3 I DEFICIENCY
286.3 II DEFICIENCY
286.3 V DEFICIENCY
286.3 VII DEFICIENCY
286.0 VIII DEFICIENCY
286.0 VIII DEFICIENCY WITH FUNCTIONAL DEFECT
286.4 VIII DEFICIENCY WITH VASCULAR DEFECT
286.0 VIII DISORDER CONGENITAL
286.0 VIII (FUNCTIONAL) DEFICIENCY
286.4 VIII WITH VASCULAR DEFECT

FACTOR (continued)
286.1 IX (FUNCTIONAL) DEFICIENCY
286.1 IX DISORDER CONGENITAL
286.3 X DEFICIENCY
286.2 XI DISORDER CONGENITAL
286.3 XII DEFICIENCY
286.3 XIII DEFICIENCY
286.0 A DEFICIENCY
286.1 B DEFICIENCY
286.2 C DEFICIENCY

403.00 FAHR VOLHARD DISEASE (MALIGNANT NEPHROSCLEROSIS)
996.4 FAILED FUSION (JOINT) (SPINAL)
659.0# FAILED INDUCTION OF LABOR - MECHANICAL (VIA SURGICAL OR INSTRUMENTAL METHODS)
659.1# FAILED INDUCTION OF LABOR - MEDICAL (NOS OR VIA DRUGS)
660.6# FAILED TRIAL LABOR

5th Digit: 659.0-1, 660.6
0. EPISODE OF CARE OR N/A
1. DELIVERED
3. ANTEPARTUM COMPLICATION

FAILURE
253.2 ADENOHYPOPHYSEAL
284.9 BONE MARROW (ANEMIA)
428.9 CARDIAC
428.9 CARDIORENAL (CHRONIC)
799.1 CARDIORESPIRATORY
0 HEART CONGESTIVE SEE 'CHF'
0 HEART SEE 'HEART FAILURE'
257.2 LEYDIGS CELL (ADULT)
799.8 MEDULLARY
661.2# TO PROGRESS COMPLICATING LABOR AND DELIVERY

5th Digit: 661.2
0. EPISODE OF CARE OR N/A
1. DELIVERED
3. ANTEPARTUM COMPLICATION

783.4 TO THRIVE
996.8# TRANSPLANT ORGAN

5th Digit: 996.8
0. ORGAN UNSPECIFIED
1. KIDNEY
2. LIVER
3. HEART
4 LUNG
5. BONE MARROW
6. PANCREAS
9. OTHER SPECIFIED ORGAN (INTESTINES)

996.52 TRANSPLANT SKIN
996.55 TRANSPLANT SKIN - ARTIFICIAL
996.55 TRANSPLANT SKIN - DECELLULARIZED ALLODERMIS
428.0 VENTRICULAR RIGHT

780.2 FAINTING
734 FALLEN ARCHES

FALLOPIAN TUBE
620.8 ABSENCE
752.19 ABSENCE CONGENITAL
752.19 ACCESSORY CONGENITAL
752.10 ANOMALY CONGENITAL
752.19 ATRESIA CONGENITAL
620.3 ATROPHY (SENILE)
620.8 CALCIFICATION
620.9 DISORDER NONINFLAMMATORY
620.8 DISORDER NONINFLAMMATORY OTHER SPECIFIED NEC
620.4 DISPLACEMENT
752.19 DISPLACEMENT CONGENITAL
620.8 HEMATOSALPINX
620.8 INFARCTION RUPTURE CYST POLYP

FALLOPIAN TUBE (continued)

867.6 INJURY TRAUMATIC
867.7 INJURY TRAUMATIC WITH OPEN WOUND INTO CAVITY
908.6 INJURY TRAUMATIC LATE EFFECT
V26.2 INSUFFLATION
752.19 OCCLUSION CONGENITAL
628.2 OCCLUSION (OBSTRUCTION)
620.4 PROLAPSE (HERNIA)
0 RUPTURE - DUE TO TUBAL PREGNANCY SEE 'TUBAL' PREGNANCY
620.3 SENILE INVOLUTION
628.2 STENOSIS
620.5 TORSION

745.2 FALLOT'S SYNDROME
746.09 FALLOT'S TRIAD
644.1# FALSE LABOR

5th Digit: 644.1

0. EPISODE OF CARE UNSPECIFIED OR N/A
3. ANTEPARTUM COMPLICATION

FALSE POSITIVE BLOOD TEST

795.79 HEPATITIS
795.6 SYPHILIS
795.5 TB

431 FALX SYNDROME

FAMILIAL

742.8 DYSAUTONOMIA
279.12 ECZEMA-THROMBOCYTOPENIA SYNDROME
333.2 ESSENTIAL MYOCLONUS
277.3 MEDITERRANEAN FEVER
277.3 PERIODIC AMYLOIDOSIS
359.3 PERIODIC PARALYSIS
211.3 POLYPOSIS

V61.9 FAMILY CIRCUMSTANCE NOS (REASON FOR ENCOUNTER)
V61.8 FAMILY CIRCUMSTANCE OTHER SPECIFIED (REASON FOR ENCOUNTER)
V61.0 FAMILY DISRUPTION (REASON FOR ENCOUNTER)

V CODES CAN EXPLAIN CIRCUMSTANCES AS TO WHY CERTAIN TESTS OR STUDIES WERE PERFORMED, SUCH AS A HISTORY OF MYOCARDIAL INFARCTION, OR FAMILY HX DIABETES.

FAMILY HISTORY

V19.6 ALLERGY DISORDER
V18.2 ANEMIA
V17.7 ARTHRITIS
V17.5 ASTHMA
V17.4 ATHEROSCLEROSIS
V19.8 BAYLOR CRETIN SYNDROME
V19.0 BLINDNESS
V18.3 BLOOD DISORDERS (OTHER)
V16.9 CA
V16.59 CA BLADDER
V16.3 CA BREAST
V16.1 CA BRONCHUS
V16.49 CA CERVIX
V16.0 CA COLON
V16.0 CA GASTROINTESTINAL TRACT
V16.40 CA GENITAL ORGANS NOS
V16.49 CA GENITAL ORGANS OTHER
V16.0 CA GI TRACT
V16.7 CA HEMATOPOIETIC
V16.2 CA INTRATHORACIC ORGANS
V16.51 CA KIDNEY
V16.1 CA LUNG
V16.7 CA LYMPHATIC AND HEMATOPOIETIC
V16.41 CA OVARY, OVIDUCT

FAMILY HISTORY (continued)

V16.49 CA PENIS
V16.42 CA PROSTATE
V16.2 CA RESPIRATORY
V16.43 CA TESTIS
V16.1 CA TRACHEA
V16.59 CA URINARY ORGANS
V16.49 CA UTERUS
V16.49 CA VAGINA
V16.49 CA VULVA
V16.8 CA OTHER SPECIFIED
V17.4 CARDIOVASCULAR DISEASES
V17.1 CEREBROVASCULAR ACCIDENT
V19.8 CONDITIONS (OTHER)
V19.5 CONGENITAL ANOMALIES
V19.7 CONSANGUINITY
V17.1 CVA
V19.2 DEAFNESS
V18.0 DIABETES MELLITUS
V18.5 DIGESTIVE DISORDERS
V19.5 DOWN'S SYNDROME (MONGOLISM)
V19.3 EAR DISORDERS (OTHER)
V18.1 ENDOCRINE AND METABOLIC DISEASES
V17.2 EPILEPSY
V19.1 EYE DISORDERS (OTHER)
V18.7 GENITOURINARY DISEASES (OTHER)
V18.69 GLOMERULONEPHRITIS
V19.2 HEARING LOSS
V17.3 HEART DISEASE (ISCHEMIC)
V16.7 HODGKIN'S DISEASE
V17.2 HUNTINGTON'S CHOREA
V17.4 HYPERTENSION
V18.8 INFECTIOUS DISEASES
V18.61 KIDNEY DISEASE - POLYCYSTIC
V18.69 KIDNEY DISEASE - OTHER
V16.6 LEUKEMIA
V16.7 LYMPHOMA
V16.7 LYMPHOSARCOMA
V18.4 MENTAL RETARDATION
V18.1 METABOLIC DISEASE
V17.8 MUSCULOSKELETAL DISEASES (OTHER)
V17.3 MYOCARDIAL INFARCTION
V17.2 NEUROLOGICAL DISEASE OTHER
V18.8 PARASITIC DISEASE
V18.61 POLYCYSTIC KIDNEY DISEASE
V17.0 PSYCHIATRIC CONDITION
V17.6 RESPIRATORY CONDITIONS (OTHER CHRONIC)
V16.7 RETICULOSARCOMA
V19.4 SKIN CONDITIONS
V17.1 STROKE
V19.0 VISION LOSS
V19.8 OTHER SPECIFIED CONDITION

V61.49 FAMILY MEMBER SICK OR HANDICAPPED (CARE OF) (PRESENCE OF)
V60.4 FAMILY MEMBER UNSUITED TO RENDER CARE (HANDICAPPED) (ILL) (OTHERWISE UNSUITED)
V25.09 FAMILY PLANNING ADVICE OTHER
994.2 FAMINE
909.4 FAMINE LATE EFFECT
301.0 FANATIC PERSONALITY DISORDER
270.0 FANCONI (-DE TONI) (-DEBRE) SYNDROME (CYSTINOSIS)
284.0 FANCONI'S ANEMIA (SYNDROME) (CONGENITAL PANCYTOPENIA)
367.0 FAR SIGHTEDNESS
272.8 FARBER UZMAN SYNDROME (DISSEMINATED LIPOGRANULOMATOSIS)
272.8 FARBER'S DISSEMINATED LIPOGRANULOMATOSIS
024 FARCY
495.0 FARMERS' LUNG
692.74 FARMERS' SKIN

F

728.89 FASCIA CALCIFICATION (CONTRACTION)
728.9 FASCIA DISORDER
728.89 FASCIA DISORDER OTHER
728.89 FASCIA LATA CONTRACTION (POSTURAL)
728.11 FASCIALIS OSSIFICANS HYPERPLASIA (PROGRESSIVE)
781.0 FASCICULATION
377.32 FASCICULITIS OPTICA

WHEN CODING AN INFECTION, USE AN ADDITIONAL CODE, [041.#(#)], TO IDENTIFY THE ORGANISM. SEE 'BACTERIAL INFECTION'.

FASCIITIS
729.4 NOS
728.89 EOSINOPHILIC
728.86 NECROTIZING
728.86 NECROTIZING WITH GANGRENE [785.4]
728.79 NODULAR
593.4 PERIRENAL
728.71 PLANTAR
728.79 TRAUMATIC PSEUDOSARCOMATOUS

121.3 FASCIOLA GIGANTICA INFECTION
121.3 FASCIOLA HEPATICA INFECTION
121.3 FASCIOLA INFECTION
121.3 FASCIOLIASIS
121.4 FASCIOLOPSIASIS
121.4 FASCIOLOPSIS BUSKI INFECTION
359.1 FASCIOSCAPULOHUMERAL MUSCULAR DYSTROPHY

FAT
958.1 EMBOLISM
908.2 EMBOLISM LATE EFFECT
673.8# EMBOLISM MATERNAL DUE TO PREGNANCY
5th Digit: 673.8
0. EPISODE OF CARE UNSPECIFIED OR N/A
1. DELIVERED
2. DELIVERED WITH POSTPARTUM COMPLICATION
3. ANTEPARTUM COMPLICATION
4. POSTPARTUM COMPLICATION

677 EMBOLISM OBSTETRICAL LATE EFFECT
792.1 IN STOOL
272.9 METABOLISM DISORDER
611.3 NECROSIS BREAST NONPUERPERAL
567.8 NECROSIS PERITONEAL
778.1 NECROSIS SUBCUTANEOUS NEONATAL
278.1 PAD
729.31 PAD KNEE (HYPERTROPHY OF)

FATIGUE
780.79 NOS
308.9 COMBAT (SEE ALSO 'STRESS REACTION')
780.79 GENERAL
300.5 PSYCHOGENIC
797 SENILE
780.71 SYNDROME CHRONIC
300.5 SYNDROME NEC

429.1 FATTY DEGENERATION HEART WITH ARTERIOSCLEROSIS [440.9]
571.8 FATTY LIVER
571.8 FATTY LIVER WITH ESOPHAGEAL VARICES [456.2#]
5th Digit: 456.2
0. WITH BLEEDING
1. WITHOUT BLEEDING

571.0 FATTY LIVER ALCOHOLIC
571.0 FATTY LIVER ALCOHOLIC WITH ESOPHAGEAL VARICES [456.2#]
5th Digit: 456.2
0. WITH BLEEDING
1. WITHOUT BLEEDING

254.8 FATTY THYMUS DEGENERATION
523.4 FAUCHARD'S PERIODONTITIS
564.7 FAULTY BOWEL HABIT SYNDROME (IDIOPATHIC MEGACOLON)
282.2 FAVISM
099.1 FAVRE-DURAND-NICOLAS CLIMATIC BUBO
701.8 FAVRE-RACOUCHOT ELASTOIDOSIS CUTANEA NODULARIS
110.9 FAVUS
757.39 FDH SYNDROME (FOCAL DERMAL HYPOPLASIA)
780.31 FEBRILE SEIZURES (CONVULSIONS)
560.39 FECAL IMPACTION
787.6 FECAL INCONTINENCE
560.39 FECAL OBSTRUCTION
0 FECAL OBSTRUCTION WITH GANGRENOUS HERNIA SEE 'HERNIA', BY SITE, GANGRENOUS
0 FECAL OBSTRUCTION WITH HERNIA SEE 'HERNIA', BY SITE, INCARCERATED
560.39 FECAL RESERVOIR SYNDROME
543.9 FECALITH APPENDIX
777.1 FECALITH CONGENITAL
787.7 FECES ABNORMAL
529.0 FEDE'S DISEASE

FEEDING PROBLEM
783.3 ELDERLY OR INFANT ORGANIC
307.59 INFANTILE PSYCHOGENIC
783.3 MISMANAGEMENT
779.3 NEONATAL
307.59 PSYCHOGENIC
779.3 REGULATION NEWBORN

985.0 FEER'S DISEASE
756.16 FEIL-KLIPPEL SYNDROME (BREVICOLLIS)
732.1 FELIX'S JUVENILE OSTEOCHONDROSIS, HIP
681.01 FELON (ANY DIGIT)
054.6 FELON HERPES SIMPLEX
714.1 FELTY'S SYNDROME (RHEUMATOID ARTHRITIS WITH SPLENOMEGALY AND LEUKOPENIA)
302.6 FEMINISM IN BOYS

INJURY OF A BLOOD VESSEL CAN BE A LACERATION, A-V FISTULA, ANEURYSM, OR HEMATOMA. USE THE "INJURY" CODE FOUND BY ANATOMICAL SITE (THE NAME OF THE BLOOD VESSEL).

FEMORAL
442.3 ARTERY ANEURYSM (A-V FISTULA) (CIRSOID) (FALSE) (VARICOSE) (RUPTURED)
440.2# ARTERY ARTERIOSCLEROSIS (DEGENERATION)
5th Digit: 440.2
0. UNSPECIFIED
1. WITH INTERMITTENT CLAUDICATION
2. WITH REST PAIN, OR REST PAIN AND (INTERMITTENT CLAUDICATION)
3. WITH ULCERATION, OR ULCERATION AND (INTERMITTENT CLAUDICATION) (REST PAIN)
4. WITH ISCHEMIC GANGRENE, OR ISCHEMIC GANGRENE AND (INTERMITTENT CLAUDICATION) (REST PAIN) (ULCERATION)
9. OTHER ATHEROSCLEROSIS EXTREMITIES

440.3# ARTERY BYPASS GRAFT ARTERIOSCLEROSIS (EXTREMITIES)
5th Digit: 440.3
0. UNSPECIFIED GRAFT
1. AUTOLOGOUS VEIN BYPASS GRAFT
2. NONAUTOLOGOUS BIOLOGICAL BYPASS GRAFT

996.62 ARTERY BYPASS GRAFT COMPLICATION - INFECTION OR INFLAMMATION
996.1 ARTERY BYPASS GRAFT COMPLICATION - MECHANICAL
996.74 ARTERY BYPASS GRAFT COMPLICATION - OTHER
444.22 ARTERY EMBOLISM (THROMBOSIS) (OCCLUSION) (INFARCTION)
904.0 ARTERY INJURY - ABOVE PROFUNDA ORIGIN
904.0 ARTERY INJURY - COMMON
908.3 ARTERY INJURY - LATE EFFECT
904.1 ARTERY INJURY - SUPERFICIAL

FEMORAL (continued)

355.2	NERVE DISORDER
355.1	NERVE DISORDER (LATERAL CUTANEOUS OF THIGH)
956.1	NERVE INJURY
907.5	NERVE INJURY LATE EFFECT
355.2	NERVE NEURITIS
355.1	NERVE NEURITIS (LATERAL CUTANEOUS OF THIGH)
355.2	NERVE OTHER LESION
904.2	VEIN INJURY
908.3	VEIN INJURY LATE EFFECT
904.2	VEIN LACERATION (RUPTURE) (HEMATOMA) (AVULSION) (ANEURYSM) TRAUMATIC
908.3	VEIN LACERATION LATE EFFECT
451.11	VEIN PHLEBITIS (DEEP) (SUPERFICIAL)

732.2	FEMORAL EPIPHYSEAL SEPARATION
0	FEMORAL EPIPHYSEAL SEPARATION TRAUMATIC SEE 'FRACTURE' FEMUR
451.19	FEMOROPOPLITEAL VEIN PHLEBITIS
755.31	FEMUR AGENESIS NEC - WITH ABSENCE COMPLETE OF DISTAL ELEMENTS
755.34	FEMUR AGENESIS NEC - WITH ABSENCE INCOMPLETE OF DISTAL ELEMENTS
755.33	FEMUR AGENESIS NEC - WITH ABSENCE TIBIA AND FIBULA (INCOMPLETE)
755.60	FEMUR ANOMALY NOS CONGENITAL
755.63	FEMUR ANTEVERSION (NECK) CONGENITAL
754.42	FEMUR BOWING CONGENITAL
595.1	FENWICK ULCER
537.89	FENWICK'S GASTRIC ATROPHY
989.5	FER DE LANCE BITE
995.0	FER DE LANCE BITE WITH ANAPHYLAXIS [989.5]
441.9	FERNELS' AORTIC ANEURYSM
257.2	FERTILE EUNUCH SYNDROME

FERTILITY

V26.4	COUNSELING AND ADVICE (GENERAL)
V26.9	MANAGEMENT
V26.8	MANAGEMENT OTHER SPECIFIED
V26.2	TEST

> *FETAL OR NEWBORN CODES (760-779), SOMETIMES REQUIRE AN ADDITIONAL CODE TO FURTHER SPECIFY THE CAUSE OF THE CONDITION, THE INFECTING ORGANISM, OR COMPLICATING DIAGNOSES. WHENEVER APPROPRIATE, DESCRIBE THE PATIENT'S MEDICAL SITUATION AS CLEARLY AND CONCISELY AS POSSIBLE USING MULTIPLE CODES.*

FETAL - INFANT'S RECORD

768.2	ACIDEMIA METABOLIC BEFORE ONSET OF LABOR - LIVEBORN INFANT
768.3	ACIDEMIA METABOLIC FIRST NOTED DURING LABOR - LIVEBORN INFANT
768.4	ACIDEMIA METABOLIC UNSPECIFIED AS TO TIME - LIVEBORN INFANT
770.8	ACIDOSIS
760.71	ALCOHOL SYNDROME
760.71	ALCOHOL SYNDROME LATE EFFECT

ANEMIA NEWBORN

773.2	UNSPECIFIED
776.5	DUE TO FETAL BLOOD LOSS
773.2	DUE TO ISOIMMUNIZATION - NOS
773.1	DUE TO ISOIMMUNIZATION - ABO
773.0	DUE TO ISOIMMUNIZATION - RH (RHESUS), ANTI-D (RH)
773.2	DUE TO ISOIMMUNIZATION - OTHER SPECIFIED
773.5	LATE DUE TO ISOIMMUNIZATION
776.5	POSTHEMORRHAGIC
776.6	PREMATURITY NEONATAL

FETAL - INFANT'S RECORD (continued)

770.8	ANOXIA
770.8	ASPHYXIA
773.#	BLOOD (GROUP) (TYPE) INCOMPATIBILITY CAUSING HEMOLYTIC DISEASE

4th Digit: 773

0. RH (RHESUS) ISOIMMUNIZATION
1. ABO ISOIMMUNIZATION
2. OTHER AND NOS ISOIMMUNIZATION

BLOOD LOSS

772.0	UNSPECIFIED
772.0	CUT END CO-TWIN'S CORD
762.3	DUE TO PLACENTAL TRANSFUSION [772.0]
772.0	EXSANGUINATION
772.0	MOTHER'S CIRCULATION
772.0	PLACENTA
772.0	RUPTURED CORD
772.0	VASA PREVIA

FETAL - INFANT'S RECORD (continued)

747.89	CIRCULATION PERSISTENT
771.8	CLOSTRIDIUM INFECTION INTRA-AMNIOTIC

DEATH

779.9	NOS
768.0	ASPHYXIA OR ANOXIA BEFORE LABOR
768.1	ASPHYXIA OR ANOXIA DURING LABOR
779.6	DUE TO INDUCED ABORTION
779.6	DUE TO TERMINATION OF PREGNANCY
798.0	INFANT SYNDROME (SIDS)
0	INFANT SYNDROME (SIDS) NEAR MISS - CODE INDIVIDUAL SYMPTOM(S)
779.9	INTRAUTERINE NOS
798.9	UNATTENDED (CAUSE UNKNOWN)

DISTRESS

768.4	LIVEBORN - UNSPECIFIED ONSET
768.2	LIVEBORN - BEFORE ONSET LABOR
768.3	LIVEBORN - DURING LABOR OR DELIVERY
768.0	STILLBORN - BEFORE ONSET OF LABOR
768.1	STILLBORN - DEATH DURING LABOR

FETAL - INFANT'S RECORD (continued)

771.8	ESCHERICHIA COLI (E. COLI) INFECTION INTRA-AMNIOTIC

> *FETAL GROWTH RETARDATION: USE AN ADDITIONAL CODE TO SPECIFY THE UNDERLYING CAUSE OF THE GROWTH RETARDATION.*

GROWTH RETARDATION

764.90	UNSPECIFIED (WEIGHT)
764.91	LESS THAN 500 GRAMS
764.92	500-749 GRAMS
764.93	750-999 GRAMS
764.94	1000-1249 GRAMS
764.95	1250-1499 GRAMS
764.96	1500-1749 GRAMS
764.97	1750-1999 GRAMS
764.98	2000-2499 GRAMS
764.99	2500 GRAMS AND OVER

FETAL - INFANT'S RECORD (continued)

763.81	HEART RATE OR RHYTHM ABNORMAL - BEFORE ONSET OF LABOR
763.82	HEART RATE OR RHYTHM ABNORMAL - DURING LABOR
763.83	HEART RATE OR RHYTHM ABNORMAL - UNSPECIFIED AS TO TIME OF ONSET
773.#	HEMOLYTIC DISEASE DUE TO ISOIMMUNIZATION

4th Digit: 773

0. RH (RHESUS) ISOIMMUNIZATION
1. ABO ISOIMMUNIZATION
2. OTHER AND NOS ISOIMMUNIZATION

770.8	HYPERCAPNIA
770.8	HYPOXIA
771.8	INFECTION INTRA-AMNIOTIC
0	JAUNDICE SEE 'JAUNDICE NEONATAL'

FETAL - INFANT'S RECORD (continued)

> *FETAL MALNUTRITION: USE AN ADDITIONAL CODE TO FURTHER SPECIFY THE CAUSE OF THE MALNUTRITION.*

MALNUTRITION

764.20 UNSPECIFIED (WEIGHT)
764.21 LESS THAN 500 GRAMS
764.22 500-749 GRAMS
764.23 750-999 GRAMS
764.24 1000-1249 GRAMS
764.25 1250-1499 GRAMS
764.26 1500-1749 GRAMS
764.27 1750-1999 GRAMS
764.28 2000-2499 GRAMS
764.29 2500 GRAMS AND OVER

FETAL - INFANT'S RECORD (continued)

747.89 PERSISTENT CIRCULATION
770.9 RESPIRATORY CONDITION
770.8 RESPIRATORY DEPRESSION
771.8 SEPSIS INTRAUTERINE
763.89 OTHER SPECIFIED COMPLICATIONS OF LABOR AND DELIVERY AFFECTING FETUS OR NEWBORN

FETAL - MOTHER'S RECORD

> ***FETUS ABNORMALITY AFFECTING MANAGEMENT OF MOTHER:*** *USE CODES FROM THIS SECTION ONLY IF THE FETAL CONDITION CAUSES A COMPLICATION THAT AFFECTS THE MANAGEMENT OF THE MOTHER. THESE CAN BE AN ADDITIONAL REASON FOR OBSERVATION, OBSTETRICAL CARE, OR ABORTION. USE THESE CODES ONLY ON THE MOTHER'S RECORD. REMEMBER, DO NOT USE THESE CODES IF THE FETAL CONDITION DOES NOT AFFECT MANAGEMENT OF THE MOTHER.*

ABNORMALITY KNOWN/SUSPECT AFFECTING MANAGEMENT OF MOTHER

655.9# UNSPECIFIED
655.4# ALCOHOLISM LISTERIOSIS TOXOPLASMOSIS
655.0# ANENCEPHALY
655.1# CHROMOSOME ABNORMALITY
655.0# CNS MALFORMATION
655.5# DAMAGE FROM DRUGS
655.8# EXPOSURE TO TOXINS OR IUD
655.8# HEART SOUNDS INAUDIBLE
655.2# HEREDITARY FAMILIAL
655.0# HYDROCEPHALUS
655.4# MATERNAL DISEASE DAMAGING FETUS
655.7# MOVEMENT DECREASED (LACK OF)
655.6# RADIATION EXPOSURE
655.3# RUBELLA MATERNAL
655.0# SPINA BIFIDA MYELOMENINGOCELE
655.4# TOXOPLASMOSIS MATERNAL
655.3# VIRAL DISEASE IN MOTHER
655.8# OTHER SPECIFIED PROBLEMS

5th Digit: 655.0-6, 8, 9
0. EPISODE OF CARE UNSPECIFIED OR N/A
1. DELIVERED
3. ANTEPARTUM COMPLICATION

FETAL - MOTHER'S RECORD (continued)

656.8# ACID-BASE IMBALANCE
656.8# ACIDOSIS INTRAUTERINE
656.3# ACIDEMIA METABOLIC FETAL
653.7# ASCITES (HYDROPS) (MYELOMENINGOCELE) (TERATOMA) (NEOPLASM UNCERTAIN BEHAVIOR) (CONJOINED TWINS)
660.1# ASCITES (HYDROPS) (MYELOMENINGOCELE) (TERATOMA) (NEOPLASM UNCERTAIN BEHAVIOR) (CONJOINED TWINS) OBSTRUCTING LABOR **[653.7#]**
656.2# BLOOD TYPE INCOMPATIBILITY COMPLICATING PREGNANCY - ABO
656.1# BLOOD TYPE INCOMPATIBILITY COMPLICATING PREGNANCY - ANTI-D ANTIBODIES (RH)
656.1# BLOOD TYPE INCOMPATIBILITY COMPLICATING PREGNANCY - RHESUS (RH)
656.2# BLOOD TYPE INCOMPATIBILITY COMPLICATING PREGNANCY - OTHER SPECIFIED
659.7# BRADYCARDIA

5th Digit: 653.7, 656.1-3, 8, 659.7, 660.1
0. EPISODE OF CARE UNSPECIFIED OR N/A
1. DELIVERED
3. ANTEPARTUM COMPLICATION

DEATH

656.4# AFTER COMPLETION OF 22 WEEKS' GESTATION

5th Digit: 656.4
0. EPISODE OF CARE UNSPECIFIED OR N/A
1. DELIVERED
3. ANTEPARTUM COMPLICATION

632 BEFORE COMPLETION OF 22 WEEKS' GESTATION (RETAINED)
669.9# DURING DELIVERY
668.9# DURING DELIVERY - ANESTHESIA NEC

5th Digit: 668.9, 669.9
0. EPISODE OF CARE NOS OR N/A
1. DELIVERED
2. WITH POSTPARTUM COMPLICATION
4. POSTPARTUM COMPLICATION

DISPROPORTION

653.5# UNSPECIFIED FETAL ABNORMALITY
660.1# UNSPECIFIED FETAL ABNORMALITY OBSTRUCTING LABOR **[653.5#]**
653.7# OTHER FETAL ABNORMALITY CAUSING DISPROPORTION

5th Digit: 653.5, 7, 660.1
0. EPISODE OF CARE UNSPECIFIED OR N/A
1. DELIVERED
3. ANTEPARTUM COMPLICATION

0 SEE ALSO 'PREGNANCY COMPLICATIONS, DISPROPORTION'

DISTRESS

656.8# NOS
656.3# ACIDEMIA METABOLIC

5th Digit: 656.3, 8
0. EPISODE OF CARE UNSPECIFIED OR N/A
1. DELIVERED
3. ANTEPARTUM COMPLICATION

GROWTH

656.6# EXCESSIVE
656.5# POOR, SMALL OR LIGHT-FOR-DATES

5th Digit: 656.5-6
0. EPISODE OF CARE UNSPECIFIED OR N/A
1. DELIVERED
3. ANTEPARTUM COMPLICATION

FETAL - MOTHER'S RECORD (continued)

659.7# HEART RATE DECELERATIONS
659.7# HEART RATE OR RHYTHM ABNORMAL
659.7# HEART TONES DEPRESSED
653.6# HYDROCEPHALUS CAUSING DISPROPORTION
660.1# HYDROCEPHALUS CAUSING DISPROPORTION OBSTRUCTING LABOR **[653.6#]**
655.0# HYDROCEPHALUS KNOWN OR SUSPECTED - CONCERN FOR FETUS
653.5# LARGE CAUSING DISPROPORTION

5th Digit: 653.5, 6, 655.0, 659.7, 660.1
0. EPISODE OF CARE UNSPECIFIED OR N/A
1. DELIVERED
3. ANTEPARTUM COMPLICATION

0 MALPOSITION OR MALPRESENTATION SEE 'PREGNANCY COMPLICATIONS, DELIVERY PROBLEMS: MALPRESENTATION / MALPOSITION'
655.4# MATERNAL DISEASE CAUSING DAMAGE TO FETUS
656.0# MATERNAL HEMORRHAGE
656.8# MECONIUM IN LIQUOR
659.7# NON-REASSURING FETAL HEART RATE OR RHYTHM
646.0# PAPYRACEOUS
653.4# PELVIC DISPROPORTION
656.1# RH INCOMPATIBILITY
659.7# TACHYCARDIA
656.8# OTHER SPECIFIED PROBLEM
656.9# PROBLEM UNSPECIFIED

5th Digit: 646.0, 653.4, 655.4, 656.0-1, 8, 9, 659.7
0. EPISODE OF CARE UNSPECIFIED OR N/A
1. DELIVERED
3. ANTEPARTUM COMPLICATION

302.81 FETISHISM
302.3 FETISHISM TRANSVESTIC
653.4# FETOPELVIC DISPROPORTION
646.0# FETUS PAPYRACEOUS

5th Digit: 646.0, 653.4
0. EPISODE OF CARE UNSPECIFIED OR N/A
1. DELIVERED
3. ANTEPARTUM COMPLICATION

0 FETUS SEE FETAL

FEVER

780.6 UNSPECIFIED
054.9 BLISTER
036.0 CEREBROSPINAL (MENINGOCOCCAL)
078.3 DUE TO CAT SCRATCH
277.3 FAMILIAL MEDITERRANEAN
V73.5 HEMORRHAGIC SCREENING EXAM
0 HEMORRHAGIC SEE 'HEMORRHAGIC FEVER'
087.0 LOUSE-BORNE RELAPSING OR RECURRENT
288.0 NEUTROPENIC
778.4 NEWBORN TRANSITORY
998.89 POSTOPERATIVE
998.59 POSTOPERATIVE DUE TO INFECTION
672.0# PUERPERAL
670.0# PUERPERAL SEPTIC

5th Digit: 670.0, 672.0
0. UNSPECIFIED
2. DELIVERED WITH POSTPARTUM COMPLICATION
4. POSTPARTUM COMPLICATION

087.9 RELAPSING OR RECURRENT UNSPECIFIED
082.0 ROCKY MOUNTAIN SPOTTED
087.1 TICK-BORNE RELAPSING OR RECURRENT
0 UNDULANT SEE 'BRUCELLOSIS'
780.6 UNKNOWN ETIOLOGY (ORIGIN)
780.6 WITH CHILLS
0 SEE ALSO 'PYREXIA'

427.31 FIBRILLATION ATRIAL (PAROXYSMAL)
427.32 FIBRILLATION-FLUTTER SYNDROME
427.41 FIBRILLATION VENTRICULAR

790.92 FIBRIN ABSENCE

286.6 FIBRINOGEN DEFICIENCY (TOTAL)
286.3 FIBRINOGEN DEFICIENCY CONGENITAL
790.92 FIBRINOGEN TITER ABNORMAL FINDINGS
286.6 FIBRINOGENOLYSIS HEMORRHAGIC

FIBRINOLYSIS

964.4 AFFECTING DRUGS
286.6 PATHOLOGIC
666.3# POSTPARTUM

5th Digit: 666.3
0. UNSPECIFIED
2. DELIVERED WITH POSTPARTUM COMPLICATION
4. POSTPARTUM COMPLICATION

CARCINOMAS AND NEOPLASMS SHOULD BE CODED BY SITE IF POSSIBLE. CODE BY CELL TYPE - "SITE NOS", IF AND ONLY IF A SITE IS NOT SPECIFIED IN THE DIAGNOSIS. OTHERWISE - REFER TO THE APPROPRIATE CATEGORY OF NEOPLASM FOR A MORE SPECIFIC CODE: SEE 'CANCER' 'CANCER METASTATIC', 'NEOPLASM UNCERTAIN BEHAVIOR', 'NEOPLASM UNSPECIFIED NATURE', OR 'BENIGN NEOPLASM'.

FIBROADENOMA

217 SITE UNSPECIFIED
0 SITE SPECIFIED SEE 'BENIGN NEOPLASM' BY SITE M9010/0

217 CELLULAR INTRACANALICULAR SITE UNSPECIFIED
0 CELLULAR INTRACANALICULAR SITE SPECIFIED SEE 'BENIGN NEOPLASM' BY SITE M9020/0

217 INTRACANALICULAR SITE UNSPECIFIED
0 INTRACANALICULAR SITE SPECIFIED SEE 'BENIGN NEOPLASM' BY SITE M9011/0

217 JUVENILE SITE UNSPECIFIED
0 JUVENILE SITE SPECIFIED SEE 'BENIGN NEOPLASM' BY SITE M9030/0

217 PERICANALICULAR SITE UNSPECIFIED
0 PERICANALICULAR SITE SPECIFIED SEE 'BENIGN NEOPLASM' BY SITE M9012/0

610.2 FIBROADENOSIS BREAST (CHRONIC) (CYSTIC) (DIFFUSE) (PERIODIC) (SEGMENTAL)

0 FIBROCASEOUS DISEASE OF LUNG SEE 'TUBERCULOSIS', PULMONARY

757.39 FIBROCUTANEOUS TAGS CONGENITAL (ANY AREA)

FIBROCYSTIC DISEASE

277.00 NOS
733.29 BONE
610.1 BREAST
526.2 JAW (BONE)
753.19 KIDNEY CONGENITAL
751.62 LIVER
518.89 LUNG
748.4 LUNG CONGENITAL
277.01 NEWBORN
277.00 PANCREAS
593.2 RENAL ACQUIRED
753.19 RENAL CONGENITAL

FIBROID UTERINE

218.9 UNSPECIFIED
654.1# MATERNAL COMPLICATING CHILDBIRTH
660.2# MATERNAL OBSTRUCTING LABOR **[654.1#]**

5th Digit: 654.1
0. EPISODE OF CARE UNSPECIFIED OR N/A
1. DELIVERED
2. DELIVERED WITH POSTPARTUM COMPLICATION
3. ANTEPARTUM COMPLICATION
4. POSTPARTUM COMPLICATION

5th Digit: 660.2
0. EPISODE OF CARE NOS OR N/A
1. DELIVERED
3. ANTEPARTUM COMPLICATION

F

FIBROID UTERINE (continued)

218.1 INTRAMURAL (INTERSTITIAL)
218.0 SUBMUCOUS
218.2 SUBSEROUS

FIBROLIPOMA

214.# SPINDLE CELL (INTRAMUSCULAR) M8851/0
4th Digit: 214
- **0. FACE SKIN AND SUBCUTANEOUS TISSUE**
- **1. SKIN AND SUBCUTANEOUS TISSUE OTHER**
- **2. INTRATHORACIC ORGANS**
- **3. INTRA-ABDOMINAL ORGANS**
- **4. SPERMATIC CORD**
- **8. OTHER SPECIFIED SITES**
- **9. SITE UNSPECIFIED**

FIBROMA

213.# AMELOBLASTIC (UPPER JAW BONE) M9330/0
4th Digit: 213
- **0. SKULL FACE UPPER JAW**
- **1. LOWER JAW**

213.# CEMENTIFYING M9274/0
213.# CHONDROMYXOID M9241/0
4th Digit: 213
- **0. SKULL FACE UPPER JAW**
- **1. LOWER JAW**
- **2. SPINE**
- **3. RIB STERNUM CLAVICLE**
- **4. UPPER LIMB LONG BONES SCAPULA**
- **5. UPPER LIMB SHORT BONES**
- **6. PELVIS SACRUM COCCYX**
- **7. LOWER LIMB LONG BONE**
- **8. LOWER LIMB SHORT BONE**
- **9. SITE UNSPECIFIED**

238.1 DESMOPLASTIC SITE UNSPECIFIED
0 DESMOPLASTIC SITE SPECIFIED SEE 'NEOPLASM UNCERTAIN BEHAVIOR' BY SITE M8823/1
215.# FASCIAL M8813/0
4th Digit: 215
- **0. HEAD FACE NECK (OR IF SITE UNSPECIFIED)**
- **2. UPPER LIMB SHOULDER**
- **3. LOWER LIMB HIP**
- **4. THORAX**
- **5. ABDOMINAL HYPOCHONDRIUM**
- **6. PELVIS BUTTOCK GROIN INGUINAL REGION PERINEUM**
- **7. TRUNK UNSPECIFIED BACK UNSPECIFIED FLANK UNSPECIFIED**
- **8. OTHER SPECIFIED SITES**
- **9. SITE UNSPECIFIED**

213.# ODONTOGENIC M9321/0
4th Digit: 213
- **0. SKULL FACE UPPER JAW**
- **1. LOWER JAW**

213.# OSSIFYING M9262/0
213.# PERIOSTEAL M8812/0
4th Digit: 213
- **0. SKULL FACE UPPER JAW**
- **1. LOWER JAW (OR IF SITE UNSPECIFIED)**
- **2. SPINE**
- **3. RIB STERNUM CLAVICLE**
- **4. UPPER LIMB LONG BONES SCAPULA**
- **5. UPPER LIMB SHORT BONES**
- **6. PELVIS SACRUM COCCYX**
- **7. LOWER LIMB LONG BONE**
- **8. LOWER LIMB SHORT BONE**
- **9. SITE UNSPECIFIED**

> *CARCINOMAS AND NEOPLASMS SHOULD BE CODED BY SITE IF POSSIBLE. CODE BY CELL TYPE - "SITE NOS", IF AND ONLY IF A SITE IS NOT SPECIFIED IN THE DIAGNOSIS. OTHERWISE - REFER TO THE APPROPRIATE CATEGORY OF NEOPLASM FOR A MORE SPECIFIC CODE: SEE 'CANCER' 'CANCER METASTATIC', 'NEOPLASM UNCERTAIN BEHAVIOR', 'NEOPLASM UNSPECIFIED NATURE', OR 'BENIGN NEOPLASM'.*

FIBROMATOSIS

238.1 SITE UNSPECIFIED
0 SITE SPECIFIED SEE 'NEOPLASM UNCERTAIN BEHAVIOR' BY SITE
238.1 ABDOMINAL SITE UNSPECIFIED
0 ABDOMINAL SITE SPECIFIED SEE 'NEOPLASM UNCERTAIN BEHAVIOR' BY SITE M8822/1
238.1 AGGRESSIVE SITE UNSPECIFIED
0 AGGRESSIVE SITE SPECIFIED SEE 'NEOPLASM UNCERTAIN BEHAVIOR' BY SITE M8821/1
728.6 DUPUYTREN'S
523.8 GINGIVAL
728.71 PLANTAR FASCIA
728.79 PROLIFERATIVE
728.79 PSEUDOSARCOMATOUS
728.79 SUBCUTANEOUS

447.8 FIBROMUSCULAR HYPERPLASIA OF ARTERY - NEC
447.3 FIBROMUSCULAR HYPERPLASIA OF ARTERY - RENAL
729.1 FIBROMYALGIA

FIBROMYOMA UTERINE

218.9 UNSPECIFIED
218.1 INTRAMURAL (INTERSTITIAL)
218.0 SUBMUCOUS
218.2 SUBSEROUS

729.1 FIBROMYOSITIS
214.# FIBROMYXOLIPOMA M8852/0
4th Digit: 214
- **0. FACE SKIN AND SUBCUTANEOUS TISSUE**
- **1. SKIN AND SUBCUTANEOUS TISSUE OTHER**
- **2. INTRATHORACIC ORGANS**
- **3. INTRA-ABDOMINAL ORGANS**
- **4. SPERMATIC CORD**
- **8. OTHER SPECIFIED SITES**
- **9. SITE UNSPECIFIED**

215.# FIBROMYXOMA M8811/0
171.# FIBROMYXOSARCOMA M8811/3
4th Digit: 171, 215
- **0. HEAD FACE NECK**
- **2. UPPER LIMB SHOULDER**
- **3. LOWER LIMB HIP**
- **4. THORAX**
- **5. ABDOMINAL HYPOCHONDRIUM**
- **6. PELVIS BUTTOCK GROIN INGUINAL REGION PERINEUM**
- **7. TRUNK UNSPECIFIED BACK UNSPECIFIED FLANK UNSPECIFIED**
- **8. OTHER SPECIFIED SITES**
- **9. SITE UNSPECIFIED**

213.# FIBRO-ODONTOMA AMELOBLASTIC M9290/0
4th Digit: 213
- **0. SKULL FACE UPPER JAW**
- **1. LOWER JAW UNSPECIFIED (OR IF SITE UNSPECIFIED)**

FIBROSARCOMA

170.# AMELOBLASTIC M9330/3
4th Digit: 170
- **0. SKULL AND FACE**
- **1. MANDIBLE (OR IF SITE UNSPECIFIED)**

FIBROSARCOMA (continued)

171.# FASCIAL M8813/3

171.# INFANTILE M8814/3

171.# UNSPECIFIED M8810/3

4th Digit: 171

0. HEAD FACE NECK
2. UPPER LIMB SHOULDER
3. LOWER LIMB HIP
4. THORAX
5. ABDOMINAL HYPOCHONDRIUM
6. PELVIS BUTTOCK GROIN INGUINAL REGION PERINEUM
7. TRUNK UNSPECIFIED BACK UNSPECIFIED FLANK UNSPECIFIED
8. OTHER SPECIFIED SITES
9. SITE UNSPECIFIED

170.# PERIOSTEAL M8812/3

4th Digit: 170

0. SKULL AND FACE
1. MANDIBLE (OR IF SITE UNSPECIFIED)
2. VERTEBRAL COLUMN
3. RIBS STERNUM CLAVICLE
4. SCAPULA LONG BONES UPPER LIMB
5. SHORT BONES UPPER LIMB
6. PELVIC BONES SACRUM COCCYX
7. LONG BONES LOWER LIMB
8. SHORT BONES LOWER LIMB
9. SITE UNSPECIFIED

159.1 SPLEEN

610.3 FIBROSCLEROSIS BREAST

FIBROSIS

607.89 CORPUS CAVERNOSA

658.8# CHORION

5th Digit: 658.8

0. EPISODE OF CARE UNSPECIFIED OR N/A
1. DELIVERED
3. ANTEPARTUM COMPLICATION

DUE TO A DEVICE, IMPLANT OR GRAFT SEE 'COMPLICATION OF A DEVICE, IMPLANT OR GRAFT - OTHER SPECIFIED'

519.3 MEDIASTINUM

349.2 MENINGES

620.8 OVARY

620.8 OVIDUCT

543.9 PERIAPPENDICEAL

423.1 PERICARDIAL

0 PERINEUM MATERNAL SEE 'VULVA, VULVAL DISORDERS COMPLICATING CHILDBIRTH', ABNORMALITY

511.0 PLEURAL

515 PULMONARY CHRONIC OR UNSPECIFIED

516.3 PULMONARY DIFFUSE (INTERSTITIAL)

503 PULMONARY DUE TO BAUXITE

587 RENAL

593.4 RETROPERITONEAL (IDIOPATHIC)

528.8 SUBMUCOSAL ORAL INCLUDING TONGUE

621.8 UTERUS

729.0 FIBROSITIS (SYNDROME)

FIBROUS

733.29 DYSPLASIA BONE OR CARTILAGE

756.54 DYSPLASIA BONE POLYOSTOTIC

756.59 DYSPLASIA DIAPHYSEAL PROGRESSIVE

526.89 DYSPLASIA JAW

0 PAPULE OF THE NOSE SITE SPECIFIED SEE 'BENIGN NEOPLASM' BY SITE M8724/0

FIBROXANTHOMA

215.# UNSPECIFIED M8831/0

4th Digit: 215

0. HEAD FACE NECK
2. UPPER LIMB SHOULDER
3. LOWER LIMB HIP
4. THORAX
5. ABDOMINAL HYPOCHONDRIUM
6. PELVIS BUTTOCK GROIN INGUINAL REGION PERINEUM
7. TRUNK UNSPECIFIED BACK NOS FLANK NOS
8. OTHER SPECIFIED SITES
9. SITE UNSPECIFIED

238.1 ATYPICAL SITE UNSPECIFIED

0 ATYPICAL SITE SPECIFIED SEE 'NEOPLASM UNCERTAIN BEHAVIOR' BY SITE M8831/1

171.# MALIGNANT M8831/3

4th Digit: 171

0. HEAD FACE NECK
2. UPPER LIMB SHOULDER
3. LOWER LIMB HIP
4. THORAX
5. ABDOMINAL HYPOCHONDRIUM
6. PELVIS BUTTOCK GROIN INGUINAL REGION PERINEUM
7. TRUNK UNSPECIFIED BACK NOS FLANK NOS
8. OTHER SPECIFIED SITES
9. SITE UNSPECIFIED

755.31 FIBULA ABSENCE - WITH ABSENCE DISTAL ELEMENTS COMPLETE CONGENITAL

755.37 FIBULA ABSENCE - WITH ABSENCE DISTAL ELEMENTS INCOMPLETE CONGENITAL

755.35 FIBULA ABSENCE - WITH ABSENCE TIBIA CONGENITAL

755.33 FIBULA ABSENCE - WITH ABSENCE TIBIA WITH FEMUR (INCOMPLETE) CONGENITAL

755.37 FIBULA AGENESIS

100.0 FIEDLER'S LEPTOSPIRAL JAUNDICE

422.91 FIEDLER'S SYNDROME (ACUTE ISOLATED MYOCARDITIS)

099.3 FIESSINGER-LEROY (-REITER) SYNDROME

099.3 FIESSINGER-LEROY (-REITER) SYNDROME WITH ARTHROPATHY **[711.1#]**

5th Digit: 711.1

0. SITE NOS
1. SHOULDER REGION
2. UPPER ARM (ELBOW) (HUMERUS)
3. FOREARM (RADIUS) (WRIST) (ULNA)
4. HAND (CARPAL) (METACARPAL) (FINGERS)
5. PELVIC REGION AND THIGH (HIP) (BUTTOCK) (FEMUR)
6. LOWER LEG (FIBULA) (KNEE) (PATELLA) (TIBIA)
7. ANKLE AND/OR FOOT (METATARSALS) (TOES) (TARSALS)
8. OTHER (HEAD) (NECK) (RIB) (SKULL) (TRUNK) (VERTEBRAE)
9. MULTIPLE

099.3 FIESSINGER-LEROY (-REITER) SYNDROME WITH CONJUNCTIVITIS [372.33]

695.1 FIESSINGER-RENDU SYNDROME (ERYTHEMA MULTIFORME EXUDATIVUM)

350.8 FIFTH CRANIAL NERVE (TRIGEMINAL) ATROPHY

350.9 FIFTH CRANIAL NERVE (TRIGEMINAL) DISORDER

951.2 FIFTH CRANIAL NERVE (TRIGEMINAL) INJURY

057.0 FIFTH DISEASE

0 FIFTH NERVE SEE 'TRIGEMINAL NERVE'

125.9 FILARIA WITH GENITAL DISEASE (MALE) [608.81]

FILARIASIS

125.9 UNSPECIFIED
125.0 BANCROFTIAN
125.1 MALAYAN
125.5 OZZARDI INFECTION
V75.6 SCREENING EXAM
125.6 OTHER SPECIFIED

075 FILATOFF'S (FILATOV'S) INFECTIOUS MONONUCLEOSIS
984.9 FILE-CUTTER'S LEAD POISONING

FILLING DEFECT

793.3 BILIARY TRACT
793.5 BLADDER
793.3 GALLBLADDER
793.5 KIDNEY
793.4 STOMACH
793.5 URETER

078.89 FILTERABLE VIRUS DISEASE NEC
752.11 FIMBRIAL CYST CONGENITAL

FINGER

V49.62 ABSENCE ACQUIRED
755.21 ABSENCE (COMPLETE OR PARTIAL) (ALL) OR (TRANSVERSE)
755.29 ABSENCE CONGENITAL
755.29 AGENESIS NEC
V49.62 AMPUTATION STATUS
736.29 CONTRACTION ACQUIRED
755.59 CONTRACTION CONGENITAL
718.44 CONTRACTION JOINT
736.20 DEFORMITY (ACQUIRED)
736.29 DEFORMITY (ACQUIRED) OTHER
736.29 DROP
959.5 INJURY
915.8 INJURY OTHER AND UNSPECIFIED SUPERFICIAL
915.9 INJURY OTHER AND UNSPECIFIED SUPERFICIAL (INFECTED)
718.94 JOINT LIGAMENT RELAXATION
0 JOINT LIGAMENT TEAR SEE 'SPRAIN'
718.14 JOINT LOOSE BODY
0 JOINT SEE ALSO 'JOINT'
681.02 NAIL ABSCESS (INFECTION)
703.8 NAIL DEFORMITY (HYPERTROPHY)
703.8 NAIL DISCOLORATION
703.0 NAIL INGROWN (INFECTED)
959.5 NAIL INJURY
703.8 NAIL OTHER SPECIFIED DISEASE
703.8 NAIL THICKENING
757.5 NAIL THICKENING CONGENITAL

989.5 FIRE ANT BITE
995.0 FIRE ANT BITE WITH ANAPHYLAXIS [989.5]

FIRST

756.0 ARCH SYNDROME
426.11 DEGREE HEART BLOCK AV
352.0 NERVE ATROPHY
352.0 NERVE DISORDERS
951.8 NERVE INJURY

537.89 FISH HOOK STOMACH
495.8 FISH MEAL WORKERS' LUNG
701.1 FISH SKIN
757.1 FISH SKIN CONGENITAL
357.0 FISHER'S SYNDROME

FISSURE

756.79 ABDOMINAL WALL (CONGENITAL)
565.0 ANAL
751.5 ANAL CONGENITAL
863.89 ANAL TRAUMATIC
863.99 ANAL TRAUMATIC WITH OPEN WOUND
908.1 ANAL TRAUMATIC LATE EFFECT
528.9 BUCCAL CAVITY

FISSURE (continued)

752.49 CLITORIS (CONGENITAL)
744.29 EAR, LOBULE (CONGENITAL)
748.3 EPIGLOTTIS (CONGENITAL)
478.79 LARYNX
748.3 LARYNX CONGENITAL
528.5 LIP
0 LIP CONGENITAL SEE 'CLEFT' LIP
611.2 NIPPLE
676.1# NIPPLE PUERPERAL, POSTPARTUM MATERNAL DUE TO PREGNANCY

5th Digit: 676.1

0. EPISODE OF CARE NOS OR N/A
1. DELIVERED
2. DELIVERED WITH POSTPARTUM COMPLICATION
3. ANTEPARTUM COMPLICATION
4. POSTPARTUM COMPLICATION

0 PALATE (CONGENITAL) SEE 'CLEFT' PALATE
565.0 POSTANAL
565.0 RECTUM
709.8 SKIN
686.9 SKIN STREPTOCOCCAL
0 SPINE (CONGENITAL) SEE 'SPINA BIFIDA'
756.3 STERNUM (CONGENITAL)
529.5 TONGUE
750.13 TONGUE CONGENITAL

FISTULA

569.81 ABDOMINAL WALL
569.81 ABDOMINOINTESTINAL
569.81 ABDOMINORECTAL
569.81 ABDOMINOSIGMOIDAL
510.0 ABDOMINOTHORACIC
619.2 ABDOMINOUTERINE
752.3 ABDOMINOUTERINE CONGENITAL
596.2 ABDOMINOVESICAL
473.9 ACCESSORY SINUSES
0 ACTINOMYCOTIC SEE 'ACTINOMYCOSIS'
473.0 ALVEOLAR ANTRUM (SEE ALSO 'SINUSITIS' MAXILLARY)
522.7 ALVEOLAR PROCESS
565.1 ANAL (TO SKIN)
751.5 ANAL CONGENITAL
565.1 ANORECTAL
619.1 ANOVAGINAL
752.49 ANOVAGINAL CONGENITAL
473.0 ANTROBUCCAL (SEE ALSO 'SINUSITIS')
473.0 ANTRUM
747.29 AORTIC SINUS
447.2 AORTODUODENAL
543.9 APPENDIX
447.0 ARTERIOVENOUS ACQUIRED
747.60 ARTERIOVENOUS VESSEL NOS (PERIPHERAL) CONGENITAL
0 ARTERIOVENOUS VESSEL SPECIFIED CONGENITAL SEE 'FISTULA' BY SITE
747.69 ARTERIOVENOUS VESSEL OTHER SPECIFIED SITES (PERIPHERAL) CONGENITAL
447.2 ARTERY
537.4 ASTROCOLIC
383.81 AURAL
744.49 AURAL CONGENITAL
383.81 AURICLE
744.49 AURICLE CONGENITAL
619.8 BARTHOLIN'S GLAND
576.4 BILE DUCT
576.4 BILIARY
751.69 BILIARY CONGENITAL
596.2 BLADDER
619.0 BLADDER AND FEMALE GENITAL TRACT
733.99 BONE
348.8 BRAIN
437.3 BRAIN ARTERIOVENOUS
747.81 BRAIN ARTERIOVENOUS CONGENITAL
430 BRAIN ARTERIOVENOUS WITH RUPTURE

F

FISTULA (continued)

744.41 BRANCHIAL (CLEFT)
744.41 BRANCHIOGENOUS
611.0 BREAST
675.1# BREAST MATERNAL DUE TO PREGNANCY
5th Digit: 675.1
0. EPISODE OF CARE NOS OR N/A
1. DELIVERED
2. DELIVERED WITH POSTPARTUM COMPLICATION
3. ANTEPARTUM COMPLICATION
4. POSTPARTUM COMPLICATION

510.0 BRONCHIAL
510.0 BRONCHOCUTANEOUS
530.89 BRONCHOESOPHAGEAL
750.3 BRONCHOESOPHAGEAL CONGENITAL
510.0 BRONCHOMEDIASTINAL
510.0 BRONCHOPLEURAL
510.0 BRONCHOVISCERAL
528.3 BUCCAL CAVITY (INFECTIVE)
747.81 CAROTID-CAVERNOUS CONGENITAL
430 CAROTID-CAVERNOUS CONGENITAL WITH HEMORRHAGE
447.0 CAROTID-CAVERNOUS NON-TRAUMATIC - ACQUIRED
430 CAROTID-CAVERNOUS NON-TRAUMATIC - ACQUIRED WITH HEMORRHAGE
900.82 CAROTID-CAVERNOUS TRAUMATIC
853.0# CAROTID-CAVERNOUS TRAUMATIC WITH HEMORRHAGE
5th Digit: 853.0
0. LEVEL OF CONSCIOUSNESS NOS
1. NO LOC
2. LOC < 1 HR
3. LOC 1 - 24 HRS
4. LOC > 24 HRS WITH RETURN TO PRIOR LEVEL
5. LOC > 24 HRS WITHOUT RETURN TO PRIOR LEVEL: OR DEATH BEFORE REGAINING CONSCIOUSNESS, REGARDLESS OF DURATION OF LOC
6. LOC DURATION NOS
9. WITH CONCUSSION NOS

908.3 CAROTID-CAVERNOUS TRAUMATIC LATE EFFECT
569.81 CECOSIGMOIDAL
569.69 CECOSTOMY
569.81 CECUM
349.81 CEREBROSPINAL (FLUID)
744.41 CERVICAL LATERAL CONGENITAL
744.49 CERVICOAURAL CONGENITAL
619.1 CERVICOSIGMOID
619.0 CERVICOVESICAL
619.8 CERVIX
510.0 CHEST WALL
575.5 CHOLECYSTOCOLIC
575.5 CHOLECYSTODUODENAL
575.5 CHOLECYSTOENTERIC
575.5 CHOLECYSTOGASTRIC
575.5 CHOLECYSTOINTESTINAL
576.4 CHOLEDOCHODUODENAL
685.1 COCCYX
685.0 COCCYX WITH ABSCESS
569.81 COLON
569.69 COLOSTOMY
619.1 COLOVAGINAL
576.4 COMMON DUCT
360.32 CORNEA, CAUSING HYPOTONY (POSTINFLAMMATORY) (POST OP) (POSTTRAUMATIC)
414.19 CORONARY ARTERIOVENOUS
746.85 CORONARY ARTERIOVENOUS CONGENITAL
510.0 COSTAL REGION
619.8 CUL-DE-SAC (DOUGLAS')
686.9 CUTANEOUS
575.5 CYSTIC DUCT
751.69 CYSTIC DUCT CONGENITAL
522.7 DENTAL
510.0 DIAPHRAGM
537.4 DUODENUM

FISTULA (continued)

380.89 EAR CANAL
569.81 ENTEROCOLIC
569.81 ENTEROCUTANEOUS
569.81 ENTEROENTERIC
569.69 ENTEROSTOMY
619.1 ENTEROUTERINE
752.3 ENTEROUTERINE CONGENITAL
619.1 ENTEROVAGINAL
752.49 ENTEROVAGINAL CONGENITAL
596.1 ENTEROVESICAL
608.89 EPIDIDYMIS
0 EPIDIDYMIS DUE TO TB SEE 'TUBERCULOSIS', EPIDIDYMIS
530.89 ESOPHAGOBRONCHIAL
750.3 ESOPHAGOBRONCHIAL CONGENITAL
530.89 ESOPHAGOCUTANEOUS
530.89 ESOPHAGOPLEUROCUTANEOUS
530.84 ESOPHAGOTRACHEAL
750.3 ESOPHAGOTRACHEAL CONGENITAL
530.89 ESOPHAGUS
750.4 ESOPHAGUS CONGENITAL
473.2 ETHMOID SINUS (SEE ALSO 'SINUSITIS', ETHMOIDAL)
747.64 EXTREMITY VESSEL (LOWER) ARTERIOVENOUS CONGENITAL
747.63 EXTREMITY VESSEL (UPPER) ARTERIOVENOUS CONGENITAL
373.11 EYELID
619.2 FALLOPIAN TUBE (EXTERNAL)
473.1 FRONTAL SINUS (SEE ALSO 'SINUSITIS', FRONTAL)
575.5 GALLBLADDER
751.69 GALLBLADDER CONGENITAL
574.2# GALLBLADDER WITH CALCULUS (SEE ALSO 'CHOLELITHIASIS')
5th Digit: 574.2
0. WITHOUT OBSTRUCTION
1. WITH OBSTRUCTION

537.4 GASTRIC
537.4 GASTROCOLIC
750.7 GASTROCOLIC CONGENITAL
537.4 GASTROENTEROCOLIC
537.4 GASTROESOPHAGEAL
747.61 GASTROINTESTINAL VESSEL ARTERIOVENOUS CONGENITAL
537.4 GASTROJEJUNAL
537.4 GASTROJEJUNOCOLIC
619.9 GENITAL TRACT FEMALE
619.1 GENITAL TRACT FEMALE - DIGESTIVE TO GENITAL
619.2 GENITAL TRACT FEMALE - GENITAL TRACT TO SKIN
619.0 GENITAL TRACT FEMALE - URINARY TRACT TO GENITAL
619.8 GENITAL TRACT FEMALE - OTHER SPECIFIED
608.89 GENITAL TRACT MALE
510.0 HEPATOPLEURAL
510.0 HEPATOPULMONARY
569.81 ILEORECTAL
569.81 ILEOSIGMOIDAL
569.69 ILEOSTOMY
596.1 ILEOVESICAL
569.81 ILEUM
386.40 INNER EAR
569.81 INTESTINE
569.81 INTESTINOCOLONIC (ABDOMINAL)
593.82 INTESTINOURETERAL
619.1 INTESTINOUTERINE
619.1 INTESTINOVAGINAL
752.49 INTESTINOVAGINAL CONGENITAL
596.1 INTESTINOVESICAL
566 ISCHIORECTAL
569.69 JEJUNOSTOMY
569.81 JEJUNUM

FISTULA (continued)

719.8# JOINT

5th Digit: 719.8

- **0. SITE NOS**
- **1. SHOULDER REGION**
- **2. UPPER ARM (ELBOW) (HUMERUS)**
- **3. FOREARM (RADIUS) (WRIST) (ULNA)**
- **4. HAND (CARPAL) (METACARPAL) (FINGERS)**
- **5. PELVIC REGION (HIP) (BUTTOCK) (FEMUR) AND THIGH**
- **6. LOWER LEG (FIBULA) (KNEE) (PATELLA) (TIBIA)**
- **7. ANKLE AND/OR FOOT (METATARSALS) (TOES) (TARSALS)**
- **8. OTHER**
- **9. MULTIPLE**

593.89 KIDNEY
619.8 LABIUM (MAJUS) (MINUS)
386.40 LABYRINTHINE
386.42 LABYRINTHINE - OVAL WINDOW
386.41 LABYRINTHINE - ROUND WINDOW
386.43 LABYRINTHINE - SEMICIRCULAR CANAL
386.48 LABYRINTHINE - COMBINED SITES
375.61 LACRIMAL
748.3 LARYNGOTRACHEAL
478.79 LARYNX
528.5 LIP
750.25 LIP CONGENITAL
510.0 LUNG
457.8 LYMPHATIC (NODE) (VESSEL)
611.0 MAMILLARY
611.0 MAMMARY GLAND
675.1# MAMMARY GLAND MATERNAL DUE TO PREGNANCY

5th Digit: 675.1

- **0. EPISODE OF CARE NOS OR N/A**
- **1. DELIVERED**
- **2. DELIVERED WITH POSTPARTUM COMPLICATION**
- **3. ANTEPARTUM COMPLICATION**
- **4. POSTPARTUM COMPLICATION**

383.1 MASTOID
473.0 MAXILLARY (SEE ALSO 'SINUSITIS', MAXILLARY)
510.0 MEDIASTINAL
510.0 MEDIASTINOBRONCHIAL
510.0 MEDIASTINOCUTANEOUS
385.89 MIDDLE EAR
528.3 MOUTH
478.1 NASAL (CAVITY) (SEPTUM)
0 NASAL SINUS SEE 'FISTULA' BY SPECIFIED SINUS
478.29 NASOPHARYNX
478.1 NOSE
360.32 OCULAR CAUSING HYPOTONY (POSTINFLAMMATORY) (POST OP) (POST TRAUMATIC)
528.3 ORAL (CUTANEOUS)
749.00 ORAL NASAL WITH CLEFT PALATE (SEE ALSO 'CLEFT' PALATE)
376.10 ORBIT
473.0 OROANTRAL
473.0 OROMAXILLARY
386.42 OVAL WINDOW
619.2 OVIDUCT (EXTERNAL)
526.89 PALATE HARD
528.9 PALATE SOFT
577.8 PANCREATIC
577.8 PANCREATICODUODENAL
527.4 PAROTID GLAND
528.3 PAROTID REGION
569.81 PELVOABDOMINOINTESTINAL
607.89 PENIS
565.1 PERIANAL
423.8 PERICARDIUM
569.81 PERICECAL

FISTULA (continued)

569.81 PERINEORECTAL
608.89 PERINEO-URETHROSCROTAL
599.1 PERINEUM PERINEAL (WITH URETHRAL INVOLVEMENT)
565.1 PERIRECTAL
567.2 PERITONEUM (SEE ALSO 'PERITONITIS')
599.1 PERIURETHRAL
478.29 PHARYNGO-ESOPHAGEAL
478.29 PHARYNX
744.41 PHARYNX BRANCHIAL CLEFT (CONGENITAL)
685.1 PILONIDAL (INFECTED) (RECTUM)
685.0 PILONIDAL WITH ABSCESS
510.0 PLEURA PLEUROCUTANEOUS
510.0 PLEUROCUTANEOUS
423.8 PLEUROPERICARDIAL
510.0 PLEUROPERITONEAL
383.81 POSTAURICULAR
998.6 POSTOPERATIVE (PERSISTENT)
744.46 PREAURICULAR CONGENITAL
602.8 PROSTATE
510.0 PULMONARY
417.0 PULMONARY VESSEL ARTERIOVENOUS
747.3 PULMONARY VESSEL ARTERIOVENOUS CONGENITAL
510.0 PULMONOPERITONEAL
565.1 RECTAL (TO SKIN)
619.1 RECTOLABIAL
569.81 RECTOSIGMOID (INTERCOMMUNICATING)
593.82 RECTOURETERAL
599.1 RECTOURETHRAL
753.8 RECTOURETHRAL CONGENITAL
619.1 RECTOUTERINE
752.3 RECTOUTERINE CONGENITAL
619.1 RECTOVAGINAL
752.49 RECTOVAGINAL CONGENITAL
596.1 RECTOVESICAL
753.8 RECTOVESICAL CONGENITAL
619.1 RECTOVESICOVAGINAL
619.1 RECTOVULVAL
752.49 RECTOVULVAL CONGENITAL
593.89 RENAL
747.62 RENAL VESSEL ARTERIOVENOUS CONGENITAL
743.58 RETINAL VESSEL ARTERIOVENOUS CONGENITAL
383.81 RETROAURICULAR
386.41 ROUND WINDOW
527.4 SALIVARY GLAND
750.24 SALIVARY GLAND CONGENITAL
360.32 SCLERA, CAUSING HYPOTONY (POSTINFLAMMATORY) (POST OP) (POSTTRAUMATIC)
608.89 SCROTUM
386.43 SEMICIRCULAR CANAL
569.81 SIGMOID
596.1 SIGMOID VESICOABDOMINAL
619.1 SIGMOIDOVAGINAL
752.49 SIGMOIDOVAGINAL CONGENITAL
747.29 SINUS OF VALSALVA CONGENITAL
686.9 SKIN (INFECTED)
593.82 SKIN - URETER
619.2 SKIN - VAGINA
473.3 SPHENOIDAL SINUS (SEE ALSO 'SINUSITIS', SPHENOIDAL)
289.59 SPLENOCOLIC
747.82 SPINAL VESSEL ARTERIOVENOUS CONGENITAL
569.81 STERCORAL
537.4 STOMACH OR DUODENUM
527.4 SUBLINGUAL GLAND
750.24 SUBLINGUAL GLAND CONGENITAL
527.4 SUBMAXILLARY GLAND
750.24 SUBMAXILLARY GLAND CONGENITAL
528.3 SUBMAXILLARY REGION
0 SURGICALLY CREATED ARTERIOVENOUS DIALYSIS CATHETER COMPLICATION SEE 'DIALYSIS'
V45.1 SURGICALLY CREATED FOR DIALYSIS (STATUS)

FISTULA (continued)

457.8	THORACIC DUCT
510.0	THORACIC REGION
510.0	THORACICOABDOMINAL
510.0	THORACICOGASTRIC
510.0	THORACICOINTESTINAL
510.0	THORACOABDOMINAL
510.0	THORACOGASTRIC
510.0	THORAX
759.2	THYROGLOSSAL DUCT CONGENITAL
246.8	THYROID
748.3	TRACHEA (CONGENITAL)
530.84	TRACHEOESOPHAGEAL
750.3	TRACHEOESOPHAGEAL CONGENITAL
519.09	TRACHEOESOPHAGEAL FOLLOWING TRACHEOSTOMY
0	TRAUMATIC ARTERIOVENOUS SEE SPECIFIED ARTERY / VEIN INJURY
0	TRAUMATIC BRAIN ARTERIOVENOUS SEE BRAIN / CEREBRAL INJURY BY TYPE
0	TUBERCULOUS SEE 'TUBERCULOUS'
002.0	TYPHOID
759.89	UMBILICAL
753.8	UMBILICO-URINARY
753.7	URACHUS CONGENITAL
593.82	URETERAL (TO SKIN)
593.82	URETEROABDOMINAL
593.82	URETEROCERVICAL
593.82	URETERORECTAL
593.82	URETEROSIGMOIDOABDOMINAL
619.0	URETEROVAGINAL
596.2	URETEROVESICAL
599.1	URETHRAL
753.8	URETHRAL CONGENITAL
599.1	URETHROPERINEAL
596.2	URETHROPERINEOVESICAL
599.1	URETHRORECTAL
753.8	URETHRORECTAL CONGENITAL
608.89	URETHROSCROTAL
619.0	URETHROVAGINAL
596.2	URETHROVESICAL
619.0	URETHROVESICOVAGINAL
599.1	URINARY NOS (PERSISTENT) (RECURRENT)
619.0	URINARY GENITAL TRACT FEMALE
619.2	UTEROABDOMINAL (ANTERIOR WALL)
752.3	UTEROABDOMINAL (ANTERIOR WALL) CONGENITAL
619.1	UTEROENTERIC
619.1	UTEROINTESTINAL
752.3	UTEROINTESTINAL CONGENITAL
619.1	UTERORECTAL
752.3	UTERORECTAL CONGENITAL
619.0	UTEROURETERIC
619.8	UTEROVAGINAL
619.0	UTEROVESICAL
752.3	UTEROVESICAL CONGENITAL
619.2	UTERUS TO ABDOMINAL WALL (SKIN)
619.8	UTERUS OTHER SPECIFIED
619.2	VAGINA (TO SKIN)
619.8	VAGINA OTHER SPECIFIED
619.1	VAGINOILEAL
619.2	VAGINOPERINEAL
596.2	VESICAL FEMALE GENITAL TRACT (BETWEEN)
596.2	VESICAL NEC (FEMALE)
596.2	VESICOABDOMINAL
619.0	VESICOCERVICOVAGINAL
596.1	VESICOCOLIC
596.2	VESICOCUTANEOUS
596.1	VESICOENTERIC
596.1	VESICOINTESTINAL
619.1	VESICOMETRORECTAL
596.2	VESICOPERINEAL
596.1	VESICORECTAL
753.8	VESICORECTAL CONGENITAL

FISTULA (continued)

596.1	VESICOSIGMOIDAL
619.1	VESICOSIGMOIDOVAGINAL
596.2	VESICOURETERAL
619.0	VESICOURETEROVAGINAL
596.2	VESICOURETHRAL
596.1	VESICOURETHRORECTAL
619.0	VESICOUTERINE
752.3	VESICOUTERINE CONGENITAL
619.0	VESICOVAGINAL
619.1	VULVORECTAL
752.49	VULVORECTAL CONGENITAL

780.39	FIT NOS
V68.0	FITNESS CERTIFICATE ISSUE
V52.8	FITTING OTHER SPECIFIED PROSTHETIC DEVICE
098.86	FITZ-HUGH AND CURTIS SYNDROME (GONOCOCCAL PERITONITIS)
577.0	FITZ'S SYNDROME (ACUTE HEMORRHAGIC PANCREATITIS)
736.79	FLACCID FOOT
736.09	FLACCID FOREARM
750.26	FLACCID PALATE CONGENITAL
807.4	FLAIL CHEST
767.3	FLAIL CHEST NEWBORN (BIRTH TRAUMA)
718.8#	FLAIL JOINT

5th Digit: 718.8

- **0. SITE NOS**
- **1. SHOULDER REGION**
- **2. UPPER ARM (ELBOW) (HUMERUS)**
- **3. FOREARM (RADIUS) (WRIST) (ULNA)**
- **4. HAND (CARPAL) (METACARPAL) (FINGERS)**
- **5. PELVIC REGION AND THIGH (HIP) (BUTTOCK) (FEMUR)**
- **6. LOWER LEG (FIBULA) (KNEE) (PATELLA) (TIBIA)**
- **7. ANKLE AND/OR FOOT (METATARSALS) (TOES) (TARSALS)**
- **8. OTHER**
- **9. MULTIPLE**

242.0#	FLAJANI (-BASEDOW) SYNDROME (EXOPHTHALMIC GOITER)

5th Digit: 242.0

- **0. WITHOUT MENTION OF THYROTOXIC CRISIS OR STORM**
- **1. WITH MENTION OF THYROTOXIC CRISIS OR STORM**

FLANK

959.1	INJURY
911.8	INJURY OTHER AND UNSPECIFIED SUPERFICIAL
911.9	INJURY OTHER AND UNSPECIFIED SUPERFICIAL (INFECTED)
789.39	MASS
789.09	PAIN
789.69	TENDERNESS

292.89	FLASHBACK DRUG INDUCED
734	FLAT FOOT ACQUIRED
754.61	FLAT FOOT CONGENITAL
754.61	FLAT FOOT RIGID (EVERTED) (SPASTIC)
341.1	FLATAU SCHILDER DISEASE
787.3	FLATULENCE
787.3	FLATUS
629.8	FLATUS VAGINALIS
504	FLAX DRESSERS' DISEASE
0	FLEA BITE SEE 'INSECT BITE NONVENOMOUS'
732.3	FLEISCHNER'S DISEASE

631 FLESHY MOLE
631 FLESHY MOLE WITH COMPLICATION DURING TREATMENT [639.#]
639.# FLESHY MOLE WITH COMPLICATION FOLLOWING TREATMENT
4th Digit: 639
0. GENITAL TRACT AND PELVIC INFECTION
1. DELAYED OR EXCESSIVE HEMORRHAGE
2. DAMAGE TO PELVIC ORGANS AND TISSUE
3. RENAL FAILURE
4. METABOLIC DISORDERS
5. SHOCK
6. EMBOLISM
8. OTHER SPECIFIED COMPLICATION
9. UNSPECIFIED COMPLICATION

300.11 FLEXIBILITAS CEREA
754.89 FLEXION CONTRACTURES OF LOWER LIMB JOINTS CONGENITAL

004.1 FLEXNERI DYSENTERY - GROUP B SHIGELLA
004.1 FLEXNER'S BACILLUS DIARRHEA DYSENTERY

FLEXOR TENDON LACERATION
727.64 TENDON HAND AND WRIST RUPTURE NONTRAUMATIC
881.22 CARPI RADIALIS
881.20 CARPI RADIALIS PROXIMAL
881.22 CARPI ULNARIS DISTAL
881.20 CARPI ULNARIS PROXIMAL
883.2 DIGITORUM PROFUNDUS FINGER
882.2 DIGITORUM PROFUNDUS HAND
881.20 DIGITORUM PROFUNDUS WRIST
883.2 DIGITORUM SUPERFICIALIS FINGER
882.2 DIGITORUM SUPERFICIALIS HAND
881.20 DIGITORUM SUPERFICIALIS WRIST
891.2 HALLUCIS ANKLE
892.2 HALLUCIS FOOT
893.2 HALLUCIS TOE
893.2 TOE
891.2 TOE ANKLE
892.2 TOE FOOT

502 FLINT DISEASE
379.24 FLOATERS (VITREOUS)

272.2 FLOATING-BETALIPOPROTEINEMIA
756.3 FLOATING RIB
781.9 FLOPPY INFANT SYNDROME
424.0 FLOPPY VALVE SYNDROME (MITRAL)
571.2 FLORID CIRRHOSIS
571.2 FLORID CIRRHOSIS WITH ESOPHAGEAL VARICES [456.2#]
5th Digit: 456.2
0. WITH BLEEDING
1. WITHOUT BLEEDING

FLU
487.# FLU
4th Digit: 487
0. WITH PNEUMONIA (ANY TYPE)
1. UNSPECIFIED OR WITH OTHER REPIRATORY MANIFESTATIONS
8. OTHER MANIFESTATIONS, (GASTROINTESTINAL)
487.1 ASIAN
008.8 GASTROENTERITIS VIRAL NEC
487.8 INTESTINAL
760.2 MATERNAL AFFECTING FETUS OR NEWBORN
771.2 MATERNAL AFFECTING FETUS OR NEWBORN - MANIFESTED IN NEWBORN
487.1 RESPIRATORY
487.0 RESPIRATORY - WITH PNEUMONIA
0 SEE ALSO 'INFLUENZA'
487.8 STOMACH
V04.8 VACCINATION
487.8 OTHER SPECIFIED

FLUID
276.9 DISORDER NEC
276.6 OVERLOAD
789.5 OVERLOAD CAUSING ASCITES
782.3 OVERLOAD WITH LOCALIZED EDEMA
276.6 RETENTION
782.3 RETENTION LOCALIZED EDEMA

FLUKE
120.9 BLOOD
121.9 DISEASE
121.3 LIVER
121.0 LIVER (CAT)
121.1 LIVER (ORIENTAL)
121.3 LIVER (SHEEP)
121.2 LUNG DISEASE (ORIENTAL)

623.5 FLUOR
131.00 FLUOR (VAGINALIS) TRICHOMONAL
V07.31 FLUORIDE ADMINISTRATION PROPHYLACTIC
0 FLUOROQUINOLONES RESISTANT INFECTION SEE 'DRUG RESISTANCE'
V72.5 FLUOROSCOPY
520.3 FLUOROSIS
259.2 FLUSH SYNDROME
782.62 FLUSHING
627.2 FLUSHING MENOPAUSAL
427.32 FLUTTER ATRIAL
427.42 FLUTTER VENTRICULAR
009.0 FLUX
134.0 FLY LARVAE INFESTATION
694.4 FOGA SELVAGEN
336.1 FOIX-ALAJOUANINE (SYNDROME)
281.2 FOLATE-MALABSORPTION CONGENITAL
266.2 FOLIC ACID DEFICIENCY
281.2 FOLIC ACID DEFICIENCY ANEMIA
297.3 FOLIE A DEUX
253.4 FOLLICLE-STIMULATING HORMONE DEFICIENCY
253.1 FOLLICLE-STIMULATING HORMONE OVERPRODUCTION

620.0 FOLLICULAR CYST ATRESIA
620.0 FOLLICULAR CYST OVARIAN

FOLLICULITIS
704.8 UNSPECIFIED
704.8 ABSCEDENS ET SUFFODIENS
704.09 DECALVANS
706.1 KELOID (KELOIDALIS)
704.8 PUSTULAR
701.8 ULERYTHEMATOSA RETICULATA
704.8 OTHER SPECIFIED DISEASES OF HAIR

270.1 FOLLING'S PHENYLKETONURIA

DO NOT CONFUSE FOLLOWUP OR ROUTINE AFTERCARE WITH "COMPLICATIONS." FOLLOWUP EXAMS AND ROUTINE AFTERCARE ARE PLANNED VISITS THAT ARE PART OF THE NORMAL COURSE OF TREATMENT. COMPLICATIONS ARE UNEXPECTED DEVELOPMENTS THAT REQUIRE SUBSEQUENT TREATMENT.

FOLLOWUP EXAM
V67.9 UNSPECIFIED
V67.2 CHEMOTHERAPY
V67.6 COMBINED TREATMENT
V67.4 FRACTURE TREATMENT - HEALED
0 FRACTURE TREATMENT - HEALING OR CURRENT SEE 'AFTERCARE', ORTHOPEDIC

FOLLOWUP EXAM (continued)

ANTIBIOTICS, COUMADIN, DIGOXIN, CHEMOTHERAPY DRUGS, AND ANY OTHER DRUGS WITH A RISK OF ADVERSE REACTIONS ARE CONSIDERED TO BE HIGH-RISK MEDICATIONS. CODES V58.61, V58.62 AND V58.69 ARE TO BE USED TO IDENTIFY PATIENTS THAT ARE CURRENTLY BEING MONITORED WHILE TAKING HIGH RISK MEDICATION. CODE V67.51 IS TO BE USED TO IDENTIFY PATIENTS THAT HAVE COMPLETED HIGH RISK MEDICATION THERAPY.

V67.51 HIGH RISK MEDICATION THERAPY - COMPLETED
V58.62 HIGH RISK MEDICATION ANTIBIOTICS - CURRENT THERAPY
V58.61 HIGH RISK MEDICATION ANTICOAGULANT - CURRENT THERAPY
V58.69 HIGH RISK MEDICATION OTHER - CURRENT THERAPY
V67.59 OTHER TREATMENT NEC
V67.3 PSYCHOTHERAPY AND OTHER TREATMENT
V67.1 RADIOTHERAPY
V67.0 SURGERY

756.89 FONG'S SYNDROME (HEREDITARY OSTEO-ONYCHODYSPLASIA)

117.2 FONSECAEA COMPACTUM INFECTION

117.2 FONSECAEA PEDROSOI INFECTION

FOOD
693.1 ALLERGY DERMATITIS
V65.3 ALLERGY DIETARY COUNSELING AND SURVEILLANCE
0 ANAPHYLACTIC SHOCK SEE 'ANAPHYLAXIS'
933.1 ASPHYXIATION (CHOKING) (ASPIRATION)
994.2 DEPRIVATION
0 INTOXICATION SEE 'FOOD POISONING'
307.59 REFUSAL

FOOD POISONING
005.9 UNSPECIFIED
005.89 BACILLUS CEREUS
005.1 BOTULISM
005.2 C WELCHII
005.2 CLOSTRIDIA PERFRINGENS
005.3 CLOSTRIDIUM
005.1 CLOSTRIDIUM BOTULINUM
989.7 FOOD CONTAMINANTS
988.9 NOXIOUS SUBSTANCE
005.89 OTHER BACTERIAL
988.8 OTHER NOXIOUS
005.89 OTHER SPECIFIED BACTERIUM NEC
003.0 SALMONELLA - GASTROENTERITIS
0 SALMONELLA - WITH OTHER MANIFESTATIONS SEE 'SALMONELLA'
005.0 STAPHYLOCOCCAL TOXEMIA
988.2 TOXIC (BERRIES) (PLANTS)
988.0 TOXIC FISH SHELLFISH
988.1 TOXIC MUSHROOMS
005.4 VIBRIO
005.4 VIBRIO PARAHAEMOLYTICUS
005.81 VIBRIO VULNIFICUS

FOOT
V49.73 ABSENCE
755.31 ABSENCE CONGENITAL
V49.73 AMPUTATION STATUS
078.4 AND MOUTH DISEASE
726.79 BURSA INFECTION
755.67 CONSTRICTION BAND CONGENITAL
736.70 DEFORMITY - NOS (ACQUIRED)
754.70 DEFORMITY - NOS CONGENITAL
736.75 DEFORMITY - CAVOVARUS (ACQUIRED)
754.59 DEFORMITY - CAVOVARUS CONGENITAL
736.79 DEFORMITY - VALGUS (ACQUIRED)
754.60 DEFORMITY - VALGUS CONGENITAL
754.69 DEFORMITY - VALGUS CONGENITAL OTHER NEC

FOOT (continued)
736.79 DEFORMITY - VARUS (ACQUIRED)
754.50 DEFORMITY - VARUS CONGENITAL
754.59 DEFORMITY - VARUS CONGENITAL OTHER NEC
736.79 DEFORMITY - OTHER ACQUIRED NEC
754.79 DEFORMITY - OTHER CONGENITAL NEC
736.79 DROP
959.7 INJURY
917.8 INJURY OTHER AND UNSPECIFIED SUPERFICIAL
917.9 INJURY OTHER AND UNSPECIFIED SUPERFICIAL INFECTED
719.87 JOINT CALCIFICATION
718.97 JOINT LIGAMENT RELAXATION
0 JOINT LIGAMENT TEAR SEE 'SPRAIN'
0 JOINT SEE ALSO 'JOINT'
718.17 LOOSE BODY (JOINT)
581.3 PROCESS DISEASE
0 SEE 'TALIPES'
845.10 SEPARATION (RUPTURE) (TEAR) (LACERATION) UNSPECIFIED SITE
845.10 STRAIN (SPRAIN) (AVULSION) (HEMARTHROSIS) UNSPECIFIED SITE

348.4 FORAMEN MAGNUM SYNDROME

742.3 FORAMEN OF LUSCHKA ATRESIA

742.3 FORAMEN OF MAGENDIE ATRESIA

742.3 FORAMEN OF MUNRO OBSTRUCTION

741.0# FORAMEN OF MUNRO OBSTRUCTION WITH SPINA BIFIDA

5th Digit: 741.0
0. REGION NOS
1. CERVICAL REGION
2. DORSAL (THORACIC REGION)
3. LUMBAR REGION

745.5 FORAMEN OVALE PATENT CONGENITAL

253.1 FORBES-ALBRIGHT SYNDROME (NONPUERPERAL AMENORRHEA AND LACTATION ASSOCIATED WITH PITUITARY TUMOR)

271.0 FORBES' GLYCOGENOSIS III

763.89 FORCED BIRTH

763.2 FORCEPS DELIVERY AFFECTING FETUS OR NEWBORN

0 FORCEPS DELIVERY SEE 'DELIVERY', FORCEPS OR VACUUM

660.7# FORCEPS OR VACUUM EXTRACTOR FAILURE

5th Digit: 660.7
0. EPISODE OF CARE UNSPECIFIED OR N/A
1. DELIVERED
3. ANTEPARTUM COMPLICATION

750.26 FORDYCE'S ECTOPIC SEBACEOUS GLANDS

705.82 FORDYCE-FOX APOCRINE MILIARIA

FOREARM
V49.65 ABSENCE (ACQUIRED)
755.21 ABSENCE CONGENITAL - INCLUDING HAND AND FINGERS
755.25 ABSENCE CONGENITAL - INCLUDING INCOMPLETE ABSENCE DISTAL ELEMENTS
V49.65 AMPUTATION STATUS
736.00 DEFORMITY ACQUIRED
959.3 INJURY
913.8 INJURY OTHER AND UNSPECIFIED SUPERFICIAL
913.9 INJURY OTHER AND UNSPECIFIED SUPERFICIAL INFECTED
841.8 SEPARATION (RUPTURE) (TEAR) (LACERATION) OTHER SPECIFIED SITES
841.8 STRAIN (SPRAIN) (AVULSION) (HEMARTHROSIS)

738.19 FOREHEAD DEFORMITY

756.0 FOREHEAD DEFORMITY CONGENITAL

959.09 FOREHEAD INJURY

FOREIGN BODIES; CAN BE SUPERFICIAL (IE. SUCH AS A SPLINTER), CAN PENETRATE THROUGH AN OPEN WOUND, CAN ENTER THROUGH AN ORIFICE, OR CAN BE OLD OR RESIDUAL. OLD OR RESIDUAL FOREIGN BODIES ARE FOUND UNDER FOREIGN BODY, "OLD". GRANULOMAS FROM A RETAINED FOREIGN BODY ARE FOUND UNDER "FOREIGN BODY", GRANULOMA AND "GRANULOMA".

FOREIGN BODY

919.6 SITE NOS SUPERFICIAL
919.7 SITE NOS SUPERFICIAL INFECTED
879.5 ABDOMINAL WALL LATERAL THROUGH OPEN WOUND
911.6 ABDOMINAL WALL SUPERFICIAL
911.7 ABDOMINAL WALL SUPERFICIAL INFECTED
879.3 ABDOMINAL WALL THROUGH OPEN WOUND
998.4 ACCIDENTALLY LEFT DURING A PROCEDURE
870.4 ADNEXA (PENETRATING)
938 ALIMENTARY TRACT NOS
916.6 ANKLE SUPERFICIAL
916.7 ANKLE SUPERFICIAL INFECTED
891.1 ANKLE THROUGH OPEN WOUND
911.6 ANUS SUPERFICIAL
911.7 ANUS SUPERFICIAL INFECTED
879.7 ANUS THROUGH OPEN WOUND
937 ANUS THROUGH ORIFICE
936 APPENDIX THROUGH ORIFICE
912.6 ARM (UPPER) SUPERFICIAL
912.7 ARM (UPPER) SUPERFICIAL INFECTED
880.13 ARM (UPPER) THROUGH OPEN WOUND
884.1 ARM MULTIPLE THROUGH OPEN WOUND
872.12 AUDITORY CANAL THROUGH OPEN WOUND
931 AUDITORY CANAL THROUGH ORIFICE
912.6 AXILLA SUPERFICIAL
912.7 AXILLA SUPERFICIAL INFECTED
880.12 AXILLA (AREA) THROUGH OPEN WOUND
911.6 BACK SUPERFICIAL
911.7 BACK SUPERFICIAL INFECTED
876.1 BACK THROUGH OPEN WOUND
939.0 BLADDER THROUGH ORIFICE
733.99 BONE - OLD
911.6 BREAST SUPERFICIAL
911.7 BREAST SUPERFICIAL INFECTED
879.1 BREAST THROUGH OPEN WOUND
934.8 BRONCHIOLE THROUGH ORIFICE
934.1 BRONCHUS THROUGH ORIFICE
873.71 BUCCAL MUCOSA THROUGH OPEN WOUND
911.6 BUTTOCK SUPERFICIAL
911.7 BUTTOCK SUPERFICIAL INFECTED
877.1 BUTTOCK THROUGH OPEN WOUND
916.6 CALF SUPERFICIAL
916.7 CALF SUPERFICIAL INFECTED
891.1 CALF THROUGH OPEN WOUND
930.1 CANTHUS (EXTERNAL) THROUGH ORIFICE
936 CECUM THROUGH ORIFICE
910.6 CHEEK SUPERFICIAL
910.7 CHEEK SUPERFICIAL INFECTED
873.51 CHEEK THROUGH OPEN WOUND
911.6 CHEST WALL SUPERFICIAL
911.7 CHEST WALL SUPERFICIAL INFECTED
875.1 CHEST WALL THROUGH OPEN WOUND
873.54 CHIN THROUGH OPEN WOUND
872.74 COCHLEA THROUGH OPEN WOUND
936 COLON THROUGH ORIFICE
930.1 CONJUNCTIVA (EXTERNAL) THROUGH ORIFICE
930.0 CORNEA (EXTERNAL) THROUGH ORIFICE
875.1 COSTAL REGION THROUGH OPEN WOUND
936 DUODENUM THROUGH ORIFICE

FOREIGN BODY (continued)

EAR

872.9 NOS THROUGH OPEN WOUND
931 NOS THROUGH ORIFICE
872.12 AUDITORY CANAL THROUGH OPEN WOUND
872.11 AURICLE THROUGH OPEN WOUND
872.71 DRUM THROUGH OPEN WOUND
872.10 EXTERNAL NOS THROUGH OPEN WOUND
385.83 MIDDLE (MASTOID) RETAINED
872.79 MULTIPLE SITES THROUGH OPEN WOUND
872.11 PINNA THROUGH OPEN WOUND
910.6 SUPERFICIAL
910.7 SUPERFICIAL INFECTED
872.79 OTHER SPECIFIED AND MULTIPLE SITES

FOREIGN BODY (continued)

881.11 ELBOW
913.6 ELBOW SUPERFICIAL
913.7 ELBOW SUPERFICIAL INFECTED
874.5 ESOPHAGUS CERVICAL THROUGH OPEN WOUND
935.1 ESOPHAGUS THROUGH ORIFICE
872.73 EUSTACHIAN TUBE

EYE

930.1 CANTHUS (EXTERNAL) THROUGH ORIFICE
930.1 CONJUNCTIVA (EXTERNAL) THROUGH ORIFICE
930.0 CORNEA (EXTERNAL) THROUGH ORIFICE
930.9 EXTERNAL THROUGH ORIFICE
930.8 EXTERNAL THROUGH ORIFICE OTHER AND COMBINED SITES
930.2 LACRIMAL PUNCTUM (EXTERNAL)

EYE MAGNETIC

871.5 ACUTE EYEBALL CURRENT PENETRATING
360.51 ANTERIOR CHAMBER (OLD)
360.50 GLOBE (OLD)
360.50 INTRAOCULAR (OLD)
360.52 IRIS OR CILIARY BODY (OLD)
360.53 LENS (OLD)
360.55 POSTERIOR WALL (OLD)
360.55 RETINA (OLD)
360.54 VITREOUS (OLD)
360.59 OTHER OR MULTIPLE SITES (OLD)

EYE NONMAGNETIC

871.6 ACUTE EYEBALL CURRENT PENETRATING
360.61 ANTERIOR CHAMBER (OLD)
360.60 GLOBE (OLD)
360.60 INTRAOCULAR (OLD)
360.62 IRIS OR CILIARY BODY (OLD)
360.63 LENS (OLD)
360.65 POSTERIOR WALL (OLD)
360.65 RETINA (OLD)
376.6 RETROBULBAR (OLD)
360.64 VITREOUS (OLD)
360.69 OTHER OR MULTIPLE SITES (OLD)

FOREIGN BODY (continued)

873.52 EYEBROW THROUGH OPEN WOUND
930.1 EYELID (EXTERNAL) THROUGH ORIFICE
918.0 EYELID AND PERIOCULAR AREA SUPERFICIAL
374.86 EYELID RETAINED
910.6 FACE SUPERFICIAL
910.7 FACE SUPERFICIAL INFECTED
873.50 FACE THROUGH OPEN WOUND
873.59 FACE OTHER AND MULTIPLE SITES THROUGH OPEN WOUND

FOREIGN BODY (continued)

883.1	FINGER
915.6	FINGER SUPERFICIAL
915.7	FINGER SUPERFICIAL INFECTED
879.5	FLANK
911.6	FLANK SUPERFICIAL
911.7	FLANK SUPERFICIAL INFECTED
892.1	FOOT
917.6	FOOT SUPERFICIAL
917.7	FOOT SUPERFICIAL INFECTED
881.10	FOREARM
913.6	FOREARM SUPERFICIAL
913.7	FOREARM SUPERFICIAL INFECTED
873.52	FOREHEAD
878.9	GENITALIA THROUGH OPEN WOUND
938	GI TRACT THROUGH ORIFICE
728.82	GRANULOMA - MUSCLE
709.4	GRANULOMA - SKIN
728.82	GRANULOMA - SOFT TISSUE NEC
709.4	GRANULOMA - SUBCUTANEOUS TISSUE
911.6	GROIN SUPERFICIAL
911.7	GROIN SUPERFICIAL INFECTED
939.9	GU TRACT SITE THROUGH ORIFICE
910.6	GUM SUPERFICIAL
910.7	GUM SUPERFICIAL INFECTED
873.72	GUM THROUGH OPEN WOUND
914.6	HAND SUPERFICIAL
914.7	HAND SUPERFICIAL INFECTED
882.1	HAND THROUGH OPEN WOUND
873.9	HEAD THROUGH OPEN WOUND
892.1	HEEL
917.6	HEEL SUPERFICIAL
917.7	HEEL SUPERFICIAL INFECTED
890.1	HIP
916.6	HIP SUPERFICIAL
916.7	HIP SUPERFICIAL INFECTED
936	ILEUM THROUGH ORIFICE
938	INGESTED
V71.8	INGESTION SUSPECTED (UNDIAGNOSED) (UNPROVEN)
0	INTERPHALANGEAL SEE 'FOREIGN BODY', FINGER
911.6	INTERSCAPULAR REGION SUPERFICIAL
911.7	INTERSCAPULAR REGION SUPERFICIAL INFECTED
936	INTESTINE THROUGH ORIFICE
871.5	INTRAOCULAR PENETRATION MAGNETIC
871.6	INTRAOCULAR PENETRATION NONMAGNETIC
934.8	INTRAPULMONARY THROUGH ORIFICE
873.54	JAW THROUGH OPEN WOUND
916.6	KNEE SUPERFICIAL
916.7	KNEE SUPERFICIAL INFECTED
891.1	KNEE THROUGH OPEN WOUND
911.6	LABIA SUPERFICIAL
911.7	LABIA SUPERFICIAL INFECTED
878.5	LABIA THROUGH OPEN WOUND
930.2	LACRIMAL PUNCTUM (EXTERNAL) THROUGH ORIFICE
874.11	LARYNX THROUGH OPEN WOUND
933.1	LARYNX THROUGH ORIFICE
874.10	LARYNX WITH TRACHEA THROUGH OPEN WOUND
908.5	LATE EFFECT IN ORIFICE
906.2	LATE EFFECT SUPERFICIAL
916.6	LEG SUPERFICIAL
916.7	LEG SUPERFICIAL INFECTED
891.1	LEG THROUGH OPEN WOUND
910.6	LIP SUPERFICIAL
910.7	LIP SUPERFICIAL INFECTED
873.53	LIP THROUGH OPEN WOUND
894.1	LOWER LIMB MULTIPLE
934.8	LUNG THROUGH ORIFICE
0	METACARPAL SEE 'FOREIGN BODY', HAND
873.79	MOUTH OTHER AND MULTIPLE SITES THROUGH OPEN WOUND
873.70	MOUTH THROUGH OPEN WOUND
935.0	MOUTH THROUGH ORIFICE

F

FOREIGN BODY (continued)

919.6	MULTIPLE SUPERFICIAL
919.7	MULTIPLE SUPERFICIAL INFECTED
879.9	MULTIPLE THROUGH OPEN WOUND
729.6	MUSCLE - OLD
728.82	MUSCLE - OLD WITH GRANULOMA
933.0	NASOPHARYNX THROUGH ORIFICE
910.6	NECK SUPERFICIAL
910.7	NECK SUPERFICIAL INFECTED
874.9	NECK THROUGH OPEN WOUND
873.32	NOSE (CAVITY) THROUGH OPEN WOUND
873.39	NOSE (MULTIPLE SITES) THROUGH OPEN WOUND
873.31	NOSE (SEPTUM) THROUGH OPEN WOUND COMPLICATED
873.33	NOSE (SINUS) THROUGH OPEN WOUND
910.6	NOSE SUPERFICIAL
910.7	NOSE SUPERFICIAL INFECTED
873.30	NOSE THROUGH OPEN WOUND
932	NOSE THROUGH ORIFICE
932	NOSTRIL THROUGH ORIFICE
870.4	OCULAR ADNEXA (PENETRATING)
376.6	OCULAR MUSCLE OLD (RESIDUAL)
733.99	OLD BONE - GRANULOMA
733.99	OLD BONE - RESIDUAL
0	OLD EYE SEE 'FOREIGN BODY', EYE
374.86	OLD EYELID - RESIDUAL
385.82	OLD MIDDLE EAR - GRANULOMA
385.83	OLD MIDDLE EAR - RESIDUAL
729.6	OLD MUSCLE
728.82	OLD MUSCLE - GRANULOMA
376.6	OLD OCULAR MUSCLE
376.6	OLD RETROBULBAR
729.6	OLD SKIN
709.4	OLD SKIN GRANULOMA
729.6	OLD SOFT TISSUE
728.82	OLD SOFT TISSUE - GRANULOMA MUSCLE
709.4	OLD SOFT TISSUE - GRANULOMA SKIN SUBCUTANEOUS TISSUE
729.6	OLD SUBCUTANEOUS
709.4	OLD SUBCUTANEOUS - GRANULOMA
870.4	ORBIT (PENETRATING)
376.6	ORBIT RETAINED / OLD (PENETRATING)
872.72	OSSICLES (EAR)
873.75	PALATE THROUGH OPEN WOUND
879.7	PELVIC AREA THROUGH OPEN WOUND
911.6	PENIS SUPERFICIAL
911.7	PENIS SUPERFICIAL INFECTED
878.1	PENIS THROUGH OPEN WOUND
939.3	PENIS THROUGH ORIFICE
911.6	PERINEUM SUPERFICIAL
911.7	PERINEUM SUPERFICIAL INFECTED
933.0	PHARYNX THROUGH ORIFICE
874.5	PHARYNX THROUGH OPEN WOUND
872.11	PINNA THROUGH OPEN WOUND
937	RECTOSIGMOID THROUGH ORIFICE
937	RECTUM THROUGH ORIFICE
376.6	OCULAR MUSCLE OLD (RESIDUAL)
733.99	RESIDUAL BONE
374.86	RESIDUAL EYELID
385.83	RESIDUAL MIDDLE EAR
729.6	RESIDUAL MUSCLE
728.82	RESIDUAL MUSCLE - GRANULOMA
376.6	RESIDUAL RETROBULBAR
729.6	RESIDUAL SKIN
709.4	RESIDUAL SKIN - GRANULOMA
729.6	RESIDUAL SOFT TISSUE
728.82	RESIDUAL SOFT TISSUE - GRANULOMA MUSCLE
709.4	RESIDUAL SOFT TISSUE - GRANULOMA SKIN SUBCUTANEOUS TISSUE
729.6	RESIDUAL SUBCUTANEOUS
709.4	RESIDUAL SUBCUTANEOUS - GRANULOMA
934.9	RESPIRATORY THROUGH ORIFICE
376.6	RETROBULBAR (PENETRATING) (OLD)

FOREIGN BODY (continued)

873.1 SCALP
910.6 SCALP SUPERFICIAL
910.7 SCALP SUPERFICIAL INFECTED
880.11 SCAPULAR AREA
912.6 SCAPULAR REGION SUPERFICIAL
912.7 SCAPULAR REGION SUPERFICIAL INFECTED
911.6 SCROTUM SUPERFICIAL
911.7 SCROTUM SUPERFICIAL INFECTED
878.3 SCROTUM THROUGH OPEN WOUND
880.10 SHOULDER
880.19 SHOULDER AND ARM MULTIPLE SITES
912.6 SHOULDER SUPERFICIAL
912.7 SHOULDER SUPERFICIAL INFECTED
932 SINUS (FRONT) (MAX) (ETHMOID) (NASAL) THROUGH ORIFICE
729.6 SKIN - OLD
709.4 SKIN - OLD WITH GRANULOMA
729.6 SOFT TISSUE - OLD (RESIDUAL)
728.82 SOFT TISSUE - OLD WITH GRANULOMA MUSCLE
709.4 SOFT TISSUE - OLD WITH GRANULOMA SKIN SUBCUTANEOUS TISSUE
935.2 STOMACH THROUGH ORIFICE
729.6 SUBCUTANEOUS - OLD
709.4 SUBCUTANEOUS - OLD WITH GRANULOMA
938 SWALLOWED
727.89 TENDON SHEATH (OLD) (RESIDUAL)
911.6 TESTIS SUPERFICIAL
911.7 TESTIS SUPERFICIAL INFECTED
890.1 THIGH
916.6 THIGH SUPERFICIAL
916.7 THIGH SUPERFICIAL INFECTED
910.6 THROAT SUPERFICIAL
910.7 THROAT SUPERFICIAL INFECTED
933.0 THROAT THROUGH ORIFICE
883.1 THUMB
915.6 THUMB SUPERFICIAL
915.7 THUMB SUPERFICIAL INFECTED
874.3 THYROID GLAND THROUGH OPEN WOUND
893.1 TOE
917.6 TOE SUPERFICIAL
917.7 TOE SUPERFICIAL INFECTED
873.74 TONGUE THROUGH OPEN WOUND
874.12 TRACHEA THROUGH OPEN WOUND
934.0 TRACHEA THROUGH ORIFICE
879.7 TRUNK
872.71 TYMPANIC MEMBRANE
939.0 URETHRA THROUGH ORIFICE
939.1 UTERUS THROUGH ORIFICE
911.6 VAGINA SUPERFICIAL
911.7 VAGINA SUPERFICIAL INFECTED
878.7 VAGINA THROUGH OPEN WOUND
939.2 VAGINA THROUGH ORIFICE
911.6 VULVA SUPERFICIAL
911.7 VULVA SUPERFICIAL INFECTED
878.5 VULVA THROUGH OPEN WOUND
939.2 VULVA THROUGH ORIFICE
881.12 WRIST
913.6 WRIST SUPERFICIAL
913.7 WRIST SUPERFICIAL INFECTED
919.6 OTHER SITES SUPERFICIAL
919.7 OTHER SITES SUPERFICIAL INFECTED

605 FORESKIN TIGHT
V20.2 FORMULA CHECK
100.89 FORT BRAGG FEVER
745.5 FOSSA OVALIS DEFECT CONGENITAL
V61.29 FOSTER CHILD PROBLEM (REASON FOR ENCOUNTER)
377.04 FOSTER KENNEDY SYNDROME
350.1 FOTHERGILL'S NEURALGIA
034.1 FOTHERGILL'S SCARLATINA ANGINOSA
V20.0 FOUNDLING SUPERVISION
079.81 FOUR CORNERS VIRUS
608.83 FOURNIER'S DISEASE
378.53 FOURTH CRANIAL NERVE DISORDER (ATROPHY) (PALSY)
951.1 FOURTH CRANIAL NERVE INJURY
664.3# FOURTH DEGREE LACERATION (PERINEAL)

5th Digit: 664.3

0. EPISODE OF CARE UNSPECIFIED OR N/A
1. DELIVERED
4. POSTPARTUM COMPLICATION

057.8 FOURTH DISEASE
743.55 FOVEA CENTRALIS ABSENCE
344.89 FOVILLE'S SYNDROME (PEDUNCULAR)
705.82 FOX FORDYCE APOCRINE MILIARIA
684 FOX'S IMPETIGO (CONTAGIOSA)

COMPOUND FRACTURE IS A FRACTURE (BONE) OPEN.

WHEN YOU HAVE A FRACTURE/DISLOCATION OF A BONE SITE, CODE ONLY THE FRACTURE. DISLOCATION OF THE FRACTURE SITE IS INCLUDED IN THE FRACTURE CODE.

FRACTURE

829.0 BONE(S) NOS CLOSED
829.1 BONE(S) NOS OPEN
808.0 ACETABULUM CLOSED
808.1 ACETABULUM OPEN
811.01 ACROMION CLOSED
811.11 ACROMION OPEN
802.8 ALVEOLUS CLOSED
802.9 ALVEOLUS OPEN

ANKLE

824.8 NOS CLOSED
824.9 NOS OPEN
824.4 BIMALLEOLAR CLOSED
824.5 BIMALLEOLAR OPEN
825.21 BONE CLOSED
825.31 BONE OPEN
824.2 LATERAL MALLEOLUS CLOSED
824.3 LATERAL MALLEOLUS OPEN
824.0 MEDIAL MALLEOLUS CLOSED
824.1 MEDIAL MALLEOLUS OPEN
824.4 POTT'S CLOSED
824.5 POTT'S OPEN
824.6 TRIMALLEOLAR CLOSED
824.7 TRIMALLEOLAR OPEN

FRACTURE (continued)

0 ANTRUM SEE 'FRACTURE' SKULL BASILAR
818.0 ARM AND FOREARM MULTIPLE SITES CLOSED
818.1 ARM AND FOREARM MULTIPLE SITES OPEN
819.0 ARMS BOTH (ANY BONES) CLOSED
819.1 ARMS BOTH (ANY BONES) OPEN
812.20 ARM(S) UPPER NOS CLOSED
812.30 ARM(S) UPPER NOS OPEN
828.0 ARM(S) WITH LEG(S) MULTIPLE CLOSED
828.1 ARM(S) WITH LEG(S) MULTIPLE OPEN
819.0 ARM(S) WITH RIB(S) AND/OR STERNUM CLOSED
819.1 ARM(S) WITH RIB(S) AND/OR STERNUM OPEN
825.21 ASTRAGALUS CLOSED
825.31 ASTRAGALUS OPEN
0 BARTON'S SEE 'FRACTURE', RADIUS DISTAL
815.01 BENNETT'S CLOSED
815.11 BENNETT'S OPEN
824.4 BIMALLEOLAR CLOSED
824.5 BIMALLEOLAR OPEN
767.3 BONE (LONG BONE) BIRTH TRAUMA

F

FRACTURE (continued)

825.0 CALCANEUS CLOSED
825.1 CALCANEUS OPEN
814.07 CAPITATE CLOSED
814.17 CAPITATE OPEN
812.49 CAPITELLUM (HUMERUS) CLOSED
812.59 CAPITELLUM (HUMERUS) OPEN
814.## CARPAL
4th Digit: 814
0. CLOSED
1. OPEN
5th Digit: 814
0. UNSPECIFIED
1. NAVICULAR (SCAPHOID)
2. LUNATE (SEMILUNAR)
3. TRIQUETRAL (CUNEIFORM)
4. PISIFORM
5. TRAPEZIUM (LARGER MULTANGULAR)
6. TRAPEZOID (SMALLER MULTANGULAR)
7. CAPITATE (OS MAGNUM)
8. HAMMATE (UNCIFORM)
9. OTHER

806.## CERVICAL WITH SPINAL CORD INJURY
4th Digit: 806
0. CLOSED
1. OPEN
5th Digit: 806
0. C1-C4 WITH CORD INJURY UNSPECIFIED
1. C1-C4 WITH COMPLETE CORD LESION
2. C1-C4 WITH ANTERIOR CORD SYNDROME
3. C1-C4 WITH CENTRAL CORD LESION
4. C1-C4 WITH INCOMPLETE CORD LESION UNSPECIFIED OR POSTERIOR CORD SYNDROME
5. C5-C7 WITH CORD INJURY UNSPECIFIED
6. C5-C7 COMPLETE LESION OF CORD
7. C5-C7 WITH ANTERIOR CORD SYNDROME
8. C5-C7 WITH CENTRAL CORD SYNDROME
9. C5-C7 WITH INCOMPLETE CORD LESION UNSPECIFIED OR POSTERIOR CORD SYNDROME

805.## CERVICAL WITHOUT SPINAL CORD INJURY
4th Digit: 805
0. CLOSED
1. OPEN
5th Digit: 805
0. LEVEL UNSPECIFIED
1. C1
2. C2
3. C3
4. C4
5. C5
6. C6
7. C7
8. MULTIPLE

813.43 CHAUFFEUR'S CLOSED
813.53 CHAUFFEUR'S OPEN
810.## CLAVICLE
4th Digit: 810
0. CLOSED
1. OPEN
5th Digit: 810
0. SITE UNSPECIFIED
1. STERNAL END
2. SHAFT
3. DISTAL OR ACROMIAL END

767.2 CLAVICLE BIRTH TRAUMA
805.6 COCCYX CLOSED
806.6# COCCYX CLOSED WITH CORD INJURY
5th Digit: 806.6
0. CORD INJURY UNSPECIFIED
1. COMPLETE CAUDA EQUINA INJURY
2. OTHER CAUDA EQUINA INJURY
9. WITH OTHER SPINAL CORD INJURY

FRACTURE (continued)

665.6# COCCYX OBSTETRICAL TRAUMA
5th Digit: 665.6
0. EPISODE OF CARE UNSPECIFIED OR N/A
1. DELIVERED
4. POSTPARTUM COMPLICATION

805.7 COCCYX OPEN
806.7# COCCYX OPEN WITH CORD INJURY
5th Digit: 806.7
0. CORD INJURY UNSPECIFIED
1. COMPLETE CAUDA EQUINA INJURY
2. OTHER CAUDA EQUINA INJURY
9. WITH OTHER SPINAL CORD INJURY

0 COLLAR BONE SEE 'FRACTURE', CLAVICLE
813.41 COLLES' CLOSED
813.51 COLLES' OPEN

COMPOUND FRACTURE IS A FRACTURE (BONE) OPEN.

0 COMPRESSION SEE 'FRACTURE', BY SITE OR 'FRACTURE', PATHOLOGICAL BY SITE
756.9 CONGENITAL
V66.4 CONVALESCENCE
811.02 CORACOID CLOSED
811.12 CORACOID OPEN
813.02 CORONOID (ULNA) CLOSED
813.12 CORONOID (ULNA) OPEN
0 COSTOCHONDRAL JUNCTION SEE 'FRACTURE' RIBS
0 COSTOSTERNAL JUNCTION SEE 'FRACTURE' RIBS
807.5 CRICOID CARTILAGE CLOSED
807.6 CRICOID CARTILAGE OPEN
825.23 CUBOID CLOSED
825.33 CUBOID OPEN
825.24 CUNEIFORM FOOT CLOSED
825.34 CUNEIFORM FOOT OPEN
814.03 CUNEIFORM WRIST CLOSED
814.13 CUNEIFORM WRIST OPEN
0 DEPRESSED SEE 'FRACTURE', BY SITE CLOSED OR OPEN
806.2# DORSAL OR DORSOLUMBAR WITH SPINAL CORD INJURY CLOSED
806.3# DORSAL OR DORSOLUMBAR WITH SPINAL CORD INJURY OPEN
5th Digit: 806.2-3
0. T1-T6 WITH CORD INJURY UNSPECIFIED
1. T1-T6 WITH COMPLETE LESION OF CORD
2. T1-T6 WITH ANTERIOR CORD SYNDROME
3. T1-T6 WITH CENTRAL CORD SYNDROME
4. T1-T6 WITH INCOMPLETE CORD LESION UNSPECIFIED OR POSTERIOR CORD SYNDROME
5. T7-T12 WITH CORD INJURY UNSPECIFIED
6. T7-T12 WITH COMPLETE LESION OF CORD
7. T7-T12 WITH ANTERIOR CORD SYNDROME
8. T7-T12 WITH CENTRAL CORD SYNDROME
9. T7-T12 WITH SPINAL CORD LESION UNSPECIFIED OR POSTERIOR CORD SYNDROME

805.2 DORSAL OR DORSOLUMBAR WITHOUT SPINAL CORD INJURY CLOSED
805.3 DORSAL OR DORSOLUMBAR WITHOUT SPINAL CORD INJURY OPEN

824.4 DUPUYTREN'S ANKLE OR FIBULA CLOSED
824.5 DUPUYTREN'S ANKLE OR FIBULA OPEN
813.42 DUPUYTREN'S RADIUS CLOSED
813.52 DUPUYTREN'S RADIUS OPEN

808.41 DUVERNEY'S CLOSED
808.51 DUVERNEY'S OPEN

812.40 ELBOW CLOSED
812.50 ELBOW OPEN

FRACTURE (continued)

812.42 EPICONDYLAR LATERAL (HUMERUS) CLOSED
812.52 EPICONDYLAR LATERAL (HUMERUS) OPEN
812.43 EPICONDYLAR MEDIAL (HUMERUS) CLOSED
812.53 EPICONDYLAR MEDIAL (HUMERUS) OPEN

0 ETHMOID SINUS SEE 'FRACTURE', SKULL BASILAR

804.## FACIAL BONES MULTIPLE

4th Digit: 804

0. CLOSED WITHOUT INTRACRANIAL INJURY
1. CLOSED WITH CEREBRAL LACERATION AND/OR CONTUSION
2. CLOSED WITH SUBARACHNOID SUBDURAL EXTRADURAL HEMORRHAGE
3. CLOSED WITH OTHER AND UNSPECIFIED INTRACRANIAL HEMORRHAGE
4. CLOSED WITH INTRACRANIAL INJURY OF OTHER AND UNSPECIFIED NATURE
5. OPEN WITHOUT MENTION OF INTRACRANIAL INJURY
6. OPEN WITH CEREBRAL LACERATION AND CONTUSION
7. OPEN WITH SUBARACHNOID SUBDURAL AND EXTRADURAL HEMORRHAGE
8. OPEN WITH OTHER AND UNSPECIFIED INTRACRANIAL HEMORRHAGE
9. OPEN WITH INTRACRANIAL INJURY OF OTHER AND UNSPECIFIED

5th Digit: 804

0. LEVEL OF CONSCIOUSNESS UNSPECIFIED
1. NO LOC
2. LOC < 1 HR
3. LOC 1 - 24 HRS
4. LOC > 24 HRS WITH RETURN TO PRIOR LEVEL
5. LOC > 24 HRS WITHOUT RETURN TO PRIOR LEVEL: OR DEATH BEFORE REGAINING CONSCIOUSNESS, REGARDLESS OF DURATION OF LOC
6. LOC DURATION UNSPECIFIED
9. WITH CONCUSSION UNSPECIFIED

802.8 FACIAL BONES OTHER CLOSED
802.9 FACIAL BONES OTHER OPEN

FEMUR CLOSED

821.00 UNSPECIFIED
820.03 CERVICOTROCHANTERIC
821.21 CONDYLE
821.20 DISTAL
821.22 DISTAL EPIPHYSIS
821.29 DISTAL MULTIPLE
820.20 EXTRACAPSULAR
820.09 HEAD
820.21 INTERTROCHANTERIC
820.00 INTRACAPSULAR
820.21 INTRATROCHANTERIC
820.02 MIDCERVICAL
820.8 NECK NOS
820.03 NECK BASE
820.09 NECK OTHER AREA
820.20 PERITROCHANTERIC
820.01 PROXIMAL EPIPHYSIS
821.01 SHAFT
820.09 SUBCAPITAL
820.22 SUBTROCHANTERIC
821.23 SUPRACONDYLAR
820.02 TRANSCERVICAL
820.01 TRANSEPIPHYSEAL
820.20 TROCHANTERIC
821.21 T-SHAPED INTO KNEE JOINT

FEMUR OPEN

821.10 UNSPECIFIED
820.13 CERVICOTROCHANTERIC
821.31 CONDYLE

FRACTURE (continued)

FEMUR OPEN (continued)

821.30 DISTAL
821.32 DISTAL EPIPHYSIS
821.39 DISTAL MULTIPLE
820.30 EXTRACAPSULAR
820.19 HEAD
820.31 INTERTROCHANTERIC
820.10 INTRACAPSULAR
820.31 INTRATROCHANTERIC
820.12 MIDCERVICAL
820.9 NECK NOS
820.13 NECK BASE
820.19 NECK OTHER AREA
820.30 PERITROCHANTERIC
820.11 PROXIMAL EPIPHYSIS
821.11 SHAFT
820.19 SUBCAPITAL
820.32 SUBTROCHANTERIC
821.33 SUPRACONDYLAR
820.12 TRANSCERVICAL
820.11 TRANSEPIPHYSEAL
820.30 TROCHANTERIC
821.31 T-SHAPED INTO KNEE JOINT

FRACTURE (continued)

823.## FIBULA AND/OR TIBIA

4th Digit: 823

0. PROXIMAL (HEAD) (PLATEAU) CLOSED
1. PROXIMAL (HEAD) (PLATEAU) OPEN
2. SHAFT CLOSED
3. SHAFT OPEN
8. SITE UNSPECIFIED CLOSED
9. SITE UNSPECIFIED OPEN

5th Digit: 823

0. TIBIA ALONE
1. FIBULA ALONE
2. TIBIA WITH FIBULA

824.8 FIBULA DISTAL END OR EPIPHYSIS CLOSED
824.9 FIBULA DISTAL END OR EPIPHYSIS OPEN
824.2 FIBULA INVOLVING ANKLE CLOSED
824.3 FIBULA INVOLVING ANKLE OPEN
816.## FINGER OR THUMB

4th Digit: 816

0. CLOSED
1. OPEN

5th Digit: 816

0. SITE UNSPECIFIED
1. MIDDLE OR PROXIMAL
2. DISTAL
3. MULTIPLE SITES

817.0 FINGER WITH METACARPAL BONES CLOSED
817.1 FINGER WITH METACARPAL BONES OPEN
807.4 FLAIL CHEST
825.## FOOT (EXCEPT TOES)

4th Digit: 825

2. CLOSED
3. OPEN

5th Digit: 825

0. UNSPECIFIED BONE(S) OF FOOT (EXCEPT TOES)
1. ASTRAGALUS
2. NAVICULAR (SCAPHOID) FOOT
3. CUBOID
4. CUNEIFORM FOOT
5. METATARSAL BONE(S)
9. OTHER

825.20 FOOT INSTEP CLOSED
825.30 FOOT INSTEP OPEN
827.0 FOOT INSTEP WITH TOE(S) CLOSED
827.1 FOOT INSTEP WITH TOE(S) OPEN
825.29 FOOT SESAMOID CLOSED
825.39 FOOT SESAMOID OPEN

FRACTURE (continued)

813.80 FOREARM NOS CLOSED
813.90 FOREARM NOS OPEN
813.40 FOREARM DISTAL CLOSED
813.50 FOREARM DISTAL OPEN
813.## FOREARM PROXIMAL (UPPER)

4th Digit: 813

0. CLOSED
1. OPEN

5th Digit: 813

0. UPPER END OF FOREARM UNSPECIFIED
1. OLECRANON PROCESS OF ULNA
2. CORONOID PROCESS OF ULNA
3. MONTEGGIA'S FRACTURE
4. OTHER AND UNSPECIFIED FRACTURES OF PROXIMAL END OF ULNA (ALONE)
5. HEAD OF RADIUS
6. NECK OF RADIUS
7. OTHER AND UNSPECIFIED FRACTURES OF PROXIMAL END OF RADIUS (ALONE)
8. RADIUS WITH ULNA UPPER END (ANY PART)

813.20 FOREARM SHAFT CLOSED
813.30 FOREARM SHAFT OPEN
0 FOSSA (ANTERIOR) (MIDDLE) (POSTERIOR) SEE 'FRACTURE', SKULL BASILAR

0 FRONTAL BONE SEE 'FRACTURE', SKULL VAULT
0 FRONTAL SINUS SEE 'FRACTURE', SKULL BASILAR

813.42 GALEAZZI'S CLOSED
813.52 GALEAZZI'S OPEN
811.03 GLENOID CLOSED
811.13 GLENOID OPEN
0 GOSSELIN'S SEE 'FRACTURE', ANKLE
0 GREENSTICK SEE 'FRACTURE' BY SITE
812.21 GRENADE-THROWERS' CLOSED
812.31 GRENADE-THROWERS' OPEN
0 GUNSHOT (DUE TO) SEE 'FRACTURE' BY SITE, OPEN
814.08 HAMATE CLOSED
814.18 HAMATE OPEN
815.## HAND (EXCEPT FINGERS)

4th Digit: 815

0. CLOSED
1. OPEN

5th Digit: 815

0. SITE UNSPECIFIED
1. BASE OF THUMB
2. BASE
3. SHAFT
4. NECK
9. MULTIPLE SITES

817.0 HAND MULTIPLE BONES WITH FINGER CLOSED
817.1 HAND MULTIPLE BONES WITH FINGER OPEN
825.0 HEEL BONE CLOSED
825.1 HEEL BONE OPEN

HIP CLOSED

820.8 UNSPECIFIED
820.21 INTERTROCHANTERIC
820.22 SUBTROCHANTERIC
820.20 TROCHANTERIC

HIP OPEN

820.9 UNSPECIFIED
820.31 INTERTROCHANTERIC
820.32 SUBTROCHANTERIC
820.30 TROCHANTERIC

HUMERUS CLOSED

812.20 SITE UNSPECIFIED
812.02 ANATOMICAL NECK
812.44 ARTICULAR PROCESS OR T-SHAPED
812.49 CAPITELLUM
812.44 CONDYLE(S) OR LOWER EPIPHYSIS

FRACTURE (continued)

HUMERUS CLOSED (continued)

812.40 DISTAL
812.49 DISTAL MULTPLE
812.49 DISTAL OTHER
812.42 EXTERNAL CONDYLE
812.03 GREATER TUBEROSITY
812.09 HEAD OR UPPER EPIPHYSIS
812.43 INTERNAL EPICONDYLE
812.42 LATERAL CONDYLE
812.09 LESSER TUBEROSITY
812.43 MEDIAL CONDYLE
812.00 PROXIMAL
812.21 SHAFT
812.41 SUPRACONDYLAR
812.01 SURGICAL NECK
812.49 TROCHLEA

HUMERUS OPEN

812.30 SITE UNSPECIFIED
812.12 ANATOMICAL NECK
812.54 ARTICULAR PROCESS OR T-SHAPED
812.59 CAPITELLUM
812.54 CONDYLE(S) OR LOWER EPIPHYSIS
812.50 DISTAL
812.59 DISTAL MULTIPLE
812.59 DISTAL OTHER
812.52 EXTERNAL CONDYLE
812.13 GREATER TUBEROSITY
812.19 HEAD OR UPPER EPIPHYSIS
812.53 INTERNAL EPICONDYLE
812.52 LATERAL CONDYLE
812.19 LESSER TUBEROSITY
812.53 MEDIAL CONDYLE
812.10 PROXIMAL
812.31 SHAFT
812.51 SUPRACONDYLAR
812.11 SURGICAL NECK
812.59 TROCHLEA

FRACTURE (continued)

807.5 HYOID CLOSED
807.6 HYOID OPEN
808.41 ILIUM CLOSED
808.51 ILIUM OPEN
0 IMPACTED SEE 'FRACTURE', BY SITE CLOSED OR OPEN
808.49 INNOMINATE BONE CLOSED
808.59 INNOMINATE BONE OPEN

825.20 INSTEP CLOSED
825.30 INSTEP OPEN
827.0 INSTEP WITH TOE(S) CLOSED
827.1 INSTEP WITH TOE(S) OPEN

808.42 ISCHIUM CLOSED
808.52 ISCHIUM OPEN

802.2# JAW LOWER (BONE) CLOSED
802.3# JAW LOWER (BONE) OPEN

5th Digit: 802.2-3

0. UNSPECIFIED
1. CONDYLAR PROCESS
2. SUBCONDYLAR
3. CORONOID PROCESS
4. RAMUS UNSPECIFIED
5. ANGLE OF JAW
6. SYMPHYSIS OF BODY
7. ALVEOLAR BORDER OF BODY
8. BODY OTHER AND UNSPECIFIED
9. MULTIPLE SITES

802.4 JAW UPPER (BONE) CLOSED
802.5 JAW UPPER (BONE) OPEN

F

FRACTURE (continued)

0 KNEE CAP SEE 'FRACTURE', PATELLA

807.5 LARYNX CLOSED
807.6 LARYNX OPEN
905.4 LATE EFFECT LOWER EXTREMITIES
905.5 LATE EFFECT MULTIPLE AND UNSPECIFIED BONES
905.3 LATE EFFECT NECK OF FEMUR
905.0 LATE EFFECT SKULL AND FACE BONES
905.1 LATE EFFECT SPINE AND TRUNK NO SPINAL CORD LESION
905.2 LATE EFFECT UPPER EXTREMITIES
812.42 LATERAL CONDYLE (HUMERUS) CLOSED
812.52 LATERAL CONDYLE (HUMERUS) OPEN
824.2 LATERAL MALLEOLUS CLOSED
824.3 LATERAL MALLEOLUS OPEN
0 LEFORT'S SEE 'FRACTURE', MAXILLA AND 'FRACTURE' EACH OTHER STRUCTURE INVOLVED (IE., 'FRACTURE' FACIAL BONE(S), NASAL CAVITY, ORBIT FLOOR, AND/OR PALATE)
827.0 LEG CLOSED
827.1 LEG OPEN
828.0 LEG CLOSED BILATERAL
828.1 LEG OPEN BILATERAL
823.8# LEG LOWER NOS CLOSED
823.9# LEG LOWER NOS OPEN

5th Digit: 823.8-9

0. TIBIA ALONE
1. FIBULA ALONE
2. TIBIA WITH FIBULA

828.0 LEG(S) WITH RIB(S) OR STERNUM CLOSED
828.1 LEG(S) WITH RIB(S) OR STERNUM OPEN
806.4 LUMBAR SPINE WITH CORD INJURY CLOSED
806.5 LUMBAR SPINE WITH CORD INJURY OPEN
805.4 LUMBAR SPINE WITHOUT CORD INJURY CLOSED
805.5 LUMBAR SPINE WITHOUT CORD INJURY OPEN
814.02 LUNATE (WRIST) CLOSED
814.12 LUNATE (WRIST) OPEN
802.4 MALAR CLOSED
802.5 MALAR OPEN
808.43 MALGAIGNE'S CLOSED
808.53 MALGAIGNE'S OPEN
824.8 MALLEOLUS CLOSED
824.9 MALLEOLUS OPEN
733.81 MALUNION

> *733.81 **FRACTURE MALUNION**-MEANS THAT HEALING HAS OCCURRED BUT THAT THE BONE(S) OR FRACTURE FRAGMENTS ARE IN POOR ALIGNMENT.*

802.## MANDIBLE

4th Digit: 802

2. CLOSED
3. OPEN

5th Digit: 802

0. UNSPECIFIED
1. CONDYLAR PROCESS
2. SUBCONDYLAR
3. CORONOID PROCESS
4. RAMUS UNSPECIFIED
5. ANGLE OF JAW
6. SYMPHYSIS OF BODY
7. ALVEOLAR BORDER OF BODY
8. BODY OTHER AND UNSPECIFIED
9. MULTIPLE SITES

825.20 MARCH CLOSED
825.30 MARCH OPEN

FRACTURE (continued)

802.2# MAXILLA INFERIOR CLOSED
802.3# MAXILLA INFERIOR OPEN

5th Digit: 802.2-3

0. UNSPECIFIED
1. CONDYLAR PROCESS
2. SUBCONDYLAR
3. CORONOID PROCESS
4. RAMUS UNSPECIFIED
5. ANGLE OF JAW
6. SYMPHYSIS OF BODY
7. ALVEOLAR BORDER OF BODY
8. BODY OTHER AND UNSPECIFIED
9. MULTIPLE SITES

802.4 MAXILLA SUPERIOR CLOSED
802.5 MAXILLA SUPERIOR OPEN
812.43 MEDIAL CONDYLE (HUMERUS) CLOSED
812.53 MEDIAL CONDYLE (HUMERUS) OPEN
824.0 MEDIAL MALLEOLUS CLOSED
824.1 MEDIAL MALLEOLUS OPEN

815.## METACARPAL

4th Digit: 815

0. CLOSED
1. OPEN

5th Digit: 815

0. SITE UNSPECIFIED
1. BASE OF THUMB
2. BASE
3. SHAFT
4. NECK
9. MULTIPLE SITES

817.0 METACARPAL MULTIPLE WITH FINGER CLOSED
817.1 METACARPAL MULTIPLE WITH FINGER OPEN
825.25 METATARSAL(S) CLOSED
825.35 METATARSAL(S) OPEN
825.29 METATARSAL(S) WITH TARSAL CLOSED
825.39 METATARSAL(S) WITH TARSAL OPEN
813.03 MONTEGGIA CLOSED
813.13 MONTEGGIA OPEN
813.42 MOORE'S CLOSED
813.52 MOORE'S OPEN
814.05 MULTANGULAR BONE LARGER CLOSED
814.15 MULTANGULAR BONE LARGER OPEN
814.06 MULTANGULAR BONE SMALLER CLOSED
814.16 MULTANGULAR BONE SMALLER OPEN

> *MULTIPLE FRACTURES SHOULD BE SEQUENCED BY SEVERITY AS LISTED BELOW;*
>
> *1. SKULL AND FACE WITH OTHER BONES*
>
> *2. PELVIS OR VERTEBRAL COLUMN WITH OTHER BONES*
>
> *3. MULTIPLE FRACTURE BOTH LIMB BONES (LOWER), LOWER WITH UPPER, AND LOWER LIMB WITH RIB OR STERNUM*
>
> *4. MULTIPLE FRACTURES BOTH UPPER LIMBS, AND UPPER LIMB WITH RIB OR STERNUM*
>
> *5. FRACTURES TRUNK (ILL-DEFINED)*

MULTIPLE BONES

829.0 NOS CLOSED
829.1 NOS OPEN

818.0 ARM NOS OR MULTIPLE BONES IN SAME UPPER LIMB CLOSED
818.1 ARM NOS OR MULTIPLE BONES IN SAME UPPER LIMB OPEN

819.0 ARM(S) WITH RIB(S), STERNUM, OR BOTH UPPER LIMBS CLOSED
819.1 ARM(S) WITH RIB(S), STERNUM, OR BOTH UPPER LIMBS OPEN

FRACTURE (continued)

MULTIPLE BONES (continued)

> *MULTIPLE FRACTURES SHOULD BE SEQUENCED BY SEVERITY AS LISTED BELOW;*
>
> *1. SKULL AND FACE WITH OTHER BONES*
>
> *2. PELVIS OR VERTEBRAL COLUMN WITH OTHER BONES*
>
> *3. MULTIPLE FRACTURE BOTH LIMB BONES (LOWER), LOWER WITH UPPER, AND LOWER LIMB WITH RIB OR STERNUM*
>
> *4. MULTIPLE FRACTURES BOTH UPPER LIMBS, AND UPPER LIMB WITH RIB OR STERNUM*
>
> *5. FRACTURES TRUNK (ILL-DEFINED)*

827.0 LEG NOS OR MULTIPLE BONES IN SAME LOWER LIMB CLOSED
827.1 LEG NOS OR MULTIPLE BONES IN SAME LOWER LIMB OPEN

828.0 LEG(S) WITH ARM(S), RIB(S), STERNUM OR BOTH LOWER LIMBS CLOSED
828.1 LEG(S) WITH ARM(S), RIB(S), STERNUM OR BOTH LOWER LIMBS OPEN

809.0 TRUNK (ILL DEFINED) CLOSED
809.1 TRUNK (ILL DEFINED) OPEN

FRACTURE (continued)

802.0 NASAL BONES (SEPTUM) CLOSED
802.1 NASAL BONES (SEPTUM) OPEN
0 NASOETHMOID BONE SEE 'FRACTURE', SKULL BASILAR
825.22 NAVICULAR FOOT CLOSED
825.32 NAVICULAR FOOT OPEN
814.01 NAVICULAR WRIST CLOSED
814.11 NAVICULAR WRIST OPEN

0 NEURAL ARCH SEE 'FRACTURE', CERVICAL, DORSAL, LUMBAR, SACRUM OR COCCYX

> *733.82 **FRACTURE NONUNION**-MEANS THAT NO HEALING HAS OCCURRED AT THE FRACTURE SITE.*

733.82 NONUNION
0 OCCIPUT BONE SEE 'FRACTURE', SKULL BASILAR

813.01 OLECRANON CLOSED
813.11 OLECRANON OPEN

802.8 ORBIT CLOSED
802.9 ORBIT OPEN
802.6 ORBIT FLOOR (BLOW OUT) CLOSED
802.7 ORBIT FLOOR (BLOW OUT) OPEN
0 ORBIT ROOF SEE 'FRACTURE' SKULL BASILAR
825.0 OS CALCIS CLOSED
825.1 OS CALCIS OPEN
802.8 PALATE CLOSED
802.9 PALATE OPEN
0 PARIETAL BONE SEE 'FRACTURE' SKULL VAULT
822.0 PATELLA CLOSED
822.1 PATELLA OPEN

> *PATHOLOGICAL FRACTURE--733.1#-NON TRAUMATIC FRACTURES-YOU SEE PATHOLOGICAL FRACTURES IN BONES WEAKENED BY DISEASE SUCH AS OSTEOPOROSIS, METASTATIC TUMORS, OSTEOMYELITIS, BONE CYSTS, PAGET'S DISEASE ETC. CODE TO 733.1# WITH AN ADDITIONAL CODE ASSIGNED IF CAUSE IS KNOWN. SEQUENCING WOULD DEPEND ON REASON FOR ENCOUNTER.*

FRACTURE (continued)

PATHOLOGICAL

733.1# UNSPECIFIED CAUSE
733.1# ABSCESS BONE [**730.2#**]
733.1# ABSCESS BONE ACUTE OR SUBACUTE [**730.0#**]
733.1# ABSCESS BONE CHRONIC (OLD) [**730.1#**]
733.1# ABSCESS PERIOSTEUM [**730.3#**]
733.1# ALGONEURODYSTROPHY [733.7]
733.1# ARTHRITIS HYPERPARATHYROID [252.0]
733.1# BUSQUET'S DISEASE [**730.1#**]
733.1# CA BONE METASTATIC BONE NOS [198.5]
733.1# CA BONE OR MARROW METASTATIC [198.5]
733.1# DISUSE ATROPHY OF BONE [733.7]
733.1# GRANULOMA BONE [**730.1#**]
733.1# HYPERPARATHYROIDISM [252.0]
733.1# OSTEITIS DEFORMANS WITH SPINE CURVATURE ABNORMALITY [731.0]
733.1# OSTEITIS DEFORMANS WITHOUT MENTION OF BONE TUMOR [731.0]
733.1# OSTEITIS FIBROSA CYSTICA GENERALISATA [252.0]
733.1# OSTEITIS FIBROSA CYSTICA WITH KYPHOSIS [252.0] [737.41]
733.1# OSTEITIS FIBROSA CYSTICA WITH LORDOSIS [252.0] [737.42]
733.1# OTEITIS FIBROSA CYSTICA WITH SCOLIOSIS [252.0] [737.42]
733.1# OSTEITIS FIBROSA CYSTICA WITH SPINE CURVATURE ABNORMALITY NOS [252.0] [737.40]
733.1# OSTEOMYELITIS ACUTE [**730.0#**]
733.1# OSTEOMYELITIS CHRONIC [**730.1#**]

5th Digit: 733.1

0. UNSPECIFIED SITE
1. HUMERUS
2. DISTAL RADIUS AND ULNA, WRIST
3. VERTEBRA
4. NECK OF FEMUR, FEMUR NOS, HIP NOS
5. OTHER SPECIFIED PART OF FEMUR
6. TIBIA OR FIBULA, ANKLE
9. OTHER SPECIFIED SITE

5th Digit: 730.0-3

0. SITE NOS
1. SHOULDER REGION
2. UPPER ARM (ELBOW) (HUMERUS)
3. FOREARM (RADIUS) (WRIST) (ULNA)
4. HAND (CARPAL) (METACARPAL) (FINGERS)
5. PELVIC REGION (HIP) (BUTTOCK) (FEMUR) AND THIGH
6. LOWER LEG (FIBULA) (KNEE) (PATELLA) (TIBIA)
7. ANKLE AND OR FOOT (METATARSALS) (TOES) (TARSALS)
8. OTHER (HEAD) (NECK) (RIB) (SKULL) (TRUNK) (VERTEBRAE)
9. MULTIPLE

F

FRACTURE (continued)

PATHOLOGICAL (continued)

733.1# OSTEOPOROSIS [**733.0#**]

5th Digit: 733.1

0. UNSPECIFIED SITE
1. HUMERUS
2. DISTAL RADIUS AND ULNA, WRIST
3. VERTEBRA
4. NECK OF FEMUR, FEMUR NOS, HIP NOS
5. OTHER SPECIFIED PART OF FEMUR
6. TIBIA OR FIBULA, ANKLE
9. OTHER SPECIFIED SITE

5th Digit: 733.0

0. NOS
1. POSTMENOPAUSAL
1. SENILE
2. IDIOPATHIC
3. DISUSE
9. DRUG INDUCED

733.1# PAGET'S DISEASE OF BONE [731.0]
733.1# PARATHYROID HYPERPLASIA [252.0]
733.1# PERIOSTITIS WITHOUT OSTEOMYELITIS [**730.3#**]

5th Digit: 733.1

0. UNSPECIFIED SITE
1. HUMERUS
2. DISTAL RADIUS AND ULNA, WRIST
3. VERTEBRA
4. NECK OF FEMUR, FEMUR NOS, HIP NOS
5. OTHER SPECIFIED PART OF FEMUR
6. TIBIA OR FIBULA, ANKLE
9. OTHER SPECIFIED SITE

5th Digit: 730.3

0. SITE NOS
1. SHOULDER REGION
2. UPPER ARM (ELBOW) (HUMERUS)
3. FOREARM (RADIUS) (WRIST) (ULNA)
4. HAND (CARPAL) (METACARPAL) (FINGERS)
5. PELVIC REGION (HIP) (BUTTOCK) (FEMUR) AND THIGH
6. LOWER LEG (FIBULA) (KNEE) (PATELLA) (TIBIA)
7. ANKLE AND OR FOOT (METATARSALS) (TOES) (TARSALS)
8. OTHER (HEAD) (NECK) (RIB) (SKULL) (TRUNK) (VERTEBRAE)
9. MULTIPLE

733.1# SUDECK'S ATROPHY (VERTEBRA) [733.7]

5th Digit: 733.1

0. UNSPECIFIED SITE
1. HUMERUS
2. DISTAL RADIUS AND ULNA, WRIST
3. VERTEBRA
4. NECK OF FEMUR, FEMUR NOS, HIP NOS
5. OTHER SPECIFIED PART OF FEMUR
6. TIBIA OR FIBULA, ANKLE
9. OTHER SPECIFIED SITE

FRACTURE (continued)

PELVIS CLOSED

808.8 UNSPECIFIED CLOSED
808.0 ACETABULUM
808.41 ILIUM
808.49 INNOMINATE BONE
808.42 ISCHIUM
808.43 MULTIPLE WITH DISRUPTION OF PELVIC CIRCLE
809.0 MULTIPLE WITH OTHER BONES
808.2 PUBIS
808.49 RIM

PELVIS OPEN

808.9 UNSPECIFIED OPEN
808.1 ACETABULUM
808.51 ILIUM

FRACTURE (continued)

PELVIS OPEN (continued)

808.59 INNOMINATE BONE
808.52 ISCHIUM
808.53 MULTIPLE WITH DISRUPTION OF PELVIC CIRCLE
809.1 MULTIPLE WITH OTHER BONES
808.3 PUBIS
808.59 RIM

FRACTURE (continued)

826.0 PHALANGES FOOT CLOSED
826.1 PHALANGES FOOT OPEN
816.00 PHALANGES HAND CLOSED
816.10 PHALANGES HAND OPEN
814.04 PISIFORM CLOSED
814.14 PISIFORM OPEN
824.4 POTT'S CLOSED
824.5 POTT'S OPEN
996.4 PROSTHETIC FIXATION DEVICE ORTHOPEDIC INTERNAL - MECHANICAL
808.2 PUBIS CLOSED
808.3 PUBIS OPEN
814.01 QUERVAIN'S CLOSED
814.11 QUERVAIN'S OPEN

> *"WITH" MEANS THAT BOTH MUST BE PRESENT. I.E. FRACTURE RADIUS WITH ULNA MEANS THAT FRACTURES OF BOTH BONES MUST OCCUR IN ORDER TO USE THIS CODE.*

RADIUS CLOSED

813.81 NOS
813.83 NOS WITH ULNA
813.42 DISTAL
813.44 DISTAL WITH ULNA
813.05 HEAD OR EPIPHYSIS
813.06 NECK
813.07 PROXIMAL OR MULTIPLE SITES
813.08 PROXIMAL OR MULTIPLE SITES WITH ULNA
813.21 SHAFT
813.23 SHAFT WITH ULNA

RADIUS OPEN

813.91 NOS
813.93 NOS WITH ULNA
813.52 DISTAL
813.54 DISTAL WITH ULNA
813.15 HEAD OR EPIPHYSIS
813.16 NECK
813.17 PROXIMAL OR MULTIPLE SITES
813.18 PROXIMAL OR MULTIPLE SITES WITH ULNA
813.31 SHAFT
813.33 SHAFT WITH ULNA

FRACTURE (continued)

807.## RIBS

4th Digit: 807

0. CLOSED
1. OPEN

5th Digit: 807

0. RIBS UNSPECIFIED
1. ONE RIB
2. TWO RIBS
3. THREE RIBS
4. FOUR RIBS
5. FIVE RIBS
6. SIX RIBS
7. SEVEN RIBS
8. EIGHT OR MORE RIBS
9. MULTIPLE RIBS UNSPECIFIED

805.6 SACRUM AND COCCYX CLOSED
805.7 SACRUM AND COCCYX OPEN

FRACTURE (continued)

806.6# SACRUM AND COCCYX WITH CORD INJURY CLOSED
806.7# SACRUM AND COCCYX WITH CORD INJURY OPEN
5th Digit: 806.6-7
0. CORD INJURY UNSPECIFIED
1. COMPLETE CAUDA EQUINA INJURY
2. OTHER CAUDA EQUINA INJURY
9. WITH OTHER SPINAL CORD INJURY

A SALTAR FRACTURE IS A FRACTURE INVOLVING A BONE'S EPIPHYSIS. CODE AS ALL OTHER FRACTURES ; BY BONE. (CLOSED) (OPEN).

825.22 SCAPHOID FOOT CLOSED
825.32 SCAPHOID FOOT OPEN
814.01 SCAPHOID WRIST CLOSED
814.11 SCAPHOID WRIST OPEN
811.0# SCAPULA CLOSED
811.1# SCAPULA OPEN
5th Digit: 811.0-1
0. SITE UNSPECIFIED
1. ACROMION
2. CORACOID
3. GLENOID OR NECK
9. BODY OF SCAPULA

0 SESAMOID SEE 'FRACTURE', BY SITE
825.21 SHEPHERD'S CLOSED
825.31 SHEPHERD'S OPEN
0 SHOULDER BLADE SEE 'FRACTURE', SCAPULA
812.00 SHOULDER CLOSED
812.10 SHOULDER OPEN
813.42 SILVERFORK CLOSED
813.52 SILVERFORK OPEN
0 SINUS BONES SEE 'FRACTURE' SKULL BASILAR
813.21 SKILLERN'S CLOSED
813.31 SKILLERN'S OPEN
803.## SKULL
801.## SKULL BASILAR
767.3 SKULL BIRTH TRAUMA
803.## SKULL MULTIPLE NOS
804.## SKULL MULTIPLE WITH OTHER BONES OF BODY
800.## SKULL VAULT
4th Digit: 800, 801, 803, 804
0. CLOSED WITHOUT INTRACRANIAL INJURY
1. CLOSED WITH CEREBRAL LACERATION AND/OR CONTUSION
2. CLOSED WITH SUBARACHNOID SUBDURAL EXTRADURAL AND EPIDURAL HEMORRHAGE
3. CLOSED WITH OTHER AND UNSPECIFIED INTRACRANIAL HEMORRHAGE
4. CLOSED WITH INTRACRANIAL INJURY OF OTHER AND UNSPECIFIED NATURE
5. OPEN WITHOUT MENTION OF INTRACRANIAL INJURY
6. OPEN WITH CEREBRAL LACERATION AND CONTUSION
7. OPEN WITH SUBARACHNOID SUBDURAL EPIDURAL AND EXTRADURAL HEMORRHAGE
8. OPEN WITH OTHER AND UNSPECIFIED INTRACRANIAL HEMORRHAGE
9. OPEN WITH INTRACRANIAL INJURY OF OTHER AND UNSPECIFIED
5th Digit: 800, 801, 803, 804
0. LEVEL OF CONSCIOUSNESS UNSPECIFIED
1. NO LOC
2. LOC < 1 HR
3. LOC 1 - 24 HRS
4. LOC > 24 HRS WITH RETURN TO PRIOR LEVEL
5. LOC > 24 HRS WITHOUT RETURN TO PRIOR LEVEL: OR DEATH BEFORE REGAINING CONSCIOUSNESS, REGARDLESS OF DURATION OF LOC
6. LOC DURATION UNSPECIFIED
9. WITH CONCUSSION UNSPECIFIED

FRACTURE (continued)

813.41 SMITH'S CLOSED
813.51 SMITH'S OPEN
0 SPHENOID BONE SEE 'FRACTURE', SKULL BASILAR
767.4 SPINE OR SPINAL CORD BIRTH TRAUMA
0 SPINE SEE 'FRACTURE', CERVICAL, DORSAL, LUMBAR, SACRUM OR COCCYX
0 SPINOUS PROCESS SEE 'FRACTURE', CERVICAL, DORSAL, LUMBAR, SACRUM OR COCCYX
0 SPONTANEOUS SEE 'FRACTURE', PATHOLOGICAL
808.41 SPRINTERS' CLOSED
808.51 SPRINTERS' OPEN
807.2 STERNUM CLOSED
807.3 STERNUM OPEN
807.4 STERNUM WITH FLAIL CHEST OPEN
821.20 STIEDA'S CLOSED
821.30 STIEDA'S OPEN
815.02 STYLOID PROCESS METACARPAL CLOSED
815.12 STYLOID PROCESS METACARPAL OPEN
813.43 STYLOID PROCESS ULNA CLOSED
813.53 STYLOID PROCESS ULNA OPEN
813.44 STYLOID PROCESS ULNA WITH RADIUS CLOSED
813.54 STYLOID PROCESS ULNA WITH RADIUS OPEN
812.41 SUPRACONDYLAR (HUMERUS) CLOSED
812.51 SUPRACONDYLAR (HUMERUS) OPEN
0 SYMPHYSIS PUBIS SEE 'FRACTURE', PUBIS
825.21 TALUS CLOSED
825.31 TALUS OPEN
825.29 TARSAL WITH METATARSAL(S) CLOSED
825.39 TARSAL WITH METATARSAL(S) OPEN
0 TEMPORAL BONE SEE 'FRACTURE', SKULL BASILAR
805.2 THORACIC VERTEBRA CLOSED
805.3 THORACIC VERTEBRA OPEN
806.2# THORACIC VERTEBRA WITH CORD INJURY CLOSED
806.3# THORACIC VERTEBRA WITH CORD INJURY OPEN
5th Digit: 806.2-3
0. T1-T6 WITH CORD INJURY UNSPECIFIED
1. T1-T6 WITH COMPLETE LESION OF CORD
2. T1-T6 WITH ANTERIOR CORD SYNDROME
3. T1-T6 WITH CENTRAL CORD SYNDROME
4. T1-T6 WITH INCOMPLETE CORD LESION UNSPECIFIED OR POSTERIOR CORD SYNDROME
5. T7-T12 WITH CORD INJURY UNSPECIFIED
6. T7-T12 WITH COMPLETE LESION OF CORD
7. T7-T12 WITH ANTERIOR CORD SYNDROME
8. T7-T12 WITH CENTRAL CORD SYNDROME
9. T7-T12 WITH SPINAL CORD LESION UNSPECIFIED OR POSTERIOR CORD SYNDROME

0 THUMB SEE 'FRACTURE', FINGER
807.5 THYROID CARTILAGE CLOSED
807.6 THYROID CARTILAGE OPEN
823.## TIBIA (AND/OR FIBULA)
4th Digit: 823
0. PROXIMAL (HEAD) (PLATEAU) CLOSED
1. PROXIMAL (HEAD) (PLATEAU) OPEN
2. SHAFT CLOSED
3. SHAFT OPEN
8. SITE UNSPECIFIED CLOSED
9. SITE UNSPECIFIED OPEN
5th Digit: 823
0. TIBIA ALONE
1. FIBULA ALONE
2. TIBIA WITH FIBULA

824.8 TIBIA DISTAL END OR EPIPHYSIS CLOSED
824.9 TIBIA DISTAL END OR EPIPHYSIS OPEN
823.00 TIBIA INTERCONDYLAR SPINE/TUBEROSITY CLOSED
823.10 TIBIA INTERCONDYLAR SPINE/TUBEROSITY OPEN
824.0 TIBIA INVOLVING ANKLE CLOSED
824.1 TIBIA INVOLVING ANKLE OPEN

	FRACTURE (continued)
823.00	TIBIAL PLATEAU CLOSED
823.10	TIBIAL PLATEAU OPEN
826.0	TOE(S) CLOSED
826.1	TOE(S) OPEN
873.63	TOOTH
873.73	TOOTH COMPLICATED
807.5	TRACHEA CLOSED
807.6	TRACHEA OPEN
0	TRANSVERSE PROCESS SEE 'FRACTURE', CERVICAL, DORSAL, LUMBAR, SACRUM OR COCCYX
814.05	TRAPEZIUM CLOSED
814.15	TRAPEZIUM OPEN
814.06	TRAPEZOID CLOSED
814.16	TRAPEZOID OPEN
V67.4	TREATMENT FOLLOWUP EXAM - HEALED
0	TREATMENT FOLLOWUP EXAM - HEALING OR CURRENT SEE 'AFTERCARE', ORTHOPEDIC
824.6	TRIMALLEOLAR CLOSED
824.7	TRIMALLEOLAR OPEN
814.03	TRIQUETRAL CLOSED
814.13	TRIQUETRAL OPEN
812.49	TROCHLEA (HUMERUS) CLOSED
812.59	TROCHLEA (HUMERUS) OPEN
	ULNA CLOSED
813.82	NOS
813.83	NOS WITH RADIUS
813.43	DISTAL
813.44	DISTAL WITH RADIUS
813.04	PROXIMAL
813.04	PROXIMAL MULTIPLE
813.08	PROXIMAL WITH RADIUS
813.22	SHAFT
813.23	SHAFT WITH RADIUS
	ULNA OPEN
813.92	NOS
813.93	NOS WITH RADIUS
813.53	DISTAL
813.54	DISTAL WITH RADIUS
813.14	PROXIMAL
813.14	PROXIMAL MULTIPLE
813.18	PROXIMAL WITH RADIUS
813.32	SHAFT
813.33	SHAFT WITH RADIUS
	FRACTURE (continued)
814.08	UNCIFORM CLOSED
814.18	UNCIFORM OPEN
767.4	VERTEBRA BIRTH TRAUMA
805.8	VERTEBRA CLOSED
805.9	VERTEBRA OPEN
809.0	VERTEBRA MULTIPLE CLOSED
809.1	VERTEBRA MULTIPLE OPEN
806.8	VERTEBRA WITH CORD INJURY CLOSED
806.9	VERTEBRA WITH CORD INJURY OPEN
802.0	VOMER CLOSED
802.1	VOMER OPEN
814.##	WRIST

4th Digit: 814
- **0. CLOSED**
- **1. OPEN**

5th Digit: 814
- **0. UNSPECIFIED**
- **1. NAVICULAR (SCAPHOID)**
- **2. LUNATE (SEMILUNAR)**
- **3. TRIQUETRAL (CUNEIFORM)**
- **4. PISIFORM**
- **5. TRAPEZIUM (LARGER MULTANGULAR)**
- **6. TRAPEZOID (SMALLER MULTANGULAR)**
- **7. CAPITATE (OS MAGNUM)**
- **8. HAMMATE (UNCIFORM)**
- **9. OTHER**

	FRACTURE (continued)
802.4	ZYGOMA CLOSED
802.5	ZYGOMA OPEN
759.83	FRAGILE X SYNDROME
704.2	FRAGILITAS CRINIUM
756.51	FRAGILITAS OSSIUM
102.0	FRAMBESIA INITIAL OR PRIMARY
102.0	FRAMBESIA INITIAL ULCER
0	FRAMBESIA SEE ALSO 'YAWS'
102.4	FRAMBESIDE GUMMATOUS
102.2	FRAMBESIDE OF EARLY YAWS
102.1	FRAMBESIOMA
756.0	FRANCESCHETTI'S SYNDROME (MANDIBULOFACIAL DYSOSTOSIS)
021.9	FRANCIS' TULAREMIA
0	FRANCISELLA (PASTURELLA) TULARENSIS SEE 'TULAREMIA'
273.2	FRANKLIN'S HEAVY CHAIN DISEASE
759.89	FRASER'S SYNDROME
709.09	FRECKLE
272.3	FREDRICKSON TYPE I OR V HYPERLIPOPROTEINEMIA
272.0	FREDRICKSON TYPE IIA HYPERLIPOPROTEINEMIA
272.2	FREDRICKSON TYPE IIB OR III HYPERLIPOPROTEINEMIA
272.1	FREDRICKSON TYPE IV HYPERLIPOPROTEINEMIA
759.89	FREEMAN SHELDON SYNDROME
099.1	FREI'S CLIMATIC BUBO
732.5	FREIBERG'S FLATTENING METATARSAL
788.41	FREQUENCY (URINARY)
350.8	FREY'S AURICULOTEMPORAL SYNDROME
	FRICTION RUB
786.7	CHEST
785.3	HEART
786.7	PLEURAL
036.3	FRIDERICHSEN-WATERHOUSE SYNDROME
041.3	FRIEDLANDER'S BACILLUS INFECTION OR ORGANISM
0	FRIEDLANDER'S ENDARTERITIS OBLITERANS SEE 'ARTERIOSCLEROSIS, ARTERIOSCLEROTIC'
334.0	FRIEDREICH'S ATAXIA
334.0	FRIEDREICH'S ATAXIA - CARDIOMYOPATHY [425.8]
756.0	FRIEDREICH'S FACIAL HEMIHYPERTROPHY
333.2	FRIEDREICH'S MYOCLONIA
757.39	FRIEDRICH-ERB-ARNOLD SYNDROME (ACROPACHYDERMA)
302.72	FRIGIDITY PSYCHOSEXUAL
253.8	FROHLICH'S ADIPOSOGENITAL DYSTROPHY (SYNDROME)
336.8	FROIN'S SYNDROME
676.6#	FROMMEL CHIARI SYNDROME MATERNAL DUE TO PREGNANCY

5th Digit: 676.6
- **0. EPISODE OF CARE UNSPECIFIED OR N/A**
- **1. DELIVERED**
- **2. DELIVERED WITH POSTPARTUM COMPLICATION**
- **3. ANTEPARTUM COMPLICATION**
- **4. POSTPARTUM COMPLICATION**

738.19	FRONTAL BONE DEFORMITY
310.0	FRONTAL LOBE SYNDROME
461.1	FRONTAL SINUS (ABSCESS) (INFECTION) (INFLAMMATION) ACUTE
473.1	FRONTAL SINUS DISEASE CHRONIC
	FROSTBITE
991.3	NOS
991.0	FACE
991.2	FOOT
991.1	HAND
909.4	LATE EFFECT
991.3	OTHER SITES

302.89 FROTTEURISM
726.0 FROZEN SHOULDER
271.2 FRUCTOSE INTOLERANCE HEREDITARY
271.2 FRUCTOSEMIA METABOLISM DISORDER
271.2 FRUCTOSURIA ESSENTIAL BENIGN
371.57 FUCHS' ENDOTHELIAL DYSTROPHY
364.21 FUCHS' HETEROCHRONIC IRIDOCYCLITIS
271.8 FUCOSIDASE ABSENCE
271.8 FUCOSIDOSIS CARBOHYDRATE TRANSPORT DISORDERS
300.13 FUGUE HYSTERICAL (DISSOCIATIVE)
300.13 FUGUE PSYCHOGENIC
308.1 FUGUES REACTION (ACUTE) (STRESS)
756.59 FULLER ALBRIGHT'S SYNDROME (OSTEITIS FIBROSA DISSEMINATA)
502 FULLER'S EARTH DISEASE
987.9 FUMES INHALATION (NOXIOUS)
780.9 FUNCTIONAL ACTIVITY DECREASE
564.9 FUNCTIONAL BOWEL SYNDROME
752.8 FUNCTIONAL PREPUBERTAL CASTRATE SYNDROME
743.52 FUNDUS COLOBOMA CONGENITAL
362.76 FUNDUS FLAVIMACULATUS HEREDITARY
0 FUNGAL SEE 'FUNGUS, FUNGAL INFECTION'
117.9 FUNGEMIA

FUNGUS, FUNGAL INFECTION
117.9 NEC
0 ASPERGILLUS SEE 'ASPERGILLOSIS'
110.0 BEARD
110.5 BODY
0 CANDIDAL SEE CANDIDIASIS
0 COCCIDIOIDES (IMMITIS) SEE 'COCCIDIOIDOMYCOSIS'
117.8 DEMATIACIOUS
110.4 FOOT
110.3 GROIN
110.2 HAND
0 HISTOPLASMA SEE 'HISTOPLASMOSIS'
110.1 NAIL (FINGER) (TOE)
118 PATHOGENIC TO COMPROMISED HOST ONLY
110.3 PERIANAL AREA
110.0 SCALP
110.8 SCROTUM
111.9 SKIN
110.4 SKIN FOOT
110.2 SKIN HAND
0 TINEA SEE 'TINEA'
110.1 TOENAIL
117.9 TRACHEA
117.8 OTHER SPECIFIED FUNGUS

754.81 FUNNEL CHEST CONGENITAL
780.6 FUO (FEVER OF UNKNOWN ORIGIN)
690.18 FURFUR
495.8 FURRIERS' LUNG
373.13 FURUNCLE EYELID
0 FURUNCLE SEE 'CARBUNCLE'

118 FUSARIUM INFECTION TO COMPROMISED HOST ONLY
0 FUSIFORM CELL TYPE TUMOR MALIGNANT SITE SPECIFIED SEE 'CANCER' BY SITE M8004/3

FUSION, FUSED
756.9 BONE CONGENITAL
V45.4 CERVICAL ARTHRODESIS STATUS
746.5 COMMISSURE MITRAL VALVE CONGENITAL
744.04 EAR OSSICLES (CONGENITAL)
996.4 FAILED (JOINT) (SPINAL)
718.54 FINGER ACQUIRED
755.12 FINGER (BONE) CONGENITAL
718.57 FOOT ACQUIRED
755.67 FOOT TALONAVICULAR CONGENITAL
718.55 HIP ACQUIRED
718.5# JOINT ACQUIRED(FIBROUS) (OSSEUS)

5th Digit: 718.5
- **0. SITE NOS**
- **1. SHOULDER REGION**
- **2. UPPER ARM (ELBOW) (HUMERUS)**
- **3. FOREARM (RADIUS) (WRIST) (ULNA)**
- **4. HAND (CARPAL) (METACARPAL) (FINGERS)**
- **5. PELVIC REGION AND THIGH (HIP) (BUTTOCK) (FEMUR)**
- **6. LOWER LEG (FIBULA) (KNEE) (PATELLA) (TIBIA)**
- **7. ANKLE AND/OR FOOT (METATARSALS) (TOES) (TARSALS)**
- **8. OTHER EXCEPT SPINE**
- **9. MULTIPLE**

755.8 JOINT CONGENITAL
996.4 JOINT FAILED
718.56 KNEE ACQUIRED
755.8 LIMB CONGENITAL
755.69 LIMB LOWER CONGENITAL
755.59 LIMB UPPER CONGENITAL
724.6 LUMBOSACRAL ACQUIRED (NONVERTEBRAL) (NONDISCOGENIC)
V45.4 LUMBOSACRAL ARTHRODESIS STATUS
756.15 LUMBOSACRAL CONGENITAL
718.58 NECK ACQUIRED
718.58 RIB ACQUIRED
756.3 RIB CONGENITAL
724.6 SACROILIAC ACQUIRED (NONVERTEBRAL) (NONDISCOGENIC)
755.69 SACROILIAC CONGENITAL
V45.4 SACROILIAC ARTHRODESIS STATUS
724.6 SACRUM ACQUIRED(NONVERTEBRAL) (NONDISCOGENIC)
V45.4 SACRUM ARTHRODESIS STATUS
755.69 SACRUM CONGENITAL
724.9 SPINE ACQUIRED (NONVERTEBRAL) (NONDISCOGENIC)
756.15 SPINE CONGENITAL
996.4 SPINE FAILED
V45.4 SPINE SURGICAL STATUS
755.67 TALONAVICULAR CONGENITAL
V45.4 THORACIC ARTHRODESIS STATUS
718.57 TOES ACQUIRED
755.14 TOES CONGENITAL
368.33 VISION WITH DEFECTIVE STEREOPSIS

085.1 GAFSA BOIL
478.29 GAG REFLEX HYPERACTIVE
289.0 GAISBOCK'S DISEASE OR SYNDROME (POLYCYTHEMIA HYPERTONICA)
289.0 GAISBOCK'S POLYCYTHEMIA HYPERTONICA

GAIT
781.2 ABNORMALITY (ATAXIC) (PARALYTIC) (SCISSOR) (SPASTIC) (STAGGERING)
719.7# DISORDER DUE TO JOINT DISORDER
5th Digit: 719.7
0. SITE NOS
5. PELVIC REGION (HIP) (BUTTOCK) (FEMUR)
6. LOWER LEG (FIBULA) (KNEE) (PATELLA) (TIBIA)
7. ANKLE AND/OR FOOT (METATARSALS)(TOES)(TARSALS)
8. OTHER
9. MULTIPLE
300.11 HYSTERICAL
V57.81 TRAINING IN THE USE OF ARTIFICIAL LIMBS

611.5 GALACTOCELE
676.8# GALACTOCELE PUERPERAL POSTPARTUM MATERNAL DUE TO PREGNANCY
5th Digit: 676.8
0. EPISODE OF CARE UNSPECIFIED OR N/A
1. DELIVERED
2. DELIVERED WITH POSTPARTUM COMPLICATION
3. ANTEPARTUM COMPLICATION
4. POSTPARTUM COMPLICATION

611.0 GALACTOPHORITIS
675.2# GALACTOPHORITIS PUERPERAL POSTPARTUM MATERNAL DUE TO PREGNANCY
5th Digit: 675.2
0. EPISODE OF CARE UNSPECIFIED OR N/A
1. DELIVERED
2. DELIVERED WITH POSTPARTUM COMPLICATION
3. ANTEPARTUM COMPLICATION
4. POSTPARTUM COMPLICATION

611.6 GALACTORRHEA
676.6# GALACTORRHEA MATERNAL DUE TO PREGNANCY
5th Digit: 676.6
0. EPISODE OF CARE UNSPECIFIED OR N/A
1. DELIVERED
2. DELIVERED WITH POSTPARTUM COMPLICATION
3. ANTEPARTUM COMPLICATION
4. POSTPARTUM COMPLICATION

271.1 GALACTOSE 1 PHOSPHATE URIDYL TRANSFERASE DEFICIENCY
271.1 GALACTOSEMIA
V77.4 GALACTOSEMIA SCREENING
271.1 GALACTOSURIA
791.1 GALACTURIA

GALLBLADDER
575.0 ABSCESS
0 ABSCESS WITH CALCULUS SEE 'CHOLECYSTITIS', ACUTE WITH CHOLELITHIASIS
V45.89 ABSENCE
751.69 ABSENCE CONGENITAL
575.8 ADHESION
751.60 ANOMALY NOS
751.69 ANOMALY OTHER SPECIFIED
751.69 ATRESIA (CONGENITAL)
575.8 ATROPHY
575.8 CALCIFICATION
0 CALCULUS SEE 'CHOLELITHIASIS'
575.6 CHOLESTEROLOSIS
575.9 DISORDER
575.8 DISORDERS OTHER SPECIFIED
793.3 FILLING DEFECT
793.3 FINDINGS ABNORMAL (NONVISUALIZATION)
575.5 FISTULA

GALLBLADDER (continued)
575.0 GANGRENOUS
0 GANGRENOUS WITH CALCULUS SEE 'CHOLECYSTITIS'
575.3 HYDROPS
575.8 HYPERTROPHY
868.02 INJURY - UNSPECIFIED
868.12 INJURY - WITH OPEN WOUND INTO CAVITY
908.1 INJURY - LATE EFFECT
575.8 NONFUNCTIONING
793.3 NONVISUALIZATION
575.2 OBSTRUCTION OR OCCLUSION
0 OBSTRUCTION OR OCCLUSION WITH CALCULUS SEE 'CHOLECYSTITIS'
575.4 PERFORATION
575.8 ULCER

GALLBLADDER CONGENITAL ANOMALIES
751.69 ABSENCE
751.60 BILE DUCTS AND LIVER
751.60 DISORDER
751.69 DUPLICATION
751.69 ECTOPIC
751.69 FLOATING
751.69 INTRAHEPATIC
751.69 OBSTRUCTION OR OCCLUSION
751.69 OBSTRUCTION OR OCCLUSION WITH JAUNDICE [774.5]

0 GALLSTONE SEE 'CHOLELITHIASIS'

086.3 GAMBIAN SLEEPING SICKNESS
312.31 GAMBLING COMPULSIVE (PATHOLOGICAL)
V69.3 GAMBLING PROBLEM
279.00 GAMMA GLOBULIN ABSENCE
V07.2 GAMMA GLOBULIN ADMINISTRATION (PROPHYLACTIC)
277.3 GAMMALOIDOSIS
273.9 GAMMOPATHY
273.1 GAMMOPATHY MONOCLONAL
273.1 GAMMOPATHY MONOCLONAL ASSOCIATED WITH LYMPHOPLASMACYTIC DYSCRASIAS
289.51 GAMNA'S SIDEROTIC SPLENOMEGALY
754.71 GAMPSODACTYLIA CONGENITAL
359.3 GAMSTORP'S DISEASE
289.51 GANDY-NANTA SIDEROTIC SPLENOMEGALY
V71.01 GANG ACTIVITY EVALUATION - ADULT SUSPECTED PSYCHIATRIC DISORDER
V71.02 GANG ACTIVITY EVALUATION - CHILD OR ADOLESCENT SUSPECTED PSYCHIATRIC DISORDER
238.9 GANGLIOGLIOMA SITE UNSPECIFIED
0 GANGLIOGLIOMA SITE SPECIFIED SEE 'NEOPLASM UNCERTAIN BEHAVIOR' BY SITE M9505/1

GANGLION
727.43 UNSPECIFIED
351.1 GENICULI SYNDROME
727.41 JOINT
333.90 SYNDROME (BASAL, BRAIN)
727.42 TENDON SHEATH

171.# GANGLIONEUROBLASTOMA M9490/3
4th Digit: 171
0. HEAD FACE NECK
2. UPPER LIMB SHOULDER
3. LOWER LIMB HIP
4. THORAX
5. ABDOMINAL HYPOCHONDRIUM
6. PELVIS BUTTOCK GROIN INGUINAL, REGION PERINEUM
7. TRUNK NOS BACK NOS FLANK NOS
8. OTHER SPECIFIED SITES
9. SITE NOS

215.# GANGLIONEUROMA M9490/0
215.# GANGLIONEUROMATOSIS M9491/0

4th Digit: 215

0. HEAD FACE NECK
2. UPPER LIMB SHOULDER
3. LOWER LIMB HIP
4. THORAX
5. ABDOMINAL HYPOCHONDRIUM
6. PELVIS BUTTOCK GROIN INGUINAL REGION PERINEUM
7. TRUNK UNSPECIFIED BACK UNSPECIFIED FLANK UNSPECIFIED
8. OTHER SPECIFIED SITES
9. SITE UNSPECIFIED

351.1 GANGLIONITIS GENICULATE UNSPECIFIED
330.1 GANGLIOSIDOSIS DISEASE

GANGRENE, 785.4 SHOULD NEVER BE SEQUENCED AS THE PRINCIPAL DIAGNOSIS IF THE CAUSE IS KNOWN. ALWAYS CODE THE UNDERLYING DISEASE FIRST. FOR EXAMPLE, DIABETIC GANGRENE OF THE LEG IS CODED WITH THE DIABETES FIRST, 250.7.# AND THE GANGRENE SECONDARY, 785.4.

GANGRENE

785.4 UNSPECIFIED
440.29 ABDOMEN ARTERIOSCLEROTIC
569.49 ANUS
440.24 ARTERIOSCLEROTIC EXTREMITIES (GENERAL)
785.4 CELLULITIS
371.40 CORNEA
707.0 DECUBITAL ULCER [785.4]
250.7# DIABETIC [785.4]

5th Digit: 250.7

0. TYPE II, ADULT-ONSET, NON-INSULIN DEPENDENT (EVEN IF REQUIRING INSULIN), OR UNSPECIFIED; CONTROLLED
1. TYPE I, JUVENILE-ONSET OR INSULIN-DEPENDENT; CONTROLLED
2. TYPE II, ADULT-ONSET, NON-INSULIN DEPENDENT (EVEN IF REQUIRING INSULIN); UNCONTROLLED
3. TYPE I, JUVENILE-ONSET OR INSULIN-DEPENDENT; UNCONTROLLED

443.0 DUE TO RAYNAUD'S [785.4]
444.22 EMBOLUS, THROMBUS ARTERIES LOWER EXTREMITIES [785.4]
444.21 EMBOLUS,THROMBUS ARTERIES UPPER EXTREMITIES [785.4]
040.0 EMPHYSEMATOUS
988.2 EPIDEMIC
785.4 EXTREMITY
440.3# EXTREMITY ARTERIOSCLEROTIC - BYPASS GRAFT

5th Digit: 440.3

0. UNSPECIFIED GRAFT
1. AUTOLOGOUS VEIN BYPASS GRAFT
2. NONAUTOLOGOUS BIOLOGICAL BYPASS GRAFT

440.24 EXTREMITY ARTERIOSCLEROTIC - NATIVE ARTERY ISCHEMIC
250.7# EXTREMITY DIABETIC [785.4]

5th Digit: 250.7

0. TYPE II, ADULT-ONSET, NON-INSULIN DEPENDENT (EVEN IF REQUIRING INSULIN), OR UNSPECIFIED; CONTROLLED
1. TYPE I, JUVENILE-ONSET OR INSULIN-DEPENDENT; CONTROLLED
2. TYPE II, ADULT-ONSET, NON-INSULIN DEPENDENT (EVEN IF REQUIRING INSULIN); UNCONTROLLED
3. TYPE I, JUVENILE-ONSET OR INSULIN-DEPENDENT; UNCONTROLLED

575.0 GALLBLADDER
0 GALLBLADDER WITH CALCULUS SEE 'CHOLECYSTITIS', ACUTE WITH CHOLELITHIASIS

GANGRENE (continued)

040.0 GAS (BACILLUS)
523.8 GINGIVAL
557.0 INTESTINAL
440.24 ISCHEMIC ARTERIOSCLEROTIC EXTREMITIES (GENERAL)
573.8 LIVER
513.0 LUNG
104.8 LUNG SPIROCHETAL
686.09 MELENEY'S (CUTANEOUS)
034.0 PHARYNX (SEPTIC)
440.24 POTT'S ISCHEMIC
443.1 PRESENILE
513.0 PULMONARY
440.24 SENILE ISCHEMIC
537.89 STOMACH

502 GANNISTER DISEASE
300.16 GANSER'S SYNDROME HYSTERICAL
287.2 GARDNER-DIAMOND SYNDROME (AUTOERYTHROCYTE SENSITIZATION)
277.5 GARGOYLISM
0 GARRE'S SEE 'OSTEOMYELITIS'
728.79 GARROD'S OR KNUCKLE PADS
752.11 GARTNER'S DUCT CYST CONGENITAL
040.0 GAS BACILLUS INFECTION
040.0 GAS GANGRENE
987.9 GAS INHALATION (NOXIOUS)
787.3 GAS PAIN
350.8 GASSERIAN GANGLION
134.0 GASTEROPHILUS (INTESTINALIS) INFESTATION
536.8 GASTRALGIA

GASTRIC

536.0 ANACIDITY
902.21 ARTERY INJURY (LACERATION) (RUPTURE) (HEMATOMA) (AVULSION) (ANEURYSM) TRAUMATIC
908.4 ARTERY INJURY LATE EFFECT
537.89 ATROPHY
094.0 CRISIS (TABETIC)
536.1 DILATATION ACUTE
536.8 DILATATION OTHER SPECIFIED
537.9 DISORDER
536.9 DISORDER FUNCTIONAL
306.4 DISORDER FUNCTIONAL PSYCHOGENIC
536.8 DISORDER (MOTILITY) (SECRETION)
536.1 DISTENTION ACUTE
537.1 DIVERTICULUM
537.89 DUODENAL RUPTURE
535.4# EROSION

5th Digit: 535.4

0. WITHOUT HEMORRHAGE
1. WITH HEMORRHAGE

537.89 LESION
536.8 MOTILITY DISORDER
537.89 MUCOSA METAPLASIA
535.20 MUCOSAL HYPERTROPHY
535.21 MUCOSAL HYPERTROPHY WITH HEMORRHAGE
537.0 OUTLET OBSTRUCTION
536.8 PAIN
536.3 PARESIS
537.89 PROLAPSE
536.8 RETENTION
537.89 REFLUX
537.89 RUPTURE
536.8 SECRETION DISORDER
536.3 STASIS
537.89 STENOSIS

GASTRIC (continued)

531.## ULCER
531.## ULCER DUE TO HELICOBACTER PYLORI [041.86]

4th Digit: 531
- **0. ACUTE WITH HEMORRHAGE**
- **1. ACUTE WITH PERFORATION**
- **2. ACUTE WITH HEMORRHAGE AND PERFORATION**
- **3. ACUTE**
- **4. CHRONIC OR UNSPECIFIED WITH HEMORRHAGE**
- **5. CHRONIC OR UNSPECIFIED WITH PERFORATION**
- **6. CHRONIC OR UNSPECIFIED WITH HEMORRHAGE AND PERFORATION**
- **7. CHRONIC**
- **9. UNSPECIFIED AS ACUTE OR CHRONIC**

5th Digit: 531
- **0. WITHOUT OBSTRUCTION**
- **1. OBSTRUCTED**

902.39 VEIN INJURY (LACERATION) (RUPTURE) (HEMATOMA) (AVULSION) (ANEURYSM) TRAUMATIC
908.4 VEIN INJURY LATE EFFECT

251.5 GASTRIN SECRETION ABNORMALITY

CARCINOMAS AND NEOPLASMS SHOULD BE CODED BY SITE IF POSSIBLE. CODE BY CELL TYPE - "SITE NOS", IF AND ONLY IF A SITE IS NOT SPECIFIED IN THE DIAGNOSIS. OTHERWISE - REFER TO THE APPROPRIATE CATEGORY OF NEOPLASM FOR A MORE SPECIFIC CODE: SEE 'CANCER' 'CANCER METASTATIC', 'NEOPLASM UNCERTAIN BEHAVIOR', 'NEOPLASM UNSPECIFIED NATURE', OR 'BENIGN NEOPLASM.'

GASTRINOMA

235.5 SITE UNSPECIFIED
0 SITE SPECIFIED SEE 'NEOPLASM UNCERTAIN BEHAVIOR' BY SITE M8153/1
157.4 MALIGNANT SITE UNSPECIFIED M8153/3
0 MALIGNANT SITE SPECIFIED SEE 'CANCER' BY SITE M8153/3

GASTRITIS

535.5# NOS
535.0# ACUTE
535.3# ALCOHOLIC
535.4# ALLERGIC
535.1# ATROPHIC
535.1# ATROPHIC (HYPERPLASTIC CHRONIC)
535.4# BILE INDUCED
535.0# CATARRHAL
535.1# CHRONIC
535.4# CIRRHOTIC (SCLEROTIC) (TOXIC)

5th Digit: 535.0-1, 3-5
- **0. WITHOUT HEMORRHAGE**
- **1. WITH HEMORRHAGE**

269.9 DUE TO DIET DEFICIENCY
535.4# DUE TO INGESTED SUBSTANCE
535.4# EOSINOPHILIC (FOLLICULAR) (GLANDULAR)
535.4# EROSIVE
535.4# GLANDULAR
535.2# HYPERTROPHIC
535.1# INFECTIOUS DUE TO HELICOBACTER PYLORI [041.86]
535.4# IRRITANT

5th Digit: 535.1, 2, 4
- **0. WITHOUT HEMORRHAGE**
- **1. WITH HEMORRHAGE**

306.4 NERVOUS (CYCLICAL)
535.0# PHLEGMONOUS
535.4# SCLEROTIC

5th Digit: 535.0, 4
- **0. WITHOUT HEMORRHAGE**
- **1. WITH HEMORRHAGE**

GASTRITIS (continued)

536.8 SPASTIC
535.0# SUBACUTE
535.4# SUPERFICIAL
535.4# SUPPURATIVE
535.4# TOXIC

5th Digit: 535.0, 4
- **0. WITHOUT HEMORRHAGE**
- **1. WITH HEMORRHAGE**

121.8 GASTRODISCOIDES HOMINIS INFECTION
442.84 GASTRODUODENAL ARTERY (ANEURYSM) (A-V FISTULA) (CIRSOID) (FALSE) (VARICOSE)
535.5# GASTRODUODENITIS

5th Digit: 535.5
- **0. WITHOUT HEMORRHAGE**
- **1. WITH HEMORRHAGE**

536.8 GASTRODYNIA

GASTROENTERITIS (COMMON TYPES)

558.9 NOS
008.8 ACUTE VIRAL
558.9 ALLERGIC NONINFECTIOUS
008.5 BACTERIAL
558.9 CHRONIC
009.0 EPIDEMIC
009.0 INFECTIOUS
487.8 INFLUENZA
003.0 SALMONELLA
004.9 SHIGELLA
004.2 SHIGELLA BOYDII
004.0 SHIGELLA DYSENTERIAE
004.1 SHIGELLA FLEXNERI (GROUP B)
004.3 SHIGELLA SONEI
004.8 SHIGELLA OTHER SPECIFIED
008.41 STAPHYLOCOCCUS

GASTROENTERITIS (OTHER INFECTIOUS)

008.62 ADENOVIRUS
008.2 AEROBACTER AEROGENES
008.1 ARIZONA GROUP OF PARACOLON BACILLI
008.66 ASTROVIRUS
008.49 BACTERIA OTHER
008.65 CALCIVIRUS
009.0 COLITIS ENTERITIS SEPTIC
009.1 COLITIS ENTERITIS OF PRESUMED INFECTIOUS ORIGIN
008.69 DUE TO SPECIFIED VIRUS
008.0# E COLI INTESTINAL INFECTION

5th Digit: 008.0
- **0. DUE TO UNSPECIFIED E. COLI**
- **1. DUE TO ENTEROPATHOGENIC E. COLI**
- **2. DUE TO ENTEROTOXIGENIC E. COLI**
- **3. DUE TO ENTEROINVASIVE E. COLI**
- **4. DUE TO ENTEROHEMORRHAGIC E. COLI**
- **9. DUE TO OTHER INTESTINAL E. COLI INFECTIONS**

008.67 ENTEROVIRUS, NEC
009.0 INFECTIOUS (SEPTIC)
009.1 INFECTIOUS ORIGIN PRESUMED
008.63 NORWALK VIRUS
008.64 OTHER SMALL ROUND VIRUSES [RSV'S]
008.69 OTHER VIRAL ENTERITIS
008.3 PROTEUS MIRABILIS
008.42 PSEUDOMONAS AERUGINOSA
008.61 ROTAVIRUS
0 SEE ALSO ENTERITIS

GASTROENTERITIS NONINFECTIOUS

558.1 DUE TO RADIATION
558.9 ALLERGIC (DIETARY)
558.9 OTHER AND UNSPECIFIED
558.2 TOXIC

442.84 GASTROEPIPLOIC ARTERY (ANEURYSM) (A-V FISTULA) (CIRSOID) (FALSE) (VARICOSE)

530.89 GASTROESOPHAGEAL INSUFFICIENCY
530.0 GASTROESOPHAGEAL JUNCTION SYNDROME
530.7 GASTROESOPHAGEAL LACERATION-HEMORRHAGE SYNDROME
530.81 GASTROESOPHAGEAL REFLUX
530.19 GASTROESOPHAGITIS

GASTROINTESTINAL TRACT

793.4 ABNORMAL (X-RAY) (ULTRASOUND) (THERMOGRAPHY)
V44.4 ARTIFICIAL OPENING STATUS OTHER
569.89 ATROPHY
578.9 BLEEDING UNSPECIFIED
277.3 DISORDER AMYLOID
536.9 DISORDER FUNCTIONAL
777.9 DISORDER PERINATAL
306.4 DISORDER PSYCHOGENIC
793.4 FILLING DEFECT
0 INFECTION SEE ALSO 'ENTERITIS'
908.1 INJURY LATE EFFECT
863.80 INJURY NOS SITE
863.90 INJURY NOS SITE WITH OPEN WOUND INTO CAVITY
863.89 INJURY OTHER SPECIFIED SITE
863.99 INJURY OTHER SPECIFIED SITE WITH OPEN WOUND INTO CAVITY
0 OBSTRUCTION SEE 'INTESTINE, INTESTINAL', OBSTRUCTION
787.99 SYMPTOMS
306.4 SYMPTOMS PSYCHOGENIC

GASTROINTESTINAL TRACT ANOMALIES

CONGENITAL

751.2 AGENESIS LOWER
751.8 AGENESIS (COMPLETE) (PARTIAL)
751.9 AGENESIS UNSPECIFIED (COMPLETE) (PARTIAL)
750.8 AGENESIS UPPER (COMPLETE) (PARTIAL)
750.8 AGENESIS UPPER ALIMENTARY TRACT
747.61 ANOMALY ARTERY PERIPHERAL VASCULAR -(ABERRANT) (ABSENCE) (AGENESIS) (ACCESSORY) (ANEURYSM) (ATRESIA) (DEFORMITY) (HYPOPLASIA) (MALPOSITION)
751.9 ANOMALY OF FIXATION
750.8 ANOMALY OTHER SPECIFIED (UGI)
751.8 ANOMALY OTHER SPECIFIED ANOMALY OF FIXATION
750.8 ANOMALY UPPER OTHER SPECIFIED
750.9 ANOMALY UNSPECIFIED UPPER ALIMENTARY TRACT
747.61 ANOMALY VEIN PERIPHERAL VASCULAR- (ABERRANT) (ABSENCE) (AGENESIS) (ACCESSORY) (ANEURYSM) (DEFORMITY) (HYPOPLASIA) (MALPOSITION)
751.2 ATRESIA LOWER (COMPLETE) (PARTIAL)
751.9 DEFORMITY
750.9 DEFORMITY UPPER ALIMENTARY TRACT
751.8 MALPOSITION DUPLICATION GI

537.89 GASTROJEJUNAL LOOP OBSTRUCTION SYNDROME
534.## GASTROJEJUNAL ULCER

4th Digit: 534

0. ACUTE WITH HEMORRHAGE
1. ACUTE WITH PERFORATION
2. ACUTE WITH HEMORRHAGE AND PERFORATION
3. ACUTE
4. CHRONIC OR UNSPECIFIED WITH HEMORRHAGE
5. CHRONIC OR UNSPECIFIED WITH PERFORATION
6. CHRONIC OR UNSPECIFIED WITH HEMORRHAGE AND PERFORATION
7. CHRONIC
9. UNSPECIFIED AS ACUTE OR CHRONIC

5th Digit: 534

0. WITHOUT OBSTRUCTION
1. OBSTRUCTED

537.89 GASTROLITHS
536.3 GASTROPARALYSIS

<u>250.6#</u> GASTROPARALYSIS <u>DIABETIC</u> [337.1]

5th Digit: 250.6

0. TYPE II, ADULT-ONSET, NON-INSULIN DEPENDENT (EVEN IF REQUIRING INSULIN), OR UNSPECIFIED; CONTROLLED
1. TYPE I, JUVENILE-ONSET OR INSULIN-DEPENDENT; CONTROLLED
2. TYPE II, ADULT-ONSET, NON-INSULIN DEPENDENT (EVEN IF REQUIRING INSULIN); UNCONTROLLED
3. TYPE I, JUVENILE-ONSET OR INSULIN-DEPENDENT; UNCONTROLLED

536.3 GASTROPARESIS
<u>250.6#</u> GASTROPARESIS <u>DIABETIC</u> [536.3]

5th Digit: 250.6

0. TYPE II, ADULT-ONSET, NON-INSULIN DEPENDENT (EVEN IF REQUIRING INSULIN), OR UNSPECIFIED; CONTROLLED
1. TYPE I, JUVENILE-ONSET OR INSULIN-DEPENDENT; CONTROLLED
2. TYPE II, ADULT-ONSET, NON-INSULIN DEPENDENT (EVEN IF REQUIRING INSULIN); UNCONTROLLED
3. TYPE I, JUVENILE-ONSET OR INSULIN-DEPENDENT; UNCONTROLLED

579.8 GASTROPATHY, EXUDATIVE
537.5 GASTROPTOSIS
569.89 GASTROSCHISIS
756.79 GASTROSCHISIS CONGENITAL
578.0 GASTROSTAXIS

MALFUNCTION OR INFECTION OF A SURGICAL PROCEDURE, IMPLANT, OR, ARTIFICIAL OPENING SHOULD BE CODED AS A "COMPLICATION."

GASTROSTOMY

V55.1 CARE
V55.1 CATHETER ADJUSTMENT OR REPOSITIONING
V55.1 CATHETER REMOVAL OR REPLACEMENT
V55.1 CLOSURE
536.40 COMPLICATION NOS
536.42 COMPLICATION MECHANICAL
536.49 COMPLICATION OTHER
V53.5 DEVICE FITTING AND ADJUSTMENT

WHEN CODING AN INFECTION OF AN OSTOMY, USE AN ADDITIONAL CODE TO SPECIFY THE ORGANISM. SEE 'BACTERIAL INFECTION'

536.41 INFECTION
<u>536.41</u> <u>INFECTION</u> WITH CELLULITIS OF ABDOMEN [682.2]
<u>536.41</u> <u>INFECTION</u> WITH SEPSIS [**038.#(#)**]

4th or 4th <u>and</u> 5th Digit Code for Organism: 038

.9 NOS
.3 ANAEROBIC
.3 BACTEROIDES
.3 CLOSTRIDIUM
.42 E COLI
.49 ENTEROBACTER AEROGENES
.40 GRAM NEGATIVE
.49 GRAM NEGATIVE OTHER
.41 HEMOPHILUS INFLUENZAE
.2 PNEUMOCOCCAL
.49 PROTEUS
.43 PSEUDOMONAS
.44 SERRATIA
.10 STAPHYLOCOCCAL NOS
.11 STAPHYLOCOCCAL AUREUS
.19 STAPHYLOCOCCAL OTHER
.0 STREPTOCOCCAL (ANAEROBIC)
.49 YERSINIA ENTEROCOLITICA
.8 OTHER SPECIFIED

536.42 MALFUNCTION
V55.1 REMOVAL OR REPLACEMENT
V44.1 STATUS
V55.1 TOILET STOMA

272.7 GAUCHER'S CEREBRAL DEGENERATION [330.2]
272.7 GAUCHER'S DISEASE (CEREBROSIDE LIPIDOSIS)
265.1 GAYET-WERNICKE'S (SUPERIOR HEMORRHAGIC POLIOENCEPHALITIS)
265.1 GAYET'S SUPERIOR HEMORRHAGIC POLIOENCEPHALITIS
0 GC SEE 'GONORRHEA'
579.0 GEE (-HERTER) (-HEUBNER) (-THAYSEN) NONTROPICAL SPRUE
347 GELINEAU'S SYNDROME
302.85 GENDER IDENTITY DISORDER ADOLESCENT OR ADULT
302.85 GENDER IDENTITY DISORDER ADULT
302.6 GENDER IDENTITY DISORDER CHILDHOOD
094.1 GENERAL PARESIS SYPHILIS
V26.3 GENETIC COUNSELING
351.1 GENICULATE GANGLIONITIS
053.11 GENICULATE GANGLIONITIS HERPETIC

GENITAL

054.10 HERPES
629.8 HYPERPLASIA FEMALE
608.89 HYPERPLASIA MALE
959.1 INJURY (EXTERNAL ORGAN)
V47.5 PROBLEM
618.9 PROLAPSE FEMALE
618.9 PROLAPSE FEMALE WITH STRESS INCONTINENCE [625.6]
618.9 PROLAPSE FEMALE WITH OTHER URINARY INCONTINENCE [788.3#]

5th Digit: 788.3
- **0. UNSPECIFIED**
- **1. URGE INCONTINENCE**
- **3. MIXED URGE AND STRESS**
- **4 WITHOUT SENSORY AWARENESS**
- **5. POST-VOID DRIBBLING**
- **6. NOCTURNAL ENURESIS**
- **7. CONTINUOUS LEAKAGE**
- **9. OTHER**

618.8 PROLAPSE FEMALE - OTHER SPECIFIED
618.8 PROLAPSE FEMALE - OTHER SPECIFIED WITH STRESS INCONTINENCE [625.6]
618.8 PROLAPSE FEMALE - OTHER SPECIFIED WITH URINARY INCONTINENCE [788.3#]

5th Digit: 788.3
- **0. UNSPECIFIED**
- **1. URGE INCONTINENCE**
- **3. MIXED URGE AND STRESS**
- **4 WITHOUT SENSORY AWARENESS**
- **5. POST-VOID DRIBBLING**
- **6. NOCTURNAL ENURESIS**
- **7. CONTINUOUS LEAKAGE**
- **9. OTHER**

760.8 TRACT OTHER LOCALIZED MATERNAL INFECTION AFFECTING FETUS OR NEWBORN
078.19 WARTS NOS SEE 'WARTS', BY TYPE

GENITAL ORGAN

752.49 ABSENCE FEMALE EXTERNAL (CERVIX, CLITORIS, VAGINA, VULVA) - CONGENITAL
752.8 ABSENCE FEMALE INTERNAL NEC - CONGENITAL
752.8 ABSENCE MALE - CONGENITAL
752.8 ACCESSORY MALE NEC (CONGENITAL)
752.9 ANOMALY CONGENITAL
752.8 ANOMALY EXTERNAL MALE
752.40 ANOMALY FEMALE EXTERNAL CONGENITAL
752.49 ANOMALY FEMALE (CONGENITAL) OTHER SPECIFIED
752.49 ATRESIA FEMALE EXTERNAL (CONGENITAL)
752.8 ATRESIA FEMALE INTERNAL (CONGENITAL)
752.8 ATRESIA MALE EXTERNAL (CONGENITAL)
752.8 ATRESIA MALE INTERNAL (CONGENITAL)
608.89 ATROPHY MALE
959.1 EXTERNAL INJURY

GENITAL ORGAN (continued)

629.9 FEMALE DISORDER
629.8 FEMALE DISORDER OTHER SPECIFIED
625.8 FEMALE OTHER SPECIFIED SYMPTOMS
625.9 FEMALE UNSPECIFIED SYMPTOMS
867.6 INJURY NEC (TRAUMATIC)
867.7 INJURY NEC (TRAUMATIC) WITH OPEN WOUND
608.9 MALE DISORDER
V13.2 HISTORY OF GENITAL SYSTEM AND OBSTETRIC DISORDER (NON GRAVID)

099.1 GENITO-ANORECTAL SYNDROME

GENITOURINARY

752.8 ABSENCE ORGANS NEC - CONGENITAL
793.5 ABNORMALITY ON X-RAY
V18.7 DISEASES OTHER FAMILY HISTORY
306.50 DISORDER (MALFUNCTION) PSYCHOGENIC
599.89 HEMORRHAGE
599.0 INFECTION NEC
V81.6 SCREENING FOR OTHER AND UNSPECIFIED CONDITONS
306.59 SYMPTOMS PSYCHOGENIC OTHER

GENU

736.5 RECURVATUM ACQUIRED
754.40 RECURVATUM CONGENITAL
736.41 VALGUM ACQUIRED
755.64 VALGUM CONGENITAL
736.42 VARUM ACQUIRED
755.64 VARUM CONGENITAL

529.1 GEOGRAPHIC TONGUE
307.52 GEOPHAGIA
117.9 GEOTRICHOSIS
300.29 GEPHYROPHOBIA
745.4 GERBODE DEFECT
530.81 GERD (GASTROESOPHAGEAL REFLUX DISEASE)
443.89 GERHARDT'S ERYTHROMELALGIA
478.30 GERHARDT'S SYNDROME (VOCAL CORD PARALYSIS)
078.81 GERLIER'S EPIDEMIC VERTIGO
056.9 GERMAN MEASLES (RUBELLA)
0 GERMAN MEASLES WITH COMPLICATIONS SEE 'RUBELLA'
606.0 GERMINAL CELL APLASIA
606.1 GERMINAL CELL DESQUAMATION
199.1 GERMINOMA SITE UNSPECIFIED
0 GERMINOMA SITE SPECIFIED SEE 'CANCER' BY SITE M9064/3
371.41 GERONTOXON
784.69 GERSTMANN'S SYNDROME (FINGER AGNOSIA)

GESTATION

651.## MULTIPLE

4th Digit: 651
- **0. TWIN**
- **1. TRIPLET**
- **2. QUADRUPLET**
- **3. TWIN WITH FETAL LOSS**
- **4. TRIPLET WITH FETAL LOSS**
- **5. QUADRUPLET WITH FETAL LOSS**
- **6. OTHER MULTIPLE PREGNANCY WITH FETAL LOSS**
- **8. OTHER SPECIFIED**
- **9. UNSPECIFIED**

5th Digit: 651
- **0. EPISODE OF CARE UNSPECIFIED OR N/A**
- **1. DELIVERED**
- **3. ANTEPARTUM COMPLICATION**

766.2 PROLONGED SYNDROME
0 SEE PREGNANCY

010.0# GHON TUBERCLE

5th Digit: 010.0

0. UNSPECIFIED
1. LAB NOT DONE
2. LABS PENDING
3. MICROSCOPY POSITIVE (IN SPUTUM)
4. CULTURE POSITIVE - MICROSCOPY NEGATIVE
5. CULTURE NEGATIVE - MICROSCOPY POSITIVE
6. CULTURE AND MICROSCOPY NEGATIVE CONFIRMED BY OTHER METHODS

370.64 GHOST VESSELS CORNEAL
102.3 GHOUL HAND
578.9 GI BLEEDING
0 GI BLEEDING SEE SPECIFIC CAUSE AND SITE
536.9 GI DISORDER (FUNCTIONAL)
863.80 GI INJURY SITE NOS
863.90 GI INJURY SITE NOS WITH OPEN WOUND
0 GI TRACT SEE 'GASTROINTESTINAL TRACT'

CARCINOMAS AND NEOPLASMS SHOULD BE CODED BY SITE IF POSSIBLE. CODE BY CELL TYPE - "SITE NOS", IF AND ONLY IF A SITE IS NOT SPECIFIED IN THE DIAGNOSIS. OTHERWISE - REFER TO THE APPROPRIATE CATEGORY OF NEOPLASM FOR A MORE SPECIFIC CODE: SEE 'CANCER' 'CANCER METASTATIC', 'NEOPLASM UNCERTAIN BEHAVIOR', 'NEOPLASM UNSPECIFIED NATURE', OR 'BENIGN NEOPLASM.'

GIANT CELL

199.1 AND SPINDLE CELL CARCINOMA SITE UNSPECIFIED
0 AND SPINDLE CELL CARCINOMA SITE SPECIFIED SEE 'CANCER' BY SITE M8030/3
446.5 ARTERITIS
648.9# ARTERITIS MATERNAL CURRENT (CO-EXISTENT) IN PREGNANCY [446.5]

5th Digit: 648.9

0. EPISODE OF CARE UNSPECIFIED OR N/A
1. DELIVERED
2. DELIVERED WITH POSTPARTUM COMPLICATION
3. ANTEPARTUM COMPLICATION
4. POSTPARTUM COMPLICATION

199.1 CARCINOMA SITE UNSPECIFIED
0 CARCINOMA SITE SPECIFIED SEE 'CANCER' BY SITE M8031/3
523.8 EPULIS
245.1 THYROIDITIS
238.0 TUMOR BONE NOS M9250/1
170.# TUMOR BONE (MALIGNANT) M9250/3

4th Digit: 170

0. SKULL AND FACE
1. MANDIBLE
2. VERTEBRAL COLUMN
3. RIBS STERNUM CLAVICLE
4. SCAPULA LONG BONES UPPER LIMB
5. SHORT BONES UPPER LIMB
6. PELVIC BONES SACRUM COCCYX
7. LONG BONES LOWER LIMB
8. SHORT BONES LOWER LIMB
9. SITE UNSPECIFIED

523.8 TUMOR GINGIVA
238.1 TUMOR SOFT AND CONNECTIVE TISSUE NOS
171.# TUMOR SOFT AND CONNECTIVE TISSUE MALIGNANT M9251/3

4th Digit: 171

0. HEAD FACE NECK
2. UPPER LIMB SHOULDER
3. LOWER LIMB HIP
4. THORAX
5. ABDOMINAL HYPOCHONDRIUM
6. PELVIS BUTTOCK GROIN INGUINAL REGION PERINEUM
7. TRUNK UNSPECIFIED BACK NOS FLANK NOS
8. OTHER SPECIFIED SITES
9. SITE UNSPECIFIED

GIANT CELL (continued)

727.02 TUMOR SYNOVIAL
727.02 TUMOR TENDON SHEATH

753.3 GIANT KIDNEY
007.1 GIARDIASIS (INTESTINAL)
696.3 GIBERT'S PITYRIASIS ROSEA
720.9 GIBNEY'S PERISPONDYLITIS
0 GIBRALTAR FEVER SEE 'BRUCELLOSIS'
780.4 GIDDINESS
271.0 GIERKE'S GLYCOGENOSIS I
213.# GIGANTIFORM CEMENTOMA

4th Digit: 213

0. SKULL FACE UPPER JAW
1. LOWER JAW UNSPECIFIED (OR IF SITE NOS)

253.0 GIGANTISM
989.5 GILA MONSTER BITE
995.0 GILA MONSTER BITE WITH ANAPHYLAXIS [989.5]
277.4 GILBERT'S SYNDROME (FAMILIAL NONHEMOLYTIC JAUNDICE)
116.0 GILCHRIST'S NORTH AMERICAN BLASTOMYCOSIS
259.8 GILFORD (-HUTCHINSON) SYNDROME (PROGERIA)
307.23 GILLES DE LA TOURETTE'S SYNDROME (MOTOR-VERBAL TIC)
759.89 GILLESPIE'S SYNDROME (DYSPLASIA OCULODENTODIGITALIS)

GINGIVAL

523.9 DISEASE NOS
523.8 FIBROMATOSIS
523.8 HYPERPLASIA
0 INFECTION SEE 'GINGIVITIS'
523.8 OCCLUSION TRAUMATIC
523.2 RECESSION
523.8 ULCER

GINGIVITIS

523.0 ACUTE
101 ACUTE NECROTIZING (ULCERATIVE)
523.1 CHRONIC
523.1 CHRONIC NONHERPETIC
054.2 HERPETIC (SIMPLEX)
101 VINCENT'S

523.1 GINGIVOSTOMATITIS
054.2 GINGIVOSTOMATITIS HERPES
117.9 GIOVANNINI'S DISEASE
024 GLANDERS
289.3 GLANDULAR ATROPHY (LYMPH)
075 GLANDULAR FEVER
752.8 GLANS PENIS DIVISION
287.1 GLANZMANN'S HEREDITARY HEMORRHAGIC THROMBASTHENIA
527.1 GLASSBLOWERS' DISEASE

GLAUCOMA

365.9 NOS
365.9 NOS WITH GLAUCOMATOUS FLECKS [366.31]
360.42 ABSOLUTE
365.22 ACUTE
365.2# ANGLE CLOSURE
365.2# ANGLE CLOSURE WITH GLAUCOMATOUS FLECKS [366.31]

5th Digit: 365.2

0. PRIMARY UNSPECIFIED
1. INTERMITTENT (SUBACUTE)
2. ACUTE
3. CHRONIC
4. RESIDUAL STAGE

GLAUCOMA (continued)

365.00 BORDERLINE
365.01 BORDERLINE OPEN ANGLE
365.01 BORDERLINE OPEN ANGLE WITH GLAUCOMATOUS FLECKS [366.31]
365.02 BORDERLINE NARROW ANGLE
365.02 BORDERLINE NARROW ANGLE WITH GLAUCOMATOUS FLECKS [366.31]
365.04 BORDERLINE OCULAR HYPERTENSION
365.04 BORDERLINE OCULAR HYPERTENSION WITH GLAUCOMATOUS FLECKS [366.31]
365.03 BORDERLINE STEROID RESPONDER
365.03 BORDERLINE STEROID RESPONDER WITH GLAUCOMATOUS FLECKS [366.31]
365.00 BORDERLINE WITH GLAUCOMATOUS FLECKS [366.31]
365.14 CHILDHOOD OR JUVENILE
365.14 CHILDHOOD OR JUVENILE WITH GLAUCOMATOUS FLECKS [366.31]
365.11 CHRONIC (SIMPLE) (NONCONGESTIVE) (NONOBSTRUCTIVE)
365.11 CHRONIC (SIMPLE) (NONCONGESTIVE) (NONOBSTRUCTIVE) WITH GLAUCOMATOUS FLECKS [366.31]
743.20 CONGENITAL INFANTILE
743.21 CONGENITAL INFANTILE SIMPLE
365.3# CORTICOSTEROID INDUCED
365.3# CORTICOSTEROID INDUCED WITH GLAUCOMATOUS FLECKS [366.31]

5th Digit: 365.3

1. GLAUCOMATOUS STAGE
2. RESIDUAL STAGE

365.60 HEMORRHAGIC
365.60 HEMORRHAGIC WITH GLAUCOMATOUS FLECKS [366.31]
365.81 HYPERSECRETION
365.81 HYPERSECRETION WITH GLAUCOMATOUS FLECKS [366.31]
365.14 INFANTILE
365.14 INFANTILE WITH GLAUCOMATOUS FLECKS [366.31]
365.14 JUVENILE
365.14 JUVENILE WITH GLAUCOMATOUS FLECKS [366.31]
365.12 LOW TENSION
365.12 LOW TENSION WITH GLAUCOMATOUS FLECKS [366.31]
365.20 MALIGNANT
365.2# NARROW ANGLE
365.2# NARROW ANGLE WITH GLAUCOMATOUS FLECKS [366.31]

5th Digit: 365.2

0. PRIMARY UNSPECIFIED
1. INTERMITTENT (SUBACUTE)
2. ACUTE
3. CHRONIC
4. RESIDUAL STAGE

365.60 NEOVASCULAR
743.20 NEWBORN
365.62 OCULAR INFLAMMATION
365.62 OCULAR INFLAMMATION WITH GLAUCOMATOUS FLECKS [366.31]
365.1# OPEN ANGLE
365.1# OPEN ANGLE WITH GLAUCOMATOUS FLECKS [366.31]

5th Digit: 365.1

0. UNSPECIFIED
1. PRIMARY (CHRONIC SIMPLE)
2. LOW TENSION
3. PIGMENTARY
4. CHILDHOOD (JUVENILE) (INFANTILE)
5. RESIDUAL STAGE

365.01 OPEN ANGLE WITH CUPPING OF OPTIC DISCS
365.01 OPEN ANGLE WITH CUPPING OF OPTIC DISCS WITH GLAUCOMATOUS FLECKS [366.31]
365.51 PHACOLYTIC
365.51 PHACOLYTIC WITH GLAUCOMATOUS FLECKS [366.31]
365.13 PIGMENTARY
365.13 PIGMENTARY WITH GLAUCOMATOUS FLECKS [366.31]

GLAUCOMA (continued)

365.60 POSTINFECTIOUS
365.60 POSTINFECTIOUS WITH GLAUCOMATOUS FLECKS [366.31]
365.52 PSEUDOEXFOLIATION
365.52 PSEUDOEXFOLIATION WITH GLAUCOMATOUS FLECKS [366.31]
V80.1 SCREENING
365.60 SECONDARY
365.60 SECONDARY WITH GLAUCOMATOUS FLECKS [366.31]
0 SUSPECT SEE 'GLAUCOMA', BORDERLINE
095.8 SYPHILITIC
365.10 WIDE ANGLE NOS
365.10 WIDE ANGLE NOS WITH GLAUCOMATOUS FLECKS [366.31]
365.82 WITH EPISCLERAL VENOUS PRESSURE INCREASED
365.82 WITH EPISCLERAL VENOUS PRESSURE INCREASED WITH GLAUCOMATOUS FLECKS [366.31]
365.89 OTHER SPECIFIED
365.89 OTHER SPECIFIED WITH GLAUCOMATOUS FLECKS [366.31]

GLAUCOMA OTHER ETIOLOGIES

250.5# DIABETIC [365.44]

5th Digit: 250.5

0. TYPE II, ADULT-ONSET, NON-INSULIN DEPENDENT (EVEN IF REQUIRING INSULIN), OR UNSPECIFIED; CONTROLLED
1. TYPE I, JUVENILE-ONSET OR INSULIN-DEPENDENT; CONTROLLED
2. TYPE II, ADULT-ONSET, NON-INSULIN DEPENDENT (EVEN IF REQUIRING INSULIN); UNCONTROLLED
3. TYPE I, JUVENILE-ONSET OR INSULIN-DEPENDENT; UNCONTROLLED

365.65 TRAUMA (OCULAR) NEC
767.8 TRAUMA (OCULAR) BIRTH TRAUMA
921.3 TRAUMA (OCULAR] (GLOBE CONTUSION) [365.65]
365.65 TRAUMA (OCULAR) WITH GLAUCOMATOUS FLECKS [366.31]
743.45 WITH ANIRIDIA [365.42]
743.44 WITH AXENFELD'S ANOMALY [365.41]
379.33 WITH DISLOCATION LENS (ANTERIOR) [365.59]
379.34 WITH DISLOCATION LENS (POSTERIOR) [365.59]
364.61 WITH EPITHELIAL DOWN GROWTH [365.64]
364.22 WITH GLAUCOMATOCYCLITIC CRISIS [365.62]
366.18 WITH HYPERMATURE CATARACT [365.51]
364.41 WITH HYPHEMA [365.63]
364.3 WITH IRIDOCYCLITIS [365.62]
364.10 WITH IRIDOCYCLITIS CHRONIC [365.62]
743.46 WITH IRIS ANOMALIES NEC [365.42]
364.51 WITH IRIS ATROPHICA [365.42]
364.74 WITH IRIS BOMBE [365.61]
364.42 WITH IRIS RUBEOSIS [365.63]
743.41 WITH MICROCORNEA [365.43]
224.# WITH NEOPLASM (BENIGN) [365.64]
190.# WITH NEOPLASM (MALIGNANT) [365.64]

4th Digit: 190, 224

0. EYE GLOBE
1. ORBIT
2. LACRIMAL GLAND
3. CONJUNCTIVA
4. CORNEA
5. RETINA
6. CHOROID
7. LACRIMAL DUCT
8. OTHER SPECIFIED
9. UNSPECIFIED

237.70 WITH NEUROFIBROMATOSIS (MULTIPLE) [365.44]
237.71 WITH NEUROFIBROMATOSIS (TYPE I) [365.44]
237.72 WITH NEUROFIBROMATOSIS (TYPE II) [365.44]
365.60 WITH OCULAR DISORDER UNSPECIFIED
365.59 WITH OTHER LENS DISORDERS
365.61 WITH PUPILLARY BLOCK

GLAUCOMA OTHER ETIOLOGIES (continued)

364.77 WITH RECESSED ANGLE [365.65]
362.35 WITH RETINAL VEIN OCCLUSION [365.63]
743.44 WITH RIEGER'S ANOMALY [365.41]
743.36 WITH SPHEROPHAKIA [365.59]
759.6 WITH STURGE WEBER [365.44]
017.3# WITH TUBERCULOSIS [365.62]

5th Digit: 017.3

- **0. NOS**
- **1. LAB NOT DONE**
- **2. LABS PENDING**
- **3. MICROSCOPY POSITIVE (IN SPUTUM)**
- **4. CULTURE POSITIVE - MICROSCOPY NEGATIVE**
- **5. CULTURE NEGATIVE - MICROSCOPY POSITIVE**
- **6. CULTURE AND MICROSCOPY NEGATIVE CONFIRMED BY OTHER METHODS**

365.64 WITH TUMORS OR CYSTS
365.63 WITH VASCULAR DISORDERS
237.71 WITH VON RECKLINGHAUSEN'S DISEASE [365.44]

364.22 GLAUCOMATOCYCLITIC CRISES
364.22 GLAUCOMATOCYCLITIC PARS PLANA HYPERPLASIA
0 GLAUCOMATOUS FLECKS (SUBCAPSULAR) SEE 'GLAUCOMA'
569.89 GLENARD'S SYNDROME (ENTEROPTOSIS)
253.2 GLINSKI-SIMMONDS SYNDROME (PITUITARY CACHEXIA)

> *CARCINOMAS AND NEOPLASMS SHOULD BE CODED BY SITE IF POSSIBLE. CODE BY CELL TYPE - "SITE NOS", IF AND ONLY IF A SITE IS NOT SPECIFIED IN THE DIAGNOSIS. OTHERWISE - REFER TO THE APPROPRIATE CATEGORY OF NEOPLASM FOR A MORE SPECIFIC CODE: SEE 'CANCER' 'CANCER METASTATIC', 'NEOPLASM UNCERTAIN BEHAVIOR', 'NEOPLASM UNSPECIFIED NATURE', OR 'BENIGN NEOPLASM.'*

GLIOBLASTOMA

191.9 SITE UNSPECIFIED
0 SITE SPECIFIED SEE 'CANCER' BY SITE M9440/3
191.9 GIANT CELL SITE UNSPECIFIED
0 GIANT CELL SITE SPECIFIED SEE 'CANCER' BY SITE M9441/3
191.9 WITH SARCOMATOUS COMPONENT SITE UNSPECIFIED
0 WITH SARCOMATOUS COMPONENT SITE SPECIFIED SEE 'CANCER' BY SITE M9442/3

GLIOMA

191.9 MALIGNANT SITE UNSPECIFIED
0 MALIGNANT SITE SPECIFIED SEE 'CANCER' BY SITE M9380/3
191.9 MIXED SITE UNSPECIFIED
0 MIXED SITE SPECIFIED SEE 'CANCER' BY SITE M9382/3
237.5 SUBEPENDYMAL SITE UNSPECIFIED
0 SUBEPENDYMAL SITE SPECIFIED SEE 'NEOPLASM UNCERTAIN BEHAVIOR' BY SITE M9383/1

191.9 GLIOMATOSIS CEREBRI SITE UNSPECIFIED
0 GLIOMATOSIS CEREBRI SITE SPECIFIED SEE 'CANCER' BY SITE M9381/3

349.89 GLIOSIS CEREBRAL
336.0 GLIOSIS SPINAL

268.0 GLISSON'S DISEASE (SEE ALSO 'RICKETS')

GLOBE

360.41 ATROPHY
360.20 DEGENERATIVE DISORDER
360.29 DEGENERATIVE DISORDER OTHER
360.9 DISORDER NOS
360.89 DISORDERS OTHER (EYE)
376.36 DISPLACEMENT (LATERAL)
360.81 LUXATION

526.1 GLOBULOMAXILLARY CYST
306.4 GLOBUS
300.11 GLOBUS HYSTERICUS
228.0# GLOMANGIOMA M8712/0

5th Digit: 228.0

- **0. SITE UNSPECIFIED**
- **1. SKIN AND SUBCUTANEOUS TISSUE**
- **2. INTRACRANIAL STRUCTURES**
- **3. RETINA**
- **4. INTRA ABDOMINAL STRUCTURES**
- **9. OTHER SITES**

171.# GLOMANGIOSARCOMA M8710/3

4th Digit: 171

- **0. HEAD FACE NECK**
- **2. UPPER LIMB SHOULDER**
- **3. LOWER LIMB HIP**
- **4. THORAX**
- **5. ABDOMINAL HYPOCHONDRIUM**
- **6. PELVIS BUTTOCK GROIN INGUINAL REGION PERINEUM**
- **7. TRUNK NOS BACK NOS FLANK NOS**
- **8. OTHER SPECIFIED SITES**
- **9. SITE NOS**

581.1 GLOMERULAR DISEASE MEMBRANOUS IDIOPATHIC
581.3 GLOMERULAR DISEASE MINIMAL CHANGE

581.3 GLOMERULITIS MINIMAL CHANGE
583.4 GLOMERULITIS PROGRESSIVE OR NECROTIZING

GLOMERULONEPHRITIS

583.# NOS

4th Digit: 583

- **0. PROLIFERATIVE (DIFFUSE)**
- **1. MEMBRANOUS**
- **2. MEMBRANOPROLIFERATIVE HYPOCOMPLEMENTEMIC PERSISTENT, LOBULAR, MESANGIOCAPILLARY, MIXED MEMBRANOUS AND PROLIFERATIVE**
- **4. RAPIDLY PROGRESSIVE, NECROTIZING, EXTRACAPILLARY WITH EPITHELIAL CRESCENTS**
- **6. WITH CORTICAL NECROSIS**
- **7. WITH MEDULLARY (PAPILLARY) NECROSIS**
- **9. UNSPECIFIED LESION IN KIDNEY**

580.# ACUTE

4th Digit: 580

- **0. PROLIFERATIVE OR POST STREPTOCOCCAL**
- **4. RAPIDLY PROGRESSIVE NECROTIZING, EXTRACAPILLARY WITH EPITHELIAL CRESCENTS**
- **9. UNSPECIFIED OR HEMORRHAGIC**

582.# CHRONIC

4th Digit: 582

- **0. PROLIFERATIVE (DIFFUSE)**
- **1. MEMBRANOUS , SCLEROSING, FOCAL, SEGMENTAL HYALINOSIS**
- **2. MEMBRANOPROLIFERATIVE, ENDOTHELIAL, HYPOCOMPLEMENTEMIC PERSISTENT, LOBULAR, MESANGIOCAPILLARY, MIXED MEMBRANOUS AND PROLIFERATIVE**
- **4. RAPIDLY PROGRESSIVE, NECROTIZING, EXTRACAPILLARY WITH EPITHELIAL CRESCENTS**
- **9. UNSPECIFIED OR HEMORRHAGIC**

581.# WITH NEPHROTIC SYNDROME

4th Digit: 581

- **0. PROLIFERATIVE,**
- **1. MEMBRANOUS , EPIMEMBRANOUS, FOCAL, SCLEROSING, SEGMENTAL HYALINOSIS**
- **2. MEMBRANOPROLIFERATIVE, LOBULAR, ENDOTHELIAL, HYPOCOMPLEMENTEMIC PERSISTENT, LOBULAR, MESANGIOCAPILLARY, MIXED MEMBRANOUS AND PROLIFERATIVE**
- **3. MINIMAL CHANGE, FOOT PROCESS, LIPOID,**
- **9. UNSPECIFIED LESION IN KIDNEY**

THE CODE IN THE LEFT MARGIN ALWAYS SEQUENCES FIRST. THE ADDITIONAL CODE IN BRACKETS TO THE RIGHT OF THE DESCRIPTION IS SEQUENCED SECONDARILY. UNDERLINING SHOWS THE CODE NUMBER THAT CORRESPONDS TO THE UNDERLINED VERBAL DESCRIPTION. UNDERLINING NEVER IMPLIES CORRECT SEQUENCING.

GLOMERULONEPHRITIS DUE TO OTHER CAUSES

277.3 AMYLOID [583.81]
277.3 AMYLOID (CHRONIC) [582.81]
403.90 ARTERIOLAR SEE ALSO 'HYPERTENSIVE RENAL DISEASE'
403.90 ARTERIOSCLEROTIC SEE ALSO 'HYPERTENSIVE RENAL DISEASE'
0 ASCENDING SEE 'PYELONEPHRITIS'
421.0 BACTERIAL ENDOCARDITIS SUBACUTE [580.81]
583.89 BASEMENT MEMBRANE NEC
446.21 BASEMENT MEMBRANE WITH PULMONARY HEMORRHAGE (GOODPASTURE'S SYNDROME) [583.81]
582.89 CHRONIC (EXUDATIVE) (FOCAL) (INTERSTITIAL)
587 CIRRHOTIC
250.4# DIABETIC [583.81]

5th Digit: 250.4

0. TYPE II, ADULT-ONSET, NON-INSULIN DEPENDENT (EVEN IF REQUIRING INSULIN), OR UNSPECIFIED; CONTROLLED
1. TYPE I, JUVENILE-ONSET OR INSULIN-DEPENDENT; CONTROLLED
2. TYPE II, ADULT-ONSET, NON-INSULIN DEPENDENT (EVEN IF REQUIRING INSULIN); UNCONTROLLED
3. TYPE I, JUVENILE-ONSET OR INSULIN-DEPENDENT; UNCONTROLLED

032.89 DIPHTHERIA [580.81]
421.0 ENDOCARDITIS BACTERIAL SUBACUTE [580.81]
581.9 EDEMA SEE ALSO 'NEPHROSIS'
583.89 EXUDATIVE NEC
580.89 EXUDATIVE ACUTE
582.89 EXUDATIVE CHRONIC
583.9 FOCAL SEE ALSO 'NEPHRITIS'
098.19 GONOCOCCAL INFECTION ACUTE [583.81]
098.39 GONOCOCCAL INFECTION CHRONIC OR LASTING 2 OR MORE MONTHS [583.81]
582.89 GRANULAR
582.89 GRANULOMATOUS
070.9 HEPATITIS (INFECTIOUS) [580.81]
070.6 HEPATITIS (INFECTIOUS) WITH HEPATIC COMA [580.81]
070.1 HEPATITIS VIRAL A (INFECTIOUS) [580.81]
070.0 HEPATITIS VIRAL A (INFECTIOUS) WITH HEPATIC COMA [580.81]
070.3# HEPATITIS VIRAL B (AUSTRALIAN ANTIGEN) [580.81]
070.2# HEPATITIS VIRAL B (AUSTRALIAN ANTIGEN) WITH HEPATIC COMA [580.81]

5th Digit: 070.2-3

0. ACUTE OR UNSPECIFIED
1. ACUTE OR UNSPECIFIED WITH DELTA
2. CHRONIC
3. CHRONIC WITH DELTA

070.5# HEPATITIS VIRAL C (D) (E) OR OTHER [580.81]
070.4# HEPATITIS VIRAL C (D) (E) OR OTHER WITH HEPATIC COMA [580.81]

5th Digit: 070.4-5

1. ACUTE OR UNSPECIFIED C
2. DELTA, OR DELTA WITH B CARRIER STATE
3. HEPATITIS E
4. CHRONIC C
9. OTHER SPECIFIED VIRAL

581.9 HYDREMIC SEE ALSO 'NEPHROSIS'
583.89 IMMUNE COMPLEX NEC
590.80 INFECTIVE SEE ALSO 'PYELONEPHRITIS'

GLOMERULONEPHRITIS DUE TO OTHER CAUSES (continued)

583.89 INTERSTITIAL NEPHRITIS (DIFFUSE) (FOCAL) NEC
580.89 INTERSTITIAL NEPHRITIS (DIFFUSE) (FOCAL) ACUTE
582.89 INTERSTITIAL NEPHRITIS (DIFFUSE) (FOCAL) CHRONIC
581.89 INTERSTITIAL NEPHRITIS (DIFFUSE) (FOCAL) WITH NEPHROTIC SYNDROME
582.9 LATENT OR QUIESCENT
710.0 LUPUS [583.81]
710.0 LUPUS (CHRONIC) (DUE TO) [582.81]
084.9 MALARIAL [581.81]
072.79 MUMPS (DUE TO) [580.81]
581.89 PARENCHYMATOUS
590.80 PURULENT SEE ALSO 'PYELONEPHRITIS'
590.80 SEPTIC SEE ALSO 'PYELONEPHRITIS'
583.89 SPECIFIED PATHOLOGY OR LESION NEC
580.89 SPECIFIED PATHOLOGY OR LESION ACUTE
582.89 SPECIFIED PATHOLOGY OR LESION CHRONIC
581.89 SPECIFIED PATHOLOGY OR LESION WITH NEPHROTIC SYNDROME
590.80 SUPPURATIVE (ACUTE) (DISSEMINATED) SEE ALSO 'PYELONEPHRITIS'
039.8 STREPTOTRICHOSIS [583.81]
095.4 SYPHILIS (LATE)
090.5 SYPHILIS CONGENITAL [583.81]
091.69 SYPHILIS EARLY [583.81]
016.0# TB [583.81]

5th Digit: 016.0

0. UNSPECIFIED
1. LAB NOT DONE
2. LABS PENDING
3. MICROSCOPY POSITIVE (IN SPUTUM)
4. CULTURE POSITIVE - MICROSCOPY NEGATIVE
5. CULTURE NEGATIVE - MICROSCOPY POSITIVE
6. CULTURE AND MICROSCOPY NEGATIVE CONFIRMED BY OTHER METHODS

002.0 TYPHOID [580.81]
581.89 WITH NEPHROTIC SYNDROME (EXUDATIVE)
277.3 WITH NEPHROTIC SYNDROME AMYLOID [581.81]
250.4# WITH NEPHROTIC SYNDROME DIABETIC [581.81]

5th Digit: 250.4

0. TYPE II, ADULT-ONSET, NON-INSULIN DEPENDENT (EVEN IF REQUIRING INSULIN), OR UNSPECIFIED; CONTROLLED
1. TYPE I, JUVENILE-ONSET OR INSULIN-DEPENDENT; CONTROLLED
2. TYPE II, ADULT-ONSET, NON-INSULIN DEPENDENT (EVEN IF REQUIRING INSULIN); UNCONTROLLED
3. TYPE I, JUVENILE-ONSET OR INSULIN-DEPENDENT; UNCONTROLLED

710.0 WITH NEPHROTIC SYNDROME LUPUS [581.81]
084.9 WITH NEPHROTIC SYNDROME MALARIAL [581.81]
446.0 WITH NEPHROTIC SYNDROME POLYARTERITIS [581.81]

250.4# GLOMERULOSCLEROSIS DIABETIC [583.81]

5th Digit: 250.4

0. TYPE II, ADULT-ONSET, NON-INSULIN DEPENDENT (EVEN IF REQUIRING INSULIN), OR UNSPECIFIED; CONTROLLED
1. TYPE I, JUVENILE-ONSET OR INSULIN-DEPENDENT; CONTROLLED
2. TYPE II, ADULT-ONSET, NON-INSULIN DEPENDENT (EVEN IF REQUIRING INSULIN); UNCONTROLLED
3. TYPE I, JUVENILE-ONSET OR INSULIN-DEPENDENT; UNCONTROLLED

237.3 GLOMUS JUGULARE TUMOR SITE UNSPECIFIED

0 GLOMUS JUGULARE TUMOR SITE SPECIFIED SEE 'NEOPLASM UNCERTAIN BEHAVIOR' BY SITE M8690/1

228.0# GLOMUS TUMOR M8711/0

5th Digit: 228.0

- **0. SITE UNSPECIFIED**
- **1. OF SKIN AND SUBCUTANEOUS TISSUE**
- **2. OF INTRACRANIAL STRUCTURES**
- **3. OF RETINA**
- **4. OF INTRABDOMINAL STRUCTURES**
- **9. OF OTHER SITES**

GLOSSITIS

529.0 NOS
529.1 AREATA EXFOLIATIVA
529.4 ATROPHIC
529.1 BENIGN MIGRATORY
529.0 GANGRENOUS
529.4 HUNTER'S (MOELLER'S)
529.2 MEDIAN RHOMBOID
529.4 MOELLER'S
265.2 PELLAGROUS
529.0 TONGUE

529.8 GLOSSOCELE
529.6 GLOSSODYNIA
529.4 GLOSSODYNIA EXFOLIATIVA

GLOSSOPHARYNGEAL

352.2 NERVE ATROPHY
352.2 NERVE DISORDERS (NEC)
951.8 NERVE INJURY
352.1 NEURALGIA
352.1 NEURITIS

529.3 GLOSSOPHYTIA
529.8 GLOSSOPTOSIS
529.6 GLOSSOPYROSIS
529.3 GLOSSOTRICHIA

748.3 GLOTTIS, GLOTTIC ATRESIA (ABSENCE) CONGENITAL
478.6 GLOTTIS, GLOTTIC EDEMA
478.79 GLOTTIS, GLOTTIC OBSTRUCTION
478.30 GLOTTIS, GLOTTIC PARALYSIS
748.2 GLOTTIS, GLOTTIC WEBBING OF LARYNX CONGENITAL

251.4 GLUCAGON EXCESS WITH HYPERPLASIA OF PANCREATIC SLIT ALPHA CELLS

251.4 GLUCAGON SECRETION ABNORMALITY

> *CARCINOMAS AND NEOPLASMS SHOULD BE CODED BY SITE IF POSSIBLE. CODE BY CELL TYPE - "SITE NOS", IF AND ONLY IF A SITE IS NOT SPECIFIED IN THE DIAGNOSIS. OTHERWISE - REFER TO THE APPROPRIATE CATEGORY OF NEOPLASM FOR A MORE SPECIFIC CODE: SEE 'CANCER' 'CANCER METASTATIC', 'NEOPLASM UNCERTAIN BEHAVIOR', 'NEOPLASM UNSPECIFIED NATURE', OR 'BENIGN NEOPLASM.'*

211.7 GLUCAGONOMA SITE UNSPECIFIED

0 GLUCAGONOMA SITE SPECIFIED SEE 'BENIGN NEOPLASM' BY SITE M8152/0

157.4 GLUCAGONOMA MALIGNANT SITE UNSPECIFIED

0 GLUCAGONOMA MALIGNANT SITE SPECIFIED SEE 'CANCER' BY SITE M8152/3

270.7 GLUCOGLYCINURIA

GLUCOSE

271.0 6 PHOSPHATASE DEFICIENCY
790.2 ABNORMAL TEST
271.3 GALACTOSE INTOLERANCE OR MALABSORPTION
790.2 TOLERANCE TEST ABNORMAL
648.8# TOLERANCE TEST ABNORMAL OF PREGNANCY

5th Digit: 648.8

- **0. EPISODE OF CARE UNSPECIFIED OR N/A**
- **1. DELIVERED**
- **2. DELIVERED WITH POSTPARTUM COMPLICATION**
- **3. ANTEPARTUM COMPLICATION**
- **4. POSTPARTUM COMPLICATION**

277.4 GLUCURONYL TRANSFERASE DEFICIENCY

305.9# GLUE SNIFFING ABUSE (NONDEPENDENT)

304.6# GLUE SNIFFING ADDICTION (DEPENDENT)

5th Digit: 304.6, 305.9

- **0. UNSPECIFIED**
- **1. CONTINUOUS**
- **2. EPISODIC**
- **3. IN REMISSION**

270.7 GLUTAMINE METABOLISM DISTURBANCES
726.5 GLUTEAL TENDINITIS
579.0 GLUTEN ENTEROPATHY
270.7 GLYCINE METABOLISM DISTURBANCES
270.7 GLYCINEMIA
270.0 GLYCINURIA (RENAL)

271.0 GLYCOGEN STORAGE METABOLISM DISORDER (NEC) - <u>CARDIAC</u> [<u>425.7</u>]

271.0 GLYCOGEN STORAGE METABOLISM DISORDER (NEC) - GENERALIZED

271.0 GLYCOGEN STORAGE METABOLISM DISORDER (NEC) - HEPATORENAL

271.0 GLYCOGEN SYNTHETASE DEFICIENCY

271.0 GLYCOGENOSIS CARDIAC - <u>CARDIOMYOPATHY</u> [<u>425.7</u>]

271.0 GLYCOGENOSIS CORI TYPES I-VII

271.0 GLYCOGENOSIS MYOPHOSPHORLASE DEFICIENCY

271.8 GLYCOLIC ACIDURIA CARBOHYDRATE TRANSPORT DISORDERS

270.8 GLYCOPROLINURIA

GLYCOSURIA

791.5 UNSPECIFIED
250.4# DIABETIC

5th Digit: 250.4

- **0. TYPE II, ADULT-ONSET, NON-INSULIN DEPENDENT (EVEN IF REQUIRING INSULIN), OR UNSPECIFIED; CONTROLLED**
- **1. TYPE I, JUVENILE-ONSET OR INSULIN-DEPENDENT; CONTROLLED**
- **2. TYPE II, ADULT-ONSET, NON-INSULIN DEPENDENT (EVEN IF REQUIRING INSULIN); UNCONTROLLED**
- **3. TYPE I, JUVENILE-ONSET OR INSULIN-DEPENDENT; UNCONTROLLED**

271.4 RENAL

277.4 GLUCURONYL TRANSFERASE SYNDROME
381.20 GLUE EAR SYNDROME
128.1 GNATHOSTOMA SPINIGERUM INFECTION
128.1 GNATHOSTOMIASIS

GOITER

240.9 UNSPECIFIED
241.9 ADENOMATOUS
246.1 CONGENITAL (DYSHORMONOGENIC)
240.9 DIFFUSE COLLOID
246.1 DUE TO ENZYME DEFECT IN SYNTHESIS OF THYROID HORMONE
246.1 DYSHORMONOGENIC
240.9 ENDEMIC
0 EXOPHTHALMIC SEE 'THYROTOXICOSIS'
0 GOITER THYROTOXIC SEE 'THYROTOXICOSIS'
240.9 HYPERPLASTIC
245.2 LYMPHADENOID
240.9 NONTOXIC DIFFUSE
241.1 NONTOXIC MULTINODULAR
241.9 NONTOXIC NODULAR
241.0 NONTOXIC UNINODULAR
240.9 PARENCHYMATOUS
240.0 SIMPLE
240.9 SPORADIC
0 TOXIC OR WITH HYPERTHYROIDISM SEE 'THYROTOXICOSIS'

257.8 GOLDBERG (-MAXWELL) (-MORRIS) SYNDROME (TESTICULAR FEMINIZATION)
440.1 GOLDBLATT'S HYPERTENSION DUE TO RENAL ARTERY OBSTRUCTION
756.0 GOLDENHAR'S SYNDROME (OCULOAURICULOVERTEBRAL DYSPLASIA)
358.0 GOLDFLAM -ERB DISEASE OR SYNDROME
757.39 GOLDSCHEIDER'S EPIDERMOLYSIS BULLOSA
448.0 GOLDSTEIN'S FAMILIAL HEMORRHAGIC TELANGIECTASIA
726.32 GOLFER'S ELBOW
757.39 GOLTZ-GORLIN SYNDROME (DERMAL HYPOPLASIA)

GONADAL

752.7 DYSGENESIS (CONGENITAL) (PURE)
758.6 DYSGENESIS (OVARIAN) (X O SYNDROME)

GONADOBLASTOMA

236.2 FEMALE SITE UNSPECIFIED
0 FEMALE SITE SPECIFIED SEE 'NEOPLASM UNCERTAIN BEHAVIOR' BY SITE M8710/3
236.4 MALE SITE UNSPECIFIED
0 MALE SITE SPECIFIED SEE 'NEOPLASM UNCERTAIN BEHAVIOR' BY SITE M8710/3

125.6 GONGYLONEMIASIS
364.73 GONIOSYNECHIAE

GONOCOCCAL

098.0 NOS
098.7 ANUSITIS
098.7 ANUS INFECTION
098.50 ARTHRITIS
098.52 BURSITIS
098.35 CERVICITIS CHRONIC
098.2 CHRONIC NEC
098.40 CONJUNCTIVITIS NEONATORUM
098.11 CYSTITIS ACUTE
098.31 CYSTITIS CHRONIC
098.89 DERMATOSIS
098.84 ENDOCARDITIS
098.36 ENDOMETRITIS CHRONIC
098.42 ENDOPHTHALMIA
098.13 EPIDIDYMO-ORCHITIS ACUTE
098.33 EPIDIDYMO-ORCHITIS CHRONIC
098.40 EYE (NEWBORN)
098.49 EYE INFECTION OTHER
098.37 FALLOPIAN TUBE (CHRONIC)
098.17 FALLOPIAN TUBE ACUTE
0 GENITOURINARY SEE 'GONORRHEA'
098.89 GONOCOCCEMIA OTHER

GONOCOCCAL (continued)

098.85 HEART DISEASE OTHER
098.41 IRIDOCYCLITIS
098.50 JOINT NOS
098.59 JOINT OTHER
098.43 KERATITIS
098.81 KERATODERMA
098.81 KERATOSIS (BLENNORRHAGICA)
098.89 LYMPHATIC (GLAND) (NODE)
098.82 MENINGITIS
098.13 ORCHITIS ACUTE
098.33 ORCHITIS CHRONIC
098.19 PELVIS (ACUTE)
098.39 PELVIS CHRONIC
098.83 PERICARDITIS
098.86 PERITONITIS
098.6 PHARYNGITIS
098.6 PHARYNX INFECTION
098.7 PROCTITIS
098.12 PROSTATITIS ACUTE
098.32 PROSTATITIS CHRONIC
098.37 PYOSALPINX (CHRONIC)
098.17 PYOSALPINX ACUTE
098.7 RECTUM INFECTION
098.59 RHEUMATISM
098.17 SALPINGITIS ACUTE
098.37 SALPINGITIS CHRONIC
098.14 SEMINAL VESICULITIS ACUTE
098.34 SEMINAL VESICULITIS CHRONIC
098.89 SEPTICEMIA
098.89 SKIN
098.53 SPONDYLITIS
098.51 SYNOVITIS
098.51 TENOSYNOVITIS
098.6 THROAT
0 URETHRA SEE 'GONORRHEA'
0 VULVA SEE 'GONORRHEA'
098.89 OTHER

'ACUTE' SEQUENCES BEFORE 'CHRONIC'.

098.89 GONOCOCCEMIA

GONORRHEA

098.0 ACUTE
098.50 ARTHRITIS
098.11 BLADDER ACUTE
098.31 BLADDER CHRONIC
098.52 BURSITIS
V02.7 CARRIER
098.35 CERVICITIS CHRONIC
098.15 CERVIX (ACUTE)
098.2 CHRONIC (LOWER GU TRACT)
098.30 CHRONIC UPPER TRACT
098.39 CHRONIC OTHER SITE
098.40 CONJUNCTIVITIS (NEONATORUM)
V65.45 COUNSELING
098.31 CYSTITIS CHRONIC
098.36 ENDOMETRITIS CHRONIC
098.33 EPIDIDYMO-ORCHITIS CHRONIC
V01.6 EXPOSURE
098.89 GONOCOCCEMIA OTHER
098.10 INFECTION (ACUTE) UPPER GENITOURINARY TRACT SITE UNSPECIFIED
098.59 INFECTION OF JOINT OTHER
098.19 INFECTION OTHER ACUTE

GONORRHEA (continued)

655.4# MATERNAL (WITH KNOWN / SUSPECTED DAMAGE TO FETUS)

5th Digit: 655.4

0. EPISODE OF CARE UNSPECIFIED OR N/A
1. DELIVERED
3. ANTEPARTUM COMPLICATION

> *647.1#: USE AN ADDITIONAL CODE TO IDENTIFY THE MATERNAL GONORRHEA.*

647.1# MATERNAL CURRENT (CO-EXISTENT) IN PREGNANCY

5th Digit: 647.1

0. EPISODE OF CARE UNSPECIFIED OR N/A
1. DELIVERED
2. DELIVERED WITH POSTPARTUM COMPLICATION
3. ANTEPARTUM COMPLICATION
4. POSTPARTUM COMPLICATION

098.6 PHARYNGITIS
098.32 PROSTATITIS CHRONIC
098.59 RHEUMATISM
098.17 SALPINGITIS ACUTE
098.37 SALPINGITIS CHRONIC
098.14 SEMINAL VESICULITIS ACUTE
098.34 SEMINAL VESICULITIS CHRONIC
098.53 SPONDYLITIS
098.51 SYNOVITIS
098.51 TENOSYNOVITIS
098.16 UTERUS (ACUTE)
098.36 UTERUS CHRONIC
098.89 OTHER SPECIFIED SITE
098.59 OTHER

078.82 GOODALL'S EPIDEMIC VOMITING

446.21 GOODPASTURE'S SYNDROME (PNEUMORENAL)
648.9# GOODPASTURE'S SYNDROME MATERNAL CURRENT (CO-EXISTENT) IN PREGNANCY [446.21]

5th Digit: 648.9

0. EPISODE OF NOS OR N/A
1. DELIVERED
2. DELIVERED WITH POSTPARTUM COMPLICATION
3. ANTEPARTUM COMPLICATION
4. POSTPARTUM COMPLICATION

446.21 GOODPASTURE'S SYNDROME WITH NEPHRITIS [583.81]

266.2 GOPALAN'S SYNDROME (BURNING FEET)
579.8 GORDON'S EXUDATIVE ENTEROPATHY
709.1 GOUGEROT BLUM DERMATITIS
701.8 GOUGEROT CARTEAUD SYNDROME OR DISEASE (CONFLUENT RETICULATE PAPILLOMATOSIS)
757.39 GOUGEROT-HAILEY-HAILEY DISEASE (BENIGN FAMILIAL CHRONIC PEMPHIGUS)
710.2 GOUGEROT (-HOUWER) -SJOGREN SYNDROME (KERATOCONJUNCTIVITIS SICCA)

423.2 GOULEY'S SYNDROME (CONSTRICTIVE PERICARDITIS)
102.6 GOUNDOU

GOUT

274.9 UNSPECIFIED
274.0 ARTHRITIS
274.89 OTHER MANIFESTATIONS
V77.5 SCREENING
274.0 SYNOVITIS
095.8 SYPHILITIC [274.9]

GOUTY

274.89 NEURITIS [357.4]
274.81 TOPHI EAR
274.82 TOPHI HEART
274.82 TOPHI OTHER SITES

359.1 GOWER'S MUSCULAR DYSTROPHY
377.04 GOWERS PATON KENNEDY SYNDROME
780.2 GOWER'S VASOVAGAL SYNDROME

620.0 GRAAFIAN FOLLICLE CYST
383.02 GRADENIGO'S SYNDROME

996.55 GRAFT SKIN ARTIFICIAL FAILURE OR REJECTION (DISLODGEMENT) (DISPLACEMENT) (NON-ADHERENCE) (POOR INCORPORATION) (SHEARING)

996.55 GRAFT SKIN DECELLULARIZED ALLODERMIS FAILURE OR REJECTION (DISLODGEMENT) (DISPLACEMENT) (NON-ADHERENCE) (POOR INCORPORATION) (SHEARING)

996.52 GRAFT SKIN FAILURE OR REJECTION
996.69 GRAFT SKIN INFECTION INFLAMMATION
996.79 GRAFT SKIN OTHER COMPLICATION
996.52 GRAFT OF OTHER TISSUE COMPLICATION NEC (MECHANICAL)
996.85 GRAFT VERSUS HOST DISEASE (BONE MARROW)

424.3 GRAHAM STEELL'S MURMUR
495.8 GRAIN HANDLERS' DISEASE OR LUNG

041.84 GRAM NEGATIVE ANAEROBES
041.85 GRAM NEGATIVE INFECTION OTHER
038.40 GRAM NEGATIVE SEPSIS

0 GRANCHER'S SPLENOPNEUMONIA SEE 'PNEUMONIA'

GRAND MAL EPILEPSY

345.10 NOS
345.11 WITH INTRACTABLE EPILEPSY
345.3 WITH STATUS

659.4# GRAND MULTIPARITY

5th Digit: 659.4

0. EPISODE OF CARE UNSPECIFIED OR N/A
1. DELIVERED
3. ANTEPARTUM COMPLICATION

GRANULAR CELL

0 CARCINOMA SITE SPECIFIED SEE 'CANCER' BY SITE M8320/3
215.# TUMOR BENIGN M9580/0
171.# TUMOR MALIGNANT M9580/3

4th Digit: 171, 215

0. HEAD FACE NECK
2. UPPER LIMB SHOULDER
3. LOWER LIMB HIP
4. THORAX
5. ABDOMINAL HYPOCHONDRIUM
6. PELVIS BUTTOCK GROIN INGUINAL REGION PERINEUM
7. TRUNK UNSPECIFIED BACK UNSPECIFIED FLANK UNSPECIFIED
8. OTHER SPECIFIED SITES
9. SITE UNSPECIFIED

701.5 GRANULATION EXCESSIVE
701.5 GRANULATION TISSUE POSTOPERATIVE

288.8 GRANULOCYTIC HYPERPLASIA
288.0 GRANULOCYTOPENIA (PRIMARY) (MALIGNANT)

GRANULOMA

568.89 ABDOMEN WALL
695.89 ANNULARE
569.49 ANUS
522.6 APICAL
543.9 APPENDIX
380.23 AURAL
503 BERYLLIUM LUNG
709.4 BERYLLIUM SKIN

GRANULOMA (continued)

730.1#	BONE

5th Digit: 730.1

0. SITE UNSPECIFIED
1. SHOULDER REGION
2. UPPER ARM (ELBOW) (HUMERUS)
3. FOREARM (RADIUS) (WRIST) (ULNA)
4. HAND (CARPAL) (METACARPAL) (FINGERS)
5. PELVIC THIGH (HIP) (BUTTOCK) (FEMUR)
6. LOWER LEG (FIBULA) (KNEE) (PATELLA) (TIBIA)
7. ANKLE AND/OR FOOT (METATARSALS) (TOES) (TARSALS)
8. OTHER (HEAD) (NECK) (RIB) (SKULL) (TRUNK) (VERTEBRAE)
9. MULTIPLE

277.8	BONE EOSINOPHILIC
526.3	BONE JAW
733.99	BONE RESIDUAL FOREIGN BODY
348.8	CEREBRAL
375.81	CANALICULUS LACRIMALIS
385.82	CHOLESTERIN MASTOID
385.82	CHOLESTERIN MIDDLE EAR
114.3	COCCIDIOIDAL (PROGRESSIVE)
114.4	COCCIDIOIDAL LUNG CHRONIC
114.0	COCCIDIOIDAL LUNG PRIMARY
114.2	COCCIDIOIDAL MENINGES
569.89	COLON
372.61	CONJUNCTIVA
522.6	DENTAL
385.82	EAR (MIDDLE) AND MASTOID (CHOLESTERIN)
0	EAR WITH OTITIS MEDIA SEE 'OTITIS MEDIA'
277.8	EOSINOPHILIC
277.8	EOSINOPHILIC - BONE
277.8	EOSINOPHILIC - LUNG
528.9	EOSINOPHILIC - ORAL MUCOSA
374.89	EYELID
701.8	FACIALE
523.8	FISSURATUM (GUM)
686.1	FOOT NEC (PYOGENIC)
733.99	FOREIGN BODY - BONE
728.82	FOREIGN BODY - MUSCLE
709.4	FOREIGN BODY - SKIN AND SUBCUTANEOUS TISSUE
728.82	FOREIGN BODY - SOFT TISSUE
0	FUNGOIDES SEE 'MYCOSIS FUNGOIDES'
446.3	GANGRAENESCENS
526.3	GIANT CELL - CENTRAL
523.8	GIANT CELL - GINGIVA
523.8	GIANT CELL - GUM
526.3	GIANT CELL - JAW
523.8	GIANT CELL - PERIPHERAL
0	HODGKIN'S SEE 'HODGKIN'S DISEASE GRANULOMA'
523.8	GUM (GIANT CELL)
569.89	ILEUM
136.9	INFECTIOUS NEC
099.2	INGUINALE
569.89	INTESTINE
364.10	IRIDOCYCLITIS
590.9	KIDNEY
375.81	LACRIMAL PASSAGES
478.79	LARYNX
446.3	LETHAL MIDLINE
277.8	LIPID
277.8	LIPOID
572.8	LIVER
515	LUNG NOS OR CHRONIC
114.4	LUNG - COCCIDIOIDAL
515	LUNG - DUE TO INORGANIC DUST
277.8	LUNG - EOSINOPHILIC
289.3	LYMPH GLAND

GRANULOMA (continued)

110.6	MAJOCCHI'S
446.3	MALIGNANT (FACE)
526.3	MANDIBLE
519.3	MEDIASTINUM
112.3	MONILIAL (OF SKIN AND NAILS)
728.82	MUSCLE
473.9	NASAL SINUS (SEE ALSO 'SINUSITIS')
998.59	OPERATION WOUND
528.9	ORAL MUCOSA (EOSINOPHILIC) (PYOGENIC)
376.11	ORBITAL
116.1	PARACOCCIDIOIDAL
099.2	PENIS VENEREAL
568.89	PERITONEAL
383.33	POSTMASTOIDECTOMY CAVITY
998.59	POSTOPERATIVE WOUND
601.8	PROSTATE
099.2	PUDENDI (ULCERATING)
522.6	PYOGENIC - MAXILLARY ALVEOLAR RIDGE
528.9	PYOGENIC - ORAL MUCOSA
686.1	PYOGENIC - SKIN
569.49	RECTAL SPHINCTER
705.89	RUBRUM NASI
135	SARCOID
686.1	SEPTIC (SKIN)
709.4	SILICA SKIN
709.4	SKIN FROM FOREIGN BODY
686.1	SKIN PYOGENIC
686.1	SKIN SEPTIC
686.1	SKIN SUPPURATIVE
094.89	SPINE SYPHILITIC (EPIDURAL)
015.0#	SPINE TUBERCULOUS [730.88]

5th Digit: 015.0

0. NOS
1. LAB NOT DONE
2. LABS PENDING
3. MICROSCOPY POSITIVE (IN SPUTUM)
4. CULTURE POSITIVE - MICROSCOPY NEGATIVE
5. CULTURE NEGATIVE - MICROSCOPY POSITIVE
6. CULTURE AND MICROSCOPY NEGATIVE CONFIRMED BY OTHER METHODS

998.89	STITCH POSTOPERATIVE - EXTERNAL
998.89	STITCH POSTOPERATIVE - INTERNAL
686.1	SUPPURATIVE (SKIN)
998.89	SUTURE POSTOPERATIVE - EXTERNAL
998.89	SUTURE POSTOPERATIVE - INTERNAL
031.1	SWIMMING POOL
728.82	TALC
998.7	TALC IN OPERATION WOUND
686.1	TELANGIECTATICUM (SKIN)
521.4	TOOTH PULP (INTERNAL)
110.6	TRICHOPHYTICUM
102.4	TROPICUM
686.1	UMBILICUS
771.4	UMBILICUS NEWBORN
599.84	URETHRAL
364.10	UVEITIS
099.2	VAGINA (VENEREUM)
099.2	VENEREUM
478.5	VOCAL CORDS
446.4	WEGENER'S (NECROTIZING RESPIRATORY GRANULOMATOSIS)

446.4	GRANULOMATOSIS (RESPIRATORY) (NECROTIZING)
288.1	GRANULOMATOUS DISEASE CHRONIC (CHILDHOOD)

CARCINOMAS AND NEOPLASMS SHOULD BE CODED BY SITE IF POSSIBLE. CODE BY CELL TYPE - "SITE NOS", IF AND ONLY IF A SITE IS NOT SPECIFIED IN THE DIAGNOSIS. OTHERWISE - REFER TO THE APPROPRIATE CATEGORY OF NEOPLASM FOR A MORE SPECIFIC CODE: SEE 'CANCER' 'CANCER METASTATIC', 'NEOPLASM UNCERTAIN BEHAVIOR', 'NEOPLASM UNSPECIFIED NATURE', OR 'BENIGN NEOPLASM'.

GRANULOSA CELL

236.2 THECA CELL TUMOR SITE UNSPECIFIED
0 THECA CELL TUMOR SITE SPECIFIED SEE 'NEOPLASM UNCERTAIN BEHAVIOR' BYSITE M8621/1
183.0 TUMOR MALIGNANT SITE UNSPECIFIED
0 TUMOR MALIGNANT SITE SPECIFIED SEE 'CANCER' BYSITE M8620/3
236.2 TUMOR SITE UNSPECIFIED
0 TUMOR SITE SPECIFIED SEE 'NEOPLASM UNCERTAIN BEHAVIOR' BY SITE M8620/1

705.89 GRANULOSIS RUBRA NASI
503 GRAPHITE LUNG DISEASE
242.00 GRAVES DISEASE (EXOPHTHALMIC GOITER)
242.01 GRAVES DISEASE (EXOPHTHALMIC GOITER) WITH CRISIS OR STORM
994.9 GRAVITATIONAL EFFECTS ABNORMAL
909.4 GRAVITATIONAL EFFECTS ABNORMAL LATE EFFECT
779.4 GRAY OR GREY SYNDROME (CHLORAMPHENICOL) (NEWBORN)
0 GREASE GUN INJURY SEE 'OPEN WOUND', BY SITE, COMPLICATED
078.89 GREEN MONKEY DISEASE
330.0 GREENFIELD'S DISEASE
309.0 GRIEF REACTION
756.0 GRIEG'S SYNDROME (HYPERTELORISM)
126.9 GRIESINGER'S DISEASE (SEE ALSO 'ANCYLOSTOMA, ANCYCLOSOMIASIS')
502 GRINDERS' DISEASE
723.5 GRISEL'S DISEASE
959.1 GROIN INJURY
911.8 GROIN INJURY OTHER AND UNSPECIFIED SUPERFICIAL
911.9 GROIN INJURY OTHER AND UNSPECIFIED SUPERFICIAL INFECTED
848.8 GROIN SPRAIN
253.3 GROWTH HORMONE DEFICIENCY
253.0 GROWTH HORMONE OVERPRODUCTION
783.4 GROWTH LACK
0 GROWTH RETARDATION FETAL SEE 'FETAL - INFANT'S RECORD', GROWTH RETARDATION
110.0 GRUBY'S DISEASE (TINEA TONSURANS)
0 GSW SEE 'OPEN WOUND' BY SITE OR ANATOMICAL INJURY
599.0 GU INFECTION NEC

646.6#: SPECIFY THE TYPE OF MATERNAL GU INFECTION WITH AN ADDITIONAL CODE.

646.6# GU INFECTION COMPLICATING PREGNANCY

5th Digit: 646.6

0. EPISODE OF CARE UNSPECIFIED OR N/A
1. DELIVERED
2. DELIVERED WITH POSTPARTUM COMPLICATION
3. ANTEPARTUM COMPLICATION
4. POSTPARTUM COMPLICATION

066.3 GUAMA FEVER (VIRAL)
344.89 GUBLER (-MILLARD) PARALYSIS (SYNDROME)
754.89 GUERIN-STERN SYNDROME (ATHROGRYPOSIS MULTPLEX CONGENITA)
049.8 GUERTIN'S DISEASE (ELECTRIC CHOREA)
357.0 GUILLAIN-BARRE (-STROHL) SYNDROME ACUTE INFECTIVE POLYNEURITIS
125.7 GUINEA WORM INFECTION
307.23 GUINON'S DISEASE (MOTOR-VERBAL TIC)
750.3 GULLET ATRESIA (CONGENITAL)
244.# GULL'S DISEASE (THYROID ATROPHY WITH MYXEDEMA)

4th Digit: 244

0. POSTSURGICAL
1. POSTABLATIVE (IRRADIATION)
2. IODINE INGESTION
3. PAS, PHENYLBUT, RESORCINOL
8. SECONDARY NEC
9. NOS

523.2 GUM ATROPHY
523.9 GUM DISEASE NEC
523.8 GUM HYPERPLASIA
959.09 GUM INJURY
910.8 GUM INJURY OTHER AND UNSPECIFIED (SUPERFICIAL)
910.9 GUM INJURY OTHER AND UNSPECIFIED (SUPERFICIAL) INFECTED
0 GUM SEE ALSO 'ALVEOLAR' OR 'GINGIVA'
102.6 GUMMA, BONE OF YAWS (LATE)
090.5 GUMMA DUE TO CONGENITAL SYPHILIS MANIFEST 2 YRS. OR MORE AFTER BIRTH
0 GUMMA SEE 'SYPHILIS'
102.6 GUMMATOUS OSTEITIS OR PERIOSTEITIS OF YAWS (LATE)
0 GUN SHOT WOUND SEE 'OPEN WOUND', BY SITE OR ANATOMICAL INJURY
742.8 GUNN'S SYNDROME (JAW-WINKING SYNDROME)
277.1 GUNTHER'S DISEASE OR SYNDROME (CONGENITAL ERYTHROPOIETIC PORPHYRIA)
350.8 GUSTATORY SWEATING SYNDROME
752.7 GYNANDRISM CONGENITAL

GYNANDROBLASTOMA

236.2 FEMALE SITE UNSPECIFIED
0 FEMALE SITE SPECIFIED SEE 'NEOPLASM UNCERTAIN BEHAVIOR' BY SITE M8632/1
236.4 MALE SITE UNSPECIFIED
0 MALE SITE SPECIFIED SEE 'NEOPLASM UNCERTAIN BEHAVIOR' BY SITE M8632/1

738.6 GYNECOID PELVIS MALE
629.9 GYNECOLOGICAL DISEASE
V72.3 GYNECOLOGICAL EXAM (ROUTINE)
611.1 GYNECOMASTIA NONPUERPERAL
300.29 GYNEPHOBIA

759.81 H 30 SYNDROME

270.0 H DISEASE

041.5 H. FLU INFECTION OR ORGANISM
0 H. INFLUENZA ARTHRITIS SEE 'ARTHRITIS OTHER SPECIFIED', PYOGENIC
V03.81 H. INFLUENZA VACCINATION
041.86 H. PYLORI INFECTION

732.3 HAAS' DISEASE
696.2 HABERMANN'S DISEASE (ACUTE PARAPSORIASIS VARIOLIFORMIS)
629.9 HABITUAL ABORTER
646.3# HABITUAL ABORTER CURRENT PREGNANCY
5th Digit: 646.3
0. EPISODE OF CARE NOS OR N/A
1. DELIVERED
3. ANTEPARTUM COMPLICATION

634.## HABITUAL ABORTER WITH CURRENT ABORTION
4th Digit: 634
0. WITH INFECTION
1. DELAYED OR EXCESSIVE
2. DAMAGE TO PELVIC ORGANS OR TISSUE
3. RENAL FAILURE
4. METABOLIC DISORDER
5. SHOCK
6. EMBOLISM
7. OTHER SPECIFIED COMPLICATIONS
8. UNSPECIFIED COMPLICATION
9. UNCOMPLICATED
5th Digit: 634
0. NOS
1. INCOMPLETE
2. COMPLETE

577.8 HADFIELD CLARKE SYNDROME PANCREATIC INFANTILISM
985.1 HAFF DISEASE
286.3 HAGEMAN FACTOR II DEFICIENCY
717.89 HAGLUND-LAWEN-FRUND SYNDROME
732.5 HAGLUND'S DISEASE (OSTEOCHONDROSIS OS TIBIALE EXTERNUM)
731.2 HAGNER'S DISEASE (HYPERTROPHIC PULMONARY OSTEOARTHROPATHY)
757.39 HAILEY-HAILEY DISEASE (BENIGN FAMILIAL CHRONIC PEMPHIGUS)

HAIR
757.4 ABSENCE (CONGENITAL)
704.9 AND HAIR FOLLICLES DISEASE
704.2 ATROPHIC
704.3 CANITIES (PREMATURE)
704.3 CIRCUMSCRIPTA ACQUIRED
704.3 COLOR VARIATION
704.3 GRAYNESS (PREMATURE)
704.3 HETEROCHROMIA
704.00 LOSS
307.9 PLUCKING
V50.0 TRANSPLANT (ELECTIVE)
704.8 AND HAIR FOLLICLES DISEASE SPECIFIED NEC

257.8 HAIRLESS WOMEN SYNDROME

202.4# HAIRY CELL LEUKEMIA M9940/3
5th Digit: 202.4
0. NOS
1. LYMPH NODES OF HEAD FACE NECK
2. LYMPH NODES INTRATHORACIC
3. LYMPH NODES ABDOMINAL
4. LYMPH NODES AXILLA AND UPPER LIMB
5. LYMPH NODES INGUINAL REGION AND LOWER LIMB
6. LYMPH NODES INTRAPELVIC
7. SPLEEN
8. LYMPH NODES MULTIPLE SITES

784.9 HALITOSIS
756.0 HALLERMANN STREIFF SYNDROME
333.0 HALLERVORDEN SPATZ DISEASE
701.0 HALLOPEAU'S DISEASE (LICHEN SCLEROSUS ET ATROPHICUS)

HALLUCINATION
780.1 NOS (AUDITORY) (GUSTATORY) (OLFACTORY) (TACTILE)
291.3 ALCOHOLIC (ACUTE) (PSYCHOTIC)
305.3# DRUG INDUCED (BAD TRIP)
5th Digit: 305.3
0. NOS
1. CONTINUOUS
2. EPISODIC
3. IN REMISSION

292.12 DRUG INDUCED (NONHALLUCINOGENIC DRUG)
780.1 NONPSYCHOTIC NONORGANIC
293.82 TRANSIENT (ORGANIC) (PSYCHOSIS)
368.16 VISUAL

305.3# HALLUCINOGEN ABUSE (NONDEPENDENT)
304.5# HALLUCINOGEN ADDICTION (DEPENDENT)
5th Digit: 304.5, 305.3
0. NOS
1. CONTINUOUS
2. EPISODIC
3. IN REMISSION

760.73 HALLUCINOGENIC TRANSMITTED VIA PLACENTA OR BREAST MILK AFFECTING FETUS OR NEWBORN

HALLUX
735.9 DEFORMITY ACQUIRED
735.3 MALLEUS
735.2 RIGIDUS
735.0 VALGUS ACQUIRED
755.66 VALGUS CONGENITAL
735.1 VARUS ACQUIRED
755.66 VARUS CONGENITAL

368.15 HALO VISUAL
757.32 HAMARTOMAS VASCULAR CONGENITAL
759.6 HAMARTOSES OTHER SPECIFIED NEC CONGENITAL
516.3 HAMMAN RICH SYNDROME
518.1 HAMMAN'S SYNDROME (SPONTANEOUS MEDIASTINAL EMPHYSEMA)
735.4 HAMMER TOE ACQUIRED
755.66 HAMMER TOE CONGENITAL
843.8 HAMSTRING SPRAIN

HAND
V49.63 ABSENCE ACQUIRED
755.28 AGENESIS
V49.63 AMPUTATION STATUS
726.4 BONE SPUR
736.00 DEFORMITY ACQUIRED
074.3 FOOT AND MOUTH DISEASE
282.61 FOOT SYNDROME
959.4 INJURY - NOS (EXCEPT FINGER)
914.8 INJURY - OTHER AND NOS SUPERFICIAL
914.9 INJURY - OTHER AND NOS SUPERFICIAL INFECTED
719.84 JOINT CALCIFICATION
842.10 SEPARATION (RUPTURE) (TEAR) (LACERATION) SITE NOS
842.10 STRAIN (SPRAIN) (AVULSION) (HEMARTHROSIS) SITE NOS

277.8 HAND SCHULLER CHRISTIAN DISEASE (CHRONIC HISTIOCYTOSIS X)
V61.49 HANDICAPPED PERSON (CARE) (PRESENCE) (PROBLEM) (IN FAMILY) (IN HOUSEHOLD)
V60.4 HANDICAPPED PERSON (FAMILY MEMBER) UNSUITED TO RENDER CARE

H

305.0# HANGOVER
5th Digit: 305.0
0. NOS
1. CONTINUOUS
2. EPISODIC
3. IN REMISSION

275.0 HANOT-CHAUFFARD (-TROISIER) (BRONZE DIABETES) SYNDROME
0 HANOT'S DISEASE SEE 'CIRRHOSIS', BILIARY
0 HANSEN'S DISEASE SEE 'LEPROSY'
079.81 HANTAAN PUUMALA VIRUS
079.81 HANTAVIRUS INFECTION
757.39 HAR HAILEY SYNDROME
363.22 HARADA'S DISEASE OR SYNDROME

749.1# HARE LIP
5th Digit: 749.1
0. NOS
1. UNILATERAL COMPLETE
2. UNILATERAL INCOMPLETE
3. BILATERAL COMPLETE
4. BILATERAL INCOMPLETE

162.3 HARE'S SYNDROME (CARCINOMA, PULMONARY APEX) M8010/3
446.0 HARKAVY'S SYNDROME
779.8 HARLEQUIN COLOR CHANGE SYNDROME
757.1 HARLEQUIN FETUS
283.2 HARLEY'S DISEASE (INTERMITTENT HEMOGLOBINURIA)
251.1 HARRIS' SYNDROME (ORGANIC HYPERINSULISM)
575.8 HARTMANN'S POUCH
270.0 HARTNUP DISEASE
270.0 HART'S SYNDROME (PELLAGRA-CEREBELLAR ATAXIA-RENAL AMINOACIDURIA)

304.3# HASHISH ADDICTION (DEPENDENT)
5th Digit: 304.3
0. NOS
1. CONTINUOUS
2. EPISODIC
3. IN REMISSION

245.2 HASHIMOTO'S THYROIDITIS (STRUMA LYMPHOMATOSA)
371.41 HASSALL HENLE BODIES
026.1 HAVERHILL FEVER

HAY FEVER
477.9 UNSPECIFIED
477.0 DUE TO POLLEN
477.8 DUE TO OTHER ALLERGEN

280.9 HAYEM-FABER SYNDROME (ACHLORHYDRIC ANEMIA)
283.9 HAYEM-WIDAL SYNDROME (ACQUIRED HEMOLYTIC JAUNDICE)
715.04 HAYGARTH'S NODULE
282.5 HB AS GENOTYPE
282.7 HB BART'S DISEASE
282.5 HB S
790.0 HCT ABNORMAL

HEAD
307.3 BANGING
900.9 BLOOD VESSEL NOS INJURY
0 BLOOD VESSEL NEC INJURY - INTRACRANIAL SEE 'INTRACRANIAL INJURY'
900.82 BLOOD VESSEL NEC INJURY - MULTIPLE
900.89 BLOOD VESSEL NEC INJURY - SPECIFIED NEC

HEAD (continued)
V48.0 DEFICIENCY
738.1# DEFORMITY OTHER ACQUIRED
5th Digit: 738.1
0. UNSPECIFIED
1. ZYGOMATIC HYPERPLASIA
2. ZYGOMATIC HYPOPLASIA
9. OTHER SPECIFIED

V48.6 DISFIGUREMENT
959.01 INJURY NOS
0 INJURY WITH CONCUSSION SEE 'CONCUSSION'
0 INJURY WITH INTRACRANIAL INJURY SEE SPECIFIED INTRACRANIAL INJURY
132.0 LICE
781.0 MOVEMENTS ABNORMAL
784.0 PAIN
V48.9 PROBLEM
V48.2 PROBLEM (MECHANICAL AND MOTOR)
V48.8 PROBLEM (OTHER)
V48.4 PROBLEM SENSORY
739.0 REGION SEGMENTAL OR SOMATIC DYSFUNCTION
784.2 SWELLING MASS OR LUMP
784.9 SYMPTOM OTHER

HEADACHE
784.0 NOS
346.2# ALLERGIC
5th Digit: 346.2
0. WITHOUT MENTION INTRACTABLE MIGRAINE
1. WITH INTRACTABLE MIGRAINE

784.0 ANALGESIC REBOUND
346.2# CLUSTER
346.2# HISTAMINE
5th Digit: 346.2
0. WITHOUT MENTION INTRACTABLE MIGRAINE
1. WITH INTRACTABLE MIGRAINE

349.0 LUMBAR PUNCTURE (DUE TO)
627.2 MENOPAUSAL
0 MIGRAINE SEE 'MIGRAINE'
625.4 PREMENSTRUAL
307.81 PSYCHOGENIC OR OF INORGANIC ORIGIN
349.0 SADDLE BLOCK (DUE TO)
346.1# SICK
5th Digit: 346.1
0. WITHOUT MENTION INTRACTABLE MIGRAINE
1. WITH INTRACTABLE MIGRAINE

349.0 SPINAL FLUID LOSS (DUE TO)
307.81 TENSION
784.0 VASCULAR
346.9# VASOMOTOR
5th Digit: 346.9
0. WITHOUT MENTION INTRACTABLE MIGRAINE
1. WITH INTRACTABLE MIGRAINE

0 HEALTH CHECK TYPE SEE 'EXAM'
0 HEALTH COUNSELING SEE 'COUNSELING'
V65.0 HEALTHY PERSON ACCOMPANYING SICK PERSON

HEARING
V53.2 AID FITTING AND ADJUSTMENT
V72.1 EXAM
V20.2 EXAM INFANT
V41.2 PROBLEM
0 SEE 'AUDITORY'

HEARING LOSS

389.9 NOS
389.14 CENTRAL
V19.2 FAMILY HISTORY OF HEARING LOSS
389.8 HIGH FREQUENCY
389.8 LOW FREQUENCY
389.12 NEURAL
388.12 NOISE INDUCED
307.6 PSYCHOGENIC
388.2 SUDDEN
388.02 TRANSIENT ISCHEMIC
951.5 TRAUMATIC
389.8 OTHER SPECIFIED FORMS

HEARING LOSS CONDUCTIVE

389.00 NOS
389.08 COMBINED TYPES
389.01 EXTERNAL EAR
389.04 INNER EAR
389.03 MIDDLE EAR
389.02 TYMPANIC MEMBRANE
389.2 WITH SENSORINEURAL LOSS

HEARING LOSS SENSORINEURAL

389.10 NOS
389.14 CENTRAL
389.18 COMBINED TYPES
389.12 NEURAL
389.11 SENSORY
389.2 WITH CONDUCTIVE LOSS

HEART

785.3 ABNORMAL HEART SOUNDS
759.89 ABSENCE CONGENITAL
746.87 AND CARDIAC APEX MALPOSITION CONGENITAL
746.9 ANOMALY CONGENITAL
746.84 ANOMALY OBSTRUCTIVE CONGENITAL NEC
429.1 ATROPHY (SEE ALSO 'MYOCARDIAL', DEGENERATION)
785.1 BEAT AWARENESS
785.0 BEAT RAPID
0 BLOCK SEE 'HEART BLOCK'
861.01 CONTUSION
861.11 CONTUSION WITH OPEN WOUND INTO THORAX
908.0 CONTUSION LATE EFFECT
0 CRISIS SEE 'HEART FAILURE'
0 DISEASE SEE 'HEART DISEASE'
746.89 DIVERTICULUM CONGENITAL
0 DYSRHYTHMIA SEE 'DYSRHYTHMIAS'
0 FAILURE SEE 'HEART FAILURE'
429.1 FATTY DEGENERATION OF HEART OR MYOCARDIUM WITH MENTION OF ARTERIOSCLEROSIS [440.9]
785.3 FRICTION RUB OR FREMITUS
746.7 HYPOPLASTIC LEFT (SYNDROME) CONGENITAL
861.00 INJURY NOS
861.10 INJURY NOS WITH OPEN WOUND INTO THORAX
908.0 INJURY NOS LATE EFFECT
861.0# LACERATION
861.1# LACERATION WITH OPEN WOUND INTO THORAX
5th Digit: 861.0-1
2. WITHOUT PENETRATION OF HEART CHAMBERS
3. WITH PENETRATION OF HEART CHAMBERS
908.0 LACERATION LATE EFFECT
785.2 MURMUR
785.1 PALPITATIONS
V43.2 REPLACEMENT STATUS (ARTIFICIAL) (PROSTHESIS)
793.2 SHADOW ABNORMAL (CXR)
785.3 SOUNDS ABNORMAL
785.3 SOUNDS INCREASED DECREASED
V15.1 SURGERY HISTORY
423.9 TAMPONADE
996.83 TRANSPLANT REJECTION (FAILURE)
V42.1 TRANSPLANT (STATUS)

HEART (continued)

746.89 VALVE ATRESIA NEC (CONGENITAL)
996.61 VALVE PROSTHESIS COMPLICATION - INFECTION OR INFLAMMATION
996.02 VALVE PROSTHESIS COMPLICATION - MECHANICAL (LEAKAGE) (OBSTRUCTION) (DISPLACEMENT)
996.71 VALVE PROSTHESIS COMPLICATION - OTHER NON-MECHANICAL (EMBOLISM) (FIBROSIS) (HEMORRHAGE) (PAIN) (STENOSIS) (THROMBUS)
V43.3 VALVE REPLACEMENT STATUS (ARTIFICIAL) (PROSTHESIS)
V42.2 VALVE TRANSPLANT STATUS
428.9 WEAK

HEART BLOCK

426.9 NOS
426.10 ATRIOVENTRICULAR BLOCK (INCOMPLETE) (PARTIAL)
426.0 ATRIOVENTRICULAR COMPLETE
426.10 AV BLOCK (INCOMPLETE) (PARTIAL)
426.0 AV BLOCK COMPLETE
0 BUNDLE BRANCH SEE 'HEART BLOCK - BUNDLE BRANCH'
746.86 CONGENITAL
426.11 FIRST DEGREE AV
426.6 INTRAVENTRICULAR NOS
426.13 MOBITZ (TYPE) I (WENCKEBACK'S)
426.12 MOBITZ (TYPE) II AV
426.13 SECOND DEGREE - MOBITZ (TYPE) I (WENCKEBACK'S)
426.12 SECOND DEGREE - MOBITZ (TYPE) II AV
426.13 SECOND DEGREE AV - OTHER
426.6 SINOATRIAL
426.6 SINOAURICULAR
426.0 THIRD DEGREE ATRIOVENTRICULAR BLOCK
426.13 WENCKEBACH'S

HEART BLOCK - BUNDLE BRANCH

426.50 NOS
426.53 BIFASCICULAR NOS
426.53 BILATERAL NOS
426.3 LEFT NOS
426.2 LEFT ANTERIOR FASCICULAR
426.3 LEFT ANTERIOR WITH LEFT POSTERIOR
426.3 LEFT COMPLETE
426.2 LEFT HEMIBLOCK
426.2 LEFT POSTERIOR FASCICULAR
0 LEFT WITH RIGHT SEE 'HEART BLOCK - BUNDLE BRANCH', RIGHT WITH LEFT
426.4 RIGHT NOS
426.53 RIGHT WITH LEFT NOS (INCOMPLETE) (MAIN STEM)
426.52 RIGHT WITH LEFT ANTERIOR FASCICULAR
426.51 RIGHT WITH LEFT POSTERIOR FASCICULAR
426.54 RIGHT WITH LEFT ANTERIOR WITH LEFT POSTERIOR
426.54 TRIFASCICULAR BLOCK

HEART DISEASE

429.9 NOS
424.1 AORTIC VALVE NOS (SEE ALSO 'AORTA, AORTIC')
395.# AORTIC VALVE RHEUMATIC (SEE ALSO 'AORTA, AORTIC')
4th Digit: 395
0. STENOSIS
1. INSUFFICIENCY
2. STENOSIS WITH INSUFFICIENCY
9. OTHER AND UNPECIFIED AORTIC DISEASE
414.0# ARTERIOSCLEROTIC
5th Digit: 414.0
0. UNSPECIFIED TYPE OF VESSEL, NATIVE OR GRAFT
1. NATIVE CORONARY VESSEL
2. AUTOLOGOUS VEIN BYPASS GRAFT
3. NONAUTOLOGOUS BIOLOGICAL BYPASS GRAFT
4. AUTOLOGOUS ARTERY BYPASS GRAFT (GASTROEPIPLOIC) (INTERNAL MAMMARY)
5. UNSPECIFIED TYPE OF BYPASS GRAFT
0 CARDIOMYOPATHY SEE 'CARDIOMYOPATHY'

HEART DISEASE (continued)

WHEN CODING A MATERNAL CARDIOVASCULAR DISEASE COMPLICATING PREGNANCY, 648.6#, USE AN ADDITIONAL CODE TO IDENTIFY THE CONDITION.

648.6# COMPLICATING PREGNANCY CURRENT (CO-EXISTENT)
5th Digit: 648.6
0. EPISODE OF CARE NOS OR N/A
1. DELIVERED
2. DELIVERED WITH POSTPARTUM COMPLICATION
3. ANTEPARTUM COMPLICATION
4. POSTPARTUM COMPLICATION

746.9 CONGENITAL NOS
760.3 CONGENITAL MATERNAL AFFECTING FETUS OR NEWBORN
746.89 CONGENITAL SPECIFIED TYPE NEC
428.0 CONGESTIVE (SEE ALSO 'CHF (CONGESTIVE HEART FAILURE)')
414.9 CORONARY (ISCHEMIC)
429.9 CRYPTOGENIC
V17.3 FAMILY HISTORY
098.85 GONOCOCCAL NEC
274.82 GOUTY
429.82 HYPERKINETIC
402.## HYPERTENSIVE
4th Digit: 402
0. MALIGNANT
1. BENIGN
9. NOS
5th Digit: 402
0. WITHOUT CHF
1. WITH CHF

414.9 ISCHEMIC
0 ISCHEMIC ACUTE - WITH MYOCARDIAL INFARCTION SEE 'MI ACUTE'
411.89 ISCHEMIC ACUTE - WITHOUT MI
411.81 ISCHEMIC ACUTE - WITHOUT MI WITH CORONARY OCCLUSION
414.9 ISCHEMIC CHRONIC
414.1# ISCHEMIC CHRONIC - ANEURYSM
5th Digit: 414.1
0. HEART WALL
1. CORONARY VESSELS (ARTERIOVENOUS)
9. OTHER

414.0# ISCHEMIC CHRONIC - ARTERIOSCLEROTIC
5th Digit: 414.0
0. UNSPECIFIED TYPE OF VESSEL, NATIVE OR GRAFT
1. NATIVE CORONARY VESSEL
2. AUTOLOGOUS VEIN BYPASS GRAFT
3. NONAUTOLOGOUS BIOLOGICAL BYPASS GRAFT
4. AUTOLOGOUS ARTERY BYPASS GRAFT (GASTROEPIPLOIC) (INTERNAL MAMMARY)
5. UNSPECIFIED TYPE OF BYPASS GRAFT

414.8 ISCHEMIC CHRONIC - OTHER
416.1 KYPHOSCOLIOTIC
394.9 MITRAL NOS (SEE ALSO 'MITRAL INSUFFICIENCY' AND 'MITRAL REGURGITATION')
396.# MITRAL AND AORTIC VALVE (NON RHEUMATIC) (RHEUMATIC)
4th Digit: 396
0. MITRAL STENOSIS AND AORTIC STENOSIS
1. MITRAL STENOSIS AND AORTIC INSUFFICIENCY
2. MITRAL INSUFFICIENCY AND AORTIC STENOSIS
3. MITRAL INSUFFICIENCY AND AORTIC INSUFFICIENCY
8. MULTIPLE INVOLVEMENT MITRAL AND AORTIC
9. UNSPECIFIED

HEART DISEASE (continued)

394.# MITRAL RHEUMATIC (SEE ALSO 'MITRAL INSUFFICIENCY' AND 'MITRAL REGURGITATION')
4th Digit: 394
0. STENOSIS
1. INSUFFICIENCY
2. STENOSIS WITH INSUFFICIENCY
9. OTHER AND UNPECIFIED MITRAL DISEASE

306.2 PSYCHOGENIC
415.0 PULMONARY ACUTE (ACUTE COR PULMONALE)
416.9 PULMONARY CHRONIC UNSPECIFIED (CHRONIC COR PULMONALE)
416.0 PULMONARY HYPERTENSION PRIMARY
416.8 PULMONARY HYPERTENSION SECONDARY
416.8 PULMONARY OTHER CHRONIC
424.3 PULMONARY VALVE
746.00 PULMONARY VALVE CONGENITAL
397.1 PULMONARY VALVE RHEUMATIC
398.90 RHEUMATIC ACUTE
392.0 RHEUMATIC ACUTE - WITH CHOREA
391.8 RHEUMATIC ACUTE - SPECIFIED NEC
398.90 RHEUMATIC CHRONIC
V81.0 SCREENING FOR ISCHEMIC HEART DISEASE
429.0 SENILE ARTERIOSCLEROTIC [440.9]
093.89 SYPHILITIC
093.1 SYPHILITIC AORTITIS
090.5 SYPHILITIC AORTITIS CONGENITAL
424.2 TRICUSPID NOS (SEE ALSO 'TRICUSPID')
397.0 TRICUSPID RHEUMATIC (SEE ALSO 'TRICUSPID')
424.90 VALVULAR CAUSE UNSPECIFIED
746.9 VALVULAR NOS CONGENITAL
746.89 VALVULAR SPECIFIED NEC CONGENITAL
429.89 OTHER SPECIFIED NEC

FOR CODING PURPOSES, CHF AND RIGHT VENTRICULAR FAILURE ARE CONSIDERED TO BE SYNONYMOUS AND BOTH ARE ASSIGNED A 4TH DIGIT OF "0". LEFT VENTRICULAR FAILURE IS NOT THE SAME AS CHF. LEFT VENTRICULAR FAILURE IS ASSIGNED A 4TH DIGIT OF "1".

HEART FAILURE

428.9 NOS
0 COMPENSATED SEE 'CHF (CONGESTIVE HEART FAILURE)'
0 COMPLICATING ABORTION SEE 'ABORTION', BY TYPE WITH OTHER SPECIFIED COMPLICATION
0 COMPLICATING PREGNANCY, LABOR, OR DELIVERY, SEE 'HEART FAILURE OBSTETRICAL'
0 CONGESTIVE SEE 'CHF (CONGESTIVE HEART FAILURE)'
429.1 DEGENERATIVE WITH ARTERIOSCLEROSIS [440.9]
997.1 DURING A PROCEDURE
0 HYPERTENSIVE SEE 'HYPERTENSIVE', CARDIOVASCULAR DISEASE
428.1 LEFT
428.1 LEFT (VENTRICULAR FAILURE)
428.1 LEFT (VENTRICULAR FAILURE) WITH PULMONARY EDEMA
997.1 POST OPERATIVE - (RESULTING FROM A PROCEDURE)
429.4 POSTOPERATIVE - DUE TO CARDIAC PROSTHESIS
997.1 POST OPERATIVE HEART SURGERY - IMMEDIATE
429.4 POST OPERATIVE HEART SURGERY - LATE

WHEN CODING A MATERNAL CARDIOVASCULAR DISEASE COMPLICATING PREGNANCY, 648.6#, USE AN ADDITIONAL CODE TO IDENTIFY THE CONDITION.

HEART FAILURE OBSTETRICAL

0 MATERNAL COMPLICATING ABORTION SEE 'ABORTION', BY TYPE WITH OTHER SPECIFIED COMPLICATION
669.4# MATERNAL COMPLICATING LABOR AND DELIVERY
648.6# MATERNAL CURRENT (CO-EXISTENT) IN PREGNANCY
5th Digit: 648.6, 669.4
0. EPISODE OF CARE NOS
1. DELIVERED WITH OR WITHOUT MENTION OF ANTEPARTUM CONDITION
2. DELIVERED WITH MENTION OF POSTPARTUM COMPLICATION
3. ANTEPARTUM CONDITION
4. POSTPARTUM COMPLICATION

668.1# MATERNAL DUE TO ANESTHESIA OR OTHER SEDATION IN L & D
5th Digit: 668.1
0. EPISODE OF CARE NOS
1. DELIVERED WITH OR WITHOUT MENTION OF ANTEPARTUM CONDITION
2. DELIVERED WITH MENTION OF POSTPARTUM COMPLICATION
3. ANTEPARTUM CONDITION
4. POSTPARTUM COMPLICATION

639.8 MATERNAL FOLLOWING ABORTION, ECTOPIC, OR MOLAR PREGNANCY

779.8 HEART FAILURE OBSTETRICAL AFFECTING FETUS OR NEWBORN
787.1 HEARTBURN

HEAT

992.1 COLLAPSE
992.2 CRAMPS
992.7 EDEMA
992.9 EFFECTS NOS
992.8 EFFECTS OTHER SPECIFIED
992.5 EXHAUSTION
992.4 EXHAUSTION - SALT (AND WATER) DEPLETION
992.3 EXHAUSTION - WATER DEPLETION
992.6 FATIGUE TRANSIENT
992.9 INJURY
V60.1 LACK (INADEQUATE HOUSING)
909.4 LATE EFFECT
0 PROSTRATION SEE 'HEAT', EXHAUSTION
992.0 PYREXIA
705.1 RASH
782.0 SENSE ABSENCE
992.0 STROKE
992.1 SYNCOPE

304.5# HEAVENLY BLUE ADDICTION
5th Digit: 304.5
0. NOS
1. CONTINUOUS
2. EPISODIC
3. IN REMISSION

273.2 HEAVY CHAIN (GAMMA G) DISEASE
766.1 HEAVY FOR DATES INFANT
796.0 HEAVY METAL ABNORMAL TOXICOLOGY
V82.5 HEAVY METAL POISONING SCREENING
626.2 HEAVY PERIODS
626.3 HEAVY PERIODS PUBERTAL

295.1# HEBEPHRENIA
5th Digit: 295.1
0. NOS
1. SUBCHRONIC
2. CHRONIC
3. SUBCHRONIC WITH ACUTE EXACERBATION
4. CHRONIC WITH ACUTE
5. IN REMISSION

715.04 HEBERDEN'S NODES (OSTEOARTHRITIS)
413.9 HEBERDEN'S SYNDROME (ANGINA PECTORIS)

HEBRA'S

695.89 DERMATITIS EXFOLIATIVA
695.1 ERYTHEMA MULTIFORME EXUDATIVUM
696.3 PITYRIASIS MACULATA ET CIRCINATA
695.89 PITYRIASIS RUBRA
696.4 PITYRIASIS RUBRA PILARIS
698.2 PRURIGO

259.2 HEDINGER'S SYNDROME (MALIGNANT CARCINOID)
135 HEERFORDT'S DISEASE (UVEOPAROTITIS)
288.2 HEGGLIN'S SYNDROME
290.1# HEIDENHAIN'S DISEASE
5th Digit: 290.1
0. UNCOMPLICATED
1. WITH DELIRIUM
2. WITH DELUSIONAL FEATURES
3. WITH DEPRESSIVE FEATURES

207.1# HEILMEYER SCHONER DISEASE
5th Digit: 207.1
0. WITHOUT MENTION OF REMISSION
1. IN REMISSION

045.9 HEINE-MEDIN DISEASE (SEE ALSO 'POLIOMYELITIS')
282.7 HEINZ-BODY ANEMIA, CONGENITAL
041.86 HELICOBACTER PYLORI INFECTION
093.1 HELLER-DOHLE DISEASE (SYPHILITIC AORTITIS)
299.1# HELLER'S DISEASE OR SYNDROME (SEE ALSO 'PSYCHOSIS CHILDHOOD')
5th Digit: 299.1
0. ACTIVE STATE
1. RESIDUAL STATE

642.5# HELLP (SYNDROME)
5th Digit: 642.5
0. EPISODE OF CARE NOS OR N/A
1. DELIVERED
2. DELIVERED WITH POSTPARTUM COMPLICATIONS
3. ANTEPARTUM COMPLICATION
4. POSTPARTUM COMPLICATIONS

0 HELMINTH INFECTION NOS SEE 'HELMINTHIASIS'

HELMINTHIASIS

128.9 NOS
126.9 ANCYLOSTOMA
126.2 ANCYLOSTOMA BRAZILIENSE
126.3 ANCYLOSTOMA CEYLANICUM
126.0 ANCYLOSTOMA DUODENALE
126.8 ANCYLOSTOMA OTHER TYPE
128.8 ANGIOSTRONGYLUS CANTONENSIS
127.1 ANISAKIS
127.0 ASCARID
127.5 CAPILLARIA
128.1 GNATHOSTOMA SPINIGERUM
127.9 INTESTINAL
V75.7 INTESTINAL SCREENING EXAM
127.8 MIXED INTESTINAL
126.9 NECATOR
126.1 NECATOR AMERICANUS

H

HELMINTHIASIS (continued)

127.4 OXYURIS VERMICULARIS (PIN WORM)
127.2 STRONGYLOID
128.0 TOXOCARA (DOG)
127.3 TRICHURIS
128.8 OTHER SPECIFIED

238.1 HEMANGIOBLASTOMA SITE NOS
0 HEMANGIOBLASTOMA SITE SPECIFIED SEE 'NEOPLASM UNCERTAIN BEHAVIOR' BY SITE M9161/1

HEMANGIOENDOTHELIOMA

238.9 SITE NOS
0 SITE SPECIFIED SEE 'NEOPLASM UNCERTAIN BEHAVIOR' BY SITE M9130/1
228.0# BENIGN M9130/0
5th Digit: 228.0
0. SITE NOS
1. SKIN AND SUBCUTANEOUS TISSUE
2. INTRACRANIAL STRUCTURES
3. RETINA
4. INTRA ABDOMINAL STRUCTURES
9. OTHER SITES

0 BONE (DIFFUSE) MALIGNANT SEE 'CANCER', BONE BY SITE
171.# MALIGNANT
4th Digit: 171
0. HEAD FACE NECK
2. UPPER LIMB SHOULDER
3. LOWER LIMB HIP
4. THORAX
5. ABDOMINAL HYPOCHONDRIUM
6. PELVIS BUTTOCK GROIN INGUINAL REGION PERINEUM
7. TRUNK NOS BACK NOS FLANK NOS
8. OTHER SPECIFIED SITES
9. SITE NOS

228.09 NERVOUS SYSTEM M9130/0

HEMANGIOMA

228.0# UNSPECIFIED M9120/0
228.0# CAPILLARY M9131/0
228.0# CAVERNOUS M9121/0
5th Digit: 228.0
0. SITE NOS
1. SKIN AND SUBCUTANEOUS TISSUE
2. INTRACRANIAL STRUCTURES
3. RETINA
4. INTRA ABDOMINAL STRUCTURES
9. OTHER SITES

228.09 CHOROID
228.09 CNS
228.09 HEART
228.0# INTRAMUSCULAR M9132/0
5th Digit: 228.0
0. SITE NOS
1. SKIN AND SUBCUTANEOUS TISSUE
2. INTRACRANIAL STRUCTURES
3. RETINA
4. INTRA ABDOMINAL STRUCTURES
9. OTHER SITES

228.09 IRIS
228.04 PERITONEUM
228.00 RACEMOSE
228.03 RETINA
228.04 RETROPERITONEAL TISSUE
228.09 SPINAL CORD
228.09 SUBGLOTTIC

HEMANGIOMA (continued)

228.0# VENOUS M9122/0
228.0# VERRUCOUS KERATOTIC M9142/0
5th Digit: 228.0
0. SITE NOS
1. SKIN AND SUBCUTANEOUS TISSUE
2. INTRACRANIAL STRUCTURES
3. RETINA
4. INTRA ABDOMINAL STRUCTURES
9. OTHER SITES

238.1 HEMANGIOPERICYTOMA NOS M9150/1
215.# HEMANGIOPERICYTOMA BENIGN M9150/0
171.# HEMANGIOPERICYTOMA MALIGNANT M9150/3
171.# HEMANGIOSARCOMA M9120/3
4th Digit: 171, 215
0. HEAD FACE NECK
2. UPPER LIMB SHOULDER
3. LOWER LIMB HIP
4. THORAX
5. ABDOMINAL HYPOCHONDRIUM
6. PELVIS BUTTOCK GROIN INGUINAL REGION PERINEUM
7. TRUNK NOS BACK NOS FLANK NOS
8. OTHER SPECIFIED SITES
9. SITE NOS

0 HEMARTHROSIS - CURRENT INJURY SEE 'SPRAIN' BY SITE
719.1# HEMARTHROSIS - OLD (NONTRAUMATIC)
5th Digit: 719.1
0. SITE NOS
1. SHOULDER REGION
2. UPPER ARM (ELBOW) (HUMERUS)
3. FOREARM (RADIUS) (WRIST) (ULNA)
4. HAND (CARPAL) (METACARPAL) (FINGERS)
5. PELVIC REGION AND THIGH (HIP) (BUTTOCK) (FEMUR)
6. LOWER LEG (FIBULA) (KNEE) (PATELLA) (TIBIA)
7. ANKLE AND/OR FOOT (METATARSALS) (TOES) (TARSALS)
8. OTHER
9. MULTIPLE

HEMATEMESIS

578.0 NOS
777.3 DUE TO SWALLOWED MATERNAL BLOOD
0 WITH ULCER SEE 'ULCER'

705.89 HEMATIDROSIS
791.2 HEMATINURIA
576.8 HEMATOBILIA

HEMATOCELE

620.7 BROAD LIGAMENT
629.0 CANAL OF NUCK
608.83 CORD MALE
620.8 FALLOPIAN TUBE
629.0 FEMALE
569.89 ISCHIORECTAL
608.83 MALE GENITALIA
629.0 OVARY
629.0 PERIUTERINE
629.0 RETROUTERINE
608.83 SCROTUM
608.83 SPERMATIC CORD
608.84 TESTIS
608.83 TUNICA VAGINALIS
621.4 UTERUS
623.6 VAGINA
624.5 VULVA

578.1 HEMATOCHEZIA
0 HEMATOCHEZIA WITH ULCER SEE 'ULCER'

H

371.12 HEMATOCORNEA
790.0 HEMATOCRIT ABNORMAL
282.7 HEMATOCRIT ELEVATED ABNORMAL FINDINGS
285.9 HEMATOCRIT LOW ABNORMAL FINDINGS
776.9 HEMATOLOGICAL DISORDER PERINATALTRANSIENT
776.8 HEMATOLOGICAL DISORDER NEONATAL TRANSIENT OTHER SPECIFIED

A HEMATOMA IS A LOCALIZED COLLECTION OF BLOOD IN AN ORGAN SPACE OR TISSUE. IN ICD-9 CODING, HEMATOMAS ARE CLASSIFIED AS TRAUMATIC OR NONTRAUMATIC. HEMATOMAS UNSPECIFIED (TRAUMATIC OR NONTRAUMATIC) SHOULD BE CODED AS TRAUMATIC HEMATOMAS, EXCEPT THOSE OF THE GENITAL ORGANS, OR THE EYE. UNSPECIFIED HEMATOMAS OF THE GENITAL ORGANS OR EYE SHOULD BE CODED AS NON-TRAUMATIC HEMATOMAS. HEMATOMAS THAT COMPLICATE PREGNANCY OR DELIVERY SHOULD BE CODED AS PREGNANCY OR LABOR AND DELIVERY COMPLICATIONS.

HEMATOMA - NONTRAUMATIC

658.8# AMNION
5th Digit: 658.8
0. EPISODE OF CARE NOS OR N/A
1. DELIVERED
3. ANTEPARTUM COMPLICATION

441.0# AORTA DISSECTING
5th Digit: 441.0
0. UNSPECIFIED SITE
1. THORACIC
2. ABDOMINAL
3. THORACOABDOMINAL

430 ARACHNOID
772.2 ARACHNOID FETUS OR NEWBORN
380.31 AURICLE (EAR)
431 BRAIN
772.9 BRAIN NEWBORN NOS
772.8 BRAIN NEWBORN NEC
611.8 BREAST
620.7 BROAD LIGAMENT
431 CEREBRAL
772.9 CEREBRAL NEWBORN NOS
772.8 CEREBRAL NEWBORN NEC
674.3# CESAREAN SECTION WOUND NOS
5th Digit: 674.3
0. EPISODE OF CARE NOS OR N/A
2. DELIVERED WITH POSTPARTUM COMPLICATION
4. POSTPARTUM COMPLICATION

656.7# CHORION (OBSTETRICAL)
5th Digit: 656.7
0. EPISODE OF CARE NOS OR N/A
1. DELIVERED
3. ANTEPARTUM COMPLICATION

998.12 COMPLICATING A PROCEDURE
607.82 CORPUS CAVERNOSUM
620.1 CORPUS LUTEUM
432.1 DURA (MATER)
767.0 DURA (MATER) FETUS OR NEWBORN
380.31 EAR EXTERNAL
608.83 EPIDIDYMIS
432.0 EPIDURAL
767.0 EPIDURAL FETUS OR NEWBORN
674.3# EPISIOTOMY
5th Digit: 674.3
0. EPISODE OF CARE NOS OR N/A
2. DELIVERED WITH POSTPARTUM COMPLICATION
4. POSTPARTUM COMPLICATION

432.0 EXTRADURAL
767.0 EXTRADURAL FETUS OR NEWBORN
374.81 EYELID
620.8 FALLOPIAN TUBE
629.8 GENITAL ORGAN FEMALE NEC
608.83 GENITAL ORGAN MALE NEC
620.0 GRAAFIAN FOLLICLE (RUPTURED)
432.9 INTRACRANIAL
767.0 INTRACRANIAL FETUS OR NEWBORN
593.81 KIDNEY CYSTIC

HEMATOMA - NONTRAUMATIC (continued)

624.5 LABIA
573.8 LIVER (SUBCAPSULAR)
430 MENINGES BRAIN
772.2 MENINGES BRAIN FETUS OR NEWBORN
620.8 MESOSALPINX
674.3# OBSTETRICAL SURGICAL WOUND
5th Digit: 674.3
0. EPISODE OF CARE NOS OR N/A
2. DELIVERED WITH POSTPARTUM COMPLICATION
4. POSTPARTUM COMPLICATION

377.42 OPTIC NERVE SHEATHS
376.32 ORBIT
620.1 OVARY
629.8 PELVIS FEMALE
608.83 PELVIS MALE
607.82 PENIS
674.3# PERINEAL WOUND (OBSTETRICAL)
5th Digit: 674.3
0. EPISODE OF CARE NOS OR N/A
2. DELIVERED WITH POSTPARTUM COMPLICATION
4. POSTPARTUM COMPLICATION

593.81 PERIRENAL CYSTIC
380.31 PINNA OR AURICLE
656.7# PLACENTAL (OBSTETRICAL)
5th Digit: 656.7
0. EPISODE OF CARE NOS OR N/A
1. DELIVERED
3. ANTEPARTUM COMPLICATION

998.12 POSTOPERATIVE
568.81 RETROPERITONEAL
568.81 RETROPUBIC MALE
608.83 SCROTUM
608.83 SEMINAL VESICLE
608.83 SPERMATIC CORD
336.1 SPINAL CORD
430 SUBARACHNOID
772.2 SUBARACHNOID FETUS OR NEWBORN
372.72 SUBCONJUNCTIVAL
432.1 SUBDURAL
767.0 SUBDURAL FETUS OR NEWBORN
267 SUBPERIOSTEAL (SYNDROME)
772.6 SUPERFICIAL FETUS OR NEWBORN
656.7# SYNCYTIUM
5th Digit: 656.7
0. EPISODE OF CARE NOS OR N/A
1. DELIVERED
3. ANTEPARTUM COMPLICATION

608.83 TESTIS
0 TRAUMATIC SEE 'HEMATOMA - TRAUMATIC'
608.83 TUNICA VAGINALIS
663.6# UMBILICAL CORD MATERNAL
5th Digit: 663.6
0. EPISODE OF CARE NOS OR N/A
1. DELIVERED
3. ANTEPARTUM COMPLICATION

762.6 UMBILICAL CORD AFFECTING FETUS OR NEWBORN
620.7 UTERINE LIGAMENT
621.4 UTERUS
623.6 VAGINAL
608.83 VAS DEFERENS
379.23 VITREOUS
624.5 VULVA

DO NOT CODE TRAUMATIC HEMATOMAS WHEN THEY ACCOMPANY A FRACTURE, DISLOCATION, LACERATION, OR A CRUSH INJURY. THEY ARE CONSIDERED TO BE INCIDENTAL TO THESE INJURIES AND ONLY A CODE FOR THE SPECIFIC INJURY IS REQUIRED.

FOR TRAUMATIC HEMATOMAS OF SITES NOT LISTED BELOW, USE THE CODE "INJURY" FOUND BY ANATOMICAL SITE.

HEMATOMA - TRAUMATIC

924.9	NOS
922.2	ABDOMEN WALL OR MUSCLE
868.00	ABDOMINAL ORGAN UNSPECIFIED
868.10	ABDOMINAL ORGAN UNSPECIFIED WITH OPEN WOUND
868.09	ABDOMINAL ORGAN OTHER OR MULTIPLE
868.19	ABDOMINAL ORGAN OTHER OR MULTIPLE WITH OPEN WOUND
921.9	ADNEXA EYE
868.01	ADRENAL GLAND
868.11	ADRENAL GLAND WITH OPEN WOUND
924.21	ANKLE
924.20	ANKLE AND FOOT
902.0	AORTA ABDOMINAL
901.0	AORTA THORACIC
852.0#	ARACHNOID
852.1#	ARACHNOID WITH OPEN INTRACRANIAL WOUND
	5th Digit: 852.0-1
	0. LEVEL OF CONSCIOUSNESS NOS
	1. NO LOC
	2. LOC < 1 HR
	3. LOC 1 - 24 HRS
	4. LOC > 24 HRS WITH RETURN TO PRIOR LEVEL
	5. LOC > 24 HRS WITHOUT RETURN TO PRIOR LEVEL: OR DEATH BEFORE REGAINING CONSCIOUSNESS, REGARDLESS OF DURATION OF LOC
	6. LOC DURATION NOS
	9. WITH CONCUSSION NOS
772.2	ARACHNOID FETUS OR NEWBORN
923.9	ARM
923.09	ARM AND SHOULDER
923.10	ARM LOWER
923.03	ARM UPPER
923.8	ARM MULTIPLE SITES
0	ARTERY SEE SPECIFIC ARTERY INJURY
920	AUDITORY CANAL (EXTERNAL) (MEATUS)
920	AURICLE EAR
923.02	AXILLARY REGION
923.09	AXILLARY REGION AND SHOULDER
923.09	AXILLARY REGION AND UPPER ARM
922.31	BACK
868.02	BILE DUCT
868.12	BILE DUCT WITH OPEN WOUND
767.1	BIRTH INJURY SKULL OR SCALP
767.8	BIRTH INJURY OTHER SPECIFIED
0	BLOOD VESSEL SEE SPECIFIC BLOOD VESSEL INJURY
924.9	BONE UNSPECIFIED
853.0#	BRAIN
853.1#	BRAIN WITH OPEN INTRACRANIAL WOUND
	5th Digit: 853.0-1
	0. LEVEL OF CONSCIOUSNESS NOS
	1. NO LOC
	2. LOC < 1 HR
	3. LOC 1 - 24 HRS
	4. LOC > 24 HRS WITH RETURN TO PRIOR LEVEL
	5. LOC > 24 HRS WITHOUT RETURN TO PRIOR LEVEL: OR DEATH BEFORE REGAINING CONSCIOUSNESS, REGARDLESS OF DURATION OF LOC
	6. LOC DURATION NOS
	9. WITH CONCUSSION NOS

HEMATOMA - TRAUMATIC (continued)

767.0	BRAIN FETUS OR NEWBORN
0	BRAIN WITH CONTUSION SEE 'CEREBRAL CONTUSION'
922.0	BREAST
867.6	BROAD LIGAMENT
867.7	BROAD LIGAMENT WITH OPEN WOUND
665.7#	BROAD LIGAMENT (OBSTETRCAL TRAUMA)
	5th Digit: 665.7
	0. EPISODE OF CARE NOS OR N/A
	1. DELIVERED
	2. DELIVERED WITH POSTPARTUM COMPLICATION
	4. POSTPARTUM COMPLICATION
920	BROW
922.32	BUTTOCK
959.9	CALCIFIED UNSPECIFIED SITE
921.1	CANTHUS
920	CAPITIS
767.1	CAPITIS DUE TO BIRTH INJURY
767.1	CAPITIS NEWBORN
861.01	CARDIAC
861.11	CARDIAC WITH OPEN WOUND INTO THORAX
952.4	CAUDA EQUINA (SPINE)
853.0#	CEREBRAL
853.1#	CEREBRAL WITH OPEN INTRACRANIAL WOUND
	5th Digit: 853.0-1
	0. LEVEL OF CONSCIOUSNESS NOS
	1. NO LOC
	2. LOC < 1 HR
	3. LOC 1 - 24 HRS
	4. LOC > 24 HRS WITH RETURN TO PRIOR LEVEL
	5. LOC > 24 HRS WITHOUT RETURN TO PRIOR LEVEL: OR DEATH BEFORE REGAINING CONSCIOUSNESS, REGARDLESS OF DURATION OF LOC
	6. LOC DURATION NOS
	9. WITH CONCUSSION NOS
767.0	CEREBRAL FETUS OR NEWBORN
0	CEREBRAL WITH CONTUSION SEE 'CEREBRAL CONTUSION'
920	CHEEK
922.1	CHEST (WALL)
920	CHIN
922.4	CLITORIS
998.12	COMPLICATING A PROCEDURE
664.5#	COMPLICATING DELIVERY PERINEUM OR VULVA (OBSTETRCAL TRAUMA)
	5th Digit: 664.5
	0. EPISODE OF CARE NOS OR N/A
	1. DELIVERED
	4. POSTPARTUM COMPLICATION
665.7#	COMPLICATING DELIVERY PELVIC OR VAGINA (OBSTETRCAL TRAUMA)
	5th Digit: 665.7
	0. EPISODE OF CARE NOS OR N/A
	1. DELIVERED
	2. DELIVERED WITH POSTPARTUM COMPLICATION
	4. POSTPARTUM COMPLICATION
921.1	CONJUNCTIVA
952.4	CONUS MEDULLARIS (SPINE)
921.3	CORNEA
922.4	CORPUS CAVERNOSUM
922.1	COSTAL REGION

HEMATOMA - TRAUMATIC (continued)

852.2# DURA (MATER)
852.3# DURA (MATER) WITH OPEN INTRACRANIAL WOUND

5th Digit: 852.2-3

0. LEVEL OF CONSCIOUSNESS NOS
1. NO LOC
2. LOC < 1 HR
3. LOC 1 - 24 HRS
4. LOC > 24 HRS WITH RETURN TO PRIOR LEVEL
5. LOC > 24 HRS WITHOUT RETURN TO PRIOR LEVEL: OR DEATH BEFORE REGAINING CONSCIOUSNESS, REGARDLESS OF DURATION OF LOC
6. LOC DURATION NOS
9. WITH CONCUSSION NOS

767.0 DURA (MATER) FETUS OR NEWBORN
920 EAR (AURICLE)
923.11 ELBOW
923.10 ELBOW WITH FOREARM
922.4 EPIDIDYMIS
852.4# EPIDURAL
852.5# EPIDURAL WITH OPEN INTRACRANIAL WOUND

5th Digit: 852.4-5

0. LEVEL OF CONSCIOUSNESS NOS
1. NO LOC
2. LOC < 1 HR
3. LOC 1 - 24 HRS
4. LOC > 24 HRS WITH RETURN TO PRIOR LEVEL
5. LOC > 24 HRS WITHOUT RETURN TO PRIOR LEVEL: OR DEATH BEFORE REGAINING CONSCIOUSNESS, REGARDLESS OF DURATION OF LOC
6. LOC DURATION NOS
9. WITH CONCUSSION NOS

767.0 EPIDURAL FETUS OR NEWBORN
922.2 EPIGASTRIC REGION
852.4# EXTRADURAL
852.5# EXTRADURAL WITH OPEN INTRACRANIAL WOUND

5th Digit: 852.4-5

0. LEVEL OF CONSCIOUSNESS NOS
1. NO LOC
2. LOC < 1 HR
3. LOC 1 - 24 HRS
4. LOC > 24 HRS WITH RETURN TO PRIOR LEVEL
5. LOC > 24 HRS WITHOUT RETURN TO PRIOR LEVEL: OR DEATH BEFORE REGAINING CONSCIOUSNESS, REGARDLESS OF DURATION OF LOC
6. LOC DURATION NOS
9. WITH CONCUSSION NOS

767.0 EXTRADURAL FETUS OR NEWBORN
924.5 EXTREMITY LOWER
924.4 EXTREMITY LOWER MULTIPLE SITES
923.9 EXTREMITY UPPER
923.8 EXTREMITY UPPER MULTIPLE SITES
921.9 EYE
921.0 EYE AND ADNEXA (BLACK EYE)
921.3 EYEBALL
921.1 EYELID
920 FACE
922.2 FEMORAL TRIANGLE
772.6 FETUS OR NEWBORN SUPERFICIAL
923.3 FINGER
923.3 FINGERNAIL
922.2 FLANK
924.20 FOOT
924.20 FOOT AND ANKLE
923.10 FOREARM
923.10 FOREARM AND ELBOW
920 FOREHEAD

HEMATOMA - TRAUMATIC (continued)

868.02 GALLBLADDER
868.12 GALLBLADDER WITH OPEN WOUND
922.4 GENITAL ORGANS EXTERNAL
921.3 GLOBE (EYE)
922.2 GROIN
920 GUM
923.20 HAND
920 HEAD
861.01 HEART
861.11 HEART WITH OPEN WOUND OF THORAX
924.20 HEEL
924.01 HIP
924.00 HIP WITH THIGH
922.2 ILIAC REGION
922.2 INGUINAL REGION
0 INTERNAL ORGANS SEE ALSO SPECIFIC ORGAN, INJURY
922.33 INTERSCAPULAR REGION
853.## INTRACRANIAL

4th Digit: 853

0. WITHOUT OPEN INTRACRANIAL WOUND
1. WITH OPEN INTRACRANIAL WOUND

5th Digit: 853

0. LEVEL OF CONSCIOUSNESS NOS
1. NO LOC
2. LOC < 1 HR
3. LOC 1 - 24 HRS
4. LOC > 24 HRS WITH RETURN TO PRIOR LEVEL
5. LOC > 24 HRS WITHOUT RETURN TO PRIOR LEVEL: OR DEATH BEFORE REGAINING CONSCIOUSNESS, REGARDLESS OF DURATION OF LOC
6. LOC DURATION NOS
9. WITH CONCUSSION NOS

767.0 INTRACRANIAL'FETUS OR NEWBORN
921.3 IRIS (EYE)
866.01 KIDNEY
866.11 KIDNEY WITH OPEN WOUND INTO CAVITY
924.11 KNEE
924.10 KNEE WITH LOWER LEG
922.4 LABIA
921.1 LACRIMAL APPARATUS, GLAND OR SAC
920 LARYNX
0 LATE EFFECT SEE 'LATE EFFECT'
924.5 LEG
924.10 LEG LOWER
924.4 LEG MULTIPLE SITES
921.3 LENS
920 LINGUAL
920 LIP
864.01 LIVER
864.11 LIVER WITH OPEN WOUND
767.8 LIVER FETUS OR NEWBORN (SUBCAPSULAR)
922.31 LUMBAR REGION
861.21 LUNG
861.31 LUNG WITH OPEN WOUND
920 MALAR REGION
920 MANDIBULAR JOINT AREA
920 MASTOID REGION
852.0# MENINGEAL BRAIN
852.1# MENINGEAL BRAIN WITH OPEN INTRACRANIAL WOUND

5th Digit: 852.0-1

0. LEVEL OF CONSCIOUSNESS NOS
1. NO LOC
2. LOC < 1 HR
3. LOC 1 - 24 HRS
4. LOC > 24 HRS WITH RETURN TO PRIOR LEVEL
5. LOC > 24 HRS WITHOUT RETURN TO PRIOR LEVEL: OR DEATH BEFORE REGAINING CONSCIOUSNESS, REGARDLESS OF DURATION OF LOC
6. LOC DURATION NOS
9. WITH CONCUSSION NOS

HEMATOMA - TRAUMATIC (continued)

772.2 MENINGEAL BRAIN FETUS OR NEWBORN
922.1 MIDTHORACIC REGION
920 MOUTH
924.8 MULTIPLE SITES
924.4 MULTIPLE SITES LOWER LIMB
922.8 MULTIPLE SITES TRUNK
923.8 MULTIPLE SITES UPPER LIMB
924.9 MUSCLE SITE UNSPECIFIED
861.01 MYOCARDIAL
861.11 MYOCARDIAL WITH OPEN WOUND OF THORAX
920 NASAL (SEPTUM)
920 NECK
920 NOSE
920 OCCIPITAL REGION
921.2 ORBITAL AREA
867.6 OVARY
867.7 OVARY WITH OPEN WOUND
920 PALATE
920 PARIETAL REGION
665.7# PELVIC COMPLICATION DELIVERY (OBSTETRICAL TRAUMA)

5th Digit: 665.7

0. EPISODE OF CARE NOS OR N/A
1. DELIVERED
2. DELIVERED WITH POSTPARTUM COMPLICATION
4. POSTPARTUM COMPLICATION

922.9 PELVIS
922.4 PENIS
861.01 PERICARDIUM
861.11 PERICARDIUM WITH OPEN WOUND OF THORAX
920 PERICRANIAL
767.1 PERICRANIAL DUE TO BIRTH INJURY
664.5# PERINEAL WOUND COMPLICATING DELIVERY (OBSTETRICAL TRAUMA)

5th Digit: 664.5

0. EPISODE OF CARE NOS OR N/A
1. DELIVERED
4. POSTPARTUM COMPLICATION

922.4 PERINEUM
921.1 PERIOCULAR
921.2 PERIORBITAL
868.03 PERITONEUM
868.13 PERITONEUM WITH OPEN WOUND
920 PHARYNX
924.11 POPLITEAL SPACE
998.12 POSTOPERATIVE
922.4 PREPUCE
922.4 PUBIC REGION
922.4 PUDENDA
861.21 PULMONARY
861.31 PULMONARY WITH OPEN WOUND
924.00 QUADRICEPS FEMORALIS
866.01 RENAL
866.11 RENAL WITH OPEN WOUND INTO CAVITY
921.2 RETROBULBAR
868.04 RETROPERITONEUM
868.14 RETROPERITONEUM WITH OPEN WOUND
922.1 RIB
922.31 SACRAL REGION
920 SALIVARY DUCTS OR GLAND
920 SCALP
767.1 SCALP FETUS OR NEWBORN
923.01 SCAPULA
923.09 SCAPULA AND SHOULDER
923.01 SCAPULAR REGION
921.3 SCLERA (EYE)
922.4 SCROTUM
923.00 SHOULDER
923.09 SHOULDER AND ARM MULTIPLE SITES
923.00 SHOULDER REGION

HEMATOMA - TRAUMATIC (continued)

924.9 SKIN UNSPECIFIED SITE
920 SKULL
922.4 SPERMATIC CORD
952.4 SPINAL CORD CAUDA EQUINA
952.4 SPINAL CORD CONUS MEDULLARIS
767.4 SPINAL CORD FETUS OR NEWBORN
865.01 SPLEEN
865.11 SPLEEN WITH OPEN WOUND INTO CAVITY
922.1 STERNAL REGION
767.8 STERNOCLEIDOMASTOID BIRTH INJURY
767.8 STERNOMASTOID BIRTH INJURY
852.0# SUBARACHNOID
852.1# SUBARACHNOID WITH OPEN INTRACRANIAL WOUND

5th Digit: 852.0-1

0. LEVEL OF CONSCIOUSNESS NOS
1. NO LOC
2. LOC < 1 HR
3. LOC 1 - 24 HRS
4. LOC > 24 HRS WITH RETURN TO PRIOR LEVEL
5. LOC > 24 HRS WITHOUT RETURN TO PRIOR LEVEL: OR DEATH BEFORE REGAINING CONSCIOUSNESS, REGARDLESS OF DURATION OF LOC
6. LOC DURATION NOS
9. WITH CONCUSSION NOS

772.2 SUBARACHNOID FETUS OR NEWBORN
921.1 SUBCONJUNCTIVAL
924.9 SUBCUTANEOUS UNSPECIFIED SITE
852.2# SUBDURAL
852.3# SUBDURAL WITH OPEN INTRACRANIAL WOUND

5th Digit: 852.2-3

0. LEVEL OF CONSCIOUSNESS NOS
1. NO LOC
2. LOC < 1 HR
3. LOC 1 - 24 HRS
4. LOC > 24 HRS WITH RETURN TO PRIOR LEVEL
5. LOC > 24 HRS WITHOUT RETURN TO PRIOR LEVEL: OR DEATH BEFORE REGAINING CONSCIOUSNESS, REGARDLESS OF DURATION OF LOC
6. LOC DURATION NOS
9. WITH CONCUSSION NOS

767.0 SUBDURAL FETUS OR NEWBORN
920 SUBMAXILLARY REGION
920 SUBMENTAL REGION
924.9 SUBPERIOSTEAL
923.3 SUBUNGUAL (FINGERNAIL OR THUMBNAIL)
924.3 SUBUNGUAL (TOENAIL)
772.6 SUPERFICIAL FETUS OR NEWBORN
920 SUPRACLAVICULAR FOSSA
920 SUPRAORBITAL
920 TEMPLE
922.4 TESTIS
767.8 TESTIS BIRTH INJURY
924.00 THIGH
924.00 THIGH AND HIP
922.1 THORAX
920 THROAT
923.3 THUMB
923.3 THUMBNAIL
924.3 TOE
924.3 TOENAIL
920 TONGUE
922.9 TRUNK
922.8 TRUNK MULTIPLE SITES
922.4 TUNICA VAGINALIS
920 TYMPANUM
920 UVULA

HEMATOMA - TRAUMATIC (continued)

922.4 VAGINA
665.7# VAGINAL COMPLICATING DELIVERY (OBSTETRICAL TRAUMA)
5th Digit: 665.7
0. EPISODE OF CARE NOS OR N/A
1. DELIVERED
2. DELIVERED WITH POSTPARTUM COMPLICATION
4. POSTPARTUM COMPLICATION

0 VEIN SEE SPECIFIC VEIN, INJURY
920 VOCAL CORD
922.4 VULVA
767.8 VULVA BIRTH TRAUMA FETUS OR NEWBORN
664.5# VULVA COMPLICATING DELIVERY (OBSTETRICAL TRAUMA)
5th Digit: 664.5
0. EPISODE OF CARE NOS OR N/A
1. DELIVERED
4. POSTPARTUM COMPLICATION

923.21 WRIST
923.20 WRIST AND HAND

621.4 HEMATOMETRA
752.3 HEMATOMETRA CONGENITAL
752.2 HEMATOMETRA CONGENITAL WITH DOUBLING OF CERVIX AND VAGINA
336.1 HEMATOMYELIA
289.9 HEMATOPOIETIC ORGAN DISORDER
277.1 HEMATOPORPHYRIA
277.1 HEMATOPORPHYRINURIA
620.8 HEMATOSALPINX OVARY OR FALLOPIAN TUBE
608.83 HEMATOSPERMIA
599.7 HEMATURIA BENIGN (ESSENTIAL)
368.60 HEMERALOPIA
781.8 HEMI-AKINESIA
781.8 HEMI-INATTENTION
740.0 HEMIANENCEPHALY CONGENITAL

HEMIANOPSIA

368.46 ALTITUDINAL
368.47 BINASAL
368.47 BITEMPORAL
368.47 HETERONYMOUS
368.46 HOMONYMOUS
095.8 SYPHILITIC

307.9 HEMIASOMATOGNOSIA

901.89 HEMIAZYGOS VEIN INJURY
908.4 HEMIAZYGOS VEIN INJURY LATE EFFECT
901.89 HEMIAZYGOS VEIN LACERATION (RUPTURE) (HEMATOMA) (AVULSION) (ANEURYSM) TRAUMATIC
908.4 HEMIAZYGOS VEIN LACERATION LATE EFFECT
333.5 HEMIBALLISM
306.8 HEMIC DISORDER PSYCHOGENIC
740.0 HEMICEPHALY CONGENITAL
754.0 HEMIFACIAL ATROPHY
759.89 HEMIHYPERTROPHY (CONGENITAL)
756.0 HEMIHYPERTROPHY CRANIAL

HEMIMELIA

755.4 HEMIMELIA
755.30 LOWER LIMB
755.31 LOWER LIMB TRANSVERSE
755.20 UPPER LIMB
755.21 UPPER LIMB TRANSVERSE

0 HEMIPARESIS SEE 'HEMIPLEGIA'

HEMIPLEGIA

342.## ACQUIRED (OLD) (CAUSE OTHER OR NOS)
436 ACQUIRED DUE TO CVA ACUTE [**342.##**]
4th Digit: 342
0. FLACCID
1. SPASTIC
8. OTHER SPECIFIED
9. UNSPECIFIED

5th Digit: 342
0. UNSPECIFIED SIDE
1. DOMINANT SIDE
2. NONDOMINANT SIDE

344.89 ALTERNANS FACIALIS
437.0 ARTERIOSCLEROTIC
344.89 ASCENDING (SPINAL) NEC
343.4 BIRTH INJURY LATE EFFECT
437.8 CEREBRAL (CURRENT EPISODE)
343.1 CONGENITAL
300.11 CONVERSION NEUROSIS (HYSTERICAL)
434.1# EMBOLIC (CURRENT)
5th Digit: 434.1
0. WITHOUT CEREBRAL INFARCTION
1. WITH CEREBRAL INFARCTION

342.0# FLACCID ACQUIRED (OLD) (CAUSE OTHER OR NOS)
5th Digit: 342.0
0. UNSPECIFIED SIDE
1. DOMINANT SIDE
2. NONDOMINANT SIDE

437.8 HYPERTENSIVE (CURRENT EPISODE)
300.11 HYSTERICAL
343.4 INFANTILE
438.2# LATE EFFECT CEREBROVASCULAR DISEASE
5th Digit: 438.2
0. UNSPECIFIED SIDE
1. DOMINANT SIDE
2. NONDOMINANT SIDE

342.## LATE EFFECT VIRAL ENCEPHALITIS [139.0]
4th Digit: 342
0. FLACCID
1. SPASTIC
8. OTHER SPECIFIED
9. UNSPECIFIED

5th Digit: 342
0. UNSPECIFIED SIDE
1. DOMINANT SIDE
2. NONDOMINANT SIDE

344.89 MIDDLE ALTERNATING NEC
767.0 NEWBORN NEC
436 SEIZURE ACUTE (CURRENT)
342.1# SPASTIC ACQUIRED (OLD) (CAUSE OTHER OR NOS)
5th Digit: 342.1
0. UNSPECIFIED SIDE
1. DOMINANT SIDE
2. NONDOMINANT SIDE

434.0# THROMBOTIC
5th Digit: 434.0
0. WITHOUT CEREBRAL INFARCTION
1. WITH CEREBRAL INFARCTION

342.## VIRAL ENCEPHALITIC (LATE) [139.0]
4th Digit: 342
0. FLACCID
1. SPASTIC
8. OTHER SPECIFIED
9. UNSPECIFIED

5th Digit: 342
0. UNSPECIFIED SIDE
1. DOMINANT SIDE
2. NONDOMINANT SIDE

781.8 HEMISPATIAL NEGLECT
117.9 HEMISPOROSIS
756.14 HEMIVERTEBRA CONGENITAL

576.8 HEMOBILIA
792.1 HEMOCCULT POSITIVE STOOL
575.8 HEMOCHOLECYST
275.0 HEMOCHROMATOSIS

HEMOGLOBIN
282.7 ELEVATED ABNORMAL FINDINGS
282.7 FETAL HEREDITARY HPFH
282.7 HEMOLYTIC DISEASE UNSTABLE
285.9 LOW ABNORMAL FINDINGS
289.7 M (HB-M) DISEASE
289.7 PATHIES
282.5 S (HB-S) TRAIT (SICKLE CELL)

HEMOGLOBINOPATHY
282.7 NOS
282.7 C HB-C
282.7 D
282.7 D HB-D
282.7 E
282.7 E HB-E
289.6 FAMILIAL
289.6 FAMILIAL POLYCYTHEMIA
289.7 HBM DISEASE
289.0 HIGH OXYGEN AFFINITY
282.7 OTHER NOS
V78.3 OTHER SCREENING
289.0 POLYCYTHEMIA
282.7 STOCKHOLM HBD
282.7 ZURICH HB-ZURICH

HEMOGLOBINURIA
791.2 NOS
283.2 ACUTE INTRAVASCULAR HEMOLYSIS
283.2 DUE TO HEMOLYSIS FROM EXTERNAL CAUSES
283.2 EXERTIONAL
283.2 INTERMITTENT
283.2 MARCH
283.2 PAROXYSMAL (COLD) (NOCTURNAL)

084.8 HEMOGLOBINURIC FEVER (BILIOUS)
999.8 HEMOLYSIS TRANSFUSION
228.1 HEMOLYMPHANGIOMA SITE NOS
0 HEMOLYMPHANGIOMA SITE SPECIFIED SEE 'BENIGN NEOPLASM', BY SITE M9175/0

HEMOLYTIC
773.2 BLOOD TYPE REACTION PERINATAL - UNSPECIFIED
773.1 BLOOD TYPE REACTION PERINATAL - ABO
773.0 BLOOD TYPE REACTION PERINATAL - RH
773.2 BLOOD TYPE REACTION PERINATAL - OTHER
773.2 DISEASE FETUS OR NEWBORN
283.0 DISEASE FETUS OR NEWBORN - AUTOIMMUNE (COLD TYPE) (WARM TYPE)
283.11 UREMIC SYNDROME (ADULT) (CHILD)

621.4 HEMOMETRA
752.3 HEMOMETRA CONGENITAL

HEMOPERICARDIUM
423.0 NOS
772.8 NEWBORN
423.0 RHEUMATIC
860.2 TRAUMATIC
860.3 TRAUMATIC WITH OPEN WOUND
908.0 TRAUMATIC LATE EFFECT

HEMOPERITONEUM
568.81 HEMOPERITONEUM
868.03 TRAUMATIC
868.13 TRAUMATIC WITH OPEN WOUND
908.1 TRAUMATIC LATE EFFECT

HEMOPHILIA
286.0 NOS
286.0 A
286.1 B
286.2 C
286.0 CLASSICAL
286.0 FAMILIAL
286.0 HEREDITARY
286.7 NONFAMILIAL
286.4 VASCULAR

041.5 HEMOPHILUS INFLUENZAE (H. INFLUENZAE) INFECTION OR ORGANISM
038.41 HEMOPHILUS INFLUENZAE SEPSIS
V03.81 HEMOPHILUS INFLUENZAE (H. INFLUENZAE) VACCINATION
616.10 HEMOPHILUS VAGINALIS VAGINITIS [041.5]
360.43 HEMOPHTHALMOS EXCEPT CURRENT INJURY

HEMOPNEUMOTHORAX
511.8 NONTRAUMATIC
860.4 TRAUMATIC
860.5 TRAUMATIC WITH OPEN WOUND
908.0 TRAUMATIC LATE EFFECT

786.3 HEMOPTYSIS

WHEN YOU CODE A HEMORRHAGIC DISORDER OR HEMORRHAGE DUE A CIRCULATING ANTI-COAGULANT SUCH AS COUMADIN OR HEPARIN, ASSIGN IT TO HEMORRHAGE BY SITE WITH AN ADDITIONAL SECONDARY E-CODE FROM THE TABLE OF DRUGS AND CHEMICALS (THERAPEUTIC USE)TO IDENTIFY THE SPECIFIC SUBSTANCE CAUSING THE ADVERSE EFFECT. FOR EXAMPLE, 578.9, HEMORRHAGE GASTROINTESTINAL DUE TO AN ADVERSE EFFECT OF COUMADIN [E934.2].

HEMORRHAGE
459.0 UNSPECIFIED NONTRAUMATIC
459.0 ABDOMEN
641.2# ABRUPTIO PLACENTA
5th Digit: 641.2
0. EPISODE OF CARE NOS OR N/A
1. DELIVERED
3. ANTEPARTUM COMPLICATION

762.1 ABRUPTIO PLACENTA AFFECTING FETUS OR NEWBORN
474.8 ADENOID
255.4 ADRENAL
772.5 ADRENAL PERINATAL
770.3 ALVEOLAR (LUNG) PERINATAL
525.8 ALVEOLAR PROCESS
998.11 AMPUTATION STUMP (SURGICAL)
997.69 AMPUTATION STUMP SECONDARY OR DELAYED
569.3 ANUS
0 ARACHNOID SEE 'HEMORRHAGE' SUBARACHNOID
459.0 ARTERY NEC
431 BASILAR ARTERY
596.8 BLADDER
596.7 BLADDER WALL
578.9 BOWEL

BRAIN
431 ANY SITE (NONTRAUMATIC)
430 ANEURYSM RUPTURED (CONGENITAL)
431 ARTERY
431 BLOOD VESSEL
767.0 FETUS OR NEWBORN NEC
772.2 FETUS OR NEWBORN SUBARACHNOID, ARACHNOID, OR MENINGEAL
0 HISTORY WITH RESIDUAL SEE 'LATE EFFECT', CEREBROVASCULAR DISEASE
V12.59 HISTORY WITHOUT RESIDUAL
997.02 IATROGENIC

HEMORRHAGE (continued)

BRAIN (continued)

674.0# MATERNAL DUE TO PREGNANCY

5th Digit: 674.0

0. EPISODE OF CARE NOS OR N/A
1. DELIVERED
2. DELIVERED WITH POSTPARTUM COMPLICATION
3. ANTEPARTUM COMPLICATION
4. POSTPARTUM COMPLICATION

0 OLD WITH RESIDUAL SEE 'LATE EFFECT', CEREBROVASCULAR DISEASE

997.02 POSTOPERATIVE

853.0# TRAUMATIC - NEC

853.1# TRAUMATIC - NEC WITH OPEN INTRACRANIAL WOUND

852.4# TRAUMATIC - EXTRADURAL OR EPIDURAL

852.5# TRAUMATIC - EXTRADURAL OR EPIDURAL WITH OPEN INTRACRANIAL WOUND

852.0# TRAUMATIC - SUBARACHNOID

852.1# TRAUMATIC - SUBARACHNOID WITH OPEN INTRACRANIAL WOUND

852.2# TRAUMATIC - SUBDURAL

852.3# TRAUMATIC - SUBDURAL WITH OPEN INTRACRANIAL WOUND

5th Digit: 852.0-5, 853.0-1

0. LEVEL OF CONSCIOUSNESS NOS
1. NO LOC
2. LOC < 1 HR
3. LOC 1 - 24 HRS
4. LOC > 24 HRS WITH RETURN TO PRIOR LEVEL
5. LOC > 24 HRS WITHOUT RETURN TO PRIOR LEVEL: OR DEATH BEFORE REGAINING CONSCIOUSNESS, REGARDLESS OF DURATION OF LOC
6. LOC DURATION NOS
9. WITH CONCUSSION NOS

HEMORRHAGE (continued)

611.79 BREAST

786.3 BRONCHUS (CAUSE UNKNOWN)

431 BULBAR ARTERY

727.89 BURSA

448.9 CAPILLARY

429.89 CARDIOVASCULAR

431 CEREBELLAR

431 CEREBRAL

767.0 CEREBRAL FETUS OR NEWBORN DUE TO BIRTH TRAUMA (INTRAPARTUM HYPOXIA / ANOXIA)

431 CEREBROMENINGEAL

431 CEREBROSPINAL

622.8 CERVIX

674.3# CESAREAN SECTION WOUND

5th Digit: 674.3

0. NOS
2. DELIVERED WITH POSTPARTUM COMPLICATION
4. POSTPARTUM COMPLICATION

363.61 CHOROID

363.62 CHOROID EXPULSIVE

386.8 COCHLEA

562.13 COLON DUE TO DIVERTICULITIS

562.12 COLON DUE TO DIVERTICULOSIS

998.11 COMPLICATING A PROCEDURE

641.9# COMPLICATING PREGNANCY, ANTEPARTUM NOS

640.9# COMPLICATING PREGNANCY, ANTEPARTUM (<22 WEEKS) NOS

640.8# COMPLICATING PREGNANCY, ANTEPARTUM (<22 WEEKS) OTHER SPECIFIED

5th Digit: 640.8-9, 641.9

0. EPISODE OF CARE NOS OR N/A
1. DELIVERED
3. ANTEPARTUM COMPLICATION

HEMORRHAGE (continued)

762.1 COMPLICATING PREGNANCY, ANTEPARTUM AFFECTING FETUS OR NEWBORN

641.3# COMPLICATING PREGNANCY, ANTEPARTUM ASSOCIATED WITH COAGULATION DEFECTS

641.8# COMPLICATING PREGNANCY, ANTEPARTUM , INTRAPARTUM - OTHER (TRAUMA, UTERINE LEIOMYOMA)

5th Digit: 641.3, 8

0. EPISODE OF CARE NOS OR N/A
1. DELIVERED
3. ANTEPARTUM COMPLICATION

372.72 CONJUNCTIVA

772.8 CONJUNCTIVA NEWBORN

607.82 CORPUS CAVERNOSUM

620.1 CORPUS LUTEUM CYST

431 CORPUS LUYSII

431 CORTICAL

782.7 CUTANEOUS

772.6 CUTANEOUS PERINATAL

286.5 DUE TO ANTITHROMBINEMIA

286.5 DUE TO ANTITHROMBOPLASTINEMIA

286.5 DUE TO ANTITHROMBOPLASTINOGENEMIA

286.5 DUE TO CIRCULATING ANTICOAGULANT

0 DUE TO ESOPHAGEAL VARICES SEE 'ESOPHAGUS, ESOPHAGEAL VARICES'

0 DUE TO GASTRODUODENITIS SEE 'GASTRITIS'

286.5 DUE TO HYPERHEPARINEMIA

286.5 DUE TO INCREASE IN ANTI-VIIIA

0 DUE TO ULCER SEE 'ULCER'

537.83 DUODENUM DUE TO ANGIODYSPLASIA

562.03 DUODENUM DUE TO DIVERTICULITIS

562.02 DUODENUM DUE TO DIVERTICULOSIS

388.69 EAR

767.1 EPICRANIAL SUBAPONEUROTIC MASSIVE

0 EPIDURAL - NONTRAUMATIC SEE 'HEMORRHAGE', EXTRADURAL

0 EPIDURAL - TRAUMATIC SEE 'HEMORRHAGE', BRAIN TRAUMATIC - EXTRADURAL

530.82 ESOPHAGUS (NONVARICEAL)

530.7 ESOPHAGUS (WEISS SYNDROME)

432.0 EXTRADURAL - NONTRAUMATIC

767.0 EXTRADURAL - FETUS OR NEWBORN DUE TO BIRTH INJURY (INTRAPARTUM HYPOXIA / ANOXIA) (TRAUMATIC)

674.0# EXTRADURAL - MATERNAL DUE TO PREGNANCY

5th Digit: 674.0

0. EPISODE OF CARE NOS OR N/A
1. DELIVERED
2. DELIVERED WITH POSTPARTUM COMPLICATION
3. ANTEPARTUM COMPLICATION
4. POSTPARTUM COMPLICATION

0 EXTRADURAL - TRAUMATIC SEE 'HEMORRHAGE', BRAIN TRAUMATIC - EXTRADURAL

360.43 EYE

364.41 EYE - CILIARY BODY

372.72 EYE - CONJUNCTIVA

362.81 EYE - FUNDUS

360.43 EYE - INTRAOCULAR

364.41 EYE - IRIS (POSTINFECTIONAL) (POSTINFLAMMATORY) (TOXIC)

362.81 EYE - RETINAL (PERIRETINAL) (SUBRETINAL)

376.89 EYE - RETROBULBAR

374.81 EYELID

921.0 EYELID (BLACK EYE NOS)

620.8 FALLOPIAN TUBE

656.0# FETAL-MATERNAL AFFECTING MANAGEMENT OF MOTHER

5th Digit: 656.0

0. EPISODE OF CARE NOS OR N/A
1. DELIVERED
3. ANTEPARTUM COMPLICATION

HEMORRHAGE (continued)

772.0 FETOMATERNAL
772.9 FETUS OR NEWBORN - NOS
772.5 FETUS OR NEWBORN - ADRENAL
767.0 FETUS OR NEWBORN - CEREBRAL OR SUBDURAL DUE TO BIRTH TRAUMA (INTRAPARTUM HYPOXIA / ANOXIA)
772.8 FETUS OR NEWBORN - CONJUNCTIVAL
772.6 FETUS OR NEWBORN - CUTANEOUS
767.1 FETUS OR NEWBORN - EPICRANIAL SUBAPONEUROTIC MASSIVE DUE TO BIRTH TRAUMA
772.0 FETUS OR NEWBORN - EXSANGUINATION
772.1 FETUS OR NEWBORN - INTRAVENTRICULAR
772.2 FETUS OR NEWBORN - SUBARACHNOID
767.0 FETUS OR NEWBORN - SUBDURAL DUE TO BIRTH TRAUMA (INTRAPARTUM HYPOXIA / ANOXIA)
772.3 FETUS OR NEWBORN - UMBILICAL AFTER BIRTH
772.8 FETUS OR NEWBORN - OTHER SPECIFIED
V73.5 FEVER SCREENING EXAM
286.6 FIBRINOLYTIC ACQUIRED
703.8 FINGERNAIL
578.9 GASTRIC (SEE ALSO 'HEMORRHAGE', GASTROINTESTINAL)
578.9 GASTROINTESTINAL UNSPECIFIED
772.4 GASTROINTESTINAL PERINATAL
0 GASTROINTESTINAL WITH ULCER SEE 'ULCER'
599.89 GENITOURINARY
0 GENITOURINARY WITH INCONTINENCE SEE 'URETHRA, URETHRAL DISORDERS WITH INCONTINENCE'
562.03 ILEUM DUE TO DIVERTICULITIS
562.02 ILEUM DUE TO DIVERTICULOSIS
626.6 INTERMENSTRUAL - IRREGULAR
626.5 INTERMENSTRUAL - REGULAR
431 INTERNAL CAPSULE (BRAIN)
578.9 INTESTINE
569.85 INTESTINE DUE TO ANGIODYSPLASIA
562.03 INTESTINE SMALL DUE TO DIVERTICULITIS
562.02 INTESTINE SMALL DUE TO DIVERTICULOSIS
431 INTRACEREBRAL
432.9 INTRACRANIAL NONTRAUMATIC NOS
998.11 INTRAOPERATIVE
431 INTRAPONTINE
431 INTRAVENTRICULAR
772.1 INTRAVENTRICULAR (PERINATAL) FETUS OR NEWBORN
562.03 JEJUNUM DUE TO DIVERTICULITIS
562.02 JEJUNUM DUE TO DIVERTICULOSIS
0 JOINT SEE 'HEMARTHROSIS'
459.0 LEG NEC
573.8 LIVER
786.3 LUNG
770.3 LUNG ALVEOLAR PERINATAL
762.1 MATERNAL AFFECTING FETUS OR NEWBORN

648.9#: USE AN ADDITIONAL CODE TO IDENTIFY THE SPECIFIC HEMORRHAGE

648.9# MATERNAL CURRENT (CO-EXISTENT) IN PREGNANCY
5th Digit: 648.9
0. EPISODE OF NOS OR N/A
1. DELIVERED
2. DELIVERED WITH POSTPARTUM COMPLICATION
3. ANTEPARTUM COMPLICATION
4. POSTPARTUM COMPLICATION

763.89 MATERNAL DUE TO COAGULATION DEFECT AFFECTING FETUS OR NEWBORN
786.3 MEDIASTINUM
431 MEDULLA
430 MENINGEAL
0 MENINGEAL MIDDLE FOLLOWING INJURY SEE 'HEMORRHAGE', BRAIN TRAUMATIC - SUBARACHNOID
0 MENSTRUAL SEE 'BLEEDING' MENSTRUAL
568.81 MESENTERY
431 MIDBRAIN
528.9 MOUTH
728.89 MUSCLE

HEMORRHAGE (continued)

784.7 NASAL
772.9 NEWBORN
776.0 NEWBORN (HEMORRHAGIC DISEASE OF NEWBORN)
0 NEWBORN SEE ALSO 'HEMORRHAGE', FETUS OR NEWBORN
611.79 NIPPLE
568.89 OMENTUM
377.42 OPTIC NERVE SHEATHS
376.32 ORBITAL
620.1 OVARY DUE TO CORPUS LUTEM CYST RUPTURED
577.8 PANCREAS
252.8 PARATHYROID GLAND
607.82 PENIS
423.0 PERICARDIUM
674.3# PERINEAL WOUND OBSTETRICAL SURGERY
5th Digit: 674.3
0. NOS
2. DELIVERED WITH POSTPARTUM COMPLICATION
4. POSTPARTUM COMPLICATION

474.8 PERITONSILLAR TISSUE
998.11 PERITONSILLAR TISSUE POST TONSILLECTOMY
253.8 PITUITARY GLAND
641.9# PLACENTA NOS
641.8# PLACENTA FROM SURGICAL OR INSTRUMENT DAMAGE
5th Digit: 641.8-9
0. EPISODE OF CARE NOS OR N/A
1. DELIVERED
3. ANTEPARTUM COMPLICATION

762.1 PLACENTA AFFECTING FETUS OR NEWBORN
641.1# PLACENTA PREVIA
5th Digit: 641.1
0. EPISODE OF CARE NOS OR N/A
1. DELIVERED
3. ANTEPARTUM COMPLICATION

762.0 PLACENTA PREVIA AFFECTING FETUS OR NEWBORN
511.8 PLEURISY
431 PONS
431 PONTINE
998.11 POSTOPERATIVE
997.02 POSTOPERATIVE BRAIN
666.1# POSTPARTUM ATONIC
666.2# POSTPARTUM SECONDARY OR DELAYED
666.0# POSTPARTUM THIRD STAGE
5th Digit: 666.0-2
0. NOS
2. DELIVERED WITH POSTPARTUM COMPLICATION
4. POSTPARTUM COMPLICATION

V23.4 PREVIOUS PREGNANCY, AFFECTING MANAGEMENT OF CURRENT PREGNANCY
602.1 PROSTATE
786.3 PULMONARY
770.3 PULMONARY PERINATAL
446.21 PULMONARY RENAL SYNDROME
569.3 RECTUM AND ANUS (NOT GI BLEEDING)
593.81 RENAL (ARTERY)
362.81 RETINAL (PERIRETINAL) (DEEP) (SUBRETINAL)
608.83 SCROTUM
562.03 SMALL INTESTINE DUE TO DIVERTICULITIS
562.02 SMALL INTESTINE DUE TO DIVERTICULOSIS
608.83 SPERMATIC CORD
459.0 SPONTANEOUS NEC
782.7 SPONTANEOUS PETECHIAL
431 STEM (BRAIN)
578.9 STOMACH
537.83 STOMACH DUE TO ANGIODYSPLASIA

HEMORRHAGE (continued)

430 SUBARACHNOID
772.2 SUBARACHNOID FETUS OR NEWBORN
674.0# SUBARACHNOID MATERNAL DUE TO PREGNANCY
5th Digit: 674.0
0. EPISODE OF CARE NOS OR N/A
1. DELIVERED
2. DELIVERED WITH POSTPARTUM COMPLICATION
3. ANTEPARTUM COMPLICATION
4. POSTPARTUM COMPLICATION

772.2 SUBARACHNOID PERINATAL (FETUS OR NEWBORN) (ANY CAUSE)
094.87 SUBARACHNOID SYPHILITIC
0 SUBARACHNOID TRAUMATIC SEE 'HEMORRHAGE', BRAIN TRAUMATIC - SUBARACHNOID
372.72 SUBCONJUNCTIVAL
431 SUBCORTICAL
432.1 SUBDURAL
767.0 SUBDURAL FETUS OR NEWBORN DUE TO BIRTH TRAUMA (INTRAPARTUM HYPOXIA / ANOXIA)
674.0# SUBDURAL MATERNAL DUE TO PREGNANCY
5th Digit: 674.0
0. EPISODE OF CARE NOS OR N/A
1. DELIVERED
2. DELIVERED WITH POSTPARTUM COMPLICATION
3. ANTEPARTUM COMPLICATION
4. POSTPARTUM COMPLICATION

0 SUBDURAL TRAUMATIC SEE 'HEMORRHAGE', BRAIN TRAUMATIC - SUBDURAL
608.83 TESTIS
784.8 THROAT
246.3 THYROID
703.8 TOENAIL
519.09 TRACHEOSTOMY STOMA
958.2 TRAUMATIC SECONDARY AND RECURRENT
608.83 TUNICA VAGINALIS
0 ULCER (DUE TO) SEE 'ULCER'
663.8# UMBILICAL CORD COMPLICATING DELIVERY
5th Digit: 663.8
0. EPISODE OF CARE NOS OR N/A
1. DELIVERED
3. ANTEPARTUM COMPLICATION

772.0 UMBILICAL CORD COMPLICATION AFFECTING FETUS OR NEWBORN
772.3 UMBILICAL CORD STUMP
772.3 UMBILICAL FETUS OR NEWBORN AFTER BIRTH
599.84 URETHRAL (NONTRAUMATIC)
626.9 UTERINE (ABNORMAL)
996.76 UTERINE - INTRAUTERINE CONTRACEPTIVE DEVICE
996.32 UTERINE - INTRAUTERINE CONTRACEPTIVE DEVICE PERFORATING UTERUS
608.83 VAS DEFERENS
663.5# VASA PREVIA
5th Digit: 663.5
0. EPISODE OF CARE NOS OR N/A
1. DELIVERED
3. ANTEPARTUM COMPLICATION

772.0 VASA PREVIA AFFECTING FETUS OR NEWBORN
431 VENTRICULAR
379.23 VITREOUS
624.8 VULVA

HEMORRHAGIC

287.9 DIATHESIS (FAMILIAL)
776.0 DIATHESIS OF NEWBORN
287.9 DISEASE NEC
286.9 DISEASE CAUSED BY COAGULATION DEFECTS
776.0 DISEASE OF NEWBORN
287.9 DISORDER NEC
286.5 DISORDER DUE TO CIRCULATING ANTICOAGULANTS
287.8 DISORDER OTHER SPECIFIED
078.6 NEPHROSONEPHRITIS
0 ULCER SEE 'ULCER'

HEMORRHAGIC FEVER

065.9 ARBOVIRUS
078.7 ARENAVIRAL
078.7 ARGENTINE
065.9 ARTHROPOD BORNE
065.8 ARTHROPOD BORNE OTHER SPECIFIED
078.7 BOLIVIAN
065.0 CENTRAL ASIAN
065.4 CHIKUNGUNYA
065.0 CRIMEAN
065.4 DENGUE
065.8 EBOLA
078.6 EPIDEMIC
078.7 JUNIN VIRUS
078.6 KOREAN
078.7 MACHUPOS VIRUS
065.8 MITE BORNE
065.4 MOSQUITO BORNE
065.1 OMSK
065.3 OTHER TICK BORNE
078.6 RUSSIAN
078.6 WITH RENAL SYNDROME

HEMORRHOIDS

UNSPECIFIED

455.6 NOS
455.8 BLEEDING

648.9#: USE AN ADDITIONAL CODE TO IDENTIFY THE SPECIFIC TYPE OF HEMORRHOIDS.

648.9# MATERNAL CURRENT (CO-EXISTENT) IN PREGNANCY
671.8# MATERNAL DUE TO PREGNANCY
5th Digit: 648.9, 671.8
0. EPISODE OF CARE NOS OR N/A
1. DELIVERED
2. DELIVERED WITH POSTPARTUM COMPLICATION
3. ANTEPARTUM COMPLICATION
4. POSTPARTUM COMPLICATION

455.8 PROLAPSED
455.8 STRANGULATED
455.7 THROMBOSED
455.8 ULCERATED
455.6 WITHOUT COMPLICATION

EXTERNAL

455.3 NOS
455.5 BLEEDING
455.5 PROLAPSED
455.5 STRANGULATED
455.4 THROMBOSED
455.5 ULCERATED
455.3 WITHOUT COMPLICATION

INTERNAL

455.0 NOS
455.2 BLEEDING
455.2 PROLAPSED
455.2 STRANGULATED
455.1 THROMBOSED
455.2 ULCERATED
455.0 WITHOUT COMPLICATION

371.11 HEMOSIDERIN DEPOSITS OF CORNEAL SCAR
275.0 HEMOSIDEROSIS
<u>275.0</u> <u>HEMOSIDEROSIS</u> IDIOPATHIC PULMONARY [516.1]
608.83 HEMOSPERMIA
286.9 HEMOSTASIS DISORDER

HEMOTHORAX

511.1 PNEUMOCOCCAL
511.8 NONTRAUMATIC
<u>998.11</u> <u>POSTOPERATIVE</u> COMPLICATING A PROCEDURE [511.8]
511.1 STAPHYLOCOCCAL
511.1 STREPTOCOCCAL

HEMOTHORAX (continued)
860.2 TRAUMATIC
860.3 TRAUMATIC WITH OPEN WOUND INTO THORAX
908.0 TRAUMATIC LATE EFFECT
012.0# TUBERCULOUS PLEURITIC
5th Digit: 012.0
0. NOS
1. LAB NOT DONE
2. LABS PENDING
3. MICROSCOPY POSITIVE (IN SPUTUM)
4. CULTURE POSITIVE - MICROSCOPY NEGATIVE
5. CULTURE NEGATIVE - MICROSCOPY POSITIVE
6. CULTURE AND MICROSCOPY NEGATIVE CONFIRMED BY OTHER METHODS
511.1 OTHER BACTERIAL

385.89 HEMOTYMPANUM
304.3# HEMP ADDICTION (DEPENDENT)
5th Digit: 304.3
0. NOS
1. CONTINUOUS
2. EPISODIC
3. IN REMISSION
719.3# HENCH ROSENBERG SYNDROME (PALINDROMIC ARTHRITIS)
5th Digit: 719.3
0. SITE NOS
1. SHOULDER REGION
2. UPPER ARM (ELBOW) (HUMERUS)
3. FOREARM (RADIUS) (WRIST) (ULNA)
4. HAND (CARPAL) (METACARPAL) (FINGERS)
5. PELVIC REGION AND THIGH (HIP) (BUTTOCK) (FEMUR)
6. LOWER LEG (FIBULA) (KNEE) (PATELLA) (TIBIA)
7. ANKLE AND/OR FOOT (METATARSALS) (TOES) (TARSALS)
8. OTHER
9. MULTIPLE
371.41 HENLE'S WARTS
287.0 HENOCH GLOSSITIS
287.0 HENOCH-SCHONLEIN (SYNDROME) (ALLERGIC PURPURA)
102.6 HENPUE

HEPATIC
442.84 ARTERY (ANEURYSM) (A-V FISTULA) (CIRSOID) (FALSE) (VARICOSE) (RUPTURED)
902.22 ARTERY INJURY
908.4 ARTERY INJURY LATE EFFECT
902.22 ARTERY LACERATION (RUPTURE) (HEMATOMA) (AVULSION) (ANEURYSM) TRAUMATIC
908.4 ARTERY LACERATION LATE EFFECT
572.2 COMA
751.69 DUCT ACCESSORY CONGENITAL
576.2 DUCT OBSTRUCTION (SEE ALSO 'BILE DUCT', OBSTRUCTION)
751.61 DUCT OBSTRUCTION CONGENITAL
572.2 ENCEPHALOPATHY
570 FAILURE
570 FAILURE ACUTE (NONINFECTIVE) (ACQUIRED)
997.4 FAILURE SPECIFIED AS DUE TO A PROCEDURE
569.89 FLEXURE SYNDROME
573.8 INSUFFICIENCY
573.8 OBSTRUCTION
902.11 VEIN INJURY
908.4 VEIN INJURY LATE EFFECT
902.11 VEIN LACERATION (RUPTURE) (HEMATOMA) (AVULSION) (ANEURYSM) TRAUMATIC
908.4 VEIN LACERATION LATE EFFECT
453.0 VEIN THROMBOSIS

HEPATITIS INFECTIOUS OR VIRAL
V02.60 CARRIER (SUSPECTED) NOS
V02.61 CARRIER (SUSPECTED) VIRAL B (HAA) (SERUM)
V02.62 CARRIER (SUSPECTED) VIRAL C
V02.69 CARRIER (SUSPECTED) VIRAL OTHER
V01.7 EXPOSURE
795.79 FALSE POSITIVE SEROLOGICAL TEST
V12.09 HISTORY
070.1 INFECTIOUS
070.3# SERUM (AUSTRALIAN ANTIGEN)
070.2# SERUM (AUSTRALIAN ANTIGEN) WITH HEPATIC COMA
5th Digit: 070.2-3
0. ACUTE OR UNSPECIFIED
1. ACUTE OR UNSPECIFIED WITH DELTA
2. CHRONIC
3. CHRONIC WITH DELTA
V02.61 SERUM (AUSTRALIAN ANTIGEN) CARRIER
V05.3 VACCINATION AND INOCULATION (PROPHYLACTIC)
070.9 VIRAL
070.6 VIRAL WITH HEPATIC COMA
070.1 VIRAL A (INFECTIOUS)
070.0 VIRAL A (INFECTIOUS) WITH HEPATIC COMA
070.3# VIRAL B (AUSTRALIAN ANTIGEN)
070.2# VIRAL B (AUSTRALIAN ANTIGEN) WITH HEPATIC COMA
5th Digit: 070.2-3
0. ACUTE OR UNSPECIFIED
1. ACUTE OR UNSPECIFIED WITH DELTA
2. CHRONIC
3. CHRONIC WITH DELTA
V02.61 VIRAL B CARRIER
V02.62 VIRAL C CARRIER
070.5# VIRAL C (D) (E) OR OTHER
070.4# VIRAL C (D) (E) OR OTHER WITH HEPATIC COMA
5th Digit: 070.4-5
1. ACUTE OR UNSPECIFIED C
2. DELTA, OR DELTA WITH B CARRIER STATE
3. HEPATITIS E
4. CHRONIC C
9. OTHER SPECIFIED VIRAL
760.8 VIRAL MATERNAL AFFECTING FETUS OR NEWBORN

647.6#: USE AN ADDITIONAL CODE TO IDENTIFY THE SPECIFIC VIRAL HEPATITIS.

647.6# VIRAL MATERNAL CURRENT (CO-EXISTENT) IN PREGNANCY
5th Digit: 647.6
0. EPISODE OF CARE UNSPECIFIED OR N/A
1. DELIVERED
2. DELIVERED WITH POSTPARTUM COMPLICATION
3. ANTEPARTUM COMPLICATION
4. POSTPARTUM COMPLICATION

HEPATITIS NON-INFECTIOUS
573.3 NOS
571.1 ACUTE ALCOHOLIC
571.1 ACUTE ALCOHOLIC WITH ESOPHAGEAL VARICES [**456.2#**]
5th Digit: 456.2
0. WITH BLEEDING
1. WITHOUT BLEEDING
570 ACUTE NON INFECTIVE
571.1 ALCOHOLIC
571.1 ALCOHOLIC WITH ESOPHAGEAL VARICES [**456.2#**]
5th Digit: 456.2
0. WITH BLEEDING
1. WITHOUT BLEEDING
573.3 CHEMICAL
573.8 CHOLANGIOLITIC
573.8 CHOLESTATIC

H

HEPATITIS NON-INFECTIOUS (continued)

571.40 CHRONIC
571.40 CHRONIC WITH ESOPHAGEAL VARICES [456.2#]
5th Digit: 456.2
0. WITH BLEEDING
1. WITHOUT BLEEDING

571.49 CHRONIC ACTIVE
571.49 CHRONIC ACTIVE WITH ESOPHAGEAL VARICES [456.2#]
5th Digit: 456.2
0. WITH BLEEDING
1. WITHOUT BLEEDING

571.41 CHRONIC PERSISTENT
571.41 CHRONIC PERSISTENT WITH ESOPHAGEAL VARICES [456.2#]
5th Digit: 456.2
0. WITH BLEEDING
1. WITHOUT BLEEDING

771.2 CONGENITAL (ACTIVE)
573.3 DIFFUSE
573.3 DRUG INDUCED
795.79 FALSE POSITIVE SEROLOGICAL TEST
774.4 GIANT CELL (NEONATAL)
573.8 HEMORRHAGIC
571.49 HYPERTROPHIC CHRONIC
571.49 HYPERTROPHIC CHRONIC WITH ESOPHAGEAL VARICES [456.2#]
5th Digit: 456.2
0. WITH BLEEDING
1. WITHOUT BLEEDING

571.49 INTERSTITIAL CHRONIC
571.49 INTERSTITIAL CHRONIC WITH ESOPHAGEAL VARICES [456.2#]
5th Digit: 456.2
0. WITH BLEEDING
1. WITHOUT BLEEDING

710.0 LUPOID [571.49]
571.49 LUPOID LUNG HEPATIZATION CHRONIC
571.49 LUPOID LUNG HEPATIZATION CHRONIC WITH ESOPHAGEAL VARICES [456.2#]
5th Digit: 456.2
0. WITH BLEEDING
1. WITHOUT BLEEDING

760.8 MATERNAL AFFECTING NEWBORN OR FETUS
646.7# MATERNAL COMPLICATING PREGNANCY
5th Digit: 646.7
0. EPISODE OF CARE NOS OR N/A
1. DELIVERED
3. ANTEPARTUM COMPLICATION

HEPATITIS (OTHER TYPES)

573.3 NOS
277.3 AMYLOID
074.8 COXSACKIE VIRUS DISEASE (DUE TO) [573.1]
078.5 CMV [573.1]
078.5 CYTOMEGALOVIRAL DISEASE (DUE TO) [573.1]
795.79 FALSE POSITIVE SEROLOGICAL TEST
774.4 FETUS OR NEWBORN
571.49 FIBROUS (CHRONIC)
0 FULMINANT SEE 'HEPATITIS INFECTIOUS OR VIRAL'
084.9 MALARIAL [573.2]
075 MONONUCLEOSIS [573.1]
072.71 MUMPS
573.3 NONINFECTIOUS
573.3 PELIOSIS
571.49 PLASMA CELL
571.49 PLASMA CELL WITH ESOPHAGEAL VARICES [456.2#]
5th Digit: 456.2
0. WITH BLEEDING
1. WITHOUT BLEEDING

HEPATITIS (OTHER TYPES) (continued)

997.4 POSTOPERATIVE ACUTE
571.49 RECURRENT
571.49 RECURRENT WITH ESOPHAGEAL VARICES [456.2#]
5th Digit: 456.2
0. WITH BLEEDING
1. WITHOUT BLEEDING

572.0 SUPPURATIVE
091.62 SYPHILIS SECONDARY
095.3 SYPHILITIC LATE
130.5 TOXOPLASMOSIS
017.9# TUBERCULOSIS
5th Digit: 017.9
0. NOS
1. LAB NOT DONE
2. LABS PENDING
3. MICROSCOPY POSITIVE (IN SPUTUM)
4. CULTURE POSITIVE - MICROSCOPY NEGATIVE
5. CULTURE NEGATIVE - MICROSCOPY POSITIVE
6. CULTURE AND MICROSCOPY NEGATIVE CONFIRMED BY OTHER METHODS

155.0 HEPATOBLASTOMA SITE NOS
0 HEPATOBLASTOMA SITE SPECIFIED SEE 'CANCER' BY SITE M8970/3

HEPATOCELLULAR

155.0 CARCINOMA SITE NOS
0 CARCINOMA SITE SPECIFIED SEE 'CANCER' BY SITE M8170/3
155.0 CHOLANGIOCARCINOMA COMBINED SITE NOS
0 CHOLANGIOCARCINOMA COMBINED SITE SPECIFIED SEE 'CANCER' BY SITE M8180/3

572.2 HEPATOCEREBRAL INTOXICATION

211.5 HEPATOCHOLANGIOMA BENIGN SITE NOS
0 HEPATOCHOLANGIOMA BENIGN SITE SPECIFIED SEE 'BENIGN NEOPLASM', BY SITE M8180/0
573.8 HEPATOCHOLANGITIS

575.1# HEPATOCYSTITIS (SEE ALSO 'CHOLECYSTITIS')
5th Digit: 575.1
0. NOS
1. CHRONIC
2. ACUTE AND CHRONIC

570 HEPATODYSTROPHY
275.1 HEPATOLENTICULAR DEGENERATION
275.1 HEPATOLENTICULAR DEGENERATION WITH DEMENTIA [294.1]
0 HEPATOLITHIASIS SEE 'CHOLEDOCHOLITHIASIS'

HEPATOMA

211.5 BENIGN M8170/0
155.0 CONGENITAL M8970/3
155.0 EMBRYONAL M8970/3
155.0 MALIGNANT M8170/3

271.0 HEPATOMEGALIA GLYCOGENIA DIFFUSA
789.1 HEPATOMEGALY
751.69 HEPATOMEGALY CONGENITAL

573.8 HEPATOPTOSIS
572.4 HEPATORENAL SYNDROME
674.8# HEPATORENAL SYNDROME MATERNAL DUE TO PREGNANCY
5th Digit: 674.8
0. NOS
2. DELIVERED WITH POSTPARTUM COMPLICATION
4. POSTPARTUM COMPLICATION

997.4 HEPATORENAL SYNDROME SPECIFIED AS DUE TO A PROCEDURE [572.4]

573.8 HEPATORRHEXIS

571.8 HEPATOSPLENOMEGALY
571.8 HEPATOSPLENOMEGALY WITH ESOPHAGEAL VARICES [456.2#]
5th Digit: 456.2
0. WITH BLEEDING
1. WITHOUT BLEEDING

572.4 HEPATOUROLOGIC SYNDROME

HEREDITARY
363.55 CHOROIDEREMIA
277.1 COPROPORPHYRIA
448.0 HEMORRHAGIC TELANGIECTASIA
282.4 LEPTOCYTOSIS
356.0 PERIPHERAL NEUROPATHY
356.2 SENSORY NEUROPATHY
334.1 SPASTIC PARAPLEGIA
282.0 SPHEROCYTOSIS WITH ANEMIA
757.0 TROPHEDEMA CONGENITAL

330.9 HEREDODEGENERATION
331.89 HEREDODEGENERATIVE DISEASE NEC - BRAIN
336.8 HEREDODEGENERATIVE DISEASE NEC - SPINAL CORD
356.3 HEREDOPATHIA ATACTICA POLYNEURITIFORMIS
752.7 HERMAPHRODITISM CONGENITAL

HERNIA
553.9 NOS
551.9 GANGRENOUS NOS (OBSTRUCTED)
552.9 INCARCERATED NOS (OBSTRUCTED) (STRANGULATED) (IRREDUCIBLE)

ABDOMINAL (WALL)
553.20 NOS
551.20 GANGRENOUS (OBSTRUCTED)
552.20 INCARCERATED (OBSTRUCTED) (STRANGULATED) (IRREDUCIBLE)
553.21 RECURRENT
551.21 RECURRENT GANGRENOUS (OBSTRUCTED)
552.21 RECURRENT INCARCERATED (OBSTRUCTED) (STRANGULATED) (IRREDUCIBLE)

BLADDER
756.71 CONGENITAL (FEMALE) (MALE)
618.0 FEMALE
618.0 FEMALE WITH STRESS INCONTINENCE [625.6]
618.0 FEMALE WITH OTHER URINARY INCONTINENCE [788.3#]
5th Digit: 788.3
0. UNSPECIFIED
1. URGE INCONTINENCE
3. MIXED URGE AND STRESS (MALE) (FEMALE)
4 WITHOUT SENSORY AWARENESS
5. POST-VOID DRIBBLING
6. NOCTURNAL ENURESIS
7. CONTINUOUS LEAKAGE
9. OTHER
596.8 MALE

HERNIA (continued)
569.69 CECOSTOMY
569.69 COLOSTOMY

DIAPHRAGMATIC
553.3 NOS
756.6 CONGENITAL
551.3 GANGRENOUS (OBSTRUCTED)
552.3 INCARCERATED (OBSTRUCTED) (STRANGULATED) (IRREDUCIBLE)
0 TRAUMATIC SEE 'DIAPHRAGM', INJURY

HERNIA (continued)
0 DISC (INTERVERTEBRAL) SEE 'HERNIATED DISC'
569.69 ENTEROSTOMY

HERNIA (continued)

EPIGASTRIC
553.29 NOS
551.29 GANGRENOUS (OBSTRUCTED)
552.29 INCARCERATED (OBSTRUCTED) (STRANGULATED) (IRREDUCIBLE)

ESOPHAGEAL
553.3 NOS
750.6 CONGENITAL
551.3 GANGRENOUS (OBSTRUCTED)
552.3 INCARCERATED (OBSTRUCTED) (STRANGULATED) (IRREDUCIBLE)

FEMORAL
553.0# NOS
551.0# GANGRENOUS (OBSTRUCTED)
552.0# INCARCERATED (OBSTRUCTED) (STRANGULATED) (IRREDUCIBLE)
5th Digit: 551.0, 552.0, 553.0
0. UNILATERAL NOS
1. UNILATERAL OR NOS RECURRENT
2. BILATERAL NOS
3. BILATERAL RECURRENT

HIATAL
553.3 NOS
750.6 CONGENITAL
551.3 GANGRENOUS (OBSTRUCTED)
552.3 INCARCERATED (OBSTRUCTED) (STRANGULATED) (IRREDUCIBLE)

HERNIA (continued)
569.69 ILEOSTOMY

INCISIONAL
553.21 NOS
551.21 GANGRENOUS (OBSTRUCTED)
552.21 INCARCERATED (OBSTRUCTED) (STRANGULATED) (IRREDUCIBLE)
553.21 RECURRENT

INGUINAL
550.9# NOS
550.0# GANGRENOUS (OBSTRUCTED)
550.1# INCARCERATED
5th Digit: 550.0-1, 9
0. UNILATERAL NOS
1. UNILATERAL OR NOS RECURRENT
2. BILATERAL NOS
3. BILATERAL RECURRENT

ISCHIATIC
553.8 NOS
551.8 GANGRENOUS (OBSTRUCTED)
552.8 INCARCERATED (OBSTRUCTED) (STRANGULATED) (IRREDUCIBLE)

ISCHIORECTAL
553.8 NOS
551.8 GANGRENOUS (OBSTRUCTED)
552.8 INCARCERATED

HERNIA (continued)
569.69 JEJUNOSTOMY

LUMBAR
553.8 NOS
551.8 GANGRENOUS (OBSTRUCTED)
552.8 INCARCERATED (OBSTRUCTED) (STRANGULATED) (IRREDUCIBLE)

LUNG
518.89 NOS
748.69 CONGENITAL

OBTURATOR
553.8 NOS
551.8 GANGRENOUS (OBSTRUCTED)
552.8 INCARCERATED (OBSTRUCTED) (STRANGULATED) (IRREDUCIBLE)

HERNIA (continued)

PARUMBILICAL

553.1 NOS
551.1 GANGRENOUS (OBSTRUCTED)
552.1 INCARCERATED (OBSTRUCTED) (STRANGULATED) (IRREDUCIBLE)

PUDENDAL

553.8 NOS
551.8 GANGRENOUS (OBSTRUCTED)
552.8 INCARCERATED (OBSTRUCTED) (STRANGULATED) (IRREDUCIBLE)

RETROPERITONEAL

553.8 NOS
551.8 GANGRENOUS (OBSTRUCTED)
552.8 INCARCERATED (OBSTRUCTED) (STRANGULATED) (IRREDUCIBLE)

SCIATIC

553.8 NOS
551.8 GANGRENOUS (OBSTRUCTED)
552.8 INCARCERATED (OBSTRUCTED) (STRANGULATED) (IRREDUCIBLE)

SCROTAL

550.9# NOS
550.0# GANGRENOUS (OBSTRUCTED)
550.1# INCARCERATED (OBSTRUCTED) (STRANGULATED) (IRREDUCIBLE)

5th Digit: 550.0-1, 9

0. UNILATERAL NOS
1. UNILATERAL OR NOS RECURRENT
2. BILATERAL NOS
3. BILATERAL RECURRENT

SPIGELIAN

553.29 NOS
551.29 GANGRENOUS (OBSTRUCTED)
552.29 INCARCERATED (OBSTRUCTED) (STRANGULATED) (IRREDUCIBLE)

UMBILICAL

553.1 NOS
551.1 GANGRENOUS (OBSTRUCTED)
552.1 INCARCERATED (OBSTRUCTED) (STRANGULATED) (IRREDUCIBLE)

VENTRAL

553.20 NOS
551.20 GANGRENOUS (OBSTRUCTED)
552.20 INCARCERATED (OBSTRUCTED) (STRANGULATED) (IRREDUCIBLE)
553.21 RECURRENT
551.21 RECURRENT GANGRENOUS (OBSTRUCTED)
552.21 RECURRENT INCARCERATED (OBSTRUCTED) (STRANGULATED) (IRREDUCIBLE)

OTHER TYPES

756.6 FORAMEN OF MORGAGNI CONGENITAL
519.3 MEDIASTINUM

OTHER SPECIFIED SITES

553.8 NOS
551.8 GANGRENOUS (OBSTRUCTED)
552.8 INCARCERATED (OBSTRUCTED) (STRANGULATED) (IRREDUCIBLE)

WHEN CODING BACK DISORDERS DUE TO DEGENERATION, DISPLACEMENT OR HNP OF THE INTERVERTEBRAL DISC, IT IS IMPORTANT TO DISTINGUISH WHETHER THESE CONDITIONS ARE WITH OR WITHOUT MYELOPATHY. MYELOPATHY REFERS TO FUNCTIONAL DISTURBANCES AND/OR PATHOLOGICAL CHANGES IN THE SPINAL CORD THAT RESULT FROM COMPRESSION.

HERNIATED DISC (HNP)

722.2 SITE UNSPECIFIED
722.70 SITE UNSPECIFIED WITH MYELOPATHY
722.0 CERVICAL
722.71 CERVICAL WITH MYELOPATHY
722.10 LUMBAR
722.73 LUMBAR WITH MYELOPATHY
722.11 THORACIC
722.72 THORACIC WITH MYELOPATHY

304.0# HEROIN ADDICTION

5th Digit: 304.0

0. NOS
1. CONTINOUS
2. EPISODIC
3. IN REMISSION

074.0 HERPANGINA

HERPES

110.5 CIRCINATUS
694.5 CIRCINATUS BULLOSUS
771.2 CONGENITAL OR PERINATAL
054.0 ECZEMA HERPETICUM
V01.7 EXPOSURE
054.6 FELON
054.10 GENITAL NOS
646.8# GESTATIONIS

5th Digit: 646.8

0. EPISODE OF CARE NOS OR N/A
1. DELIVERED
2. DELIVERED WITH POSTPARTUM COMPLICATION
3. ANTEPARTUM COMPLICATION
4. POSTPARTUM COMPLICATION

054.2 GINGIVOSTOMATITIS
695.1 IRIS
054.43 KERATOCONJUNCTIVITIS SIMPLEX
054.3 MENINGOENCEPHALITIS
054.13 PENILE INFECTION
054.10 PROGENITALIS
054.2 STOMATITIS
054.12 VULVAL ULCERATION
054.11 VULVOVAGINITIS
054.6 WHITLOW
054.19 OTHER GENITAL HERPES INFECTION (SCROTUM)
054.49 OTHER OPHTHALMIC COMPLICATION
054.8 OTHER SPECIFIED COMPLICATION

HERPES SIMPLEX

054.9 NOS
054.8 WITH COMPLICATION NOS
054.19 ANUS
771.2 CONGENITAL OR PERINATAL
054.43 CONJUNCTIVITIS
054.43 CORNEA
054.43 CORNEA DISCIFORM
054.41 DERMATITIS OF EYELID
054.0 ECZEMA HERPETICUM
054.3 ENCEPHALITIS
054.6 FELON
0 GENITAL SEE 'HERPES'
054.2 GINGIVOSTOMATITIS
054.44 IRIDOCYCLITIS
054.42 KERATITIS DENDRITIC
054.43 KERATITIS DISCIFORM
054.9 LIP

HERPES SIMPLEX (continued)
054.72 MENINGITIS
054.3 MENINGOENCEPHALITIS
054.40 OPHTHALMIC COMPLICATION
054.73 OTITIS EXTERNA
054.5 SEPSIS
054.71 VISCERAL
054.6 WHITLOW
054.79 OTHER COMPLICATION
054.49 OTHER OPHTHALMIC COMPLICATION

HERPES ZOSTER
053.9 NOS
053.8 WITH COMPLICATION NOS
053.21 CONJUNCTIVITIS
053.21 CORNEA
053.20 DERMATITIS EYELID
053.11 GENICULATE
053.11 GENICULATE GANGLIONITIS
053.22 IRIDOCYCLITIS
053.21 KERATOCONJUNCTIVITIS
053.0 MENINGITIS
053.10 NERVOUS SYSTEM COMPLICATION UNSPECIFIED
053.20 OPHTHALMICUS
053.71 OTITIS EXTERNA
053.13 POLYNEUROPATHY POST HERPETIC
053.12 TRIGEMINAL NEURALGIA POSTHERPETIC
053.19 OTHER NERVOUS SYSTEM COMPLICATION
053.29 OTHER OPHTHALMIC COMPLICATION
053.79 OTHER SPECIFIED COMPLICATION

053.11 HERPETIC GENICULATE GANGLIONITIS

HERPETIC KERATITIS
090.3 CONGENITAL SYPHILIS INTERSTITIAL
054.42 DENDRITIC HERPES SIMPLEX
054.43 DISCIFORM HERPES SIMPLEX
053.21 HERPES ZOSTER

282.61 HERRICK'S ANEMIA SYNDROME
271.0 HERS' DISEASE (GLYCOGENOSIS VI)
579.0 HERTER (-GEE) DISEASE OR SYNDROME (NONTROPICAL SPRUE)
579.0 HERTER'S INFANTILISM
701.8 HERXHEIMER'S DISEASE (DIFFUSE IDIOPATHIC CUTANEOUS ATROPHY)
995.0 HERXHEIMER'S REACTION
909.9 HERXHEIMER'S REACTION LATE EFFECT
364.53 HETEROCHROMIA IRIS (ACQUIRED)

HETEROPHORIA
378.40 NOS
378.45 ALTERNATING HYPERPHORIA
378.44 CYCLOPHORIA
378.41 ESOPHORIA
378.42 EXOPHORIA
378.43 VERTICAL

121.6 HETEROPHYIASIS INFECTION
368.8 HETEROPSIA
742.4 HETEROTOPIA CEREBRALIS
742.59 HETEROTOPIA SPINALIS
728.13 HETEROTOPIC CALCIFICATION POSTOPERATIVE

HETEROTROPIA
378.2# INTERMITTENT
5th Digit: 378.2
0. NOS
1. ESOTROPIC INTERMITTENT MONOCULAR
2. ESOTROPIC INTERMITTENT ALTERNATING
3. EXOTROPIC INTERMITTENT MONOCULAR
4. EXOTROPIC INTERMITTENT ALTERNATING

378.3# OTHER OR UNSPECIFIED
5th Digit: 378.3
0. NOS
1. VERTICAL
2. HYPOTROPIC
3. CYCLOTROPIC
4. MICROTROPIC (MONOFIXATION)
5. ACCOMMODATIVE ESOTROPIC

579.0 HEUBNER HERTER DISEASE OR SYNDROME (NONTROPICAL SPRUE)
094.89 HEUBNER'S DISEASE
755.00 HEXADACTYLISM
572.4 HEYD'S SYNDROME (HEPATORENAL)
759.81 HHHO SYNDROME
0 HIATAL HERNIA SEE 'HERNIA', HIATAL
V03.81 HIB VACCINATION
214.# HIBERNOMA M8880/0
4th Digit: 214
0. FACE SKIN AND SUBCUTANEOUS TISSUE
1. SKIN AND SUBCUTANEOUS TISSUE OTHER
2. INTRATHORACIC ORGANS
3. INTRA ABDOMINAL ORGANS
4. SPERMATIC CORD
8. OTHER SPECIFIED SITES
9. UNSPECIFIED SITE

786.8 HICCOUGH
306.1 HICCOUGH PSYCHOGENIC
644.1# HICKS (BRAXTON) CONTRACTIONS
5th Digit: 644.1
0. EPISODE OF CARE NOS OR N/A
3. ANTEPARTUM COMPLICATION

752.65 HIDDEN PENIS CONGENITAL
705.83 HIDRADENITIS
705.83 HIDRADENITIS SUPPURATIVA
0 HIDROCYSTOMA SEE 'BENIGN NEOPLASM', SKIN BY SITE M8404/0
786.8 HIGH COMPLIANCE BLADDER
282.4 HIGH FETAL GENE DISEASE

HIGH HEAD
652.5# AT TERM
660.0# AT TERM OBSTRUCTING LABOR **[652.5#]**
652.6# AT TERM WITH MULTIPLE GESTATION
660.0# AT TERM WITH MULTIPLE GESTATION OBSTRUCTING LABOR **[652.6#]**
5th Digit: 652.5-6, 660.0
0. EPISODE OF CARE NOS OR N/A
1. DELIVERED
3. ANTEPARTUM COMPLICATION

ANTIBIOTICS, COUMADIN, DIGOXIN, CHEMOTHERAPY DRUGS, AND ANY OTHER DRUGS WITH A RISK OF ADVERSE REACTIONS ARE CONSIDERED TO BE HIGH-RISK MEDICATIONS. CODES V58.61, V58.62 AND V58.69 ARE TO BE USED TO IDENTIFY PATIENTS THAT ARE CURRENTLY BEING MONITORED WHILE TAKING HIGH RISK MEDICATION. CODE V67.51 IS TO BE USED TO IDENTIFY PATIENTS THAT HAVE COMPLETED HIGH RISK MEDICATION THERAPY.

V67.51 HIGH RISK MEDICATION FOLLOWUP - COMPLETED THERAPY
V58.62 HIGH RISK MEDICATION MANAGEMENT - ANTIBIOTICS CURRENT THERAPY
V58.61 HIGH RISK MEDICATION MANAGEMENT - ANTICOAGULANT CURRENT THERAPY
V58.69 HIGH RISK MEDICATION MANAGEMENT - OTHER CURRENT THERAPY
0 HIGH RISK PREGNANCY SUPERVISION SEE 'PREGNANCY SUPERVISION', HIGH RISK
220 HILAR CELL TUMOR SITE NOS
0 HILAR CELL TUMOR SITE SPECIFIED SEE 'BENIGN NEOPLASM', BY SITE M8660/0
081.9 HILDENBRAND'S DISEASE (TYPHUS)
337.0 HILGER'S SYNDROME
579.1 HILL DIARRHEA
017.0# HILLIARD'S LUPUS

5th Digit: 017.0

- **0. NOS**
- **1. LAB NOT DONE**
- **2. LABS PENDING**
- **3. MICROSCOPY POSITIVE (IN SPUTUM)**
- **4. CULTURE POSITIVE - MICROSCOPY NEGATIVE**
- **5. CULTURE NEGATIVE - MICROSCOPY POSITIVE**
- **6. CULTURE AND MICROSCOPY NEGATIVE CONFIRMED BY OTHER ETHODS**

744.29 HILLOCK EAR CONGENITAL

HIP

V49.77 AMPUTATION STATUS
736.30 DEFORMITY - ACQUIRED
736.39 DEFORMITY - ACQUIRED OTHER NEC
755.63 DEFORMITY - CONGENITAL OTHER (SEE ALSO 'HIP', JOINT DISORDER CONGENITAL)
754.32 FLEXION DEFORMITY CONGENITAL
959.6 INJURY
916.8 INJURY OTHER AND NOS SUPERFICIAL
916.9 INJURY OTHER AND NOS SUPERFICIAL INFECTED
719.85 JOINT CALCIFICATION
0 JOINT DISORDER SEE ALSO 'JOINT'
719.95 JOINT DISORDER
755.63 JOINT DISORDER - CONGENITAL
754.3# JOINT DISORDER - CONGENITAL DISLOCATION OR SUBLUXATION

5th Digit: 754.3

- **0. DISLOCATION UNILATERAL OR UNSPECIFIED**
- **1. DISLOCATION BILATERAL**
- **2. SUBLUXATION UNILATERAL**
- **3. SUBLUXATION BILATERAL**
- **5. DISLOCATION ONE HIP, SUBLUXATION OTHER HIP**

V82.3 JOINT DISORDER - CONGENITAL DISLOCATION OR SUBLUXATION SCREENING
711.05 JOINT DISORDER - SUPPURATIVE (PYOGENIC)
015.1# JOINT DISORDER - TUBERCULOUS [730.85]

5th Digit: 015.1

- **0. NOS**
- **1. LAB NOT DONE**
- **2. LABS PENDING**
- **3. MICROSCOPY POSITIVE (IN SPUTUM)**
- **4. CULTURE POSITIVE - MICROSCOPY NEGATIVE**
- **5. CULTURE NEGATIVE - MICROSCOPY POSITIVE**
- **6. CULTURE AND MICROSCOPY NEGATIVE CONFIRMED BY OTHER METHODS**

HIP (continued)

718.85 JOINT INSTABILITY (OLD)
718.15 JOINT LOOSE BODY
718.95 JOINT LIGAMENT RELAXATION
0 JOINT LIGAMENT TEAR SEE 'SPRAIN'
0 JOINT SEE ALSO 'JOINT'
754.32 PREDISLOCATION STATUS AT BIRTH
754.32 PRELUXATION CONGENITAL
739.5 REGION SEGMENTAL OR SOMATIC DYSFUNCTION
V43.64 REPLACEMENT STATUS
V82.3 SCREENING FOR CONGENITAL DISLOCATION OR SUBLUXATION
843.9 SEPARATION (RUPTURE) (TEAR) (LACERATION) SITE NOS
843.8 SEPARATION (RUPTURE) (TEAR) (LACERATION) OTHER SPECIFIED SITES
843.9 STRAIN (SPRAIN) (AVULSION) (HEMARTHROSIS) SITE NOS
843.8 STRAIN (SPRAIN) (AVULSION) (HEMARTHROSIS) OTHER SPECIFIED SITES

759.6 HIPPEL'S DISEASE (RETINOCEREBRAL ANGIOMATOSIS)
379.49 HIPPUS DYSFUNCTION (PUPIL)
250.0# HIRSCHFELD'S (ACUTE DIABETES MELLITUS)

5th Digit: 250.0

- **0. TYPE II, ADULT-ONSET, NON-INSULIN DEPENDENT (EVEN IF REQUIRING INSULIN), OR UNSPECIFIED; CONTROLLED**
- **1. TYPE I, JUVENILE-ONSET OR INSULIN-DEPENDENT; CONTROLLED**
- **2. TYPE II, ADULT-ONSET, NON-INSULIN DEPENDENT (EVEN IF REQUIRING INSULIN); UNCONTROLLED**
- **3. TYPE I, JUVENILE-ONSET OR INSULIN-DEPENDENT; UNCONTROLLED**

751.3 HIRSCHSPRUNG'S DISEASE (CONGENITAL MEGACOLON)
704.1 HIRSUTISM
134.2 HIRUDINIASIS
134.2 HIRUDINIASIS EXTERNAL INTERNAL
083.1 HIS-WERNER DISEASE (TRENCH FEVER)
004.1 HISS RUSSELL DYSENTERY
270.5 HISTIDINE METABOLISM DISTURBANCES
270.5 HISTIDINEMIA
270.5 HISTIDINURIA

HISTIOCYTIC

202.3# MEDULLARY RETICULOSIS M9721/3

5th Digit: 202.3

- **0. NOS**
- **1. LYMPH NODES OF HEAD FACE NECK**
- **2. LYMPH NODES INTRATHORACIC**
- **3. LYMPH NODES ABDOMINAL**
- **4. LYMPH NODES AXILLA AND UPPER LIMB**
- **5. LYMPH NODES INGUINAL REGION AND LOWER LIMB**
- **6. LYMPH NODES INTRAPELVIC**
- **7. SPLEEN**
- **8. LYMPH NODES MULTIPLE SITES**

HISTIOCYTOMA

216.# FIBROUS ATYPICAL M8830/1

4th Digit: 216

0. LIP (SKIN OF)
1. EYELID INCLUDING CANTHUS
2. EAR (EXTERNAL) (AURICLE) (PINNA)
3. FACE (CHEEK) (NOSE) (TEMPLE) (EYEBROW)
4. SCALP NECK
5. TRUNK BACK EXCEPT SCROTUM
6. UPPER LIMB INCLUDING SHOULDER
7. LOWER LIMB INCLUDING HIP
8. OTHER SPECIFIED SITES
9. SKIN NOS

171.# FIBROUS MALIGNANT M8830/3

4th Digit: 171

0. HEAD FACE NECK
2. UPPER LIMB SHOULDER
3. LOWER LIMB HIP
4. THORAX
5. ABDOMINAL HYPOCHONDRIUM
6. PELVIS BUTTOCK GROIN INGUINAL REGION PERINEUM
7. TRUNK NOS BACK NOS FLANK NOS
8. OTHER SPECIFIED SITES
9. SITE NOS

HISTIOCYTOSIS

277.8 ACUTE CHRONIC
202.5# DIFFERENTIATED PROGRESSIVE ACUTE M9722/3
202.3# MALIGNANT M9720/3
202.5# X ACUTE (PROGRESSIVE) M9722/3

5th Digit: 202.3, 5

0. NOS
1. LYMPH NODES OF HEAD FACE NECK
2. LYMPH NODES INTRATHORACIC
3. LYMPH NODES ABDOMINAL
4. LYMPH NODES AXILLA AND UPPER LIMB
5. LYMPH NODES INGUINAL REGION AND LOWER LIMB
6. LYMPH NODES INTRAPELVIC
7. SPLEEN
8. LYMPH NODES MULTIPLE SITES

277.8 X (CHRONIC)

795.4 HISTOLOGICAL FINDINGS OTHER NOS ABNORMAL

115.9# HISTOPLASMOSIS

115.0# HISTOPLASMOSIS CAPSULATUM (AMERICAN) (SMALL FORM)

115.1# HISTOPLASMOSIS DUBOISII (AFRICAN) (LARGE FORM)

5th Digit: 115.0-9

0. UNSPECIFIED
1. MENINGITIS
2. RETINITIS
3. PERICARDITIS
4. ENDOCARDITIS
5. PNEUMONIA
9. OTHER SITE

THE V-CODES FOR HISTORY ARE NOT ASSIGNED IF THE CONDITION IS STILL PRESENT OR STILL BEING TREATED. THEY ARE FURTHER EXPLANATORY, HOWEVER, AS ADDITIONAL CODES IN SHOWING THE MEDICAL COMPLEXITY OF A PATIENT.

HISTORY

V15.4# ABUSE (EMOTIONAL) (PHYSICAL)

5th Digit: V15.4

1. PHYSICAL ABUSE, RAPE
2. EMOTIONAL ABUSE, NEGLECT
9. OTHER

V11.8 ADDICTION TO DRUGS
V11.8 ADJUSTMENT REACTION
V11.1 AFFECTIVE DISORDERS
V11.1 AFFECTIVE DISORDER (NOT IN REMISSION)
V11.3 ALCOHOLISM
V14.6 ALLERGY ANALGESIC AGENT
V14.4 ALLERGY ANESTHETIC AGENT
V14.5 ALLERGY CODEINE
V14.0 ALLERGY PENICILLIN
V14.9 ALLERGY MEDICINAL AGENT
V14.5 ALLERGY NARCOTIC
V14.1 ALLERGY OTHER ANTIBIOTIC AGENT
V15.0 ALLERGY OTHER THAN TO MEDICINAL AGENTS
V14.3 ALLERGY TO OTHER ANTI-INFECTIVE AGENT
V14.7 ALLERGY SERUM
V14.2 ALLERGY SULFA
V14.7 ALLERGY VACCINE
V14.8 ALLERGY OTHER SPECIFIED MEDICINAL AGENTS
V12.3 ANEMIA
V13.4 ARTHRITIS
V15.84 ASBESTOS EXPOSURE
V11.8 AUTISM
V12.41 BENIGN NEOPLASM BRAIN
V11.1 BIPOLAR PSYCHOSIS
V12.3 BLOOD DISORDER
V12.3 BLOOD FORMING ORGAN DISORDER
V15.85 BODY FLUIDS EXPOSURE (POTENTIALLY HAZARDOUS)
V10.9 CANCER
V10.51 CANCER BLADDER
V10.81 CANCER BONE
V10.85 CANCER BRAIN
V10.3 CANCER BREAST
V10.11 CANCER BRONCHUS AND LUNG
V10.05 CANCER CECUM
V10.41 CANCER CERVIX
V10.05 CANCER COLON
V10.89 CANCER CONNECTIVE TISSUE
V10.88 CANCER ENDOCRINE GLANDS (OTHER SPECIFIED GLANDS)
V10.48 CANCER EPIDIDYMIS
V10.03 CANCER ESOPHAGUS
V10.84 CANCER EYE
V10.40 CANCER FEMALE GENITAL ORGAN
V10.44 CANCER GENITAL ORGANS (FEMALE) OTHER SPECIFIED
V10.45 CANCER GENITAL ORGAN (MALE)
V10.00 CANCER GI TRACT
V10.09 CANCER GI TRACT (OTHER SPECIFIED SITES)
V10.52 CANCER KIDNEY
V10.05 CANCER LARGE INTESTINE
V10.21 CANCER LARYNX
V10.02 CANCER LIP
V10.07 CANCER LIVER
V10.11 CANCER LUNG AND BRONCHUS
V10.79 CANCER LYMPHATIC AND HEMATOPOIETIC OTHER
V10.49 CANCER MALE GENITAL ORGANS (OTHER SPECIFIED)
V10.82 CANCER MELANOMA SKIN (MALIGNANT)
V10.22 CANCER NASAL CAVITIES MIDDLE EAR ACCESSORY
V10.86 CANCER NERVOUS SYSTEM OTHER PARTS
V10.02 CANCER ORAL CAVITY INCLUDING LIP
V10.43 CANCER OVARY

HISTORY (continued)

V10.02	CANCER PHARYNX
V10.46	CANCER PROSTATE
V10.06	CANCER RECTUM (RECTOSIGMOID JUNCTION) (ANUS)
V10.29	CANCER RESPIRATORY AND INTRATHORACIC ORGANS
V10.20	CANCER RESPIRATORY ORGAN
V10.83	CANCER SKIN
V10.09	CANCER SMALL INTESTINE
V10.89	CANCER SOFT TISSUE
V10.04	CANCER STOMACH
V10.47	CANCER TESTIS
V10.87	CANCER THYROID
V10.29	CANCER THYMUS
V10.01	CANCER TONGUE
V10.12	CANCER TRACHEA
V10.50	CANCER URINARY TRACT
V10.59	CANCER URINARY TRACT (OTHER SPECIFIED)
V10.42	CANCER UTERUS (EXCLUDING CERVIX)
V10.89	CANCER (OTHER SITES)
V10.09	CANCER (OTHER SPECIFIED)
V12.50	CARDIOVASCULAR DISEASE UNSPECIFIED
V12.59	CARDIOVASCULAR DISEASE OTHER SPECIFIED
V12.50	CIRCULATORY DISEASE UNSPECIFIED
V12.59	CIRCULATORY DISEASE OTHER SPECIFIED
V14.5	CODEINE ALLERGY
V12.72	COLON POLYPS
V13.61	CONGENITAL MALFORMATION - HYPOSPADIAS
V13.69	CONGENITAL MALFORMATION - OTHER
V15.7	CONTRACEPTION
V12.59	CVA
V11.8	DEMENTIA
V11.1	DEPRESSIVE PSYCHOSIS
V15.42	DESERTION
V12.70	DIGESTIVE SYSTEM DISEASE
V12.79	DIGESTIVE SYSTEM DISEASE OTHER SPECIFIED
V13.8	DISEASE OTHER SPECIFIED
V13.9	DISEASE UNSPECIFIED
V11.8	DRUG ABUSE
V12.51	EMBOLISM (PULMONARY)
V15.42	EMOTIONAL ABUSE
V12.2	ENDOCRINE DISORDER
V12.49	EPILEPSY
V15.84	EXPOSURE ASBESTOS
V15.85	EXPOSURE BODY FLUIDS - POTENTIALLY HAZARDOUS
V15.86	EXPOSURE LEAD

FAMILY

V19.6	ALLERGY DISORDER
V18.2	ANEMIA
V17.7	ARTHRITIS
V17.5	ASTHMA
V17.4	ATHEROSCLEROSIS
V19.8	BAYLOR CRETIN SYNDROME
V19.0	BLINDNESS
V18.3	BLOOD DISORDERS (OTHER)
V16.9	CA
V16.59	CA BLADDER
V16.3	CA BREAST
V16.1	CA BRONCHUS
V16.49	CA CERVIX
V16.0	CA COLON
V16.0	CA GASTROINTESTINAL TRACT
V16.40	CA GENITAL ORGANS NOS
V16.49	CA GENITAL ORGANS OTHER
V16.0	CA GI TRACT
V16.7	CA HEMATOPOIETIC
V16.2	CA INTRATHORACIC ORGANS
V16.51	CA KIDNEY
V16.1	CA LUNG
V16.7	CA LYMPHATIC AND HEMATOPOIETIC
V16.41	CA OVARY, OVIDUCT
V16.49	CA PENIS
V16.42	CA PROSTATE

HISTORY (continued)

FAMILY (continued)

V16.2	CA RESPIRATORY
V16.43	CA TESTIS
V16.1	CA TRACHEA
V16.59	CA URINARY ORGANS
V16.49	CA UTERUS
V16.49	CA VAGINA
V16.49	CA VULVA
V16.8	CA OTHER SPECIFIED
V17.4	CARDIOVASCULAR DISEASES
V17.1	CEREBROVASCULAR ACCIDENT
V19.8	CONDITIONS (OTHER)
V19.5	CONGENITAL ANOMALIES
V19.7	CONSANGUINITY
V17.1	CVA
V19.2	DEAFNESS
V18.0	DIABETES MELLITUS
V18.5	DIGESTIVE DISORDERS
V19.5	DOWN'S SYNDROME (MONGOLISM)
V19.3	EAR DISORDERS (OTHER)
V18.1	ENDOCRINE AND METABOLIC DISEASES
V17.2	EPILEPSY
V19.1	EYE DISORDERS (OTHER)
V18.7	GENITOURINARY DISEASES (OTHER)
V18.69	GLOMERULONEPHRITIS
V19.2	HEARING LOSS
V17.3	HEART DISEASE (ISCHEMIC)
V16.7	HODGKIN'S DISEASE
V17.2	HUNTINGTON'S CHOREA
V17.4	HYPERTENSION
V18.8	INFECTIOUS DISEASES
V18.61	KIDNEY DISEASE - POLYCYSTIC
V18.69	KIDNEY DISEASE - OTHER
V16.6	LEUKEMIA
V16.7	LYMPHOMA
V16.7	LYMPHOSARCOMA
V18.4	MENTAL RETARDATION
V18.1	METABOLIC DISEASE
V17.8	MUSCULOSKELETAL DISEASES (OTHER)
V17.3	MYOCARDIAL INFARCTION
V17.2	NEUROLOGICAL DISEASE OTHER
V19.8	OTHER SPECIFIED CONDITION
V18.8	PARASITIC DISEASE
V17.0	PSYCHIATRIC CONDITION
V17.6	RESPIRATORY CONDITIONS (OTHER CHRONIC)
V16.7	RETICULOSARCOMA
V19.4	SKIN CONDITIONS
V17.1	STROKE
V19.0	VISION LOSS

HISTORY (continued)

V13.2	GENITAL SYSTEM DISORDER (NONGRAVID)
V15.9	HEALTH HAZARDS
V15.89	HEALTH HAZARDS OTHER SPECIFIED
V15.1	HEART AND/OR GREAT VESSELS SURGERY
V15.1	HEART SURGERY
V12.09	HEPATITIS
V23.89	HIGH RISK PREGNANCY OTHER (SEE ALSO 'PREGNANCY SUPERVISION', HIGH RISK)
V10.72	HODGKIN'S DISEASE
V23.1	HYDATIDIFORM MOLE AFFECTING PREGNANCY SUPERVISION
V12.59	HYPERTENSION
V12.2	IMMUNITY DISORDER
V12.00	INFECTIOUS AND PARASITIC DISEASE UNSPECIFIED OTHER
V12.09	INFECTIOUS AND PARASITIC DISEASE OTHER SPECIFIED
V15.5	INJURY
V15.86	LEAD EXPOSURE
V10.60	LEUKEMIA
V10.61	LEUKEMIA (LYMPHOID)
V10.63	LEUKEMIA (MONOCYTIC)
V10.62	LEUKEMIA (MYELOID)
V10.69	LEUKEMIA (OTHER TYPE)

HISTORY (continued)

V10.61	LYMPHOID LEUKEMIA
V10.71	LYMPHOSARCOMA NOT IN REMISSION
V10.71	LYMPHOSARCOMA AND RETICULOSARCOMA NOT IN REMISSION
V12.03	MALARIA
0	MATERNAL AFFECTING MANAGEMENT OF PREGNANCY SEE 'PREGNANCY SUPERVISION'
V10.82	MELANOMA SKIN (MALIGNANT)
V11.#	MENTAL DISORDER (NOT IN REMISSION)

4th Digit: V11

0. SCHIZOPHRENIA
1. AFFECTIVE DISORDER
2. NEUROSIS
8. OTHER MENTAL DISORDERS
9. MENTAL DISORDER NOS

V23.89	MENTAL DISORDER MATERNAL AFFECTING SUPERVISION OF PREGNANCY
V12.2	METABOLIC DISORDER
V10.63	MONOCYTIC LEUKEMIA
V13.5	MUSCULOSKELETAL DISORDER
V10.62	MYELOID LEUKEMIA
412	MYOCARDIAL INFARCTION
V15.42	NEGLECT (ABUSE)
V12.40	NERVOUS SYSTEM DISORDER NOS
V12.49	NERVOUS SYSTEM DISORDER OTHER
V11.2	NEUROSIS
V15.81	NONCOMPLIANCE WITH MEDICAL TREATMENT
V12.1	NUTRITIONAL DEFICIENCY
V13.2	OBSTETRIC DISORDER (NONGRAVID)
0	OBSTETRIC DISORDER AFFECTING MANAGEMENT OF CURRENT PREGNANCY SEE 'PREGNANCY SUPERVISION', HIGH RISK
V12.00	PARASITIC DISEASE UNSPECIFIED OTHER
V12.09	PARASITIC DISEASE OTHER SPECIFIED
V12.71	PEPTIC ULCER
V13.7	PERINATAL PROBLEMS
V15.41	PHYSICAL ABUSE
V15.6	POISONING
V12.02	POLIOMYELITIS
V12.72	POLYPS COLON
V15.4#	PSYCHOLOGICAL TRAUMA

5th Digit: V15.4

1. PHYSICAL ABUSE, RAPE
2. EMOTIONAL ABUSE, NEGLECT
9. OTHER

V11.8	PSYCHOSIS
V12.51	PULMONARY EMBOLISM
V15.3	RADIATION EXPOSURE
V15.41	RAPE
V13.01	RENAL CALCULUS
V13.00	RENAL DISEASE
V12.6	RESPIRATORY DISEASE
V10.71	RETICULOSARCOMA NOT IN REMISSION
V11.0	SCHIZOPHRENIA
V12.40	SENSE ORGAN DISORDER NOS
V12.49	SENSE ORGAN DISORDER OTHER
V14.7	SERUM ALLERGY
V13.3	SKIN DISEASE
V12.59	STROKE
V14.2	SULFA ALLERGY
V14.2	SULFONAMIDES ALLERGY
V15.2	SURGERY MAJOR ORGANS (OTHER SPECIFIED)
V15.82	TOBACCO USE
V12.52	THROMBOPHLEBITIS
V12.51	THROMBOSIS
V13.1	TROPHOBLASTIC DISEASE (NONGRAVID)
V12.01	TUBERCULOSIS
V13.00	URINARY SYSTEM DISORDER
V13.01	URINARY CALCULI
V13.09	URINARY SYSTEM DISORDER OTHER SPECIFIED
V14.7	VACCINE ALLERGY

301.50 HISTRIONIC PERSONALITY DISORDER

> *AIDS, ARC AND SYMPTOMATIC HIV INFECTIONS ALL CODE TO 042. THIS CODE SHOULD BE SEQUENCED AS THE PRINCIPAL DIAGNOSIS WITH AN ADDITIONAL CODE FOR ANY MANIFESTATION. EXCEPTION: IF THE ENCOUNTER IS FOR AN UNRELATED CONDITION SUCH AS A TRAUMA, SEQUENCE THE TRAUMA AS THE PRINCIPAL DIAGNOSIS, FOLLOWED BY THE 042 AND THEN THE ADDITIONAL CODES FOR THE MANIFESTATIONS.*

HIV

V08	CARRIER WITH CONFIRMED HIV POSITIVE STATUS (NO HIV SYMPTOMS PRESENT)
V65.44	COUNSELING (ADVICE) (EDUCATION) (INSTRUCTION ON PREVENTION)
V01.7	EXPOSURE
079.51	HTLV I
079.52	HTLV II
V08	INFECTION ASYMPTOMATIC
647.6#	INFECTION ASYMPTOMATIC - MATERNAL CURRENT (CO-EXISTENT) IN PREGNANCY [V08]

5th Digit: 647.6

0. EPISODE OF CARE UNSPECIFIED OR N/A
1. DELIVERED
2. DELIVERED WITH POSTPARTUM COMPLICATION
3. ANTEPARTUM COMPLICATION
4. POSTPARTUM COMPLICATION

042	INFECTION SYMPTOMATIC
647.6#	INFECTION SYMPTOMATIC - MATERNAL CURRENT (CO-EXISTENT) IN PREGNANCY [042]

5th Digit: 647.6

0. EPISODE OF CARE UNSPECIFIED OR N/A
1. DELIVERED
2. DELIVERED WITH POSTPARTUM COMPLICATION
3. ANTEPARTUM COMPLICATION
4. POSTPARTUM COMPLICATION

042	INFECTION DUE TO HIV II [079.53]
795.71	NONSPECIFIC SEROLOGIC EVIDENCE
V08	POSITIVE (ASYMPTOMATIC)
V08	STATUS (ASYMPTOMATIC)
V73.89	TEST
V73.89	TEST HIGH RISK GROUP INDIVIDUAL [V69.8]
V65.44	TEST RESULTS ENCOUNTER - NEGATIVE TEST

708.9 HIVES

> *WHEN CODING BACK DISORDERS DUE TO DEGENERATION, DISPLACEMENT OR HNP OF THE INTERVERTEBRAL DISC, IT IS IMPORTANT TO DISTINGUISH WHETHER THESE CONDITIONS ARE WITH OR WITHOUT MYELOPATHY. MYELOPATHY REFERS TO FUNCTIONAL DISTURBANCES AND/OR PATHOLOGICAL CHANGES IN THE SPINAL CORD THAT RESULT FROM COMPRESSION.*

HNP

722.2	SITE UNSPECIFIED
722.70	SITE UNSPECIFIED WITH MYELOPATHY
722.0	CERVICAL
722.71	CERVICAL WITH MYELOPATHY
722.10	LUMBAR
722.73	LUMBAR WITH MYELOPATHY
722.11	THORACIC
722.72	THORACIC WITH MYELOPATHY

784.49 HOARSENESS

V60.0 HOBO (HOMELESS PERSON)

HODGKIN'S DISEASE
201.9# NOS M9650/3
201.1# GRANULOMA M9661/3
201.7# LYMPHOCYTIC DEPLETION M9653/3
201.7# LYMPHOCYTIC DEPLETION DIFFUSE FIBROSIS M9654/3
201.7# LYMPHOCYTIC DEPLETION RETICULAR TYPE M9655/3
201.4# LYMPHOCYTIC PREDOMINANCE M9651/3
201.9# LYMPHOGRANULOMA M9650/3
201.9# LYMPHOMA M9650/3
201.6# MIXED CELLULARITY M9652/3
201.5# NODULAR SCLEROSIS M9656/3
201.5# NODULAR SCLEROSIS CELLULAR PHASE M9657/3
201.0# PARAGRANULOMA M9660/3
201.2# SARCOMA M9662/3
5th Digit: 201.0-2, 4-7, 9
0. UNSPECIFIED SITE, EXTRANODAL AND SOLID ORGAN SITES
1. LYMPH NODES OF HEAD FACE NECK
2. LYMPH NODES INTRATHORACIC
3. LYMPH NODES ABDOMINAL
4. LYMPH NODES AXILLA AND UPPER LIMB
5. LYMPH NODES INGUINAL REGION AND LOWER LIMB
6. LYMPH NODES INTRAPELVIC
7. SPLEEN
8. LYMPH NODES MULTIPLE SITES

441.9 HODGSON'S DISEASE
441.5 HODGSON'S DISEASE - RUPTURED
272.8 HOFFA'S (-KASTERT) DISEASE OR SYNDROME (LIPOSYNOVITIS PREPATELLARIS)
244.9 HOFFMANN'S SYNDROME (MYXEDEMA WITH MYOPATHY) [359.5]
427.2 HOFFMANN-BOUVERET SYNDROME (PAROXYSMAL TACHYCARDIA)
335.0 HOFFMANN-WERDNIG SYNDROME
V60.5 HOLIDAY RELIEF CARE
282.0 HOLLA DISEASE (SEE ALSO 'SPHEROCYTOSIS')
272.6 HOLLANDER-SIMONS SYNDROME (PROGRESSIVE LIPODYSTROHY)
362.33 HOLLENHORST PLAQUE
736.73 HOLLOW FOOT
754.71 HOLLOW FOOT CONGENITAL
379.46 HOLMES-ADIE SYNDROME
368.16 HOLMES' SYNDROME (VISUAL DISORIENTATION)
742.2 HOLOPROSENCEPHALY CONGENITAL
V60.1 HOME INADEQUATE FOR CARE DUE TO TECHNICAL DEFECTS
V60.0 HOMELESS PERSON
270.4 HOMOCYSTINE METABOLISM DISTURBANCES
270.4 HOMOCYSTINURIA
270.2 HOMOGENTISIC ACID DEFECTS
302.0 HOMOSEXUAL CONFLICT DISORDER
302.2 HOMOSEXUAL PEDOPHILIA
302.0 HOMOSEXUALITY
282.61 HOMOZYGOUS - HB-S DISEASE
518.89 HONEYCOMB LUNG
748.4 HONEYCOMB LUNG CONGENITAL
117.3 HONG KONG EAR
752.49 HOODED CLITORIS
752.69 HOODED PENIS CONGENITAL
078.4 HOOF AND MOUTH DISEASE
126.9 HOOKWORM
358.0 HOPPE GOLDFLAM SYNDROME

HORDEOLUM
373.11 NOS
373.11 EXTERNUM
373.12 INTERNUM

259.9 HORMONE ABNORMAL FINDINGS
259.9 HORMONE DISORDER (DISTURBANCE)
259.8 HORMONE DISORDER (DISTURBANCE) - OTHER SPECIFIED
V07.4 HORMONE REPLACEMENT THERAPY, POSTMENOPAUSAL
259.2 HORMONE SECRETION BY CARCINOID TUMORS
702.8 HORN CUTANEOUS

HORNER'S
337.2# SYNDROME
5th Digit: 337.2
0. UNSPECIFIED
1. UPPER LIMB
2. LOWER LIMB
9. OTHER SPECIFIED SITE
954.0 SYNDROME TRAUMATIC
520.4 TEETH

753.3 HORSESHOE KIDNEY
361.32 HORSESHOE TEAR RETINAL DEFECT WITHOUT DETACHMENT
446.5 HORTON'S DISEASE (TEMPORAL ARTERITIS)
346.2# HORTON'S NEURALGIA
5th Digit: 346.2
0. WITHOUT MENTION INTRACTABLE MIGRAINE
1. WITH INTRACTABLE MIGRAINE

WHEN USING CODE V66.7, CODE THE TERMINAL ILLNESS FIRST.

V66.7 HOSPICE CARE ENCOUNTER
301.51 HOSPITAL ADDICTION SYNDROME
309.83 HOSPITALISM

HOST-VERSUS-GRAFT REJECTION (IMMUNE) (NON-IMMUNE)
996.80 ORGAN UNSPECIFIED
996.85 BONE MARROW
996.51 CORNEA
996.55 DECELLULARIZED ALLODERMIS
996.83 HEART
996.89 INTESTINES
996.81 KIDNEY
996.82 LIVER
996.84 LUNG
996.86 PANCREAS
996.52 SKIN
996.55 SKIN - ARTIFICIAL
996.89 OTHER SPECIFIED NEC

627.2 HOT FLASHES (MENOPAUSAL)
537.6 HOURGLASS STRICTURE STOMACH

HOUSING
V60.9 CIRCUMSTANCE
V60.8 CIRCUMSTANCE OTHER SPECIFIED
V60.0 HOMELESS
V60.1 INADEQUATE
V60.0 LACK OF

282.7 HPFH (HEREDITARY PERSISTENCE FETAL HEMOGLOBIN)
079.4 HPV
078.1# HPV (HUMAN PAPILLOMAVIRUS) WART
5th Digit: 078.1
0. UNSPECIFIED, CONDYLOMA NOS, VERRUCA NOS, VERRUCA VULGARIS, WARTS (INFECTIOUS)
1. CONDYLOMA ACUMINATUM
9. OTHER SPECIFIED VIRAL, GENITAL NOS, VERRUCA: PLANA, PLANTARIS

079.51 HTLV I
079.52 HTLV II
0 HTLV III SEE 'HIV' INFECTION
0 HTN (HYPERTENSION) SEE 'HYPERTENSION'

401.9 HUCHARD'S DISEASE (CONTINUED ARTERIAL HYPERTENSION)
371.11 HUDSON STAHLI LINES
218.9 HUGUIER'S DISEASE (UTERINE FIBROMA)
0 HUMAN BITE SEE 'OPEN WOUND', BY SITE, COMPLICATED
253.3 HUMAN GROWTH HORMONE DEFICIENCY
253.0 HUMAN GROWTH HORMONE OVERPRODUCTION
0 HUMAN IMMUNODEFICIENCY VIRUS SEE 'HIV' INFECTION
079.4 HUMAN PAPILLOMAVIRUS INFECTION
078.1# HUMAN PAPILLOMAVIRUS WART

5th Digit: 078.1

0. UNSPECIFIED, CONDYLOMA NOS, VERRUCA NOS, VERRUCA VULGARIS, WARTS (INFECTIOUS)
1. CONDYLOMA ACUMINATUM
9. OTHER SPECIFIED VIRAL, GENITAL NOS, VERRUCA: PLANA, PLANTARIS

755.21 HUMERUS ABSENCE WITH ABSENCE COMPLETE DISTAL ELEMENTS - CONGENITAL
755.24 HUMERUS ABSENCE WITH ABSENCE INCOMPLETE DISTAL ELEMENTS - CONGENITAL
755.23 HUMERUS ABSENCE WITH ABSENCE RADIUS AND ULNA (INCOMPLETE) - CONGENITAL
736.89 HUMERUS DEFORMITY
755.50 HUMERUS DEFORMITY CONGENITAL
737.9 HUNCHBACK ACQUIRED
994.2 HUNGER
909.4 HUNGER LATE EFFECT
595.1 HUNNER'S ULCER
334.2 HUNT'S DISEASE (DYSSYNERGIA CEREBELLARIS MYOCLONICA)
053.11 HUNT'S SYNDROME (HERPETIC GENICULATE GANGLIONITIS)
529.4 HUNTERIAN GLOSSITIS SYNDROME

HUNTER'S

277.5 CEREBRAL DEGENERATION DISEASE OF CHILDHOOD [330.3]
529.4 GLOSSITIS
277.5 SYNDROME (MUCOPOLYSACCHARIDOSIS I)

333.4 HUNTINGTON'S CHOREA
333.4 HUNTINGTON'S CHOREA WITH DEMENTIA [294.1]
V17.2 HUNTINGTON'S CHOREA FAMILY HISTORY
203.0# HUPPERT'S DISEASE (MULTIPLE MYELOMA) M9730/3

5th Digit: 203.0

0. WITHOUT MENTION OF REMISSION
1. IN REMISSION

277.5 HURLER'S SYNDROME (MUCOPOLYSACCHARIDOSIS I)

HUTCHINSON'S

709.1 ANGIOMA SERPEGINOSUM
705.81 CHEIROPOMPHOLYX
090.5 INCISORS OR TEETH SYNDROME

HUTCHINSON'S (continued)

173.# MELANOTIC FRECKLE MALIGNANT M8742/2

4th Digit: 173

0. SKIN OF LIP
1. EYELID INCLUDING CANTHUS
2. SKIN OF EAR AURICULAR CANAL (EXTERNAL) EXTERNAL MEATUS PINNA
3. SKIN OF UNSPECIFIED PARTS OF FACE CHEEK (EXTERNAL) CHIN EYEBROW FOREHEAD NOSE (EXT)
4. SCALP AND SKIN OF NECK
5. ALL SKIN TRUNK AXILLARY FOLD PERIANAL ABDOMINAL WALL ANUS BACK BREAST (OR MASTECTOMY SITE) BUTTOCK
6. ALL SKIN UPPER LIMB SHOULDER ARM FINGER FOREARM HAND
7. ALL SKIN LOWER LIMB HIP ANKLE FOOT HEEL KNEE LEG THIGH TOE POPITEAL AREA
8. OTHER SPECIFIED SKIN SITES CONTIGUOUS OVERLAPPING SITES UNDETERMINED POINT OF ORIGIN
9. SITE UNSPECIFIED

692.72 PRURIGO ESTIVALIS (ACUTE)
692.72 SUMMER ERUPTION (ACUTE)
090.5 TEETH MANIFEST 2 YRS. OR MORE AFTER BIRTH

135 HUTCHINSON-BOECK SYNDROME (SARCOIDOSIS)
259.8 HUTCHINSON-GILFORD DISEASE OR SYNDROME (PROGERIA)
728.9 HYALINE DISEASE (DIFFUSE) (GENERALIZED)
371.49 HYALINE FORMATION CORNEA
769 HYALINE MEMBRANE DISEASE (PULMONARY) NEWBORN
581.1 HYALINOSIS SEGMENTAL
379.22 HYALITIS (ASTEROID)
0 HYDATID DISEASE SEE 'ECHINOCOCCUS'

HYDATIDIFORM MOLE

236.1 NOS M9100/1
630 BENIGN
630 BENIGN WITH COMPLICATION DURING TREATMENT [639.#]
639.# BENIGN WITH COMPLICATION FOLLOWING TREATMENT

4th Digit: 639

0. GENITAL TRACT AND PELVIC INFECTION
1. DELAYED OR EXCESSIVE HEMORRHAGE
2. DAMAGE TO PELVIC ORGANS AND TISSUE
3. RENAL FAILURE
4. METABOLIC DISORDERS
5. SHOCK
6. EMBOLISM
8. OTHER SPECIFIED COMPLICATION
9. UNSPECIFIED COMPLICATION

630 COMPLICATING PREGNANCY (DELIVERY) (UNDELIVERED)
630 COMPLICATING PREGNANCY (DELIVERY) (UNDELIVERED) WITH COMPLICATION DURING TREATMENT [639.#]
639.# COMPLICATING PREGNANCY (DELIVERY) (UNDELIVERED) WITH COMPLICATION FOLLOWING TREATMENT

4th Digit: 639

0. GENITAL TRACT AND PELVIC INFECTION
1. DELAYED OR EXCESSIVE HEMORRHAGE
2. DAMAGE TO PELVIC ORGANS AND TISSUE
3. RENAL FAILURE
4. METABOLIC DISORDERS
5. SHOCK
6. EMBOLISM
8. OTHER SPECIFIED COMPLICATION
9. UNSPECIFIED COMPLICATION

V23.1 HISTORY AFFECTING PREGNANCY SUPERVISION
236.1 INVASIVE M9100/1
186.9 MALE CHORIOCARCINOMA
236.1 MALIGNANT M 9100/1

0 HYDATIDOSIS SEE 'ECHINOCOCCUS'
698.3 HYDE'S DISEASE (PRURIGO NODULARIS)

HYDRAMNIOS
761.3 ACUTE (CHRONIC) AFFECTING FETUS OR NEWBORN
657.0# HYDRAMNIOS
5th Digit: 657.0
0. EPISODE OF CARE NOS OR N/A
1. DELIVERED
3. ANTEPARTUM COMPLICATION
0 SEE 'POLYHYDRAMNIOS'

742.3 HYDRANENCEPHALY
102.6 HYDRARTHROSIS OF YAWS, (EARLY) (LATE)
868.00 HYDRAULIC CONCUSSION SYNDROME (ABDOMEN)
285.9 HYDREMIA

HYDROA
694.0 HYDROA
692.72 AESTIVALE
646.8# GESTATIONIS
5th Digit: 646.8
0. EPISODE OF CARE NOS OR N/A
1. DELIVERED
2. DELIVERED WITH POSTPARTUM COMPLICATION
3. ANTEPARTUM COMPLICATION
4. POSTPARTUM COMPLICATION
694.0 HERPETIFORMIS
694.0 PRURIGINOSA
692.72 VACCINIFORME

0 HYDROADENITIS SEE 'HIDRADENITIS'
719.0# HYDROARTHROSIS
719.3# HYDROARTHROSIS INTERMITTENT
5th Digit: 719.0, 3
0. SITE NOS
1. SHOULDER REGION
2. UPPER ARM (ELBOW) (HUMERUS)
3. FOREARM (RADIUS) (WRIST) (ULNA)
4. HAND (CARPAL) (METACARPAL) (FINGERS)
5. PELVIC REGION AND THIGH (HIP) (BUTTOCK) (FEMUR)
6. LOWER LEG (FIBULA) (KNEE) (PATELLA) (TIBIA)
7. ANKLE AND/OR FOOT (METATARSALS) (TOES) (TARSALS)
8. OTHER
9. MULTIPLE
591 HYDROCALYCOSIS
753.29 HYDROCALYCOSIS CONGENITAL

HYDROCELE
629.1 CANAL OF NUCK
752.41 CANAL OF NUCK CONGENITAL
778.6 CONGENITAL
603.0 ENCYSTED (TESTES) (TUNICA) (SPERMATIC CORD)
603.1 INFECTED (TESTES) (TUNICA) (SPERMATIC CORD)
603.1 INFECTED E. COLI [041.4]
603.1 INFECTED H. FLU [041.5]
603.1 INFECTED KLEBSIELLA [041.3]
603.1 INFECTED PNEUMOCOCCUS [041.2]
603.1 INFECTED PNEUMONIAE [041.89]
603.1 INFECTED PROTEUS [041.6]
603.1 INFECTED STAPH [**041.1#**]
5th Digit: 041.1
0. NOS
1. AUREUS
9. OTHER STAPH

HYDROCELE (continued)
603.1 INFECTED STREP [**041.0#**]
5th Digit: 041.0
0. NOS
1. GROUP A
2. GROUP B
3. GROUP C
4. GROUP D (ENTEROCOCCUS)
5. GROUP G
9. OTHER STREP

603.1 INFECTED OTHER SPECIFIED [**041.8#**]
5th Digit: 041.8
1. MYCOPLASMA, EATON'S AGENT, PPLO
2. BACILLUS FRAGILIS
3. CLOSTRIDIUM PERFRINGENS
4. OTHER ANAEROBES
5. AEROBACTER AEROGENES, MIMA POLYMORPHA, SERRATIA, (OTHER GRAM-NEGATIVE)
9. OTHER SPECIFIED BACTERIA
603.9 TESTES (TUNICA) (SPERMATIC CORD)
603.8 OTHER SPECIFIED TYPES MALE GENITAL

HYDROCEPHALUS
331.4 ACQUIRED
742.3 CEREBRAL DEGENERATION (CONGENITAL) [331.7]
741.0# CEREBRAL DEGENERATION (CONGENITAL) (SPINA BIFIDA) [331.7]
5th Digit: 741.0
0. REGION NOS
1. CERVICAL REGION
2. DORSAL (THORACIC REGION)
3. LUMBAR REGION
331.3 COMMUNICATING (ACQUIRED)
742.3 CONGENITAL
742.3 DUE TO AQUEDUCT SYLVIUS ANOMALY (CONGENITAL)
742.3 DUE TO ATRESIA FORAMINA OF MAGENDIE AND LUSCHKA (CONGENITAL)
771.2 DUE TO TOXOPLASMOSIS (CONGENITAL)
655.0# FETALIS AFFECTING PREGNANCY MANAGEMENT
653.6# FETALIS CAUSING DISPROPORTION
660.1# FETALIS OBSTRUCTING LABOR [**653.6#**]
5th Digit: 653.6, 655.0, 660.1
0. EPISODE OF CARE NOS OR N/A
1. DELIVERED
3. ANTEPARTUM COMPLICATION
742.3 NEWBORN CONGENITAL
331.4 OBSTRUCTIVE
741.0# WITH SPINA BIFIDA
5th Digit: 741.0
0. REGION NOS
1. CERVICAL REGION
2. DORSAL (THORACIC REGION)
3. LUMBAR REGION

623.8 HYDROCOLPOS CONGENITAL
216.# HYDROCYSTOMA M8404/0
4th Digit: 216
0. LIP (SKIN OF)
1. EYELID INCLUDING CANTHUS
2. EAR (EXTERNAL) (AURICLE) (PINNA)
3. FACE (CHEEK) (NOSE) (EYEBROW) (TEMPLE)
4. SCALP NECK EXCEPT SCROTUM
5. TRUNK BACK
6. UPPER LIMB INCLUDING SHOULDER
7. LOWER LIMB INCLUDING HIP
8. OTHER SPECIFIED SITES
9. SKIN NOS

742.0 HYDROENCEPHALOCELE CONGENITAL

HYDROMENINGOCELE
741.91 CERVICAL SPINAL REGION CONGENITAL
741.01 CERVICAL SPINAL REGION CONGENITAL WITH HYDROCEPHALUS CONGENITAL
742.0 CRANIAL CONGENITAL
741.92 DORSAL [THORACIC] REGION CONGENITAL
741.02 DORSAL [THORACIC] REGION CONGENITAL WITH HYDROCEPHALUS
741.93 LUMBAR REGION CONGENITAL
741.03 LUMBAR REGION CONGENITAL WITH HYDROCEPHALUS
741.90 SPINAL REGION CONGENITAL
741.00 SPINAL REGION CONGENITAL WITH HYDROCEPHALUS

621.8 HYDROMETRA
742.1 HYDROMICROCEPHALY CONGENITAL
742.53 HYDROMYELIA SPINAL CORD CONGENITAL

HYDROMYELOCELE
741.91 CERVICAL SPINAL REGION CONGENITAL
741.01 CERVICAL SPINAL REGION CONGENITAL WITH HYDROCEPHALUS CONGENITAL
741.92 DORSAL [THORACIC] REGION CONGENITAL
741.02 DORSAL [THORACIC] REGION CONGENITAL WITH HYDROCEPHALUS
741.93 LUMBAR REGION CONGENITAL
741.03 LUMBAR REGION CONGENITAL WITH HYDROCEPHALUS
741.90 SPINAL REGION CONGENITAL
741.00 SPINAL REGION CONGENITAL WITH HYDROCEPHALUS

591 HYDRONEPHROSIS
753.29 HYDRONEPHROSIS CONGENITAL
071 HYDROPHOBIA
511.8 HYDROPNEUMOTHORAX
782.3 HYDROPS
773.3 HYDROPS FETALIS DUE TO BLOOD TYPE REACTION [773.#]

4th Digit: 773
0. RH (RHESUS) ISOIMMUNIZATION
1. ABO ISOIMMUNIZATION
2. OTHER AND NOS ISOIMMUNIZATION

778.0 HYDROPS FETALIS IDIOPATHIC
575.3 HYDROPS GALLBLADDER
742.53 HYDRORHACHIS SPINAL CORD CONGENITAL
614.1 HYDROSALPINX
511.8 HYDROTHORAX
593.5 HYDROURETER
753.22 HYDROURETER CONGENITAL
591 HYDROURETERONEPHROSIS
599.84 HYDROURETHRA
270.2 HYDROXYKYNURENINURIA
255.2 HYDROXYLASE 21 DEFICIENCY
270.8 HYDROXYPROLINEMIA
255.2 HYDROXYSTEROID 18 DEHYDROGENASE DEFICIENCY
228.1 HYGROMA CYSTIC
727.3 HYGROMA PREPATELLAR
0 HYGROMA SUBDURAL SEE 'HEMATOMA', SUBDURAL

HYMEN
752.49 ABSENCE (CONGENITAL)
752.49 ACCESSORY (CONGENITAL)
623.3 ATRESIA (POSTINFECTIVE)
752.42 ATRESIA CONGENITAL
752.49 DIVISION
752.49 HYPERPLASIA CONGENITAL
752.42 IMPERFORATE CONGENITAL
623.3 OCCLUSION
752.42 OCCLUSION CONGENITAL
0 PERSISTENT MATERNAL SEE 'VULVA, VULVAL DISORDERS COMPLICATING CHILDBIRTH'
623.3 RIGID ACQUIRED OR CONGENITAL
623.3 TIGHT ACQUIRED OR CONGENITAL

123.6 HYMENOLEPIASIS
123.6 HYMENOLEPIS DIMINUTA NANA INFECTION
782.0 HYPALGESIA
447.8 HYPERABDUCTION SYNDROME
536.8 HYPERACIDITY STOMACH
596.51 HYPERACTIVE BLADDER
0 HYPERACTIVE BLADDER WITH INCONTINENCE SEE 'BLADDER DISORDERS WITH INCONTINENCE'
787.5 HYPERACTIVE BOWEL SOUNDS
564.1 HYPERACTIVE BOWEL SYNDROME
314.01 HYPERACTIVITY (ADULT) (CHILD)
388.42 HYPERACUSIS
255.1 HYPERALDOSTERONISM WITH HYPOKALEMIC ALKALOSIS (SYNDROME)
783.6 HYPERALIMENTATION ORGANIC
278.8 HYPERALIMENTATION OTHER (EXCESSIVE INTAKE)
270.6 HYPERAMMONEMIA
791.9 HYPERAZOTEMIA
V46.8 HYPERBARIC CHAMBER DEPENDENCE
272.0 HYPERBETALIPOPROTEINEMIA
272.2 HYPERBETALIPOPROTEINEMIA WITH PREBETALIPOPROTEINEMIA

HYPERBILIRUBINEMIA
782.4 NOS
277.4 CONGENITAL
277.4 DISORDERS OF BILIRUBIN EXCRETION
774.6 NEONATAL NOS (TRANSIENT)
774.1 NEONATAL BIRTH TRAUMA
774.30 NEONATAL DELAYED CONJUGATION NOS
774.39 NEONATAL DELAYED CONJUGATION DISEASE OTHER
774.4 NEONATAL DUE TO LIVER DAMAGE
277.4 NEONATAL GILBERT'S SYNDROME [774.31]
774.1 NEONATAL HEMOLYTIC
282.# NEONATAL HEREDITARY HEMOLYTIC [774.0]

4th Digit: 282
0. SPHEROCYTIC
1. ELLIPTOCYTOTIC
2. G6PD (GLUTATHIONE REDUCTASE)
3. HEXOKINASE (PK) (TPI) DEFICIENCY NONSPHEROCYTIC TYPE II
4. THALASSEMIA (MEDITERRANEAN) (COOLEY'S)
5. SICKLE CELL TRAIT
7. HEMOGLOBINOPATHY (HB-C) (HB-D) (HB-E) (FETAL) OR NOS
8. OTHER SPECIFIED (STOMACYTOSIS)
9. NOS

243 NEONATAL HYPOTHYROIDISM CONGENITAL [774.31]
774.2 NEONATAL PREMATURITY
0 SEE ALSO 'JAUNDICE'

275.42 HYPERCALCEMIA DISORDER OR SYNDROME
275.40 HYPERCALCINURIA
786.09 HYPERCAPNIA
770.8 HYPERCAPNIA FETAL
276.4 HYPERCAPNIA WITH MIXED ACID-BASE DISORDER
278.3 HYPERCAROTINEMIA
276.9 HYPERCHLOREMIA
272.0 HYPERCHOLESTEROLEMIA
272.2 HYPERCHOLESTEROLEMIA AND HYPERGLYCERIDEMIA
V65.3 HYPERCHOLESTEROLEMIA DIETARY COUNSELING AND SURVEILLANCE
289.8 HYPERCOAGULATION SYNDROME

536.2 HYPEREMESIS
643.0# HYPEREMESIS GRAVIDARUM MILD
643.1# HYPEREMESIS GRAVIDARUM WITH METABOLIC DISTURBANCE
5th Digit: 643.0-1
0. EPISODE OF CARE NOS OR N/A
1. DELIVERED
3. ANTEPARTUM COMPLICATION

374.82 HYPEREMIA EYELID
362.89 HYPEREMIA RETINA
288.3 HYPEREOSINOPHILIC SYNDROME (IDIOPATHIC)
782.0 HYPERESTHESIA SKIN
256.0 HYPERESTROGENISM

718.8# HYPEREXTENSION OF JOINT
5th Digit: 718.8
0. SITE NOS
1. SHOULDER REGION
2. UPPER ARM (ELBOW) (HUMERUS)
3. FOREARM (RADIUS) (WRIST) (ULNA)
4. HAND (CARPAL) (METACARPAL) (FINGERS)
5. PELVIC REGION AND THIGH (HIP) (BUTTOCK) (FEMUR)
6. LOWER LEG (FIBULA) (KNEE) (PATELLA) (TIBIA)
7. ANKLE AND/OR FOOT (METATARSALS) (TOES) (TARSALS)
8. OTHER
9. MULTIPLE

256.0 HYPERFUNCTION OVARY ESTROGEN
256.1 HYPERFUNCTION OVARY OTHER

289.8 HYPERGAMMAGLOBULINEMIA
273.1 HYPERGAMMAGLOBULINEMIA [BMH] BENIGN MONOCLONAL
273.0 HYPERGAMMAGLOBULINEMIA BENIGN PRIMARY
273.0 HYPERGAMMAGLOBULINEMIA POLYCLONAL WALDENSTROM'S
273.8 HYPERGLOBULINEMIA
790.6 HYPERGLYCEMIA
251.3 HYPERGLYCEMIA POSTPANCREATECTOMY
0 HYPERGLYCEMIA WITH DIABETES SEE 'DIABETES, DIABETIC' UNCOMPLICATED, UNCONTROLLED
272.3 HYPERGLYCERIDEMIA MIXED
272.1 HYPERGLYCERIDEMIA PURE
270.7 HYPERGLYCINEMIA

286.5 HYPERHEPARINEMIA HEMORRHAGIC DUE TO CIRCULATING ANTICOAGULANTS
780.8 HYPERHIDROSIS
270.5 HYPERHISTIDINEMIA

251.1 HYPERINSULIN ECTOPIC (FUNCTIONAL)
775.0 HYPERINSULIN INFANTILE (OF DIABETIC MOTHER)
775.6 HYPERINSULIN NEONATAL CAUSING HYPOGLYCEMIA

251.1 HYPERINSULINISM
251.1 HYPERINSULINISM HYPERPLASIA PANCREATIC ISLET BETA CELLS
251.0 HYPERINSULINISM IATROGENIC

276.9 HYPERIODEMIA
276.7 HYPERKALEMIA (HYPERKALEMIC SYNDROME)

701.1 HYPERKERATOSIS (FOLLICULARIS) (PALMOPLANTARIS)
371.89 HYPERKERATOSIS CORNEA (LIMBIC)
702.0 HYPERKERATOSIS SENILE

HYPERKINETIC
314.2 CONDUCT DISORDER
314.1 CONDUCT DISORDER WITH DEVELOPMENT DELAY
314.9 SYNDROME - NOS
314.00 SYNDROME - WITH ATTENTION DEFICIT
314.01 SYNDROME - WITH ATTENTION DEFICIT AND HYPERACTIVITY
314.1 SYNDROME - WITH DEVELOPMENTAL DELAY
314.8 SYNDROME - WITH OTHER SPECIFIED MANIFESTATIONS
429.82 SYNDROME, HEART

375.20 HYPERLACRIMATION
571.1 HYPERLIPEMIA-HEMOLYTIC ANEMIA-ICTERUS SYNDROME

HYPERLIPIDEMIA
272.4 HYPERLIPIDEMIA
272.0 GROUP A
272.1 GROUP B
272.3 GROUP D
272.2 MIXED
272.4 OTHER SPECIFIED

272.7 HYPERLIPIDOSIS

HYPERLIPOPROTEINEMIA
272.4 NOS
272.3 FREDRICKSON TYPE I OR V
272.0 FREDRICKSON TYPE IIA
272.2 FREDRICKSON TYPE IIB OR III
272.1 FREDRICKSON TYPE IV

492.8 HYPERLUCENT LUNG UNILATERAL
491.21 HYPERLUCENT LUNG WITH ACUTE BRONCHITIS
491.20 HYPERLUCENT LUNG WITH CHRONIC BRONCHITIS
491.21 HYPERLUCENT LUNG WITH CHRONIC BRONCHITIS WITH EXACERBATION
256.1 HYPERLUTEINIZATION
270.7 HYPERLYSINEMIA

275.2 HYPERMAGNESEMIA
275.2 HYPERMAGNESEMIA METABOLISM DISORDERS
775.5 HYPERMAGNESEMIA NEONATAL

626.2 HYPERMENORRHEA
627.0 HYPERMENORRHEA PREMENOPAUSAL
626.3 HYPERMENORRHEA PUBERTY

794.7 HYPERMETABOLISM
270.4 HYPERMETHIONINEMIA
367.0 HYPERMETROPIA

HYPERMOBILITY
564.1 CECUM
724.71 COCCYX
564.1 COLON
306.4 COLON PSYCHOGENIC
564.89 ILEUM
564.89 INTESTINAL
718.8# JOINT (ACQUIRED)
5th Digit: 718.8
0. SITE
1. SHOULDER REGION
2. UPPER ARM (ELBOW) (HUMERUS)
3. FOREARM (RADIUS) (WRIST) (ULNA)
4. HAND (CARPAL) (METACARPAL) (FINGERS)
5. PELVIC REGION (HIP) (BUTTOCK) (FEMUR)
6. LOWER LEG (FIBULA) (KNEE) (PATELLA) (TIBIA)
7. ANKLE AND/OR FOOT (METATARSALS) (TOES) (TARSALS)
8. OTHER
9. MULTIPLE

753.3 KIDNEY, CONGENITAL
717.5 KNEE MENISCUS
718.81 SCAPULA
536.8 STOMACH
306.4 STOMACH PSYCHOGENIC
728.5 SYNDROME
752.52 TESTIS CONGENITAL
599.81 URETHRAL

784.49 HYPERNASALITY
276.0 HYPERNATREMIA (SYNDROME)

238.9 HYPERNEPHROID TUMOR SITE NOS
0 HYPERNEPHROID TUMOR SITE SPECIFIED SEE 'NEOPLASM UNCERTAIN BEHAVIOR' BY SITE M8311/1

367.0 HYPEROPIA
270.6 HYPERORNITHINEMIA
276.0 HYPEROSMOLALITY
276.0 HYPEROSMOLALITY SODIUM [NA] EXCESS
276.0 HYPEROSMOLARITY SYNDROME
733.99 HYPEROSTEOGENESIS

HYPEROSTOSIS
733.90 NOS
733.3 CALVARIAL
733.3 CORTICAL
756.59 CORTICAL INFANTILE
733.3 FRONTAL, INTERNAL OF SKULL
733.3 INTERNA FRONTALIS
733.99 MONOMELIC
733.3 SKULL
756.0 SKULL CONGENITAL
721.8 VERTEBRAL
721.6 VERTEBRAL ANKYLOSING

271.8 HYPEROXALURIA (PRIMARY) CARBOHYDRATE TRANSPORT DISORDERS
987.8 HYPEROXIA
252.0 HYPERPARATHYROIDISM
259.3 HYPERPARATHYROIDISM ECTOPIC HORMONE SECRETION
588.8 HYPERPARATHYROIDISM RENAL
787.4 HYPERPERISTALSIS
270.1 HYPERPHENYLALANINEMIA
378.45 HYPERPHORIA ALTERNATING
275.3 HYPERPHOSPHATEMIA
709.00 HYPERPIGMENTATION
0 HYPERPLASIA / HYPERPLASTIC SEE ANATOMICAL SITE
272.1 HYPERPREBETALIPOPROTEINEMIA
272.3 HYPERPREBETALIPOPROTEINEMIA WITH CHYLOMICRONEMIA
272.1 HYPERPREBETALIPOPROTEINEMIA FAMILIAL
253.1 HYPERPROLACTINEMIA
270.8 HYPERPROLINEMIA
273.8 HYPERPROTEINEMIA
289.8 HYPERPROTHROMBINEMIA
780.6 HYPERPYREXIA
995.86 HYPERPYREXIA MALIGNANT DUE TO ANESTHESIA
909.9 HYPERPYREXIA MALIGNANT DUE TO ANESTHESIA - LATE EFFECT
344.61 HYPERREFLEXIA DETRUSOR
0 HYPERREFLEXIA DETRUSOR WITH INCONTINENCE SEE 'BLADDER DISORDERS WITH INCONTINENCE'
527.7 HYPERSALIVATION
270.8 HYPERSARCOSINEMIA
288.2 HYPERSEGMENTATION LEUKOCYTES HEREDITARY

HYPERSENSITIVITY
995.3 NOS
909.9 LATE EFFECT
478.8 REACTION UPPER RESPIRATORY
V72.7 SCREENING EXAM

HYPERSOMNIA
780.54 NOS
307.43 ASSOCIATED WITH ACUTE OR INTERMITTENT EMOTIONAL REACTIONS OR CONFLICTS
307.44 ASSOCIATED WITH DEPRESSION
349.89 BULIMIA SYNDROME
307.44 PERSISTENT
307.43 TRANSIENT
780.53 WITH SLEEP APNEA
780.54 OTHER

289.4 HYPERSPLENIC SYNDROME
289.4 HYPERSPLENISM
288.0 HYPERSPLENISM PRIMARY NEUTROPENIA
0 HYPERSYMPATHETIC SYNDROME SEE 'NEUROPATHY PERIPHERAL', AUTONOMIC
246.8 HYPER-TBG-NEMIA
756.0 HYPERTELORISM CONGENITAL
376.41 HYPERTELORISM ORBIT
756.0 HYPERTELORISM ORBIT CONGENITAL

HYPERTENSION
401.9 NOS
401.0 ACCELERATED
401.1 BENIGN
401.# ESSENTIAL
  4th Digit: 401
    0. MALIGNANT, ACCELERATED
    1. BENIGN
    9. NOS
V12.59 HISTORY
348.2 INTRACRANIAL (BENIGN)
401.# LABILE
  4th Digit: 401
    0. MALIGNANT, ACCELERATED
    1. BENIGN
    9. NOS
401.0 MALIGNANT
760.0 MATERNAL AFFECTING FETUS OR NEWBORN
0 MATERNAL COMPLICATING PREGNANCY SEE 'HYPERTENSION COMPLICATING PREGNANCY'
365.04 OCULAR
572.3 PORTAL
572.3 PORTAL WITH ESOPHAGEAL VARICES [**456.2#**]
  5th Digit: 456.2
    0. WITH BLEEDING
    1. WITHOUT BLEEDING
997.91 POSTOPERATIVE (DUE TO A PROCEDURE)
306.2 PSYCHOGENIC
416.0 PULMONARY CHRONIC PRIMARY
416.8 PULMONARY CHRONIC SECONDARY
747.89 PULMONARY PERSISTENT CONGENITAL
405.91 RENOVASCULAR SECONDARY
405.11 RENOVASCULAR SECONDARY - BENIGN
405.01 RENOVASCULAR SECONDARY - MALIGNANT
V81.1 SCREENING
405.## SECONDARY
  4th Digit: 405
    0. MALIGNANT, ACCELERATED
    1. BENIGN
    9. NOS
  5th Digit: 405
    1. RENOVASCULAR
    9. OTHER
796.2 TRANSIENT

HYPERTENSION COMPLICATING PREGNANCY
642.9# UNSPECIFIED
642.0# BENIGN
642.2# MALIGNANT
642.6# ECLAMPSIA
642.7# ECLAMPSIA OR PRE-ECLAMPSIA WITH PRE-EXISTING HYPERTENSION
642.0# ESSENTIAL- NOS OR BENIGN
642.7# ESSENTIAL- NOS OR BENIGN WITH SUPERIMPOSED PRE-ECLAMPSIA OR ECLAMPSIA
  5th Digit: 642
    0. EPISODE OF CARE NOS OR N/A
    1. DELIVERED
    2. DELIVERED WITH POSTPARTUM COMPLICATIONS
    3. ANTEPARTUM COMPLICATION
    4. POSTPARTUM COMPLICATIONS

HYPERTENSION COMPLICATING PREGNANCY (continued)

642.3# GESTATIONAL- NOS
642.0# PRE-EXISTING (CHRONIC) - NOS
642.0# PRE-EXISTING (CHRONIC) - BENIGN
642.2# PRE-EXISTING (CHRONIC) - MALIGNANT
642.7# PRE-EXISTING (CHRONIC) - WITH SUPERIMPOSED PRE-ECLAMPSIA OR ECLAMPSIA

642.1# SECONDARY TO RENAL DISEASE
642.7# SECONDARY TO RENAL DISEASE WITH SUPERIMPOSED PRE-ECLAMPSIA OR ECLAMPSIA

642.3# TRANSIENT- NOS

642.4# WITH EDEMA AND/OR ALBUMINURIA - MILD
642.5# WITH EDEMA AND/OR ALBUMINURIA - SEVERE
642.2# WITH RENAL AND/OR HEART DISEASE

5th Digit: 642
- **0. EPISODE OF CARE NOS OR N/A**
- **1. DELIVERED**
- **2. DELIVERED WITH POSTPARTUM COMPLICATIONS**
- **3. ANTEPARTUM COMPLICATION**
- **4. POSTPARTUM COMPLICATIONS**

HYPERTENSIVE

402.## CARDIOVASCULAR DISEASE (HEART)

4th Digit: 402
- **0. MALIGNANT**
- **1. BENIGN**
- **9. NOS**

5th Digit: 402
- **0. WITHOUT CHF**
- **1. WITH CHF**

0 CRISIS SEE 'HYPERTENSION'
760.0 DISORDER AFFECTING FETUS OR NEWBORN
437.2 ENCEPHALOPATHY
404.## HEART AND RENAL DISEASE

4th Digit: 404
- **0. MALIGNANT**
- **1. BENIGN**
- **9. NOS**

5th Digit: 404
- **0. WITHOUT CHF OR RENAL FAILURE**
- **1. WITH CHF**
- **2. WITH RENAL FAILURE**
- **3. WITH CHF AND RENAL FAILURE**

403.## RENAL DISEASE

4th Digit: 403
- **0. MALIGNANT**
- **1. BENIGN**
- **9. NOS**

5th Digit: 403
- **0. WITHOUT RENAL FAILURE**
- **1. WITH RENAL FAILURE**

HYPERTENSIVE (continued)

WHEN YOU HAVE A PATIENT WITH BOTH RENAL FAILURE AND HYPERTENSION, ICD 9-CM DOES PRESUME A CAUSE AND EFFECT RELATIONSHIP AND YOU SHOULD ASSIGN CODES FROM 403.##, (HYPERTENSIVE RENAL DISEASE). HOWEVER, IF YOU HAVE ACUTE RENAL FAILURE THAT IS NOT DUE TO HYPERTENSION, ALONG WITH HYPERTENSIVE RENAL DISEASE, TWO CODES ARE REQUIRED. ONE IS FOR THE ACUTE RENAL FAILURE (584.#), AND ONE IS FOR THE HYPERTENSIVE RENAL DISEASE.

584.# RENAL DISEASE WITH ACUTE NON-HYPERTENSIVE RENAL FAILURE **[403.##]**

4th Digit: 584
- **5. WITH TUBULAR NECROSIS**
- **6. RENAL CORTICAL NECROSIS**
- **7. MEDULLARY (PAPILLARY) NECROSIS**
- **8. SPECIFIED PATHOLOGICAL LESION**
- **9. RENAL FAILURE UNSPECIFIED**

4th Digit: 403
- **0. MALIGNANT**
- **1. BENIGN**
- **9. NOS**

5th Digit: 403
- **0. WITHOUT RENAL FAILURE**
- **1. WITH RENAL FAILURE**

362.11 RETINOPATHY

HYPERTENSION AND HEART DISEASE: UNLESS THE CAUSE OF THE HEART DISEASE IS STATED AS "DUE TO HYPERTENSION", "HYPERTENSIVE HEART DISEASE", OR "HYPERTENSIVE CARDIOVIASCULAR DISEASE" DO NOT ASSUME A CAUSE AND EFFECT RELATIONSHIP. CODE THE CONDITIONS SEPARATELY. EXAMPLE: CHF - 428.0, HYPERTENSION - 401.9.

780.6 HYPERTHERMIA NOS
995.86 HYPERTHERMIA MALIGNANT (DUE TO ANESTHESIA)
909.9 HYPERTHERMIA MALIGNANT DUE TO ANESTHESIA - LATE EFFECT
778.4 HYPERTHERMIA NEWBORN
301.11 HYPERTHYMIC PERSONALITY DISORDER
254.8 HYPERTHYMISM

242.## HYPERTHYROIDISM

4th Digit: 242
- **0. DIFFUSE**
- **1. UNINODULAR**
- **2. MULTINODULAR**
- **3. NODULAR UNSPECIFIED**
- **4. ECTOPIC THYROID NODULAR**
- **8. OTHER SPECIFIED**
- **9. NOS**

5th Digit: 242
- **0. WITHOUT MENTION OF THYROTOXIC CRISIS OR STORM**
- **1. WITH MENTION OF THYROTOXIC CRISIS OR STORM**

775.3 HYPERTHYROIDISM NEONATAL
763.7 HYPERTONIC LABOR AFFECTING FETUS OR NEWBORN
661.4# HYPERTONIC UTERINE CONTRACTIONS (INCOORDINATE) OR (PROLONGED)

5th Digit: 661.4

0. EPISODE OF CARE NOS OR N/A
1. DELIVERED
3. ANTEPARTUM COMPLICATION

596.51 HYPERTONICITY BLADDER
0 HYPERTONICITY BLADDER WITH INCONTINENCE SEE 'BLADDER DISORDERS WITH INCONTINENCE'
728.85 HYPERTONICITY MUSCLE
779.8 HYPERTONICITY NEWBORN
776.4 HYPERTRANSFUSION SYNDROME, NEWBORN

HYPERTRICHOSIS
704.1 NOS
757.4 CONGENITAL
374.54 EYELID

272.1 HYPERTRIGLYCERIDEMIA, ESSENTIAL
701.4 HYPERTROPHIC SCAR
569.49 HYPERTROPHY ANAL PAPILLAE
729.31 HYPERTROPHY FAT PAD KNEE
599.89 HYPERTROPHY VERUMONTANUM
270.2 HYPERTYROSINEMIA AMINO ACID METABOLISM (AROMATIC) DISTURBANCES
790.6 HYPERURICEMIA
270.3 HYPERVALINEMIA

HYPERVENTILATION
786.01 NOS
306.1 PSYCHOGENIC
306.1 SYNDROME, PSYCHOGENIC

273.3 HYPERVISCOSITY SYNDROME (OF SERUM)
289.0 HYPERVISCOSITY SYNDROME (OF SERUM) POLYCYTHEMIC
282.8 HYPERVISCOSITY SYNDROME (OF SERUM) SCLEROTHYMIC

HYPERVITAMINOSIS
278.2 A
963.5 A DUE TO POISONING
278.4 D
963.5 D DUE TO POISONING
278.8 NEC

276.6 HYPERVOLEMIA
364.41 HYPHEMA
273.8 HYPOALBUMINEMIA
272.5 HYPOALPHALIPOPROTEINEMIA
993.2 HYPOBAROPATHY
909.4 HYPOBAROPATHY LATE EFFECT
272.5 HYPOBETALIPOPROTEINEMIA (FAMILIAL)

HYPOCALCEMIA
275.41 NOS
775.4 COW'S MILK NEWBORN
269.3 DIETARY
775.4 NEWBORN
775.4 PHOSPHATE-LOADING NEONATAL

276.9 HYPOCHLOREMIA
536.8 HYPOCHLORHYDRIA STOMACH
300.7 HYPOCHONDRIASIS
782.0 HYPOESTHESIA
280.9 HYPOFERREMIA
280.0 HYPOFERREMIA DUE TO BLOOD LOSS CHRONIC
286.6 HYPOFIBRINOGENEMIA
286.3 HYPOFIBRINOGENEMIA CONGENITAL

HYPOGAMMAGLOBULINEMIA
279.00 UNSPECIFIED
279.06 ACQUIRED PRIMARY
279.06 CONGENITAL
279.04 CONGENITAL SEX-LINKED
279.09 INFANCY TRANSIENT
279.06 SPORADIC

HYPOGASTRIC
902.51 ARTERY INJURY
908.4 ARTERY INJURY LATE EFFECT
902.51 ARTERY LACERATION (RUPTURE) (HEMATOMA) (AVULSION) (ANEURYSM) TRAUMATIC
908.4 ARTERY LACERATION LATE EFFECT
908.4 BLOOD VESSELS OTHER INJURY LATE EFFECT
902.52 VEIN INJURY
908.4 VEIN INJURY LATE EFFECT

352.5 HYPOGLOSSAL NERVE ATROPHY
352.5 HYPOGLOSSAL NERVE DISORDERS
951.7 HYPOGLOSSAL NERVE INJURY

HYPOGLYCEMIA
251.2 NOS
251.0 ADMINISTERED INSULIN OR ORAL AGENT
250.8# DIABETIC
250.3# DIABETIC COMA

5th Digit: 250.3, 8

0. TYPE II, ADULT-ONSET, NON-INSULIN DEPENDENT (EVEN IF REQUIRING INSULIN), OR UNSPECIFIED; CONTROLLED
1. TYPE I, JUVENILE-ONSET OR INSULIN-DEPENDENT; CONTROLLED
2. TYPE II, ADULT-ONSET, NON-INSULIN DEPENDENT (EVEN IF REQUIRING INSULIN); UNCONTROLLED
3. TYPE I, JUVENILE-ONSET OR INSULIN-DEPENDENT; UNCONTROLLED

V65.3 DIETARY COUNSELING AND SURVEILLANCE
251.2 FAMILIAL IDIOPATHIC
579.3 FOLLOWING GI SURGERY
251.1 HYPERINSULINISM (ECTOPIC) (FUNCTIONAL)
251.1 HYPERPLASTIC PANCREATIC ISLET BETA CELLS
251.0 IATROGENIC
270.3 LEUCINE INDUCED
775.6 NEONATAL
775.0 NEONATAL CAUSED BY MATERNAL DIABETES
251.2 REACTIVE
251.2 REACTIVE SPONTANEOUS OR DUE TO DIABETES TREATMENT
251.2 SYNDROME (FAMILIAL) (NEONATAL)
251.1 SYNDROME FUNCTIONAL (FAMILIAL) (NEONATAL)
962.3 THERAPEUTIC MISADVENTURE
251.0 WITH COMA (IATROGENIC)
251.1 OTHER SPECIFIED NEC

HYPOGONADISM
256.3 FEMALE
253.4 GONADOTROPIC (ISOLATED)
253.4 HYPOGONADOTROPIC WITH ANOSMIA
257.2 MALE
256.3 OVARIAN
253.4 PITUITARY (SECONDARY)
257.2 TESTICULAR

705.0 HYPOHIDROSIS
251.3 HYPOINSULINEMIA POSTSURGICAL
276.8 HYPOKALEMIA (SYNDROME)
588.8 HYPOKALEMIA RENAL
359.3 HYPOKALEMIC FAMILIAL PERIODIC PARALYSIS
588.8 HYPOKALEMIC NEPHROPATHY
272.5 HYPOLIPOPROTEINEMIA
275.2 HYPOMAGNESEMIA
775.4 HYPOMAGNESEMIA NEWBORN

HYPOMANIA

301.11 HYPOMANIC PERSONALITY DISORDER CHRONIC
296.0# MILD
296.0# SINGLE EPISODE
296.1# RECURRENT
296.4# CIRCULAR

5th Digit: 296.0-1, 4

1. MILD
2. MODERATE
3. SEVERE WITHOUT MENTION OF PSYCHOTIC BEHAVIOR
4. SEVERE SPECIFIED AS WITH PSYCHOTIC BEHAVIOR
5. IN PARTIAL OR NOS REMISSION
6. IN FULL REMISSION

626.1 HYPOMENORRHEA
783.9 HYPOMETABOLISM
784.49 HYPONASALITY
276.1 HYPONATREMIA SODIUM [NA] DEFICIENCY
252.1 HYPOPARATHYROIDISM
775.4 HYPOPARATHYROIDISM TRANSIENT NEONATAL
275.3 HYPOPHOSPHATASIA
275.3 HYPOPHOSPHATEMIA FAMILIAL
433.8# HYPOPHYSEAL ARTERY OBSTRUCTION OR OCCLUSION (THROMBOSIS)

5th Digit: 433.8

0. WITHOUT CEREBRAL INFARCTION
1. WITH CEREBRAL INFARCTION

253.8 HYPOPHYSEAL SYNDROME
253.8 HYPOPHYSEOTHALAMIC SYNDROME
253.9 HYPOPHYSIS DISORDER
253.1 HYPOPHYSIS HYPERFUNCTION
253.2 HYPOPHYSIS HYPOFUNCTION
709.00 HYPOPIGMENTATION

HYPOPITUITARISM

253.2 NOS
253.7 HORMONE INDUCED
253.7 HYPOPHYSECTOMY-INDUCED
253.7 POSTABLATIVE
253.7 POSTSURGICAL
253.7 RADIOTHERAPY INDUCED
253.2 SYNDROME

0 HYPOPLASIA / HYPOPLASTIC SEE ANATOMICAL SITE
746.7 HYPOPLASTIC LEFT HEART SYNDROME
276.8 HYPOPOTASSEMIA SYNDROME
286.3 HYPOPROCONVERTINEMIA
273.8 HYPOPROTEINEMIA
286.7 HYPOPROTHROMBINEMIA ACQUIRED
364.05 HYPOPYON
370.04 HYPOPYON ULCER (CORNEAL)
790.99 HYPORENINISM EXTREME
288.2 HYPOSEGMENTATION LEUKOCYTES HEREDITARY
307.42 HYPOSOMNIA PERSISTENT ASSOCIATED WITH EMOTIONAL REACTIONS OR CONFLICTS
307.41 HYPOSOMNIA TRANSIENT ASSOCIATED WITH EMOTIONAL REACTIONS OR CONFLICTS
276.1 HYPOSOMOLALITY AND/OR HYPONATREMIA (SYNDROME)
753.8 HYPOSPADIAS CONGENITAL - FEMALE
V13.61 HYPOSPADIAS CONGENITAL - HISTORY
752.61 HYPOSPADIAS CONGENITAL - MALE
606.1 HYPOSPERMATOGENESIS
372.72 HYPOSPHAGMA
246.8 HYPO-TBG-NEMIA

HYPOTENSION

458.9 NOS
458.1 CHRONIC
458.2 IATROGENIC

> *648.9#: USE AN ADDITIONAL CODE TO IDENTIFY THE SPECIFIC TYPE OF HYPOTENSION.*

648.9# MATERNAL CURRENT (CO-EXISTENT) IN PREGNANCY

5th Digit: 648.9

0. EPISODE OF NOS OR N/A
1. DELIVERED
2. DELIVERED WITH POSTPARTUM COMPLICATION
3. ANTEPARTUM COMPLICATION
4. POSTPARTUM COMPLICATION

669.2# MATERNAL SYNDROME

5th Digit: 669.2

0. EPISODE OF CARE NOS OR N/A
1. DELIVERED
2. DELIVERED WITH POSTPARTUM COMPLICATION
3. ANTEPARTUM COMPLICATION
4. POSTPARTUM COMPLICATION

458.0 ORTHOSTATIC
333.0 ORTHOSTATIC WITH PARKINSONIAN SYNDROME IDIOPATHIC
333.0 ORTHOSTATIC WITH PARKINSONIAN SYNDROME SYMPTOMATIC
458.1 PERMANENT IDIOPATHIC
458.2 POSTOPERATIVE
458.0 POSTURAL
458.8 OTHER SPECIFIED

HYPOTHERMIA

780.9 NOS
991.6 ACCIDENTAL
909.4 ACCIDENTAL LATE EFFECT
995.89 DUE TO ANESTHESIA
909.9 DUE TO ANESTHESIA LATE EFFECT
778.3 NEWBORN OTHER
780.9 NOT ASSOCIATED WITH LOW ENVIRONMENTAL TEMPERATURE

HYPOTHYROIDISM

244.9 NOS
244.8 ACQUIRED OTHER SPECIFIED
243 CONGENITAL
246.1 CONGENITAL DYSHORMONOGENIC GOITER
244.3 IATROGENIC
244.0 POSTSURGICAL
244.0 POSTSURGICAL WITH MYOPATHY [359.5]
244.1 POST IRRADIATION
244.2 RESULTING FROM ADMINISTRATION OR INGESTION OF IODIDE
244.8 SECONDARY NEC

301.12 HYPOTHYMIC PERSONALITY DISORDER
781.3 HYPOTONIA
779.8 HYPOTONIA AFFECTING FETUS OR NEWBORN
759.81 HYPOTONIA-HYPOMENTIA-HYPOGONADISM-OBESITY SYNDROME
728.9 HYPOTONIA MUSCLE

HYPOTONIC UTERINE DYSFUNCTION

763.7 AFFECTING FETUS OR NEWBORN
661.0# PRIMARY
661.1# SECONDARY
661.2# OTHER AND UNSPECIFIED

5th Digit: 661.0-2

0. EPISODE OF CARE NOS OR N/A
1. DELIVERED
3. ANTEPARTUM COMPLICATION

H

HYPOTONY

360.34 EYE ANTERIOR CHAMBER FLAT (POSTINFLAMMATORY) (POST OP) (POSTTRAUMATIC)
360.33 EYE ASSOCIATED WITH OTHER OCULAR DISORDERS
360.32 EYE DUE TO OCULAR FISTULA (POSTINFLAMMATORY) (POST OP) (POSTTRAUMATIC)
360.32 EYE FOLLOWING LOSS OF AQUEOUS OR VITREOUS
360.30 EYE NOS (POSTINFLAMMATORY) (POST OP) (POSTTRAUMATIC)
360.31 EYE PRIMARY (POSTINFLAMMATORY) (POST OP) (POSTTRAUMATIC)

704.09 HYPOTRICHOSIS
704.09 HYPOTRICHOSIS POSTINFECTION
378.32 HYPOTROPIA
786.09 HYPOVENTILATION
264.9 HYPOVITAMINOSIS A NOS

HYPOVOLEMIA

276.5 DEHYDRATION
998.0 POSTOPERATIVE
958.4 TRAUMATIC
908.6 TRAUMATIC LATE EFFECT

277.2 HYPOXANTHINE GUANINE PHOSPHORIBOSYLTRANSFERASE DEFICIENCY [HG PRT DEFICIENCY]

799.0 HYPOXEMIA

HYPOXIA

799.0 NOS
768.9 BIRTH - UNSPECIFIED
768.6 BIRTH - MILD
768.6 BIRTH - MODERATE
768.5 BIRTH - SEVERE
768.5 BIRTH - SEVERE WITH NEUROLOGIC INVOLVEMENT
348.1 CEREBRAL
997.01 CEREBRAL RESULTING FROM A PROCEDURE
770.8 FETAL
993.2 HIGH ALTITUDE
909.4 HIGH ALTITUDE LATE EFFECT
0 INTRAUTERINE SEE 'FETAL', DISTRESS
770.8 NEWBORN

V45.89 HYSTERECTOMY STATUS

300.10 HYSTERIA
300.11 HYSTERIA CONVERSION
301.50 HYSTERICAL PERSONALITY
300.11 HYSTERICAL TETANY

272.7 I CELL DISEASE
255.0 IATROGENIC SYNDROME OF EXCESS CORTISOL
049.8 ICELAND DISEASE (EPIDEMIC NEUROMYASTHENIA)
286.6 ICF SYNDROME (INTRAVASCULAR COAGULATION-FIBRINOLYSIS)
701.1 ICHTHYOSIS
757.1 ICHTHYOSIS CONGENITAL

ICTERUS
782.4 NOS
646.7# GRAVIS OF PREGNANCY
5th Digit: 646.7
0. EPISODE OF CARE NOS OR N/A
1. DELIVERED
3. ANTEPARTUM COMPLICATION

774.6 NEONATORUM
576.8 OBSTRUCTION
751.61 OBSTRUCTION CONGENITAL

992.0 ICTUS SOLARIS
909.4 ICTUS SOLARIS LATE EFFECT

692.89 ID REACTION
0 IDDM (INSULIN DEPENDENT DIABETES MELLITUS) SEE 'DIABETES'
0 IDENTITY CRISIS SEE 'IDENTITY DISORDER'

IDENTITY DISORDER
313.82 NOS
300.14 DISSOCIATIVE
313.82 EMOTIONAL DISTURBANCE CHILDHOOD OR ADOLESCENCE
302.85 GENDER - ADULT
302.6 GENDER - CHILDHOOD
302.85 PSYCHOSEXUAL - ADULT
302.6 PSYCHOSEXUAL - CHILDHOOD

IDIOPATHIC
769 CARDIORESPIRATORY DISTRESS SYNDROME, NEWBORN
516.3 FIBROSING ALVEOLITIS
425.1 HYPERTROPHIC SUBAORTIC STENOSIS
425.2 MURAL CARDIOMYOPATHY
581.9 NEPHROTIC SYNDROME (INFANTILE)
337.0 PERIPHERAL AUTONOMIC NEUROPATHY
356.4 PROGRESSIVE POLYNEUROPATHY
275.0 PULMONARY HEMOSIDEROSIS [516.1]
769 RESPIRATORY DISTRESS SYNDROME NEWBORN
593.4 RETROPERITONEAL FIBROSIS
579.0 STEATORRHEA
238.7 THROMBOCYTHEMIA SITE NOS
0 THROMBOCYTHEMIA SITE SPECIFIED SEE 'NEOPLASM UNCERTAIN BEHAVIOR' BY SITE M9962/1
287.3 THROMBOCYTOPENIC PURPURA
333.6 TORSION DYSTONIA

318.2 IDIOT IQ LESS THAN 20
279.01 IGA SELECTIVE IMMUNODEFICIENCY
279.03 IGG OTHER SELECTIVE IMMUNOGLOBULIN DEFICIENCY
279.02 IGM IMMUNODEFICIENCY SELECTIVE
279.05 IGM INCREASED IMMUNODEFICIENCY

IHD (ISCHEMIC HEART DISEASE)
414.9 NOS
0 ACUTE, WITH MI SEE 'MI ACUTE'
411.89 ACUTE, WITHOUT MI
411.81 ACUTE, WITHOUT MI, WITH CORONARY (ARTERY) OCCLUSION
411.89 ACUTE SUBENDOCARDIAL
414.10 ANEURYSM (MURAL) (VENTRICULAR)
414.11 ANEURYSM CORONARY VESSELS
414.19 ANEURYSM OTHER

IHD (ISCHEMIC HEART DISEASE) (continued)
414.0# ARTERIOSCLEROTIC
5th Digit: 414.0
0. UNSPECIFIED TYPE OF VESSEL, NATIVE OR GRAFT
1. NATIVE CORONARY VESSEL
2. AUTOLOGOUS VEIN BYPASS GRAFT
3. NONAUTOLOGOUS BIOLOGICAL BYPASS GRAFT
4. AUTOLOGOUS ARTERY BYPASS GRAFT (GASTROEPIPLOIC) (INTERNAL MAMMARY)
5. UNSPECIFIED TYPE OF BYPASS GRAFT

414.9 CHRONIC
414.1# CHRONIC - ANEURYSM
5th Digit: 414.1
0. HEART WALL
1. CORONARY VESSELS (ARTERIOVENOUS)
9. OTHER

414.0# CHRONIC - ARTERIOSCLEROTIC
5th Digit: 414.0
0. UNSPECIFIED TYPE OF VESSEL, NATIVE OR GRAFT
1. NATIVE CORONARY VESSEL
2. AUTOLOGOUS VEIN BYPASS GRAFT
3. NONAUTOLOGOUS BIOLOGICAL BYPASS GRAFT
4. AUTOLOGOUS ARTERY BYPASS GRAFT (GASTROEPIPLOIC) (INTERNAL MAMMARY)
5. UNSPECIFIED TYPE OF BYPASS GRAFT

414.8 CHRONIC - MYOCARDIAL
414.8 CHRONIC - OTHER
411.89 CORONARY INSUFFICIENCY ACUTE
V17.3 FAMILY HISTORY
411.89 SUBACUTE
411.89 OTHER SPECIFIED - ACUTE
414.8 OTHER SPECIFIED - CHRONIC

425.1 IHSS (IDIOPATHIC HYPERTROPHIC SUBAORTIC STENOSIS)

558.9 ILEITIS NONINFECTIOUS (ALLERGIC) (DIETARY)
558.9 ILEITIS NONINFECTIOUS (OTHER AND NOS)
555.0 ILEITIS REGIONAL (SEGMENTAL) (TERMINAL)
560.9 ILEOCECAL COIL OBSTRUCTION (SEE ALSO 'INTESTINE, INTESTINAL', OBSTRUCTION)
564.89 ILEOCECAL COIL STASIS
902.26 ILEO-COLIC ARTERY INJURY
908.4 ILEO-COLIC ARTERY INJURY LATE EFFECT
902.31 ILEO-COLIC VEIN INJURY
908.4 ILEO-COLIC VEIN INJURY LATE EFFECT
556.1 ILEOCOLITIS ULCERATIVE (CHRONIC)

ILEOSTOMY
V53.5 BELT FITTING AND ADJUSTMENT
V55.2 CARE
V55.2 CATHETER ADJUSTMENT OR REPOSITIONING
V55.2 CATHETER REMOVAL OR REPLACEMENT
V55.2 CLOSURE
569.60 COMPLICATION - NOS
569.62 COMPLICATION - MECHANICAL
569.69 COMPLICATION - OTHER
569.69 FISTULA
569.69 HERNIA

I-J-K

I-J-K

ILEOSTOMY (continued)

> *WHEN CODING AN INFECTION OF AN OSTOMY, USE AN ADDITIONAL CODE TO SPECIFY THE ORGANISM. SEE 'BACTERIAL INFECTION'*

569.61 INFECTION
569.61 INFECTION WITH CELLULITIS OF ABDOMEN [682.2]
569.61 INFECTION WITH SEPSIS [038.#(#)]

4th or 4th and 5th Digit Code for Organism: 038

- .9 NOS
- .3 ANAEROBIC
- .3 BACTEROIDES
- .3 CLOSTRIDIUM
- .42 E COLI
- .49 ENTEROBACTER AEROGENES
- .40 GRAM NEGATIVE
- .49 GRAM NEGATIVE OTHER
- .41 HEMOPHILUS INFLUENZAE
- .2 PNEUMOCOCCAL
- .49 PROTEUS
- .43 PSEUDOMONAS
- .44 SERRATIA
- .10 STAPHYLOCOCCAL NOS
- .11 STAPHYLOCOCCAL AUREUS
- .19 STAPHYLOCOCCAL OTHER
- .0 STREPTOCOCCAL (ANAEROBIC)
- .49 YERSINIA ENTEROCOLITICA
- .8 OTHER SPECIFIED

569.62 MALFUNCTION
569.69 PROLAPSE
V44.3 STATUS
V55.3 TOILET STOMA

ILEUM, ILEAL

V45.72 ABSENCE POSTSURGICAL
751.1 ATRESIA (ABSENCE) CONGENITAL
564.89 DILATATION
306.4 DILATATION PSYCHOGENIC
562.00 DIVERTICULA
863.29 INJURY (TRAUMATIC)
863.39 INJURY (TRAUMATIC) WITH OPEN WOUND
564.89 IRRITABILITY
560.9 OBSTRUCTION (SEE ALSO 'INTESTINE, INTESTINAL', OBSTRUCTION)
569.83 PERFORATION
211.3 POLYP
564.89 STASIS

ILEUS

560.1 ADYNAMIC
537.2 CHRONIC DUODENAL
560.31 GALLSTONE
751.3 HIRSCHSPRUNG'S
777.1 MECONIUM
277.01 MECONIUM DUE TO CYSTIC FIBROSIS
564.89 MYXEDEMA
777.4 NEWBORN TRANSITORY
560.1 PARALYTIC
997.4 POSTOPERATIVE

062.8 ILHEUS VIRAL ENCEPHALITIS

> *INJURY OF A BLOOD VESSEL CAN BE A LACERATION, A-V FISTULA, ANEURYSM, OR HEMATOMA. USE THE "INJURY" CODE FOUND BY ANATOMICAL SITE (THE NAME OF THE BLOOD VESSEL).*

ILIAC

444.81 ARTERY (EMBOLISM) (THROMBOSIS) (OCCLUSION) (INFARCTION)
902.53 ARTERY INJURY
902.59 ARTERY INJURY SPECIFIED BRANCH NEC
908.4 ARTERY INJURY OR LACERATION LATE EFFECT
902.53 ARTERY LACERATION (RUPTURE) (HEMATOMA) (AVULSION) (ANEURYSM) TRAUMATIC

ILIAC (continued)

902.59 BLOOD VESSELS OTHER INJURY
908.4 BLOOD VESSELS OTHER INJURY LATE EFFECT
726.5 BONE SPUR
902.54 VEIN INJURY
902.54 VEIN LACERATION (RUPTURE) (HEMATOMA) (AVULSION) (ANEURYSM) TRAUMATIC
908.4 VEIN INJURY OR LACERATION LATE EFFECT
902.50 VESSEL INJURY VESSEL UNSPECIFIED (ANEURYSM) TRAUMATIC
908.4 VESSEL OTHER INJURY LATE EFFECT

444.81 ILIOFEMORAL ARTERY OBSTRUCTION
843.0 ILIOFEMORAL STRAIN (SPRAIN) (AVULSION) (HEMARTHROSIS) (SEPARATION)

355.79 ILIOHYPOGASTRIC MONONEUROPATHY
355.79 ILIOHYPOGASTRIC NERVE COMPRESSION (ENTRAPMENT)
355.79 ILIOHYPOGASTRIC NERVE DISORDER (LESION)

355.79 ILIOINGUINAL MONONEUROPATHY
355.79 ILIOINGUINAL NERVE COMPRESSION (ENTRAPMENT)
355.79 ILIOINGUINAL NERVE DISORDER (LESION)
355.79 ILIOINGUINAL NEURITIS

728.89 ILIOTIBIAL BAND FRICTION SYNDROME
V61.6 ILLEGITIMACY CAUSING FAMILY PROBLEM (REASON FOR ENCOUNTER)

318.0 IMBECILE
281.1 IMERSLUND GRASBECK SYNDROME (ANEMIA DUE TO FAMILIAL SELECTIVE VITAMIN B-12 MALABSORPTION)
270.5 IMIDAZOLE AMINO ACID DISORDER
270.8 IMIDOGLYCINURIA FAMILIAL
270.8 IMINOACIDOPATHY
301.89 IMMATURE PERSONALITY DISORDER
994.1 IMMERSION (NON FATAL DROWNING)
909.4 IMMERSION (NON FATAL DROWNING) LATE EFFECT
991.4 IMMERSION FOOT
728.3 IMMOBILITY SYNDROME

IMMUNE

279.3 DEFICIENCY
279.10 DISORDER CELL MEDIATED DEFICIENCY UNSPECIFIED
279.19 DISORDER CELL MEDIATED DEFICIENCY OTHER SPECIFIED NEC
V12.2 DISORDER HISTORY
V77.9 DISORDERS SCREENING
279.9 MECHANISM DISORDER
279.8 MECHANISM DISORDER SPECIFIED NEC
V07.2 SERA [GAMMA GLOBULIN] PROPHYLACTIC ADMINISTRATION
760.79 SERA TRANSMITTED VIA PLACENTA OR BREAST MILK AFFECTING FETUS OR NEWBORN

279.2 IMMUNITY DEFICIENCY SYNDROME, COMBINED
0 IMMUNIZATION SEE 'VACCINATION'

IMMUNODEFICIENCY

279.3 NOS
279.2 AGAMMAGLOBULINEMIA AUTOSOMAL RECESSIVE
279.04 AGAMMAGLOBULINEMIA BRUTON'S TYPE
279.2 AGAMMAGLOBULINEMIA SWISS-TYPE
279.04 AGAMMAGLOBULINEMIA X-LINKED
279.2 AGAMMAGLOBULINEMIA X-LINKED RECESSIVE
279.2 APLASIA OR DYSPLASIA
334.8 ATAXIA TELANGIECTASIA (LOUIS-BAR)
279.2 AUTOSOMAL RECESSIVE SWISS-TYPE
279.00 B-CELL
279.13 CELLULAR WITH ABNORMAL IMMUNOGLOBULIN DEFICIENCY
279.2 COMBINED SEVERE
279.8 COMPLEMENT C1-C9 DEFICIENCY
279.06 DYSGAMMAGLOBULINEMIA ACQUIRED (CONGENITAL) (PRIMARY)

IMMUNODEFICIENCY (continued)

0 HUMAN VIRUS SEE 'HIV' INFECTION
279.00 HYPOGAMMAGLOBULINEMIA
279.06 HYPOGAMMAGLOBULINEMIA ACQUIRED PRIMARY
279.06 HYPOGAMMAGLOBULINEMIA CONGENITAL
279.04 HYPOGAMMAGLOBULINEMIA CONGENITAL SEX-LINKED
279.09 HYPOGAMMAGLOBULINEMIA INFANCY TRANSIENT
279.06 HYPOGAMMAGLOBULINEMIA SPORADIC
279.01 IGA SELECTIVE
279.03 IGG
279.05 IGM INCREASED
279.02 IGM SELECTIVE
279.9 IMMUNE MECHANISM DISORDER
279.19 OTHER CELL MEDIATED DEFICIENCY
334.8 OTHER CELL MEDIATED DEFICIENCY CAUSING ATAXIA TELANGIECTASIA
279.2 SYNDROME COMBINED
279.10 T-CELL
279.2 THYMIC
279.05 WITH HYPER IGM AUTOSOMAL RECESSIVE
279.05 WITH HYPER IGM X-LINKED

795.79 IMMUNOGLOBULINS ELEVATED

795.79 IMMUNOLOGICAL FINDINGS ABNORMAL OTHER AND UNSPECIFIED

203.8# IMMUNOPROLIFERATIVE NEOPLASM OTHER

203.1# IMMUNOPROLIFERATIVE PLASMA CELL LEUKEMIA

5th Digit: 203.1, 8

0. WITHOUT MENTION OF REMISSION
1. IN REMISSION

380.4 IMPACTED CERUMEN

560.30 IMPACTION COLON
560.39 IMPACTION FECAL
560.30 IMPACTION INTESTINE

411.1 IMPENDING CORONARY SYNDROME
752.42 IMPERFORATE HYMEN CONGENITAL

IMPETIGO

684 NOS
684 BULLOUS
684 CIRCINATE
684 EAR (EXTERNAL) [380.13]
684 EYELID [373.5]
694.3 HERPETIFORMIS
684 NEONATORUM
684 PINNA [380.13]
684 SIMPLEX
686.8 ULCERATIVE
684 VULGARIS

726.2 IMPINGEMENT SHOULDER SYNDROME
724.4 IMPINGEMENT VERTEBRAL BODIES SYNDROME

IMPOTENCE

250.6# DIABETIC (DUE TO PERIPHERAL NEUROPATHY) [607.84]
250.7# DIABETIC PERIPHERAL (DUE TO VASCULAR DISEASE) [607.84]

5th Digit: 250.6-7

0. TYPE II, ADULT-ONSET, NON-INSULIN DEPENDENT (EVEN IF REQUIRING INSULIN), OR UNSPECIFIED; CONTROLLED
1. TYPE I, JUVENILE-ONSET OR INSULIN-DEPENDENT; CONTROLLED
2. TYPE II, ADULT-ONSET, NON-INSULIN DEPENDENT (EVEN IF REQUIRING INSULIN); UNCONTROLLED
3. TYPE I, JUVENILE-ONSET OR INSULIN-DEPENDENT; UNCONTROLLED

607.84 ORGANIC
997.99 ORGANIC POSTPROSTATECTOMY [607.84]
302.72 PSYCHOSEXUAL

V62.5 IMPRISONMENT
312.30 IMPULSE CONTROL DISORDER

INANITION

263.9 INANITION
994.2 DUE TO DEPRIVATION OF FOOD
263.9 DUE TO MALNUTRITION
780.6 FEVER

253.6 INAPPROPRIATE ADH (SYNDROME)

V68.0 INCAPACITY CERTIFICATE ISSUE

654.3# INCARCERATED UTERUS RETROVERTED COMPLICATING CHILDBIRTH

5th Digit: 654.3

0. EPISODE OF CARE NOS OR N/A
1. DELIVERED
2. DELIVERED WITH POSTPARTUM COMPLICATION
3. ANTEPARTUM COMPLICATION
4. POSTPARTUM COMPLICATION

526.1 INCISOR CANAL CYST

077.0 INCLUSION CONJUNCTIVITIS
078.5 INCLUSION DISEASE
078.5 INCLUSION DISEASE SALIVARY GLAND

761.0 INCOMPETENT CERVIX AFFECTING FETUS OR NEWBORN
756.0 INCOMPLETE MANDIBULOFACIAL SYNDROME

WHEN CODING URINARY INCONTINENCE, CODE THE UNDERLYING CAUSE OF THE INCONTINENCE, SUCH AS THE CYSTOCELE, RECTOCELE, PROSTATITIS, BLADDER DISORDERS, ETC.) THE CAUSE WOULD BE SEQUENCED FIRST. THE INCONTINENCE WOULD BE SEQUENCED SECOND.

INCONTINENCE

787.6 FECAL
787.6 SPHINCTER ANI
599.84 URETHRAL SPHINCTER
788.30 URINE NOS
788.37 URINE - CONTINUOUS LEAKAGE
788.30 URINE - MALE, NOS
788.39 URINE - NEUROGENIC
788.36 URINE - NOCTURNAL ENURESIS
788.39 URINE - OVERFLOW
788.39 URINE - PARADOXICAL
788.35 URINE - POST-VOID DRIBBLING
625.6 URINE - STRESS, FEMALE
788.32 URINE - STRESS, MALE
788.33 URINE - URGE AND STRESS MIXED (MALE) (FEMALE)
788.31 URINE - URGE INCONTINENCE
788.34 URINE - WITHOUT SENSORY AWARENESS
788.39 URINE - SPECIFIED NEC
788.39 URINE OTHER
0 WITH BLADDER DISORDERS SEE 'BLADDER DISORDERS WITH INCONTINENCE'
0 WITH URETHRAL DISORDERS SEE 'URETHRA, URETHRAL DISORDERS WITH INCONTINENCE'
0 WITH URINARY OBSTRUCTION SEE 'URINARY' OBSTRUCTION WITH INCONTINENCE

781.3 INCOORDINATION MUSCULAR

385.24 INCUS ABSENCE
744.04 INCUS ABSENCE CONGENITAL

082.1 INDIAN TICK TYPHUS
270.2 INDICANURIA AMINO ACID METABOLISM AROMATIC DISTURBANCES
536.8 INDIGESTION

791.9 INDOLACETIC ACID ELEVATED ABNORMAL
791.9 INDOLACETIC ACID URINARY ELEVATION
099.8 INDOLENT BUBO

I-J-K

763.89 INDUCTION OF LABOR (MEDICAL) AFFECTING FETUS OR NEWBORN
607.81 INDURATIO PENIS PLASTICA
782.8 INDURATION SKIN
305.0# INEBRIETY NOS

5th Digit: 305.0

0. NOS
1. CONTINUOUS
2. EPISODIC
3. IN REMISSION

INFANT

798.0 DEATH SUDDEN SYNDROME (SIDS)
0 DEATH SUDDEN SYNDROME (SIDS) NEAR MISS - CODE INDIVIDUAL SYMPTOM(S)
0 EVALUATION FOR SUSPECTED CONDITION NOT FOUND SEE 'OBSERVATION NEWBORN / INFANT SUSPECTED CONDITION (UNDIAGNOSED) (UNPROVEN) NOT FOUND'
766.1 HEAVY FOR DATES
766.0 LARGE EXCEPTIONALLY (BIRTHWEIGHT > 4500 GRAMS)
766.1 LARGE FOR DATES OTHER (REGARDLESS OF GESTATION)
0 LIGHT FOR DATES SEE 'LIGHT FOR DATES'
255.2 HERCULES SYNDROME
766.2 POST TERM (>42 WEEKS)

> *765.##: USE AN ADDITIONAL CODE IF NECESSARY, TO FURTHER SPECIFY THE CONDITION OF THE PREMATURE INFANT.*

PREMATURE

765.10 >28 WEEKS AND/OR WEIGHT UNSPECIFIED
765.14 >28 WEEKS AND/OR 1000-1249 GRAMS
765.15 >28 WEEKS AND/OR 1250-1499 GRAMS
765.16 >28 WEEKS AND/OR 1500-1749 GRAMS
765.17 >28 WEEKS AND/OR 1750-1999 GRAMS
765.18 >28 WEEKS AND/OR 2000-2499 GRAMS
765.19 >28 WEEKS AND/OR 2500 GRAMS AND OVER

PREMATURE EXTREME

765.00 <28 WEEKS AND/OR WEIGHT UNSPECIFIED
765.01 <28 WEEKS AND/OR LESS THAN 500 GRAMS
765.02 <28 WEEKS AND/OR 500-749 GRAMS
765.03 <28 WEEKS AND/OR 750-999 GRAMS

INFANT (continued)

995.55 SHAKEN SYNDROME
775.0 SYNDROME OF DIABETIC MOTHER

INFANTILE

261 ATROPHY (MALNUTRITION SEVERE)
288.0 GENETIC AGRANULOCYTOSIS
330.8 NECROTIZING ENCEPHALOMYELOPATHY
345.6# SPASMS

5th Digit: 345.6

0. WITHOUT MENTION OF INTRACTABLE EPILEPSY
1. WITH INTRACTABLE EPILEPSY

335.0 SPINAL MUSCULAR ATROPHY

259.9 INFANTILISM
253.3 INFANTILISM SYNDROME

INFARCTION

0 SEE ALSO SPECIFIED ORGAN
557.0 APPENDICES EPIPLOICAE
410.8# ATRIAL

5th Digit: 410.8

0. EPISODE NOS
1. INITIAL EPISODE
2. SUBSEQUENT EPISODE

557.0 BOWEL

INFARCTION (continued)

434.91 BRAIN STEM
434.11 BRAIN STEM EMBOLIC
V12.59 BRAIN STEM HISTORY WITHOUT RESIDUAL
997.02 BRAIN STEM IATROGENIC
997.02 BRAIN STEM POSTOPERATIVE
434.01 BRAIN STEM THROMBOTIC
0 BRAIN STEM WITH RESIDUAL SEE 'LATE EFFECT', CEREBROVASCULAR DISEASE
611.8 BREAST
434.91 CEREBELLUM
434.11 CEREBELLUM EMBOLIC
434.01 CEREBELLUM THROMBOTIC
434.91 CEREBRAL
434.11 CEREBRAL EMBOLIC
997.02 CEREBRAL POSTOPERATIVE
434.01 CEREBRAL THROMBOTIC
620.8 FALLOPIAN TUBE
575.8 GALLBLADDER
573.4 HEPATIC
415.19 LUNG
415.11 LUNG IATROGENIC
415.11 LUNG POSTOPERATIVE
457.8 LYMPHATIC
557.0 MESENTERIC
0 MYOCARDIAL SEE 'MYOCARDIAL INFARCTION ACUTE'
620.8 OVARY
577.8 PANCREAS
252.8 PARATHYROID
253.8 PITUITARY
762.2 PLACENTA AFFECTING FETUS OR NEWBORN
656.7# PLACENTA AFFECTING MANAGEMENT OF MOTHER

5th Digit: 656.7

0. EPISODE OF CARE NOS OR N/A
1. DELIVERED
3. ANTEPARTUM COMPLICATION

602.8 PROSTATE
415.19 PULMONARY
415.11 PULMONARY IATROGENIC
415.11 PULMONARY POSTOPERATIVE
593.81 RENAL
362.84 RETINAL
336.1 SPINAL CORD
289.59 SPLEEN
608.83 TESTICULAR
246.3 THYROID

> *WHEN CODING AN INFECTION, USE AN ADDITIONAL CODE, [041.#], TO IDENTIFY THE ORGANISM. SEE 'BACTERIAL INFECTION'.*

INFECTION

997.62 AMPUTATION STUMP (CHRONIC)
0 AMPUTATION STUMP ORIGINAL ADMISSION SEE 'AMPUTATION' BY SITE, 'TRAUMATIC COMPLICATED'
0 SEE ALSO ANATOMICAL SITE, ORGAN OR ORGANISM
0 BACTERIA SEE 'BACTERIAL INFECTION'
996.64 CATHETER (INDWELLING) (URINARY)
997.62 CHRONIC OF STUMP FOLLOWING AMPUTATION
0 COMPLICATION OF INTERNAL PROSTHESIS IMPLANT OR GRAFT SEE 'COMPLICATION OF AN INTERNAL PROSTHESIS IMPLANT OR GRAFT - INFECTION OR INFLAMMATION' BY SPECIFIED DEVICE
771.8 FETAL INTRA-AMNIOTIC
999.3 FOLLOWING INFUSION INJECTION TRANSFUSION OR VACCINATION

INFECTION (continued)

760.2 MATERNAL AFFECTING FETUS OR NEWBORN NOT MANIFESTED IN FETUS OR NEWBORN
647.9# MATERNAL CURRENT (CO-EXISTENT) IN PREGNANCY NOS
646.6# MATERNAL GENITOURINARY COMPLICATING PREGNANCY

5th Digit: 646.6, 647.9
0. EPISODE OF CARE NOS OR N/A
1. DELIVERED
2. DELIVERED WITH POSTPARTUM COMPLICATION
3. ANTEPARTUM COMPLICATION
4. POSTPARTUM COMPLICATION

760.1 MATERNAL RENAL OR URINARY AFFECTING FETUS OR NEWBORN
647.6# MATERNAL VIRAL CURRENT (CO-EXISTENT) IN PREGNANCY
647.8# MATERNAL OTHER SPECIFIED CURRENT (CO-EXISTENT) IN PREGNANCY

5th Digit: 647.6, 8
0. EPISODE OF CARE NOS OR N/A
1. DELIVERED
2. DELIVERED WITH POSTPARTUM COMPLICATION
3. ANTEPARTUM COMPLICATION
4. POSTPARTUM COMPLICATION

771.4 NAVEL CORD OR PERINATAL
0 OSTOMY SEE SPECIFIED OSTOMY
771.8 PERINATAL OTHER
998.59 POSTOPERATIVE
998.51 POSTOPERATIVE SEROMA
771.4 UMBILICAL STUMP
079.#(#) VIRAL AND CHLAMYDIAL IN CONDITIONS CLASSIFIED ELSEWHERE, SITE NOS

4th or 4th <u>and</u> 5th Digit: 079
0. ADENOVIRUS
1. ECHO VIRUS
2. COXSACKIE VIRUS
3. RHINOVIRUS
6. RESPIRATORY SYNCYTIAL VIRUS (RSV)
8#. OTHER SPECIFIED VIRAL AND CHLAMYDIAL
88. OTHER SPECIFIED CHLAMYDIAL
89. OTHER SPECIFIED VIRAL
9#. UNSPECIFIED VIRAL AND CHLAMYDIAL
98. UNSPECIFIED CHLAMYDIAL
99. UNSPECIFIED VIRAL

0 SEE ALSO ANATOMICAL SITE, ORGAN OR ORGANISM
958.3 WOUND, POSTTRAUMATIC NEC FOLLOWING TRAUMA
908.6 WOUND, POSTTRAUMATIC NEC FOLLOWING TRAUMA LATE EFFECT

INFECTIOUS

139.8 AND PARASITIC DISEASE LATE EFFECTS

647.8#: USE AN ADDITIONAL CODE TO IDENTIFY THE MATERNAL INFECTION OR PARASITIC DISEASE.

647.8# AND PARASITIC DISEASES MATERNAL CURRENT (CO-EXISTENT) IN PREGNANCY OTHER SPECIFIED

5th Digit: 647.8
0. EPISODE OF CARE NOS OR N/A
1. DELIVERED
2. DELIVERED WITH POSTPARTUM COMPLICATION
3. ANTEPARTUM COMPLICATION
4. POSTPARTUM COMPLICATION

462 ANGINA THROAT
136.9 DISEASE UNSPECIFIED
V12.00 DISEASE UNSPECIFIED HISTORY
V12.09 DISEASE OTHER HISTORY
V75.9 DISEASE SCREENING EXAM
0 SEE ALSO ORGAN

INFERIOR MESENTERIC

954.1 PLEXUS INJURY
902.32 VEIN INJURY
908.4 VEIN INJURY LATE EFFECT
902.32 VEIN LACERATION (RUPTURE) (HEMATOMA) (AVULSION) (ANEURYSM) TRAUMATIC
908.4 VEIN LACERATION LATE EFFECT

747.40 INFERIOR VENA CAVA ANOMALY CONGENITAL
902.10 INFERIOR VENA CAVA INJURY
902.19 INFERIOR VENA CAVA INJURY OTHER SITE
908.4 INFERIOR VENA CAVA INJURY LATE EFFECT
459.2 INFERIOR VENA CAVA SYNDROME

CODE V26.2 IS TO BE USED FOR COUPLES UNDERGOING INFERTILITY TESTING AND MANAGEMENT. V26.2 IS ASSIGNED FOR BOTH THE MALE AND THE FEMALE. ASSIGN THE CODE FOR THE CAUSE OF THE INFERTILITY AS A SECONDARY CODE TO V26.2 ON THE INFERTILE PARTNER'S RECORD. REMEMBER, DO NOT USE A MALE DIAGNOSIS CODE ON A FEMALE'S RECORD OR A FEMALE DIAGNOSIS CODE ON A MALE'S RECORD.

INFERTILITY FEMALE

628.9 UNSPECIFIED
628.0 ASSOCIATED WITH ANNOVULATION
628.4 ASSOCIATED WITH ANOMALY OF CERVICAL MUCUS
628.4 ASSOCIATED WITH CONGENITAL STRUCTURAL ANOMALY
628.4 CERVICAL OR VAGINAL ORIGIN
628.4 DYSMUCORRHEA
V23.0 HISTORY AFFECTING PREGNANCY SUPERVISION
V26.2 INVESTIGATION, MANAGEMENT AND TESTING
628.3 NON IMPLANTATION
628.1 PITUITARY-HYPOTHALAMIC ORIGIN
628.2 TUBAL ORIGIN (BLOCK) (STENOSIS) (OCCLUSION)
628.3 UTERINE ORIGIN
628.8 OTHER SPECIFIED ORIGIN

INFERTILITY FEMALE OTHER CAUSES

<u>253.0</u> DUE TO <u>ACROMEGALY</u> [628.1]
<u>253.8</u> DUE TO <u>ADIPOSOGENITAL DYSTROPHY</u> [628.1]
<u>253.1</u> DUE TO <u>FORBES-ALBRIGHT</u> [628.1]
<u>256.3</u> DUE TO <u>OVARIAN FAILURE</u> [628.0]
<u>253.2</u> DUE TO <u>PANHYPOPITUITARISM</u> [628.1]
<u>614.6</u> DUE TO <u>PERITUBULAR ADHESIONS</u> (POSTOPERATIVE) (POSTINFECTION) [628.2]
<u>253.3</u> DUE TO <u>PITUITARY DWARFISM</u> [628.1]
<u>253.4</u> DUE TO <u>PROLACTIN DEFICIENCY</u> [628.1]
<u>256.4</u> DUE TO <u>STEIN LEVENTHAL</u> [628.0]

CODE V26.2 IS TO BE USED FOR COUPLES UNDERGOING INFERTILITY TESTING AND MANAGEMENT. V26.2 IS ASSIGNED FOR BOTH THE MALE AND THE FEMALE. ASSIGN THE CODE FOR THE CAUSE OF THE INFERTILITY AS A SECONDARY CODE TO V26.2 ON THE INFERTILE PARTNER'S RECORD. REMEMBER, DO NOT USE A MALE DIAGNOSIS CODE ON A FEMALE'S RECORD OR A FEMALE DIAGNOSIS CODE ON A MALE'S RECORD.

INFERTILITY MALE

606.9 UNSPECIFIED
606.0 AZOOSPERMIA
606.8 DUE TO INFECTION (RADIATION) (DRUGS) (DISEASE)
606.8 EXTRATESTICULAR CAUSES (DRUGS DISEASE INFECTION RADIATION ETC.)
606.0 GERMINAL CELL APLASIA
606.1 GERMINAL CELL DESQUAMATION
606.1 HYPOSPERMATOGENESIS
V26.2 INVESTIGATION, MANAGEMENT AND TESTING
606.8 OBSTRUCTION EFFERENT DUCTS
606.1 OLIGOSPERMIA
606.0 SPERMATOGENIC ARREST COMPLETE
606.1 SPERMATOGENIC ARREST INCOMPLETE
606.8 SYSTEMIC DISEASE

I-J-K

I-J-K

134.9 INFESTATION (SKIN) NOS

INFILTRATING

174.9 DUCT CARCINOMA SITE NOS
0 DUCT CARCINOMA SITE SPECIFIED SEE 'CANCER' BY SITE M8500/3
174.9 DUCTULAR CARCINOMA SITE NOS
0 DUCTULAR CARCINOMA SITE SPECIFIED SEE 'CANCER' BY SITE M8521/3

996.60 INFLAMMATION COMPLICATION OF INTERNAL PROSTHESIS IMPLANT OR GRAFT
174.9 INFLAMMATORY CARCINOMA SITE NOS
0 INFLAMMATORY CARCINOMA SITE SPECIFIED SEE 'CANCER' BY SITE M8530/3

INFLUENZA

487.1 NOS
487.1 ASIAN
487.8 ENCEPHALITIS
487.8 GASTROENTERITIS
487.8 GASTROINTESTINAL INVOLVEMENT
487.1 LARYNGITIS
760.2 MATERNAL AFFECTING FETUS OR NEWBORN
771.2 MATERNAL AFFECTING FETUS OR NEWBORN - MANIFESTED IN NEWBORN
487.8 MYOCARDITIS
487.8 OTITIS MEDIA [382.02]
487.1 PHARYNGITIS
487.0 PNEUMONIA
487.1 RESPIRATORY INVOLVEMENT
487.0 RESPIRATORY INVOLVEMENT - WITH PNEUMONIA
487.1 SINUSITIS
487.1 SYNDROME
V04.8 VACCINATION

726.69 INFRAPATELLAR BURSITIS
840.3 INFRASPINATUS SEPARATION (RUPTURE) (TEAR) (LACERATION)
840.3 INFRASPINATUS STRAIN (SPRAIN) (AVULSION) (HEMARTHROSIS)
746.83 INFUNDIBULAR PULMONIC STENOSIS CONGENITAL
996.62 INFUSION PUMP COMPLICATION - INFECTION OR INFLAMMATION
996.1 INFUSION PUMP COMPLICATION - MECHANICAL
996.74 INFUSION PUMP COMPLICATION - OTHER
703.0 INGROWN FINGERNAIL (WITH INFECTION)
703.0 INGROWN TOENAIL (WITH INFECTION)
0 INHALATION FLAME SEE 'BURN', INTERNAL ORGANS
740.2 INIENCEPHALY CONGENITAL

INJURY TO INTERNAL ORGANS - LUNG, SPLEEN, LIVER, KIDNEY, ETC., CAN BE A CONTUSION, LACERATION, TEAR, OR RUPTURE. YOU MAY FIND THE CODE UNDER THE CONDITION OR UNDER THE ANATOMICAL SITE.

INJURY

959.9 SITE NOS
959.8 NOS (OTHER SPECIFIED SITES) INCLUDING MULTIPLE
919.8 SITE NOS SUPERFICIAL
919.9 SITE NOS SUPERFICIAL INFECTED
V71.3 EVALUATION WORK RELATED WITH NO APPARENT INJURY
V15.5 HISTORY

INJURY (continued)

869.0 INTERNAL - UNSPECIFIED OR ILL-DEFINED ORGANS
869.1 INTERNAL - UNSPECIFIED OR ILL-DEFINED ORGANS WITH OPEN WOUND INTO CAVITY
868.00 INTERNAL - INTRAABDOMINAL UNSPECIFIED ORGAN
868.10 INTERNAL - INTRAABDOMINAL UNSPECIFIED ORGAN WITH OPEN WOUND INTO CAVITY
868.09 INTERNAL - INTRAABDOMINAL OTHER AND/OR MULTIPLE ORGAN(S)
868.19 INTERNAL - INTRAABDOMINAL OTHER AND/OR MULTIPLE ORGAN(S) WITH OPEN WOUND INTO CAVITY
0 INTERNAL - FOR SPECIFIC INJURY SEE ANATOMICAL SITE
908.0 INTERNAL - LATE EFFECT (CHEST)
908.1 INTERNAL - LATE EFFECT (INTRA ABDOMINAL ORGANS)
908.2 INTERNAL - LATE EFFECT (OTHER INTERNAL ORGANS)
908.9 LATE EFFECT (NOS)
760.5 MATERNAL AFFECTING FETUS OR NEWBORN
648.9# MATERNAL NON-OBSTETRICAL CURRENT (CO-EXISTENT) IN PREGNANCY

5th Digit: 648.9

0. EPISODE OF CARE UNSPECIFIED OR N/A
1. DELIVERED
2. DELIVERED WITH POSTPARTUM COMPLICATION
3. ANTEPARTUM COMPLICATION
4. POSTPARTUM COMPLICATION

V71.4 MVA, EVALUATION WITH NO APPARENT INJURY
V65.43 PREVENTION COUNSELING
0 SEE ALSO ANATOMICAL SITE INJURED OR TYPE OF INJURY

V61.3 IN-LAW PROBLEM
653.2# INLET CONTRACTION PELVIS
660.1# INLET CONTRACTION PELVIS OBSTRUCTING LABOR [653.2#]

5th Digit: 653.2, 660.1

0. EPISODE OF CARE NOS OR N/A
1. DELIVERED
3. ANTEPARTUM COMPLICATION

INJURY OF A BLOOD VESSEL CAN BE A LACERATION, A-V FISTULA, ANEURYSM, OR HEMATOMA. USE THE "INJURY" CODE FOUND BY ANATOMICAL SITE (THE NAME OF THE BLOOD VESSEL).

INNOMINATE

747.69 ARTERY ORIGIN ANOMALY (ABERRANT) (ABSENCE) (AGENESIS) (ACCESSORY) (ANEURYSM) (DEFORMITY) (HYPOPLASIA) (MALPOSITION)
901.1 ARTERY INJURY
908.4 ARTERY INJURY LATE EFFECT
901.1 ARTERY LACERATION (RUPTURE) (HEMATOMA) (AVULSION) (ANEURYSM) TRAUMATIC
908.4 ARTERY LACERATION LATE EFFECT
901.3 VEIN INJURY
908.4 VEIN INJURY LATE EFFECT
901.3 VEIN LACERATION (RUPTURE) (HEMATOMA) (AVULSION) (ANEURYSM) TRAUMATIC
908.4 VEIN LACERATION LATE EFFECT

0 INOCULATION SEE 'VACCINATION (NEED FOR)'

WHEN CODING FOR AN INSECT BITE OR STING, THE IMPORTANT DISTINCTION TO BE MADE IS WHETHER THE INSECT IS VENOMOUS OR NONVENOMOUS, NOT WHETHER THE CONTACT IS A "BITE" OR A "STING". BELOW ARE THE NONVENOMOUS CODES. LOOK UNDER "STING VENOMOUS" FOR THE VENOMOUS CODES.

INSECT BITE NONVENOMOUS

919.4 NOS
919.5 NOS INFECTED
911.4 ABDOMINAL WALL
911.5 ABDOMINAL WALL INFECTED
916.4 ANKLE
916.5 ANKLE INFECTED

WHEN CODING FOR AN INSECT BITE OR STING, THE IMPORTANT DISTINCTION TO BE MADE IS WHETHER THE INSECT IS VENOMOUS OR NONVENOMOUS, NOT WHETHER THE CONTACT IS A "BITE" OR A "STING". BELOW ARE THE NONVENOMOUS CODES. LOOK UNDER "STING VENOMOUS" FOR THE VENOMOUS CODES.

INSECT BITE NONVENOMOUS (continued)

911.4 ANUS
911.5 ANUS INFECTED
912.4 ARM (UPPER)
912.5 ARM (UPPER) INFECTED
912.4 AXILLA
912.5 AXILLA INFECTED
911.4 BACK
911.5 BACK INFECTED
911.4 BREAST
911.5 BREAST INFECTED
911.4 BUTTOCK
911.5 BUTTOCK INFECTED
916.4 CALF
916.5 CALF INFECTED
910.4 CHEEK
910.5 CHEEK INFECTED
911.4 CHEST WALL
911.5 CHEST WALL INFECTED
910.4 EAR
910.5 EAR INFECTED
913.4 ELBOW
913.5 ELBOW INFECTED
918.0 EYELID AND PERIOCULAR AREA
919.5 EYELID AND PERIOCULAR AREA INFECTED
910.4 FACE
910.5 FACE INFECTED
915.4 FINGER
915.5 FINGER INFECTED
911.4 FLANK
911.5 FLANK INFECTED
917.4 FOOT
917.5 FOOT INFECTED
913.4 FOREARM
913.5 FOREARM INFECTED
911.4 GROIN
911.5 GROIN INFECTED
910.4 GUM
910.5 GUM INFECTED
914.4 HAND
914.5 HAND INFECTED
917.4 HEEL
917.5 HEEL INFECTED
916.4 HIP
916.5 HIP INFECTED
911.4 INTERSCAPULAR REGION
911.5 INTERSCAPULAR REGION INFECTED
916.4 KNEE
916.5 KNEE INFECTED
911.4 LABIA
911.5 LABIA INFECTED
906.2 LATE EFFECT
916.4 LEG
916.5 LEG INFECTED
910.4 LIP
910.5 LIP INFECTED
919.4 MULTIPLE
919.5 MULTIPLE INFECTED
910.4 NECK
910.5 NECK INFECTED
910.4 NOSE
910.5 NOSE INFECTED
911.4 PENIS
911.5 PENIS INFECTED
911.4 PERINEUM
911.5 PERINEUM INFECTED

INSECT BITE NONVENOMOUS (continued)

910.4 SCALP
910.5 SCALP INFECTED
912.4 SCAPULAR REGION
912.5 SCAPULAR REGION INFECTED
911.4 SCROTUM
911.5 SCROTUM INFECTED
912.4 SHOULDER
912.5 SHOULDER INFECTED
911.4 TESTIS
911.5 TESTIS INFECTED
916.4 THIGH
916.5 THIGH INFECTED
910.4 THROAT
910.5 THROAT INFECTED
915.4 THUMB
915.5 THUMB INFECTED
917.4 TOE
917.5 TOE INFECTED
911.4 TRUNK
911.5 TRUNK INFECTED
911.4 VAGINA
911.5 VAGINA INFECTED
911.4 VULVA
911.5 VULVA INFECTED
913.4 WRIST
913.5 WRIST INFECTED
919.4 OTHER SITES
919.5 OTHER SITES INFECTED

989.5 INSECT BITE VENOMOUS (SPIDER)
134.9 INSECT INFESTATION
134.8 INSECT INFESTATION OTHER SPECIFIED
V26.1 INSEMINATION ARTIFICIAL

INSOMNIA

780.52 NOS
307.42 CHRONIC ASSOCIATED WITH (ANXIETY) (DEPRESSION) (PSYCHOSIS)
307.42 PERSISTENT PSYCHOGENIC
307.49 SUBJECTIVE COMPLAINT
307.41 TRANSIENT PSYCHOGENIC
780.51 WITH SLEEP APNEA
0 SEE ALSO 'SLEEP DISORDER / DISTURBANCE'
780.52 OTHER

774.4 INSPISSATED BILE SYNDROME, NEWBORN

INSTABILITY

596.59 DETRUSOR
0 DETRUSOR WITH INCONTINENCE SEE 'BLADDER DISORDERS WITH INCONTINENCE'
718.8# JOINT (OLD) (POSTTRAUMATIC)

5th Digit: 718.8

0. SITE NOS
1. SHOULDER REGION
2. UPPER ARM, ELBOW
3. FOREARM, WRIST
4. HAND
5. PELVIC REGION AND THIGH, HIP
6. LOWER LEG KNEE
7. ANKLE AND/OR FOOT
8. OTHER
9. MULTIPLE

724.6 JOINT - LUMBOSACRAL
724.6 JOINT - SACROILIAC
599.83 URETHRAL

I-J-K

251.0 INSULIN COMA

250.3# INSULIN COMA DIABETIC

5th Digit: 250.3

- **0. TYPE II, ADULT-ONSET, NON-INSULIN DEPENDENT (EVEN IF REQUIRING INSULIN), OR UNSPECIFIED; CONTROLLED**
- **1. TYPE I, JUVENILE-ONSET OR INSULIN-DEPENDENT; CONTROLLED**
- **2. TYPE II, ADULT-ONSET, NON-INSULIN DEPENDENT (EVEN IF REQUIRING INSULIN); UNCONTROLLED**
- **3. TYPE I, JUVENILE-ONSET OR INSULIN-DEPENDENT; UNCONTROLLED**

251.3 INSULIN DEFICIENCY POSTSURGICAL

INSULINOMA

211.7 SITE NOS
0 SITE SPECIFIED SEE 'BENIGN NEOPLASM', BY SITE M8151/0
157.4 MALIGNANT SITE NOS
0 MALIGNANT SITE SPECIFIED SEE 'CANCER' BY SITE M8151/3

INTEGUMENT

757.9 ANOMALY CONGENITAL
757.8 ANOMALIES OTHER SPECIFIED CONGENITAL
778.9 CONDITION NOS INVOLVING TEMPERATURE REGULATION (PERINATAL)

0 INTERACTIONAL (CHILDHOOD) DISORDER PSYCHOTIC SEE 'PSYCHOSIS CHILDHOOD'

INTERCOSTAL

901.81 ARTERY INJURY
908.4 ARTERY INJURY LATE EFFECT
901.81 ARTERY LACERATION (RUPTURE) (HEMATOMA) (AVULSION) (ANEURYSM) TRAUMATIC
908.4 ARTERY LACERATION LATE EFFECT
786.59 MUSCLE PAIN
353.8 NERVE DISORDER (LESION)
901.81 VEIN INJURY
908.4 VEIN INJURY LATE EFFECT
901.81 VEIN LACERATION (RUPTURE) (HEMATOMA) (AVULSION) (ANEURYSM) TRAUMATIC
908.4 VEIN LACERATION LATE EFFECT

279.4 INTERFERON DEFICIENCY
411.1 INTERMEDIATE CORONARY (ARTERY) SYNDROME
626.6 INTERMENSTRUAL BLEEDING IRREGULAR
626.5 INTERMENSTRUAL BLEEDING REGULAR
625.2 INTERMENSTRUAL PAIN
279.4 INTERFERON DEFICIENCY
443.9 INTERMITTENT CLAUDICATION NOS
453.8 INTERMITTENT CLAUDICATION VENOUS
431 INTERNAL CAPSULE HEMORRHAGE (CEREBRAL)

433.1# INTERNAL CAROTID ARTERY SYNDROME

5th Digit: 433.1

- **0. WITHOUT CEREBRAL INFARCTION**
- **1. WITH CEREBRAL INFARCTION**

INTERNAL FIXATION DEVICE ORTHOPEDIC

996.67 (PIN) (ROD) (SCREW) - INFECTION OR INFLAMMATION
996.4 (PIN) (ROD) (SCREW) - MECHANICAL COMPLICATION
996.78 (PIN) (ROD) (SCREW) - OTHER SPECIFIED COMPLICATION
V54.0 AFTERCARE OR REMOVAL

INTERNAL INJURY

869.0 UNSPECIFIED OR ILL-DEFINED ORGANS
869.1 UNSPECIFIED OR ILL-DEFINED ORGANS WITH OPEN WOUND INTO CAVITY

INTERNAL INJURY (continued)

868.00 INTRA-ABDOMINAL UNSPECIFIED ORGAN
868.10 INTRA-ABDOMINAL UNSPECIFIED ORGAN WITH OPEN WOUND INTO CAVITY
868.09 INTRA-ABDOMINAL OTHER AND/OR MULTIPLE ORGAN(S)
868.19 INTRA-ABDOMINAL OTHER AND/OR MULTIPLE ORGAN(S) WITH OPEN WOUND INTO CAVITY
0 FOR SPECIFIC INJURY SEE ANATOMICAL SITE
908.0 LATE EFFECT (CHEST)
908.1 LATE EFFECT (INTRA ABDOMINAL ORGANS)
908.2 LATE EFFECT (OTHER INTERNAL ORGANS)

900.1 INTERNAL JUGULAR VEIN INJURY
908.3 INTERNAL JUGULAR VEIN INJURY LATE EFFECT
901.82 INTERNAL MAMMARY ARTERY OR VEIN INJURY
908.4 INTERNAL MAMMARY ARTERY OR VEIN INJURY LATE EFFECT
V47.9 INTERNAL ORGAN PROBLEM
V47.0 INTERNAL ORGANS DEFICIENCIES
V47.1 INTERNAL ORGANS MECHANICAL AND MOTOR PROBLEM

INTERPHALANGEAL

842.13 HAND SEPARATION (RUPTURE) (TEAR) (LACERATION)
842.13 HAND STRAIN (SPRAIN) (AVULSION) (HEMARTHROSIS)
845.13 FOOT SEPARATION (RUPTURE) (TEAR) (LACERATION)
845.13 FOOT STRAIN (SPRAIN) (AVULSION) (HEMARTHROSIS)

INTERSCAPULAR REGION

911.8 INJURY OTHER AND NOS SUPERFICIAL
911.9 INJURY OTHER AND NOS SUPERFICIAL INFECTED
959.1 REGION INJURY

724.8 INTERSPINOUS LIGAMENT SYNDROME
253.4 INTERSTITIAL CELL-STIMULATING HORMONE DEFICIENCY
253.1 INTERSTITIAL CELL-STIMULATING HORMONE OVERPRODUCTION
695.89 INTERTRIGO
112.3 INTERTRIGO CANDIDAL
0 INTERTRIGO MYCOTIC SEE SPECIFIC MYCOSIS
745.4 INTERVENTRICULAR SEPTAL DEFECT

WHEN CODING BACK DISORDERS DUE TO DEGENERATION, DISPLACEMENT OR HNP OF THE INTERVERTEBRAL DISC, IT IS IMPORTANT TO DISTINGUISH WHETHER THESE CONDITIONS ARE WITH OR WITHOUT MYELOPATHY. MYELOPATHY REFERS TO FUNCTIONAL DISTURBANCES AND/OR PATHOLOGICAL CHANGES IN THE SPINAL CORD THAT RESULT FROM COMPRESSION.

INTERVERTEBRAL DISC

CALCIFICATION OR DISCITIS

722.90 NOS
722.91 CERVICAL
722.93 LUMBAR (LUMBOSACRAL)
722.92 THORACIC (THORACOLUMBAR)

DEGENERATIVE DISEASE (DEGENERATION)

722.6 SITE NOS
722.70 SITE NOS WITH MYELOPATHY
722.4 CERVICAL
722.71 CERVICAL WITH MYELOPATHY
722.52 LUMBAR (LUMBOSACRAL)
722.73 LUMBAR (LUMBOSACRAL)WITH MYELOPATHY
722.51 THORACIC (THORACOLUMBAR)
722.72 THORACIC (THORACOLUMBAR) WITH MYELOPATHY

DISORDER

722.90 UNSPECIFIED
722.70 UNSPECIFIED WITH MYELOPATHY

INTERVERTEBRAL DISC (continued)

DISPLACEMENT (RUPTURE)

722.2	SITE NOS
722.70	SITE NOS WITH MYELOPATHY
722.0	CERVICAL
722.71	CERVICAL WITH MYELOPATHY
722.10	LUMBAR
722.73	LUMBAR WITH MYELOPATHY
722.11	THORACIC
722.72	THORACIC WITH MYELOPATHY

HERNIATION

722.2	SITE NOS
722.70	SITE NOS WITH MYELOPATHY
722.0	CERVICAL
722.71	CERVICAL WITH MYELOPATHY
722.10	LUMBAR
722.73	LUMBAR WITH MYELOPATHY
722.11	THORACIC
722.72	THORACIC WITH MYELOPATHY

INTESTINE, INTESTINAL

751.2	ABSENCE CONGENITAL - LARGE
751.1	ABSENCE CONGENITAL - SMALL
V45.72	ABSENCE POSTSURGICAL - LARGE OR SMALL
V45.3	ANASTOMOSIS STATUS
557.1	ANGINA
V53.5	APPLIANCE OR DEVICE OTHER FITTING AND ADJUSTMENT
564.89	ATONY
751.2	ATRESIA LARGE (CONGENITAL)
751.1	ATRESIA SMALL (CONGENITAL)
569.89	ATROPHY
V45.3	BYPASS STATUS
259.2	CARCINOID SYNDROME
560.39	CONCRETION
789.0#	CRAMP

5th Digit: 789.0

0. UNSPECIFIED SITE
1. UPPER RIGHT QUADRANT
2. UPPER LEFT QUADRANT
3. LOWER RIGHT QUADRANT
4. LOWER LEFT QUADRANT
5. PERIUMBILIC
6. EPIGASTRIC
7. GENERALIZED
9. OTHER SPECIFIED SITE (MULTIPLE)

306.4	CRAMP PSYCHOGENIC
123.4	DIPHYLLOBOTHRIASIS
569.9	DISORDER
564.9	DISORDER FUNCTIONAL
751.3	DISORDER FUNCTIONAL - CONGENITAL
564.81	DISORDER FUNCTIONAL - NEUROGENIC
564.4	DISORDER FUNCTIONAL - POSTOPERATIVE
306.4	DISORDER FUNCTIONAL - PSYCHOGENIC
564.89	DISORDER FUNCTIONAL - OTHER SPECIFIED
562.10	DIVERTICULUM (LARGE)
562.00	DIVERTICULUM (SMALL)
751.5	DIVERTICULUM CONGENITAL (SMALL) (LARGE)
751.5	DUPLICATION CONGENITAL
569.89	ENTEROPTOSIS
793.4	FILLING DEFECT
557.0	GANGRENE
787.3	GAS SYNDROME
569.89	GRANULOMA
564.89	HYPERMOBILITY
569.89	HYPERPLASIA LYMPHOID
564.89	HYPOFUNCTION
564.89	HYPOMOTILITY
564.89	IMMOBILITY
560.30	IMPACTION
560.39	IMPACTION BY CALCULUS
560.31	IMPACTION BY GALLSTONE
0	INFECTION SEE 'GASTROENTERITIS'

INTESTINE, INTESTINAL (continued)

863.89	INJURY NOS
863.99	INJURY NOS WITH OPEN WOUND INTO CAVITY
863.4#	INJURY - LARGE INTESTINE (TRAUMATIC)
863.5#	INJURY - LARGE INTESTINE (TRAUMATIC) WITH OPEN WOUND

5th Digit: 863.4, 5

0. LARGE UNSPECIFIED SITE
1. ASCENDING [RIGHT] COLON
2. TRANSVERSE COLON
3. DESCENDING [LEFT] COLON
4. SIGMOID COLON
5. RECTUM
6. MULTIPLE SITES IN COLON AND RECTUM
9. OTHER

908.1	INJURY - LATE EFFECT
863.2#	INJURY - SMALL INTESTINE (TRAUMATIC)
863.3#	INJURY - SMALL INTESTINE (TRAUMATIC) WITH OPEN WOUND

5th Digit: 863.2-3

0. UNSPECIFIED SITE
1. DUODENUM
9. OTHER SPECIFIED SITE

560.0	INVAGINATION
557.1	ISCHEMIA
560.2	KNOT SYNDROME
569.89	LESION
040.2	LIPODYSTROPHY
751.4	MALROTATION CONGENITAL
557.0	NECROSIS

OBSTRUCTION (DUE TO) / OCCLUSION (DUE TO)

560.9	NOS
560.1	ADYNAMIC
560.81	ADHESIONS (POSTOPERATIVE)
127.0	ASCARIS LUMBRICOIDES
560.81	BAND
560.39	CALCULUS
560.30	COLON IMPACTION
751.2	CONGENITAL - LARGE
751.1	CONGENITAL - SMALL
997.4	DUE TO A PROCEDURE
997.5	DUE TO A PROCEDURE INVOLVING URINARY TRACT
560.39	FECAL IMPACTION
560.31	GALLSTONES
0	HERNIA SEE 'HERNIA', BY SITE, INCARCERATED
0	HERNIA GANGRENOUS SEE 'HERNIA', BY SITE, GANGRENOUS
751.2	INFANTILE - LARGE
751.1	INFANTILE - SMALL
560.89	MURAL THICKENING
777.2	NEWBORN DUE TO INSPISSATED MILK PERINATAL
777.1	NEWBORN DUE TO MECONIUM
277.01	NEWBORN DUE TO MECONIUM IN MUCOVISCIDOSIS
777.4	NEWBORN TRANSITORY
560.81	POSTOPERATIVE (DUE TO ADHESIONS)
560.2	VOLVULUS
560.89	OTHER SPECIFIED CAUSE

INTESTINE, INTESTINAL (continued)

569.83	PERFORATION
569.89	PERICOLITIS
569.89	PERISIGMOIDITIS
569.89	PROLAPSE
564.1	SPASM
306.4	SPASM PSYCHOGENIC
564.89	STASIS
996.89	TRANSPLANT REJECTION (FAILURE)
V42.89	TRANSPLANT STATUS
751.5	TRANSPOSITION CONGENITAL
557.9	VASCULAR INSUFFICIENCY NOS
557.0	VASCULAR INSUFFICIENCY ACUTE
557.1	VASCULAR INSUFFICIENCY CHRONIC
569.89	VISCEROPTOSIS

IN-TOEING (DUE TO)

755.64 BOWLEG (GENU VARUM)
755.63 FEMORAL ANTEVERSION
754.53 METATARSUS VARUS
755.69 TIBIA TORSION, INTERNAL

303.0# INTOXICATION ALCOHOL ACUTE - DEPENDENT
305.0# INTOXICATION ALCOHOL ACUTE - NON DEPENDENT

5th Digit: 303.0, 305.0
0. NOS
1. CONTINUOUS
2. EPISODIC
3. IN REMISSION

291.4 INTOXICATION ALCOHOL ACUTE - PATHOLOGIC (IDIOSYNCRATIC)
291.0 INTOXICATION DELIRIUM ALCOHOL
292.81 INTOXICATION DELIRIUM DRUG
0 INTOXICATION DRUG SEE 'DRUG', ABUSE
292.81 INTOXICATION DRUG WITH DELIRIUM
431 INTRACEREBRAL HEMORRHAGE (RUPTURED ANEURYSM)
853.## INTRACEREBRAL HEMORRHAGE TRAUMATIC

4th Digit: 853
0. WITHOUT MENTION OF OPEN INTRACRANIAL WOUND
1. WITH MENTION OF OPEN INTRACRANIAL WOUND

5th Digit: 853
0. LEVEL OF CONSCIOUSNESS NOS
1. NO LOC
2. LOC < 1 HR
3. LOC 1 - 24 HRS
4. LOC > 24 HRS WITH RETURN TO PRIOR LEVEL
5. LOC > 24 HRS WITHOUT RETURN TO PRIOR LEVEL: OR DEATH BEFORE REGAINING CONSCIOUSNESS, REGARDLESS OF DURATION OF LOC
6. LOC DURATION NOS
9. WITH CONCUSSION NOS

907.0 INTRACEREBRAL INJURY LATE EFFECT
905.0 INTRACEREBRAL INJURY LATE EFFECT WITH MENTION OF SKULL FRACTURE
854.## INTRACRANIAL INJURY TRAUMATIC

4th Digit: 854
0. WITHOUT MENTION OF OPEN INTRACRANIAL WOUND
1. WITH MENTION OF OPEN INTRACRANIAL WOUND

5th Digit: 854
0. LEVEL OF CONSCIOUSNESS NOS
1. NO LOC
2. LOC < 1 HR
3. LOC 1 - 24 HRS
4. LOC > 24 HRS WITH RETURN TO PRIOR LEVEL
5. LOC > 24 HRS WITHOUT RETURN TO PRIOR LEVEL: OR DEATH BEFORE REGAINING CONSCIOUSNESS, REGARDLESS OF DURATION OF LOC
6. LOC DURATION NOS
9. WITH CONCUSSION NOS

907.0 INTRACRANIAL INJURY LATE EFFECT
905.0 INTRACRANIAL INJURY LATE EFFECT WITH MENTION OF SKULL FRACTURE
781.9 INTRACRANIAL PRESSURE INCREASED
348.2 INTRACRANIAL PRESSURE INCREASED DUE TO BENIGN INTRACRANIAL HYPERTENSION
0 INTRACRANIAL PRESSURE INCREASED DUE TO HYDROCEPHALUS SEE 'HYDROCEPHALUS'
767.8 INTRACRANIAL PRESSURE INCREASED DUE TO INJURY AT BIRTH

INTRADUCTAL CARCINOMA IN SITU

233.0 NONINFILTRATING SITE NOS
0 NONINFILTRATING SITE SPECIFIED SEE 'CARCINOMA IN SITU', BY SITE M8500/2

216.# INTRAEPIDERMAL EPITHELIOMA OF JODASSOHN M8096/0

4th Digit: 216
0. LIP (SKIN OF)
1. EYELID INCLUDING CANTHUS
2. EAR (EXTERNAL) (AURICLE) (PINNA)
3. FACE (CHEEK) (NOSE) (EYEBROW) (TEMPLE)
4. SCALP NECK
5. TRUNK BACK EXCEPT SCROTUM
6. UPPER LIMB INCLUDING SHOULDER
7. LOWER LIMB INCLUDING HIP
8. OTHER SPECIFIED SITES
9. SKIN NOS

365.00 INTRAOCULAR PRESSURE INCREASED
V53.09 INTRATHECAL INFUSION PUMP DEVICE FITTING AND ADJUSTMENT
862.8 INTRATHORACIC ORGANS INJURY MULTIPLE OR UNSPECIFIED
862.9 INTRATHORACIC ORGANS INJURY MULTIPLE OR UNSPECIFIED WITH OPEN WOUND
862.2# INTRATHORACIC ORGANS INJURY OTHER SPECIFIED
862.3# INTRATHORACIC ORGANS INJURY OTHER SPECIFIED WITH OPEN WOUND INTO CAVITY

5th Digit: 862.2-3
1. BRONCHUS
2. ESOPHAGUS
9. OTHER

908.0 INTRATHORACIC ORGANS INJURY LATE EFFECT
0 INTRAUTERINE CONTRACEPTIVE DEVICE SEE 'IUD'
286.6 INTRAVASCULAR COAGULATION-FIBRINOLYSIS SYNDROME (ICF)
286.6 INTRAVASCULAR COAGULOPATHY SYNDROME (ICF)
639.1 INTRAVASCULAR HEMOLYSIS POST ABORTION OR ECTOPIC/MOLAR PREGNANCY
426.6 INTRAVENTRICULAR BLOCK NOS (HEART)
313.22 INTROVERSION OF CHILDHOOD
313.22 INTROVERTED DISORDER OF CHILDHOOD OR ADOLESCENCE
301.21 INTROVERTED PERSONALITY

INTUSSUSCEPTION

543.9 APPENDIX
560.0 COLON ANY PART
560.0 INTESTINE ANY PART
560.0 RECTUM

560.0 INVAGINATION COLON
560.0 INVAGINATION INTESTINE
759.89 INVERTED MARFAN'S SYNDROME
296.2# INVOLUTIONAL MELANCHOLIA (PSYCHOSIS)
296.3# INVOLUTIONAL MELANCHOLIA (PSYCHOSIS) RECURRENT

5th Digit: 296.2-3
0. NOS
1. MILD
2. MODERATE
3. SEVERE WITHOUT MENTION OF PSYCHOTIC BEHAVIOR
4. SEVERE SPECIFIED AS WITH PSYCHOTIC BEHAVIOR
5. IN PARTIAL OR NOS REMISSION
6. IN FULL REMISSION

269.3 IODINE DEFICIENCY (DIETARY)
0 IODINE THERAPY RADIOACTIVE, CODE THE UNDERLYING DISEASE

IQ
318.2 <20 (PROFOUND RETARDATION)
318.1 20-34 (SEVERE RETARDATION)
318.0 35-49 (MODERATE RETARDATION)
317 50-70 (MILD RETARDATION)

769 IRDS NEWBORN (IDIOPATHIC RESPIRATORY DISTRESS)

IRIDOCYCLITIS
364.3 NOS
364.00 ACUTE SUBACUTE
364.04 ALLERGIC
364.10 CHRONIC
098.41 GONOCOCCAL
364.23 LENS INDUCED
363.21 POSTERIOR (CYCLITIS)
364.01 PRIMARY
364.02 RECURRENT
364.04 SECONDARY
364.03 SECONDARY INFECTIOUS
054.44 HERPES SIMPLEX
053.22 HERPES ZOSTER

IRIDOCYCLITIS ASSOCIATED WITH OTHER DISORDERS
135 CHRONIC DUE TO SARCOID [364.11]
017.3# CHRONIC DUE TO TB [364.11]
5th Digit: 017.3
0. NOS
1. LAB NOT DONE
2. LABS PENDING
3. MICROSCOPY POSITIVE (IN SPUTUM)
4. CULTURE POSITIVE - MICROSCOPY NEGATIVE
5. CULTURE NEGATIVE - MICROSCOPY POSITIVE
6. CULTURE AND MICROSCOPY NEGATIVE CONFIRMED BY OTHER METHODS

364.21 FUCHS' HETEROCHROMIC
0 SEE ALSO 'IRITIS'
360.11 SYMPATHETIC (UVEITIS)
091.52 SYPHILITIC SECONDARY
017.3# TUBERCULOUS [364.11]
5th Digit: 017.3
0. NOS
1. LAB NOT PENDING
2. LABS PENDING
3. MICROSCOPY POSITIVE (IN SPUTUM)
4. CULTURE POSITIVE - MICROSCOPY NEGATIVE
5. CULTURE NEGATIVE - MICROSCOPY POSITIVE
6. CULTURE AND MICROSCOPY NEGATIVE CONFIRMED BY OTHER METHODS

364.76 IRIDODIALYSIS
379.49 IRIDOPLEGIA (COMPLETE) (PARTIAL) (REFLEX)
364.52 IRIDOSCHISIS

IRIS
743.45 ABSENCE (CONGENITAL)
364.70 ADHESIONS
364.9 AND CILIARY BODY DISORDER NOS
364.77 AND CILIARY BODY RECESSION OF CHAMBER ANGLE
743.20 ATRESIA, FILTRATION ANGLE
364.59 ATROPHY (GENERALIZED) (SECTOR SHAPED)
364.54 ATROPHY (SPHINCTER)
364.51 ATROPHY ESSENTIAL OR PROGRESSIVE
364.51 ATROPHY ESSENTIAL OR PROGRESSIVE WITH CONGENITAL GLAUCOMA [365.42]
364.74 BOMBE
365.62 BOMBE WITH GLAUCOMA [364.22]
743.46 COLOBOMA CONGENITAL
364.55 CYST PUPILLARY MARGIN (MIOTIC)
364.56 DEGENERATION (CHAMBER ANGLE)
364.57 DEGENERATION (CHANGES OF CILIARY BODY)
364.53 DEGENERATION PIGMENTARY
364.54 DEGENERATION PUPILLARY MARGIN
364.9 DISORDER

IRIS (continued)
364.54 ECTROPION OF PIGMENT EPITHELIUM
364.41 HEMORRHAGE
364.53 HETEROCHROMIA ACQUIRED
364.42 NEOVASCULARIZATION
364.53 PIGMENT DISPERSION SYNDROME
364.8 PROLAPSE
871.1 PROLAPSE TRAUMATIC
364.53 TRANSLUCENCY

IRITIS
364.3 NOS
364.01 ACUTE PRIMARY
364.02 ACUTE RECURRENT
364.00 ACUTE SUBACUTE
364.04 SECONDARY
364.03 SECONDARY INFECTIOUS
0 SEE ALSO 'IRIDOCYCLITIS'
0 SEE ALSO 'UVEITIS'
091.52 SYPHILITIC (SECONDARY)

IRITIS OTHER
098.41 GONOCOCCAL
274.89 GOUTY [364.11]
054.44 HERPES SIMPLEX
053.22 HERPES ZOSTER
364.10 RHEUMATIC

790.6 IRON ABNORMAL BLOOD LEVEL
V46.1 IRON LUNG DEPENDENCE
285.0 IRON METABOLIC DISORDERS SIDEROBLASTIC ANEMIA
275.0 IRON METABOLISM DISORDERS
799.2 IRRITABILITY
564.1 IRRITABLE BOWEL SYNDROME
316 IRRITABLE COLON PSYCHOGENIC [564.1]
306.2 IRRITABLE HEART SYNDROME
300.5 IRRITABLE WEAKNESS SYNDROME
0 ISAMBERT'S DISEASE SEE 'TUBERCULOSIS', LARYNGITIS
435.9 ISCHEMIC ATTACK CEREBRAL TRANSIENT (TIA)
557.9 ISCHEMIC BOWEL SYNDROME (TRANSIENT)
557.1 ISCHEMIC BOWEL SYNDROME CHRONIC
557.1 ISCHEMIC BOWEL SYNDROME DUE TO MESENTERIC ARTERY SYNDROME

ISCHEMIC HEART DISEASE
414.9 NOS
411.89 ACUTE
411.89 ACUTE SUBENDOCARDIAL
411.81 ACUTE WITH CORONARY OCCLUSION (ARTERY)
0 ACUTE WITH MI SEE 'MI (MYOCARDIAL INFARCTION) ACUTE'
414.10 ANEURYSM (MURAL) (VENTRICULAR)
414.11 ANEURYSM CORONARY VESSELS
414.19 ANEURYSM OTHER
414.0# ARTERIOSCLEROTIC
5th Digit: 414.0
0. UNSPECIFIED TYPE OF VESSEL, NATIVE OR GRAFT
1. NATIVE CORONARY VESSEL
2. AUTOLOGOUS VEIN BYPASS GRAFT
3. NONAUTOLOGOUS BIOLOGICAL BYPASS GRAFT
4. AUTOLOGOUS ARTERY BYPASS GRAFT (GASTROEPIPLOIC) (INTERNAL MAMMARY)
5. UNSPECIFIED TYPE OF BYPASS GRAFT

ISCHEMIC HEART DISEASE (continued)
414.9 CHRONIC
414.1# CHRONIC - ANEURYSM
5th Digit: 414.1
0. HEART WALL
1. CORONARY VESSELS (ARTERIOVENOUS)
9. OTHER

414.0# CHRONIC - ARTERIOSCLEROTIC
5th Digit: 414.0
0. UNSPECIFIED TYPE OF VESSEL, NATIVE OR GRAFT
1. NATIVE CORONARY VESSEL
2. AUTOLOGOUS VEIN BYPASS GRAFT
3. NONAUTOLOGOUS BIOLOGICAL BYPASS GRAFT
4. AUTOLOGOUS ARTERY BYPASS GRAFT (GASTROEPIPLOIC) (INTERNAL MAMMARY)
5. UNSPECIFIED TYPE OF BYPASS GRAFT

414.8 CHRONIC - MYOCARDIAL
414.8 CHRONIC - OTHER
411.89 CORONARY INSUFFICIENCY ACUTE
V17.3 FAMILY HISTORY
411.89 SUBACUTE
411.89 OTHER SPECIFIED - ACUTE
414.8 OTHER SPECIFIED - CHRONIC

553.8 ISCHIATIC HERNIA
843.1 ISCHIOCAPSULAR SEPARATION (RUPTURE) (TEAR) (LACERATION)
843.1 ISCHIOCAPSULAR STRAIN (SPRAIN) (AVULSION) (HEMARTHROSIS)
732.1 ISCHIOPUBIC SYNCHONDROSIS (OF VAN NECK) HIP AND PELVIS JUVENILE
553.8 ISCHIORECTAL HERNIA
599.82 ISD - INTRINSIC (URETHRAL) SPHINCTER DEFICIENCY
732.5 ISELIN'S DISEASE (OSTEOCHONDROSIS FIFTH METATARSAL)
081.2 ISLAND DISEASE (SCRUB TYPHUS)
251.1 ISLANDS OF LANGERHANS HYPERPLASIA
157.4 ISLET CELL CARCINOMA SITE NOS
0 ISLET CELL CARCINOMA SITE SPECIFIED SEE 'CANCER' BY SITE M8150/3
251.9 ISLET CELL (PANCREATIC) HYPERPLASIA
251.5 ISLET CELL (PANCREATIC) HYPERPLASIA - ALPHA CELLS WITH EXCESS GASTRIN
251.4 ISLET CELL (PANCREATIC) HYPERPLASIA - ALPHA CELLS WITH EXCESS GLUCAGON
251.1 ISLET CELL (PANCREATIC) HYPERPLASIA - BETA CELLS
V28.5 ISOIMMUNIZATION SCREENING ANTENATAL
0 ISOIMMUNIZATION SEE 'BLOOD', TYPE
253.3 ISOLATED DEFICIENCY HGH
253.3 ISOLATED DEFICIENCY OF HUMAN GROWTH HORMONE [HGH]
V07.0 ISOLATION (FOR INFECTION PROPHYLAXIS)
V62.4 ISOLATION SOCIAL
270.3 ISOLEUCINE METABOLISM DISTURBANCES
256.4 ISOSEXUAL VIRILIZATION
007.2 ISOSPORA (BELLI) (HOMINIS) INTESTINAL INFECTION
007.2 ISOSPORIASIS
985.5 ITAI-ITAI DISEASE

ITCH
698.9 UNSPECIFIED
698.0 ANUS
110.3 DHOBIE
698.9 EAR
379.99 EYE
698.1 GENITAL ORGANS

ITCH (continued)
110.3 JOCK
306.3 PSYCHOGENIC
V61.10 SEVEN-YEAR
698.8 UREMIC
698.8 OTHER SPECIFIED
0 SEE ALSO 'PRURITUS'

287.3 ITP - IDIOPATHIC THROMBOCYTOPENIC PURPURA
255.0 ITSENKO-CUSHING SYNDROME (PITUITARY BASOPHILISM)

IUD
996.65 COMPLICATION - INFECTION OR INFLAMMATION
996.32 COMPLICATION - MECHANICAL
996.76 COMPLICATION - OTHER
V25.1 INSERTION
V25.42 REINSERTION CHECKING
V25.42 REMOVAL
V25.42 ROUTINE CARE
V45.51 STATUS (OR PRESENCE)

286.6 IVC SYNDROME (INTRAVASCULAR COAGULOPATHY)
759.0 IVEMARK'S SYNDROME (ASPLENIA WITH CONGENITAL HEART DISEASE)
362.62 IWANOFF'S CYSTS

714.4 JACCOUD'S SYNDROME
751.4 JACKSON'S MEMBRANE
344.89 JACKSON'S PARALYSIS (SYNDROME)
751.4 JACKSON'S MEMBRANE (COLON) CONGENITAL
757.5 JADASSOHN-LEWANDOWSKI SYNDROME (PACHYONYCHIA CONGENITA)
701.3 JADASSOHN-PELLIZARI'S DISEASE (ANETODERMA)
252.0 JAFFE-LICHTENSTEIN (-UEHLINGER) SYNDROME
759.6 JAHNKE'S SYNDROME (ENCEPHALOCUTANEOUS ANGIOMATOSIS)
046.1 JAKOB CREUTZFELDT DISEASE OR SYNDROME
046.1 JAKOB CREUTZFELDT DISEASE OR SYNDROME WITH DEMENTIA [294.1]
285.8 JAKSCH (-LUZET) (-HAYEM) DISEASE OR SYNDROME (PSEUDOLEUKEMIA INFANTUM)
300.89 JANET'S DISEASE
330.1 JANSKY BIELSCHOWSKY DISEASE
062.0 JAPANESE ENCEPHALITIS
321.8 JAPANESE MENINGITIS
081.2 JAPANESE RIVER FEVER
100.89 JAPANESE SEVEN DAY FEVER

JAUNDICE
782.4 NOS
277.4 BILIRUBIN EXCRETION DISORDERS
282.0 FAMILIAL ACHOLURIC
100.0 LEPTOSPIRAL (HEMORRHAGIC)
576.8 OBSTRUCTIVE
100.0 SPIROCHETAL (HEMORRHAGIC)

JAUNDICE NEONATAL
774.6 NOS
774.2 NOS ASSOCIATED WITH PRETERM DELIVERY
773.1 ABO REACTION PERINATAL
774.1 BRUISING PERINATAL
774.30 CONJUGATION DELAYED NOS
774.39 CONJUGATION DELAYED BREAST MILK INHIBITORS
774.39 CONJUGATION DELAYED DEVELOPMENTAL
774.2 CONJUGATION DELAYED PRE-TERM DELIVERY
774.39 CONJUGATION OTHER
774.2 DELIVERY PRE-TERM
774.1 DRUGS TRANSMITTED FROM MOTHER

JAUNDICE NEONATAL (continued)

774.1 HEMOLYTIC PERINATAL
774.1 INFECTION
773.# ISOIMMUNIZATION MATERNAL (DUE TO)
4th Digit: 773
0. RH (RHESUS) ISOIMMUNIZATION
1. ABO ISOIMMUNIZATION
2. OTHER AND NOS ISOIMMUNIZATION

774.4 LIVER DAMAGE
773.0 RH REACTION PERINATAL
774.1 SWALLOWED MATERNAL BLOOD
774.1 TOXINS TRANSMITTED FROM MOTHER

JAUNDICE NEONATAL OTHER

282.# ANEMIA HEMOLYTIC HEREDITARY [774.0]
4th Digit: 282
0. SPHEROCYTIC
1. ELLIPTOCYTOTIC
2. G6PD (GLUTATHIONE REDUCTASE)
3. HEXOKINASE (PK) (TPI) DEFICIENCY NONSPHEROCYTOTIC TYPEII
4. THALASSEMIA (MEDITERRANEAN) (COOLEY'S)
5. SICKLE CELL TRAIT
7. HEMOGLOBINOPATHY (HB-C) (HB-D) (HB- E) (FETAL) OR NOS
8. OTHER SPECIFIED (STOMATOCYTOSIS)
9. NOS

751.61 BILE DUCT OBSTRUCTION (CONGENITAL) [774.5]
277.4 CRIGLER NAJJAR [774.31]
277.00 CYSTIC FIBROSIS [774.5]
277.01 CYSTIC FIBROSIS WITH MECONIUM ILEUS [774.5]
271.1 GALACTOSEMIC [774.5]
277.4 GILBERT'S [774.31]
243 HYPOTHYROID (CONGENITAL) [774.31]
277.01 MUCOVISCIDOSIS [774.5]

JAW

0 ANOMALY SEE 'JAW ANOMALIES'
374.43 BLINKING
524.5 CLOSURE ABNORMAL
526.9 DISEASE NEC
526.2 DISEASE FIBROCYSTIC
526.89 DISEASE OTHER SPECIFIED
526.89 FIBROUS DYSPLASIA
524.09 HYPOPLASIA
959.09 INJURY
848.1 SEPARATION (RUPTURE) (TEAR) (LACERATION)
848.1 STRAIN (SPRAIN) (AVULSION) (HEMARTHROSIS)
742.8 WINKING SYNDROME
0 SEE ALSO 'MANDIBLE, MANDIBULAR'
0 SEE ALSO 'MAXILLA, MAXILLARY'

JAW ANOMALIES

524.7# DENTOALVEOLAR
5th Digit: 524.7
0. UNSPECIFIED ALVEOLAR ANOMALY
1. ALVEOLAR MAXILLARY HYPERPLASIA
2. ALVEOLAR MANDIBULAR HYPERPLASIA
3. ALVEOLAR MAXILLARY HYPOPLASIA
4. ALVEOLAR MANDIBULAR HYPOPLASIA
9. OTHER SPECIFIED ALVEOLAR ANOMALY

524.1# JAW RELATIONSHIP TO CRANIAL BASE
5th Digit: 524.1
0. UNSPECIFIED ANOMALY
1. MAXILLARY ASYMMETRY
2. OTHER JAW ASYMMETRY
9. OTHER SPECIFIED ANOMALY

JAW ANOMALIES (continued)

524.0# JAW SIZE (MAJOR ANOMALIES)
5th Digit: 524.0
0. UNSPECIFIED ANOMALY
1. MAXILLARY HYPERPLASIA
2. MANDIBULAR HYPERPLASIA
3. MAXILLARY HYPOPLASIA
4. MANDIBULAR HYPOPLASIA
5. MACROGENIA
6. MICROGENIA
9. OTHER SPECIFIED ANOMALY

291.5 JEALOUSY ALCOHOLIC PSYCHOTIC
0 JEJUNAL SEE 'JEJUNUM, JEJUNAL'
558.9 JEJUNITIS NONINFECTIOUS (ALLERGIC) (DIETARY) SEE ALSO 'ENTERITIS'

JEJUNOSTOMY

V53.5 BELT FITTING AND ADJUSTMENT
V55.3 CARE
V55.3 CATHETER ADJUSTMENT OR REPOSITIONING
V55.3 CATHETER REMOVAL OR REPLACEMENT
V55.3 CLOSURE
569.60 COMPLICATION - NOS
569.62 COMPLICATION - MECHANICAL
569.69 COMPLICATION - OTHER
569.69 FISTULA
569.69 HERNIA

WHEN CODING AN INFECTION OF AN OSTOMY, USE AN ADDITIONAL CODE TO SPECIFY THE ORGANISM. SEE 'BACTERIAL INFECTION'

569.61 INFECTION
569.61 INFECTION WITH CELLULITIS OF ABDOMEN [682.2]
569.61 INFECTION WITH SEPSIS [**038.#(#)**]
4th or 4th and 5th Digit Code for Organism: 038
.9 NOS
.3 ANAEROBIC
.3 BACTEROIDES
.3 CLOSTRIDIUM
.42 E COLI
.49 ENTEROBACTER AEROGENES
.40 GRAM NEGATIVE
.49 GRAM NEGATIVE OTHER
.41 HEMOPHILUS INFLUENZAE
.2 PNEUMOCOCCAL
.49 PROTEUS
.43 PSEUDOMONAS
.44 SERRATIA
.10 STAPHYLOCOCCAL NOS
.11 STAPHYLOCOCCAL AUREUS
.19 STAPHYLOCOCCAL OTHER
.0 STREPTOCOCCAL (ANAEROBIC)
.49 YERSINIA ENTEROCOLITICA
.8 OTHER SPECIFIED

569.62 MALFUNCTION
569.69 PROLAPSE
V44.3 STATUS
V55.3 TOILET STOMA

JEJUNUM, JEJUNAL

751.1 ABSENCE CONGENITAL
V45.72 ABSENCE POSTSURGICAL
751.1 ATRESIA (CONGENITAL)
562.00 DIVERTICULUM
564.89 DILATATION
306.4 DILATATION PSYCHOGENIC

JEJUNUM, JEJUNAL (continued)

751.1 IMPERFORATE CONGENITAL
863.29 INJURY TRAUMATIC
863.39 INJURY TRAUMATIC WITH OPEN WOUND
564.89 IRRITABILITY
0 JEJUNITIS SEE 'ENTERITIS'
560.9 OBSTRUCTION (SEE ALSO 'INTESTINE, INTESTINAL', OBSTRUCTION)
564.89 STASIS
564.2 SYNDROME

363.05 JENSEN'S DISEASE
307.45 JET LAG SYNDROME
756.4 JEUNE'S DISEASE OR SYNDROME CONGENITAL (ASPHYXIATING THORACIC DYSTROPHY)
134.1 JIGGER DISEASE
779.5 JITTERY BABY
V62.2 JOB DISSATISFACTION
288.1 JOB'S SYNDROME (CHRONIC GRANULOMATOUS DISEASE)
110.3 JOCK ITCH
695.1 JOHNSON-STEVENS DISEASE (ERYTHEMA MULTIFORME EXUDATIVUM)

JOINT

755.8 ABSENCE NEC CONGENITAL
718.5# ANKYLOSIS
719.8# CALCIFICATION
718.4# CONTRACTURE
719.6# CREPITUS

5th Digit: 718.4, 5, 719.6, 8

0. SITE NOS
1. SHOULDER REGION
2. UPPER ARM (ELBOW) (HUMERUS)
3. FOREARM (RADIUS) (WRIST) (ULNA)
4. HAND (CARPAL) (METACARPAL) (FINGERS)
5. PELVIC REGION AND THIGH (HIP) (BUTTOCK) (FEMUR)
6. LOWER LEG (FIBULA) (KNEE) (PATELLA) (TIBIA)
7. ANKLE AND/OR FOOT (METATARSALS) (TOES) (TARSALS)
8. OTHER
9. MULTIPLE

718.9# DERANGEMENT (OLD)

5th Digit: 718.9

0. SITE NOS
1. SHOULDER REGION
2. UPPER ARM (ELBOW) (HUMERUS)
3. FOREARM (RADIUS) (WRIST) (ULNA)
4. HAND (CARPAL) (METACARPAL) (FINGERS)
5. PELVIC REGION AND THIGH (HIP) (BUTTOCK) (FEMUR)
7. ANKLE AND/OR FOOT (METATARSALS) (TOES) (TARSALS)
8. OTHER
9. MULTIPLE

717.9 DERANGEMENT (OLD) - KNEE
724.9 DERANGEMENT (OLD) - SPINE
718.3# DERANGEMENT (OLD) - RECURRENT
724.9 DERANGEMENT (OLD) - RECURRENT SPINE
718.8# DERANGEMENT (OLD) - OTHER NEC
0 DISLOCATION SEE 'DISLOCATION'
719.9# DISORDER

5th Digit: 718.3, 8, 719.9

0. SITE NOS
1. SHOULDER REGION
2. UPPER ARM (ELBOW) (HUMERUS)
3. FOREARM (RADIUS) (WRIST) (ULNA)
4. HAND (CARPAL) (METACARPAL) (FINGERS)
5. PELVIC REGION AND THIGH (HIP) (BUTTOCK) (FEMUR)
6. LOWER LEG (FIBULA) (KNEE) (PATELLA) (TIBIA)
7. ANKLE AND/OR FOOT (METATARSALS) (TOES) (TARSALS)
8. OTHER
9. MULTIPLE

JOINT (continued)

306.0 DISORDER PSYCHOGENIC (ARTICULATION DISORDER)
724.9 DISORDER SPINE
719.7# DISORDER WITH DIFFICULTY WALKING

5th Digit: 719.7

0. SITE NOS
5. PELVIC REGION (HIP) (BUTTOCK) (FEMUR)
6. LOWER LEG (FIBULA) (KNEE) (PATELLA) (TIBIA)
7. ANKLE AND/OR FOOT (METATARSALS)(TOES)(TARSALS)
8. OTHER
9. MULTIPLE

719.0# EFFUSION
719.3# EFFUSION INTERMITTENT
719.8# FISTULA
718.8# FLAIL
719.1# HEMARTHROSIS
0 HEMARTHROSIS CURRENT INJURY SEE 'SPRAIN'
719.1# HEMORRHAGE (NONTRAUMATIC)
719.0# HYDRARTHROSIS
719.3# HYDRARTHROSIS INTERMITTENT
718.8# HYPEREXTENSION (OLD)
716.9# INFLAMMATION
718.8# INSTABILITY (OLD)

5th Digit: 716.9, 718.8, 719.0-1, 3, 8

0. SITE NOS
1. SHOULDER REGION
2. UPPER ARM (ELBOW) (HUMERUS)
3. FOREARM (RADIUS) (WRIST) (ULNA)
4. HAND (CARPAL) (METACARPAL) (FINGERS)
5. PELVIC REGION AND THIGH (HIP) (BUTTOCK) (FEMUR)
6. LOWER LEG (FIBULA) (KNEE) (PATELLA) (TIBIA)
7. ANKLE AND/OR FOOT (METATARSALS) (TOES) (TARSALS)
8. OTHER
9. MULTIPLE

724.6 INSTABILITY LUMBOSACRAL (OLD) - (NONVERTEBRAL) (NONDISCOGENIC)
724.6 INSTABILITY SACROILIAC (OLD) - (NONVERTEBRAL) (NONDISCOGENIC)
719.9# LIGAMENT RELAXATION

5th Digit: 719.9

0. SITE NOS
1. SHOULDER REGION
2. UPPER ARM (ELBOW) (HUMERUS)
3. FOREARM (RADIUS) (WRIST) (ULNA)
4. HAND (CARPAL) (METACARPAL) (FINGERS)
5. PELVIC REGION AND THIGH (HIP) (BUTTOCK) (FEMUR)
7. ANKLE AND/OR FOOT (METATARSALS) (TOES) (TARSALS)
8. OTHER
9. MULTIPLE

717.9 LIGAMENT RELAXATION - KNEE
0 LIGAMENT TEAR SEE 'SPRAIN'
0 MENISCUS TEAR SEE 'MENISCUS'
718.1# MICE

5th Digit: 718.1

0. SITE NOS
1. SHOULDER REGION
2. UPPER ARM (ELBOW) (HUMERUS)
3. FOREARM (RADIUS) (WRIST) (ULNA)
4. HAND (CARPAL) (METACARPAL) (FINGERS)
5. PELVIC REGION AND THIGH (HIP) (BUTTOCK) (FEMUR)
7. ANKLE AND/OR FOOT (METATARSALS) (TOES) (TARSALS)
8. OTHER SPECIFIED SITES
9. MULTIPLE

717.6 MICE KNEE
724.9 MICE VERTEBRAL (FACET)

JOINT (continued)

719.4# PAIN

5th Digit: 719.4

0. SITE NOS
1. SHOULDER REGION
2. UPPER ARM (ELBOW) (HUMERUS)
3. FOREARM (RADIUS) (WRIST) (ULNA)
4. HAND (CARPAL) (METACARPAL)
5. PELVIC REGION AND THIGH (HIP) (BUTTOCK) (FEMUR)
6. LOWER LEG (FIBULA) (PATELLA) (TIBIA)
7. ANKLE AND/OR FOOT (METATARSALS) (TOES) (TARSALS)
8. OTHER

996.66 PROSTHESIS INFECTION OR INFLAMMATION
V43.60 REPLACEMENT STATUS
V43.66 REPLACEMENT STATUS - ANKLE
V43.62 REPLACEMENT STATUS - ELBOW
V43.69 REPLACEMENT STATUS - FINGER
V43.64 REPLACEMENT STATUS - HIP
V43.65 REPLACEMENT STATUS - KNEE
V43.61 REPLACEMENT STATUS - SHOULDER
V43.63 REPLACEMENT STATUS - WRIST
V43.69 REPLACEMENT STATUS - OTHER
719.6# SNAPPING

5th Digit: 719.6

0. SITE NOS
1. SHOULDER REGION
2. UPPER ARM (ELBOW) (HUMERUS)
3. FOREARM (RADIUS) (WRIST) (ULNA)
4. HAND (CARPAL) (METACARPAL)
5. PELVIC REGION AND THIGH (HIP) (BUTTOCK) (FEMUR)
6. LOWER LEG (FIBULA) (PATELLA) (TIBIA)
7. ANKLE AND/OR FOOT (METATARSALS) (TOES) (TARSALS)
8. OTHER
9. MULTIPLE

727.05 SNAPPING FINGER OR THUMB
524.69 SNAPPING JAW
717.9 SNAPPING KNEE
0 SPRAIN OR STRAIN SEE 'SPRAIN'
719.5# STIFFNESS
724.6 STIFFNESS LUMBOSACRAL
724.6 STIFFNESS SACROILIAC
719.0# SWELLING
0 TEAR SEE 'SPRAIN'
719.6# OTHER SYMPTOMS REFERABLE TO JOINT
719.8# OTHER DISORDERS OF JOINT

5th Digit: 719.0, 5-6, 8

0. SITE NOS
1. SHOULDER REGION
2. UPPER ARM (ELBOW) (HUMERUS)
3. FOREARM (RADIUS) (WRIST) (ULNA)
4. HAND (CARPAL) (METACARPAL) (FINGERS)
5. PELVIC REGION AND THIGH (HIP) (BUTTOCK) (FEMUR)
6. LOWER LEG (FIBULA) (KNEE) (PATELLA) (TIBIA)
7. ANKLE AND/OR FOOT (METATARSALS) (TOES) (TARSALS)
8. OTHER
9. MULTIPLE

288.2 JORDAN'S SYNDROME
284.0 JOSEPH-DIAMOND-BLACKFAN SYNDROME (CONGENITAL HYPOPLASTIC ANEMIA)
523.0 JOURDAIN'S DISEASE (ACUTE GINGIVITIS)
352.6 JUGULAR FORAMEN SYNDROME

JUGULAR VEIN

900.81 INJURY SITE NOS
900.81 INJURY - EXTERNAL
900.1 INJURY - INTERNAL
908.3 INJURY - LATE EFFECT
451.89 PHLEBITIS

427.60 JUNCTIONAL PREMATURE CONTRACTION
135 JUNGLING'S DISEASE (SARCOIDOSIS)
286.4 JURGENS' DISEASE
174.9 JUVENILE BREAST CARCINOMA SITE NOS
0 JUVENILE BREAST CARCINOMA SITE SPECIFIED SEE 'CANCER' BY SITE M8502/3
312.9 JUVENILE DELINQUENCY
090.40 JUVENILE GENERAL PARESIS
102.7 JUXTA-ARTICULAR NODULE
593.89 JUXTAGLOMERULAR HYPERPLASIA (COMPLEX) (KIDNEY)
236.91 JUXTAGLOMERULAR TUMOR SITE NOS
0 JUXTAGLOMERULAR TUMOR SITE SPECIFIED SEE 'NEOPLASM UNCERTAIN BEHAVIOR' BY SITE M8361/1

203.0# KAHLER'S DISEASE OR SYNDROME (MULTIPLE MYELOMA)

5th Digit: 203.0

0. WITHOUT MENTION OF REMISSION
1. IN REMISSION

759.6 KALISCHER'S DISEASE OR SYNDROME (ENCEPHALOCUTANEOUS ANGIOMATOSIS)
253.4 KALLMANN'S SYNDROME (HYPOGONADOTROPIC HYPOGONADISM WITH ANOSMIA)
299.0# KANNER'S SYNDROME (AUTISM)

5th Digit: 299.0

0. ACTIVE
1. RESIDUAL

KAPOSI'S

757.33 DISEASE CONGENITAL
697.8 LICHEN RUBER
696.4 LICHEN RUBER ACUMINATUS
697.8 LICHEN RUBER MONILIFORMIS
176.# SARCOMA M9140/3

4th Digit: 176

0. SKIN
1. SOFT TISSUE
2. SOFT PALATE
3. GASTROINTESTINAL
4. LUNG
5. LYMPH NODES
8. OTHER SPECIFIED SITES (EXTERNAL GENITALIA) (SCROTUM) (VULVA)
9. SITE UNSPECIFIED

054.0 VARICELLIFORM ERUPTION HERPES SIMPLEX
757.33 XERODERMA PIGMENTOSUM

759.3 KARTAGENER'S SYNDROME (SINUSISTIS, BRONCHIECTASIS, SITUS INVERSUS)
795.2 KARYOTYPE ABNORMAL
287.3 KASABACH-MERRITT SYNDROME (CAPILLARY HEMANGIOMA ASSOCIATED WITH THROMBOCYTOPENIC PURPURA)

716.0#	KASCHIN BECK DISEASE (ENDEMIC POLYARTHRITIS)
	5th Digit: 716.0
	0. SITE NOS
	1. SHOULDER REGION
	2. UPPER ARM (ELBOW) (HUMERUS)
	3. FOREARM (RADIUS) (WRIST) (ULNA)
	4. HAND (CARPAL) (METACARPAL) (FINGERS)
	5. PELVIC REGION AND THIGH (HIP) (BUTTOCK) (FEMUR)
	6. LOWER LEG (FIBULA) (KNEE) (PATELLA) (TIBIA)
	7. ANKLE AND/OR FOOT (METATARSALS) (TOE) (TARSALS)
	8. OTHER (HEAD) (NECK) (RIB) (SKULL) ((TRUNK) (VERTEBRAE)
	9. MULTIPLE
756.4	KAST'S SYNDROME (DYSCHONDROPLASIA WITH HEMANGIOMA)
120.2	KATAYAMA DISEASE OR FEVER
446.1	KAWASAKI DISEASE
275.1	KAYSER FLEISCHER RING (CORNEA) [371.14]
284.0	KAZNELSON'S SYNDROME (CONGENITAL HYPOPLASTIC ANEMIA)
081.2	KEDANI FEVER (SCRUB TYPHUS)
280.8	KELLY'S SYNDROME (SIDEROPENIC DYSPHAGIA)
701.4	KELOID
371.00	KELOID CORNEA
066.1	KEMEROVO TICK BORNE FEVER
335.11	KENNEDY SYNDROME
082.1	KENYA TICK TYPHUS
706.2	KERATIN CYST
	KERATITIS
370.9	NOS
370.24	ACTINIC
370.22	AREOLAR
370.23	FILAMENTARY
370.50	INTERSTITIAL
370.52	INTERSTITIAL DIFFUSE
370.59	INTERSTITIAL OTHER
370.22	MACULAR
370.22	NUMMULAR
370.21	PUNCTATE
370.54	SCLEROSING
370.22	STELLATE
370.22	STRIATE
370.20	SUPERFICIAL
370.40	SUPERFICIAL (WITH CONJUNCTIVITIS)
370.00	ULCERATED
370.24	WELDERS'
370.8	OTHER FORMS
	KERATITIS OTHER
054.42	ARBORESCENS
054.42	DENDRITIC
052.7	DISCIFORM VARICELLA [370.44]
372.13	EPITHELIALIS VERNALIS [370.32]
098.43	GONOCOCCAL
055.71	MEASLES (RUBEOLA MOBILLI)
055.71	RUBEOLA
050.9	SMALLPOX [370.44]
090.3	SYPHILITIC
017.3#	TUBERCULOUS INTERSTITIAL [370.59]
	5th Digit: 017.3
	0. NOS
	1. LAB NOT DONE
	2. LABS PENDING
	3. MICROSCOPY POSITIVE (IN SPUTUM)
	4. CULTURE POSITIVE - MICROSCOPY NEGATIVE
	5. CULTURE NEGATIVE - MICROSCOPY POSITIVE
	6. CULTURE AND MICROSCOPY NEGATIVE CONFIRMED BY OTHER METHODS
0	SEE ALSO 'KERATOCONJUNCTIVITIS'
238.2	KERATOACANTHOMA
	KERATOCONJUNCTIVITIS
370.40	NOS
052.7	CHICKENPOX [370.44]
051.0	COWPOX [370.44]
077.1	EPIDEMIC
370.34	EXPOSURE (DUE TO)
054.42	HERPES SIMPLEX DENDRITIC
054.43	HERPES SIMPLEX DISCIFORM
053.21	HERPETIC (ZOSTER)
372.13	LIMBAR AND CORNEAL INVOLVEMENT IN VERNAL CONJUNCTIVITIS [370.32]
055.71	MEASLES (RUBEOLA MOBILLI)
370.35	NEUROTROPHIC
370.49	OTHER
370.31	PHLYCTENULAR
055.71	RUBEOLA
370.33	SICCA
710.2	SICCA (SJOGRENS)
050.9	SMALLPOX [370.44]
372.13	VERNAL WITH CORNEAL INVOLVEMENT [370.32]
	KERATOCONJUNCTIVITIS OTHER TYPES
017.3#	TB [370.31]
	5th Digit: 017.3
	0. NOS
	1. LAB NOT DONE
	2. LABS PENDING
	3. MICROSCOPY POSITIVE (IN SPUTUM)
	4. CULTURE POSITIVE - MICROSCOPY NEGATIVE
	5. CULTURE NEGATIVE - MICROSCOPY POSITIVE
	6. CULTURE AND MICROSCOPY NEGATIVE CONFIRMED BY OTHER METHODS
052.8	VARICELLA (DUE TO)
053.21	ZOSTER (DUE TO)
	KERATOCONUS
371.60	NOS
371.62	ACUTE HYDROPS
371.61	STABLE CONDITION
	KERATODERMA
701.1	ACQUIRED
701.1	CLIMACTERICUM
757.39	CONGENITAL
701.1	PALMARIS ET PLANTARIS
701.1	TYLODES PROGRESSIVE
695.89	KERATOLYSIS EXFOLIATIVA
757.39	KERATOLYSIS EXFOLIATIVA CONGENITAL, NEONATORUM
	KERATOMA
701.1	NOS
757.39	CONGENITAL
757.1	MALIGNUM CONGENITALE
702.0	SENILE
	KERATOMALACIA
371.45	NOS
264.4	VITAMIN A DEFICIENCY
111.1	KERATOMYCOSIS NIGRICANS
	KERATOPATHY
371.43	BAND-SHAPED
371.40	DEGENERATIVE
371.49	DISCRETE COLLIQUATIVE
371.50	HEREDITARY

KERATOSIS

701.1 NOS
702.0 ACTINIC
702.0 ACTINIC SOLAR
692.4 ARSENICAL
701.1 BLENNORRHAGICA
098.81 BLENNORRHAGICA GONOCOCCAL
757.39 CONGENITAL (ANY TYPE)
264.8 FOLLICULAR DUE TO VITAMIN A DEFICIENCY
701.1 FOLLICULARIS ACQUIRED
757.39 FOLLICULARIS CONGENITAL
264.8 FOLLICULARIS DUE TO VITAMIN A DEFICIENCY
757.39 FOLLICULARIS SPINULOSA
608.89 GENITALIA MALE EXTERNAL
607.89 GENITALIA MALE PENILE
098.81 GONOCOCCAL
701.2 NIGRICANS
380.21 OBTURANS OF EXTERNAL EAR (CANAL)
757.39 PALMARIS ET PLANTARIS
607.89 PENILE
757.39 PILARIS
701.1 PILARIS ACQUIRED
701.1 PUNCTATA
608.89 SCROTAL
702.1# SEBORRHEIC

5th Digit: 702.1

1. INFLAMED
9. OTHER

702.0 SENILE
702.0 SOLAR
757.39 SPINULOSA DECALVANS
757.39 SUPRAFOLLICULARIS
478.29 TONSILLARIS
623.1 VAGINA
757.39 VEGETANS

110.0 KERION

KERNICTERUS

773.4 DUE TO BLOOD TYPE REACTION PERINATAL [773.#]

4th Digit: 773

0. RH (RHESUS) ISOIMMUNIZATION
1. ABO ISOIMMUNIZATION
2. OTHER AND NOS ISOIMMUNIZATION

774.7 NOT DUE TO ISOIMMUNIZATION PERINATAL
774.7 NEWBORN

276.2 KETOACIDOSIS
0 KETOACIDOSIS DIABETIC SEE 'DIABETES, DIABETIC', KETOACIDOSIS

791.6 KETONURIA
270.3 KETONURIA BRANCHED CHAIN
791.9 KETOSTEROIDS (17) ELEVATED

KIDNEY

V45.73 ABSENCE POSTSURGICAL
593.89 ADHESIONS
587 ATROPHY (CONTRACTION) (CIRRHOSIS) (FIBROSIS)
593.89 CALCIFICATION
592.0 CALCULUS
788.0 COLIC
0 CONGENITAL DISORDER SEE 'KIDNEY CONGENITAL'
587 CONTRACTED
866.01 CONTUSION
866.11 CONTUSION WITH OPEN WOUND INTO CAVITY
908.1 CONTUSION LATE EFFECT
593.89 DILATATION
V18.61 DISEASE FAMILY HISTORY - POLYCYSTIC
V18.69 DISEASE FAMILY HISTORY - OTHER

KIDNEY (continued)

593.9 DISORDER
593.81 DISORDER VASCULAR
593.89 DISORDER OTHER SPECIFIED
588.9 DISORDER FUNCTIONAL
588.8 DISORDER FUNCTIONAL OTHER SPECIFIED
593.89 DIVERTICULUM
V59.4 DONOR NON-AUTOGENOUS
654.4# ECTOPIC COMPLICATING PREGNANCY
660.2# ECTOPIC OBSTRUCTING LABOR [**654.4#**]

5th Digit: 654.4

0. EPISODE OF CARE UNSPECIFIED OR N/A
1. DELIVERED
2. DELIVERED WITH POSTPARTUM COMPLICATION
3. ANTEPARTUM COMPLICATION
4. POSTPARTUM COMPLICATION

5th Digit: 660.2

0. EPISODE OF CARE UNSPECIFIED OR N/A
1. DELIVERED
3. ANTEPARTUM COMPLICATION

0 FAILURE SEE 'RENAL FAILURE'
793.5 FILLING DEFECT
593.0 FLOATING
794.4 FUNCTION STUDY ABNORMAL
593.89 HYPERPLASIA
593.1 HYPERTROPHY
590.9 INFECTION
866.## INJURY

4th Digit: 866

0. CLOSED
1. WITH OPEN WOUND INTO CAVITY

5th Digit: 866

0. INJURY NOS
1. CONTUSION/HEMATOMA
2. LACERATION
3. RUPTURE

908.1 INJURY LATE EFFECT
866.02 LACERATION
866.12 LACERATION WITH OPEN WOUND INTO CAVITY
908.1 LACERATION LATE EFFECT
593.89 OBSTRUCTION
593.89 OCCLUSION
0 RENAL CYST SEE 'CYST', RENAL
794.4 SCAN ABNORMAL
584.5 SHOCK SYNDROME
958.5 SHOCK SYNDROME FOLLOWING CRUSH INJURY
908.6 SHOCK SYNDROME FOLLOWING CRUSH INJURY LATE EFFECT
589.9 SMALL
589.1 SMALL BILATERAL
589.0 SMALL UNILATERAL
592.0 STAGHORN CALCULUS
592.0 STONE
274.11 STONE URIC ACID
996.81 TRANSPLANT REJECTION (FAILURE)
V42.0 TRANSPLANT (STATUS)
589.9 UNDERSIZED
589.1 UNDERSIZED BILATERAL
589.0 UNDERSIZED UNILATERAL

KIDNEY CONGENITAL

753.0 ABSENCE
753.3 ACCESSORY
753.3 ATRESIA
753.0 ATROPHY
753.0 ATROPHY INFANTILE
753.3 CALCULUS
753.3 CONTRACTED
753.11 CYST
753.11 CYST SINGLE
753.10 CYSTIC DISEASE
753.19 CYSTIC DISEASE OTHER SPECIFIED

I-J-K

KIDNEY CONGENITAL (continued)

753.3 DISCOID
753.3 DISPLACED
753.3 DOUBLE WITH DOUBLE PELVIS
753.15 DYSPLASIA
753.3 ECTOPIC
753.19 FIBROCYSTIC
753.3 FUSION
753.3 GIANT
753.3 HORSESHOE
753.3 HYPERPLASIA
753.0 HYPOPLASIA
753.3 LOBULATION
753.3 MALROTATION
753.16 MEDULLARY CYSTIC
753.17 MEDULLARY SPONGE
753.19 MULTICYSTIC
753.12 POLYCYSTIC (DISEASE OF)
753.13 POLYCYSTIC AUTOSOMAL DOMINANT
753.14 POLYCYSTIC AUTOSOMAL RECESSIVE
753.12 POLYCYSTIC TYPE UNSPECIFIED
753.17 SPONGIFORM
0 SEE ALSO 'RENAL'

732.3 KIENBOCK'S DISEASE (CARPAL LUNATE) (WRIST)
289.3 KIKUCHI DISEASE
250.4# KIMMELSTIEL WILSON SYNDROME DIABETIC [581.81]

5th Digit: 250.4

0. TYPE II, ADULT-ONSET, NON-INSULIN DEPENDENT (EVEN IF REQUIRING INSULIN), OR UNSPECIFIED; CONTROLLED

1. TYPE I, JUVENILE-ONSET OR INSULIN-DEPENDENT; CONTROLLED

2. TYPE II, ADULT-ONSET, NON-INSULIN DEPENDENT (EVEN IF REQUIRING INSULIN); UNCONTROLLED

3. TYPE I, JUVENILE-ONSET OR INSULIN-DEPENDENT; UNCONTROLLED

275.1 KINNIER WILSON'S DISEASE (HEPATOLENTICULAR DEGENERATION)
798.1 KIROSHI SYNDROME
V54.8 KIRSCHNER WIRE REMOVAL
075 KISSING DISEASE
721.5 KISSING SPINE
695.1 KLAUDER'S SYNDROME (ERYTHEMA MULTIFORME EXUDATIVUM)
583.9 KLEBS DISEASE
041.3 KLEBSIELLA PNEUMONIAE INFECTION OR ORGANISM
270.2 KLEIN-WAARDENBURG SYNDROME (PTOSIS-EPICANTHUS)
349.89 KLEINE LEVIN SYNDROME
312.32 KLEPTOMANIA
758.7 KLINEFELTER'S SYNDROME
446.4 KLINGER'S DISEASE
756.16 KLIPPEL FEIL SYNDROME (BREVICOLLIS)
759.89 KLIPPEL TRENAUNAY SYNDROME
723.8 KLIPPEL'S DISEASE (CERVICAL)
767.6 KLUMPKE DEJERINE PALSY, PARALYSIS OR SYNDROME (INJURY TO BRACHIAL PLEXUS AT BIRTH)
310.0 KLUVER-BUCY (-TERZIAN) SYNDROME

KNEE

736.5 BACK (GENU RECURVATUM)
719.86 CALCIFICATION
0 CAP SEE 'PATELLA, PATELLAR'
844.0 COLLATERAL LIGAMENTS SPRAIN - LATERAL
844.1 COLLATERAL LIGAMENTS SPRAIN - MEDIAL

KNEE (continued)

717.89 COLLATERAL LIGAMENTS SPRAIN OLD - NOS
717.81 COLLATERAL LIGAMENTS SPRAIN OLD - LATERAL
717.82 COLLATERAL LIGAMENTS SPRAIN OLD - MEDIAL
718.46 CONTRACTURE
719.66 CREPITUS
844.2 CRUCIATE LIGAMENT SPRAIN ACUTE
717.89 CRUCIATE LIGAMENT SPRAIN- NOS OLD
717.83 CRUCIATE LIGAMENT SPRAIN- ANTERIOR OLD
717.84 CRUCIATE LIGAMENT SPRAIN- POSTERIOR OLD
736.6 DEFORMITY ACQUIRED
755.64 DEFORMITY (JOINT) CONGENITAL
736.6 DEFORMITY OTHER (ACQUIRED)
717.9 DERANGEMENT INTERNAL (OLD)
717.89 DERANGEMENT INTERNAL (OLD) - OTHER
719.06 EFFUSION
719.36 EFFUSION INTERMITTENT
719.86 FISTULA
718.86 FLAIL
719.16 HEMARTHROSIS
0 HEMARTHROSIS CURRENT INJURY SEE 'SPRAIN'
719.06 HYDRARTHROSIS
719.36 HYDRARTHROSIS INTERMITTENT
718.86 HYPEREXTENSION (OLD)
716.96 INFLAMMATION
959.7 INJURY
916.8 INJURY OTHER AND UNSPECIFIED SUPERFICIAL
916.9 INJURY OTHER AND UNSPECIFIED SUPERFICIAL INFECTED
718.86 INSTABILITY (OLD)
719.86 JOINT CALCIFICATION
736.41 KNOCK
755.64 KNOCK CONGENITAL
836.1 LATERAL MENISCUS TEAR ACUTE
717.41 LATERAL MENISCUS BUCKET HANDLE TEAR (OLD)
717.40 LATERAL MENISCUS DERANGEMENT (OLD)
717.42 LATERAL MENISCUS DERANGEMENT ANTERIOR HORN (OLD)
717.43 LATERAL MENISCUS DERANGEMENT POSTERIOR HORN (OLD)
717.49 LATERAL MENISCUS DERANGEMENT OTHER (OLD)

717.89 LIGAMENT DISRUPTION (OLD)
717.85 LIGAMENT DISRUPTION (OLD) - CAPSULAR
717.83 LIGAMENT DISRUPTION (OLD) - CRUCIATE ANTERIOR
717.84 LIGAMENT DISRUPTION (OLD) - CRUCIATE POSTERIOR
717.81 LIGAMENT DISRUPTION (OLD) - LATERAL COLLATERAL
717.82 LIGAMENT DISRUPTION (OLD) - MEDIAL COLLATERAL
717.85 LIGAMENT DISRUPTION (OLD) - OTHER LIGAMENT
717.89 LIGAMENT RELAXATION
0 LIGAMENT SPRAIN SEE 'SPRAIN', KNEE
717.6 LOOSE BODY OLD
836.0 MEDIAL MENISCUS - TEAR ACUTE
836.0 MEDIAL MENISCUS - BUCKET HANDLE TEAR ACUTE
717.0 MEDIAL MENISCUS - BUCKET HANDLE TEAR OLD
717.1 MEDIAL MENISCUS DERANGEMENT - ANTERIOR HORN (OLD)
717.2 MEDIAL MENISCUS DERANGEMENT - POSTERIOR HORN (OLD)
717.3 MEDIAL MENISCUS DERANGEMENT - OTHER OR UNSPECIFIED (OLD)
844.8 PATELLAR SPRAIN
717.89 PATELLAR SPRAIN - OLD
V43.65 REPLACEMENT STATUS
717.9 SNAPPING
0 SPRAIN SEE ALSO 'SPRAIN', KNEE
719.56 STIFFNESS
719.06 SWELLING
0 TEAR SEE 'SPRAIN'
719.66 OTHER SYMPTOMS REFERABLE TO JOINT
719.86 OTHER DISORDERS OF JOINT

911.1 KNIGHT'S DISEASE (INFECTED ABRASION)
736.41 KNOCK KNEE
755.64 KNOCK KNEE CONGENITAL
794.19 KOBIYASHI ABNORMAL FUNCTION STUDY
757.39 KOBNER'S DISEASE (EPIDERMYLOSIS BULLOSA)
694.4 KOENIG-WICHMANN DISEASE (PEMPHIGUS)

KOHLER
732.4 DISEASE PATELLAR
732.5 DISEASE TARSAL NAVICULAR (BONE) (OSTEOARTHROSIS JUVENILIS)
732.5 FREIBERG DISEASE (INFRACTION METATARSAL HEAD)
732.5 MOUCHET DISEASE (OSTEOARTHROSIS JUVENILIS)
726.62 PELLEGRINI-STIEDA SYNDROME (CALCIFICATION KNEE JOINT)

703.8 KOILONYCHIA
757.5 KOILONYCHIA CONGENITAL
345.7# KOJEVNIKOV'S EPILEPSY
5th Digit: 345.7
0. WITHOUT MENTION OF INTRACTABLE EPILEPSY
1. WITH INTRACTABLE EPILEPSY

747.21 KOMMERELL'S DIVERTICULUM CONGENITAL
732.7 KONIG'S DISEASE (OSTEOCHONDRITIS DISSECANS)
564.89 KONIG'S SYNDROME
294.0 KORSAKOFF'S (-WERNICKE) PSYCHOSIS OR SYNDROME
291.1 KORSAKOFF'S (-WERNICKE) PSYCHOSIS OR SYNDROME ALCOHOLIC
288.0 KOSTMANN'S SYNDROME (INFANTILE GENETIC AGRANULOCYTOSIS)

KRABBE'S
756.89 CONGENITAL MUSCLE HYPOPLASIA (SYNDROME)
759.6 CUTANEOCEREBRAL ANGIOMA (SYNDROME)
330.0 DISEASE

0 KRAEPELIN-MOREL DISEASE SEE 'SCHIZOPHRENIA'
759.6 KRAFT-WEBER-DIMITRI DISEASE
607.0 KRAUROSIS PENIS
371.13 KRUKENBERG SPINDLE
198.6 KRUKENBERG'S TUMOR OVARY M8490/6
793.5 KUB ABNORMAL
330.1 KUFS' DISEASE
335.11 KUGELBERG WELANDER DISEASE
362.52 KUHNT JUNIUS DEGENERATION
721.7 KUMMELL'S (-VERNEUIL) (SPONDYLITIS) DISEASE
0 KUNDRAT'S DISEASE SEE 'LYMPHOSARCOMA'
571.49 KUNKEL SYNDROME (LUPOID HEPATITIS)
046.0 KURU
446.0 KUSSMAUL (-MEIER) DISEASE (POLYARTERITIS NODOSA)
V82.8 KVEIM TEST
260 KWASHIORKOR
065.2 KYASANUR FOREST DISEASE
270.2 KYNURENINASE DEFECTS

KYPHOSCOLIOSIS, KYPHOSCOLOLIOTIC
737.30 ACQUIRED
737.30 AND SCOLIOSIS IDIOPATHIC
756.19 CONGENITAL
737.33 DUE TO RADIATION
737.30 IDIOPATHIC
737.32 IDIOPATHIC - INFANTILE PROGRESSIVE
737.31 IDIOPATHIC - INFANTILE RESOLVING
416.1 HEART DISEASE
268.1 LATE EFFECT OF RICKET'S [737.43]
737.34 THORACOGENIC

KYPHOSCOLIOSIS, KYPHOSCOLOLIOTIC (continued)
015.0# TUBERCULOUS [737.43]
5th Digit: 015.0
0. UNSPECIFIED
1. LAB NOT DONE
2. LABS PENDING
3. MICROSCOPY POSITIVE (IN SPUTUM)
4. CULTURE POSITIVE - MICROSCOPY NEGATIVE
5. CULTURE NEGATIVE - MICROSCOPY POSITIVE
6. CULTURE AND MICROSCOPY NEGATIVE CONFIRMED BY OTHER METHODS

737.39 OTHER SPECIFIED NEC

KYPHOSIS, KYPHOTIC
737.10 ACQUIRED (POSTURAL)
737.19 ACQUIRED OTHER
737.0 ADOLESCENT POSTURAL
737.41 ASSOCIATED WITH OTHER CONDITIONS
356.1 CHARCOT MARIE TOOTH [737.41]
756.19 CONGENITAL
737.11 DUE TO RADIATION
277.5 MUCOPOLYSACCHARIDOSIS [737.41]
237.7# NEUROFIBROMATOSIS [737.41]
5th Digit: 237.7
0. UNSPECIFIED
1. TYPE I
2. TYPE II
731.0 OSTEITIS DEFORMANS [737.41]
252.0 OSTEITIS FIBROSA CYSTICA [737.41]
733.0# OSTEOPOROTIC [737.41]
5th Digit: 733.0
0. UNSPECIFIED
1. SENILE
2. IDIOPATHIC
3. DISUSE
9. DRUG INDUCED

045.## POLIOMYELITIS [737.41]
4th Dgit: 045
0. ACUTE BULBAR PARALYTIC
1. ACUTE WITH OTHER PARALYSIS
2. ACUTE NON PARALYTIC
9. ACUTE UNSPECIFIED
5th Dgit: 045
0. POLIOVIRUS UNSPECIFIED
1. POLIOVIRUS TYPE I
2. POLIOVIRUS TYPE II
3. POLIOVIRUS TYPE III

138 POLIOMYELITIS LATE EFFECT [737.41]
737.12 POSTLAMINECTOMY
737.11 RADIATION
015.0# TUBERCULOUS [737.41]
5th Digit: 015.0
0. UNSPECIFIED
1. LAB NOT DONE
2. LABS PENDING
3. MICROSCOPY POSITIVE (IN SPUTUM)
4. CULTURE POSITIVE - MICROSCOPY NEGATIVE
5. CULTURE NEGATIVE - MICROSCOPY POSITIVE
6. CULTURE AND MICROSCOPY NEGATIVE CONFIRMED BY OTHER METHODS

237.7# VON RECKLINGHAUSEN'S DISEASE [737.41]
5th Digit: 237.7
0. UNSPECIFIED OR MULTIPLE
1. TYPE I
2. TYPE II

737.19 OTHER SPECIFIED CAUSE NEC

701.1 KYRLE'S DISEASE (HYPERKERATOSIS FOLLICULARIS IN CUTEM PENETRANS)

307.23 LA TOURETTE'S DISORDER
796.2 LABILE BLOOD PRESSURE
301.59 LABILE PERSONALITY DISORDER

LABIUM, LABIAL (MAJUS) (MINUS)

752.49 ABSENCE CONGENITAL
624.4 ADHERENT (MINUS)
752.49 ADHESION CONGENITAL
624.8 CYST
616.9 DISEASE INFLAMMATORY
616.8 DISEASE INFLAMMATORY - OTHER NEC
624.9 DISEASE NONINFLAMMATORY
624.8 DISEASE NONINFLAMMATORY - OTHER NEC
616.9 DISORDER INFLAMMATORY
616.8 DISORDER INFLAMMATORY - OTHER NEC
624.9 DISORDER NONINFLAMMATORY
624.8 DISORDER NONINFLAMMATORY - OTHER NEC
752.49 FUSION CONGENITAL
624.3 HYPERTROPHY
911.8 INJURY OTHER AND UNSPECIFIED SUPERFICIAL
911.9 INJURY OTHER AND UNSPECIFIED SUPERFICIAL - INFECTED
749.1# LEPORINUM
5th Digit: 749.1
0. CLEFT UNSPECIFIED
1. CLEFT UNILATERAL COMPLETE
2. CLEFT UNILATERAL INCOMPLETE
3. CLEFT BILATERAL COMPLETE
4. CLEFT BILATERAL INCOMPLETE

752.49 MINORA DIVISION CONGENITAL
624.6 POLYP

LABOR ABNORMALITIES

661.9# UNSPECIFIED
5th Digit: 661.9
0. EPISODE OF CARE UNSPECIFIED OR N/A
1. DELIVERED
3. ANTEPARTUM COMPLICATION

669.9# COMPLICATION UNSPECIFIED
669.4# COMPLICATION OTHER OF OBSTETRICAL SURGERY AND PROCEDURES
669.8# COMPLICATION OTHER SPECIFIED
5th Digit: 669.4, 8-9
0. EPISODE OF CARE UNSPECIFIED OR N/A
1. DELIVERED
2. DELIVERED WITH POSTPARTUM COMPLICATION
3. ANTEPARTUM COMPLICATION
4. POSTPARTUM COMPLICATION

LABOR ABNORMALITIES (continued)

0 DESULTORY SEE 'UTERUS, UTERINE DISORDERS COMPLICATING PREGNANCY', INERTIA OTHER
661.4# DYSCOORDINATE
659.1# FAILED INDUCTION NOS (DRUGS)
659.0# FAILED INDUCTION MECHANICAL
660.6# FAILED TRIAL
5th Digit: 659.0-1, 660.6, 661.4
0. EPISODE OF CARE UNSPECIFIED OR N/A
1. DELIVERED
3. ANTEPARTUM COMPLICATION

644.1# FALSE >37 WEEKS
644.0# FALSE >22 AND <37 WEEKS
5th Digit: 644.0-1
0. EPISODE OF CARE UNSPECIFIED OR N/A
3. ANTEPARTUM COMPLICATION

0 IRREGULAR SEE 'UTERUS, UTERINE DISORDERS COMPLICATING PREGNANCY', INERTIA OTHER
661.3# PRECIPITATE
5th Digit: 661.3
0. EPISODE OF CARE UNSPECIFIED OR N/A
1. DELIVERED
3. ANTEPARTUM COMPLICATION

644.2# PREMATURE WITH ONSET OF DELIVERY <37 WEEKS
5th Digit: 644.2
0. EPISODE OF CARE UNSPECIFIED OR N/A
1. DELIVERED

644.0# PREMATURE WITHOUT DELIVERY >22 AND <37 WEEKS
5th Digit: 644.0
0. EPISODE OF CARE UNSPECIFIED OR N/A
3. ANTEPARTUM COMPLICATION

662.1# PROLONGED
662.0# PROLONGED FIRST STAGE
662.2# PROLONGED SECOND STAGE
5th Digit: 662.0-2
0. EPISODE OF CARE UNSPECIFIED OR N/A
1. DELIVERED
3. ANTEPARTUM COMPLICATION

644.1# THREATENED >37 WEEKS
644.0# THREATENED >22 AND <37 WEEKS (DUE TO IRRITABLE UTERUS)
5th Digit: 644.0-1
0. EPISODE OF CARE UNSPECIFIED OR N/A
3. ANTEPARTUM COMPLICATION

0 SEE ALSO 'UTERUS, UTERINE DISORDERS COMPLICATING PREGNANCY', INERTIA

LABOR AND DELIVERY COMPLICATIONS

ABNORMALITIES OF PELVIC ORGANS OR TISSUE

OBSTRUCTING LABOR

660.9# OBSTRUCTED LABOR NOS
660.2# BLADDER DILATATION OBSTRUCTING LABOR **[654.4#]**
660.2# CERVICAL INCOMPETENCE OBSTRUCTING LABOR **[654.5#]**
660.2# CERVICAL POLYP OBSTRUCTING LABOR **[654.6#]**
660.2# CERVICAL STENOSIS OBSTRUCTING LABOR **[654.6#]**
660.2# CERVIX ABNORMALITY OBSTRUCTING LABOR **[654.6#]**
660.2# CERVIX CICATRIX OBSTRUCTING LABOR **[654.6#]**
660.2# CERVIX RIGID OBSTRUCTING LABOR **[654.6#]**
660.2# CERVIX TUMOR OBSTRUCTING LABOR **[654.6#]**
660.2# CESAREAN SECTION (PREVIOUS) OBSTRUCTING LABOR **[654.2#]**
660.2# CYSTOCELE OBSTRUCTING LABOR **[654.4#]**
660.9# DYSTOCIA NOS OBSTRUCTING LABOR
660.2# KIDNEY ECTOPIC OBSTRUCTING LABOR **[654.4#]**
660.5# LOCKED TWINS OBSTRUCTING LABOR **[652.6#]**
660.0# MALPOSITION OF FETUS AT ONSET OBSTRUCTING LABOR **[652.9#]**
660.8# OTHER CAUSES OBSTRUCTING LABOR
660.2# PELVIC OR SOFT TISSUE OBSTRUCTING LABOR **[654.9#]**
660.2# PERINEAL FIBROSIS OBSTRUCTING LABOR **[654.8#]**
660.2# PERSISTENT HYMEN OBSTRUCTING LABOR **[654.8#]**
660.2# PREVIOUS C SECTION OBSTRUCTING LABOR **[654.2#]**
660.2# RECTOCELE OBSTRUCTING LABOR **[654.4#]**
660.2# SEPTATE VAGINA OBSTRUCTING LABOR **[654.7#]**
660.2# SHIRODKAR SUTURE OBSTRUCTING LABOR **[654.5#]**
660.0# SHOULDER DYSTOCIA OBSTRUCTING LABOR **[652.8#]**
660.4# SHOULDER GIRDLE DYSTOCIA OBSTRUCTING LABOR
660.3# TRANSVERSE AND PERSISTENT OCCIPITO-POSTERIOR POSITION OBSTRUCTING LABOR **[652.8#]**
660.2# UTERINE ABNORMALITY CONGENITAL OBSTRUCTING LABOR **[654.0#]**
660.2# UTERINE FIBROID OBSTRUCTING LABOR **[654.1#]**
660.2# UTERINE SACCULATION OBSTRUCTING LABOR **[654.4#]**
660.2# UTERUS PROLAPSE OBSTRUCTING LABOR **[654.4#]**
660.2# UTERUS RETROVERTED (INCARCERATED) OBSTRUCTING LABOR **[654.3#]**
660.2# UTERUS BICORNIS OBSTRUCTING LABOR **[654.0#]**
660.2# VAGINA ABNORMALITY OBSTRUCTING LABOR **[654.7#]**
660.2# VAGINAL PROLAPSE OBSTRUCTING LABOR **[654.7#]**
660.2# VAGINAL STENOSIS OBSTRUCTING LABOR **[654.7#]**
660.2# VAGINAL TUMOR OBSTRUCTING LABOR **[654.7#]**
660.2# VULVA ABNORMALITY OBSTRUCTING LABOR **[654.8#]**
660.2# VULVA TUMOR OBSTRUCTING LABOR **[654.8#]**
660.2# VULVA VARICOSE VEINS OBSTRUCTING LABOR **[671.1#]**
660.8# OTHER OBSTRUCTED LABOR

5th Digit: 652.6, 8 -9, 654.0-9, 660.0-9,

0. EPISODE OF CARE UNSPECIFIED OR N/A
1. DELIVERED
3. ANTEPARTUM COMPLICATION

5th Digit: 654.0-1, 3-9, 671.1

0. EPISODE OF CARE UNSPECIFIED OR N/A
1. DELIVERED
2. DELIVERED WITH POSTPARTUM COMPLICATION
3. ANTEPARTUM COMPLICATION
4. POSTPARTUM COMPLICATION

LABOR AND DELIVERY COMPLICATIONS

DISPROPORTIONS

653.9# DISPROPORTION UNSPECIFIED
660.1# DISPROPORTION UNSPECIFIED OBSTRUCTING LABOR **[653.9#]**
653.0# BONY PELVIS ABNORMALITY NOS
660.1# BONY PELVIS ABNORMALITY NOS OBSTRUCTING LABOR **[653.0#]**
655.0# CEPHALOPELVIC DISPROPORTION DUE TO ANENCEPHALY, HYDROCEPHALY, SPINA BIFIDA (SUSPECTED / KNOWN) AFFECTING MANAGEMENT OF MOTHER
653.4# CEPHALOPELVIC DISPROPORTION NOS
660.1# CEPHALOPELVIC DISPROPORTION NOS OBSTRUCTING LABOR **[653.4#]**
653.7# CONJOINED TWINS
660.1# CONJOINED TWINS OBSTRUCTING LABOR **[653.7#]**
653.7# FETAL ASCITES
660.1# FETAL ASCITES OBSTRUCTING LABOR **[653.7#]**
655.0# FETAL CNS MALFORMATION (SUSPECTED / KNOWN) AFFECTING MANAGEMENT OF MOTHER
653.5# FETAL DISPROPORTION NOS
660.1# FETAL DISPROPORTION NOS OBSTRUCTING LABOR **[653.5#]**
656.6# FETAL GROWTH EXCESSIVE
653.6# FETAL HYDROCEPHALUS
660.1# FETAL HYDROCEPHALUS OBSTRUCTING LABOR **[653.6#]**
653.7# FETAL HYDROPS
660.1# FETAL HYDROPS OBSTRUCTING LABOR **[653.7#]**
653.7# FETAL MYELOMENINGOCELE
660.1# FETAL MYELOMENINGOCELE OBSTRUCTING LABOR **[653.7#]**
653.7# FETAL SACRAL TUMOR
660.1# FETAL SACRAL TUMOR OBSTRUCTING LABOR **[653.7#]**
653.7# FETAL TUMOR
660.1# FETAL TUMOR OBSTRUCTING LABOR **[653.7#]**
653.4# FETOPELVIC DISPROPORTION
660.1# FETOPELVIC DISPROPORTION OBSTRUCTING LABOR **[653.4#]**
655.0# FETOPELVIC DISPROPORTION DUE TO ANENCEPHALY, HYDROCEPHALY, SPINA BIFIDA (SUSPECTED / KNOWN) AFFECTING MANAGEMENT OF MOTHER
653.5# FETUS UNUSUALLY LARGE
660.1# FETUS UNUSUALLY LARGE OBSTRUCTING LABOR **[653.5#]**
653.2# INLET CONTRACTION (PELVIS)
660.1# INLET CONTRACTION (PELVIS) OBSTRUCTING LABOR **[653.2#]**
656.6# LARGE FOR DATES
653.0# PELVIC DEFORMITY NOS
660.1# PELVIC DEFORMITY NOS OBSTRUCTING LABOR **[653.0#]**
653.1# PELVIS CONTRACTED
660.1# PELVIS CONTRACTED OBSTRUCTING LABOR **[653.1#]**
660.4# SHOULDER (GIRDLE) DYSTOCIA
653.8# DISPROPORTION OTHER
660.1# DISPROPORTION OTHER OBSTRUCTING LABOR **[653.8#]**

5th Digit: 653.0-2, 4-9, 655.0, 656.6, 660.1, 4

0. EPISODE OF CARE UNSPECIFIED OR N/A
1. DELIVERED
3. ANTEPARTUM COMPLICATION

LABOR AND DELIVERY COMPLICATIONS

FETAL ABNORMALITY (KNOWN / SUSPECTED) AFFECTING MANAGEMENT OF MOTHER

655.9#	ABNORMALITY UNSPECIFIED
655.4#	ALCOHOL ADDICTION MATERNAL
655.0#	ANENCEPHALY
655.1#	CHROMOSOMAL ABNORMALITY
655.5#	DRUG DAMAGE
655.8#	ENVIRONMENTAL TOXINS
655.8#	HEART SOUNDS INAUDIBLE
655.2#	HEREDITARY DISEASE IN FAMILY
655.0#	HYDROCEPHALUS
655.8#	IUD
655.4#	MATERNAL
655.7#	MOVEMENT (ABSENT) (DECREASED)
655.8#	OTHER ABNORMALITY NEC
655.6#	RADIATION
655.3#	RUBELLA MATERNAL
655.0#	SPINA BIFIDA (WITH MYELOMENINGOCELE)
655.4#	TOXOPLASMOSIS MATERNAL
655.3#	VIRAL DISEASE MATERNAL
655.8#	OTHER SPECIFIED FETAL ABNORMALITY

5th Digit: 655.0-9

0. EPISODE OF CARE UNSPECIFIED OR N/A
1. DELIVERED
3. ANTEPARTUM COMPLICATION

LABOR AND DELIVERY COMPLICATIONS

FETAL AND PLACENTAL PROBLEMS AFFECTING MANAGEMENT OF MOTHER

656.2#	ABO ISOIMMUNIZATION
0	ABORTION MISSED SEE 'ABORTION', MISSED
656.1#	ANTI-D (RH) ANTIBODIES
659.7#	DEPRESSED FETAL HEART TONES
656.8#	FETAL ACID-BASE BALANCE ABNORMAL
656.9#	FETAL AND PLACENTAL PROBLEM UNSPECIFIED
656.0#	FETAL BLOOD LEAKAGE INTO MATERNAL CIRCULATION
659.7#	FETAL BRADY/TACHYCARDIA
0	FETAL DEATH < 22 WEEKS SEE 'ABORTION', MISSED
656.4#	FETAL DEATH >22 WEEKS
656.4#	FETAL DEATH, INTRAUTERINE
656.8#	FETAL DISTRESS NOS
656.3#	FETAL DISTRESS - METABOLIC ACIDEMIA
659.7#	FETAL HEART RATE OR RHYTHM DECELERATION
656.0#	FETAL-MATERNAL HEMORRHAGE
656.3#	FETAL METABOLIC ACIDEMIA
656.8#	INTRAUTERINE ACIDOSIS
656.6#	LARGE FOR DATES
656.5#	LIGHT FOR DATES
656.8#	LITHOPEDIAN
656.8#	MECONIUM IN LIQUOR
659.7#	NON-REASSURING FETAL HEART RATE OR RHYTHM
656.7#	PLACENTA ABNORMAL
656.7#	PLACENTAL CONDITION OTHER
656.7#	PLACENTAL INFARCT
656.5#	PLACENTAL INSUFFICIENCY

5th Digit: 656.0-9, 659.7

0. EPISODE OF CARE UNSPECIFIED OR N/A
1. DELIVERED
3. ANTEPARTUM COMPLICATION

674.4#	PLACENTAL POLYP

5th Digit: 674.4

0. EPISODE OF CARE UNSPECIFIED OR N/A
2. DELIVERED WITH POSTPARTUM COMPLICATION
4. POSTPARTUM COMPLICATION

LABOR AND DELIVERY COMPLICATIONS

FETAL AND PLACENTAL PROBLEMS AFFECTING MANAGEMENT OF MOTHER (continued)

658.4#	PLACENTITIS
656.1#	RH INCOMPATIBILITY
656.1#	RHESUS ISOIMMUNIZATION
656.5#	SMALL FOR DATES
656.8#	PLACENTA AND FETAL PROBLEMS OTHER SPECIFIED

5th Digit: 656.1, 5, 8, 658.4

0. EPISODE OF CARE UNSPECIFIED OR N/A
1. DELIVERED
3. ANTEPARTUM COMPLICATION

LABOR AND DELIVERY COMPLICATIONS

MALPOSITION / MALPRESENTATION

652.9#	NOS OF FETUS AT ONSET
660.0#	NOS OF FETUS AT ONSET OBSTRUCTING LABOR [652.9#]
652.2#	BREECH DELIVERY
660.0#	BREECH DELIVERY OBSTRUCTING LABOR [652.2#]
652.1#	BREECH PRESENTATION WITH VERSION
660.0#	BREECH PRESENTATION WITH VERSION OBSTRUCTING LABOR [652.1#]
652.2#	BREECH PRESENTATION
660.0#	BREECH PRESENTATION OBSTRUCTING LABOR [652.2#]
652.6#	BREECH PRESENTATION WITH MULTIPLE GESTATION
660.0#	BREECH PRESENTATION WITH MULTIPLE GESTATION OBSTRUCTING LABOR [652.6#]
652.4#	BROW PRESENTATION
660.0#	BROW PRESENTATION OBSTRUCTING LABOR [652.4#]
652.2#	BUTTOCKS PRESENTATION
660.0#	BUTTOCKS PRESENTATION OBSTRUCTING LABOR [652.2#]
652.1#	CEPHALIC VERSION
660.0#	CEPHALIC VERSION OBSTRUCTING LABOR [652.1#]
652.4#	CHIN PRESENTATION
660.0#	CHIN PRESENTATION OBSTRUCTING LABOR [652.4#]
652.2#	COMPLETE BREECH PRESENTATION
660.0#	COMPLETE BREECH PRESENTATION OBSTRUCTING LABOR [652.2#]
652.8#	COMPOUND PRESENTATION
660.0#	COMPOUND PRESENTATION OBSTRUCTING LABOR [652.8#]
652.4#	EXTENDED HEAD PRESENTATION
660.0#	EXTENDED HEAD PRESENTATION OBSTRUCTING LABOR [652.4#]
652.4#	FACE PRESENTATION
660.0#	FACE PRESENTATION OBSTRUCTING LABOR [652.4#]
652.8#	FACE TO PUBES PRESENTATION
660.0#	FACE TO PUBES PRESENTATION OBSTRUCTING LABOR [652.8#]
652.8#	FOOTLING PRESENTATION
660.0#	FOOTLING PRESENTATION OBSTRUCTING LABOR [652.8#]
652.2#	FRANK BREECH PRESENTATION
660.0#	FRANK BREECHPRESENTATION OBSTRUCTING LABOR [652.2#]
652.5#	HIGH HEAD AT TERM
660.0#	HIGH HEAD AT TERM OBSTRUCTING LABOR [652.5#]
652.6#	HIGH HEAD AT TERM WITH MULTIPLE GESTATION
660.0#	HIGH HEAD AT TERM WITH MULTIPLE GESTATION OBSTRUCTING LABOR [652.6#]

5th Digit: 652.1-2, 4-6, 8-9, 660.0

0. EPISODE OF CARE UNSPECIFIED OR N/A
1. DELIVERED
3. ANTEPARTUM COMPLICATION

MALPOSITION / MALPRESENTATION (continued)

652.8# INCOMPLETE BREECH PRESENTATION
660.0# INCOMPLETE BREECH PRESENTATION OBSTRUCTING LABOR **[652.8#]**
652.6# LOCKED TWINS
660.0# LOCKED TWINS OBSTRUCTING LABOR **[652.6#]**
652.8# MALPRESENTATION OTHER SPECIFIED
660.0# MALPRESENTATION OTHER SPECIFIED OBSTRUCTING LABOR **[652.8#]**
652.6# MALPRESENTATION WITH MULTIPLE GESTATION
660.0# MALPRESENTATION WITH MULTIPLE GESTATION OBSTRUCTING LABOR **[652.6#]**
652.1# MALPRESENTATION WITH VERSION
660.0# MALPRESENTATION WITH VERSION OBSTRUCTING LABOR **[652.1#]**
652.3# OBLIQUE LIE
660.0# OBLIQUE LIE OBSTRUCTING LABOR **[652.3#]**
652.6# OBLIQUE LIE WITH MULTIPLE GESTATION
660.0# OBLIQUE LIE WITH MULTIPLE GESTATION OBSTRUCTING LABOR **[652.6#]**
652.7# PROLAPSE ARM
660.0# PROLAPSE ARM OBSTRUCTING LABOR **[652.7#]**
652.6# PROLAPSE ARM WITH MULTIPLE GESTATION
660.0# PROLAPSE ARM WITH MULTIPLE GESTATION OBSTRUCTING LABOR **[652.6#]**
652.8# PROLAPSE FOOT
660.0# PROLAPSE FOOT OBSTRUCTING LABOR **[652.8#]**
652.8# PROLAPSE LEG
660.0# PROLAPSE LEG OBSTRUCTING LABOR **[652.8#]**
660.3# TRANSVERSE ARREST OF FETAL HEAD
652.3# TRANSVERSE AND PERSISTENT OCCIPITO-POSTERIOR POSITION
660.0# TRANSVERSE AND PERSISTENT OCCIPITO-POSTERIOR POSITION OBSTRUCTING LABOR **[652.3#]**
652.3# TRANSVERSE LIE
660.0# TRANSVERSE LIE OBSTRUCTING LABOR **[652.3#]**
652.6# TRANSVERSE LIE WITH MULTIPLE GESTATION
660.0# TRANSVERSE LIE WITH MULTIPLE GESTATION OBSTRUCTING LABOR **[652.6#]**
652.0# UNSTABLE LIE
660.0# UNSTABLE LIE OBSTRUCTING LABOR **[652.0#]**
652.6# UNSTABLE LIE WITH MULTIPLE GESTATION
660.0# UNSTABLE LIE WITH MULTIPLE GESTATION OBSTRUCTING LABOR **[652.6#]**

5th Digit: 652.0-1, 3, 6-8, 660.0, 3

0. EPISODE OF CARE UNSPECIFIED OR N/A
1. DELIVERED
3. ANTEPARTUM COMPLICATION

LABOR AND DELIVERY COMPLICATIONS

IN ORDER TO USE THE FOLLOWING CODES, THE MEDICAL RECORD MUST SPECIFY THAT THE MATERNAL CONDITION IS A CAUSE OF MORBIDITY OR MORTALITY IN THE FETUS OR NEWBORN. THE MERE FACT THAT THE CONDITION EXISTED IN THE MOTHER OR COMPLICATED THE PREGNANCY DOES NOT WARRANT THE USE OF THESE CODES ON THE NEWBORN'S RECORD. REMEMBER, CODES 760-763 APPLY ONLY TO THE INFANT AND ARE NEVER ASSIGNED TO THE MOTHER'S RECORD. CONVERSELY, NEVER CODE THE MOTHER'S CONDITION WITH THESE FETAL/NEWBORN CODES.

MATERNAL DISORDERS AFFECTING FETUS OR NEWBORN

762.9 UNSPECIFIED ABNORMALITIES OF CHORION AND AMNION
761.9 UNSPECIFIED COMPLICATIONS - DUE TO CURRENT PREGNANCY
760.9 UNSPECIFIED CONDITIONS - UNRELATED TO CURRENT PREGNANCY
762.6 UNSPECIFIED CONDITIONS OF UMBILICAL CORD
763.9 UNSPECIFIED DISORDER - DUE TO LABOR AND DELIVERY

LABOR AND DELIVERY COMPLICATIONS

MATERNAL DISORDERS AFFECTING FETUS OR NEWBORN (continued)

761.4 ABDOMINAL PREGNANCY
763.1 ABNORMALITY BONY
763.89 ABNORMALITY SOFT TISSUES
761.8 ABORTION SPONTANEOUS
762.1 ABRUPTIO PLACENTAE
760.79 ADRENOGENITAL IATROGENIC SYNDROME AFFECTING FETUS OR NEWBORN
760.71 ALCOHOL TRANSMITTED VIA PLACENTA OR BREAST MILK
762.1 AMNIOCENTESIS DAMAGE TO PLACENTA
762.8 AMNION ADHESION TO FETUS
762.7 AMNIONITIS
763.5 ANALGESICS ADMINISTERED DURING LABOR AND DELIVERY
763.5 ANESTHETICS ADMINISTERED DURING LABOR AND DELIVERY
760.74 ANTIBIOTICS (ANTI-INFECTIVES) TRANSMITTED VIA PLACENTA OR BREAST MILK
760.1 BACTERIURIA
763.1 BLADDER DILATATION
762.1 BLOOD LOSS MATERNAL
763.0 BREECH DELIVERY AND EXTRACTION
761.7 BREECH MALPRESENTATION BEFORE LABOR AND DELIVERY
760.8 CERVICITIS
763.89 CERVIX ABNORMALITY
761.0 CERVIX INCOMPETENT
763.89 CERVIX SCAR
763.1 CERVIX SCAR OBSTRUCTING LABOR
763.89 CERVIX STENOSIS/STRICTURE
763.1 CERVIX STENOSIS/STRICTURE OBSTRUCTING LABOR
763.4 CESAREAN DELIVERY
763.89 CESAREAN SCAR PREVIOUS
762.1 CESAREAN SECTION DAMAGE (SEPARATION) (HEMORRHAGE) TO PLACENTA
762.7 CHORIOAMNIONITIS
762.9 CHORION AND AMNION ABNORMALITY
762.8 CHORION AND AMNION ABNORMALITIES OTHER SPECIFIED
760.3 CIRCULATORY DISEASE MATERNAL CHRONIC
763.89 CLEIDOTOMY FETAL
760.75 COCAINE TRANSMITTED VIA PLACENTA OR BREAST MILK
763.7 CONTRACTION RING
760.75 CRACK (COCAINE) TRANSMITTED VIA PLACENTA OR BREAST MILK
763.89 CRANIOCLASIS, FETAL
763.89 CRANIOTOMY, FETAL
763.89 CYSTOCELE
763.1 CYSTOCELE OBSTRUCTING LABOR
761.6 DEATH (MATERNAL)
763.89 DELAYED BIRTH OR DELIVERY NEC
763.89 DELAYED BIRTH OR DELIVERY SECOND TWIN, TRIPLET ETC.
763.0 DELIVERY AND EXTRACTION
763.6 DELIVERY RAPID SECOND STAGE
760.76 DES (DIETHYLSTILBESTROL) TRANSMITTED VIA PLACENTA OR BREAST MILK
763.89 DESTRUCTIVE OPERATION OR PROCEDURE ON LIVE FETUS TO FACILITATE DELIVERY
775.0 DIABETES CAUSING FETAL HYPOGLYCEMIA
760.76 DIETHYLSTILBESTROL (DES) TRANSMITTED VIA PLACENTA OR BREAST MILK
763.5 DRUG REACTION MATERNAL
761.4 ECTOPIC PREGNANCY
763.89 ENDOCERVICAL OS STENOSIS/STRICTURE
763.1 ENDOCERVICAL OS STENOSIS/STRICTURE OBSTRUCTING LABOR
760.8 ENDOMETRITIS
763.89 EXHAUSTION MATERNAL
761.7 EXTERNAL VERSION MALPRESENTATION BEFORE LABOR AND DELIVERY
763.89 EXTRACTION FETAL MANUAL OR WITH HOOK

LABOR AND DELIVERY COMPLICATIONS

MATERNAL DISORDERS AFFECTING FETUS OR NEWBORN (continued)

IN ORDER TO USE THE FOLLOWING CODES, THE MEDICAL RECORD MUST SPECIFY THAT THE MATERNAL CONDITION IS A CAUSE OF MORBIDITY OR MORTALITY IN THE FETUS OR NEWBORN. THE MERE FACT THAT THE CONDITION EXISTED IN THE MOTHER OR COMPLICATED THE PREGNANCY DOES NOT WARRANT THE USE OF THESE CODES ON THE NEWBORN'S RECORD. REMEMBER, CODES 760-763 APPLY ONLY TO THE INFANT AND ARE NEVER ASSIGNED TO THE MOTHER'S RECORD. CONVERSELY, NEVER CODE THE MOTHER'S CONDITION WITH THESE FETAL/NEWBORN CODES.

762.3 FETAL BLOOD LOSS DUE TO PLACENTAL TRANSFUSION [772.0]
763.89 FORCED BIRTH
763.2 FORCEPS DELIVERY
760.73 HALLUCINOGENIC TRANSMITTED VIA PLACENTA OR BREAST MILK
762.1 HEMORRHAGE COMPLICATING PREGNANCY, ANTEPARTUM
763.89 HEMORRHAGE DUE TO COAGULATION DEFECT
760.8 HEPATITIS MATERNAL
761.3 HYDRAMNIOS ACUTE (CHRONIC)
760.0 HYPERTENSIVE DISORDERS MATERNAL
760.79 IMMUNE SERA TRANSMITTED VIA PLACENTA OR BREAST MILK
763.89 INDUCTION OF LABOR (MEDICAL)
760.8 INFECTION GENITAL TRACT OTHER LOCALIZED MATERNAL
760.2 INFECTION MATERNAL NOT MANIFESTED IN FETUS OR NEWBORN
760.1 INFECTION URINARY TRACT
760.2 INFLUENZA
763.89 INJURY DUE TO OBSTETRICAL TRAUMA
760.5 INJURY MATERNAL
761.4 INTRAPERITONEAL PREGNANCY
760.1 KIDNEY NECROSIS
760.8 LIVER NECROSIS
761.7 MALPRESENTATION/MALPOSITION BEFORE LABOR
763.1 MALPRESENTATION/MALPOSITION DURING LABOR
761.6 MATERNAL DEATH
760.79 MEDICINAL AGENTS NEC TRANSMITTED VIA PLACENTA OR BREAST MILK
762.7 MEMBRANITIS
763.89 MULTIPARITY
761.5 MULTIPLE PREGNANCY
763.5 NARCOSIS DUE TO DRUG (CORRECTLY ADMINISTERED)
763.5 NARCOTIC REACTION (INTOXICATION) MATERNAL DURING L&D
760.72 NARCOTIC TRANSMITTED VIA PLACENTA OR BREAST MILK
760.70 NOXIOUS SUBSTANCE UNSPECIFIED TRANSMITTED VIA PLACENTA OR BREAST MILK
760.79 NOXIOUS SUBSTANCE OTHER SPECIFIED TRANSMITTED VIA PLACENTA OR BREAST MILK
760.4 NUTRITIONAL DEFICIENCY DISORDERS MATERNAL
761.7 OBLIQUE LIE BEFORE LABOR AND DELIVERY
761.2 OLIGOHYDRAMNIOS
763.5 OPIATE REACTION (INTOXICATION) MATERNAL DURING L&D
763.89 OS UTERI STRICTURE
763.1 OS UTERI STRICTURE OBSTRUCTING LABOR
763.89 OVARIAN CYST
763.1 OVARIAN CYST OBSTRUCTING LABOR
763.1 PELVIS BONY
763.1 PELVIS CONTRACTED
763.89 PELVIS CYST
763.1 PELVIS CYST OBSTRUCTING LABOR
763.89 PELVIS DEFORMITY
760.8 PELVIS INFLAMMATORY DISEASE
763.89 PELVIS ORGANS OR SOFT TISSUE ABNORMALITY
763.89 PELVIS ORGANS SURGERY PREVIOUS
763.1 PELVIS ROBERT'S

LABOR AND DELIVERY COMPLICATIONS

MATERNAL DISORDERS AFFECTING FETUS OR NEWBORN (continued)

763.89 PENDULOUS ABDOMEN
761.4 PERITONEAL PREGNANCY
763.1 PERSISTENT OCCIPITOPOSTERIOR POSITION
762.1 PLACENTA DAMAGE
762.2 PLACENTA INFARCTION
762.0 PLACENTA PREVIA
762.3 PLACENTA TRANSFUSION SYNDROMES
762.7 PLACENTITIS
762.3 POLYCYTHEMIA NEONATORUM PLACENTAL TRANSFUSION [776.4]
761.3 POLYHYDRAMNIOS
763.6 PRECIPITATE DELIVERY
760.0 PRE-ECLAMPSIA
761.1 PREMATURE RUPTURE OF MEMBRANES
760.3 RESPIRATORY DISEASE MATERNAL CHRONIC
762.1 RUPTURE MARGINAL SINUS
760.8 SALPINGITIS
763.1 SHOULDER DYSTOCIA
763.1 SHOULDER PRESENTATION
763.1 SPONDYLOLISTHESIS
763.1 SPONDYLOLYSIS
760.6 SURGERY MATERNAL
762.1 SURGICAL INDUCTION WITH DAMAGE TO PLACENTA
760.70 TOXIC SUBSTANCE NOS TRANSMITTED VIA PLACENTA OR BREAST MILK
760.79 TOXIC SUBSTANCE NEC TRANSMITTED VIA PLACENTA OR BREAST MILK
763.5 TRANQUILIZER REACTION (MATERNAL)
761.7 TRANSVERSE LIE BEFORE LABOR AND DELIVERY
763.1 TRANSVERSE LIE-PRESENTATION DURING LABOR AND DELIVERY
761.5 TRIPLET PREGNANCY
761.4 TUBAL PREGNANCY
761.5 TWIN PREGNANCY
762.5 UMBILICAL CORD ENTANGLEMENT (CORD AROUND NECK, KNOT, TORSION)
762.4 UMBILICAL CORD PROLAPSE (PRESENTATION)
762.6 UMBILICAL CORD OTHER AND UNSPECIFIED CONDITIONS
761.7 UNSTABLE LIE BEFORE LABOR AND DELIVERY
760.1 URINARY TRACT DISEASES MATERNAL
763.89 UTERUS ABNORMALITY
763.89 UTERUS ABSCESS (TO ABDOMINAL WALL)
763.89 UTERUS ADHESION
763.89 UTERUS BICORNIS/DOUBLE
763.89 UTERUS BODY POLYP (CORPUS) (MUCOUS)
763.7 UTERUS CONTRACTIONS ABNORMAL
763.7 UTERUS HYPERTONIC/HYPOTONIC
763.7 UTERUS INERTIA-DYSFUNCTION
763.89 UTERUS PERFORATION WITH OBSTETRICAL TRAUMA
763.1 UTERUS PROLAPSE
763.89 UTERUS RUPTURE
763.1 UTERUS SACCULATION
763.89 UTERUS SHAPE ABNORMALITY
763.89 UTERUS SURGERY PREVIOUS
763.89 UTERUS VERSION
763.3 VACUUM EXTRACTOR DELIVERY
763.3 VACUUM RUPTURE
763.89 VAGINA ABNORMALITY
763.89 VAGINA STENOSIS/STRICTURE
763.1 VAGINA STENOSIS/STRICTURE OBSTRUCTING LABOR
760.8 VAGINITIS
763.89 VULVA ABNORMALITY
762.8 OTHER SPECIFIED ABNORMALITIES OF CHORION AND AMNION
761.8 OTHER SPECIFIED COMPLICATIONS - DUE TO CURRENT PREGNANCY
760.8 OTHER SPECIFIED CONDITIONS - UNRELATED TO CURRENT PREGNANCY
762.6 OTHER SPECIFIED CONDITIONS OF UMBILICAL CORD
763.89 OTHER SPECIFIED DISORDER - DUE TO LABOR AND DELIVERY

LABOR AND DELIVERY COMPLICATIONS

TRAUMA OBSTETRICAL

664.9# UNSPECIFIED TRAUMA , VULVA AND PERINEUM (DELIVERY)
664.0# FIRST DEGREE PERINEAL LACERATION (DELIVERY)
664.1# SECOND DEGREE PERINEAL LACERATION (DELIVERY)
664.2# THIRD DEGREE PERINEAL LACERATION (DELIVERY)
664.3# FOURTH DEGREE PERINEAL LACERATION (DELIVERY)
664.4# UNSPECIFIED PERINEAL LACERATION (DELIVERY)
664.5# HEMATOMA, VULVA AND PERINEUM (DELIVERY)
664.8# TRAUMA OTHER SPECIFIED, VULVA AND PERINEUM (DELIVERY)

5th Digit: 664.0-5, 8-9
- **0. EPISODE OF CARE UNSPECIFIED OR N/A**
- **1. DELIVERED**
- **4. POSTPARTUM COMPLICATION**

665.0# UTERINE RUPTURE BEFORE ONSET

5th Digit: 665.0
- **0. EPISODE OF CARE UNSPECIFIED OR N/A**
- **1. DELIVERED**
- **3. ANTEPARTUM COMPLICATION**

665.1# UTERINE RUPTURE
665.1# UTERINE RUPTURE DURING LABOR

5th Digit: 665.1
- **0. EPISODE OF CARE UNSPECIFIED OR N/A**
- **1. DELIVERED**

LABOR AND DELIVERY COMPLICATIONS

OTHER COMPLICATIONS

ELDERLY MULTIGRAVIDA: SECOND OR MORE PREGNANCY IN A WOMAN WHO WILL BE 35 YEARS OF AGE OR OLDER AT EXPECTED DATE OF DELIVERY.

659.6# AGE ADVANCED MATERNAL - ELDERLY MULTIGRAVIDA

ELDERLY PRIMIGRAVIDA: FIRST PREGNANCY IN A WOMAN WHO WILL BE 35 YEARS OF AGE OR OLDER AT EXPECTED DATE OF DELIVERY.

659.5# AGE ADVANCED MATERNAL - ELDERLY PRIMIGRAVIDA

YOUNG MATERNAL AGE: PREGNANCY IN FEMALE WHO IS LESS THAN 16 YEARS OLD AT EXPECTED DATE OF DELIVERY.

659.8# AGE YOUNG MATERNAL COMPLICATING LABOR AND DELIVERY
659.3# BACTEREMIA DURING LABOR

5th Digit: 659.3, 5-6, 8
- **0. EPISODE OF CARE NOS OR N/A**
- **1. DELIVERED**
- **3. ANTEPARTUM COMPLICATION**

644.1# FALSE LABOR >37 WEEKS
644.0# FALSE LABOR >22 AND <37 WEEKS

5th Digit: 644.0-1
- **0. EPISODE OF CARE UNSPECIFIED OR N/A**
- **3. ANTEPARTUM COMPLICATION**

648.9#: USE AN ADDITIONAL CODE TO IDENTIFY THE SPECIFIC NONOBSTETRICAL TRAUMA.

648.9# INJURY-TRAUMA NON-OBSTETRICAL CURRENT (CO-EXISTENT) IN PREGNANCY
669.9# LABOR AND DELIVERY COMPLICATION
669.4# LABOR AND DELIVERY COMPLICATION OTHER OF OBSTETRICAL SURGERY AND PROCEDURES
669.8# LABOR AND DELIVERY COMPLICATION OTHER SPECIFIED

5th Digit: 648.9, 669.4, 8-9
- **0. EPISODE OF CARE UNSPECIFIED OR N/A**
- **1. DELIVERED**
- **2. DELIVERED WITH POSTPARTUM COMPLICATION**
- **3. ANTEPARTUM COMPLICATION**
- **4. POSTPARTUM COMPLICATION**

677 LATE EFFECT

LABOR AND DELIVERY COMPLICATIONS

OTHER COMPLICATIONS (continued)

ELDERLY MULTIGRAVIDA: SECOND OR MORE PREGNANCY IN A WOMAN WHO WILL BE 35 YEARS OF AGE OR OLDER AT EXPECTED DATE OF DELIVERY.

659.6# MULTIGRAVIDA ELDERLY

5th Digit: 659.6
- **0. EPISODE OF CARE NOS OR N/A**
- **1. DELIVERED**
- **3. ANTEPARTUM COMPLICATION**

644.2# PREMATURE LABOR WITH ONSET OF DELIVERY <37 WEEKS

5th Digit: 644.2
- **0. EPISODE OF CARE UNSPECIFIED OR N/A**
- **1. DELIVERED**

644.0# PREMATURE LABOR WITHOUT DELIVERY >22 AND <37 WEEKS

5th Digit: 644.0
- **0. EPISODE OF CARE UNSPECIFIED OR N/A**
- **3. ANTEPARTUM COMPLICATION**

ELDERLY PRIMIGRAVIDA: FIRST PREGNANCY IN A WOMAN WHO WILL BE 35 YEARS OF AGE OR OLDER AT EXPECTED DATE OF DELIVERY.

659.5# PRIMIGRAVIDA ELDERLY
659.2# PYREXIA OR FEVER DURING LABOR

5th Digit: 659.2, 5
- **0. EPISODE OF CARE UNSPECIFIED OR N/A**
- **1. DELIVERED**
- **3. ANTEPARTUM COMPLICATION**

669.1# SHOCK DURING LABOR AND DELIVERY

5th Digit: 669.1
- **0. EPISODE OF CARE NOS OR N/A**
- **1. DELIVERED**
- **2. DELIVERED WITH POSTPARTUM COMPLICATION**
- **3. ANTEPARTUM COMPLICATION**
- **4. POSTPARTUM COMPLICATION**

644.1# THREATENED LABOR >37 WEEKS
644.0# THREATENED LABOR >22 AND <37 WEEKS (DUE TO IRRITABLE UTERUS)

5th Digit: 644.0-1
- **0. EPISODE OF CARE UNSPECIFIED OR N/A**
- **3. ANTEPARTUM COMPLICATION**

648.9#: USE AN ADDITIONAL CODE TO IDENTIFY THE SPECIFIC NONOBSTETRICAL TRAUMA.

648.9# TRAUMA-INJURY NON-OBSTETRICAL CURRENT (CO-EXISTENT) IN PREGNANCY
665.9# TRAUMA -INJURY OBSTETRICAL

5th Digit: 648.9, 665.9
- **0. EPISODE OF CARE NOS OR N/A**
- **1. DELIVERED**
- **2. DELIVERED WITH POSTPARTUM COMPLICATION**
- **3. ANTEPARTUM COMPLICATION**
- **4. POSTPARTUM COMPLICATION**

663.0# UMBILICAL CORD PROLAPSE
659.9# UNSPECIFIED INDICATION FOR CARE OR INTERVENTION OF L AND D
659.8# UNSPECIFIED INDICATION FOR CARE OR INTERVENTION OF L AND D OTHER SPECIFIED

5th Digit: 659.8-9, 663.0
- **0. EPISODE OF CARE UNSPECIFIED OR N/A**
- **1. DELIVERED**
- **3. ANTEPARTUM COMPLICATION**

V72.6 LABORATORY EXAM OR TEST (ROUTINE)

LABYRINTH, LABYRINTHINE

744.05 ABSENCE CONGENITAL
386.9 DISORDER
386.8 DISORDER OTHER
386.50 DYSFUNCTION
386.58 DYSFUNCTION OTHER FORMS AND COMBINATIONS
386.51 HYPERACTIVE UNILATERAL
386.52 HYPERACTIVE BILATERAL
386.53 HYPOACTIVE UNILATERAL
386.54 HYPOACTIVE BILATERAL
959.09 INJURY
386.55 LOSS OF REACTIVITY UNILATERAL
386.56 LOSS OF REACTIVITY BILATERAL
386.50 SYNDROME
386.9 VERTIGINOUS SYNDROMES

LABYRINTHITIS

386.30 UNSPECIFIED
386.31 DIFFUSE
386.31 SEROUS
386.32 CIRCUMSCRIBED
386.32 FOCAL
386.33 PURULENT
386.33 SUPPURATIVE
386.34 TOXIC
386.35 VIRAL

WHEN AN OPEN WOUND OR LACERATION IS ACCOMPANIED BY CELLULITIS, TWO CODES ARE NEEDED, THE CODE FOR THE __COMPLICATED__ OPEN WOUND OR LACERATION AND A CODE FOR THE CELLULITIS. SEQUENCING DEPENDS ON WHICH DIAGNOSIS REQUIRED THE MAJOR WORK AND EFFORT.

LACERATION

0 SEE ALSO 'OPEN WOUND', BY SITE

879.8 NOS
879.9 NOS COMPLICATED

879.2 ABDOMEN WALL ANTERIOR
879.3 ABDOMEN WALL ANTERIOR COMPLICATED

879.4 ABDOMEN WALL LATERAL
879.5 ABDOMEN WALL LATERAL COMPLICATED

998.2 ACCIDENTAL DURING A PROCEDURE
892.2 ACHILLES TENDON (OPEN)
V58.3 AFTERCARE

873.62 ALVEOLAR (GUM)
873.72 ALVEOLAR (GUM) COMPLICATED

891.0 ANKLE
891.1 ANKLE COMPLICATED
891.2 ANKLE WITH TENDON INVOLVEMENT

879.6 ANUS
879.7 ANUS COMPLICATED
863.89 ANUS (SPHINCTER) INTERNAL
565.0 ANUS NONTRAUMATIC
664.2# ANUS OBSTETRICAL (DURING DELIVERY)
664.3# ANUS OBSTETRICAL (DURING DELIVERY) INCLUDING MUCOSA (ANAL) (RECTAL)

5th Digit: 664.2-3

0. EPISODE OF CARE UNSPECIFIED OR N/A
1. DELIVERED
4. POSTPARTUM COMPLICATION

884.0 ARM NOS
884.1 ARM NOS COMPLICATED
884.2 ARM NOS WITH TENDON INVOLVEMENT

0 ARM LOWER SEE 'LACERATION' FOREARM

IN ICD-9, A COMPLICATED LACERATION OR OPEN WOUND IS DEFINED AS THAT WHICH IS INFECTED, CONTAINS A FOREIGN BODY, OR IS GROSSLY CONTAMINATED.

LACERATION (continued)

884.0 ARM MULTIPLE SITES
884.1 ARM MULTIPLE SITES COMPLICATED
884.0 ARM MULTIPLE SITES OF ONE UPPER LIMB
884.2 ARM MULTIPLE SITES WITH TENDON INVOLVEMENT

880.03 ARM UPPER
880.13 ARM UPPER COMPLICATED
880.23 ARM UPPER WITH TENDON INVOLVEMENT

0 ARTERY SEE SPECIFIC ARTERY

872.02 AUDITORY CANAL
872.12 AUDITORY CANAL COMPLICATED

872.01 AURICLE (PINNA)
872.11 AURICLE (PINNA) COMPLICATED

880.02 AXILLA
880.12 AXILLA COMPLICATED
880.22 AXILLA WITH TENDON INVOLVEMENT

880.09 AXILLA WITH OTHER SITES OF UPPER ARM
880.19 AXILLA WITH OTHER SITES OF UPPER ARM COMPLICATED
880.29 AXILLA WITH OTHER SITES OF UPPER ARM WITH TENDON INVOLVEMENT

876.0 BACK
876.1 BACK COMPLICATED

0 BLOOD VESSEL SEE 'BLOOD VESSEL INJURY', BY SITE

665.5# BOWEL OBSTETRICAL

5th Digit: 665.5

0. EPISODE OF CARE UNSPECIFIED OR N/A
1. DELIVERED
4. POSTPARTUM COMPLICATION

851.8# BRAIN - NOS AND NEC
851.9# BRAIN - NOS AND NEC WITH OPEN INTRACRANIAL WOUND
851.6# BRAIN - CEREBELLUM
851.7# BRAIN - CEREBELLUM WITH OPEN INTRACRANIAL WOUND
851.2# BRAIN - CEREBRAL CORTEX
851.3# BRAIN - CEREBRAL CORTEX WITH OPEN INTRACRANIAL WOUND
851.6# BRAIN STEM
851.7# BRAIN STEM WITH OPEN INTRACRANIAL WOUND

5th Digit: 851.2-3, 6-9

0. LEVEL OF CONSCIOUSNESS NOS
1. NO LOC
2. LOC < 1 HR
3. LOC 1 - 24 HRS
4. LOC > 24 HRS WITH RETURN TO PRIOR LEVEL
5. LOC > 24 HRS WITHOUT RETURN TO PRIOR LEVEL: OR DEATH BEFORE REGAINING CONSCIOUSNESS, REGARDLESS OF DURATION OF LOC
6. LOC DURATION NOS
9. WITH CONCUSSION NOS

879.0 BREAST
879.1 BREAST COMPLICATED

620.6 BROAD LIGAMENT SYNDROME

0 BROW SEE 'LACERATION', EYEBROW

873.61 BUCCAL MUCOSA
873.71 BUCCAL MUCOSA COMPLICATED

877.0 BUTTOCK
877.1 BUTTOCK COMPLICATED

L

*WHEN AN OPEN WOUND OR LACERATION IS ACCOMPANIED BY CELLULITIS, TWO CODES ARE NEEDED, THE CODE FOR THE **COMPLICATED** OPEN WOUND OR LACERATION AND A CODE FOR THE CELLULITIS. SEQUENCING DEPENDS ON WHICH DIAGNOSIS REQUIRED THE MAJOR WORK AND EFFORT.*

LACERATION (continued)

891.0 CALF
891.1 CALF COMPLICATED
891.2 CALF WITH TENDON INVOLVEMENT

870.8 CANALICULUS LACRIMALIS
870.2 CANALICULUS LACRIMALIS WITH LACERATION OF EYELID

870.8 CANTHUS, EYE

0 CEREBELLUM SEE 'LACERATION' BRAIN - CEREBELLUM
0 CEREBRAL CORTEX SEE 'LACERATION' BRAIN - CEREBRAL CORTEX

622.3 CERVIX NONPUERPERAL NONTRAUMATIC
665.3# CERVIX OBSTETRICAL

5th Digit: 665.3

0. EPISODE OF CARE UNSPECIFIED OR N/A
1. DELIVERED
4. POSTPARTUM COMPLICATION

873.41 CHEEK EXTERNAL
873.51 CHEEK EXTERNAL COMPLICATED

873.61 CHEEK INTERNAL
873.71 CHEEK INTERNAL COMPLICATED

875.0 CHEST WALL
875.1 CHEST WALL COMPLICATED

873.44 CHIN
873.54 CHIN COMPLICATED

429.5 CHORDAE HEART
363.63 CHOROID

878.8 CLITORIS
878.9 CLITORIS COMPLICATED

872.64 COCHLEA
872.74 COCHLEA COMPLICATED

871.9 CONJUNCTIVA (ALONE)
0 CORNEA SEE 'LACERATION', EYEBALL

875.0 COSTAL REGION
875.1 COSTAL REGION COMPLICATED

0 DESCEMET'S MEMBRANE SEE 'LACERATION', EYEBALL

862.0 DIAPHRAGM
862.1 DIAPHRAGM WITH OPEN WOUND INTO CAVITY
908.0 DIAPHRAGM LATE EFFECT

872.8 EAR
872.9 EAR COMPLICATED

872.01 EAR AURICLE (PINNA)
872.11 EAR AURICLE (PINNA) COMPLICATED

872.02 EAR CANAL
872.12 EAR CANAL COMPLICATED

872.61 EAR DRUM
872.71 EAR DRUM COMPLICATED

872.00 EAR EXTERNAL NOS
872.10 EAR EXTERNAL NOS COMPLICATED

872.62 EAR OSSICLES (INCUS) (MALLEUS) (STAPES)
872.72 EAR OSSICLES (INCUS) (MALLEUS) (STAPES) COMPLICATED

*WHEN AN OPEN WOUND OR LACERATION IS ACCOMPANIED BY CELLULITIS, TWO CODES ARE NEEDED, THE CODE FOR THE **COMPLICATED** OPEN WOUND OR LACERATION AND A CODE FOR THE CELLULITIS. SEQUENCING DEPENDS ON WHICH DIAGNOSIS REQUIRED THE MAJOR WORK AND EFFORT.*

LACERATION (continued)

872.69 EAR OTHER AND MULTIPLE SITES
872.79 EAR OTHER AND MULTIPLE SITES COMPLICATED

881.01 ELBOW
881.11 ELBOW COMPLICATED
881.21 ELBOW WITH TENDON INVOLVEMENT

878.2 EPIDIDYMIS
878.3 EPIDIDYMIS COMPLICATED

879.2 EPIGASTRIC REGION
879.3 EPIGASTRIC REGION COMPLICATED

874.01 EPIGLOTTIS
874.11 EPIGLOTTIS COMPLICATED

874.4 ESOPHAGUS CERVICAL
874.5 ESOPHAGUS CERVICAL COMPLICATED

862.22 ESOPHAGUS THORACIC
862.32 ESOPHAGUS THORACIC WITH OPEN WOUND INTO CAVITY
908.0 ESOPHAGUS THORACIC LATE EFFECT
530.7 ESOPHAGUS MALLORY WEISS TEAR

872.63 EUSTACHIAN TUBE
872.73 EUSTACHIAN TUBE COMPLICATED

871.4 EYE
870.9 EYE (OCULAR ADNEXA)
870.8 EYE (OCULAR ADNEXA) OTHER SPECIFIED
870.3 EYE (ORBIT) PENETRATING
0 EYE WITH FOREIGN BODY SEE 'FOREIGN BODY', EYE

871.4 EYEBALL NOS
871.7 EYEBALL PENETRATING NOS
871.2 EYEBALL WITH PARTIAL LOSS OF INTRAOCULAR TISSUE
0 EYEBALL WITH FOREIGN BODY SEE 'FOREIGN BODY', EYE
871.1 EYEBALL WITH PROLAPSE OF INTRAOCULAR TISSUE
871.0 EYEBALL WITHOUT PROLAPSE OF INTRAOCULAR TISSUE

873.42 EYEBROW
873.52 EYEBROW COMPLICATED

870.8 EYELID NEC
870.0 EYELID AND PERIOCULAR AREA
870.1 EYELID FULL THICKNESS
870.2 EYELID INVOLVING LACRIMAL PASSAGES

873.40 FACE
873.50 FACE COMPLICATED

873.49 FACE OTHER AND MULTIPLE SITES
873.59 FACE OTHER AND MULTIPLE SITES COMPLICATED

883.0 FINGER (NAIL)
883.1 FINGER (NAIL) COMPLICATED
883.2 FINGER (NAIL) WITH TENDON INVOLVEMENT

879.4 FLANK
879.5 FLANK COMPLICATED

892.0 FOOT
892.1 FOOT COMPLICATED
892.2 FOOT WITH TENDON INVOLVEMENT

881.00 FOREARM
881.10 FOREARM COMPLICATED
881.20 FOREARM WITH TENDON INVOLVEMENT

873.42 FOREHEAD
873.52 FOREHEAD COMPLICATED

IN ICD-9, A COMPLICATED LACERATION OR OPEN WOUND IS DEFINEDAS THAT WHICH IS INFECTED, CONTAINS A FOREIGN BODY, OR IS GROSSLY CONTAMINATED.

LACERATION (continued)

878.8 GENITALIA
878.9 GENITALIA COMPLICATED

873.62 GINGIVA
873.72 GINGIVA COMPLICATED

0 GLOBE SEE 'LACERATION', EYEBALL

879.4 GROIN
879.5 GROIN COMPLICATED

873.62 GUM
873.72 GUM COMPLICATED

882.0 HAND
882.1 HAND COMPLICATED
882.2 HAND WITH TENDON INVOLVEMENT

873.8 HEAD
873.9 HEAD COMPLICATED

861.02 HEART
861.03 HEART WITH PENETRATION OF CHAMBER
861.12 HEART WITH OPEN WOUND INTO THORAX
861.13 HEART WITH OPEN WOUND INTO THORAX AND PENETRATION OF CHAMBER
908.0 HEART LATE EFFECT

0 HEEL SEE 'LACERATION', FOOT

890.0 HIP
890.1 HIP COMPLICATED
890.2 HIP WITH TENDON INVOLVEMENT

878.6 HYMEN
878.7 HYMEN COMPLICATED

879.4 HYPOCHONDRIUM
879.5 HYPOCHONDRIUM COMPLICATED

879.2 HYPOGASTRIC REGION
879.3 HYPOGASTRIC REGION COMPLICATED

879.4 ILIAC REGION
879.5 ILIAC REGION COMPLICATED

879.4 INGUINAL REGION
879.5 INGUINAL REGION COMPLICATED

892.0 INSTEP
892.1 INSTEP COMPLICATED
892.2 INSTEP WITH TENDON INVOLVEMENT

0 INTERNAL ORGAN SEE SPECIFIC ORGAN

876.0 INTERSCAPULAR REGION
876.1 INTERSCAPULAR REGION COMPLICATED

0 IRIS SEE 'LACERATION', EYEBALL

873.44 JAW
873.54 JAW COMPLICATED

866.02 KIDNEY
866.03 KIDNEY WITH COMPLETE DISRUPTION OF PARENCHYMA
866.13 KIDNEY WITH COMPLETE DISRUPTION OF PARENCHYMA AND OPEN WOUND INTO CAVITY
866.12 KIDNEY WITH OPEN WOUND INTO CAVITY
908.1 KIDNEY LATE EFFECT

891.0 KNEE
891.1 KNEE COMPLICATED
891.2 KNEE WITH TENDON INVOLVEMENT

*WHEN AN OPEN WOUND OR LACERATION IS ACCOMPANIED BY CELLULITIS, TWO CODES ARE NEEDED, THE CODE FOR THE **COMPLICATED** OPEN WOUND OR LACERATION AND A CODE FOR THE CELLULITIS. SEQUENCING DEPENDS ON WHICH DIAGNOSIS REQUIRED THE MAJOR WORK AND EFFORT.*

LACERATION (continued)

878.4 LABIA
878.5 LABIA COMPLICATED
664.0# LABIA OBSTETRICAL (DURING DELIVERY)
5th Digit: 664.0
0. EPISODE OF CARE UNSPECIFIED OR N/A
1. DELIVERED
4. POSTPARTUM COMPLICATION

870.8 LACRIMAL APPARATUS, GLAND OR SAC
870.2 LACRIMAL APPARATUS, GLAND OR SAC WITH LACERATION OF EYELID

874.## LARYNX
4th Digit: 874
0. UNSPECIFIED
1. COMPLICATED
5th Digit: 874
0. LARYNX WITH TRACHEA
1. LARYNX

908.0 LATE EFFECT DIAPHRAGM
908.0 LATE EFFECT ESOPHAGUS
906.1 LATE EFFECT EXTREMITIES
906.0 LATE EFFECT HEAD, NECK OR TRUNK
908.0 LATE EFFECT HEART
908.1 LATE EFFECT KIDNEY
908.1 LATE EFFECT LIVER
908.0 LATE EFFECT LUNG
908.0 LATE EFFECT MYOCARDIUM
908.0 LATE EFFECT PULMONARY
908.1 LATE EFFECT RENAL
908.1 LATE EFFECT SPLEEN
908.2 LATE EFFECT URETHRA
905.8 LATE EFFECT WITH TENDON INVOLVEMENT

891.0 LEG NOS OR LOWER
891.1 LEG NOS OR LOWER COMPLICATED
891.2 LEG NOS OR LOWER WITH TENDON INVOLVEMENT

890.0 LEG UPPER
890.1 LEG UPPER COMPLICATED
890.2 LEG UPPER WITH TENDON INVOLVEMENT

894.0 LIMB LOWER NOS OR MULTIPLE SITES
894.1 LIMB LOWER NOS OR MULTIPLE SITES COMPLICATED
894.2 LIMB LOWER NOS OR MULTIPLE SITES WITH TENDON INVOLVEMENT

884.0 LIMB UPPER NOS OR MULTIPLE SITES
884.1 LIMB UPPER NOS OR MULTIPLE SITES COMPLICATED
884.2 LIMB UPPER NOS OR MULTIPLE SITES WITH TENDON INVOLVEMENT

873.43 LIP
873.53 LIP COMPLICATED

864.0# LIVER
864.1# LIVER WITH OPEN WOUND INTO CAVITY
5th Digit: 864.0-1
0. INJURY UNSPECIFIED
1. HEMATOMA, CONTUSION
2. MINOR (< 1 CM. DEEP)
3. MODERATE (< 10 CM. LONG - < 3 CM. DEEP)
4. MAJOR (10 CM. LONG - 3 CM. DEEP, MULTIPLE MODERATES OR STELLATE)
5. LACERATION UNSPECIFIED
9. OTHER

IN ICD-9, A COMPLICATED LACERATION OR OPEN WOUND IS DEFINED AS THAT WHICH IS INFECTED, CONTAINS A FOREIGN BODY, OR IS GROSSLY CONTAMINATED.

LACERATION (continued)

908.1 LIVER LATE EFFECT

876.0 LOIN
876.1 LOIN COMPLICATED

876.0 LUMBAR REGION
876.1 LUMBAR REGION COMPLICATED

861.22 LUNG
861.32 LUNG WITH OPEN WOUND
908.0 LUNG LATE EFFECT

873.41 MALAR
873.51 MALAR COMPLICATED

873.44 MANDIBLE
873.54 MANDIBLE COMPLICATED

873.49 MASTOID
873.59 MASTOID COMPLICATED

0 MENINGES SEE 'LACERATION' BRAIN

0 MENISCUS SEE 'MENISCUS' TEAR

875.0 MIDTHORACIC REGION
875.1 MIDTHORACIC REGION COMPLICATED

873.60 MOUTH
873.70 MOUTH COMPLICATED

873.64 MOUTH FLOOR
873.74 MOUTH FLOOR COMPLICATED

873.69 MOUTH OTHER AND MULTIPLE SITES
873.79 MOUTH OTHER AND MULTIPLE SITES COMPLICATED

879.8 MULTIPLE
879.9 MULTIPLE COMPLICATED

894.0 MULTIPLE LOWER LIMB
894.1 MULTIPLE LOWER LIMB COMPLICATED
894.2 MULTIPLE LOWER LIMB WITH TENDON INVOLVEMENT

884.0 MULTIPLE UPPER LIMB
884.1 MULTIPLE UPPER LIMB COMPLICATED
884.2 MULTIPLE UPPER LIMB WITH TENDON INVOLVEMENT

618.7 MUSCLES PELVIC FLOOR (OLD)
618.7 MUSCLES PELVIC FLOOR (OLD) WITH STRESS INCONTINENCE [625.6]
618.7 MUSCLES PELVIC FLOOR (OLD) WITH OTHER URINARY INCONTINENCE [788.3#]

5th Digit: 788.3

0. UNSPECIFIED
1. URGE INCONTINENCE
3. MIXED URGE AND STRESS (MALE) (FEMALE)
4 WITHOUT SENSORY AWARENESS
5. POST-VOID DRIBBLING
6. NOCTURNAL ENURESIS
7. CONTINUOUS LEAKAGE
9. OTHER

861.02 MYOCARDIUM
861.03 MYOCARDIUM WITH PENETRATION OF CHAMBER
861.12 MYOCARDIUM WITH OPEN WOUND INTO THORAX
861.13 MYOCARDIUM WITH OPEN WOUND INTO THORAX AND PENETRATION OF CHAMBER
908.0 MYOCARDIUM LATE EFFECT

*WHEN AN OPEN WOUND OR LACERATION IS ACCOMPANIED BY CELLULITIS, TWO CODES ARE NEEDED, THE CODE FOR THE **COMPLICATED** OPEN WOUND OR LACERATION AND A CODE FOR THE CELLULITIS. SEQUENCING DEPENDS ON WHICH DIAGNOSIS REQUIRED THE MAJOR WORK AND EFFORT.*

LACERATION (continued)

0 NAIL SEE 'LACERATION', FINGER, THUMB OR TOE

0 NASAL SEE 'LACERATION', NOSE

873.22 NASOPHARYNX
873.32 NASOPHARYNX COMPLICATED

874.8 NECK
874.9 NECK COMPLICATED

874.8 NECK NAPE
874.9 NECK NAPE COMPLICATED

874.8 NECK OTHER AND UNSPECIFIED
874.9 NECK OTHER AND UNSPECIFIED COMPLICATED

NERVE

957.9 UNSPECIFIED
956.4 CUTANEOUS SENSORY LOWER LIMB
955.5 CUTANEOUS SENSORY UPPER LIMB
957.0 HEAD AND NECK SUPERFICIAL
957.8 MULTIPLE UNSPECIFIED
956.8 PELVIC GIRDLE AND LOWER LIMB MULTIPLE
956.5 PELVIC GIRDLE AND LOWER LIMB OTHER SPECIFIED
956.9 PELVIC GIRDLE AND LOWER LIMB UNSPECIFIED
907.3 ROOT INJURY LATE EFFECT
953.8 ROOT INJURY MULTIPLE SITES
953.9 ROOT INJURY SITE UNSPECIFIED
955.8 SHOULDER GIRDLE AND UPPER LIMB MULTIPLE INJURY
955.7 SHOULDER GIRDLE AND UPPER LIMB OTHER SPECIFIED
955.9 SHOULDER GIRDLE AND UPPER LIMB UNSPECIFIED
954.9 TRUNK UNSPECIFIED
954.8 TRUNK OTHER SPECIFIED
957.1 OTHER SPECIFIED
0 SEE ALSO 'NERVE INJURY'

LACERATION (continued)

873.20 NOSE
873.30 NOSE COMPLICATED

873.22 NOSE CAVITY
873.32 NOSE CAVITY COMPLICATED

873.29 NOSE MULTIPLE SITES
873.39 NOSE MULTIPLE SITES COMPLICATED

873.21 NOSE SEPTUM
873.31 NOSE SEPTUM COMPLICATED

873.23 NOSE SINUS
873.33 NOSE SINUS COMPLICATED

0 OCCIPITAL REGION SEE 'LACERATION', SCALP

870.8 ORBIT
870.3 ORBIT PENETRATING
870.4 ORBIT PENETRATING WITH FOREIGN BODY
870.9 ORBITAL REGION

0 ORGAN INTERNAL SEE SPECIFIC ORGAN

872.62 OSSICLES EAR
872.72 OSSICLES EAR COMPLICATED

873.65 PALATE
873.75 PALATE COMPLICATED

0 PALM SEE 'LACERATION', HAND

IN ICD-9, A COMPLICATED LACERATION OR OPEN WOUND IS DEFINED AS THAT WHICH IS INFECTED, CONTAINS A FOREIGN BODY, OR IS GROSSLY CONTAMINATED.

LACERATION (continued)

874.2 PARATHYROID GLAND
874.3 PARATHYROID GLAND COMPLICATED

0 PARIETAL REGION SEE 'LACERATION', SCALP

879.6 PELVIC REGION
879.7 PELVIC REGION COMPLICATED

618.7 PELVIC FLOOR MUSCLES (OLD)
618.7 PELVIC FLOOR MUSCLES (OLD) WITH STRESS INCONTINENCE [625.6]
618.7 PELVIC FLOOR MUSCLES (OLD) WITH OTHER URINARY INCONTINENCE **[788.3#]**

5th Digit: 788.3
0. UNSPECIFIED
1. URGE INCONTINENCE
3. MIXED URGE AND STRESS (MALE) (FEMALE)
4 WITHOUT SENSORY AWARENESS
5. POST-VOID DRIBBLING
6. NOCTURNAL ENURESIS
7. CONTINUOUS LEAKAGE
9. OTHER

664.1# PELVIC FLOOR MUSCLES OBSTETRICAL (DURING DELIVERY)

5th Digit: 664.1
0. EPISODE OF CARE UNSPECIFIED OR N/A
1. DELIVERED
4. POSTPARTUM COMPLICATION

878.0 PENIS
878.1 PENIS COMPLICATED

0 PERINEAL (OLD) (POSTPARTAL) SEE 'LACERATION', PELVIC FLOOR MUSCLES
664.4# PERINEAL OBSTETRICAL NOS
664.0# PERINEAL 1ST DEGREE OBSTETRICAL INVOLVING : (FOURCHETTE) (HYMEN) (LABIA) (SKIN) (VAGINA) (VULVA)
664.1# PERINEAL 2ND DEGREE OBSTETRICAL INVOLVING : (PELVIC FLOOR) (PERINEAL MUSCLES) (VAGINAL MUSCLES)
664.2# PERINEAL 3RD DEGREE OBSTETRICAL INVOLVING : (ANAL SPHINCTER) (RECTOVAGINAL SEPTUM) (SPHINCTER NOS)
664.3# PERINEAL 4TH DEGREE OBSTETRICAL INVOLVING : 3RD DEGREE AND (ANAL MUCOSA) (RECTAL MUCOSA)

5th Digit: 664.0-4
0. EPISODE OF CARE UNSPECIFIED OR N/A
1. DELIVERED
4. POSTPARTUM COMPLICATION

879.6 PERINEUM
879.7 PERINEUM COMPLICATED

870.8 PERIOCULAR AREA
870.0 PERIOCULAR AREA WITH LACERATION OF SKIN

665.5# PERITONEUM OBSTETRICAL (DURING DELIVERY)
665.5# PERIURETHRAL OBSTETRICAL (DURING DELIVERY)

5th Digit: 665.5
0. EPISODE OF CARE UNSPECIFIED OR N/A
1. DELIVERED
4. POSTPARTUM COMPLICATION

874.4 PHARYNX
874.5 PHARYNX COMPLICATED

872.01 PINNA
872.11 PINNA COMPLICATED

891.0 POPLITEAL
891.1 POPLITEAL COMPLICATED
891.2 POPLITEAL WITH TENDON INVOLVEMENT

*WHEN AN OPEN WOUND OR LACERATION IS ACCOMPANIED BY CELLULITIS, TWO CODES ARE NEEDED, THE CODE FOR THE **COMPLICATED** OPEN WOUND OR LACERATION AND A CODE FOR THE CELLULITIS. SEQUENCING DEPENDS ON WHICH DIAGNOSIS REQUIRED THE MAJOR WORK AND EFFORT.*

LACERATION (continued)

0 PREPUCE SEE 'LACERATION', PENIS

879.2 PUBIC REGION
879.3 PUBIC REGION COMPLICATED

878.8 PUDENDA
878.9 PUDENDA COMPLICATED

861.22 PULMONARY
861.32 PULMONARY WITH OPEN WOUND OF THORAX
908.0 PULMONARY LATE EFFECT

623.4 RECTOVAGINAL (SEPTUM) OLD
878.8 RECTOVAGINAL (SEPTUM)
878.9 RECTOVAGINAL (SEPTUM) COMPLICATED

665.4# RECTOVAGINAL (SEPTUM) OBSTETRICAL

5th Digit: 665.4
0. EPISODE OF CARE UNSPECIFIED OR N/A
1. DELIVERED
4. POSTPARTUM COMPLICATION

866.02 RENAL
866.12 RENAL WITH OPEN WOUND INTO CAVITY
908.1 RENAL LATE EFFECT

877.0 SACRAL REGION
877.1 SACRAL REGION COMPLICATED

0 SACROILIAC REGION SEE 'LACERATION', SACRAL REGION

873.69 SALIVARY (DUCTS) (GLAND)
873.79 SALIVARY (DUCTS) (GLAND) COMPLICATED

873.0 SCALP
873.1 SCALP COMPLICATED

880.01 SCAPULAR
880.11 SCAPULAR AREA COMPLICATED
880.21 SCAPULAR WITH TENDON INVOLVEMENT

871.9 SCLERA

878.2 SCROTUM
878.3 SCROTUM COMPLICATED

891.0 SHIN
891.1 SHIN COMPLICATED
891.2 SHIN WITH TENDON INVOLVEMENT

880.00 SHOULDER
880.10 SHOULDER COMPLICATED
880.20 SHOULDER WITH TENDON INVOLVEMENT

880.09 SHOULDER AND ARM MULTIPLE SITES
880.19 SHOULDER AND ARM MULTIPLE SITES COMPLICATED
880.29 SHOULDER AND ARM MULTIPLE SITES WITH TENDON INVOLVEMENT

879.8 SKIN NOS
879.9 SKIN NOS COMPLICATED

0 SPERMATIC CORD (SCROTAL) SEE 'LACERATION', SCROTUM

0 SPINAL CORD SEE 'SPINAL CORD INJURY', BY SITE
767.4 SPINE OR SPINAL CORD DUE TO BIRTH TRAUMA

865.09 SPLEEN
865.19 SPLEEN WITH OPEN WOUND INTO CAVITY
865.04 SPLEEN WITH DISRUPTION OF PARENCHYMA
865.14 SPLEEN WITH DISRUPTION OF PARENCHYMA WITH OPEN WOUND INTO CAVITY
908.1 SPLEEN LATE EFFECT

L

IN ICD-9, A COMPLICATED LACERATION OR OPEN WOUND IS DEFINED AS THAT WHICH IS INFECTED, CONTAINS A FOREIGN BODY, OR IS GROSSLY CONTAMINATED.

LACERATION (continued)

865.02 SPLEEN CAPSULE
865.12 SPLEEN CAPSULE WITH OPEN WOUND INTO CAVITY
908.1 SPLEEN CAPSULE LATE EFFECT

865.03 SPLEEN INTO PARENCHYMA
865.13 SPLEEN INTO PARENCHYMA WITH OPEN WOUND INTO CAVITY
908.1 SPLEEN INTO PARENCHYMA LATE EFFECT

875.0 STERNAL REGION
875.1 STERNAL REGION COMPLICATED

0 SUBMAXILLARY REGION SEE 'LACERATION', JAW
0 SUBMENTAL REGION SEE 'LACERATION', JAW

0 SUBUNGUAL SEE 'LACERATION', FINGER, THUMB OR TOE

874.8 SUPRACLAVICULAR REGION
874.9 SUPRACLAVICULAR REGION COMPLICATED

0 SUPRAORBITAL SEE 'LACERATION', FOREHEAD

873.49 TEMPLE
873.59 TEMPLE COMPLICATED

0 TEMPORAL REGION SEE 'LACERATION', TEMPLE

TENDON

881.20 ABDUCTOR POLLICIS FOREARM
882.2 ABDUCTOR POLLICIS HAND
883.2 ABDUCTOR POLLICIS THUMB
881.22 ABDUCTOR POLLICIS WRIST
845.09 ACHILLES
892.2 ACHILLES WITH OPEN WOUND
881.20 BICEPS DISTAL
891.2 BICEPS FEMORIS
880.23 BICEPS PROXIMAL
883.2 EXTENSOR DIGITI MINIMUMI FINGER
882.2 EXTENSOR DIGITI MINIMUMI HAND
891.2 EXTENSOR HALLUCIS ANKLE
892.2 EXTENSOR HALLUCIS FOOT
893.2 EXTENSOR HALLUCIS TOE
883.2 EXTENSOR INDICUS PROPRIUS FINGER
882.2 EXTENSOR INDICUS PROPRIUS HAND
882.2 EXTENSOR POLLICIS BREVIS HAND
883.2 EXTENSOR POLLICIS BREVIS THUMB
881.20 EXTENSOR POLLICIS LONGUS FOREARM
882.2 EXTENSOR POLLICIS LONGUS HAND
883.2 EXTENSOR POLLICIS LONGUS THUMB
881.22 EXTENSOR POLLICIS LONGUS WRIST
893.2 EXTENSOR TOE
891.2 EXTENSOR TOE ANKLE
892.2 EXTENSOR TOE FOOT
881.22 FLEXOR CARPI RADIALIS
881.20 FLEXOR CARPI RADIALIS PROXIMAL
881.22 FLEXOR CARPI ULNARIS DISTAL
881.20 FLEXOR CARPI ULNARIS PROXIMAL
883.2 FLEXOR DIGITORUM PROFUNDUS FINGER
882.2 FLEXOR DIGITORUM PROFUNDUS HAND
881.22 FLEXOR DIGITORUM PROFUNDUS WRIST
883.2 FLEXOR DIGITORUM SUPERFICIALIS FINGER
882.2 FLEXOR DIGITORUM SUPERFICIALIS HAND
881.22 FLEXOR DIGITORUM SUPERFICIALIS WRIST

WHEN AN OPEN WOUND OR LACERATION IS ACCOMPANIED BY CELLULITIS, TWO CODES ARE NEEDED, THE CODE FOR THE __COMPLICATED__ OPEN WOUND OR LACERATION AND A CODE FOR THE CELLULITIS. SEQUENCING DEPENDS ON WHICH DIAGNOSIS REQUIRED THE MAJOR WORK AND EFFORT.

LACERATION (continued)

TENDON (continued)

891.2 FLEXOR HALLUCIS ANKLE
892.2 FLEXOR HALLUCIS FOOT
893.2 FLEXOR HALLUCIS TOE
893.2 FLEXOR TOE
891.2 FLEXOR TOE ANKLE
892.2 FLEXOR TOE FOOT
905.8 LATE EFFECT
844.9 LOWER LIMB NEC
894.2 LOWER LIMB WITH OPEN WOUND
891.2 PATELLAR
890.2 QUADRICEPS
891.2 QUADRICEPS IN KNEE
881.20 TRICEPS DISTAL
880.21 TRICEPS PROXIMAL
840.9 UPPER LIMB NEC
884.2 UPPER LIMB WITH OPEN WOUND

LACERATION (continued)

878.2 TESTIS
878.3 TESTIS COMPLICATED

890.0 THIGH
890.1 THIGH COMPLICATED
890.2 THIGH WITH TENDON INVOLVEMENT

875.0 THORAX EXTERNAL
875.1 THORAX EXTERNAL COMPLICATED

874.8 THROAT
874.9 THROAT COMPLICATED

883.0 THUMB (NAIL)
883.1 THUMB (NAIL) COMPLICATED
883.2 THUMB (NAIL) WITH TENDON INVOLVEMENT

874.2 THYROID GLAND
874.3 THYROID GLAND COMPLICATED

893.0 TOE (NAIL)
893.1 TOE (NAIL) COMPLICATED
893.2 TOE (NAIL) WITH TENDON INVOLVEMENT

873.64 TONGUE
873.74 TONGUE COMPLICATED

873.64 TONGUE AND FLOOR OF MOUTH
873.74 TONGUE AND FLOOR OF MOUTH COMPLICATED

874.## TRACHEA
4th Digit: 874
0. UNSPECIFIED
1. COMPLICATED
5th Digit: 874
0. LARYNX WITH TRACHEA
2. TRACHEA

879.6 TRUNK
879.7 TRUNK COMPLICATED

878.2 TUNICA VAGINALIS
878.3 TUNICA VAGINALIS COMPLICATED

872.61 TYMPANIC MEMBRANE
872.71 TYMPANIC MEMBRANE COMPLICATED

WHEN AN OPEN WOUND OR LACERATION IS ACCOMPANIED BY CELLULITIS, TWO CODES ARE NEEDED, THE CODE FOR THE COMPLICATED OPEN WOUND OR LACERATION AND A CODE FOR THE CELLULITIS. SEQUENCING DEPENDS ON WHICH DIAGNOSIS REQUIRED THE MAJOR WORK AND EFFORT.

LACERATION (continued)

879.2 UMBILICAL REGION
879.3 UMBILICAL REGION COMPLICATED

599.84 URETHRA NONTRAUMATIC
665.5# URETHRA OBSTETRICAL (DURING DELIVERY)
5th Digit: 665.5
0. EPISODE OF CARE UNSPECIFIED OR N/A
1. DELIVERED
4. POSTPARTUM COMPLICATION

867.0 URETHRA TRAUMATIC
908.2 URETHRA TRAUMATIC LATE EFFECT
867.1 URETHRA TRAUMATIC WITH OPEN WOUND INTO CAVITY

665.1# UTERUS OBSTETRICAL NEC DURING LABOR
5th Digit: 665.1
0. EPISODE OF CARE UNSPECIFIED OR N/A
1. DELIVERED

621.8 UTERUS OLD (POSTPARTUM)

873.69 UVULA
873.79 UVULA COMPLICATED

878.6 VAGINA
878.7 VAGINA COMPLICATED
665.4# VAGINA OBSTETRICAL
5th Digit: 665.4
0. EPISODE OF CARE UNSPECIFIED OR N/A
1. DELIVERED
4. POSTPARTUM COMPLICATION

623.4 VAGINA OLD
618.7 VAGINA OLD INVOLVING MUSCLES
618.7 VAGINA OLD INVOLVING MUSCLES WITH STRESS INCONTINENCE [625.6]
618.7 VAGINA OLD INVOLVING MUSCLES WITH OTHER URINARY INCONTINENCE [788.3#]
5th Digit: 788.3
0. UNSPECIFIED
1. URGE INCONTINENCE
3. MIXED URGE AND STRESS (MALE) (FEMALE)
4 WITHOUT SENSORY AWARENESS
5. POST-VOID DRIBBLING
6. NOCTURNAL ENURESIS
7. CONTINUOUS LEAKAGE
9. OTHER

0 VEIN SEE SPECIFIC VEIN, INJURY
871.2 VITREOUS (HUMOR)

878.4 VULVA
878.5 VULVA COMPLICATED
664.0# VULVA OBSTETRICAL (DURING DELIVERY)
5th Digit: 664.0
0. EPISODE OF CARE UNSPECIFIED OR N/A
1. DELIVERED
4. POSTPARTUM COMPLICATION

624.4 VULVA OLD OR SCARRING

881.02 WRIST
881.12 WRIST COMPLICATED
881.22 WRIST WITH TENDON INVOLVEMENT

LACRIMAL

743.65 ANOMALIES (APPARATUS) (PASSAGES) (SPECIFIED) CONGENITAL
743.65 ATRESIA (CONGENITAL)
375.13 ATROPHY PRIMARY
375.14 ATROPHY SECONDARY
375.53 CANALICULI OBSTRUCTION OR OCCLUSION
375.53 CANALICULI STENOSIS
375.31 CANALICULITIS ACUTE
375.61 FISTULA
743.64 GLAND ANOMALIES (SPECIFIED) CONGENITAL
375.12 GLAND CYSTIC DEGENERATION
375.16 GLAND DISLOCATION
375.00 GLAND DISORDER
375.03 GLAND ENLARGEMENT CHRONIC
375.89 GLAND DISORDER - OTHER
375.81 GRANULOMA (PASSAGES)
375.43 MUCOCELE
743.65 OBSTRUCTION OR OCCLUSION CONGENITAL
375.69 PASSAGES CHANGES OTHER
375.51 PUNCTUM EVERSION
375.52 PUNCTUM OBSTRUCTION OR OCCLUSION
375.52 PUNCTUM STENOSIS
375.54 SAC OBSTRUCTION OR OCCLUSION
375.54 STENOSIS (SAC)
375.9 SYSTEM DISORDER
375.89 SYSTEM DISORDERS OTHER

LACTATION

676.9# DISORDER (LACTATING) MATERNAL DUE TO PREGNANCY
676.8# DISORDERS OTHER SPECIFIED MATERNAL DUE TO PREGNANCY
676.4# FAILURE MATERNAL DUE TO PREGNANCY
676.5# SUPPRESSED MATERNAL DUE TO PREGNANCY
5th Digit: 676.4-5, 8-9
0. EPISODE OF CARE UNSPECIFIED OR N/A
1. DELIVERED
2. DELIVERED WITH POSTPARTUM COMPLICATION
3. ANTEPARTUM COMPLICATION
4. POSTPARTUM COMPLICATION

579.2 LACTEAL OBSTRUCTION WITH STEATORRHEA
790.4 LACTIC ACID DEHYDROGENASE ABNORMAL BLOOD LEVEL
271.3 LACTOSE (INTOLERANCE) (MALABSORPTION) (METABOLISM DISORDER)
434.91 LACUNAR INFARCT
571.2 LAENNEC'S CIRRHOSIS (LIVER)
571.5 LAENNEC'S CIRRHOSIS (LIVER) WITH ESOPHAGEAL VARICES [456.2#]
5th Digit: 456.2
0. WITH BLEEDING
1. WITHOUT BLEEDING

333.2 LAFORA'S DISEASE
759.6 LAGLEYZE-VON HIPPEL DISEASE CONGENITAL

LAGOPHTHALMOS

374.20 UNSPECIFIED
374.23 CICATRICIAL
374.22 MECHANICAL
374.21 PARALYTIC

286.3 LAKI LORAND DEFICIENCY
307.9 LALLING
007.1 LAMBLIASIS
704.1 LANUGINOSA ACQUIRED
100.0 LANCERAUX-MATHIEU DISEASE (LEPTOSPIRAL JAUNDICE)

L

359.1 LANDOUZY DEJERINE MUSCULAR DYSTROPHY
357.0 LANDRY'S DISEASE
569.89 LANE'S DISEASE
063.8 LANGAT ENCEPHALITIS
758.0 LANGDON DOWN SYNDROME (MONGOLISM)
315.31 LANGUAGE DISORDER DEVELOPMENTAL - EXPRESSIVE
315.32 LANGUAGE DISORDER DEVELOPMENTAL - RECEPTIVE (EXPRESSIVE - RECEPTIVE) (MIXED)
438.1# LANGUAGE DISORDER LATE EFFECT OF CEREBROVASCULAR DISEASE
5th Digit: 438.1
0. UNSPECIFIED
1. APHASIA
2. DYSPHASIA
9. OTHER
757.4 LANUGO PERSISTENT CONGENITAL
V64.4 LAPAROSCOPIC SURGICAL PROCEDURE CONVERTED TO OPEN PROCEDURE
277.3 LARDACEOUS DISEASE (ANY SITE)
766.0 LARGE BABY EXCEPTIONALLY (BIRTHWEIGHT >4500 GRAMS)
199.1 LARGE CELL CARCINOMA SITE NOS
0 LARGE CELL CARCINOMA SITE SPECIFIED SEE 'CANCER' BY SITE M8012/3
656.6# LARGE FOR DATES AFFECTING MANAGEMENT OF MOTHER
5th Digit: 656.6
0. EPISODE OF CARE UNSPECIFIED OR N/A
1. DELIVERED
3. ANTEPARTUM COMPLICATION
766.1 LARGE FOR DATES INFANT (REGARDLESS OF GESTATION PERIOD)
115.1# LARGE FORM HISTOPLASMOSIS
5th Digit: 115.1
0. WITHOUT MENTION OF MANIFESTATION
1. MENINGITIS
2. RETINITIS
3. PERICARDITIS
4. ENDOCARDITIS
5. PNEUMONIA
9. OTHER
751.2 LARGE INTESTINE (ABSENCE) (ATRESIA) (STENOSIS) (OBSTRUCTION) CONGENITAL
100.0 LARREY-WEIL DISEASE (LEPTOSPIRAL JAUNDICE)
732.4 LARSEN (-JOHANSSON) DISEASE (JUVENILE OSTEOPATHIA PATELLAE)
755.8 LARSEN'S SYNDROME (FLATTENED FACIES AND MULTIPLE CONGENITAL DISLOCATIONS)
126.9 LARVA MIGRANS CUTANEOUS
128.0 LARVA MIGRANS VISCERALIS INFECTION
0 LARYNGEAL SEE 'LARYNX, LARYNGEAL'

LARYNGITIS
464.0 ACUTE
464.0 ACUTE H. FLU
487.1 ACUTE INFLUENZAL
034.0 ACUTE STREPTOCOCCAL
464.0 ACUTE PNEUMOCOCCAL
476.0 CATARRHAL
476.0 CHRONIC
476.0 CHRONIC ATROPHIC
476.1 CHRONIC WITH TRACHEITIS
476.0 HYPERTROPHIC
487.1 INFLUENZA
464.0 OBSTRUCTIVE
476.0 SICCA
464.0 ULCERATIVE

748.3 LARYNGOCELE CONGENITAL
465.0 LARYNGOPHARYNGITIS ACUTE
478.30 LARYNGOPLEGIA
478.75 LARYNGOSPASM

LARYNGOTRACHEITIS
464.20 ACUTE
464.21 ACUTE WITH OBSTRUCTION
476.1 CHRONIC
032.3 DIPHTHERITIC

LARYNX, LARYNGEAL
478.79 ABSCESS
748.3 ABSENCE OR AGENESIS CONGENITAL
748.3 ATRESIA CONGENITAL
478.79 ATROPHY
478.79 CALCIFICATION
478.71 CELLULITIS AND PERICHONDRITIS
925.2 CRUSHING INJURY
478.70 DISEASE
478.6 EDEMA
478.79 GRANULOMA
959.09 INJURY
478.79 LEUKOPLAKIA
478.79 NECROSIS
352.3 NERVE DISORDER RECURRENT
478.79 NODULE
478.79 OBSTRUCTION
748.3 OBSTRUCTION CONGENITAL
478.79 PACHYDERMA
478.30 PARALYSIS
478.33 PARALYSIS BILATERAL PARTIAL
478.34 PARALYSIS BILATERAL COMPLETE
478.31 PARALYSIS UNILATERAL PARTIAL
478.32 PARALYSIS UNILATERAL COMPLETE
478.4 POLYP
212.1 POLYP (ADENOMATOUS)
V43.81 REPLACEMENT (PROSTHESIS) STATUS
478.75 SPASM
478.74 STENOSIS
748.3 STENOSIS CONGENITAL
748.3 STRIDOR CONGENITAL
748.2 SUBGLOTTIC CONGENITAL
478.79 ULCER
748.2 WEB
748.2 WEB GLOTTIC

297.9 LASEGUE'S DISEASE (PERSECUTION MANIA)
780.79 LASSITUDE

LATE EFFECTS ARE RECOGNIZED TO BE THOSE RESIDUAL PROBLEMS STEMMING FROM AN OLD INJURY OR DISORDER (SUCH AS PARALYSIS FROM AN OLD STROKE). USE THIS CATEGORY ONLY AS A SECONDARY DIAGNOSIS.

LATE EFFECT
326 ABSCESS INTRACRANIAL OR INTRASPINAL
909.5 ADVERSE EFFECT OF DRUG, MEDICINAL OR BIOLOGICAL SUBSTANCE
909.9 ALLERGIC REACTION
997.6# AMPUTATION POSTOPERATIVE STUMP
5th Digit: 997.6
0. NOS
1. NEUROMA OF STUMP
2. INFECTION (CHRONIC)
9. OTHER
905.9 AMPUTATION TRAUMATIC
909.5 BIOLOGICAL SUBSTANCE ADVERSE EFFECT
906.9 BURN - SITE NOS
906.5 BURN - EYE FACE HEAD AND NECK
906.6 BURN - WRIST AND HAND
906.7 BURN - OTHER EXTREMITIES
906.8 BURN - OTHER SPECIFIED SITES

LATE EFFECT (continued)

CEREBROVASCULAR DISEASE

> *WHEN THE LATE EFFECT OR RESIDUAL CONDITION IS NOT IDENTIFIED IN THE 438.## CODE-USE AN ADDITIONAL CODE TO SPECIFY THAT CONDITION. IE CODES 438.5 AND 438.89*

438.9 UNSPECIFIED
438.81 APRAXIA
438.0 COGNITIVE DEFECT
438.82 DYSPHAGIA
438.2# PARALYTIC - HEMIPLEGIA OR HEMIPARESIS
438.4# PARALYTIC - MONOPLEGIA LOWER LIMB
438.3# PARALYTIC - MONOPLEGIA UPPER LIMB
5th Digit: 438.2-4
0. UNSPECIFIED SIDE
1. DOMINANT SIDE
2. NONDOMINANT SIDE

438.5# PARALYTIC - OTHER SYNDROME
5th Digit: 438.5
0. UNSPECIFIED SIDE
1. DOMINANT SIDE
2. NONDOMINANT SIDE
3. BILATERAL

438.1# SPEECH AND LANGUAGE DEFICIT
5th Digit: 438.1
0. UNSPECIFIED
1. APHASIA
2. DYSPHASIA
9. OTHER

438.89 OTHER SPECIFIED

LATE EFFECT (continued)

677 COMPLICATIONS CHILDBIRTH, DELIVERY, PREGNANCY OR PUERPERIUM
909.3 COMPLICATIONS OF SURGICAL AND MEDICAL CARE
908.6 COMPLICATIONS EARLY OF TRAUMA OTHER SPECIFIED
906.3 CONTUSION
906.4 CRUSH INJURY
0 CVA SEE 'LATE EFFECT', CEREBROVASCULAR DISEASE
677 DELIVERY COMPLICATION
905.6 DISLOCATION (ANY SITE)
909.5 DRUG ADVERSE EFFECT
326 ENCEPHALITIS NOS AND NEC
326 ENCEPHALITIS POSTIMMUNIZATION
139.0 ENCEPHALITIS VIRAL
326 ENCEPHALOMYELITIS POSTIMMUNIZATION
909.4 ENVIRONMENTAL CAUSES
908.5 FOREIGN BODY IN ORIFICE
905.0 FRACTURE FACE AND SKULL BONES
905.4 FRACTURE OF LOWER EXTREMITIES
905.5 FRACTURE OF MULTIPLE AND UNSPECIFIED BONES
905.3 FRACTURE OF NECK OF FEMUR
905.2 FRACTURE OF UPPER EXTREMITIES
905.0 FRACTURE SKULL AND FACE BONES
905.1 FRACTURE SPINE AND TRUNK WITHOUT SPINAL CORD LESION
907.2 FRACTURE SPINE AND TRUNK WITH SPINAL CORD LESION
906.3 HEMATOMA TRAUMATIC
326 INFECTION INTRACRANIAL PYOGENIC
139.8 INFECTIOUS AND PARASITIC DISEASE
908.3 INJURY BLOOD VESSEL OF HEAD NECK AND EXTREMITIES
908.4 INJURY BLOOD VESSEL OF THORAX ABDOMEN AND PELVIS
908.6 INJURY CERTAIN COMPLICATIONS OF TRAUMA
908.1 INJURY INTERNAL ABDOMINAL ORGANS
908.0 INJURY INTERNAL CHEST
908.2 INJURY INTERNAL ORGANS (OTHER)
907.0 INJURY INTRACRANIAL
905.0 INJURY INTRACRANIAL WITH SKULL FRACTURE

LATE EFFECT (continued)

907.1 INJURY NERVE CRANIAL
907.5 INJURY NERVE OF PELVIC GIRDLE AND LOWER LIMB PERIPHERAL
907.4 INJURY NERVE OF SHOULDER GIRDLE AND UPPER LIMB PERIPHERAL
907.9 INJURY NERVE OTHER AND UNSPECIFIED
907.3 INJURY NERVE ROOT(S) SPINAL PLEXUS(ES) AND OTHER NERVES OF TRUNK (INJURY)
907.2 INJURY SPINAL CORD
907.3 INJURY SPINAL NERVE ROOT AND PLEXUS(ES)
906.2 INJURY SUPERFICIAL
905.8 INJURY TENDON
908.9 INJURY UNSPECIFIED
909.5 MEDICINE ADVERSE EFFECT
139.8 MEASLES
326 MYELITIS
905.8 OPEN WOUND OF EXTREMITIES WITH TENDON INJURY
906.1 OPEN WOUND OF EXTREMITIES WITHOUT TENDON INJURY
906.0 OPEN WOUND OF HEAD NECK AND TRUNK
139.8 PARASITIC DISEASE
326 PHLEBITIS OF INTRACRANIAL VENOUS SINUSES
138 POLIOMYELITIS
909.0 POISONING DUE TO DRUG MEDICINAL OR BIOLOGICAL SUBSTANCE
677 PREGNANCY, CHILDBIRTH OR PUERPERAL COMPLICATION
326 PYOGENIC INTRACRANIAL INFECTION
909.2 RADIATION
268.1 RICKETS
905.7 SPRAIN AND STRAIN
905.8 SPRAIN AND STRAIN WITH TENDON INJURY
0 STROKE SEE 'LATE EFFECT', CEREBROVASCULAR DISEASE
326 THROMBOPHLEBITIS OF INTRACRANIAL VENOUS SINUSES
137.0 TB (RESPIRATORY OR NOS)
137.3 TB BONES AND JOINTS
137.1 TB CENTRAL NERVOUS SYSTEM
137.2 TB GENITOURINARY
137.4 TB OTHER ORGANS
909.0 TOXIC EFFECTS OF DRUGS, MEDICINAL OR BIOLOGICAL SUBSTANCES
909.1 TOXIC EFFECTS OF NONMEDICAL SUBSTANCES
139.1 TRACHOMA
909.9 OTHER AND UNSPECIFIED EXTERNAL CAUSES
909.4 OTHER EXTERNAL ENVIRONMENTAL CAUSES

LATERAL

717.81 COLLATERAL LIGAMENT DISRUPTION (OLD)
717.9 COLLATERAL LIGAMENT RELAXATION
844.0 COLLATERAL LIGAMENT SPRAIN STRAIN OR TEAR
355.1 CUTANEOUS NERVE OF THIGH SYNDROME
726.32 EPICONDYLITIS
355.1 FEMORAL CUTANEOUS NERVE (THIGH) (COMPRESSION) (SYNDROME)
436 MEDULLARY SYNDROME
836.1 MENISCUS TEAR (KNEE) ACUTE
717.41 MENISCUS BUCKET HANDLE TEAR (KNEE) (OLD)
717.40 MENISCUS DERANGEMENT (KNEE) (OLD)
717.42 MENISCUS DERANGEMENT (KNEE) ANTERIOR HORN (OLD)
717.43 MENISCUS DERANGEMENT (KNEE) POSTERIOR HORN (OLD)
717.49 MENISCUS DERANGEMENT (KNEE) OTHER (OLD)

989.82 LATEX POISONING OR REACTION
362.63 LATTICE DEGENERATION RETINAL
272.8 LAUNOIS BENSAUDE'S LIPOMATOSIS
253.8 LAUNOIS-CLERET SYNDROME (ADIPOSOGENITAL DYSTROPHY)
253.0 LAUNOIS' SYNDROME (PITUITARY GIGANTISM)
759.89 LAURENCE-MOON (-BARDET) -BIEDL SYNDROME (OBESITY, POLYDACTYLY AND MENTAL RETARDATION)
0 LAV (LYMPHADENOPATHY- ASSOCIATED VIRUS) SEE 'HIV' INFECTION

759.6 LAWFORD'S SYNDROME (ENCEPHALOCUTANEOUS ANGIOMATOSIS)

305.9# LAXATIVE ABUSE NONDEPENDENT

5th Digit: 305.9

0. UNSPECIFIED
1. CONTINUOUS
2. EPISODIC
3. IN REMISSION

288.0 LAZY LEUKOCYTE SYNDROME
728.3 LAZY POSTURE SYNDROME
426.3 LBBB
790.4 LDH ELEVATED
272.0 LDL ELEVATED
V82.5 LEAD, HEAVY METAL SCREENING
V15.86 LEAD EXPOSURE HISTORY
371.15 LEAD INCRUSTATION CORNEA
0 LEARNING DIFFICULTIES (DELAY IN DEVELOPMENT) SEE 'DEVELOPMENTAL DISORDER'
V40.0 LEARNING PROBLEM
377.16 LEBER'S OPTIC ATROPHY
283.19 LEDERER-BRILL SYNDROME (ACQUIRED INFECTIOUS HEMOLYTIC ANEMIA)
283.19 LEDERER'S ANEMIA OR DISEASE (ACQUIRED INFECTIOUS HEMOLYTIC ANEMIA)
134.2 LEECHE INFESTATION (AQUATIC) (LAND)
802.4 LEFORT'S FRACTURE CLOSED
802.5 LEFORT'S FRACTURE OPEN
781.8 LEFT SIDED NEGLECT
746.89 LEFT VENTRICLE DIVERTICULUM CONGENITAL
428.1 LEFT VENTRICULAR FAILURE
398.91 LEFT VENTRICULAR FAILURE RHEUMATIC CHRONIC
429.3 LEFT VENTRICULAR HYPERTROPHY
745.4 LEFT VENTRICULAR RIGHT ATRIAL COMMUNICATION CONGENITAL

LEG

736.89 ABSENCE ACQUIRED
755.31 ABSENCE CONGENITAL - WITH COMPLETE ABSENCE OF DISTAL ELEMENTS (FOOT AND TOES)
755.35 ABSENCE CONGENITAL - WITH INCOMPLETE ABSENCE OF DISTAL ELEMENTS
0 AMPUTATION STATUS SEE 'AMPUTATION' STATUS - LOWER LIMB
904.8 BLOOD VESSEL NEC INJURY
904.7 BLOOD VESSEL NEC INJURY MULTIPLE
904.7 BLOOD VESSEL INJURY SPECIFIED NEC
736.42 BOWING ACQUIRED
754.44 BOWING LONG BONES CONGENITAL
732.1 CALVE PERTHES
736.89 DEFORMITY (ACQUIRED) NEC
959.7 INJURY
916.8 INJURY OTHER AND UNSPECIFIED SUPERFICIAL
916.9 INJURY OTHER AND UNSPECIFIED SUPERFICIAL INFECTED
736.81 LENGTH DISCREPANCY (ACQUIRED)
755.30 LENGTH DISCREPANCY CONGENITAL
V52.1 PROSTHESIS (FITTING AND ADJUSTMENT) (REMOVAL)
755.30 SHORTENING CONGENITAL

V62.5 LEGAL PROBLEM (REASON FOR ENCOUNTER)
732.1 LEGG (-CALVE) (-PERTHES) DISEASE (CAPITAL FEMORAL OSTEOCHONDROSIS)
482.84 LEGIONNAIRES' DISEASE
757.0 LEGS HEREDITARY EDEMA CONGENITAL
330.8 LEIGH'S DISEASE
695.89 LEINER'S DISEASE (EXFOLIATIVE DERMATITIS)

LEIOMYOMA

215.9 SITE NOS
0 SITE SPECIFIED SEE 'BENIGN NEOPLASM', CONNECTIVE TISSUE (SOFT TISSUE) BY SITE M8890/0

LEIOMYOMA (continued)

215.# BIZARRE M8893/0

4th Digit: 215

0. HEAD FACE NECK
2. UPPER LIMB SHOULDER
3. LOWER LIMB HIP
4. THORAX
5. ABDOMINAL HYPOCHONDRIUM
6. PELVIS BUTTOCK GROIN INGUINAL REGION PERINEUM
7. TRUNK NOS BACK NOS FLANK NOS
8. OTHER SPECIFIED SITES
9. SITE UNSPECIFIED

238.1 CELLULAR SITE NOS
0 CELLULAR SITE SPECIFIED SEE 'NEOPLASM UNCERTAIN BEHAVIOR' BY SITE M8892/1
238.1 EPITHELIOID SITE NOS
0 EPITHELIOID SITE SPECIFIED SEE 'NEOPLASM UNCERTAIN BEHAVIOR' BY SITE M8891/1
218.9 UTERINE
218.1 UTERINE INTRAMURAL (INTERSTITIAL)
0 UTERINE SEE 'FIBROID UTERINE'
218.0 UTERINE SUBMUCOUS
218.2 UTERINE SUBPERITONEAL
218.2 UTERINE SUBSEROUS

238.1 LEIOMYOMATOSIS INTRAVASCULAR SITE NOS
0 LEIOMYOMATOSIS INTRAVASCULAR SITE SPECIFIED SEE 'NEOPLASM UNCERTAIN BEHAVIOR' BY SITE M8890/1

LEIOMYOSARCOMA

171.# UNSPECIFIED M8890/3
171.# EPITHELIOID M8891/3

4th Digit: 171

0. HEAD FACE NECK
2. UPPER LIMB SHOULDER
3. LOWER LIMB HIP
4. THORAX
5. ABDOMINAL HYPOCHONDRIUM
6. PELVIS BUTTOCK GROIN INGUINAL REGION PERINEUM
7. TRUNK NOS BACK NOS FLANK NOS
8. OTHER SPECIFIED SITES
9. SITE UNSPECIFIED

LEISHMANIASIS

085.9 UNSPECIFIED

CUTANEOUS

085.2 ACUTE NECROTIZING
085.4 AMERICAN
085.2 ASIAN DESERT
085.3 DIFFUSE
085.1 DRY FORM
085.3 ETHIOPIAN
085.1 LATE
085.3 LEPROMATOUS
085.1 RECURRENT
085.2 RURAL
085.1 ULCERATING
085.1 URBAN
085.2 WET FORM
085.2 ZOONOTIC FORM

LEISHMANIASIS (continued)

085.0 DERMAL, POST-KALA-AZAR
085.5 EYELID [373.6]
085.5 LEISHMANIA BRAZILIENSIS
085.0 LEISHMANIA DONOVANI
085.3 LEISHMANIA ETHIOPICA
085.0 LEISHMANIA INFANTUM
085.4 LEISHMANIA MEXICANA
085.1 LEISHMANIA TROPICA (MINOR)
085.2 LEISHMANIA TROPICA MAJOR

LEISHMANIASIS (continued)

085.0 MEDITERRANEAN
085.5 MUCOCUTANEOUS (AMERICAN) CONJUNCTIVITIS [372.15]
V75.2 SCREENING EXAM
085.4 TEGUMENTARIA DIFFUSA
V05.2 VACCINATION
085.0 VISCERAL (KALA-AZAR) (INDIAN)

695.4 LELOIR'S DISEASE (LUPUS ERYTHEMATOSUS)
426.0 LENEGRE'S DISEASE
345.0# LENNOX'S SYNDROME (SEE ALSO 'EPILEPSY, EPILEPTIC')
5th Digit: 345.0
0. WITHOUT MENTION OF INTRACTABLE EPILEPSY
1. WITH INTRACTABLE EPILEPSY

LENS

379.31 ABSENCE
743.35 ABSENCE CONGENITAL
V45.61 ABSENCE STATUS POST CATARACT EXTRACTION
743.9 ANOMALY
743.36 ANOMALY - SHAPE
743.39 ANOMALY - SPECIFIED NEC
366.8 CALCIFICATION
743.36 DEFECT (SHAPE) CONGENITAL
743.37 ECTOPIC CONGENITAL
379.39 OTHER DISORDERS NONSURGICAL
996.53 PROLAPSE (OCULAR)
V43.1 REPLACEMENT (ARTIFICIAL) (PROSTHESIS) (MECHANICAL)
V45.61 REPLACEMENT STATUS (ARTIFICIAL) (PROSTHESIS) FOLLOWING CATARACT EXTRACTION [V43.1]

275.1 LENTICULAR SYNDROME
709.09 LENTIGO (JUVENILE) (SENILE)
0 LENTIGO MALIGNA SEE 'MELANOMA'
733.3 LEONTIASIS OSSIUM
242.9# LEOPOLD-LEVI'S SYNDROME (PAROXYSMAL THYROID INSTABILITY)
5th Digit: 242.9
0. WITHOUT MENTION OF THYROTOXIC CRISIS OR STORM
1. WITH MENTION OF THYROTOXIC CRISIS OR STORM

282.4 LEPORE HEMOGLOBIN SYNDROME

LEPROSY

030.9 UNSPECIFIED
030.3 BORDERLINE (GROUP B)
030.9 CORNEA [371.89]
030.3 DIMORPHOUS
030.0 EYELID [373.4]
030.2 INDETERMINATE (GROUP I)
030.0 LEPROMATOUS (TYPE L)
030.1 TUBERCULOID (TYPE T)
030.8 OTHER SPECIFIED
V74.2 SCREENING EXAM

322.9 LEPTOMENINGITIS NOS (SEE ALSO 'MENINGITIS')

LEPTOSPIROSIS

100.9 UNSPECIFIED
100.89 AUSTRALIS
100.89 BATAVIAE
100.0 ICTEROHEMORRHAGICA
100.81 MENINGITIS
100.89 PYROGENES
V74.8 SCREENING EXAM

756.59 LERI WEILL SYNDROME
444.0 LERICHE'S SYNDROME (AORTIC OCCLUSION)
733.7 LERICHE'S DISEASE (POSTTRAUMATIC OSTEOPOROSIS)
386.00 LERMOYEZ'S SYNDROME
302.0 LESBIANISM
277.2 LESCH-NYHAN SYNDROME (HYPOXANTHINE-GUANINE PHOSPHROIBOSYLTRANSFERASE DEFICIENCY)

TO CODE A LESION OF A SITE NOT LISTED BELOW, SEE DISORDER UNDER SPECIFIED ANATOMICAL SITE.

LESION

378.54 ABDUCENS NERVE
103.2 ACHROMIC OF PINTA
525.8 ALVEOLAR PROCESS
569.49 ANORECTAL
0 AORTIC (VALVE) SEE 'ENDOCARDITIS', AORTIC
388.5 AUDITORY NERVE
333.90 BASAL GANGLION
576.8 BILE DUCT
596.9 BLADDER
733.90 BONE
353.0 BRACHIAL PLEXUS
348.8 BRAIN
742.9 BRAIN CONGENITAL
0 BRAIN VASCULAR SEE 'LESION' CEREBROVASCULAR
528.9 BUCCAL
373.9 CANTHUS
0 CARATE SEE 'PINTA'
537.89 CARDIA
0 CARDIAC SEE 'HEART DISEASE'
103.2 CARDIOVASCULAR OF PINTA
344.60 CAUDA EQUINA
344.61 CAUDA EQUINA WITH NEUROGENIC BLADDER
569.89 CECUM

CEREBROVASCULAR

437.9 NOS
437.1 DEGENERATIVE
V12.59 HEALED
0 HEALED WITH RESIDUAL SEE 'LATE EFFECT', CEREBROVASCULAR DISEASE
437.2 HYPERTENSIVE
437.8 SPECIFIED TYPE NEC

LESION (continued)

353.2 CERVICAL ROOT (NERVE) NEC
377.54 CHIASMAL
377.54 CHIASMAL WITH INFLAMMATORY DISORDER
377.52 CHIASMAL NEOPLASM NEC
377.51 CHIASMAL NEOPLASM PITUITARY
377.51 CHIASMAL PITUITARY DISORDER
377.53 CHIASMAL VASCULAR DISORDER
351.8 CHORDA TYMPANI
103.2 CICATRICIAL OF PINTA
793.1 COIN, LUNG
569.89 COLON
372.9 CONJUNCTIVA
0 CORONARY ARTERY SEE 'CAD (CORONARY ARTERY DISEASE)'

CRANIAL NERVE

352.9 NOS
352.0 FIRST
377.49 SECOND
378.51 THIRD PARTIAL
378.52 THIRD TOTAL
378.53 FOURTH
350.9 FIFTH
378.54 SIXTH
351.9 SEVENTH
388.5 EIGHTH
352.2 NINTH
352.3 TENTH
352.4 ELEVENTH
352.5 TWELFTH

TO CODE A LESION OF A SITE NOT LISTED BELOW, SEE DISORDER UNDER SPECIFIED ANATOMICAL SITE.

TO CODE A LESION OF A SITE NOT LISTED BELOW, SEE DISORDER UNDER SPECIFIED ANATOMICAL SITE.

LESION (continued)

0	CYSTIC SEE 'CYST' BY SITE
709.9	DERMAL (SKIN)
537.89	DUODENUM
537.3	DUODENUM WITH OBSTRUCTION
103.2	DYSCHROMIC OF PINTA
373.9	EYELID
350.8	GASSERIAN GANGLION
537.89	GASTRIC
537.89	GASTRODUODENAL
569.89	GASTROINTESTINAL
352.2	GLOSSOPHARYNGEAL NERVE
0	HEART (ORGANIC) SEE 'HEART DISEASE'
0	HEART VASCULAR SEE 'CARDIOVASCULAR DISEASE'
709.9	HELIX (EAR)
103.1	HYPERCHROMIC, DUE TO PINTA (CARATE)
701.1	HYPERKERATOTIC SEE ALSO 'KERATOSIS'
352.5	HYPOGLOSSAL NERVE
478.29	HYPOPHARYNX
253.9	HYPOTHALAMIC
569.89	ILEOCECAL COIL
569.89	ILEUM
355.79	ILIOHYPOGASTRIC NERVE
355.79	ILIOINGUINAL NERVE
0	IN CONTINUITY SEE 'NERVE INJURY' BY SITE
569.89	INTESTINE
0	INTRACEREBRAL SEE 'LESION' CEREBROVASCULAR
0	INTRACHIASMAL SEE 'LESION' CHIASMAL
784.2	INTRACRANIAL, SPACE-OCCUPYING NEC
0	JOINT SEE 'JOINT', DISORDER
701.1	KERATOTIC SEE ALSO 'KERATOSIS'
593.9	KIDNEY NOS
352.3	LARYNGEAL NERVE (RECURRENT)
030.0	LEONINE
528.5	LIP
573.8	LIVER
353.1	LUMBOSACRAL PLEXUS
353.4	LUMBOSACRAL ROOT (NERVE) NEC
518.89	LUNG
793.1	LUNG COIN
473.0	MAXILLARY SINUS
0	MITRAL SEE 'ENDOCARDITIS', MITRAL
348.8	MOTOR CORTEX
0	NERVE SEE SPECIFIED NERVE BY SITE, DISORDER
349.9	NERVOUS SYSTEM
742.9	NERVOUS SYSTEM, CONGENITAL
	NONALLOPATHIC
739.9	ABDOMEN
739.7	ACROMIOCLAVICULAR
739.1	CERVICAL, CERVICOTHORACIC
739.8	COSTOCHONDRAL
739.8	COSTOVERTEBRAL
739.6	EXTREMITY, LOWER
739.7	EXTREMITY, UPPER
739.0	HEAD
739.5	HIP
739.6	LOWER EXTREMITY
739.3	LUMBAR, LUMBOSACRAL
739.0	OCCIPITOCERVICAL
739.5	PELVIC
739.5	PUBIC
739.8	RIB CAGE
739.4	SACRAL, SACROCOCCYGEAL, SACROILIAC
739.8	STERNOCHONDRAL
739.7	STERNOCLAVICULAR
739.2	THORACIC, THORACOLUMBAR
739.7	UPPER EXTREMITY

LESION (continued)

478.1	NOSE (INTERNAL)
0	OBSTRUCTIVE SEE 'OBSTRUCTION' BY SITE
355.79	OBTURATOR NERVE
0	OCCLUSIVE ARTERY SEE 'EMBOLISM' BY SITE
0	ORGAN OR SITE NEC SEE ORGAN BY SITE, DISEASE
733.90	OSTEOLYTIC
620.8	OVARY
363.32	PARAMACULAR OF RETINA
537.89	PEPTIC
523.8	PERIODONTAL, DUE TO TRAUMATIC OCCLUSION
569.49	PERIRECTAL
568.89	PERITONEUM (GRANULOMATOUS)
709.00	PIGMENTED (SKIN)
0	PINTA SEE 'PINTA'
0	POLYPOID SEE 'POLYP' BY SITE
0	PRECHIASMAL SEE 'LESION' CHIASMAL
0	PRIMARY SEE 'SYPHILIS PRIMARY'
103.0	PRIMARY CARATE
103.0	PRIMARY PINTA
102.0	PRIMARY YAWS
518.89	PULMONARY
793.1	PULMONARY COIN
537.89	PYLORUS
990	RADIATION NEC
990	RADIUM NEC
569.89	RECTOSIGMOID
0	RETINA, RETINAL SEE 'RETINOPATHY'
362.17	RETINA VASCULAR
568.89	RETROPERITONEAL
720.1	ROMANUS
724.6	SACROILIAC (JOINT)
527.8	SALIVARY GLAND
527.8	SALIVARY GLAND BENIGN LYMPHOEPITHELIAL
355.79	SAPHENOUS NERVE
0	SECONDARY SYPHILIS SEE 'SYPHILIS SECONDARY'
569.89	SIGMOID
473.9	SINUS (ACCESSORY) (NASAL) SEE ALSO 'SINUSITIS'
709.9	SKIN
686.00	SKIN SUPPURATIVE
784.2	SPACE-OCCUPYING, INTRACRANIAL NEC
336.9	SPINAL CORD
742.9	SPINAL CORD CONGENITAL
0	SPINAL CORD, TRAUMATIC SEE 'SPINAL CORD INJURY' BY SITE
289.50	SPLEEN
537.89	STOMACH
0	SYPHILITIC SEE 'SYPHILIS'
0	TERTIARY SEE 'SYPHILIS TERTIARY'
353.3	THORACIC ROOT (NERVE)
474.9	TONSILLAR FOSSA
525.8	TOOTH, TEETH
521.0	TOOTH, TEETH WHITE SPOT
0	TRICUSPID SEE 'ENDOCARDITIS', TRICUSPID
350.9	TRIGEMINAL NERVE
0	ULCERATED OR ULCERATIVE SEE 'ULCER' BY SITE
621.9	UTERUS NEC
623.8	VAGINA
352.3	VAGUS NERVE
424.90	VALVULAR NOS
	VASCULAR
459.9	NOS
0	AFFECTING CENTRAL NERVOUS SYSTEM SEE 'LESION' CEREBROVASCULAR
904.9	FOLLOWING TRAUMA SEE ALSO SPECIFIED BLOOD VESSEL, INJURY
362.17	RETINA

TO CODE A LESION OF A SITE NOT LISTED BELOW, SEE DISORDER UNDER SPECIFIED ANATOMICAL SITE.

LESION (continued)

VASCULAR (continued)

663.6# UMBILICAL CORD

5th Digit: 663.6

0. EPISODE OF CARE NOS OR N/A

1. DELIVERED

3. ANTEPARTUM COMPLICATION

762.6 UMBILICAL CORD AFFECTING FETUS OR NEWBORN

LESION (continued)

377.73 VISUAL CORTEX NEC

377.63 VISUAL PATHWAY NEC

0 WARTY SEE 'VERRUCA'

521.0 WHITE SPOT, ON TEETH

990 X-RAY NEC

446.3 LETHAL MIDLINE GRANULOMA

648.9# LETHAL MIDLINE GRANULOMA MATERNAL CURRENT (CO-EXISTENT) IN PREGNANCY [446.3]

5th Digit: 648.9

0. EPISODE OF NOS OR N/A

1. DELIVERED

2. DELIVERED WITH POSTPARTUM COMPLICATION

3. ANTEPARTUM COMPLICATION

4. POSTPARTUM COMPLICATION

780.79 LETHARGY

202.5# LETTERER SIWE DISEASE M9722/3

5th Digit: 202.5

0. UNSPECIFIED

1. LYMPH NODES OF HEAD FACE NECK

2. LYMPH NODES INTRATHORACIC

3. LYMPH NODES ABDOMINAL

4. LYMPH NODES AXILLA AND UPPER LIMB

5. LYMPH NODES INGUINAL REGION AND LOWER LIMB

6. LYMPH NODES INTRAPELVIC

7. SPLEEN

8. LYMPH NODES MULTIPLE SITES

270.3 LEUCINE METABOLISM DISTURBANCES

270.3 LEUCINOSIS

360.44 LEUCOCORIA EYE

371.04 LEUCOMA ADHERENT (CORNEA)

LEUKEMIA QUICK REFERENCE

208.9# NOS M9800/3

208.0# ACUTE NOS M9801/3

208.0# ALEUKEMIC NOS M9804/3

205.1# BASOPHILIC M9870/3

208.0# BLAST CELL M9801/3

208.1# CHRONIC NOS M9803/3

207.8# COMPOUND M9810/3

205.1# EOSINOPHILIC M9880/3

207.0# ERYTHREMIA ACUTE M9841/3

207.1# ERYTHREMIA CHRONIC M9842/3

207.0# ERYTHREMIA ERYTHROLEUKEMIA ACUTE M9801/3

202.4# HAIRY CELL M9940/3

204.9# LYMPHOID NOS M9820/3

204.0# LYMPHOID ACUTE M9821/3

204.8# LYMPHOID ALEUKEMIC M9824/3

204.1# LYMPHOID CHRONIC M9823/3

204.2# LYMPHOID SUBACUTE M9822/3

207.8# LYMPHOSARCOMA CELL M9850/3

5th Digit: 202, 204, 205, 207, 208

0. WITHOUT MENTION OF REMISSION

1. IN REMISSION

LEUKEMIA QUICK REFERENCE (continued)

207.8# MAST CELL M9900/3

207.2# MEGAKARYOCYTIC M9910/3

206.9# MONOCYTIC NOS M9890/3

206.0# MONOCYTIC ACUTE M9891/3

206.8# MONOCYTIC ALEUKEMIC M9894/3

206.1# MONOCYTIC CHRONIC M9893/3

206.2# MONOCYTIC SUBACUTE M9892/3

205.9# MYELOID NOS M9860/3

205.0# MYELOID ACUTE M9861/3

205.8# MYELOID ALEUKEMIC SUBLEUKEMIC M9864/3

205.1# MYELOID CHRONIC M9863/3

205.2# MYELOID SUBACUTE M9862/3

205.1# NAEGELI-TYPE MONOCYTIC M9863/3

205.1# NEUTROPHILIC M9865/3

203.1# PLASMA CELL M9830/3

204.9# PROLYMPHOCYTIC SITE NOS M9825/3

0 PROLYMPHOCYTIC SITE SPECIFIED SEE 'LEUKEMIA QUICK REFERENCE', LYMPHOID

205.0# PROMYELOCYTIC ACUTE M9866/3

0 SCHILLING TYPE MONOCYTIC SEE 'LEUKEMIA QUICK REFERENCE', MONOCYTIC

208.0# STEM CELL M9801/3

208.2# SUBACUTE NOS M9802/3

208.8# SUBLEUKEMIC NEC M9804/3

207.2# THROMBOCYTIC M9910/3

208.0# UNDIFFERENTIATED M9801/3

5th Digit: 203, 204, 205, 206, 207, 208

0. WITHOUT MENTION OF REMISSION

1. IN REMISSION

LEUKEMIA

208.## NOS CELL TYPE

4th Digit: 208

0. ACUTE M9801/3

1. CHRONIC (ACUTE EXACERBATION OF CHRONIC) M9803/3

2. SUBACUTE M9802/3

8. OTHER LEUKEMIA OF UNSPECIFIED CELL TYPE M9800/3

9. UNSPECIFIED M9800/3

5th Digit: 208

0. WITHOUT MENTION OF REMISSION

1. IN REMISSION

V16.6 FAMILY HISTORY

205.## GRANULOCYTIC (MYELOID)

4th Digit: 205

0. ACUTE M9800/3

1. CHRONIC (ACUTE EXACERBATION OF CHRONIC) M9863/3

2. SUBACUTE M9862/3

8. ALEUKEMIC LEUKEMIA (GRANULOCYTIC) MYELOGENOUS MYELOID MYELOSIS M9864/3

9. UNSPECIFIED M9860/3

5th Digit: 205

0. WITHOUT MENTION OF REMISSION

1. IN REMISSION

206.9# HISTIOCYTIC M9890/3

5th Digit: 206.9

0. WITHOUT MENTION OF REMISSION

1. IN REMISSION

V10.60 HISTORY

V10.63 HISTORY MONOCYTIC

V10.69 HISTORY OTHER TYPE

LEUKEMIA (continued)

204.## LYMPHATIC
204.0# LYMPHOBLASTIC M9821/3
204.## LYMPHOCYTIC
204.## LYMPHOGENOUS
204.## LYMPHOID
4th Digit: 204
0. ACUTE (BLASTIC) M9821/3
1. CHRONIC M9823/3
2. SUBACUTE M9822/3
8. ALEUKEMIC LEUKEMIA M9824/3
9. UNSPECIFIED M9820/3
5th Digit: 204
0. WITHOUT MENTION OF REMISSION
1. IN REMISSION

207.8# LYMPHOSARCOMA CELL M9850/3
207.8# MAST CELL M9900/3
207.2# MEGAKARYOCYTIC M9910/3
5th Digit: 207.2, 8
0. WITHOUT MENTION OF REMISSION
1. IN REMISSION
206.0# MONOBLASTIC M9891/3
206.## MONOCYTIC
206.## MONOCYTOID
4th Digit: 206
0. ACUTE M9891/3
1. CHRONIC (ACUTE EXACERBATION OF CHRONIC) M9893/3
2. SUBACUTE M9892/3
8. ALEUKEMIC LEUKEMIA (MONOCYTIC MONOCYTOID) M9894/3
9. UNSPECIFIED M9890/3
5th Digit: 206
0. WITHOUT MENTION OF REMISSION
1. IN REMISSION

205.0# MYELOBLASTIC (MYELOID) M9861/3
205.## MYELOCYTIC (MYELOID)
205.## MYELOGENOUS (MYELOID)
205.## MYELOID
205.3# MYELOID SARCOMA M9930/3
205.## MYELOMONOCYTIC (MYELOID)
205.## MYELOSCLEROTIC (MYELOID)
205.## MYELOSIS (MYELOID)
4th Digit: 205
0. ACUTE M9861/3
1. CHRONIC (ACUTE EXACERBATION OF CHRONIC) M9863/3
2. SUBACUTE M9862/3
3. MYELOID SARCOMA M9930/3
8. ALEUKEMIC LEUKEMIA (GRANULOCYTIC) MYELOGENOUS MYELOID, ALEUKEMIC MYELOSIS M9864/3
9. UNSPECIFIED M9860/3
5th Digit: 205
0. WITHOUT MENTION OF REMISSION
1. IN REMISSION

203.1# PLASMA CELL M9830/3
5th Digit: 203.1
0. WITHOUT MENTION OF REMISSION
1. IN REMISSION

202.4# LEUKEMIC RETICULOENDOTHELIOSIS M9940/3
5th Digit: 202.4
0. UNSPECIFIED
1. LYMPH NODES OF HEAD FACE NECK
2. LYMPH NODES INTRATHORACIC
3. LYMPH NODES ABDOMINAL
4. LYMPH NODES AXILLA AND UPPER LIMB
5. LYMPH NODES INGUINAL REGION AND LOWER LIMB
6. LYMPH NODES INTRAPELVIC
7. SPLEEN
8. LYMPH NODES MULTIPLE SITES

288.8 LEUKEMOID REACTION
288.8 LEUKEMOID REACTION LYMPHOCYTIC MONOCYTIC MYELOCYTIC
446.29 LEUKOCLASTIC VASCULITIS
288.2 LEUKOCYTIC ANOMALY HEREDITARY
288.8 LEUKOCYTOSIS
288.3 LEUKOCYTOSIS EOSINOPHILIC
709.09 LEUKODERMA

LEUKODYSTROPHY

330.0 UNSPECIFIED
330.0 GLOBOID CELL
330.0 LIPIDOSIS
330.0 METACHROMATIC
330.0 SUDANOPHILIC

528.7 LEUKOEDEMA ORAL (MOUTH) (TONGUE)
323.9 LEUKOENCEPHALOPATHY (SEE ALSO 'ENCEPHALITIS')
046.3 LEUKOENCEPHALOPATHY MULTIFOCAL
702.8 LEUKOKERATOSIS NEC
528.6 LEUKOKERATOSIS ORAL MUCOSA
288.2 LEUKOMELANOPATHY HEREDITARY
703.8 LEUKONYCHIA (PUNCTATA) (STRIATA)
757.5 LEUKONYCHIA CONGENITAL
288.0 LEUKOPENIA
776.7 LEUKOPENIA NEONATAL TRANSITORY

LEUKOPLAKIA

569.49 ANUS
622.2 CERVIX
530.83 ESOPHAGUS
528.6 GINGIVA
478.79 LARYNX
528.6 LIPS
528.6 ORAL MUCOSA INCLUDING TONGUE
607.0 PENIS
702.8 SKIN NEC
528.6 TONGUE
478.29 TONSIL
599.84 URETHRA (POST INFECTIONAL)
621.8 UTERUS
623.1 VAGINA
596.8 VESICAL
0 VESICAL WITH INCONTINENCE SEE 'BLADDER DISORDERS WITH INCONTINENCE'
478.5 VOCAL CORD
624.0 VULVA

LEUKORRHEA

623.5 NOS
623.5 NONINFECTIVE
131.00 TRICHOMONAL

426.0 LEV'S HEART BLOCK (SYNDROME)
253.3 LEVI'S DWARFISM (SYNDROME)
746.87 LEVOCARDIA (ISOLATED)
334.3 LEVY-ROUSSY SYNDROME
078.19 LEWANDOWSKI-LUTZ DISEASE
017.0# LEWANDOWSKI'S DISEASE (TUBERCULOSIS)
5th Digit: 017.0
0. UNSPECIFIED
1. LAB NOT DONE
2. LABS PENDING
3. MICROSCOPY POSITIVE (IN SPUTUM)
4. CULTURE POSITIVE - MICROSCOPY NEGATIVE
5. CULTURE NEGATIVE - MICROSCOPY POSITIVE
6. CULTURE AND MICROSCOPY NEGATIVE CONFIRMED BY OTHER METHODS

536.2 LEYDEN'S DISEASE (PERIODIC VOMITING)
257.2 LEYDIG'S CELL FAILURE (ADULT)

LEYDIG CELL TUMOR
236.2 FEMALE SITE NOS
0 FEMALE SITE SPECIFIED SEE 'NEOPLASM UNCERTAIN BEHAVIOR' BY SITE M8650/1
236.4 MALE SITE NOS
0 MALE SITE SPECIFIED SEE 'NEOPLASM UNCERTAIN BEHAVIOR' BY SITE M8650/1
220 BENIGN FEMALE SITE NOS
0 BENIGN FEMALE SITE SPECIFIED SEE 'BENIGN NEOPLASM', BY SITE M8650/0
222.0 BENIGN MALE SITE NOS
0 BENIGN MALE SITE SPECIFIED SEE 'BENIGN NEOPLASM', BY SITE M8650/0
183.0 MALIGNANT FEMALE SITE NOS
0 MALIGNANT FEMALE SITE SPECIFIED SEE 'CANCER' BY SITE M8630/3
186.9 MALIGNANT MALE SITE NOS
0 MALIGNANT MALE SITE SPECIFIED SEE 'CANCER' BY SITE M8650/3

099.1 LGV
647.2# LGV MATERNAL CURRENT (CO-EXISTENT) IN PREGNANCY
5th Digit: 647.2
0. EPISODE OF CARE UNSPECIFIED OR N/A
1. DELIVERED
2. DELIVERED WITH POSTPARTUM COMPLICATION
3. ANTEPARTUM COMPLICATION
4. POSTPARTUM COMPLICATION

710.0 LIBMAN SACKS DISEASE (VERRUCOUS ENDOCARDITIS) [424.91]

LICE
132.9 UNSPECIFIED
132.0 HEAD
132.1 BODY
132.2 PUBIC
0 SEE 'PEDICULOSIS'

LICHEN
697.9 NOS
698.3 LICHENIFICATION
697.1 NITIDUS
698.3 OBTUSUS CORNEUS
757.39 PILARIS (CONGENITAL)
697.0 PLANOPILARIS (RUBER PLANUS)
697.0 PLANUS
696.4 RUBER ACUMINATUS
697.8 RUBER MONILIFORME STRIATA
701.0 SCLEROSUS ET ATROPHICUS
017.0# SCROFULOSUS (TUBERCULOUS)
5th Digit: 017.0
0. UNSPECIFIED
1. LAB NOT DONE
2. LABS PENDING
3. MICROSCOPY POSITIVE (IN SPUTUM)
4. CULTURE POSITIVE - MICROSCOPY NEGATIVE
5. CULTURE NEGATIVE - MICROSCOPY POSITIVE
6. CULTURE AND MICROSCOPY NEGATIVE CONFIRMED BY OTHER METHODS
698.3 SIMPLEX CHRONICUS
757.39 SPINULOSUS (CONGENITAL)
697.8 STRIATA
698.2 URTICATUS
697.8 OTHER

281.0 LICHTHEIM'S DISEASE OR SYNDROME (SUBACUTE COMBINED SCLEROSIS WITH PERNICIOUS ANEMIA) [336.2]
374.41 LID RETRACTION OR LAG
289.59 LIEN MIGRANS

CODES V69.#, LIFESTYLE PROBLEMS, MAY BE USED TO IDENTIFY RISK FACTORS SUCH AS LACK OF PHYSICAL EXERCISE, HIGH RISK SEXUAL BEHAVIOR, ETC. THESE CODES SHOULD BE ASSIGNED AS ADDITIONAL DIAGNOSES WHEN THE PHYSICIAN DOCUMENTS THE PRESENCE OF RISK FACTORS IN THE MEDICAL RECORD. THESE CODES ARE CLINICALLY IMPORTANT BECAUSE THEY SHOW THE PRESENCE OF RISK FACTORS THAT NEED SURVEILLANCE AND PREVENTION PROGRAMS. THESE CODES, HOWEVER, SHOULD NOT BE USED AS THE PRINCIPAL DIAGNOSIS WHEN THE REASON FOR ENCOUNTER IS FOR COUNSELING OF THE RISK FACTORS.

LIFESTYLE PROBLEM
V69.9 PROBLEM NOS
V69.1 DIET AND EATING HABITS INAPPROPRIATE
V69.3 GAMBLING AND BETTING
V69.0 PHYSICAL EXERCISE (LACK OF)
V69.8 SELF-DAMAGING BEHAVIOR
V69.2 SEXUAL BEHAVIOR HIGH RISK
V69.8 OTHER LIFESTYLE PROBLEMS

LIGAMENT
728.89 CALCIFICATION
717.89 CALCIFICATION KNEE (MEDIAL COLLATERAL)
756.89 CONTRACTION CONGENITAL
728.9 DISORDER
728.89 DISORDER OTHER
0 DIVISION SEE 'SPRAIN' BY SITE
0 DIVISION WITH OPEN WOUND SEE 'LACERATION'
728.4 LAXITY
728.89 OSSIFICATION
718.9# RELAXATION JOINT
5th Digit: 718.9
0. SITE NOS
1. SHOULDER REGION
2. UPPER ARM (ELBOW) (HUMERUS)
3. FOREARM (RADIUS) (WRIST) (ULNA)
4. HAND (CARPAL) (METACARPAL) (FINGERS)
5. PELVIC REGION AND THIGH (HIP) (BUTTOCK) (FEMUR)
7. ANKLE AND/OR FOOT (METATARSALS) (TOES) (TARSALS)
8. OTHER
9. MULTIPLE
717.9 RELAXATION JOINT - KNEE
724.6 RELAXATION JOINT - LUMBOSACRAL
724.6 RELAXATION JOINT - SACROILIAC

203.0# LIGHT CHAIN DISEASE
5th Digit: 203.0
0. WITHOUT MENTION OF REMISSION
1. IN REMISSION

LIGHT FOR DATES
656.5# AFFECTING MANAGEMENT OF MOTHER
5th Digit: 656.5
0. EPISODE OF CARE UNSPECIFIED OR N/A
1. DELIVERED
3. ANTEPARTUM COMPLICATION

LIGHT FOR DATES WITH FETAL MALNUTRITION
764.10 WEIGHT UNSPECIFIED
764.11 < 500 GRAMS
764.12 500 - 749 GRAMS
764.13 750 - 999 GRAMS
764.14 1000 - 1249 GRAMS
764.15 1250 - 1499 GRAMS
764.16 1500 - 1749 GRAMS
764.17 1750 - 1999 GRAMS
764.18 2000-2499 GRAMS
764.19 2500 GRAMS AND OVER

L

LIGHT FOR DATES WITHOUT MENTION OF FETAL MALNUTRITION

764.00 WEIGHT UNSPECIFIED
764.01 < 500 GRAMS
764.02 500 - 749 GRAMS
764.03 750 - 999 GRAMS
764.04 1000 - 1249 GRAMS
764.05 1250 - 1499 GRAMS
764.06 1500 - 1749 GRAMS
764.07 1750 - 1999 GRAMS
764.08 2000- 2499 GRAMS
764.09 2500 GRAMS AND OVER

780.4 LIGHT HEADEDNESS
362.13 LIGHT REFLEX INCREASED RETINA
994.0 LIGHTNING (STRUCK BY)
909.4 LIGHTNING (STRUCK BY) LATE EFFECT
0 LIGHTNING BURN SEE 'BURN'
588.8 LIGHTWOOD'S SYNDROME (RENAL TUBULAR ACIDOSIS)
270.0 LIGNAC'S (-DE TONI) (-FANCONI) (-DEBRE) DISEASE OR SYNDROME (CYSTINOSIS)
413.9 LIKOFF'S SYNDROME (ANGINA IN MENOPAUSAL WOMEN)

LIMB

755.4 ABSENCE - NOS (COMPLETE) (PARTIAL) - CONGENITAL
755.30 ABSENCE LOWER - NOS CONGENITAL (ACQUIRED)
755.31 ABSENCE LOWER - COMPLETE/TRANSVERSE CONGENITAL (ACQUIRED)
755.32 ABSENCE LOWER - INCOMPLETE CONGENITAL (ACQUIRED)
755.20 ABSENCE UPPER - NOS CONGENITAL (ACQUIRED)
755.21 ABSENCE UPPER - COMPLETE/TRANSVERSE CONGENITAL (ACQUIRED)
755.22 ABSENCE UPPER - INCOMPLETE CONGENITAL (ACQUIRED)
0 AMPUTATION (ABSENCE) STATUS SEE 'AMPUTATION', STATUS
755.9 ANOMALY CONGENITAL - LIMB UNSPECIFIED
755.60 ANOMALY CONGENITAL - LOWER LIMB
755.50 ANOMALY CONGENITAL - UPPER LIMB
755.8 ANOMALY OTHER SPECIFIED CONGENITAL - LIMB UNSPECIFIED
729.82 CRAMP
V49.0 DEFICIENCY
736.9 DEFORMITY ACQUIRED SITE NOS
736.89 DEFORMITY ACQUIRED NEC, ARM LEG SHOULDER
V49.4 DISFIGUREMENT
729.9 DISORDER - SOFT TISSUE
729.89 DISORDER - MUSCULOSKELETAL
306.0 DISORDER PSYCHOGENIC (MUSCULOSKELETAL)
754.89 FLEXION CONTRACTURES OF JOINTS (LOWER LIMB) CONGENITAL
359.1 GIRDLE MUSCULAR DYSTROPHY
729.5 PAIN
V49.9 PROBLEM
V49.1 PROBLEM MECHANICAL
V49.2 PROBLEM MOTOR
V49.3 PROBLEM SENSORY
V49.5 PROBLEM (OTHER)
V49.8 PROBLEM OTHER SPECIFIED
V43.7 REPLACEMENT STATUS (ARTIFICIAL) (PROSTHESIS)
729.81 SWELLING
747.64 VESSEL LOWER ATRESIA
747.63 VESSEL UPPER ATRESIA

759.6 LINDAU'S DISEASE (RETINOCEREBRAL ANGIOMATOSIS)
529.3 LINGUA VILLOSA NIGRA
151.9 LINITIS PLASTICA SITE NOS
0 LINITIS PLASTICA SITE SPECIFIED SEE 'CANCER' BY SITE M8142/3

LIP

528.5 ABSCESS
750.26 ABSENCE CONGENITAL
528.5 ATROPHY
528.9 BITING
528.5 CYST
528.5 DISEASE NEC
054.9 FEVER BLISTER
749.1# FISSURE (CONGENITAL)

5th Digit: 749.1

0. CLEFT UNSPECIFIED
1. CLEFT UNILATERAL COMPLETE
2. CLEFT UNILATERAL INCOMPLETE
3. CLEFT BILATERAL COMPLETE
4. CLEFT BILATERAL INCOMPLETE

528.5 FISTULA
750.25 FISTULA CONGENITAL
528.5 HYPERTROPHY
744.81 HYPERTROPHY CONGENITAL
959.09 INJURY
910.8 INJURY OTHER AND UNSPECIFIED (SUPERFICIAL)
910.9 INJURY OTHER AND UNSPECIFIED (SUPERFICIAL) INFECTED
750.25 PITS (MUCUS) CONGENITAL
709.2 SCAR
528.5 ULCER

790.5 LIPASE ABNORMAL BLOOD LEVEL
272.3 LIPEMIA RETINALIS

LIPID, LIPOID

272.9 ABNORMAL FINDINGS NEC
220 CELL TUMOR OF OVARY
272.8 DERMATOARTHRITIS [713.0]
272.9 DISORDER (METABOLISM) - NOS
272.7 DISORDER (METABOLISM) - STORAGE
272.8 DISORDER (METABOLISM) - SPECIFIED NEC
272.5 HIGH-DENSITY DEFICIENCY
581.3 NEPHROSIS
507.1 PNEUMONIA
516.8 PNEUMONIA ENDOGENOUS
507.1 PNEUMONIA EXOGENOUS
272.7 STORAGE DISEASE
272.8 METABOLISM DISORDER OTHER

LIPIDOSIS

272.7 NOS
330.1 CEREBRAL (TAY SACH'S)
272.7 CHEMICALLY INDUCED
330.0 SULFATIDE

229.9 LIPOADENOMA SITE NOS
0 LIPOADENOMA SITE SPECIFIED SEE 'BENIGN NEOPLASM', BY SITE M8324/0
229.9 LIPOBLASTOMATOSIS SITE NOS
0 LIPOBLASTOMATOSIS SITE SPECIFIED SEE 'BENIGN NEOPLASM', BY SITE M8881/0
277.5 LIPOCHONDRODYSTROPHY
288.1 LIPOCHROME HISTIOCYTOSIS (FAMILIAL)

LIPODYSTROPHY

272.6 NOS
040.2 INTESTINAL
272.6 PROGRESSIVE

272.8 LIPOGRANULOMATOSIS DISSEMINATED
0 LIPOID SEE 'LIPID, LIPOID'

LIPOMA

214.# NOS M8850/0
214.# INTRAMUSCULAR M8856/0
214.# SPINDLE CELL M8857/0

4th Digit: 214

0. FACE SKIN AND SUBCUTANEOUS TISSUE
1. SKIN AND SUBCUTANEOUS TISSUE OTHER
2. INTRATHORACIC ORGANS
3. INTRA-ABDOMINAL ORGANS
4. SPERMATIC CORD
8. OTHER SPECIFIED SITES MUSCLE, FASCIA M8856/0
9. UNSPECIFIED SITE M8850/0

272.5 LIPOPROTEIN DISORDER (DEFICIENCY) (METABOLISM)

LIPOSARCOMA

171.# UNSPECIFIED M8850/3
171.# MIXED TYPE M8855/3
171.# MYXOID M8855/3
171.# PLEOMORPHIC M8854/3
171.# ROUND CELL M8853/3
171.# WELL DIFFERENTIATED TYPE M8851/3

4th Digit: 171

0. HEAD FACE NECK
2. UPPER LIMB SHOULDER
3. LOWER LIMB HIP
4. THORAX
5. ABDOMINAL HYPOCHONDRIUM
6. PELVIS BUTTOCK GROIN INGUINAL REGION PERINEUM
7. TRUNK NOS BACK NOS FLANK NOS
8. OTHER SPECIFIED SITES
9. SITE UNSPECIFIED

272.8 LIPOSYNOVITIS PREPATELLARIS

616.50 LIPSCHUTZ'S DISEASE OR ULCER
307.9 LISPING
027.0 LISTERIA MONOCYTOGENES INFECTION (SEPTICEMIA)

027.0 LISTERIOSIS
771.2 LISTERIOSIS CONGENITAL OR PERINATAL
655.4# LISTERIOSIS MATERNAL WITH SUSPECTED DAMAGE TO FETUS

5th Digit: 655.4

0. EPISODE OF CARE UNSPECIFIED OR N/A
1. DELIVERED
3. ANTEPARTUM COMPLICATION

780.79 LISTLESSNESS
790.6 LITHIUM ABNORMAL BLOOD LEVEL
656.8# LITHOPEDIAN FETUS AFFECTING MOTHER

5th Digit: 656.8

0. EPISODE OF CARE UNSPECIFIED OR N/A
1. DELIVERED
3. ANTEPARTUM COMPLICATION

V62.5 LITIGATION PROBLEM (REASON FOR ENCOUNTER)
0 LITTLE'S DISEASE SEE 'CEREBRAL PALSY'

LIVER

0 SEE ALSO 'HEPATIC'
751.69 ABSENCE (LOBE) CONGENITAL
751.69 ACCESSORY CONGENITAL
571.0 ALCOHOLIC FATTY
277.3 AMYLOID DEGENERATION
751.60 ANOMALY NOS
751.69 ANOMALY OTHER SPECIFIED
570 ATROPHY (SEE ALSO 'NECROSIS', LIVER)
639.8 ATROPHY POST ABORTIVE (ECTOPIC) (MOLAR) PREGNANCY
571.2 CIRRHOSIS ALCOHOLIC
571.5 CIRRHOSIS OBSTRUCTIVE (SEE ALSO 'CIRRHOSIS', LIVER)
573.0 CONGESTION, CHRONIC PASSIVE
0 CONTUSION SEE 'LIVER TRAUMA', CONTUSION

LIVER (continued)

573.8 CYST
751.62 CYST CONGENITAL
122.8 CYST ECHINOCOCCAL
122.0 CYST ECHINOCOCCAL GRANULOSIS
127.4 CYST OXYURIS VERMICULARIS
570 DEGENERATION (PARENCHYMATOUS)
571.3 DISEASE ALCOHOLIC
571.1 DISEASE ALCOHOLIC - ACUTE
571.3 DISEASE ALCOHOLIC - CHRONIC
571.9 DISEASE CHRONIC
571.3 DISEASE CHRONIC ALCOHOLIC
571.8 DISEASE CHRONIC NONALCOHOLIC OTHER
572.8 DISEASE CHRONIC OTHER SEQUELAE
573.3 DISEASE DRUG INDUCED
573.9 DISORDER

646.7#: SPECIFY THE MATERNAL LIVER DISORDER WITH AN ADDITIONAL CODE.

646.7# DISORDER IN PREGNANCY

5th Digit: 646.7

0. EPISODE OF CARE UNSPECIFIED OR N/A
1. DELIVERED
3. ANTEPARTUM COMPLICATION

573.8 DISORDERS OTHER SPECIFIED
V59.6 DONOR NON-AUTOGENOUS
751.69 DUPLICATION OF CONGENITAL
573.9 ENGORGEMENT
789.1 ENLARGEMENT
572.8 FAILURE SEQUELAE OF OTHER DISEASE
997.4 FAILURE SPECIFIED AS DUE TO A PROCEDURE
571.0 FATTY ALCOHOLIC
571.8 FATTY NONALCOHOLIC
272.8 FLAP
751.69 FLOATING CONGENITAL
121.3 FLUKE
121.0 FLUKE (CAT)
121.1 FLUKE (CHINESE) (ORIENTAL)
790.4 FUNCTION STUDY ABNORMAL-BLOOD
794.8 FUNCTION STUDY ABNORMAL-RADIOLOGIC
271.0 GLYCOGEN INFILTRATION
271.0 GLYCOGENOSIS
0 HEMATOMA TRAUMATIC SEE 'LIVER TRAUMA', HEMATOMA
674.8# HEPATORENAL SYNDROME MATERNAL DUE TO PREGNANCY

5th Digit: 674.8

0. UNSPECIFIED
2. DELIVERED WITH POSTPARTUM COMPLICATION
4. POSTPARTUM COMPLICATION

751.69 HYPERPLASIA (CONGENITAL)
0 INJURY TRAUMATIC SEE 'LIVER TRAUMA'
572.4 KIDNEY SYNDROME
0 LACERATION SEE 'LIVER TRAUMA', LACERATION
570 NECROSIS ACUTE SUBACUTE MASSIVE

646.7#: SPECIFY THE MATERNAL NECROSIS WITH AN ADDITIONAL CODE.

646.7# NECROSIS OF PREGNANCY

5th Digit: 646.7

0. EPISODE OF CARE UNSPECIFIED OR N/A
1. DELIVERED
3. ANTEPARTUM COMPLICATION

639.8 NECROSIS POST ABORTIVE (ECTOPIC) (MOLAR) PREGNANCY
573.8 OBSTRUCTION
751.62 POLYCYSTIC DISEASE CONGENITAL
573.8 PROLAPSE
573.8 PTOSIS
767.8 RUPTURE - BIRTH TRAUMA FETUS
573.8 RUPTURE - NONTRAUMATIC
0 RUPTURE - TRAUMATIC SEE 'LIVER TRAUMA', RUPTURE

LIVER (continued)
794.8 SCAN ABNORMAL
709.09 SPOTS
V42.7 TRANSPLANT (STATUS)
996.82 TRANSPLANT REJECTION (FAILURE)

INJURY TO INTERNAL ORGANS - LUNG, SPLEEN, LIVER, KIDNEY, ETC., CAN BE A CONTUSION, LACERATION, TEAR, OR RUPTURE. YOU MAY FIND THE CODE UNDER THE CONDITION OR UNDER THE ANATOMICAL SITE.

LIVER TRAUMA
864.00 UNSPECIFIED
864.10 UNSPECIFIED WITH OPEN WOUND INTO CAVITY
864.01 CONTUSION
864.11 CONTUSION WITH OPEN WOUND INTO CAVITY
864.01 HEMATOMA
864.11 HEMATOMA WITH OPEN WOUND INTO CAVITY
864.00 INJURY
864.## LACERATION
4th Digit: 864
0. CLOSED
1. WITH OPEN WOUND INTO CAVITY
5th Digit: 864
2. MINOR (< 1CM. DEEP)
3. MODERATE (<10 CM. LONG - <3 CM. DEEP)
4. MAJOR 10 CM. LONG - 3 CM. DEEP, MULTIPLE, MODERATE OR STELLATE)
5. UNSPECIFIED
908.1 LATE EFFECT
864.04 RUPTURE
864.14 RUPTURE WITH OPEN WOUND INTO CAVITY
864.09 OTHER
864.19 OTHER WITH OPEN WOUND INTO CAVITY

989.5 LIZARD BITE
995.0 LIZARD BITE WITH ANAPHYLAXIS [989.5]
258.1 LLOYD'S SYNDROME
125.2 LOA LOA INFECTION
V45.89 LOBECTOMY STATUS
116.2 LOBO'S DISEASE (KELOID BLASTOMYCOSIS)
116.2 LOBOA (BLASTOMYCES) LOBOI INFECTION
116.2 LOBOMYCOSIS
310.0 LOBOTOMY SYNDROME
756.51 LOBSTEIN'S DISEASE (BRITTLE BONES AND BLUE SCLERA)
755.58 LOBSTER-CLAW HAND CONGENITAL

LOBULAR
174.9 CARCINOMA SITE NOS
0 CARCINOMA SITE SPECIFIED SEE 'CANCER' BY SITE M8520/3
233.0 CARCINOMA IN SITU SITE NOS
0 CARCINOMA IN SITU SITE SPECIFIED SEE 'CA IN SITU' BY SITE M8520/2

344.81 LOCKED IN STATE
438.53 LOCKED IN STATE LATE EFFECT OF CEREBROVASCULAR DISEASE [344.81]
652.6# LOCKED TWINS COMPLICATING PREGNANCY
660.5# LOCKED TWINS OBSTRUCTING LABOR **[652.6#]**
5th Digit: 660.5, 652.6
0. EPISODE OF CARE UNSPECIFIED OR N/A
1. DELIVERED
3. ANTEPARTUM COMPLICATION
334.9 LOCOMOTOR SYSTEM DISEASE
518.3 LOFFLER'S SYNDROME (EOSINOPHILIC PNEUMONITIS)
135 LOFGREN'S SYNDROME (SARCOIDOSIS)
125.2 LOIASIS BANCROFTIAN
125.2 LOIASIS EYELID [373.6]

082.8 LONE STAR FEVER
758.3 LONG ARM 18 OR 21 DELETION SYNDROME
754.0 LONG FACE SYNDROME
0 LOOSE BODY JOINT SEE 'JOINT', MICE
525.8 LOOSE TEETH
268.2 LOOSER (-DEBRAY) - MILKMAN SYNDROME (OSTEOMALACIA WITH PSEUDOFRACTURES)
253.3 LORAIN LEVI SYNDROME (PITUITARY DWARFISM)

THE CODE IN THE LEFT MARGIN ALWAYS SEQUENCES FIRST. THE ADDITIONAL CODE IN BRACKETS TO THE RIGHT OF THE DESCRIPTION IS SEQUENCED SECONDARILY. UNDERLINING SHOWS THE CODE NUMBER THAT CORRESPONDS TO THE UNDERLINED VERBAL DESCRIPTION. UNDERLINING NEVER IMPLIES CORRECT SEQUENCING.

LORDOSIS
737.20 ACQUIRED (POSTURAL)
737.29 ACQUIRED OTHER
737.22 ACQUIRED OTHER POSTSURGICAL
737.42 ASSOCIATED WITH OTHER CONDITIONS
356.1 CHARCOT MARIE TOOTH [737.42]
277.5 MUCOPOLYSACCHARIDOSIS [737.42]
237.7# NEUROFIBROMATOSIS [737.42]
5th Digit: 237.7
0. UNSPECIFIED
1. TYPE I
2. TYPE II
252.0 OSTEITIS FIBROSA CYSTICA [737.42]
733.0# OSTEOPOROTIC [737.42]
5th Digit: 733.0
0. UNSPECIFIED
1. SENILE
2. IDIOPATHIC
3. DISUSE
9. OTHER
138 POLIOMYELITIS LATE EFFECT [737.42]
045.## POLIOMYELITIS [737.42]
4th Dgit: 045
0. ACUTE BULBAR PARALYTIC
1. ACUTE WITH OTHER PARALYSIS
2. ACUTE NON PARALYTIC
9. ACUTE UNSPECIFIED
5th Digit: 045
0. UNSPECIFIED
1. TYPE I
2. TYPE II
3. TYPE III
737.21 POSTLAMINECTOMY
754.2 POSTURAL CONGENITAL
237.7# VON RECKLINGHAUSEN'S DISEASE [737.42]
5th Digit: 237.7
0. UNSPECIFIED
1. TYPE I
2. TYPE II

729.89 LOSS OF FUNCTION MUSCULOSKELETAL NEC
335.20 LOU GEHRIG'S DISEASE
334.8 LOUIS-BAR SYNDROME (ATAXIA-TELANGIECTASIA)
993.2 LOW ATMOSPHERIC PRESSURE SYNDROME
724.2 LOW BACK PAIN SYNDROME (NONVERTEBRAL) (NONDISCOGENIC)
306.0 LOW BACK PAIN SYNDROME PSYCHOGENIC
596.52 LOW COMPLIANCE BLADDER
0 LOW COMPLIANCE BLADDER WITH INCONTINENCE SEE 'BLADDER DISORDERS WITH INCONTINENCE'
428.9 LOW OUTPUT SYNDROME (CARDIAC)

270.8 LOWE'S SYNDROME (OCULOCEREBRORENAL DYSTROPHY)

270.8 LOWE-TERREY-MCLACHLAN SYNDROME (OCULOCEREBRORENAL DYSTROPHY)

739.6 LOWER EXTREMITIES SEGMENTAL OR SOMATIC DYSFUNCTION

755.31 LOWER LIMB ABSENCE CONGENITAL

755.60 LOWER LIMB ANOMALY NOS CONGENITAL

767.4 LOWER RADICULAR SYNDROME, NEWBORN

426.81 LOWN (-GANONG) - LEVINE SYNDROME (SHORT P-R INTERVAL, NORMAL QRS COMPLEX AND SUPRAVENTRICULAR TACHYCARDIA)

305.3# LSD ABUSE (NONDEPENDENT)

304.5# LSD ADDICTION (DEPENDENT)

5th Digit: 304.5, 305.3

- **0. UNSPECIFIED**
- **1. CONTINUOUS**
- **2. EPISODIC**
- **3. IN REMISSION**

466.0 LUCAS-CHAMPIONNIERE DISEASE (FIBRINOUS BRONCHITIS)

774.30 LUCEY-DRISCOLL SYNDROME (JAUNDICE DUE TO DELAYED CONJUGATION)

528.3 LUDORICI ANGINA

528.3 LUDWIG'S ANGINA

528.3 LUDWIG'S DISEASE (SUBMAXILLARY CELLULITIS)

0 LUETIC DISEASE SEE 'SYPHILIS'

276.5 LUETSCHER'S DEHYDRATION SYNDROME

724.2 LUMBAGO NONVERTEBRAL (NONDISCOGENIC)

724.2 LUMBALGIA

> *WHEN CODING BACK DISORDERS DUE TO DEGENERATION, DISPLACEMENT OR HNP OF THE INTERVERTEBRAL DISC, IT IS IMPORTANT TO DISTINGUISH WHETHER THESE CONDITIONS ARE WITH OR WITHOUT MYELOPATHY. MYELOPATHY REFERS TO FUNCTIONAL DISTURBANCES AND/OR PATHOLOGICAL CHANGES IN THE SPINAL CORD THAT RESULT FROM COMPRESSION.*

LUMBAR

756.13 ABSENCE (CONGENITAL) (VERTEBRA)

756.11 ABSENCE (CONGENITAL) (VERTEBRA) - ISTHMUS

756.11 ABSENCE (CONGENITAL) (VERTEBRA) - PARS ARTICULARIS

721.3 ARTHRITIS

722.93 DISC CALCIFICATION OR DISCITIS

722.52 DISC DISEASE/DEGENERATION

722.73 DISC DISEASE/DEGENERATION - WITH MYELOPATHY

722.93 DISC DISORDER

722.73 DISC DISORDER WITH MYELOPATHY

722.10 DISC DISPLACEMENT

722.73 DISC DISPLACEMENT WITH MYELOPATHY

722.10 DISC HERNIATION

722.73 DISC HERNIATION WITH MYELOPATHY

722.73 DISC SYNDROME

553.8 HERNIA

722.10 NERVE COMPRESSION - DISCOGENIC

722.73 NERVE COMPRESSION - DISCOGENIC WITH MYELOPATHY

724.4 NERVE COMPRESSION - ROOT (BY SCAR TISSUE) NEC

722.83 NERVE COMPRESSION - ROOT POSTOPERATIVE

721.3 OSTEOARTHRITIS

997.09 PUNCTURE FLUID LEAKAGE

349.0 PUNCTURE REACTION (HEADACHE)

724.4 RADICULITIS (NONVERTEBRAL) (NONDISCOGENIC)

739.3 REGION SEGMENTAL OR SOMATIC DYSFUNCTION

953.2 ROOT INJURY (NERVE)

847.2 SEPARATION (RUPTURE) (TEAR) (LACERATION)

724.02 STENOSIS

847.2 STRAIN (SPRAIN) (AVULSION) (HEMARTHROSIS)

721.3 SPONDYLARTHRITIS

721.3 SPONDYLOSIS

721.42 SPONDYLOSIS WITH MYELOPATHY (CORD COMPRESSION)

LUMBAR (continued)

721.3 SPONDYLOSIS WITH OSTEOPOROSIS **[733.0#]**

721.7 SPONDYLOSIS TRAUMATIC WITH OSTEOPOROSIS **[733.0#]**

5th Digit: 733.0

- **0. UNSPECIFIED**
- **1. SENILE**
- **2. IDIOPATHIC**
- **3. DISUSE**
- **9. DRUG INDUCED**

724.4 VERTEBRAL SYNDROME

LUMBOSACRAL

724.6 ANKYLOSIS (NONVERTEBRAL) (NONDISCOGENIC)

724.6 DISORDER (NONVERTEBRAL) (NONDISCOGENIC)

0 DISORDER DISCOGENIC SEE 'INTERVERTEBRAL DISC'

724.6 INSTABILITY (NONVERTEBRAL) (NONDISCOGENIC)

353.1 PLEXUS DISORDER (LESION) (NONDISCOGENIC)

953.5 PLEXUS INJURY (NERVE)

739.3 REGION SEGMENTAL OR SOMATIC DYSFUNCTION

353.4 ROOT (NERVE) DISORDER (LESION) NEC (NONDISCOGENIC)

846.0 SEPARATION (RUPTURE) (TEAR) (LACERATION)

721.3 SPONDYLOSIS

721.42 SPONDYLOSIS WITH MYELOPATHY (CORD COMPRESSION)

721.3 SPONDYLOSIS WITH OSTEOPOROSIS **[733.0#]**

721.7 SPONDYLOSIS TRAUMATIC WITH OSTEOPOROSIS **[733.0#]**

5th Digit: 733.0

- **0. UNSPECIFIED**
- **1. SENILE**
- **2. IDIOPATHIC**
- **3. DISUSE**
- **9. DRUG INDUCED**

846.0 STRAIN (SPRAIN) (AVULSION) (HEMARTHROSIS)

724.6 STRAIN (SPRAIN) CHRONIC (NONVERTEBRAL) (NONDISCOGENIC)

LUNG

518.89 ABSENCE ACQUIRED (ANY PART)

748.5 AGENESIS HYPOPLASIA OR DYSPLASIA CONGENITAL

748.60 ANOMALY CONGENITAL

748.69 ANOMALY CONGENITAL OTHER

748.5 ATRESIA (CONGENITAL)

518.89 ATROPHY (SENILE)

748.69 ATROPHY CONGENITAL

748.69 AZYGOS LOBE (FISSURE) CONGENITAL

503 BARIUM DISEASE

492.0 BLEB

770.5 BLEB CONGENITAL

518.89 CALCIFICATION

515 CIRRHOSIS

518.0 COLLAPSE SEE ALSO ATELECTASIS

514 CONGESTION

861.21 CONTUSION

861.31 CONTUSION WITH OPEN WOUND INTO CAVITY

908.0 CONTUSION LATE EFFECT

518.89 CYSTIC ACQUIRED

748.4 CYSTIC CONGENITAL

518.89 DISEASE NEC

748.60 DISEASE CONGENITAL

748.4 DISEASE CONGENITAL CYSTIC (POLYCYSTIC)

508.0 DISORDERS DUE TO RADIATION ACUTE

508.1 DISORDERS DUE TO RADIATION CHRONIC

508.8 DISORDERS DUE TO OTHER EXTERNAL AGENTS

508.9 DISORDERS DUE TO UNSPECIFIED EXTERNAL AGENTS

V59.8 DONOR NON-AUTOGENOUS

748.5 DYSPLASIA CONGENITAL

515 FIBROSIS (ATROPHIC) (MASSIVE) (CONFLUENT) (PERIBRONCHIAL) (PERIALVEOLAR)

121.2 FLUKE (ORIENTAL)

518.89 HERNIA

748.5 HYPOPLASIA CONGENITAL

LUNG (continued)

515 INDURATION
415.19 INFARCTION
415.11 INFARCTION IATROGENIC
415.11 INFARCTION POSTOPERATIVE
518.3 INFILTRATE
793.1 INFILTRATE X-RAY FINDING
861.20 INJURY NOS
861.30 INJURY NOS WITH OPEN WOUND INTO THORAX
908.0 INJURY NOS LATE EFFECT
515 INTERSTITIAL LUNG DISEASE CHRONIC
277.3 INVOLVEMENT AMYLOIDOSIS [517.8]
710.4 INVOLVEMENT POLYMYOSITIS [517.8]
135 INVOLVEMENT SARCOID [517.8]
710.2 INVOLVEMENT SJOGREN'S DISEASE [517.8]
095.1 INVOLVEMENT SYPHILITIC
710.0 INVOLVEMENT SYSTEMIC LUPUS ERYTHEMATOSUS [517.8]
710.1 INVOLVEMENT SYSTEMIC SCLEROSIS [517.2]
861.22 LACERATION
861.32 LACERATION WITH OPEN WOUND INTO THORAX
908.0 LACERATION LATE EFFECT
748.69 LOBE ACCESSORY CONGENITAL
492.8 NODULE EMPHYSEMATOUS
518.89 NODULE SOLITARY
518.89 OBSTRUCTION OR OCCLUSION NOS
496 OBSTRUCTION AIRWAY CHRONIC
0 OBSTRUCTION CHRONIC SEE 'COPD'
0 OBSTRUCTION WITH ASTHMA SEE 'ASTHMA'
491.2# OBSTRUCTION WITH CHRONIC BRONCHITIS

5th Digit: 491.2

0.WITHOUT MENTION OF ACUTE EXACERBATION
1.WITH ACUTE EXACERBATION

492.8 OBSTRUCTION WITH EMPHYSEMA
518.89 POLYCYSTIC
493.2# POLYCYSTIC ASTHMA

5th Digit: 493.2

0. WITHOUT MENTION OF STATUS ASTHMATICUS
1. WITH STATUS ASTHMATICUS

748.4 POLYCYSTIC CONGENITAL
518.89 PSEUDOCYST
513.0 PURULENT (CAVITARY)
V45.89 RESECTION STATUS
518.89 RESTRICTIVE
714.81 RHEUMATOID
794.2 SCAN ABNORMAL
748.5 SEQUESTRATION CONGENITAL
793.1 SHADOW (RADIOLOGICAL FINDING)
V42.6 TRANSPLANT (STATUS)
996.84 TRANSPLANT REJECTION (FAILURE)
492.0 VANISHING

135 LUPOID OF BOECK (MILIARY)

LUPUS

710.0 NOS
695.4 DISCOID (LOCAL)
695.4 ERYTHEMATOSUS
373.34 ERYTHEMATOSUS (DISCOID) (LOCAL) EYELID
710.0 ERYTHEMATOSUS DISSEMINATED
710.0 ERYTHEMATOSUS DISSEMINATED POLYNEUROPATHY [357.1]
710.0 ERYTHEMATOSUS ENDOCARDITIS [424.91]
286.5 ERYTHEMATOSUS INHIBITOR
710.0 ERYTHEMATOSUS NEPHRITIS [583.81]
710.0 ERYTHEMATOSUS NEPHRITIS ACUTE [580.81]
710.0 ERYTHEMATOSUS NEPHRITIS CHRONIC [582.81]
710.0 ERYTHEMATOSUS NEPHROTIC SYNDROME [581.81]
710.0 ERYTHEMATOSUS RENAL DISEASE [583.81]

LUPUS (continued)

710.0 ERYTHEMATOSUS SYSTEMIC
286.5 ERYTHEMATOSUS SYSTEMIC [SLE] INHIBITOR INCREASE
710.0 ERYTHEMATOSUS SYSTEMIC WITH ENCEPHALITIS [323.8]
710.0 ERYTHEMATOSUS SYSTEMIC WITH LUNG INVOLVEMENT [517.8]
017.0# EXEDENS TUBERCULOUS
017.0# HILLIARD'S TUBERCULOUS
017.0# MILIARIS DISSEMINATUS FACIEI TUBERCULOUS

5th Digit: 017.0

0. UNSPECIFIED
1. LAB NOT DONE
2. LABS PENDING
3. MICROSCOPY POSITIVE (IN SPUTUM)
4. CULTURE POSITIVE - MICROSCOPY NEGATIVE
5. CULTURE NEGATIVE - MICROSCOPY POSITIVE
6. CULTURE AND MICROSCOPY NEGATIVE CONFIRMED BY OTHER METHODS

135 PERNIO (BESNIER)
017.0# VULGARIS TUBERCULOUS
017.0# VULGARIS TUBERCULOUS EYELID DERMATITIS [373.4]

5th Digit: 017.0

0. UNSPECIFIED
1. LAB NOT DONE
2. LABS PENDING
3. MICROSCOPY POSITIVE (IN SPUTUM)
4. CULTURE POSITIVE - MICROSCOPY NEGATIVE
5. CULTURE NEGATIVE - MICROSCOPY POSITIVE
6. CULTURE AND MICROSCOPY NEGATIVE CONFIRMED BY OTHER METHODS

620.1 LUTEIN CYST
253.4 LUTEINIZING HORMONE DEFICIENCY
253.1 LUTEINIZING HORMONE OVERPRODUCTION
745.5 LUTEMBACHER'S SYNDROME (ATRIAL SEPTAL DEFECT WITH MITRAL STENOSIS)
220 LUTEOMA SITE NOS
0 LUTEOMA SITE SPECIFIED SEE 'BENIGN NEOPLASM', BY SITE M8610/0
620.1 LUTEUM CORPUS RUPTURE (INFECTED) (OVARY)
701.1 LUTZ MIESCHER DISEASE (ELASTOSIS PERFORANS SERPIGINOSA)
116.1 LUTZ- SPLENDORE-DE ALMEIDA DISEASE (BRAZILIAN BLASTOMYCOSIS)
360.81 LUXATION EYE (GLOBE)
429.3 LVH
695.1 LYELL'S SYNDROME (TOXIC EPIDERMAL NECROLYSIS) DUE TO DRUG PROPERLY ADMINISTERED
977.9 LYELL'S SYNDROME (TOXIC EPIDERMAL NECROLYSIS) DUE TO OVERDOSE (WRONG DRUG GIVEN OR TAKEN)

LYME DISEASE

088.81 NOS
088.81 WITH ARTHRITIS **[711.8#]**

5th Digit: 711.8

0. SITE UNSPECIFIED
1. SHOULDER REGION
2. UPPER ARM
3. FOREARM
4. HAND
5. PELVIC REGION AND THIGH
6. LOWER LEG
7. ANKLE AND FOOT
8. OTHER SPECIFIED SITES
9. MULTIPLE SITES

088.81 WITH MENINGIOENCEPHALITIS [320.7]
088.81 WITH MENINGITIS [320.7]
088.81 WITH MYOCARDITIS [422.0]

LYMPH, LYMPHATIC

648.9#: USE AN ADDITIONAL CODE TO IDENTIFY LYMPHATIC CHANNEL DISORDER.

648.9# CHANNELS DISORDER MATERNAL CURRENT (CO-EXISTENT) IN PREGNANCY
5th Digit: 648.9
0. EPISODE OF NOS OR N/A
1. DELIVERED
2. DELIVERED WITH POSTPARTUM COMPLICATION
3. ANTEPARTUM COMPLICATION
4. POSTPARTUM COMPLICATION

457.9 CHANNELS DISORDER NONINFECTIOUS
457.1 CHANNELS OBSTRUCTION
457.8 CHANNELS OTHER DISORDER NONINFECTIOUS
289.9 GLAND (SYSTEM) DISORDER
306.8 GLAND (SYSTEM) DISORDER PSYCHOGENIC
289.3 NODE - CALCIFICATION
785.6 NODE - ENLARGEMENT
457.8 NODE - FISTULA
785.6 NODE - HYPERPLASIA
457.8 NODE - INFARCTION
228.1 NODE - LYMPHANGIOMA
457.8 NODE - RUPTURE
457.1 OBSTRUCTION OR OCCLUSION
289.9 SYSTEM (GLAND) DISORDER
306.8 SYSTEM (GLAND) DISORDER PSYCHOGENIC
457.9 VESSEL - DISORDER NONINFECTIOUS
457.8 VESSEL - DISORDER OTHER SPECIFIED NONINFECTIOUS
457.8 VESSEL - FISTULA
457.8 VESSEL - INFARCTION
457.1 VESSEL - OBSTRUCTION
457.8 VESSEL - RUPTURE

LYMPHADENITIS

289.3 UNSPECIFIED
683 ACUTE
289.2 ACUTE MESENTERIC
675.2# BREAST MATERNAL DUE TO PREGNANCY
5th Digit: 675.2
0. EPISODE OF NOS OR N/A
1. DELIVERED
2. DELIVERED WITH POSTPARTUM COMPLICATION
3. ANTEPARTUM COMPLICATION
4. POSTPARTUM COMPLICATION

289.3 CERVICAL
099.0 CHANCROIDAL
289.1 CHRONIC
289.2 CHRONIC MESENTERIC
695.89 DERMATOPATHIC
500 DUE TO ANTHRACOSIS (OCCUPATIONAL)
125.1 DUE TO BRUGIA (WUCHERERIA) MALAYI
032.89 DUE TO DIPHTHERIA (TOXIN)
099.1 DUE TO LYMPHOGRANULOMA VENEREUM
125.0 DUE TO WUCHERERIA BANCROFTI
289.3 GENERALIZED
098.89 GONORRHEAL
289.1 GRANULOMATOUS
683 INFECTIONAL (PURULENT) (PYOGENIC) (STREPTOCOCCAL)
289.2 MESENTERIC ACUTE, CHRONIC OR SUBACUTE
002.0 MESENTERIC DUE BACILLUS TYPHI
027.2 MESENTERIC DUE PASTEURELLA MULTOCIDA
078.3 REGIONAL
683 SEPTIC
289.1 SUBACUTE
289.2 SUBACUTE MESENTERIC
683 SUPPURATIVE
091.4 SYPHILITIC (EARLY) (SECONDARY)
095.8 SYPHILITIC LATE
0 TB SEE 'TUBERCULOSIS', LYMPH NODES
099.1 VENEREAL

LYMPHADENOPATHY

785.6 NOS
0 -ASSOCIATED VIRUS (LAV) SEE 'HIV' INFECTION
785.6 UNKNOWN ETIOLOGY

372.8 LYMPHANGIECTASIS CONJUNCTIVA

LYMPHANGIOMA

228.1 NOS M9170/0
228.1 ANY SITE
228.1 CAPILLARY ANY SITE M9171/0
228.1 CAVERNOUS NEVUS ANY SITE M9172/0
228.1 CONGENITAL ANY SITE M9170/0
228.1 CYSTIC ANY SITE M9173/0

228.1 LYMPHANGIOMYOMA M9174/0
238.1 LYMPHANGIOMYOMATOSIS SITE NOS
0 LYMPHANGIOMYOMATOSIS SITE SPECIFIED SEE 'NEOPLASM UNCERTAIN BEHAVIOR' BY SITE M9174/1
171.# LYMPHANGIOSARCOMA M9170/3
4th Digit: 171
0. HEAD FACE NECK
2. UPPER LIMB SHOULDER
3. LOWER LIMB HIP
4. THORAX
5. ABDOMINAL HYPOCHONDRIUM
6. PELVIS BUTTOCK GROIN INGUINAL REGION PERINEUM
7. TRUNK NOS BACK NOS FLANK NOS
8. OTHER SPECIFIED SITES
9. SITE NOS

LYMPHANGITIS

457.2 NOS
682.9 ACUTE
0 ACUTE SEE 'CELLULITIS'
682.3 ACUTE ARM AND FOREARM MAXILLA SHOULDER
682.5 ACUTE BUTTOCK (GLUTEAL)
682.0 ACUTE FACE NOSE SUBMANDIBULAR
682.7 ACUTE FOOT (EXCEPT TOES)
682.4 ACUTE HAND (EXCEPT FINGERS)
682.8 ACUTE HEAD AND SCALP
682.1 ACUTE NECK
682.9 ACUTE SITE UNSPECIFIED
682.6 ACUTE THIGH (LEG) ANKLE
682.2 ACUTE TRUNK AND GROIN
675.2# BREAST DUE TO PREGNANCY
5th Digit: 675.2
0. EPISODE OF CARE UNSPECIFIED OR N/A
1. DELIVERED
2. DELIVERED WITH POSTPARTUM COMPLICATION
3. ANTEPARTUM COMPLICATION
4. POSTPARTUM COMPLICATION

457.2 CHRONIC (SUBACUTE)
125.1 DUE TO BRUGIA (WUCHERERIA) MALAYI
125.0 DUE TO WUCHERERIA BANCROFTI
682.2 GROIN

648.9#: USE AN ADDITIONAL CODE TO IDENTIFY LYMPHANGITIS.

648.9# MATERNAL CURRENT (CO-EXISTENT) IN PREGNANCY
5th Digit: 648.9
0. EPISODE OF NOS OR N/A
1. DELIVERED
2. DELIVERED WITH POSTPARTUM COMPLICATION
3. ANTEPARTUM COMPLICATION
4. POSTPARTUM COMPLICATION

0 LYMPHATIC SEE 'LYMPH, LYMPHATIC'

LYMPHEDEMA

457.1 ACQUIRED (PRAECOX) (SECONDARY) (OBLITERANS) NOS

> *648.9#: USE AN ADDITIONAL CODE TO IDENTIFY LYMPHEDEMA ACQUIRED.*

648.9# ACQUIRED (PRAECOX) (SECONDARY) (OBLITERANS) MATERNAL CURRENT (CO-EXISTENT) IN PREGNANCY

5th Digit: 648.9

0. EPISODE OF NOS OR N/A
1. DELIVERED
2. DELIVERED WITH POSTPARTUM COMPLICATION
3. ANTEPARTUM COMPLICATION
4. POSTPARTUM COMPLICATION

997.99 ACQUIRED (PRAECOX) (SECONDARY) (OBLITERANS) SURGICAL NEC

757.0 CONGENITAL

457.0 POSTMASTECTOMY SYNDROME

200.1# LYMPHOBLASTOMA M9630/3

5th Digit: 200.1

0. UNSPECIFIED SITE, EXTRANODAL AND SOLID ORGAN SITES
1. LYMPH NODES OF HEAD FACE NECK
2. LYMPH NODES INTRATHORACIC
3. LYMPH NODES ABDOMINAL
4. LYMPH NODES AXILLA AND UPPER LIMB
5. LYMPH NODES INGUINAL REGION AND LOWER LIMB
6. LYMPH NODES INTRAPELVIC
7. SPLEEN
8. LYMPH NODES MULTIPLE SITES

V59.8 LYMPHOCYTE DONOR NON-AUTOGENOUS

049.0 LYMPHOCYTIC CHORIOMENINGITIS

201.4# LYMPHOCYTIC HISTIOCYTIC PREDOMINANCE HODGKINS M9651/3

200.1# LYMPHOCYTOMA

5th Digit: 200.1, 201.4

0. UNSPECIFIED SITE, EXTRANODAL AND SOLID ORGAN SITES
1. LYMPH NODES OF HEAD FACE NECK
2. LYMPH NODES INTRATHORACIC
3. LYMPH NODES ABDOMINAL
4. LYMPH NODES AXILLA AND UPPER LIMB
5. LYMPH NODES INGUINAL REGION AND LOWER LIMB
6. LYMPH NODES INTRAPELVIC
7. SPLEEN
8. LYMPH NODES MULTIPLE SITES

288.8 LYMPHOCYTOPENIA

288.8 LYMPHOCYTOSIS SYMPTOMATIC

199.1 LYMPHOEPITHELIAL CARCINOMA SITE NOS

0 LYMPHOEPITHELIAL CARCINOMA SITE SPECIFIED SEE 'CANCER' BY SITE M8082/3

099.1 LYMPHOGRANULOMA INGUINALE

201.9# LYMPHOGRANULOMA MALIGNANT M9650/3

5th Digit: 201.9

0. UNSPECIFIED SITE, EXTRANODAL AND SOLID ORGAN SITES
1. LYMPH NODES OF HEAD FACE NECK
2. LYMPH NODES INTRATHORACIC
3. LYMPH NODES ABDOMINAL
4. LYMPH NODES AXILLA AND UPPER LIMB
5. LYMPH NODES INGUINAL REGION AND LOWER LIMB
6. LYMPH NODES INTRAPELVIC
7. SPLEEN
8. LYMPH NODES MULTIPLE SITES

099.1 LYMPHOGRANULOMA VENEREUM

647.2# LYMPHOGRANULOMA VENEREUM MATERNAL CURRENT (CO-EXISTENT) IN PREGNANCY [099.1]

5th Digit: 647.2

0. EPISODE OF CARE UNSPECIFIED OR N/A
1. DELIVERED
2. DELIVERED WITH POSTPARTUM COMPLICATION
3. ANTEPARTUM COMPLICATION
4. POSTPARTUM COMPLICATION

655.4# LYMPHOGRANULOMA VENEREUM MATERNAL WITH KNOWN/SUSPECTED FETAL DAMAGE

5th Digit: 655.4

0. EPISODE OF CARE UNSPECIFIED OR N/A
1. DELIVERED
3. ANTEPARTUM COMPLICATION

135 LYMPHOGRANULOMATOSIS BENIGN (SCHAUMANN'S) M9650/3

201.9# LYMPHOGRANULOMATOSIS MALIGNANT M9650/3

5th Digit: 201.9

0. UNSPECIFIED SITE, EXTRANODAL AND SOLID ORGAN SITES
1. LYMPH NODES OF HEAD FACE NECK
2. LYMPH NODES INTRATHORACIC
3. LYMPH NODES ABDOMINAL
4. LYMPH NODES AXILLA AND UPPER LIMB
5. LYMPH NODES INGUINAL REGION AND LOWER LIMB
6. LYMPH NODES INTRAPELVIC
7. SPLEEN
8. LYMPH NODES MULTIPLE SITES

V10.61 LYMPHOID LEUKEMIA HISTORY

LYMPHOMA

202.8# NOS (MALIGNANT) M9590/3

0 BENIGN SEE 'BENIGN NEOPLASM', BY SITE M9590/0

200.2# BURKITT'S LYMPHOMA M9750/3

202.0# CENTROBLASTIC TYPE FOLLICULAR MALIGNANT M9697/3

202.8# CENTROBLASTIC TYPE MALIGNANT M9632/3

202.8# CENTROBLASTIC-CENTROCYTIC DIFFUSE MALIGNANT M9614/3

202.8# CENTROCYTIC MALIGNANT M9622/3

202.8# CONVOLUTED CELL TYPE MALIGNANT M9602/3

202.8# DIFFUSE NEC M9590/3

202.0# FOLLICULAR (GIANT) M9690/3

202.0# FOLLICULAR CENTER CELL CLEAVED M9695/3

202.8# FOLLICULAR CENTER CELL CLEAVED MALIGNANT M9623/3

202.0# FOLLICULAR CENTER CELL NONCLEAVED M9698/3

202.8# FOLLICULAR CENTER CELL NONCLEAVED MALIGNANT M9633/3

202.8# FOLLICULAR CENTER CELL MALIGNANT M9615/3

202.0# FOLLICULAR CENTROBLASTIC-CENTROCYTIC MALIGNANT M9692/3

202.0# FOLLICULAR LYMPHOCYTIC INTERMEDIATE DIFFERENTIATION M9694/3

200.0# HISTIOCYTIC (DIFFUSE) M9640/3

200.0# HISTIOCYTIC (DIFFUSE) NODULAR M9642/3

200.0# HISTIOCYTIC (DIFFUSE) PLEOMORPHIC CELL TYPE M9641/3

200.8# IMMUNOBLASTIC TYPE MALIGNANT M9612/3

200.1# LYMPHOBLASTIC (DIFFUSE) M9630/3

5th Digit: 200.0-2, 8 202.0, 8

0. UNSPECIFIED SITE, EXTRANODAL AND SOLID ORGAN SITES
1. LYMPH NODES OF HEAD FACE NECK
2. LYMPH NODES INTRATHORACIC
3. LYMPH NODES ABDOMINAL
4. LYMPH NODES AXILLA AND UPPER LIMB
5. LYMPH NODES INGUINAL REGION AND LOWER LIMB
6. LYMPH NODES INTRAPELVIC
7. SPLEEN
8. LYMPH NODES MULTIPLE SITES

LYMPHOMA (continued)

200.1# LYMPHOCYTIC INTERMEDIATE DIFFERENTIATION M9621/3
202.0# LYMPHOCYTIC INTERMEDIATE DIFFERENTIATION NODULAR MALIGNANT M9694/3
202.0# LYMPHOCYTIC, NODULAR M9690/3
202.0# LYMPHOCYTIC POORLY DIFFERENTIATED M9696/3
202.0# LYMPHOCYTIC POORLY DIFFERENTIATED NODULAR MALIGNANT M9696/3
200.1# LYMPHOCYTIC POORLY DIFFERENTIATED MALIGNANT M9630/3
200.1# LYMPHOCYTIC WELL DIFFERENTIATED MALIGNANT M9620/3
202.0# LYMPHOCYTIC WELL DIFFERENTIATED NODULAR MALIGNANT M9693/3
202.8# LYMPHOCYTIC-HISTIOCYTIC MIXED MALIGNANT M9613/3
200.8# LYMPHOPLASMACYTOID TYPE MALIGNANT M9611/3
200.1# LYMPHOSARCOMA TYPE M9610/3
202.8# MALIGNANT NOS M9590/3
200.8# MIXED LYMPHOCYTIC-HISTIOCYTIC (DIFFUSE) M9613/3
202.0# MIXED LYMPHOCYTIC-HISTIOCYTIC NODULAR MALIGNANT M9691/3
202.0# NODULAR MALIGNANT M9690/3
202.8# NON HODGKIN'S TYPE MALIGNANT M9591/3
200.0# RETICULUM CELL TYPE M9640/3
202.8# STEM CELL TYPE MALIGNANT M9601/3
202.1# T CELL
202.8# UNDIFFERENTIATED CELL TYPE MALIGNANT M9600/3

5th Digit: 200.0, 1, 8, 202.0, 1, 8

0. UNSPECIFIED SITE, EXTRANODAL AND SOLID ORGAN SITES
1. LYMPH NODES OF HEAD FACE NECK
2. LYMPH NODES INTRATHORACIC
3. LYMPH NODES ABDOMINAL
4. LYMPH NODES AXILLA AND UPPER LIMB
5. LYMPH NODES INGUINAL REGION AND LOWER LIMB
6. LYMPH NODES INTRAPELVIC
7. SPLEEN
8. LYMPH NODES MULTIPLE SITES

229.9 LYMPHOMATOUS TUMOR BENIGN SITE NOS
0 LYMPHOMATOUS TUMOR BENIGN SITE SPECIFIED SEE 'BENIGN NEOPLASM', BY SITE M9590/0
288.8 LYMPHOPENIA

LYMPHOPROLIFERATIVE

238.7 DISEASE CHRONIC SITE NOS
0 DISEASE CHRONIC SITE SPECIFIED SEE 'NEOPLASM UNCERTAIN BEHAVIOR' BY SITE M9970/1

078.3 LYMPHORETICULOSIS BENIGN (OF INOCULATION)

LYMPHOSARCOMA

200.1# LYMPHOSARCOMA M9610/3
200.2# BURKITT'S TUMOR LYMPHOMA M9750/3
200.1# DIFFUSE NOS M9610/3
202.0# FOLLICULAR (GIANT) M9690/3
V10.71 HISTORY
200.1# LYMPHOBLASTIC (DIFFUSE) M9630/3
200.1# LYMPHOCYTIC (DIFFUSE) M9610/3
200.8# MIXED (DIFFUSE) M9613/3
202.0# NODULAR M9690/3
200.1# PROLYMPHOCYTIC M9631/3

5th Digit: 200.1, 2, 8, 202.0

0. UNSPECIFIED SITE, EXTRANODAL AND SOLID ORGAN SITES
1. LYMPH NODES OF HEAD FACE NECK
2. LYMPH NODES INTRATHORACIC
3. LYMPH NODES ABDOMINAL
4. LYMPH NODES AXILLA AND UPPER LIMB
5. LYMPH NODES INGUINAL REGION AND LOWER LIMB
6. LYMPH NODES INTRAPELVIC
7. SPLEEN
8. LYMPH NODES MULTIPLE SITES

270.7 LYSINE METABOLISM DISTURBANCES
071 LYSSA

031.2 MAC BACTEREMIA (MYCOBACTERIUM AVIUM-INTRACELLULARE COMPLEX)
V46.9 MACHINE DEPENDENCE

MACLEOD'S SYNDROME
492.8 MACLEOD'S SYNDROME
491.21 WITH ACUTE BRONCHITIS
491.20 WITH CHRONIC BRONCHITIS
491.21 WITH CHRONIC BRONCHITIS WITH EXACERBATION

756.0 MACROCEPHALY
744.81 MACROCHEILIA CONGENITAL
751.3 MACROCOLON CONGENITAL
289.8 MACROCYTOSIS (MACROCYTHEMIA)
755.57 MACRODACTYLIA FINGERS
755.65 MACRODACTYLIA TOES
520.2 MACRODONTIA
742.4 MACROENCEPHALY CONGENITAL
524.05 MACROGENIA
259.8 MACROGENITOSOMIA PRAECOX (SYNDROME)
255.2 MACROGENITOSOMIA PRAECOX MALE
273.3 MACROGLOBULINEMIA (SYNDROME)
750.15 MACROGLOSSIA CONGENITAL

MACROGNATHIA
524.00 UNSPECIFIED
524.02 MANDIBULAR
524.72 MANDIBULAR ALVEOLAR
524.01 MAXILLARY
524.71 MAXILLARY ALVEOLAR

742.4 MACROGYRIA CONGENITAL
V09.2 MACROLIDES RESISTANT INFECTION (SEE 'DRUG RESISTANCE')
368.14 MACROPSIA
744.83 MACROSTOMIA CONGENITAL
744.22 MACROTIA CONGENITAL

MACULAR
743.55 CHANGES CONGENITAL
362.83 EDEMA
362.53 EDEMA CYSTOID
250.5# EDEMA DIABETIC [362.01]

5th Digit: 250.5

0. TYPE II, ADULT-ONSET, NON-INSULIN DEPENDENT (EVEN IF REQUIRING INSULIN), OR UNSPECIFIED; CONTROLLED

1. TYPE I, JUVENILE-ONSET OR INSULIN-DEPENDENT; CONTROLLED

2. TYPE II, ADULT-ONSET, NON-INSULIN DEPENDENT (EVEN IF REQUIRING INSULIN); UNCONTROLLED

3. TYPE I, JUVENILE-ONSET OR INSULIN-DEPENDENT; UNCONTROLLED

362.56 PUCKERING
363.32 SCAR (OTHER)
V80.2 SENILE LESIONS (SCREENING FOR)
362.55 TOXIC MACULOPATHY

MACULAR DEGENERATION
362.50 UNSPECIFIED
362.75 CONGENITAL
362.54 CYST HOLE OR PSEUDOHOLE
362.53 CYSTOID
362.52 EXUDATIVE (SENILE)
362.75 JUVENILE
362.56 PUCKERING
362.50 SENILE
362.51 SENILE ATROPHIC DRY
362.52 SENILE DISCIFORM WET
362.52 SENILE EXUDATIVE
362.51 SENILE NONEXUDATIVE
362.55 TOXIC

362.55 MACULOPATHY TOXIC
374.55 MADAROSIS EYELID
755.54 MADELUNG'S DEFORMITY
272.8 MADELUNG'S DISEASE (LIPOMATOSIS)

MADURA
117.4 FOOT
039.4 FOOT ACTINOMYCOTIC

117.4 MADURELLA GRISEA INFECTION
117.4 MADURELLA MYCETOMII INFECTION
039.9 MADUROMYCOSIS NOS (SEE ALSO 'ACTINOMYCOSIS')
117.4 MADUROMYCOSIS MYCOTIC INFECTION
756.4 MAFFUCCI'S SYNDROME (DYSCHONDROPLASIA WITH HEMANGIOMAS)
306.4 MAGENBLASE SYNDROME
134.0 MAGGOT INFECTION ORBIT (EYE) [376.13]
134.0 MAGGOT INFESTATION
526.4 MAGITOT'S DISEASE
790.6 MAGNESIUM ABNORMAL BLOOD LEVEL
781.7 MAGNESIUM DEFICIENCY SYNDROME
275.2 MAGNESIUM METABOLISM DISORDER
031.0 MAI (MYCOBACTERIUM AVIUM INTRACELLULARE)
709.1 MAJOCCHI'S DISEASE (PURPURA ANNULARIS TELANGIECTODES)
110.6 MAJOCCHI'S GRANULOMA

MALABSORPTION
579.8 CALCIUM
579.8 CARBOHYDRATE
579.8 DRUG INDUCED
579.8 DUE TO BACTERIAL OVERGROWTH
579.8 FAT
579.9 INTESTINAL
579.3 POSTSURGICAL SYNDROME
579.8 PROTEIN
331.3 SPINAL FLUID SYNDROME
579.9 SYNDROME

MALACOPLAKIA
596.8 BLADDER
0 BLADDER WITH INCONTINENCE SEE 'BLADDER DISORDERS WITH INCONTINENCE'
569.89 COLON
593.89 PELVIS (KIDNEY)
593.89 URETER
599.84 URETHRA

V62.4 MALADJUSTMENT SOCIAL (REASON FOR ENCOUNTER)
780.79 MALAISE

MALARIA
084.6 NOS
084.9 ALGID
084.9 CARDIAC
V02.9 CARRIER (SUSPECTED)
084.9 CEREBRAL
771.2 CONGENITAL OR PERINATAL
084.0 FALCIPARUM [MALIGNANT TERTIAN]
084.6 FEVER NOS
084.5 FEVER BY MORE THAN ONE PARASITE
084.0 FEVER BY PLASMODIUM FALCIPARUM
084.2 FEVER BY PLASMODIUM MALARIAE
084.3 FEVER BY PLASMODIUM OVALE
084.1 FEVER BY PLASMODIUM VIVAX
084.8 HEMOGLOBINURIC
084.9 HEPATITIS [573.2]
V12.03 HISTORY

M

MALARIA (continued)
084.7 INDUCED (THERAPEUTICALLY)
084.2 MALARIAE
655.4# MATERNAL (WITH KNOWN / SUSPECTED DAMAGE TO FETUS)
5th Digit: 655.4
0. EPISODE OF CARE UNSPECIFIED OR N/A
1. DELIVERED
3. ANTEPARTUM COMPLICATION

> *647.4#: USE AN ADDITIONAL CODE TO IDENTIFY THE MATERNAL MALARIA.*

647.4# MATERNAL CURRENT (CO-EXISTENT) IN PREGNANCY
5th Digit: 647.4
0. EPISODE OF CARE UNSPECIFIED OR N/A
1. DELIVERED
2. DELIVERED WITH POSTPARTUM COMPLICATION
3. ANTEPARTUM COMPLICATION
4. POSTPARTUM COMPLICATION

084.5 MIXED
084.4 MONKEY
084.9 NEPHROTIC SYNDROME [581.81]
084.3 OVALE
084.2 QUARTAN
V75.1 SCREENING
084.0 SUBTERTIAN
084.1 VIVAX (BENIGN TERTIAN)

608.89 MALASSEZ'S DISEASE (CYSTIC)
111.0 MALASSEZIA (PITYROSPORUM) FURFUR INFECTION
607.84 MALE ERECTILE DISORDER ORGANIC
302.72 MALE ERECTILE DISORDER PSYCHOSEXUAL
608.9 MALE GENITAL ORGAN DISORDER
919.8 MALIBU DISEASE
919.9 MALIBU DISEASE INFECTED
259.2 MALIGNANT CARCINOID SYNDROME
0 MALIGNANT NEOPLASM SEE 'CANCER' BY SITE
199.0 MALIGNANT NEOPLASM UNSPECIFIED SITE
0 MALIGNANT SEE SPECIFIED CONDITION
V65.2 MALINGERER
024 MALLEOMYCES MALLEI INFECTION
025 MALLEOMYCES PSEUDOMALLEI
736.1 MALLET FINGER
024 MALLEUS
385.21 MALLEUS IMPAIRED MOBILITY
530.7 MALLORY WEISS SYNDROME

MALNUTRITION
263.9 NOS (CALORIE)
263.9 CALORIE
261 CALORIE DEFICIENCY SEVERE
269.9 DEFICIENCY UNSPECIFIED
995.84 DUE TO NEGLECT - ADULT
995.52 DUE TO NEGLECT - CHILD
269.9 DUE TO NUTRITIONAL DEFICIENCY
263.9 DYSTROPHY
579.3 FOLLOWING GI SURGERY
263.2 PHYSICAL RETARDATION
263.9 PROTEIN-CALORIE
263.1 PROTEIN-CALORIE MILD
263.0 PROTEIN-CALORIE MODERATE
263.8 PROTEIN-CALORIE WEIGHT FOR AGE
263.8 PROTEIN-CALORIE OTHER
262 PROTEIN-CALORIE OTHER SEVERE
V77.2 SCREENING
263.9 WEIGHT FOR AGE

MALNUTRITION FETAL
764.20 WEIGHT UNSPECIFIED
764.21 <500 GRAMS
764.22 500-749 GRAMS
764.23 750-999 GRAMS
764.24 1000-1249 GRAMS
764.25 1250-1499 GRAMS
764.26 1500-1749 GRAMS
764.27 1750-1999 GRAMS
764.28 2000-2499 GRAMS
764.29 2500 GRAMS

MALNUTRITION FETAL - LIGHT FOR DATES
764.10 WEIGHT UNSPECIFIED
764.11 < 500 GRAMS
764.12 500 - 749 GRAMS
764.13 750 - 999 GRAMS
764.14 1000 - 1249 GRAMS
764.15 1250 - 1499 GRAMS
764.16 1500 - 1749 GRAMS
764.17 1750 - 1999 GRAMS
764.18 2000-2499 GRAMS
764.19 2500 GRAMS AND OVER

MALOCCLUSION
524.4 NOS
524.5 ABNORMAL SWALLOWING
524.5 MOUTH BREATHING
524.69 TEMPOROMANDIBULAR
524.5 TONGUE LIP OR FINGER HABITS

MALOCCLUSION DUE TO JAW ANOMALIES
524.7# DENTOALVEOLAR
5th Digit: 524.7
0. UNSPECIFIED ALVEOLAR ANOMALY
1. ALVEOLAR MAXILLARY HYPERPLASIA
2. ALVEOLAR MANDIBULAR HYPERPLASIA
3. ALVEOLAR MAXILLARY HYPOPLASIA
4. ALVEOLAR MANDIBULAR HYPOPLASIA
9. OTHER SPECIFIED ALVEOLAR ANOMALY

524.1# JAW RELATIONSHIP TO CRANIAL BASE
5th Digit: 524.1
0. UNSPECIFIED ANOMALY
1. MAXILLARY ASYMMETRY
2. OTHER JAW ASYMMETRY
9. OTHER SPECIFIED ANOMALY

524.0# JAW SIZE
5th Digit: 524.0
0. UNSPECIFIED ANOMALY
1. MAXILLARY HYPERPLASIA
2. MANDIBULAR HYPERPLASIA
3. MAXILLARY HYPOPLASIA
4. MANDIBULAR HYPOPLASIA
5. MACROGENIA
6. MICROGENIA
9. OTHER SPECIFIED ANOMALY

MALPOSITION/MALPRESENTATION
652.9# NOS
660.0# NOS OBSTRUCTING LABOR **[652.9#]**
5th Digit: 652.9, 660.0
0. EPISODE OF CARE UNSPECIFIED OR N/A
1. DELIVERED
3. ANTEPARTUM COMPLICATION

761.7 AFFECTING FETUS OR NEWBORN BEFORE LABOR
763.1 AFFECTING FETUS OR NEWBORN DURING LABOR

MALPOSITION/MALPRESENTATION (continued)

652.4# BROW PRESENTATION
660.0# BROW PRESENTATION OBSTRUCTING LABOR [652.4#]
652.2# BUTTOCKS PRESENTATION
660.0# BUTTOCKS PRESENTATION OBSTRUCTING LABOR [652.2#]
652.4# CHIN PRESENTATION
660.0# CHIN PRESENTATION OBSTRUCTING LABOR [652.4#]
652.2# COMPLETE BREECH PRESENTATION
660.0# COMPLETE BREECH PRESENTATION OBSTRUCTING LABOR [652.2#]
652.8# COMPOUND PRESENTATION
660.0# COMPOUND PRESENTATION OBSTRUCTING LABOR [652.8#]
652.4# EXTENDED HEAD PRESENTATION
660.0# EXTENDED HEAD PRESENTATION OBSTRUCTING LABOR [652.4#]
652.4# FACE PRESENTATION
660.0# FACE PRESENTATION OBSTRUCTING LABOR [652.4#]
652.8# FACE TO PUBES PRESENTATION
660.0# FACE TO PUBES PRESENTATION OBSTRUCTING LABOR [652.8#]
652.8# FOOTLING PRESENTATION
660.0# FOOTLING PRESENTATION OBSTRUCTING LABOR [652.8#]
652.2# FRANK BREECH PRESENTATION
660.0# FRANK BREECH PRESENTATION OBSTRUCTING LABOR [652.2#]
652.5# HIGH HEAD AT TERM
660.0# HIGH HEAD AT TERM OBSTRUCTING LABOR[652.5#]
652.8# INCOMPLETE BREECH PRESENTATION
660.0# INCOMPLETE BREECH PRESENTATION OBSTRUCTING LABOR [652.8#]
652.9# MALPOSITION OF FETUS AT ONSET COMPLICATING PREGNANCY
660.0# MALPOSITION OF FETUS AT ONSET OBSTRUCTING LABOR [652.9#]
652.7# PROLAPSED ARM
660.0# PROLAPSED ARM OBSTRUCTING LABOR [652.7#]
0 SEE ALSO 'PREGNANCY COMPLICATIONS, DELIVERY PROBLEMS: MALPRESENTATION / MALPOSITION'
652.3# TRANSVERSE LIE (OBLIQUE LIE)
660.0# TRANSVERSE LIE (OBLIQUE LIE) OBSTRUCTING LABOR [652.3#]
652.0# UNSTABLE LIE
660.0# UNSTABLE LIE OBSTRUCTING LABOR [652.0#]
652.6# WITH MULTIPLE GESTATION
660.0# WITH MULTIPLE GESTATION OBSTRUCTING LABOR [652.6#]
652.1# WITH VERSION
660.0# WITH VERSION OBSTRUCTING LABOR [652.1#]
652.8# OTHER SPECIFIED
660.0# OTHER SPECIFIED OBSTRUCTING LABOR [652.8#]

5th Digit: 652.0-9, 660.0
- **0. EPISODE OF CARE UNSPECIFIED OR N/A**
- **1. DELIVERED**
- **3. ANTEPARTUM COMPLICATION**

495.4 MALT WORKERS' LUNG
0 MALTA FEVER SEE 'BRUCELLA'
733.81 MALUNION FRACTURE

MAMMARY

901.82 ARTERY INTERNAL INJURY
908.4 ARTERY INTERNAL INJURY LATE EFFECT
901.82 ARTERY INTERNAL LACERATION (RUPTURE)(HEMATOMA) (AVULSION) (ANEURYSM) TRAUMATIC
908.4 ARTERY INTERNAL LACERATION LATE EFFECT
610.4 DUCT ECTASIA
611.8 DUCT OCCLUSION
610.9 DYSPLASIA BENIGN
611.1 GLAND HYPERTROPHY (ENLARGEMENT)
901.82 VEIN INTERNAL INJURY
908.4 VEIN INTERNAL INJURY LATE EFFECT
901.82 VEIN INTERNAL LACERATION (RUPTURE) (HEMATOMA) (AVULSION) (ANEURYSM) TRAUMATIC
908.4 VEIN INTERNAL LACERATION LATE EFFECT

MAMMOGRAM

793.8 ABNORMAL FINDING
V71.1 EVALUATION SUSPECTED MALIGNANT NEOPLASM, NONE FOUND
V72.5 ROUTINE EXAM
V76.11 SCREENING BREAST CANCER FOR HIGH RISK PATIENT
V76.12 SCREENING BREAST CANCER OTHER

MANDIBLE, MANDIBULAR

526.4 ABSCESS (OSTEITIS) (PERIOSTITIS) ACUTE SUPPURATIVE
524.09 ABSENCE (CONGENITAL)
524.72 ALVEOLAR HYPERPLASIA
524.74 ALVEOLAR HYPOPLASIA
526.89 CONDYLAR UNILATERAL HYPERPLASIA
526.89 DISEASE (OTHER SPECIFIED)
524.02 HYPERPLASIA
524.04 HYPOPLASIA
526.4 NECROSIS
524.2 TEETH POSTERIOR LINGUAL OCCLUSION

756.0 MANDIBULOFACIAL DYSOSTOSIS SYNDROME

MANIC DEPRESSIVE PSYCHOSIS

296.80 NOS
296.82 ATYPICAL DEPRESSED
296.81 ATYPICAL MANIC
296.89 MIXED TYPE
296.80 REACTION
296.80 SYNDROME

MANIC DEPRESSIVE PSYCHOSIS BIPOLAR

296.7 CIRCULAR (ALTERNATING) - NOS
296.5# CIRCULAR (ALTERNATING) - DEPRESSED
296.4# CIRCULAR (ALTERNATING) - MANIC
296.6# CIRCULAR (ALTERNATING) - MIXED

5th Digit: 296.4-6
- **0. UNSPECIFIED**
- **1. MILD**
- **2. MODERATE**
- **3. SEVERE WITHOUT MENTION OF PSYCHOTIC BEHAVIOR**
- **4. SEVERE SPECIFIED AS WITH PSYCHOTIC BEHAVIOR**
- **5. IN PARTIAL OR UNSPECIFIED REMISSION**
- **6. IN FULL REMISSION**

296.7 TYPE I
296.89 TYPE II
296.8# OTHER AND UNSPECIFIED

5th Digit: 296.8
- **0. UNSPECIFIED**
- **1. ATYPICAL MANIC**
- **2. ATYPICAL DEPRESSIVE**
- **9. OTHER (MIXED)**

MANIC DEPRESSIVE PSYCHOSIS MONOPOLAR

296.0# HYPOMANIC SINGLE EPISODE OR UNSPECIFIED
296.1# HYPOMANIC RECURRENT
296.0# MANIC SINGLE EPISODE OR UNSPECIFIED
296.1# MANIC RECURRENT
296.2# DEPRESSED SINGLE EPISODE OR UNSPECIFIED
296.3# DEPRESSED RECURRENT

5th Digit: 296.0-3
- **0. UNSPECIFIED**
- **1. MILD**
- **2. MODERATE**
- **3. SEVERE WITHOUT MENTION OF PSYCHOTIC BEHAVIOR**
- **4. SEVERE SPECIFIED AS WITH PSYCHOTIC BEHAVIOR**
- **5. IN PARTIAL OR UNSPECIFIED REMISSION**
- **6. IN FULL REMISSION**

731.2 MANKOWSKY'S FAMILIAL DYSPLASTIC OSTEOPATHY (SYNDROME)
271.8 MANNOSIDOSIS CARBOHYDRATE TRANSPORT DISORDERS
125.5 MANSONELLA OZZARDI INFECTION
120.1 MANSON'S DISEASE (SCHISTOSOMA)
V74.1 MANTOUX TEST (TB)
795.5 MANTOUX TEST ABNORMAL
495.6 MAPLE BARK STRIPPERS' LUNG
270.3 MAPLE SYRUP (URINE) DISEASE OR SYNDROME
447.4 MARABLE'S SYNDROME (CELIAC ARTERY COMPRESSION)
261 MARASMUS
078.89 MARBURG DISEASE
759.89 MARCHESANI WEILL BRADYMORPHISM ECTOPIA LENTIS (SYNDROME)
341.8 MARCHIAFAVA BIGNAMI DISEASE OR SYNDROME
283.2 MARCHIAFAVA-MICHELI SYNDROME (PAROXYSMAL NOCTURNAL HEMOGLOBINURIA)
742.8 MARCUS GUNN'S SYNDROME (JAW-WINKING SYNDROME)
759.82 MARFAN'S SYNDROME (ARACHNODACTYLY)
090.49 MARFAN'S SYNDROME, CONGENITAL SYPHILIS
090.49 MARFAN'S SYNDROME, CONGENITAL SYPHILIS WITH LUXATION OF LENS [379.32]
731.2 MARIE-BAMBERGER DISEASE (HYPERTROPHIC PULMONARY OSTEOARTHROPATHY)
757.39 MARIE-BAMBERGER DISEASE PRIMARY (ACROPACHYDERMA)
720.0 MARIE STRUMPELL SPONDYLITIS
334.2 MARIE'S CEREBELLAR ATAXIA
253.0 MARIE'S SYNDROME (ACROMEGALY)
757.39 MARIE'S SYNDROME PRIMARY OR IDIOPATHIC (ACROPACHYDERMA)
731.2 MARIE'S SYNDROME SECONDARY (HYPERTROPHIC PULMONARY OSTEOARTHROPATHY)
305.2# MARIJUANA ABUSE (NONDEPENDENT)
304.3# MARIJUANA ADDICTION (DEPENDENT)

5th Digit: 304.3, 305.2

0. UNSPECIFIED
1. CONTINUOUS
2. EPISODIC
3. IN REMISSION

379.46 MARKUS-ADIE SYNDROME
596.0 MARION'S DISEASE (BLADDER NECK OBSTRUCTION)
V61.10 MARITAL PROBLEMS (REASON FOR ENCOUNTER)
277.5 MAROTEAUX LAMY SYNDROME (MUCOPOLYSACCHARIDOSIS VI)
277.5 MARQUIO BRAILSFORD DISEASE
082.1 MARSEILLES FEVER
242.0# MARSH'S DISEASE (EXOPHTHALMIC GOITER)

5th Digit: 242.0

0. WITHOUT MENTION OF THYROTOXIC CRISIS OR STORM
1. WITH MENTION OF THYROTOXIC CRISIS OR STORM

715.27 MARTIN'S DISEASE SYNDROME (OSTEOARTHRITIS)
275.49 MARTIN-ALBRIGHT SYNDROME (PSEUDOHYPOPARATHYROIDISM)
446.7 MARTORELL-FABRE SYNDROME (PULSELESS DISEASE)
302.83 MASOCHISM SEXUAL
301.89 MASOCHISTIC PERSONALITY

TO CODE A MASS OF A SITE NOT LISTED BELOW, SEE DISORDER OR DISEASE BY ANATOMICAL SITE.

MASS
789.3# ABDOMEN

5th Digit: 789.3

0. UNSPECIFIED SITE
1. UPPER RIGHT QUADRANT
2. UPPER LEFT QUADRANT
3. LOWER RIGHT QUADRANT
4. LOWER LEFT QUADRANT
5. PERIUMBILIC
6. EPIGASTRIC
7. GENERALIZED
9. OTHER SPECIFIED SITE (MULTIPLE)

787.99 ANAL
733.90 BONE
348.8 BRAIN
611.72 BREAST
784.2 CHEEK
786.6 CHEST
569.89 COLON
0 CYSTIC SEE 'CYST'
388.8 EAR
789.36 EPIGASTRIC
379.92 EYE
625.8 GENITAL ORGANS FEMALE
784.2 GUM
784.2 HEAD
784.2 INTRACRANIAL
719.6# JOINT

5th Digit: 719.6

0. SITE NOS
1. SHOULDER REGION
2. UPPER ARM (ELBOW) (HUMERUS)
3. FOREARM (RADIUS) (WRIST) (ULNA)
4. HAND (CARPAL) (METACARPAL) (FINGERS)
5. PELVIC REGION AND THIGH (HIP) (BUTTOCK) (FEMUR)
6. LOWER LEG (FIBULA) (KNEE) (PATELLA) (TIBIA)
7. ANKLE AND/OR FOOT (METATARSALS) (TOES) (TARSALS)
8. OTHER
9. MULTIPLE

593.9 KIDNEY
786.6 LUNG
785.6 LYMPH NODE
786.6 MEDIASTINUM
784.2 MOUTH
729.89 MUSCLE (LIMB)
784.2 NASAL SINUS
784.2 NECK
784.2 NOSE
784.2 PALATE
789.39 PELVIC
607.89 PENIS
625.8 PERINEUM
789.35 PERIUMBILIC
787.99 RECTAL
593.9 RENAL
789.39 RETROPERITONEAL
608.89 SCROTUM
782.2 SKIN
729.9 SOFT TISSUE
789.2 SPLEEN
782.2 SUBCUTANEOUS
786.6 SUBSTERNAL
240.9 SUBSTERNAL THYROID
782.2 SUPERFICIAL LOCALIZED

M

MASS (continued)

608.89 TESTES
784.2 THROAT
784.2 TONGUE
789.35 UMBILICUS
625.8 UTERUS
625.8 VAGINA
625.8 VULVA

770.1 MASSIVE ASPIRATION OF NEWBORN SYNDROME

MAST CELL

757.33 DISEASE CONGENITAL
202.6# SARCOMA M9740/3
202.6# SYSTEMIC TISSUE MAST CELL DISEASE M974103
202.6# TUMOR MALIGNANT M9740/3

5th Digit: 202.6

0. UNSPECIFIED SITE, EXTRANODAL AND SOLID ORGAN SITES
1. LYMPH NODES OF HEAD FACE NECK
2. LYMPH NODES INTRATHORACIC
3. LYMPH NODES ABDOMINAL
4. LYMPH NODES AXILLA AND UPPER LIMB
5. LYMPH NODES INGUINAL REGION AND LOWER LIMB
6. LYMPH NODES INTRAPELVIC
7. SPLEEN
8. LYMPH NODES MULTIPLE SITES

238.5 TUMOR UNCERTAIN BEHAVIOR SITE NOS M9740/1

620.6 MASTERS ALLEN SYNDROME
V41.6 MASTICATION PROBLEM

MASTITIS

611.0 ACUTE
610.1 CHRONIC CYSTIC
771.5 NEONATAL INFECTIVE
778.7 NEONATAL NONINFECTIVE
610.4 PERIDUCTAL
610.4 PLASMA CELL
611.0 RETROMAMMARY
611.0 SUBMAMMARY

MASTITIS OBSTETRICAL

675.2# MATERNAL DUE TO PREGNANCY NOS (INTERSTITIAL) (PARENCHYMATOUS)
675.1# MATERNAL DUE TO PREGNANCY - PURULENT (RETROMAMMARY) (SUBMAMMARY)

5th Digit: 675.1-2

0. EPISODE OF CARE UNSPECIFIED OR N/A
1. DELIVERED
2. DELIVERED WITH POSTPARTUM COMPLICATION
3. ANTEPARTUM COMPLICATION
4. POSTPARTUM COMPLICATION

238.5 MASTOCYTOMA SITE NOS
0 MASTOCYTOMA SITE SPECIFIED SEE 'NEOPLASM UNCERTAIN BEHAVIOR' BY SITE M9740/1
202.6# MASTOCYTOMA MALIGNANT M9740/3
202.6# MASTOCYTOSIS M9741/3

5th Digit: 202.6

0. UNSPECIFIED SITE, EXTRANODAL AND SOLID ORGAN SITES
1. LYMPH NODES OF HEAD FACE NECK
2. LYMPH NODES INTRATHORACIC
3. LYMPH NODES ABDOMINAL
4. LYMPH NODES AXILLA AND UPPER LIMB
5. LYMPH NODES INGUINAL REGION AND LOWER LIMB
6. LYMPH NODES INTRAPELVIC
7. SPLEEN
8. LYMPH NODES MULTIPLE SITES

757.33 MASTOCYTOSIS SYNDROME
611.71 MASTODYNIA

383.1 MASTOID CARIES
383.9 MASTOID DISEASE
959.09 MASTOID INJURY
385.9 MASTOID PROCESS DISEASE
383.89 MASTOID DISORDERS OTHER
383.89 MASTOID PERFORATION (ANTRUM) CELL

MASTOIDECTOMY COMPLICATION

383.30 UNSPECIFIED
383.33 CHRONIC INFLAMMATION CAVITY
383.33 GRANULATIONS OF POSTMASTOIDECTOMY CAVITY
383.31 MUCOSAL CYST
383.32 RECURRENT CHOLESTEATOMA

MASTOIDITIS

383.9 UNSPECIFIED SUPPURATIVE (HEMORRHAGIC) (PNEUMOCCOCAL) (STREPTOCCAL) (ACUTE)
383.00 ACUTE
383.01 ACUTE WITH SUBPERIOSTIAL ABSCESS
383.02 ACUTE WITH OTHER COMPLICATIONS
383.1 CHRONIC
015.6# TUBERCULOUS

5th Digit: 015.6

0. UNSPECIFIED SITE, EXTRANODAL AND SOLID ORGAN SITES
1. LAB NOT DONE
2. LABS PENDING
3. MICROSCOPY POSITIVE (IN SPUTUM)
4. CULTURE POSITIVE - MICROSCOPY NEGATIVE
5. CULTURE NEGATIVE - MICROSCOPY POSITIVE
6. CULTURE AND MICROSCOPY NEGATIVE CONFIRMED BY OTHER METHODS

307.9 MASTURBATION

0 MATERNAL DISORDERS SEE 'PREGNANCY COMPLICATIONS, MATERNAL CONDITIONS'

MATERNAL DISORDERS AFFECTING FETUS OR NEWBORN

IN ORDER TO USE THE FOLLOWING CODES, THE MEDICAL RECORD MUST SPECIFY THAT THE MATERNAL CONDITION IS A CAUSE OF MORBIDITY OR MORTALITY IN THE FETUS OR NEWBORN. THE MERE FACT THAT THE CONDITION EXISTED IN THE MOTHER OR COMPLICATED THE PREGNANCY DOES NOT WARRANT THE USE OF THESE CODES ON THE NEWBORN'S RECORD. REMEMBER, CODES 760-763 APPLY ONLY TO THE INFANT AND ARE NEVER ASSIGNED TO THE MOTHER'S RECORD. CONVERSELY, NEVER CODE THE MOTHER'S CONDITION WITH THESE FETAL/NEWBORN CODES.

762.9 UNSPECIFIED ABNORMALITIES OF CHORION AND AMNION
761.9 UNSPECIFIED COMPLICATIONS - DUE TO CURRENT PREGNANCY
760.9 UNSPECIFIED CONDITIONS - UNRELATED TO CURRENT PREGNANCY
762.6 UNSPECIFIED CONDITIONS OF UMBILICAL CORD
763.9 UNSPECIFIED DISORDER - DUE TO LABOR AND DELIVERY
761.4 ABDOMINAL PREGNANCY
763.1 ABNORMALITY BONY
763.89 ABNORMALITY SOFT TISSUES
761.8 ABORTION SPONTANEOUS
762.1 ABRUPTIO PLACENTAE
760.79 ADRENOGENITAL IATROGENIC SYNDROME AFFECTING FETUS OR NEWBORN
760.71 ALCOHOL TRANSMITTED VIA PLACENTA OR BREAST MILK
762.1 AMNIOCENTESIS DAMAGE TO PLACENTA
762.8 AMNION ADHESION TO FETUS
762.7 AMNIONITIS
763.5 ANALGESICS ADMINISTERED DURING LABOR AND DELIVERY
763.5 ANESTHETICS ADMINISTERED DURING LABOR AND DELIVERY
760.74 ANTIBIOTICS (ANTI-INFECTIVES) TRANSMITTED VIA PLACENTA OR BREAST MILK

M

MATERNAL DISORDERS AFFECTING FETUS OR NEWBORN (continued)

IN ORDER TO USE THE FOLLOWING CODES, THE MEDICAL RECORD MUST SPECIFY THAT THE MATERNAL CONDITION IS A CAUSE OF MORBIDITY OR MORTALITY IN THE FETUS OR NEWBORN. THE MERE FACT THAT THE CONDITION EXISTED IN THE MOTHER OR COMPLICATED THE PREGNANCY DOES NOT WARRANT THE USE OF THESE CODES ON THE NEWBORN'S RECORD. REMEMBER, CODES 760-763 APPLY ONLY TO THE INFANT AND ARE NEVER ASSIGNED TO THE MOTHER'S RECORD. CONVERSELY, NEVER CODE THE MOTHER'S CONDITION WITH THESE FETAL/NEWBORN CODES.

760.1 BACTERIURIA
763.1 BLADDER DILATATION
762.1 BLOOD LOSS MATERNAL
763.0 BREECH DELIVERY AND EXTRACTION
761.7 BREECH MALPRESENTATION BEFORE LABOR AND DELIVERY
760.8 CERVICITIS
763.89 CERVIX ABNORMALITY
761.0 CERVIX INCOMPETENT
763.89 CERVIX SCAR
763.1 CERVIX SCAR OBSTRUCTING LABOR
763.89 CERVIX STENOSIS/STRICTURE
763.1 CERVIX STENOSIS/STRICTURE OBSTRUCTING LABOR
763.4 CESAREAN DELIVERY
763.89 CESAREAN SCAR PREVIOUS
762.1 CESAREAN SECTION DAMAGE (SEPARATION) (HEMORRHAGE) TO PLACENTA
762.7 CHORIOAMNIONITIS
762.9 CHORION AND AMNION ABNORMALITY
762.8 CHORION AND AMNION ABNORMALITIES OTHER SPECIFIED
760.3 CIRCULATORY DISEASE MATERNAL CHRONIC
763.89 CLEIDOTOMY FETAL
760.75 COCAINE TRANSMITTED VIA PLACENTA OR BREAST MILK
763.7 CONTRACTION RING
760.75 CRACK (COCAINE) TRANSMITTED VIA PLACENTA OR BREAST MILK
763.89 CRANIOCLASIS, FETAL
763.89 CRANIOTOMY, FETAL
763.89 CYSTOCELE
763.1 CYSTOCELE OBSTRUCTING LABOR
761.6 DEATH (MATERNAL)
763.89 DELAYED BIRTH OR DELIVERY NEC
763.89 DELAYED BIRTH OR DELIVERY SECOND TWIN, TRIPLET ETC.
763.0 DELIVERY AND EXTRACTION
763.6 DELIVERY RAPID SECOND STAGE
760.76 DES (DIETHYLSTILBESTROL) TRANSMITTED VIA PLACENTA OR BREAST MILK
763.89 DESTRUCTIVE OPERATION OR PROCEDURE ON LIVE FETUS TO FACILITATE DELIVERY
775.0 DIABETES CAUSING FETAL HYPOGLYCEMIA
760.76 DIETHYLSTILBESTROL (DES) TRANSMITTED VIA PLACENTA OR BREAST MILK
763.5 DRUG REACTION MATERNAL
761.4 ECTOPIC PREGNANCY
763.89 ENDOCERVICAL OS STENOSIS/STRICTURE
763.1 ENDOCERVICAL OS STENOSIS/STRICTURE OBSTRUCTING LABOR
760.8 ENDOMETRITIS
763.89 EXHAUSTION MATERNAL
761.7 EXTERNAL VERSION MALPRESENTATION BEFORE LABOR AND DELIVERY
763.89 EXTRACTION FETAL MANUAL OR WITH HOOK
762.3 FETAL BLOOD LOSS DUE TO PLACENTAL TRANSFUSION [772.0]
763.89 FORCED BIRTH
763.2 FORCEPS DELIVERY

MATERNAL DISORDERS AFFECTING FETUS OR NEWBORN (continued)

760.73 HALLUCINOGENIC TRANSMITTED VIA PLACENTA OR BREAST MILK
762.1 HEMORRHAGE COMPLICATING PREGNANCY, ANTEPARTUM
763.89 HEMORRHAGE DUE TO COAGULATION DEFECT
760.8 HEPATITIS MATERNAL
761.3 HYDRAMNIOS ACUTE (CHRONIC)
760.0 HYPERTENSIVE DISORDERS MATERNAL
760.79 IMMUNE SERA TRANSMITTED VIA PLACENTA OR BREAST MILK
763.89 INDUCTION OF LABOR (MEDICAL)
760.8 INFECTION GENITAL TRACT OTHER LOCALIZED MATERNAL
760.2 INFECTION MATERNAL NOT MANIFESTED IN FETUS OR NEWBORN
760.1 INFECTION URINARY TRACT
760.2 INFLUENZA
763.89 INJURY DUE TO OBSTETRICAL TRAUMA
760.5 INJURY MATERNAL
761.4 INTRAPERITONEAL PREGNANCY
760.1 KIDNEY NECROSIS
760.8 LIVER NECROSIS
761.7 MALPRESENTATION/MALPOSITION BEFORE LABOR
763.1 MALPRESENTATION/MALPOSITION DURING LABOR
761.6 MATERNAL DEATH
760.79 MEDICINAL AGENTS NEC TRANSMITTED VIA PLACENTA OR BREAST MILK
762.7 MEMBRANITIS
763.89 MULTIPARITY
761.5 MULTIPLE PREGNANCY
763.5 NARCOSIS DUE TO DRUG (CORRECTLY ADMINISTERED)
763.5 NARCOTIC REACTION (INTOXICATION) MATERNAL DURING L&D
760.72 NARCOTIC TRANSMITTED VIA PLACENTA OR BREAST MILK
760.70 NOXIOUS SUBSTANCE UNSPECIFIED TRANSMITTED VIA PLACENTA OR BREAST MILK
760.79 NOXIOUS SUBSTANCE OTHER SPECIFIED TRANSMITTED VIA PLACENTA OR BREAST MILK
760.4 NUTRITIONAL DEFICIENCY DISORDERS MATERNAL
761.7 OBLIQUE LIE BEFORE LABOR AND DELIVERY
761.2 OLIGOHYDRAMNIOS
763.5 OPIATE REACTION (INTOXICATION) MATERNAL DURING L&D
763.89 OS UTERI STRICTURE
763.1 OS UTERI STRICTURE OBSTRUCTING LABOR
763.89 OVARIAN CYST
763.1 OVARIAN CYST OBSTRUCTING LABOR
763.1 PELVIS BONY
763.1 PELVIS CONTRACTED
763.89 PELVIS CYST
763.1 PELVIS CYST OBSTRUCTING LABOR
763.89 PELVIS DEFORMITY
760.8 PELVIS INFLAMMATORY DISEASE
763.89 PELVIS ORGANS OR SOFT TISSUE ABNORMALITY
763.89 PELVIS ORGANS SURGERY PREVIOUS
763.1 PELVIS ROBERT'S
763.89 PENDULOUS ABDOMEN
761.4 PERITONEAL PREGNANCY
763.1 PERSISTENT OCCIPITOPOSTERIOR POSITION
762.1 PLACENTA DAMAGE
762.2 PLACENTA INFARCTION
762.0 PLACENTA PREVIA
762.3 PLACENTA TRANSFUSION SYNDROMES
762.7 PLACENTITIS
762.3 POLYCYTHEMIA NEONATORUM PLACENTAL TRANSFUSION [776.4]
761.3 POLYHYDRAMNIOS
763.6 PRECIPITATE DELIVERY
760.0 PRE-ECLAMPSIA
761.1 PREMATURE RUPTURE OF MEMBRANES
760.3 RESPIRATORY DISEASE MATERNAL CHRONIC
762.1 RUPTURE MARGINAL SINUS

MATERNAL DISORDERS AFFECTING FETUS OR NEWBORN (continued)

IN ORDER TO USE THE FOLLOWING CODES, THE MEDICAL RECORD MUST SPECIFY THAT THE MATERNAL CONDITION IS A CAUSE OF MORBIDITY OR MORTALITY IN THE FETUS OR NEWBORN. THE MERE FACT THAT THE CONDITION EXISTED IN THE MOTHER OR COMPLICATED THE PREGNANCY DOES NOT WARRANT THE USE OF THESE CODES ON THE NEWBORN'S RECORD. REMEMBER, CODES 760-763 APPLY ONLY TO THE INFANT AND ARE NEVER ASSIGNED TO THE MOTHER'S RECORD. CONVERSELY, NEVER CODE THE MOTHER'S CONDITION WITH THESE FETAL/NEWBORN CODES.

760.8 SALPINGITIS
763.1 SHOULDER DYSTOCIA
763.1 SHOULDER PRESENTATION
763.1 SPONDYLOLISTHESIS
763.1 SPONDYLOLYSIS
760.6 SURGERY MATERNAL
762.1 SURGICAL INDUCTION WITH DAMAGE TO PLACENTA
760.70 TOXIC SUBSTANCE NOS TRANSMITTED VIA PLACENTA OR BREAST MILK
760.79 TOXIC SUBSTANCE NEC TRANSMITTED VIA PLACENTA OR BREAST MILK
763.5 TRANQUILIZER REACTION (MATERNAL)
761.7 TRANSVERSE LIE BEFORE LABOR AND DELIVERY
763.1 TRANSVERSE LIE-PRESENTATION DURING LABOR AND DELIVERY
761.5 TRIPLET PREGNANCY
761.4 TUBAL PREGNANCY
761.5 TWIN PREGNANCY
762.5 UMBILICAL CORD ENTANGLEMENT (CORD AROUND NECK, KNOT, TORSION)
762.4 UMBILICAL CORD PROLAPSE (PRESENTATION)
762.6 UMBILICAL CORD OTHER AND UNSPECIFIED CONDITIONS
761.7 UNSTABLE LIE BEFORE LABOR AND DELIVERY
760.1 URINARY TRACT DISEASES MATERNAL
763.89 UTERUS ABNORMALITY
763.89 UTERUS ABSCESS (TO ABDOMINAL WALL)
763.89 UTERUS ADHESION
763.89 UTERUS BICORNIS/DOUBLE
763.89 UTERUS BODY POLYP (CORPUS) (MUCOUS)
763.7 UTERUS CONTRACTIONS ABNORMAL
763.7 UTERUS HYPERTONIC/HYPOTONIC
763.7 UTERUS INERTIA-DYSFUNCTION
763.89 UTERUS PERFORATION WITH OBSTETRICAL TRAUMA
763.1 UTERUS PROLAPSE
763.89 UTERUS RUPTURE
763.1 UTERUS SACCULATION
763.89 UTERUS SHAPE ABNORMALITY
763.89 UTERUS SURGERY PREVIOUS
763.89 UTERUS VERSION
763.3 VACUUM EXTRACTOR DELIVERY
763.3 VACUUM RUPTURE
763.89 VAGINA ABNORMALITY
763.89 VAGINA STENOSIS/STRICTURE
763.1 VAGINA STENOSIS/STRICTURE OBSTRUCTING LABOR
760.8 VAGINITIS
763.89 VULVA ABNORMALITY
762.8 OTHER SPECIFIED ABNORMALITIES OF CHORION AND AMNION
761.8 OTHER SPECIFIED COMPLICATIONS - DUE TO CURRENT PREGNANCY
760.8 OTHER SPECIFIED CONDITIONS - UNRELATED TO CURRENT PREGNANCY
762.6 OTHER SPECIFIED CONDITIONS OF UMBILICAL CORD
763.89 OTHER SPECIFIED DISORDER - DUE TO LABOR AND DELIVERY

315.1 MATHEMATICS DEVELOPMENTAL DELAY

100.0 MATHIEU'S DISEASE (LEPTOSPIRAL JAUNDICE)

732.3 MAUCLAIRE'S DISEASE

091.3 MAURIAC'S DISEASE (ERYTHEMA NODOSUM SYPHILITICUM)

081.0 MAXCY'S DISEASE

MAXILLA, MAXILLARY
524.09 ABSENCE (CONGENITAL)
524.71 ALVEOLAR HYPERPLASIA
524.73 ALVEOLAR HYPOPLASIA
524.11 ASYMMETRY
524.01 HYPERPLASIA
524.03 HYPOPLASIA
959.09 INJURY
461.0 SINUS (ABSCESS) (INFECTION) (INFLAMMATION) ACUTE

288.2 MAY HEGGLIN SYNDROME
066.3 MAYARO FEVER (VIRAL)
610.8 MAZOPLASIA (MAMMARY)
271.0 MCARDLE'S (-SCHMID) (-PEARSON) DISEASE OR SYNDROME (GLYCOGENOSIS V)
756.59 MCCUNE-ALBRIGHT SYNDROME (OSTEITIS FIBROSA DISSEMINATA)
446.1 MCLS
648.9# MCLS MATERNAL CURRENT (CO-EXISTENT) IN PREGNANCY [446.1]

5th Digit: 648.9
0. EPISODE OF NOS OR N/A
1. DELIVERED
2. DELIVERED WITH POSTPARTUM COMPLICATION
3. ANTEPARTUM COMPLICATION
4. POSTPARTUM COMPLICATION

251.2 MCQUARRIE'S SYNDROME (IDIOPATHIC FAMILIAL HYPOGLYCEMIA)

MEASLES
055.9 NOS WITHOUT COMPLICATION
055.79 COMPLICATION OTHER (RUBEOLA MOBILLI)
055.8 COMPLICATION UNSPECIFIED (RUBEOLA MOBILLI)
055.0 ENCEPHALITIS (RUBEOLA)
V01.7 EXPOSURE
0 GERMAN SEE 'RUBELLA'
055.71 KERATITIS (RUBEOLA MOBILLI)
055.71 KERATOCONJUNCTIVITIS (RUBEOLA MOBILLI)
139.8 LATE EFFECT
647.6# MATERNAL COMPLICATING PREGNANCY **[055.#]**

5th Digit: 647.6
0. EPISODE OF CARE UNSPECIFIED OR N/A
1. DELIVERED
2. DELIVERED WITH POSTPARTUM COMPLICATION
3. ANTEPARTUM COMPLICATION
4. POSTPARTUM COMPLICATION

4th or 4th and 5th Digit: 055
0. POSTMEASLES ENCEPHALITIS
1. POSTMEASLES PNEUMONIA
2. POSTMEASLES OTITIS MEDIA
7#. OTHER SPECIFIED COMPLICATIONS
1. MEASLES KERATOCONJUNCTIVITIS
9. OTHER SPECIFIED COMPLICATION
8. UNSPECIFIED COMPLICATION
9. WITHOUT MENTION OF COMPLICATION

055.2 OTITIS MEDIA (RUBEOLA)
055.1 PNEUMONIA (RUBEOLA)
V73.2 SCREENING EXAM
V04.2 VACCINATION MEASLES ALONE
V06.4 VACCINATION MEASLES, MUMPS, RUBELLA (MMR)

753.6 MEATUS URINARIUS ATRESIA (CONGENITAL)
751.0 MECKEL'S DIVERTICULUM CONGENITAL

MECONIUM
770.1 ASPIRATION SYNDROME
777.1 ILEUS NEWBORN
277.01 ILEUS WITH CYSTIC FIBROSIS

MECONIUM (continued)

792.3 IN LIQUOR
656.8# IN LIQUOR FETAL AFFECTING MANAGEMENT OF MOTHER
5th Digit: 656.8
0. EPISODE OF CARE UNSPECIFIED OR N/A
1. DELIVERED
3. ANTEPARTUM COMPLICATION

777.1 OBSTRUCTION NEWBORN DUE TO FECALITHS
277.01 OBSTRUCTION NEWBORN IN MUCOVISCIDOSIS
792.3 PASSAGE
777.1 PASSAGE DELAYED, NEWBORN
777.6 PERITONITIS
777.1 PLUG SYNDROME

440.20 MEDIAL CALCIFICATION

MEDIAL COLLATERAL LIGAMENT

717.82 DISRUPTION (OLD)
717.9 RELAXATION
844.1 TEAR (STRAIN)(RUPTURE) ACUTE

726.31 MEDIAL EPICONDYLITIS

MEDIAL MENISCUS

836.0 TEAR KNEE ACUTE
836.0 BUCKET HANDLE TEAR ACUTE
717.0 BUCKET HANDLE TEAR OLD
717.1 DERANGEMENT (KNEE) ANTERIOR HORN (OLD)
717.2 DERANGEMENT (KNEE) POSTERIOR HORN (OLD)
717.3 DERANGEMENT (KNEE) OTHER OR UNSPECIFIED (OLD)

MEDIAN

526.1 ANTERIOR MAXILLARY CYST
447.4 ARCUATE LIGAMENT SYNDROME
526.1 PALATAL CYST

MEDIAN NERVE

526.1 ANTERIOR MAXILLARY CYST
447.4 ARCUATE LIGAMENT SYNDROME
354.0 CARPAL TUNNEL NEURITIS (NEURALGIA) (RADICULITIS)
354.1 DISORDER NEC
354.0 ENTRAPMENT
955.1 INJURY
354.1 NEURITIS

0 MEDIASTINAL SEE 'MEDIASTINUM, MEDIASTINAL'
519.2 MEDIASTINITIS

MEDIASTINOPERICARDITIS

420.90 ACUTE
391.0 ACUTE RHEUMATIC
393 CHRONIC RHEUMATIC

MEDIASTINUM, MEDIASTINAL

785.6 ADENOPATHY
442.89 ARTERY (ANEURYSM) (A-V FISTULA) (CIRSOID) (FALSE) (VARICOSE) (RUPTURED)
519.3 DISEASE NEC
519.3 FIBROSIS SYNDROME
519.3 HERNIA
862.29 INJURY TRAUMATIC
862.39 INJURY TRAUMATIC WITH OPEN WOUND
519.3 OBSTRUCTION
519.3 RETRACTION
793.2 SHIFT (CXR)

MEDICAL

V68.0 CERTIFICATE ISSUE OF
V70.0 EXAM ROUTINE GENERAL
0 EXAM SEE 'EXAM'
V15.81 TREATMENT NONCOMPLIANCE HISTORY

MEDICAL CARE UNAVAILABLE

V63.9 UNSPECIFIED
V63.2 AWAITING CARE ELSEWHERE
V60.4 HOUSEHOLD MEMBER UNABLE TO RENDER CARE
V63.1 IN HOME
V63.0 NO OTHER FACILITY
V63.8 OTHER SPECIFIED REASON
V63.0 RESIDENCE TOO REMOTE

0 MEDICATION ERROR SEE 'POISONING'

ANTIBIOTICS, COUMADIN, DIGOXIN, CHEMOTHERAPY DRUGS, AND ANY OTHER DRUGS WITH A RISK OF ADVERSE REACTIONS ARE CONSIDERED TO BE HIGH-RISK MEDICATIONS. CODES V58.61, V58.62 AND V58.69 ARE TO BE USED TO IDENTIFY PATIENTS THAT ARE CURRENTLY BEING MONITORED WHILE TAKING HIGH RISK MEDICATION. CODE V67.51 IS TO BE USED TO IDENTIFY PATIENTS THAT HAVE COMPLETED HIGH RISK MEDICATION THERAPY.

V67.51 MEDICATION HIGH RISK FOLLOWUP - COMPLETED THERAPY
V58.62 MEDICATION HIGH RISK MANAGEMENT - ANTIBIOTICS CURRENT THERAPY
V58.61 MEDICATION HIGH RISK MANAGEMENT - ANTICOAGULANT CURRENT THERAPY
V58.69 MEDICATION HIGH RISK MANAGEMENT - OTHER CURRENT THERAPY

V68.1 MEDICATION REPEAT PRESCRIPTION
760.79 MEDICINAL AGENTS NEC TRANSMITTED VIA PLACENTA OR BREAST MILK AFFECTING FETUS OR NEWBORN

045.9# MEDIN'S DISEASE (POLIOMYELITIS)
5th Digit: 045.9
0. UNSPECIFIED
1. TYPE I
2. TYPE II
3. TYPE III

MEDITERRANEAN

282.4 ANEMIA
282.4 DISEASE WITH HEMOGLOBINOPATHY
0 FEVER SEE 'BRUCELLA'
082.1 TICK FEVER

MEDULLARY

193 CARCINOMA SITE NOS
0 CARCINOMA SITE SPECIFIED SEE 'CANCER' BY SITE M8510/3
193 CARCINOMA WITH AMYLOID STROMA SITE NOS
0 CARCINOMA WITH AMYLOID STROMA SITE SPECIFIED SEE 'CANCER' BY SITE M8511/3
174.9 CARCINOMA WITH LYMPHOID STROMA SITE NOS
0 CARCINOMA WITH LYMPHOID STROMA SITE SPECIFIED SEE 'CANCER' BY SITE M8512/3
348.8 CENTER DISEASE (IDIOPATHIC) (RESPIRATORY)
255.8 HYPERPLASIA (ADRENAL)
284.9 HYPOPLASIA NOS
344.89 PARALYSIS (TEGMENTAL)

MEDULLOBLASTOMA

191.6 SITE NOS
0 SITE SPECIFIED SEE 'CANCER' BY SITE M9470/3
191.6 DESMOPLASTIC SITE NOS
0 DESMOPLASTIC SITE SPECIFIED SEE 'CANCER' BY SITE M9471/3

MEDULLOEPITHELIOMA

199.1 SITE NOS
0 SITE SPECIFIED SEE 'CANCER' BY SITE M9501/3
199.1 TERATOID SITE NOS
0 TERATOID SITE SPECIFIED SEE 'CANCER' BY SITE M9502/3

M

191.6 MEDULLOMYOBLASTOMA SITE NOS

0 MEDULLOMYOBLASTOMA SITE SPECIFIED SEE 'CANCER' BY SITE M9472/3

756.83 MEEKEREN-EHLERS-DANLOS SYNDROME

MEGACOLON

564.7 NOS

751.3 CONGENITAL

564.7 FUNCTIONAL

751.3 HIRSCHSPRUNG'S

556.5 TOXIC

530.0 MEGAESOPHAGUS

MEGAKARYOCYTIC

287.3 HYPOPLASIA

238.7 MYELOSCLEROSIS UNCERTAIN BEHAVIOR

207.2# MYELOSIS M9920/3

5th Digit: 207.2

0. WITHOUT MENTION OF REMISSION

1. IN REMISSION

742.4 MEGALENCEPHALY CONGENITAL

751.5 MEGALOAPPENDIX CONGENITAL

751.5 MEGALODUODENUM CONGENITAL

750.7 MEGALOGASTRIA DUPLICATION CONGENITAL

753.22 MEGALOURETER CONGENITAL

MEIBOMIAN

373.2 GLAND CYST

373.12 GLAND CYST INFECTED

373.12 GLAND INFECTION

757.0 MEIGE-MILROY DISEASE OR SYNDROME (CHRONIC HEREDITARY EDEMA)

333.82 MEIGE SYNDROME (BELPHAROSPASM-OROMANDIBULAR DYSTONIA)

296.90 MELANCHOLIA (PSYCHOSIS)

648.4# MELANCHOLIA MATERNAL CURRENT (CO-EXISTENT) IN PREGNANCY RECURRENT (PSYCHOSIS) [**296.3#**]

648.4# MELANCHOLIA MATERNAL CURRENT (CO-EXISTENT) IN PREGNANCY SINGLE EPISODE (PSYCHOSIS) [**296.2#**]

5th Digit: 648.4

0. EPISODE OF CARE UNSPECIFIED OR N/A

1. DELIVERED

2. DELIVERED WITH POSTPARTUM COMPLICATION

3. ANTEPARTUM COMPLICATION

4. POSTPARTUM COMPLICATION

5th Digit: 296.2, 3

0. UNSPECIFIED

1. MILD

2. MODERATE

3. SEVERE WITHOUT MENTION OF PSYCHOTIC BEHAVIOR

4. SEVERE SPECIFIED AS WITH PSYCHOTIC BEHAVIOR

5. IN PARTIAL OR UNSPECIFIED REMISSION

6. IN FULL REMISSION

791.9 MELANIN URINE ABNORMAL

172.# MELANOCARCINOMA M8720/3

4th Digit: 172

0. LIP

1. EYELID CANTHUS

2. EAR (AURICLE) AURICULAR CANAL (EXTERNAL) EXTERNAL (ACOUSTIC) MEATUS PINNA

3. UNSPECIFIED PARTS OF FACE CHEEK (EXTERNAL) CHIN EYEBROW FOREHEAD NOSE (EXT) TEMPLE

4. SCALP AND NECK

5. TRUNK AXILLA BREAST BUTTOCK GROIN PERIANAL SKIN PERINEUM UMBILICUS

6. UPPER LIMB SHOULDER

7. LOWER LIMB HIP

8. OTHER SPECIFIED SKIN SITES CONTIGUOUS OR OVERLAPPING UNDETERMINED POINT OF ORIGIN

9. SITE UNSPECIFIED

253.4 MELANOCYTE-STIMULATING HORMONE DEFICIENCY

253.1 MELANOCYTE-STIMULATING HORMONE OVERPRODUCTION

709.09 MELANODERMA

521.0 MELANODONTIA INFANTILE

MELANOMA BY CELL TYPE

172.# MELANOMA M8720/3

172.# AMELANOTIC M8730/3

172.# BALLOON CELL M8722/3

172.# EPITHELIOID AND SPINDLE CELL (MIXED) M8775/3

172.# EPITHELIOID CELL M8771/3

172.# IN GIANT PIGMENTED NEVUS M8761/3

172.# IN HUTCHINSON'S MELANOTIC FRECKLE M8742/3

172.# IN JUNCTIONAL NEVUS (MALIGNANT) M8740/3

172.# IN PRECANCEROUS MELANOSIS M8741/3 (MALIGNANT)

0 JUVENILE SEE 'BENIGN NEOPLASM', SKIN, BY SITE M8770/0

172.# NODULAR M8721/3

172.# SPINDLE CELL M8772/3

4th Digit: 172

0. LIP

1. EYELID CANTHUS

2. EAR (AURICLE) AURICULAR CANAL (EXTERNAL) (ACOUSTIC) MEATUS PINNA

3. UNSPECIFIED PARTS OF FACE CHEEK (CHIN EYEBROW FOREHEAD NOSE (EXT) TEMPLE

4. SCALP AND NECK

5. TRUNK AXILLA BREAST GROIN PERIANAL SKIN PERINEUM UMBILICUS

6. UPPER LIMB SHOULDER

7. LOWER LIMB HIP

8. OTHER SPECIFIED SKIN SITES CONTIGUOUS OR OVERLAPPING UNDETERMINED POINT OF ORIGIN

9. SITE UNSPECIFIED

190.0 SPINDLE CELL TYPE A SITE NOS M8773/3

190.0 SPINDLE CELL TYPE B SITE NOS M8774/3

172.# SUPERFICIAL SPREADING M8743/3

4th Digit: 172

0. LIP

1. EYELID CANTHUS

2. EAR (AURICLE) AURICULAR CANAL (EXTERNAL) (ACOUSTIC) MEATUS PINNA

3. UNSPECIFIED PARTS OF FACE CHEEK (CHIN EYEBROW FOREHEAD NOSE (EXT) TEMPLE

4. SCALP AND NECK

5. TRUNK AXILLA BREAST GROIN PERIANAL SKIN PERINEUM UMBILICUS

6. UPPER LIMB SHOULDER

7. LOWER LIMB HIP

8. OTHER SPECIFIED SKIN SITES CONTIGUOUS OR OVERLAPPING UNDETERMINED POINT OF ORIGIN

9. SITE UNSPECIFIED

MELANOMA BY SITE

172.5 ABDOMINAL WALL

172.7 ANKLE SKIN

154.3 ANUS

154.2 ANUS CANAL

172.5 ANUS SKIN

172.6 ARM SKIN

172.2 AURICLE CANAL

172.5 AXILLA SKIN

172.5 BACK SKIN

172.5 BREAST SKIN

172.5 BUTTOCK SKIN

172.3 CHEEK (EXTERNAL) (SKIN)

172.5 CHEST WALL

172.3 CHIN (SKIN)

172.2 EAR MEATUS EXTERNAL

172.2 EAR SKIN

172.2 EXTERNAL AUDITORY CANAL SKIN

0 EYE SEE 'CANCER' EYE

172.3 EYEBROW (SKIN)

MELANOMA BY SITE (continued)

172.1 EYELID
172.1 EYELID INCLUDING CANTHUS SKIN
172.3 FACE SKIN
172.6 FINGER SKIN
172.6 FINGERNAIL NEC
172.5 FLANK
172.7 FOOT SKIN
172.6 FOREARM SKIN
172.3 FOREHEAD (SKIN)
187.1 FORESKIN
184.4 GENITALS FEMALE EXTERNAL
187.9 GENTALS MALE
172.5 GROIN
172.6 HAND SKIN
172.7 HEEL SKIN
172.2 HELIX
172.7 HIP SKIN
172.5 INTRASCAPULAR
172.3 JAW
172.7 KNEE SKIN
184.1 LABIUM MAJUS
184.2 LABIUM MINUS
172.7 LEG SKIN
140.1 LIP LOWER VERMILION BORDER
140.0 LIP NOS VERMILION BORDER
140.0 LIP UPPER VERMILION BORDER
172.0 LIP SKIN
172.7 LOWER LIMB SKIN
172.1 MEIBOMIAN GLAND
172.4 NECK (SKIN)
172.3 NOSE (EXTERNAL) (SKIN)
172.8 OVERLAPPING SITES SKIN
187.4 PENIS
172.5 PERIANAL SKIN
172.5 PERINEUM SKIN
172.2 PINNA (SKIN)
172.7 POPLITEAL AREA SKIN
187.1 PREPUCE
172.5 PUBIS
184.4 PUDENDUM
172.4 SCALP (SKIN)
187.7 SCROTUM
172.3 SEPTUM NASAL
172.6 SHOULDER SKIN
172.8 SKIN OTHER
172.5 SUBMAMMARY FOLD
172.9 SUPERFICIAL SPREADING SITE UNSPECIFIED
172.3 TEMPLE (SKIN)
172.7 THIGH SKIN
172.7 TOENAIL
172.7 TOE SKIN
172.5 TRUNK SKIN
172.5 UMBILICUS SKIN
172.6 UPPER LIMB SKIN
184.0 VAGINAL VAULT
184.4 VULVA

528.9 MELANOPLAKIA

MELANOSIS

255.4 ADDISONIAN
017.6# ADDISONIAN TUBERCULOUS

5th Digit: 017.6

0. NOS
1. LAB NOT DONE
2. LABS PENDING
3. MICROSCOPY POSITIVE (IN SPUTUM)
4. CULTURE POSITIVE - MICROSCOPY NEGATIVE
5. CULTURE NEGATIVE - MICROSCOPY POSITIVE
6. CULTURE AND MICROSCOPY NEGATIVE CONFIRMED BY OTHER METHODS

MELANOSIS (continued)

255.4 ADRENAL
569.89 COLON
372.55 CONJUNCTIVA
743.49 CONJUNCTIVA CONGENITAL
757.33 CORII DEGENERATIVA
371.12 CORNEA
743.43 CORNEA CONGENITAL
743.42 CORNEA CONGENITAL INTERFERING WITH VISION
743.43 CORNEA PRENATAL
743.42 CORNEA PRENATAL INTERFERING WITH VISION
372.55 EYE
743.49 EYE CONGENITAL
709.09 JUTE SPINNERS'
757.33 LENTICULARIS PROGRESSIVA
573.8 LIVER
232.9 PRECANCEROUS SITE NOS
0 PRECANCEROUS SITE SPECIFIED SEE 'CA IN SITU' SKIN BY SITE M8741/2
709.09 RIEHL'S
379.19 SCLERA
743.47 SCLERA CONGENITAL
255.4 SUPRARENAL
709.09 TAR
709.09 TOXIC

229.9 MELANOTIC NEUROECTODERMAL TUMOR SITE NOS
0 MELANOTIC NEUROECTODERMAL TUMOR SITE SPECIFIED SEE 'BENIGN NEOPLASM', BY SITE M9363/0

791.9 MELANURIA

758.89 MELAS SYNDROME
709.09 MELASMA

578.1 MELENA
777.3 MELENA DUE TO SWALLOWED MATERNAL BLOOD
772.4 MELENA PERINATAL

686.09 MELENEY'S GANGRENE OR ULCER (CHRONIC UNDERMINING)
025 MELIOIDOSIS
351.8 MELKERSSON'S (-ROSENTHAL) SYNDROME

762.7 MEMBRANITIS AFFECTING FETUS OR NEWBORN
0 MEMBRANITIS SEE 'AMNIONITIS'

464.4 MEMBRANOUS ANGINA
581.1 MEMBRANOUS GLOMERULAR DISEASE IDIOPATHIC

780.9 MEMORY DISTURBANCE (LOSS)
310.1 MEMORY DISTURBANCE MILD ORGANIC

270.2 MENDE'S SYNDROME (PTOSIS-EPICANTHUS)
668.0# MENDELSON'S SYNDROME DURING LABOR

5th Digit: 668.0

0. EPISODE OF CARE NOS OR N/A
1. DELIVERED
2. DELIVERED WITH POSTPARTUM COMPLICATION
3. ANTEPARTUM COMPLICATION
4. POSTPARTUM COMPLICATION

997.3 MENDELSON'S SYNDROME RESULTING FROM A PROCEDURE
535.2 MENETRIER'S SYNDROME (HYPERTROPHIC GASTRITIS)

MENIERE'S DISEASE (SYNDROME)

386.00 ACTIVE NOS
386.02 ACTIVE COCHLEAR
386.01 ACTIVE COCHLEOVESTIBULAR
386.03 ACTIVE VESTIBULAR
386.04 IN REMISSION

349.2 MENINGEAL ADHESIONS (CEREBRAL) (SPINAL)
349.2 MENINGEAL CALCIFICATION (CEREBRAL)
0 MENINGEAL DISEASE SEE 'MENINGITIS'

088.81 MENINGIOENCEPHALITIS DUE TO LYME DISEASE [320.7]

MENINGIOMA

225.2 SITE NOS
0 SITE SPECIFIED SEE 'BENIGN NEOPLASM', BY SITE M9530/0

225.2 ANGIOMATOUS SITE NOS
0 ANGIOMATOUS SITE SPECIFIED SEE 'BENIGN NEOPLASM', BY SITE M9534/0

225.2 FIBROUS SITE NOS
0 FIBROUS SITE SPECIFIED SEE 'BENIGN NEOPLASM', BY SITE M9532/0

225.2 HEMANGIOBLASTIC SITE NOS
0 HEMANGIOBLASTIC SITE SPECIFIED SEE 'BENIGN NEOPLASM', BY SITE M9535/0
225.2 HEMANGIOPERICYTIC SITE NOS
0 HEMANGIOPERICYTIC SITE SPECIFIED SEE 'BENIGN NEOPLASM', BY SITE M9536/0

192.1 MALIGNANT SITE NOS
0 MALIGNANT SITE SPECIFIED SEE 'CANCER' BY SITE M9530/3
225.2 MENINGOTHELIOMATOUS SITE NOS
0 MENINGOTHELIOMATOUS SITE SPECIFIED SEE 'BENIGN NEOPLASM', BY SITE M9531/0

237.6 PAPILLARY SITE NOS
0 PAPILLARY SITE SPECIFIED SEE 'NEOPLASM UNCERTAIN BEHAVIOR' BY SITE M9538/1
225.2 PSAMMOMATOUS SITE NOS
0 PSAMMOMATOUS SITE SPECIFIED SEE 'BENIGN NEOPLASM', BY SITE M9533/0

225.2 TRANSITIONAL SITE NOS
0 TRANSITIONAL SITE SPECIFIED SEE 'BENIGN NEOPLASM', BY SITE M9537/0

237.6 MENINGIOMATOSIS SITE NOS
0 MENINGIOMATOSIS SITE SPECIFIED SEE 'NEOPLASM UNCERTAIN BEHAVIOR' BY SITE M9530/1

781.6 MENINGISM

781.6 MENINGISMUS (INFECTIONAL) (PNEUMOCOCCAL)
997.09 MENINGISMUS (INFECTIONAL) (PNEUMOCOCCAL) DUE TO SERUM OR VACCINE [321.8]

THE CODE IN THE LEFT MARGIN ALWAYS SEQUENCES FIRST. THE ADDITIONAL CODE IN BRACKETS TO THE RIGHT OF THE DESCRIPTION IS SEQUENCED SECONDARILY. UNDERLINING SHOWS THE CODE NUMBER THAT CORRESPONDS TO THE UNDERLINED VERBAL DESCRIPTION. UNDERLINING NEVER IMPLIES CORRECT SEQUENCING.

MENINGITIS

322.9 UNSPECIFIED
047.9 ABACTERIAL SEE ALSO 'MENINGITIS', BY SPECIFIC VIRUS
049.1 ADENOVIRUS
320.82 AEROBACTER AEROGENES
320.81 ANAEROBIC (GRAM-NEGATIVE)
047.9 ASEPTIC
088.81 ASEPTIC DUE TO LYME DISEASE [320.7]
322.0 ASEPTIC NONINFECTIVE
320.89 BACILLUS PYOCYANEUS
320.9 BACTERIAL
320.81 BACTEROIDES (FRAGILIS) (ORALIS) (MALANINOGENICUS)
036.0 CEREBROSPINAL
V02.59 CEREBROSPINAL CARRIER (SUSPECTED OF)
322.2 CHRONIC, CAUSE UNSPECIFIED
320.81 CLOSTRIDIUM (HAEMOLYTICUM) (NOVYI) NEC
047.0 COXSACKIE VIRUS
997.09 DUE TO VACCINATION [321.8]

MENINGITIS (continued)

320.82 E COLI [041.4]
047.1 ECHO VIRUS
320.82 ENTEROBACTER AEROGENES
322.1 EOSINOPHILIC
036.0 EPIDEMIC
320.81 EUBACTERIUM
320.89 EUBACTERIUM FIBRINOPURULENT SPECIFIED NEC
320.89 FIBRINOPURULENT NEC
320.82 FRIEDLANDER BACILLUS [041.3]
320.81 FUSOBACTERIUM
098.82 GONOCOCCAL
320.81 GRAM-NEGATIVE ANAEROBES [041.84]
320.82 GRAM-NEGATIVE BACTERIA NEC [041.85]
036.0 GRAM-NEGATIVE COCCI
320.82 GRAM-NEGATIVE COCCI SPECIFIED NEC
320.0 HEMOPHILUS [041.5]
054.72 HERPES SIMPLEX
053.0 HERPES ZOSTER
320.82 KLEBSIELLA PNEUMONIAE [041.3]
326 LATE EFFECT
100.81 LEPTOSPIRAL (ASEPTIC)
027.0 LISTERIOSIS [320.7]
049.0 LYMPHOCYTIC
036.0 MENINGOCOCCAL
047.1 MENINGO -ERUPTIVE SYNDROME
320.82 MIMA POLYMORPHA
072.1 MUMPS
321.8 NONBACTERIAL ORGANISMS CLASSIFIED ELSEWHERE [100.81]
322.0 NONPYOGENIC
320.81 PEPTOCOCCUS
320.81 PEPTOSTREPTOCOCCUS
033.0 PERTUSSIS [320.7]
320.1 PNEUMOCOCCAL [041.2]
320.81 PROPRIONIBACTERIUM
320.82 PROTEUS MORGANII [041.6]
320.82 PSEUDOMONAS [041.7]
320.89 PURULENT SPECIFIED ORGANISM NEC
320.89 PYOGENIC SPECIFIED ORGANISM NEC
003.21 SALMONELLA
135 SARCOID [321.4]
320.89 SEPTIC SPECIFIED ORGANISM NEC
320.82 SERRATIA (MARCESCENS)
320.3 STAPHYLOCOCCAL **[041.1#]**

5th Digit: 041.1

0. NOS
1. AUREUS
9. OTHER STAPH

997.09 STERILE
320.2 STREPTOCOCCAL **[041.0#]**

5th Digit: 041.0

0. NOS
1. GROUP A
2. GROUP B
3. GROUP C
4. GROUP D (ENTEROCOCCUS)
5. GROUP G
9. OTHER STREP

320.89 SUPPURATIVE SPECIFIED ORGANISM NEC
094.2 SYPHILITIC
091.81 SYPHILITIC ACUTE SECONDARY
090.42 SYPHILITIC (CONGENITAL)
094.2 SYPHILITIC MENINGOVASCULAR
111.2 TINEA BLANCA [321.1]
111.1 TINEA NIGRA [321.1]
111.0 TINEA VERSICOLOR [321.1]
320.81 TREPONEMA (DENTICOLA) (MACRODENTICUM)
110.8 TRICHOPHYTON [321.1]
086.9 TRYPANASOMAL [321.3]

MENINGITIS (continued)

013.0# TUBERCULOSIS
- **5th Digit: 013.0**
  - **0. UNSPECIFIED**
  - **1. LAB NOT DONE**
  - **2. LABS PENDING**
  - **3. MICROSCOPY POSITIVE (IN SPUTUM)**
  - **4. CULTURE POSITIVE - MICROSCOPY NEGATIVE**
  - **5. CULTURE NEGATIVE - MICROSCOPY POSITIVE**
  - **6. CULTURE AND MICROSCOPY NEGATIVE CONFIRMED BY OTHER METHODS**

002.0 TYPHOID [320.7]
997.09 VACCINATION COMPLICATION [321.8]
320.81 VEILLONELLA
320.82 VIBRIO VULNIFICUS
047.9 VIRAL UNSPECIFIED
321.2 VIRAL NOT ELSEWHERE CLASSIFIED
047.8 VIRAL OTHER SPECIFIED
033.0 WHOOPING COUGH [320.7]
322.0 WITH CLEAR CEREBROSPINAL FLUID

MENINGITIS OTHER SPECIFIED

039.8 ACTINOMYCOTIC [320.7]
117.6 ALLESCHERIOSIS [321.1]
117.3 ASPERGILLOSIS [321.1]
111.3 BLACK PIEDRA [321.1]
116.0 BLASTOMYCOTIC [321.1]
112.83 CANDIDAL
117.2 CHROMOBLASTOMYCOTIC [321.1]
117.5 CRYPTOCOCCAL [321.0]
114.2 COCCIDIOIDOMYCOSIS
117.8 DEMATIACIOUS FUNGI [321.1]
111.9 DERMATOMYCOSIS [321.1]
110.# DERMATOPHYTOSIS [321.1]
- **4th Digit: 110**
  - **0. SCALP AND BEARD**
  - **1. NAIL (UNGUIUM)**
  - **2. HAND (MANUUM)**
  - **3. GROIN AND PERIANAL (CRURIS)**
  - **4. FOOT (PEDIS)**
  - **5. BODY (CORPORUS)**
  - **6. DEEP SEATED (GRANULOMA TRICHOPHYTICUM)**
  - **8. OTHER SPECIFIED SITE**
  - **9. UNSPECIFIED SITE**

110.8 EPIDERMOPHYTON [321.1]
115.91 HISTOPLASMA
115.01 HISTOPLASMA CAPSULATUM
115.11 HISTOPLASMA DUBOISII
116.2 LOBOMYCOTIC [321.1]
110.8 MICROSPORUM [321.1]
117.9 MYCOTIC NOS [321.1]
117.4 MYCOTIC MYCETOMAS [321.1]
110.1 NAIL FUNGAL DISEASE [321.1]
116.1 PARACOCCIDIOIDOMYCOTIC [321.1]
117.8 PHAEHYPHOMYCOTIC [321.1]
111.0 PITYRIASIS VERSICOLOR [321.1]
045.2# POLIOVIRUS ACUTE NONPARALYTIC [321.2]
- **5th Digit: 045.2**
  - **0. POLIOVIRUS UNSPECIFIED**
  - **1. POLIOVIRUS TYPE I**
  - **2. POLIOVIRUS TYPE II**
  - **3. POLIOVIRUS TYPE III**

117.0 RHINOSPORIDIOSIS [321.1]
117.1 SPOROTRICHOSIS [321.1]

MENINGITIS OTHER SPECIFIED (continued)

086.# TRYPANASOMAL [321.3]
- **4th Digit: 086**
  - **0. AMERICAN WITH HEART INVOLVEMENT**
  - **1. AMERICAN WITH INVOLVEMENT OF ORGAN OTHER THAN HEART**
  - **2. AMERICAN NOS**
  - **3. GAMBIAN**
  - **4. RHODESIAN**
  - **5. AFRICAN NOS**
  - **9. NOS**

117.7 ZYGOMATIC (PHYCOMOSIS) (MUCORMYCOSIS) [321.1]

047.1 MENINGO ERUPTIVE SYNDROME

MENINGOCELE

349.2 ACQUIRED
742.0 CEREBRAL CONGENITAL
741.9# SPINAL
741.0# WITH HYDROCEPHALUS
741.9# WITHOUT HYDROCEPHALUS
- **5th Digit: 741.0,9**
  - **0. REGION NOS**
  - **1. CERVICAL**
  - **2. DORSAL**
  - **3. LUMBAR**

MENINGOCOCCAL

036.3 ADRENAL SYNDROME
036.82 ARTHRITIS
036.40 CARDITIS
V02.59 CARRIER (SUSPECTED OF)
036.1 ENCEPHALITIS
036.42 ENDOCARDITIS
V01.8 EXPOSURE
036.3 HEMORRHAGIC ADRENALITIS
036.0 MENINGITIS
036.2 MENINGOCOCCEMIA
036.43 MYOCARDITIS
036.81 OPTIC NEURITIS
036.41 PERICARDITIS
036.2 SEPSIS
036.3 WATERHOUSE FRIDERICHSEN SYNDROME
036.9 INFECTION
036.89 INFECTIONS OTHER

036.2 MENINGOCOCCEMIA

MENINGOENCEPHALITIS

323.9 NOS
048 ACUTE NEC
039.8 ACTINOMYCOSIS [320.7]
0 BACTERIAL, PURULENT, PYOGENIC, OR SEPTIC SEE 'MENINGITIS'
116.0 BLASTOMYCOSIS [323.4]
094.1 CHRONIC NEC
094.1 DIFFUSE NEC
063.2 DIPHASIC
036.0 EPIDEMIC
136.2 FREE LIVING AMEBAE
054.3 HERPES
048 INFECTIOUS (ACUTE)
320.0 INFLUENZAL
027.0 LISTERIA MONOCYTOGENES [320.7]
088.81 LYME DISEASE [320.7]
049.0 LYMPHOCYTIC (SEROUS) (BENIGN)
072.2 MUMPS
136.2 NAEGLERIA
123.9 PARASITIC [323.4]
320.1 PNEUMOCOCCAL
136.2 PRIMARY AMEBIC
056.01 RUBELLA

M

MENINGOENCEPHALITIS (continued)

048 SEROUS
049.0 SEROUS LYMPHOCYTIC
094.2 SPECIFIC
117.1 SPOROTRICHOSIS [321.1]
320.3 STAPHYLOCOCCAL
320.2 STREPTOCOCCAL
094.2 SYPHILITIC
013.0# TB

5th Digit: 013.0

0. NOS
1. LAB NOT DONE
2. LABS PENDING
3. MICROSCOPY POSITIVE (IN SPUTUM)
4. CULTURE POSITIVE - MICROSCOPY NEGATIVE
5. CULTURE NEGATIVE - MICROSCOPY POSITIVE
6. CULTURE AND MICROSCOPY NEGATIVE CONFIRMED BY OTHER METHODS

989.9 TOXIC NEC [323.7]
987.8 TOXIC DUE TO CARBON TETRACHLORIDE [323.7]
961.3 TOXIC DUE TO HYDROXYQUINOLINE DERIVATIVES [323.7]
984.9 TOXIC DUE TO LEAD [323.7]
985.0 TOXIC DUE TO MERCURY [323.7]
985.8 TOXIC DUE TO THALLIUM [323.7]
130.0 TOXOPLASMOSIS (ACQUIRED)
771.2 TOXOPLASMOSIS CONGENITAL (ACTIVE) [323.4]
086.1 TRYPANOSOMIC [323.2]
048 VIRUS NEC
0 SEE ALSO 'ENCEPHALITIS'

742.0 MENINGOENCEPHALOCELE CONGENITAL
0 MENINGOMYELITIS SEE 'MENINGITIS'

MENINGOMYELOCELE

741.0# WITH HYDROCEPHALUS
741.9# WITHOUT HYDROCEPHALUS

5th Digit: 741.0, 9

0. REGION NOS
1. CERVICAL
2. DORSAL
3. LUMBAR

MENISCUS

0 CHONDROCALCINOSIS SEE 'CHONDROCALCINOSIS'
717.5 DISCOID OLD
718.0# DISORDER (DERANGEMENT) (TEAR) (RUPTURE) - OLD

5th Digit: 718.0

0. SITE UNSPECIFIED
1. SHOULDER REGION
2. UPPER ARM (ELBOW) (HUMERUS)
3. FOREARM (RADIUS) (WRIST) (ULNA)
4. HAND (CARPAL) (METACARPAL) (FINGERS)
5. PELVIC REGION AND THIGH (HIP) (BUTTOCK) (FEMUR)
7. ANKLE AND/OR FOOT (METATARSALS) (TOES) (TARSALS)
8. OTHER
9. MULTIPLE

270.2 DISORDER IN OCHRONOSIS
717.5 DISORDER KNEE (DERANGEMENT) (TEAR) (RUPTURE) - OLD (SEE ALSO 'MENISCUS', KNEE TEAR - OLD)
717.5 KNEE CONGENITAL DISCOID
717.5 KNEE CYST - SEMILUNAR CARTILAGE
717.5 KNEE DERANGEMENT - SEMILUNAR CARTILAGE
717.5 KNEE DERANGEMENT NEC - OLD

MENISCUS (continued)

KNEE TEAR - ACUTE

836.2 UNSPECIFIED MEDIAL OR LATERAL
836.1 LATERAL NOS
836.0 MEDIAL NOS
836.1 ANTERIOR HORN (LATERAL)
836.0 ANTERIOR HORN (MEDIAL)
836.1 BUCKET HANDLE (LATERAL)
836.0 BUCKET HANDLE (MEDIAL)
836.1 POSTERIOR HORN (LATERAL)
836.0 POSTERIOR HORN (MEDIAL)
836.1 OTHER SPECIFIED (LATERAL)
836.0 OTHER SPECIFIED (MEDIAL)

KNEE TEAR - OLD

717.5 UNSPECIFIED NEC
717.40 LATERAL NOS
717.3 MEDIAL NOS
717.42 ANTERIOR HORN (LATERAL)
717.1 ANTERIOR HORN (MEDIAL)
717.41 BUCKET HANDLE (LATERAL)
717.0 BUCKET HANDLE (MEDIAL)
717.43 POSTERIOR HORN (LATERAL)
717.2 POSTERIOR HORN (MEDIAL)
717.49 OTHER SPECIFIED (LATERAL)
717.3 OTHER SPECIFIED (MEDIAL)

759.89 MENKES' SYNDROME (GLUTAMIC ACID)
270.3 MENKES' SYNDROME-MAPLE SYRUP (URINE) DISEASE

MENOMETRORRHAGIA

626.2 MENOMETRORRHAGIA
627.0 MENOPAUSAL
626.3 PUBERTAL

MENOPAUSE, MENOPAUSAL

627.2 NOS
627.9 AND POSTMENOPAUSAL DISORDER
627.8 AND POSTMENOPAUSAL DISORDERS OTHER SPECIFIED
716.3# ARTHRITIS

5th Digit: 716.3

0. SITE NOS
1. SHOULDER REGION
2. UPPER ARM
3. FOREARM
4. HAND
5. PELVIC REGION AND THIGH
6. LOWER LEG
7. ANKLE AND/OR FOOT
8. OTHER
9. MULTIPLE

627.4 ARTIFICIAL
627.0 BLEEDING
627.2 CLIMACTERIC STATES
627.2 CRISIS
296.2# DEPRESSION (MELANCHOLIA) - SINGLE EPISODE
296.3# DEPRESSION (MELANCHOLIA) - RECURRENT

5th Digit: 296.2-3

0. NOS
1. MILD
2. MODERATE
3. SEVERE WITHOUT MENTION OF PSYCHOTIC BEHAVIOR
4. SEVERE SPECIFIED AS WITH PSYCHOTIC BEHAVIOR
5. IN PARTIAL OR NOS REMISSION
6. IN FULL REMISSION

627.4 POSTARTIFICIAL SYNDROME

M

MENOPAUSE, MENOPAUSAL (continued)

256.3 PREMATURE
256.2 PREMATURE - POSTIRRADIATION
256.2 PREMATURE - POSTSURGICAL
627.4 STATES (ARTIFICIAL)
627.4 SURGICAL
627.2 SYMPTOMS
627.2 SYNDROME

MENORRHAGIA

626.2 NOS
626.2 PRIMARY
627.0 CLIMACTERIC
627.0 PRECLIMACTERIC
627.0 PREMENOPAUSAL
627.0 MENOPAUSAL
627.1 POSTMENOPAUSAL
626.3 PUBERTAL

626.2 MENORRHEA
626.3 MENORRHEA PUBERTAL

MENSTRUATION, MENSTRUAL

626.0 ABSENCE
625.3 CRAMPS
626.9 DISORDER
306.52 DISORDER PSYCHOGENIC
626.8 DISORDER OTHER
626.2 EXCESSIVE HEAVY PERIODS
627.0 EXCESSIVE MENOPAUSAL
626.3 EXCESSIVE ONSET OF PUBERTY
627.0 EXCESSIVE PREMENOPAUSAL
V25.3 EXTRACTION
626.1 INFREQUENT
626.4 IRREGULAR
625.4 MENSTRUAL MOLIMEN
625.3 PAIN
627.1 POSTMENOPAUSAL BLEEDING
V25.3 REGULATION
626.8 SUPPRESSION
625.4 SYNDROME
626.8 OTHER SPECIFIED DISORDER NEC

MENTAL DISORDER

291.9 ALCOHOLIC PSYCHOSIS (SEE ALSO 'PSYCHOSIS ALCOHOLIC')
V66.3 CONVALESCENCE
292.9 DRUG INDUCED (PSYCHOSIS) (SEE ALSO 'PSYCHOSIS DRUG INDUCED')
293.9 DUE TO OR ASSOCIATED WITH PHYSICAL CONDITION
310.# DUE TO ORGANIC BRAIN DAMAGE (NONPSYCHOTIC)

4th Digit: 310

0. FRONTAL LOBE SYNDROME
1. ORGANIC PERSONALITY SYNDROME
2. POSTCONCUSSION SYNDROME
8. OTHER SPECIFIED NONPSYCHOTIC DISORDER NEC
9. UNSPECIFIED NONPSYCHOTIC DISORDER

V11.8 HISTORY

648.4#: USE AN ADDITIONAL CODE TO IDENTIFY THE SPECIFIC MATERNAL MENTAL DISORDER.

648.4# MATERNAL CURRENT (CO-EXISTENT) IN PREGNANCY

5th Digit: 648.4

0. EPISODE OF CARE UNSPECIFIED OR N/A
1. DELIVERED
2. DELIVERED WITH POSTPARTUM COMPLICATION
3. ANTEPARTUM COMPLICATION
4. POSTPARTUM COMPLICATION

MENTAL DISORDER (continued)

V23.89 MATERNAL PREVIOUS AFFECTING MANAGEMENT OF PREGNANCY
0 NEUROTIC SEE 'NEUROSIS, NEUROTIC'
310.9 NONPSYCHOTIC FOLLOWING ORGANIC BRAIN DAMAGE
310.1 PRESENILE NON PSYCHOTIC
0 PSYCHOTIC SEE 'PSYCHOSIS'
V79.9 SCREENING (AND DEVELOPMENTAL HANDICAPS)
V79.8 SCREENING (AND DEVELOPMENTAL HANDICAPS) - OTHER SPECIFIED

MENTAL PROBLEM

V40.9 UNSPECIFIED
V40.2 OTHER SPECIFIED

MENTAL RETARDATION

319 UNSPECIFIED
317 MILD IQ 50-70
318.0 MODERATE IQ 35-49
318.1 SEVERE IQ 20-34
318.2 PROFOUND
V18.4 FAMILY HISTORY
V79.2 SCREENING

780.9 MENTAL STATUS ALTERED
304.0# MEPERIDINE DEPENDENCE

5th Digit: 304.0

0. UNSPECIFIED
1. CONTINUOUS
2. EPISODIC
3. IN REMISSION

355.1 MERALGIA PARESTHETICA
758.89 MERFF SYNDROME
330.0 MERZBACHER-PELIZAEUS DISEASE

305.3# MESCALINE ABUSE (NONDEPENDENT)
304.5# MESCALINE ADDICTION (DEPENDENT)

5th Digit: 304.5, 305.3

0. UNSPECIFIED
1. CONTINUOUS
2. EPISODIC
3. IN REMISSION

344.89 MESENCEPHALIC PARALYSIS NEC
710.9 MESENCHYMAL DISEASE

MESENCHYMOMA

238.9 SITE NOS
0 SITE SPECIFIED SEE 'NEOPLASM UNCERTAIN BEHAVIOR' BY SITE M8990/1
215.# BENIGN M8990/0

4th Digit: 215

0. HEAD FACE NACK
2. UPPER LIMB SHOULDER
3. LOWER LIMB HIP
4. THORAX
5. ABDOMINAL HYPOCHONDRIUM
6. PELVIS BUTTOCK GROIN INGUINAL REGION PERINEUM
7. TRUNK NOS BACK NOS FLANK NOS
8. OTHER SPECIFIED SITES
9. SITE UNSPECIFIED

199.1 MALIGNANT SITE NOS
0 MALIGNANT SITE SPECIFIED SEE 'CANCER' BY SITE M8990/3

M

INJURY OF A BLOOD VESSEL CAN BE A LACERATION, A-V FISTULA, ANEURYSM, OR HEMATOMA. USE THE "INJURY" CODE FOUND BY ANATOMICAL SITE (THE NAME OF THE BLOOD VESSEL).

MESENTERY, MESENTERIC

027.2 ADENITIS BY PASTEURELLA MULTOCIDA
557.1 ARTERITIS
442.84 ARTERY (SUPERIOR) ANEURYSM OR A-V FISTULA (CIRSOID) (FALSE) (VARICOSE)
557.1 ARTERY ARTERIOSCLEROSIS
557.0 ARTERY EMBOLISM
557.0 ARTERY INFARCTION
557.0 ARTERY INFARCTION (EMBOLIC) (THROMBOTIC)

902.20 ARTERY INJURY - BRANCH UNSPECIFIED
902.27 ARTERY INJURY - INFERIOR
908.4 ARTERY INJURY - LATE EFFECT
902.25 ARTERY INJURY - SUPERIOR
902.26 ARTERY INJURY - SUPERIOR PRIMARY BRANCHES
902.29 ARTERY INJURY - OTHER ARTERY

557.0 ARTERY INSUFFICIENCY (ACUTE)
557.1 ARTERY INSUFFICIENCY (CHRONIC)

902.20 ARTERY LACERATION NOS (RUPTURE) (HEMATOMA) (AVULSION) (ANEURYSM) TRAUMATIC
902.27 ARTERY LACERATION INFERIOR (RUPTURE) (HEMATOMA) (AVULSION) (ANEURYSM) (EMBOLISM) (THROMBOSIS) TRAUMATIC
902.25 ARTERY LACERATION SUPERIOR (RUPTURE) (HEMATOMA) (AVULSION) (ANEURYSM) (EMBOLISM) (THROMBOSIS) TRAUMATIC

557.0 ARTERY OCCLUSION
557.1 ARTERY SUPERIOR SYNDROME

863.89 INJURY (TRAUMATIC)
863.99 INJURY (TRAUMATIC) WITH OPEN WOUND

751.4 UNIVERSAL CONGENITAL
557.1 VASCULAR INSUFFICIENCY SYNDROME (WITH GANGRENE)
902.39 VEIN INJURY
902.32 VEIN INJURY - INFERIOR
902.31 VEIN INJURY - SUPERIOR

996.59 MESH EXTRUSION (REINFORCING)
524.2 MESIO-OCCLUSION
746.87 MESOCARDIA
199.1 MESODERMAL MIXED TUMOR SITE NOS
0 MESODERMAL MIXED TUMOR SITE SPECIFIED SEE 'CANCER' BY SITE M8951/3

MESONEPHRIC

752.8 DUCT AGENESIS (CONGENITAL)
238.9 TUMOR SITE NOS
0 TUMOR SITE SPECIFIED SEE 'NEOPLASM UNCERTAIN BEHAVIOR' BY SITE M9110/1

MESONEPHROMA

229.9 BENIGN SITE NOS
0 BENIGN SITE SPECIFIED SEE 'BENIGN NEOPLASM', BY SITE M9110/0
199.1 MALIGNANT SITE NOS
0 MALIGNANT SITE SPECIFIED SEE 'CANCER' BY SITE M9110/3

867.6 MESOSALPINX INJURY TRAUMATIC
867.7 MESOSALPINX INJURY TRAUMATIC WITH OPEN WOUND

MESOTHELIOMA

229.9 BENIGN SITE NOS
0 BENIGN SITE SPECIFIED SEE 'BENIGN NEOPLASM', BY SITE M9050/0
229.9 BIPHASIC TYPE - BENIGN SITE NOS
0 BIPHASIC TYPE - BENIGN SITE SPECIFIED SEE 'BENIGN NEOPLASM', BY SITE M9050/0
199.1 BIPHASIC TYPE - MALIGNANT SITE NOS
0 BIPHASIC TYPE - MALIGNANT SITE SPECIFIED SEE 'CANCER' BY SITE M9053/3

MESOTHELIOMA (continued)

229.9 EPITHELIOID - BENIGN SITE NOS
0 EPITHELIOID - BENIGN SITE SPECIFIED SEE 'BENIGN NEOPLASM', BY SITE M9052/0
199.1 EPITHELIOID - MALIGNANT SITE NOS
0 EPITHELIOID - MALIGNANT SITE SPECIFIED SEE 'CANCER' BY SITE M9052/3

229.9 FIBROUS - BENIGN SITE NOS
0 FIBROUS - BENIGN SITE SPECIFIED SEE 'BENIGN NEOPLASM', BY SITE M9051/0
199.1 FIBROUS - MALIGNANT SITE NOS
0 FIBROUS - MALIGNANT SITE SPECIFIED SEE 'CANCER' BY SITE M9051/3

199.1 MALIGNANT SITE NOS
0 MALIGNANT SITE SPECIFIED SEE 'CANCER' BY SITE M9050/3

METABOLIC

276.2 ACIDOSIS
V77.9 DISEASE SCREENING
277.9 DISORDER
669.0# DISORDER COMPLICATING LABOR AND DELIVERY

5th Digit: 669.0

0. EPISODE OF CARE UNSPECIFIED OR N/A
1. DELIVERED
2. DELIVERED WITH POSTPARTUM COMPLICATION
3. ANTEPARTUM COMPLICATION
4. POSTPARTUM COMPLICATION

639.4 DISORDER FOLLOWING ABORTION, ECTOPIC, MOLAR PREGNANCY
V12.2 DISORDER HISTORY
275.9 DISORDER MINERAL
275.8 DISORDER MINERAL OTHER
277.8 DISORDER OTHER SPECIFIED
775.9 DISTURBANCES FETUS AND NEWBORN
775.8 DISTURBANCES NEONATAL OTHER TRANSITORY
656.3# FETAL ACIDEMIA AFFECTING MANAGEMENT MOTHER

5th Digit: 656.3

0. EPISODE OF CARE UNSPECIFIED OR N/A
1. DELIVERED
3. ANTEPARTUM COMPLICATION

783.9 PROBLEM
V77.9 SCREENING FOR DISEASE
V77.7 SCREENING FOR OTHER INBORN ERRORS

277.9 METABOLISM DISORDER
783.9 METABOLISM SYMPTOM OTHER
755.28 METACARPALS AGENESIS
755.21 METACARPALS AGENESIS WITH ALL FINGERS COMPLETE
842.12 METACARPOPHALANGEAL SEPARATION (RUPTURE) (TEAR) (LACERATION)
842.12 METACARPOPHALANGEAL STRAIN (SPRAIN) (AVULSION)(HEMARTHROSIS)
121.5 METAGONIMIASIS
121.5 METAGONIMUS YOKOGAWAI INFECTION
709.00 METAL PIGMENTATION
502 METAL POLISHERS' DISEASE
360.24 METALLOSIS OTHER (GLOBE)
368.14 METAMORPHOPSIA
537.89 METAPLASIA GASTRIC MUCOSA
289.8 METAPLASIA MYELOID
275.40 METASTATIC CALCIFICATION

METASTATIC CANCER M8010/6

199.1 UNSPECIFIED SITE
198.5 COCCYX
198.89 COCCYGEAL BODY
198.89 HIP
196.# LYMPH NODE METASTATIC
4th Digit: 196
0. HEAD, FACE, NECK, CERVICAL, SUPRACLAVICULAR, CERVICOFACIAL, SCALENE
1. INTRATHORACIC, INTERCOSTAL, BRONCHOPULMONARY, MEDIASTINAL, TRACHEOBRONCHIAL
2. INTRABDOMINAL, MESENTERIC, RETROPERITONEAL, INTESTINAL
3. AXILLA, UPPER LIMB, BRACHIAL, INFRACLAVICULAR, PECTORAL, EPITROCHLEAR
5. LOWER LIMB, INGUINAL, FEMORAL, GROIN, POPLITEAL, TIBIAL
6. INTRAPELVIC, HYPOGASTRIC, ILIAC, PARAMETRIAL, OBTURATOR
8. MULTIPLE SITES
9. LYMPH NODES NOS

197.# RESPIRATORY AND DIGESTIVE
4th Digit: 197
0. LUNG, BRONCHUS
1. MEDIASTINUM
2. PLEURA
3. TRACHEA OR OTHER RESPIRATORY ORGANS
4. SMALL INTESTINE, DUODENUM
5. LARGE INTESTINE, RECTUM
6. RETROPERITONEUM AND PERITONEUM
7. LIVER, SPECIFIED AS SECONDARY
8. OTHER DIGESTIVE ORGANS AND SPLEEN

198.#(#) OTHER SPECIFIED SITES
4th or 4th and 5th Digit: 198
0. KIDNEY
1. OTHER URINARY ORGANS
2. SKIN AND SKIN OF BREAST OR MASTECTOMY SITE SKIN
3. BRAIN AND SPINAL CORD
4. OTHER PARTS OF NERVOUS SYSTEM, MENINGES (CEREBRAL) (SPINAL)
5. BONE AND BONE MARROW
6. OVARY
7. ADRENAL GLAND, SUPRARENAL GLAND
8#. OTHER SPECIFIED
81. BREAST (SOFT) (CONNECTIVE) OR BREAST TISSUE MASTECTOMY SITE
82. GENITAL ORGANS
89. OTHER

259.2 METASTATIC CARCINOID SYNDROME

726.70 METATARSALGIA
355.6 METATARSALGIA MORTON'S

755.38 METATARSALS AGENESIS (COMPLETE) (PARTIAL)
755.31 METATARSALS AGENESIS (COMPLETE) (PARTIAL) WITH COMPLETE ABSENCE OF DISTAL ELEMENTS
845.12 METATARSOPHALANGEAL SEPARATION (RUPTURE) (TEAR) (LACERATION)
845.12 METATARSOPHALANGEAL STRAIN (SPRAIN) (AVULSION)(HEMARTHROSIS)

754.53 METATARSUS ABDUCTUS VARUS (CONGENITAL)
754.60 METATARSUS ADDUCTUS VALGUS (CONGENITAL)
754.52 METATARSUS PRIMUS VARUS CONGENITAL
754.53 METATARSUS VARUS (CONGENITAL)

173.# METATYPICAL CARCINOMA M8095/3
4th Digit: 173
0. SKIN OF LIP
1. EYELID INCLUDING CANTHUS
2. SKIN OF EAR AURICULAR CANAL (EXTERNAL) EXTERNAL MEATUS PINNA
3. SKIN OF UNSPECIFIED PARTS OF FACE CHEEK (EXTERNAL) CHIN EYEBROW FOREHEAD NOSE (EXT)
4. SCALP AND SKIN OF NECK
5. ALL SKIN TRUNK AXILLARY FOLD PERIANAL ABDOMINAL WALL ANUS BACK BREAST (OR MASTECTOMY SITE) BUTTOCK
6. ALL SKIN UPPER LIMB SHOULDER ARM FINGER FOREARM HAND
7. ALL SKIN LOWER LIMB HIP ANKLE FOOT HEEL KNEE LEG THIGH TOE POPITEAL AREA
8. OTHER SPECIFIED SKIN SITES CONTIGUOUS OVERLAPPING SITES UNDETERMINED POINT OF ORIGIN
9. SITE UNSPECIFIED

V09.0 METHACILLIN RESISTANT INFECTION
304.0# METHADONE ADDICTION (DEPENDENT)
5th Digit: 304.0
0. UNSPECIFIED
1. CONTINUOUS
2. EPISODIC
3. IN REMISSION

METHEMOGLOBINEMIA

289.7 ACQUIRED
289.7 ACQUIRED WITH SULFHEMOGLOBINEMIA
289.7 CONGENITAL
289.7 HEREDITARY
289.7 TOXIC

270.4 METHIONINEMIA
270.4 METHIONINE METABOLISM DISTURBANCES
304.4# METHYLPHENIDATE DEPENDENCE
5th Digit: 304.4
0. UNSPECIFIED
1. CONTINUOUS
2. EPISODIC
3. IN REMISSION

METRITIS (SEE ALSO 'ENDOMETRITIS')

615.9 NOS
615.0 ACUTE
615.1 CHRONIC

626.6 METRORRHAGIA
733.99 MEYENBURG-ALTHERR-UEHLINGER SYNDROME
759.89 MEYER-SCHWICKERATH AND WEYERS SYNDROME (DYSPLASIA OCULODENTODIGITALIS)

ACUTE MYOCARDIAL INFARCTION - 410.## - THE FOLLOWING 5th DIGIT SUBCLASSIFICATION IS TO BE USED WITH CATEGORY 410.

0 - "EPISODE OF CARE UNSPECIFIED" - USE ONLY WHEN YOU HAVE INSUFFICIENT INFORMATION TO DETERMINE WHETHER EPISODE OF CARE IS INITIAL OR SUBSEQUENT.

1 - "INITIAL EPISODE OF CARE" - USE TO DESIGNATE THE ACUTE PHASE OF CARE, REGARDLESS OF THE LOCATION OF TREATMENT. THIS INCLUDES: 1) CASES ADMITTED TO INITIAL HOSPITAL 2) CASES TRANSFERRED FOR CARE OR TREATMENT OR BOTH 3) IF TRANSFERRED BACK TO INITIAL HOSPITAL DURING ACUTE PHASE OF CARE. EXAMPLE: ACUTE MI ADMITTED HOSPITAL II - 410.91, ACUTE MI FOR HEART CATHETER HOSPITAL II - 410.91, ACUTE MI RETURNED TO HOSPITAL I POST, HEART CATH DURING ACUTE PHASE OF CARE - 410.91, NOT DURING ACUTE PHASE - 410.92.

2 - "SUBSEQUENT EPISODE OF CARE" - USE TO DESIGNATE OBSERVATION, TREATMENT OR EVALUATION OF MI WITHIN 8 WEEKS OF ONSET, BUT FOLLOWING THE ACUTE PHASE, OR IN THE HEALING STATE WHERE THE EPISODE OF CARE MAY BE FOR RELATED OR UNRELATED CONDITION. EXAMPLE: PATIENT ADMITTED TO HOSPITAL 4 WEEKS POST ACUTE MI FOR (PTCA) - 410.92. PATIENT RETURNED TO HOSPITAL I AFTER (PTCA) ANGIOPLASTY WITH STABILIZATION OF HER MI. SHE HAS PICKED UP VIRUS INFECTION IN HOSPITAL II. DIAGNOSIS WOULD BE VIRUS INFECTION 079.99, ACUTE MI, SUBSEQUENT 410.92.

MI (MYOCARDIAL INFARCTION) ACUTE

410.9# UNSPECIFIED
410.0# ANTEROLATERAL
410.1# ANTERIOR OTHER
410.1# ANTERIOR (WALL)
410.1# ANTEROAPICAL
410.1# ANTEROSEPTAL
410.5# BASOLATERAL
410.2# INFEROLATERAL
410.3# INFEROPOSTERIOR
410.4# INFERIOR WALL
410.4# INFERIOR OTHER
410.5# LATERAL APICAL
410.5# LATERAL OTHER
410.7# NON-Q WAVE
410.7# NONTRANSMURAL
410.5# POSTEROLATERAL
410.6# POSTERIOR (POSTEROBASAL)
410.7# SUBENDOCARDIAL
410.8# ATRIUM PAPILLARY OR SEPTUM ALONE

5th Digit: 410.0-9

0. EPISODE UNSPECIFIED
1. INITIAL EPISODE
2. SUBSEQUENT EPISODE

MI (MYOCARDIAL INFARCTION) ASSOCIATED DIAGNOSES

412 DIAGNOSED ON EKG BUT PRESENTING NO SYMPTOMS
V71.7 EVALUATION NO MI FOUND
412 HISTORY
411.1 IMPENDING
412 OLD
411.0 POST MYOCARDIAL INFARCTION SYNDROME

757.39 MIBELLI'S DISEASE

MICE (JOINT)

718.1# NEC

5th Digit: 718.1

0. SITE NOS
1. SHOULDER REGION
2. UPPER ARM (ELBOW) (HUMERUS)
3. FOREARM (RADIUS) (WRIST) (ULNA)
4. HAND (CARPAL) (METACARPAL) (FINGERS)
5. PELVIC REGION AND THIGH (HIP) (BUTTOCK) (FEMUR)
7. ANKLE AND/OR FOOT (METATARSALS) (TOES) (TARSALS)
8. OTHER SPECIFIED SITES
9. MULTIPLE

MICE (JOINT) (continued)

717.6 KNEE
724.9 VERTEBRAL (FACET)

282.4 MICHELI-RIETTE SYNDROME (THALASSEMIA MINOR)
721.5 MICHOTTE'S SYNDROME
742.1 MICRENCEPHALY CONGENITAL
362.14 MICROANEURYSMS RETINAL
795.3 MICROBIOLOGIC NEC ABNORMAL
742.1 MICROCEPHALUS
744.82 MICROCHEILIA CONGENITAL
751.5 MICROCOLON CONGENITAL
743.41 MICROCORNEA
743.22 MICROCORNEA ASSOCIATED WITH BUPHTHALMOS
362.62 MICROCYSTOID DEGENERATION (RETINA)
520.2 MICRODONTIA
282.4 MICRODREPANOCYTOSIS
750.7 MICROGASTRIA DUPLICATION CONGENITAL
524.06 MICROGENIA
191.9 MICROGLIOMA SITE NOS
0 MICROGLIOMA SITE SPECIFIED SEE 'CANCER' BY SITE M9710/3
750.16 MICROGLOSSIA CONGENITAL

MICROGNATHIA

524.00 UNSPECIFIED
756.0 GLOSSOPTOSIS SYNDROME
524.04 MANDIBULAR
524.74 MANDIBULAR ALVEOLAR
524.03 MAXILLARY
524.73 MAXILLARY ALVEOLAR

742.2 MICROGYRIA CONGENITAL
516.2 MICROLITHIASIS PULMONARY ALVEOLAR
0 MICROORGANISMS RESISTANT TO DRUGS SEE 'DRUG RESISTANCE'
752.64 MICROPENIS CONGENITAL
743.36 MICROPHAKIA CONGENITAL

MICROPHTHALMOS

743.10 NOS (CONGENITAL)
743.11 SIMPLE (CONGENITAL)
743.12 WITH OTHER ANOMALIES OF EYE AND ADNEXA (CONGENITAL)

368.14 MICROPSIA
744.89 MICROSOMIA
110.9 MICROSPORIC TINEA
136.8 MICROSPORIDIA
111.1 MICROSPOROSIS NIGRA
110.# MICROSPORUM INFECTIONS

4th Digit: 110

0. SCALP AND BEARD
1. NAIL (UNGUIUM)
2. HAND (MANUUM)
3. GROIN AND PERIANAL (CRURIS)
4. FOOT (PEDIS)
5. BODY (CORPORUS)
6. DEEP SEATED (GRANULOMA TRICHOPHYTICUM)
8. OTHER SPECIFIED SITE
9. UNSPECIFIED SITE

744.84 MICROSTOMIA CONGENITAL
744.23 MICROTIA CONGENITAL
378.34 MICROTROPIA

MICTURITION

788.69 DISORDER NEC
306.53 DISORDER PSYCHOGENIC
788.41 FREQUENCY
788.43 FREQUENCY NOCTURNAL
788.1 PAINFUL
306.53 PAINFUL - PSYCHOGENIC

M

348.8 MIDBRAIN SYNDROME

344.89 MIDDLE ALTERNATING PARALYSIS

385.9 MIDDLE EAR AND MASTOID DISORDER

385.89 MIDDLE EAR AND MASTOID DISORDER OTHER

959.09 MIDDLE EAR INJURY

382.2 MIDDLE EAR PERSISTENT MUCOSAL DISEASE (WITH POSTERIOR OR SUPERIOR MARGINAL PERFORATION OF EAR DRUM)

518.0 MIDDLE LOBE SYNDROME (LUNG) (RIGHT)

353.0 MIDDLE RADICULAR SYNDROME

524.2 MIDLINE DEVIATION

709.3 MIESCHER'S DISEASE OR SYNDROME-GRANULOMATOSIS DISCIFORMIS

701.2 MIESCHER'S SYNDROME-FAMILIAL ACANTHOSIS NIGRICANS

759.89 MIETEN'S SYNDROME

MIGRAINE

346.9# MIGRAINE
346.2# ABDOMINAL
346.1# ATYPICAL
346.2# BASILAR
346.2# BING HORTON
346.0# CLASSIC
346.2# CLUSTER
346.1# COMMON
346.8# HEMIPLEGIC
346.2# HISTAMINE
346.2# LOWER HALF
625.4 MENSTRUAL
346.8# OPHTHALMOPLEGIC
346.2# RETINAL
346.0# SYNDROME
346.2# VARIANT
346.0# WITH AURA
346.0# WITH TRANSIENT FOCAL NEUROLOGICAL PHENOMENA
346.8# OTHER

5th Digit: 346.0-2, 8-9

0. WITHOUT MENTION INTRACTABLE MIGRAINE
1. WITH INTRACTABLE MIGRAINE

V60.0 MIGRANT SOCIAL (HOMELESS PERSON)

770.7 MIKITY-WILSON SYNDROME (PULMONARY DYSMATURITY)

527.1 MIKULICZ'S DISEASE OR SYNDROME (DRYNESS OF MOUTH, DECREASED LACRIMATION)

783.4 MILESTONE DELAYED

705.1 MILIARIA RUBRA (TROPICALIS)

078.2 MILIARY FEVER

709.3 MILIA (UM) COLLOID

374.84 MILIA (UM) EYELID

706.2 MILIA (UM) SEBACEOUS SEE ALSO 'SEBACEOUS' CYST

999.9 MILK ALKALI SYNDROME (MILK DRINKERS')

690.11 MILK CRUST

423.1 MILK SPOTS PERICARDIUM

051.1 MILKERS' NODE

268.2 MILKMAN (-LOOSER) DISEASE OR SYNDROME (OSTEOMALACIA WITH PSEUDOFRACTURES)

344.89 MILLARD-GUBLER (MILLARD-GUBLER-FOVILLE) SYNDROME

357.0 MILLER FISHER'S SYNDROME

268.2 MILLER'S DISEASE (OSTEOMALACIA)

335.29 MILL'S DISEASE

759.6 MILLES' SYNDROME (ENCEPHALOCUTANEOUS ANGIOMATOSIS)

757.0 MILROY'S DISEASE CONGENITAL (CHRONIC HEREDITARY EDEMA)

041.85 MIMA POLYMORPHA INFECTION OR ORGANISM

985.0 MINAMATA DISEASE

500 MINERS' ASTHMA

727.2 MINER'S ELBOW

727.2 MINER'S KNEE

MINERAL

790.6 ABNORMAL BLOOD LEVEL
269.3 DEFICIENCY NEC
275.9 METABOLISM DISORDER
275.8 METABOLISM DISORDERS OTHER SPECIFIED

282.0 MINKOWSKI CHAUFFARD SYNDROME

336.1 MINOR'S DISEASE

776.0 MINOT'S DISEASE (HEMORRHAGIC DISEASE NEWBORN)

379.42 MIOSIS PERSISTENT NOT DUE TO MIOTICS

576.2 MIRIZZI'S SYNDROME (HEPATIC DUCT STENOSIS)

0 MIRIZZI'S SYNDROME WITH CALCULUS, CHOLELITHIASIS OR STONES SEE 'CHOLEDOCHOLITHIASIS'

999.9 MISADVENTURE OF MEDICAL CARE

998.2 MISADVENTURE OF SURGERY (ACCIDENTAL PUNCTURE) OF ORGAN

0 MISCARRIAGE SEE 'ABORTION', SPONTANEOUS

313.1 MISERY OF CHILDHOOD AND ADOLESCENCE

632 MISSED ABORTION

632 MISSED ABORTION WITH COMPLICATION DURING TREATMENT [**639.#**]

639.# MISSED ABORTION WITH COMPLICATION FOLLOWING TREATMENT

4th Digit: 639

0. GENITAL TRACT AND PELVIC INFECTION
1. DELAYED OR EXCESSIVE HEMORRHAGE
2. DAMAGE TO PELVIC ORGANS AND TISSUE
3. RENAL FAILURE
4. METABOLIC DISORDERS
5. SHOCK
6. EMBOLISM
8. OTHER SPECIFIED COMPLICATION
9. UNSPECIFIED COMPLICATION

656.4# MISSED DELIVERY (FETAL DEATH AFTER 22 WEEKS)

5th Digit: 656.4

0. EPISODE OF CARE NOS
1. DELIVERED WITH OR WITHOUT MENTION OF ANTEPARTUM CONDITION
3. ANTEPARTUM CONDITION

443.89 MITCHELL'S DISEASE (ERYTHROMELALGIA)

133.9 MITE INFESTATION

758.9 MITOCHONDRIAL CHROMOSOME ANOMALIES

396.9 MITRAL AND AORTIC VALVE DISEASE

396.8 MITRAL AND AORTIC VALVE DISEASE MULTIPLE INSUFFICIENCY AND STENOSIS

785.2 MITRAL CLICK (-MURMUR) SYNDROME

0 MITRAL INCOMPETENCE SEE 'MITRAL INSUFFICIENCY'

MITRAL INSUFFICIENCY

424.0 NOS
396.3 AND AORTIC INSUFFICIENCY
396.3 AND AORTIC INSUFFICIENCY RHEUMATIC
396.2 AND AORTIC STENOSIS
396.2 AND AORTIC STENOSIS RHEUMATIC
421.0 BACTERIAL (ACUTE) (CHRONIC)
746.6 CONGENITAL
394.1 RHEUMATIC
093.21 SYPHILITIC
396.3 WITH AORTIC VALVE DISEASE

0 MITRAL REGURGITATION SEE 'MITRAL INSUFFICIENCY'

M

MITRAL STENOSIS

394.0 NOS
396.1 AND AORTIC INSUFFICIENCY
396.1 AND AORTIC INSUFFICIENCY RHEUMATIC
396.0 AND AORTIC STENOSIS
396.0 AND AORTIC STENOSIS RHEUMATIC
421.0 BACTERIAL (ACUTE) (CHRONIC)
746.5 CONGENITAL
394.0 RHEUMATIC
396.1 WITH AORTIC VALVE DISEASE
394.2 WITH INSUFFICIENCY
421.0 WITH INSUFFICIENCY BACTERIAL (ACUTE) (CHRONIC)
394.2 WITH INSUFFICIENCY RHEUMATIC
093.21 WITH INSUFFICIENCY SYPHILITIC
394.2 WITH REGURGITATION
093.21 SYPHILITIC
424.0 SPECIFIED CAUSE NON RHEUMATIC

746.89 MITRAL VALVE ATRESIA
746.7 MITRAL VALVE ATRESIA OR HYPOPLASIA OF AORTIC ORIFICE OR VALVE, WITH HYPOPLASIA OF ASCENDING AORTA AND DEFECTIVE DEVELOPMENT OF LEFT VENTRICLE
424.0 MITRAL VALVE DISEASE (PROLAPSE)
394.9 MITRAL VALVE DISEASE CHRONIC
424.0 MITRAL VALVE PROLAPSE SYNDROME

625.2 MITTELSCHMERZ

041.89 MIXED FLORA INFECTION

199.1 MIXED TUMOR MALIGNANT SITE NOS
0 MIXED TUMOR MALIGNANT SITE SPECIFIED SEE 'CANCER' BY SITE M8940/3
757.39 MLJET DISEASE (MAL DE MELEDA)
V06.4 MMR VACCINATION

426.13 MOBITZ (TYPE) I HEART BLOCK
426.12 MOBITZ (TYPE) II HEART BLOCK AV
346.8# MOBIUS' DISEASE OR SYNDROME (OPHTHALMOPLEGIC MIGRAINE)

5th Digit: 346.8
0. WITHOUT MENTION INTRACTABLE MIGRAINE
1. WITH INTRACTABLE MIGRAINE

352.6 MOBIUS' SYNDROME (CONGENITAL OCULOFACIAL PARALYSIS)
267 MOELLER'S DISEASE (VITAMIN C DEFICIENCY)
529.4 MOELLER'S GLOSSITIS
759.89 MOHR'S SYNDROME (TYPES I AND II)

MOLAR PREGNANCY

631 NOS
631 NOS WITH COMPLICATION DURING TREATMENT [**639.#**]
639.# NOS WITH COMPLICATION FOLLOWING TREATMENT

4th Digit: 639
0. GENITAL TRACT AND PELVIC INFECTION
1. DELAYED OR EXCESSIVE HEMORRHAGE
2. DAMAGE TO PELVIC ORGANS AND TISSUE
3. RENAL FAILURE
4. METABOLIC DISORDERS
5. SHOCK
6. EMBOLISM
8. OTHER SPECIFIED COMPLICATION
9. UNSPECIFIED COMPLICATION

MOLAR PREGNANCY (continued)

631 BLIGHTED OVUM
631 BLIGHTED OVUM WITH COMPLICATION DURING TREATMENT [**639.#**]
639.# BLIGHTED OVUM WITH COMPLICATION FOLLOWING TREATMENT

4th Digit: 639
0. GENITAL TRACT AND PELVIC INFECTION
1. DELAYED OR EXCESSIVE HEMORRHAGE
2. DAMAGE TO PELVIC ORGANS AND TISSUE
3. RENAL FAILURE
4. METABOLIC DISORDERS
5. SHOCK
6. EMBOLISM
8. OTHER SPECIFIED COMPLICATION
9. UNSPECIFIED COMPLICATION

631 CARNEOUS MOLE
631 CARNEOUS MOLE WITH COMPLICATION DURING TREATMENT [**639.#**]
639.# CARNEOUS MOLE WITH COMPLICATION FOLLOWING TREATMENT
639.# COMPLICATION FOLLOWING MOLAR PREGNANCY

4th Digit: 639
0. GENITAL TRACT AND PELVIC INFECTION
1. DELAYED OR EXCESSIVE HEMORRHAGE
2. DAMAGE TO PELVIC ORGANS AND TISSUE
3. RENAL FAILURE
4. METABOLIC DISORDERS
5. SHOCK
6. EMBOLISM
8. OTHER SPECIFIED COMPLICATION
9. UNSPECIFIED COMPLICATION

631 FLESHY MOLE
631 FLESHY MOLE WITH COMPLICATION DURING TREATMENT [**639.#**]
639.# FLESHY MOLE WITH COMPLICATION FOLLOWING TREATMENT

4th Digit: 639
0. GENITAL TRACT AND PELVIC INFECTION
1. DELAYED OR EXCESSIVE HEMORRHAGE
2. DAMAGE TO PELVIC ORGANS AND TISSUE
3. RENAL FAILURE
4. METABOLIC DISORDERS
5. SHOCK
6. EMBOLISM
8. OTHER SPECIFIED COMPLICATION
9. UNSPECIFIED COMPLICATION

630 HYDATIDIFORM MOLE
630 HYDATIDIFORM MOLE WITH COMPLICATION DURING TREATMENT [**639.#**]
639.# HYDATIDIFORM MOLE WITH COMPLICATION FOLLOWING TREATMENT

4th Digit: 639
0. GENITAL TRACT AND PELVIC INFECTION
1. DELAYED OR EXCESSIVE HEMORRHAGE
2. DAMAGE TO PELVIC ORGANS AND TISSUE
3. RENAL FAILURE
4. METABOLIC DISORDERS
5. SHOCK
6. EMBOLISM
8. OTHER SPECIFIED COMPLICATION
9. UNSPECIFIED COMPLICATION

MOLAR PREGNANCY (continued)

631 MOLE NOS
631 MOLE NOS WITH COMPLICATION DURING TREATMENT [639.#]
639.# MOLE NOS WITH COMPLICATION FOLLOWING TREATMENT
4th Digit: 639
- **0. GENITAL TRACT AND PELVIC INFECTION**
- **1. DELAYED OR EXCESSIVE HEMORRHAGE**
- **2. DAMAGE TO PELVIC ORGANS AND TISSUE**
- **3. RENAL FAILURE**
- **4. METABOLIC DISORDERS**
- **5. SHOCK**
- **6. EMBOLISM**
- **8. OTHER SPECIFIED COMPLICATION**
- **9. UNSPECIFIED COMPLICATION**

631 STONE MOLE
631 STONE MOLE WITH COMPLICATION DURING TREATMENT [639.#]
639.# STONE MOLE WITH COMPLICATION FOLLOWING TREATMENT
4th Digit: 639
- **0. GENITAL TRACT AND PELVIC INFECTION**
- **1. DELAYED OR EXCESSIVE HEMORRHAGE**
- **2. DAMAGE TO PELVIC ORGANS AND TISSUE**
- **3. RENAL FAILURE**
- **4. METABOLIC DISORDERS**
- **5. SHOCK**
- **6. EMBOLISM**
- **8. OTHER SPECIFIED COMPLICATION**
- **9. UNSPECIFIED COMPLICATION**

630 TROPHOBLASTIC DISEASE NOS
630 TROPHOBLASTIC DISEASE NOS WITH COMPLICATION DURING TREATMENT [639.#]
639.# TROPHOBLASTIC DISEASE NOS WITH COMPLICATION FOLLOWING TREATMENT
4th Digit: 639
- **0. GENITAL TRACT AND PELVIC INFECTION**
- **1. DELAYED OR EXCESSIVE HEMORRHAGE**
- **2. DAMAGE TO PELVIC ORGANS AND TISSUE**
- **3. RENAL FAILURE**
- **4. METABOLIC DISORDERS**
- **5. SHOCK**
- **6. EMBOLISM**
- **8. OTHER SPECIFIED COMPLICATION**
- **9. UNSPECIFIED COMPLICATION**

630 VESICULAR MOLE
630 VESICULAR MOLE WITH COMPLICATION DURING TREATMENT [639.#]
639.# VESICULAR MOLE WITH COMPLICATION FOLLOWING TREATMENT
4th Digit: 639
- **0. GENITAL TRACT AND PELVIC INFECTION**
- **1. DELAYED OR EXCESSIVE HEMORRHAGE**
- **2. DAMAGE TO PELVIC ORGANS AND TISSUE**
- **3. RENAL FAILURE**
- **4. METABOLIC DISORDERS**
- **5. SHOCK**
- **6. EMBOLISM**
- **8. OTHER SPECIFIED COMPLICATION**
- **9. UNSPECIFIED COMPLICATION**

236.1 MOLE INVASIVE

0 MOLE PRODUCT OF CONCEPTION SEE 'MOLAR PREGNANCY'

0 MOLE SKIN BENIGN SEE 'BENIGN NEOPLASM', SKIN
0 MOLE SKIN MALIGNANT SEE 'MELANOMA BY SITE'

267 MOLLER'S DISEASE (INFANTILE SCURVY)
078.0 MOLLUSCUM CONTAGIOSUM

440.2# MONCKEBERG'S MEDIAL SCLEROSIS
5th Digit: 440.2
- **0. UNSPECIFIED**
- **1. WITH INTERMITTENT CLAUDICATION**
- **2. WITH REST PAIN, OR REST PAIN AND (INTERMITTENT CLAUDICATION)**
- **3. WITH ULCERATION, OR ULCERATION AND (INTERMITTENT CLAUDICATION) (REST PAIN)**
- **4. WITH ISCHEMIC GANGRENE, OR ISCHEMIC GANGRENE AND (INTERMITTENT CLAUDICATION) (REST PAIN) (ULCERATION)**
- **9. OTHER ATHEROSCLEROSIS EXTREMITIES**

440.3# MONCKEBERG'S MEDIAL SCLEROSIS BYPASS GRAFT
5th Digit: 440.3
- **0. UNSPECIFIED GRAFT**
- **1. AUTOLOGOUS VEIN BYPASS GRAFT**
- **2. NONAUTOLOGOUS BIOLOGICAL BYPASS GRAFT**

744.05 MONDINI'S MALFORMATION (COCHLEA)
451.89 MONDOR'S DISEASE (THROMBOPHLEBITIS OF BREAST)
993.2 MONGE'S DISEASE
757.33 MONGOLIAN SPOT
758.0 MONGOLISM
757.4 MONILETHRIX CONGENITAL

MONILIASIS

771.7 NEONATAL
112.1 VULVOVAGINITIS
0 SEE ALSO 'CANDIDIASIS"

368.54 MONOCHROMATISM (CONE) (ROD)
075 MONOCYTIC ANGINA
V10.63 MONOCYTIC LEUKEMIA HISTORY
288.8 MONOCYTOSIS (SYMPTOMATIC)
378.34 MONOFIXATION SYNDROME

MONONEURITIS

355.9 NOS
378.54 ABDUCENS (NERVE)
352.4 ACCESSORY NERVE
388.5 ACOUSTIC (8TH NERVE)
094.86 ACOUSTIC (SYPHILITIC)
353.0 AXILLARY NERVE (NONDISCOGENIC)
353.8 COSTAL REGION (NONDISCOGENIC)
388.5 EIGHTH NERVE
351.8 FACIAL NERVE
352.1 GLOSSOPHARYNGEAL
274.89 GOUTY [357.4]
355.79 ILIOHYPOGASTRIC
355.79 ILIOINGUINAL
355.8 LOWER LIMB
355.79 LOWER LIMB OTHER
354.1 MEDIAN NERVE
354.5 MULTIPLEX
377.30 OPHTHALMIC
377.41 OPTIC (ISCHEMIC)
341.0 OPTIC IN MYELITIS
377.30 OPTIC NERVE
377.33 OPTIC NUTRITIONAL
377.34 OPTIC TOXIC
355.5 PERITONEAL
723.4 RADIAL (NERVE)
094.85 RETROBULBAR SYPHILITIC
355.79 SAPHENOUS
724.3 SCIATIC (NERVE)
351.8 SEVENTH NERVE
723.4 SUBSCAPULAR (NERVE)
357.7 TOXIC
350.8 TRIGEMINAL
053.12 TRIGEMINAL POST HERPETIC
723.4 ULNAR (NERVE)
354.9 UPPER LIMB
354.8 UPPER LIMB OTHER
352.3 VAGUS (NERVE)
386.12 VESTIBULAR
0 SEE ALSO 'NEUROPATHY'

MONONUCLEOSIS
V01.7 EXPOSURE
075 INFECTIOUS
075 INFECTIOUS WITH ENCEPHALITIS [323.0]
075 INFECTIOUS WITH HEPATITIS [573.1]

MONOPLEGIA
344.5 NOS
306.0 DISORDER PSYCHOGENIC
344.3# LOWER LIMB (OLD)
438.4# LOWER LIMB (OLD) LATE EFFECT OF CEREBROVASCULAR DISEASE
344.4# UPPER LIMB (OLD)
438.3# UPPER LIMB (OLD) LATE EFFECT OF CEREBROVASCULAR DISEASE
5th Digit: 344.3-4, 438.3-4
0. UNSPECIFIED SIDE
1. DOMINANT SIDE
2. NONDOMINANT SIDE
781.4 TRANSIENT

752.8 MONORCHISM CONGENITAL

MONSTER
740.0 ACEPHALIC
759.4 COMPOSITE
759.4 COMPOUND
759.4 DOUBLE
759.7 SINGLE
759.4 TWIN
759.89 SPECIFIED TYPE NEC

813.03 MONTEGGIA'S FOREARM FRACTURE - CLOSED
813.13 MONTEGGIA'S FOREARM FRACTURE - OPEN
835.## MONTEGGIA'S HIP DISLOCATION
4th Digit: 835
0. CLOSED
1. OPEN
5th Digit: 835
0. UNSPECIFIED
1. POSTERIOR
2. OBTURATOR
3. ANTERIOR
296.99 MOOD SWINGS (PSYCHOSIS)
345.5# MOORE'S SYNDROME
5th Digit: 345.5
0. WITHOUT MENTION OF INTRACTABLE EPILEPSY
1. WITH INTRACTABLE EPILEPSY
370.07 MOOREN'S ULCER (CORNEAL)
278.01 MORBID OBESTIY
799.9 MORBIDITY OR MORTALITY UNKNOWN CAUSE
0 MORBILLI SEE 'MEASLES'
429.9 MORBUS CORDIS
295.9# MOREL-KRAEPELIN DISEASE (SEE ALSO 'SCHIZOPHRENIA')
5th Digit: 295.9
0. NOS
1. SUBCHRONIC
2. CHRONIC
3. SUBCHRONIC WITH ACUTE EXACERBATION
4. CHRONIC WITH ACUTE
5. IN REMISSION
733.3 MOREL-MOORE SYNDROME (HYPEROSTOSIS FRONTALIS INTERNA)
733.3 MOREL-MORGAGNI SYNDROME (HYPEROSTOSIS FRONTALIS INTERNA)
426.9 MORGAGNI-ADAMS-STOKES SYNDROME (SYNCOPE WITH HEART BLOCK)
366.18 MORGAGNI CATARACT SENILE
733.3 MORGAGNI'S DISEASE (SYNDROME) (HYPEROSTOSIS FRONTALIS INTERNA)
607.3 MORNING PRIAPISM
643.0# MORNING SICKNESS
5th Digit: 643.0
0. EPISODE OF CARE UNSPECIFIED OR N/A
1. DELIVERED
3. ANTEPARTUM COMPLICATION

317 MORON
701.0 MORPHEA
304.0# MORPHINE ADDICTION (DEPENDENT)
5th Digit: 304.0
0. NOS
1. CONTINUOUS
2. EPISODIC
3. IN REMISSION
277.5 MORQUIO (-BRAILSFORD) (-ULLRICH) DISEASE OR SYNDROME (MUCOPOLYSACCHARIDOSIS IV)
257.8 MORRIS SYNDROME (TESTICULAR FEMINIZATION)
355.6 MORTON'S NEUROMA OR SYNDROME
336.0 MORVAN'S DISEASE
758.9 MOSAICISM, MOSAIC (CHROMOSOMAL)
758.5 MOSAICISM, MOSAIC AUTOSOMAL
758.81 MOSAICISM, MOSAIC SEX
446.6 MOSCHCOWITZ'S (-SINGER-SYMMERS) SYNDROME (THROMBOTIC THROMBOCYTOPENIC PURPURA)
0 MOSQUITO BITE SEE 'INSECT BITE NONVENOMOUS', BY SITE
V73.5 MOSQUITO BORNE DISEASE SCREENING EXAM

MOTION
0 RANGE (JOINT) LIMITATION SEE 'STIFF, STIFFNESS', JOINT
994.6 SICKNESS - NOS
909.4 SICKNESS - LATE EFFECT

315.4 MOTOR DEVELOPMENT DISORDER SPECIFIC
307.9 MOTOR DISORDER PSYCHOGENIC
335.20 MOTOR NEURON DISEASE (BULBAR) (MIXED TYPE)
335.29 MOTOR NEURON DISEASE OTHER
520.3 MOTTLED TEETH
732.5 MOUCHET'S DISEASE (JUVENILE OSTEOCHONDROSIS FOOT)
494 MOUNIER-KUHN SYNDROME
993.2 MOUNTAIN SICKNESS
909.4 MOUNTAIN SICKNESS LATE EFFECT

MOUTH
528.3 ABSCESS
750.26 ANOMALIES OTHER SPECIFIED CONGENITAL
784.9 BREATHING
524.5 BREATHING MALOCCLUSION
528.2 CANKER SORE ULCER
528.3 CELLULITIS
528.9 DENTURE SORE
528.9 DISEASE (SOFT TISSUE)
528.9 DISEASE (SOFT TISSUE) OTHER SPECIFIED
523.8 HYPERPLASIA - GUM
529.8 HYPERPLASIA - TONGUE
528.9 HYPERPLASIA - SOFT TISSUE NEC (INFLAMMATORY) (IRRITATIVE) (MUCOSA)
959.09 INJURY

MOVEMENT
781.0 ABNORMAL (DYSTONIC) (INVOLUNTARY)
655.7# DECREASE FETAL
5th Digit: 655.7
0. EPISODE OF CARE UNSPECIFIED OR N/A
1. DELIVERED
3. ANTEPARTUM COMPLICATION

333.90 DISORDER NEC
300.11 DISORDER HYSTERICAL
307.3 DISORDER STEREOTYPIC (REPETITIVE)
333.99 DISORDER OTHER
374.43 PARADOXICAL FACIAL

437.5 MOYAMOYA DISEASE

V72.5 MRI

V09.0 MRSA (METHACILLIN RESISTANT STAPHYLOCOCCUS AUREUS)

340 MS

340 MS WITH DEMENTIA [294.1]

066.3 MUCAMBO FEVER (VIRAL)

696.2 MUCHA'S (-HABERMAN) DISEASE OR SYNDROME (ACUTE PARAPSORIASIS VARIOLIFORMIS)

701.8 MUCINOSIS (CUTANEOUS) (PAPULAR)

199.1 MUCOCARCINOID TUMOR MALIGNANT SITE NOS

0 MUCOCARCINOID TUMOR MALIGNANT SITE SPECIFIED SEE 'CANCER' BY SITE M8243/3

MUCOCELE

543.9 APPENDIX
528.9 BUCCAL CAVITY
575.3 GALLBLADDER
375.43 LACRIMAL
375.43 ORBIT
527.6 SALIVARY GLAND
478.1 SINUS (NASAL)
478.1 SINUS (NASAL) ACCESSORY
478.1 TURBINATE (MIDDLE) (NASAL)
621.8 UTERUS

446.1 MUCOCUTANEOUS LYMPH NODE SYNDROME (ACUTE) (FEBRILE) (INFANTILE) (MCLS)

MUCOEPIDERMOID

199.1 CARCINOMA SITE NOS
0 CARCINOMA SITE SPECIFIED SEE 'CANCER' BY SITE M8430/3
238.9 TUMOR SITE NOS
0 TUMOR SITE SPECIFIED SEE 'NEOPLASM UNCERTAIN BEHAVIOR' BY SITE M8430/1

272.7 MUCOLIPIDOSIS (I)(II)(III) DISEASE

277.5 MUCOPOLYSACCHARIDE METABOLISM DISORDER

277.5 MUCOPOLYSACCHARIDOSIS

277.5 MUCOPOLYSACCHARIDOSIS CARDIOMYOPATHY [425.7]

277.5 MUCOPOLYSACCHARIDOSIS CEREBRAL DEGENERATION DISEASE OF CHILDHOOD [330.3]

117.7 MUCOR INFECTION

288.0 MUCOSITIS NECROTICANS AGRANULOCYTICA

0 MUCOUS SEE 'MUCUS'

0 MUCOVISCIDOSIS SEE 'CYSTIC', FIBROSIS

792.1 MUCUS IN STOOL

933.1 MUCUS PLUG (SEE ALSO 'ASPHYXIATION FOOD, MUCUS OR FOREIGN BODY INHALATION')

770.1 MUCUS PLUG ASPIRATION OF NEWBORN

519.1 MUCUS PLUG BRONCHIAL

519.1 MUCUS PLUG TRACHEOBRONCHIAL

079.81 MUERTO CANYON VIRUS

752.8 MULLERIAN DUCT CYST CONGENITAL

199.1 MULLERIAN MIXED TUMOR SITE NOS

0 MULLERIAN MIXED TUMOR SITE SPECIFIED SEE 'CANCER' BY SITE M8950/3

710.8 MULTIFOCAL FIBROSCLEROSIS (IDIOPATHIC) NEC

046.3 MULTIFOCAL LEUKOENCEPHALOPATHY

ELDERLY MULTIGRAVIDA: SECOND OR MORE PREGNANCY IN A WOMAN WHO WILL BE 35 YEARS OF AGE OR OLDER AT EXPECTED DATE OF DELIVERY.

659.6# MULTIGRAVIDA ELDERLY

5th Digit: 659.6

0. EPISODE OF CARE UNSPECIFIED OR N/A
1. DELIVERED
3. ANTEPARTUM COMPLICATION

763.89 MULTIPARITY AFFECTING FETUS OR NEWBORN

V61.5 MULTIPARITY CAUSING FAMILY CIRCUMSTANCE PROBLEM (REASON FOR ENCOUNTER)

V82.6 MULTIPHASIC SCREENING

MULTIPLE

919.0 ABRASION
919.1 ABRASIONS INFECTED
260 DEFICIENCY SYNDROME
258.0 ENDOCRINE ADENOMATOSIS
258.0 ENDOCRINE ADENOMATOSIS WITH POLYGLANDULAR ACTIVITY
0 GESTATION SEE 'GESTATION', MULTIPLE
919.8 INJURY OTHER AND UNSPECIFIED SUPERFICIAL
919.9 INJURY OTHER AND UNSPECIFIED SUPERFICIAL INFECTED
203.0# MYELOMA M9730/3

5th Digit: 203.0

0. WITHOUT MENTION OF REMISSION
1. IN REMISSION

301.51 OPERATIONS SYNDROME
300.14 PERSONALITY DISORDER
0 PREGNANCY SEE 'GESTATION', MULTIPLE
761.5 PREGNANCY AFFECTING FETUS OR NEWBORN
340 SCLEROSIS
340 SCLEROSIS WITH DEMENTIA [294.1]

MUMPS

072.9 UNSPECIFIED
072.2 ENCEPHALITIS
V01.7 EXPOSURE
072.71 HEPATITIS
072.1 MENINGITIS
072.2 MENINGOENCEPHALITIS
072.0 ORCHITIS
072.3 PANCREATITIS
072.9 PAROTITIS
072.72 POLYNEUROPATHY
072.9 UNCOMPLICATED
V04.6 VACCINATION ALONE
072.8 WITH UNSPECIFIED COMPLICATION
072.79 WITH OTHER SPECIFIED COMPLICATION

301.51 MUNCHAUSEN SYNDROME

728.11 MUNCHMEYER'S DISEASE OR SYNDROME (EXOSTOSIS LUXURIANS)

429.79 MURAL THROMBUS (ATRIAL) (VENTRICULAR) ACQUIRED FOLLOWING MYOCARDIAL INFARCTION <8 WEEKS [410.##]

4th Digit: 410

0. ANTEROLATERAL
1. ANTERIOR (WALL) ANTEROAPICAL ANTEROSEPTAL OTHER ANTERIOR
2. INFEROLATERAL
3. INFEROPOSTERIOR
4. INFERIOR OTHER
5. LATERAL APICAL, BASOLATERAL, POSTEROLATERAL, LATERAL OTHER
6. POSTERIOR (PSTEROBASAL)
7. SUBENDOCARDIAL
8. ATRIUM PAPILLARY OR SEPTUM ALONE
9. UNSPECIFIED

5th Digit: 410

0. EPISODE UNSPECIFIED
1. INITIAL EPISODE
2. SUBSEQUENT EPISODE

M

429.79 MURAL THROMBUS (ATRIAL) (VENTRICULAR) ACQUIRED FOLLOWING MYOCARDIAL INFARCTION >8 WEEKS [414.8]
093.89 MURAL THROMBUS DUE TO SYPHILIS
412 MURAL THROMBUS HEALED OR OLD
0 MURCHISON-SANDERSON SYNDROME SEE 'HODGKIN'S DISEASE'
785.2 MURMUR HEART
283.2 MURRI'S DISEASE (INTERMITTENT HEMOGLOBINURIA)
062.4 MURRAY VALLEY ENCEPHALITIS

MUSCLE, MUSCULAR
756.81 ABSENCE (PECTORAL) CONGENITAL
743.69 ABSENCE EYE (ACCESSORY) CONGENITAL
756.81 ABSENCE WITH TENDON ABSENCE CONGENITAL
756.82 ACCESSORY CONGENITAL

ATROPHY
728.2 NOS (DISUSE)
335.21 DUCHENNE-ARAN
728.2 EXTREMITIES
335.11 FAMILIAL SPINAL (JUVENILE)
728.2 GENERAL
335.0 INFANTILE SPINAL
356.1 NEUROPATHIC
356.1 PERONEAL
335.0 PROGRESSIVE OF INFANCY
335.21 PROGRESSIVE PURE
335.10 SPINAL NOS
335.19 SPINAL ADULT
335.0 SPINAL INFANTILE (PROGRESSIVE OF INFANCY)
335.11 SPINAL JUVENILE
335.19 SPINAL OTHER
095.6 SYPHILITIC

MUSCLE, MUSCULAR (continued)
728.10 CALCIFICATION AND OSSIFICATION
728.13 CALCIFICATION HETEROTOPIC POSTOPERATIVE
275.49 CALCIUM SALT INFILTRATE
756.89 CONTRACTION CONGENITAL
958.6 CONTRACTURE POSTTRAUMATIC
908.6 CONTRACTURE POSTTRAUMATIC - LATE EFFECT
729.82 CRAMP (LIMB) (GENERAL)
994.1 CRAMP DUE TO IMMERSION
300.11 CRAMP HYSTERICAL
728.84 DIASTASIS
359.9 DISEASE
728.9 DISEASE INFLAMMATORY
728.9 DISORDER
306.0 DISORDER PSYCHOGENIC
728.3 DISORDER OTHER SPECIFIED
0 DIVISION SEE 'SPRAIN', BY SITE
0 DIVISION WITH OPEN WOUND SEE 'LACERATION'

DYSTROPHY
359.1 NOS
359.0 BENIGN CONGENITAL MYOPATHY
359.0 CONGENITAL HEREDITARY
359.1 DISTAL
359.1 DUCHENNE
359.1 ERB'S
359.1 FASCIOSCAPULOHUMERAL
359.1 GOWER'S
359.1 LANDOUZY DEJERINE
359.1 LIMB GIRDLE
359.1 OCULAR
359.1 OCULOPHARYNGEAL

MUSCLE, MUSCULAR (continued)
781.3 INCOORDINATION
275.49 INFILTRATE CALCAREOUS
728.83 RUPTURE NONTRAUMATIC
728.85 SPASM
728.9 WEAKNESS

955.4 MUSCULOCUTANEOUS NERVE INJURY

MUSCULOSKELETAL
729.89 LOSS OF FUNCTION NEC
729.89 SYMPTOMS IN LIMBS OTHER
781.9 SYMPTOMS OTHER
793.7 SYSTEM ABNORMAL (X-RAY) (ULTRASOUND) (THERMOGRAPHY)
756.9 SYSTEM ANOMALY (ABSENCE) CONGENITAL NEC
729.9 SYSTEM DISORDER NEC
306.0 SYSTEM DISORDER PSYCHOGENIC

495.5 MUSHROOM WORKERS' LUNG

MUTISM
309.83 ELECTIVE - ADJUSTMENT REACTION
313.23 ELECTIVE - EMOTIONAL DISTURBANCE OF CHILDHOOD
300.11 HYSTERICAL

V71.4 MVA EVALUATION NO APPARENT INJURY
424.0 MVP
751.3 MYA'S DISEASE (CONGENITAL DILATION COLON)
729.1 MYALGIA
710.5 MYALGIA EOSINOPHILIA SYNDROME
074.1 MYALGIA EPIDEMIC

MYASTHENIA
005.1 BOTULANI [358.1]
250.6# DIABETIC [358.1]

5th Digit: 250.6

0. TYPE II, ADULT-ONSET, NON-INSULIN DEPENDENT (EVEN IF REQUIRING INSULIN), OR UNSPECIFIED; CONTROLLED

1. TYPE I, JUVENILE-ONSET OR INSULIN-DEPENDENT; CONTROLLED

2. TYPE II, ADULT-ONSET, NON-INSULIN DEPENDENT (EVEN IF REQUIRING INSULIN); UNCONTROLLED

3. TYPE I, JUVENILE-ONSET OR INSULIN-DEPENDENT; UNCONTROLLED

358.0 GRAVIS
775.2 GRAVIS NEONATAL
244.# HYPOTHYROID [358.1]

4th Digit: 244

0. POSTSURGICAL
1. POSTABLATIVE (IRRADIATION)
2. IODINE INGESTION
3. PAS, PHENYLBUT, RESORCINOL
8. SECONDARY NEC
9. NOS

243 HYPOTHYROID CONGENITAL
358.1 NEOPLASTIC
281.0 PERNICIOUS ANEMIA [358.1]
536.8 STOMACH
306.4 STOMACH PSYCHOGENIC
242.## THYROTOXIC [358.1]

4th Digit: 242

0. TOXIC DIFFUSE GOITER
1. TOXIC UNINODULAR GOITER
2. TOXIC MULTINODULAR GOITER
3. TOXIC NODULAR GOITER UNSPECIFIED
4. FROM ECTOPIC THYROID NODULE
8. OF OTHER SPECIFIED ORIGIN
9. WITHOUT GOITER OR OTHER CAUSE

5th Digit: 242

0. WITHOUT STORM
1. WITH STORM

117.4 MYCETOMAS MYCOTIC

M

MYCOBACTERIA

031.9 ATYPICAL INFECTION NOS
031.0 AVIUM INFECTION PULMONARY
031.2 AVIUM INTRACELLULARE COMPLEX INFECTION DISSEMINATED (DMAC)
031.9 DISEASES
031.1 DISEASES CUTANEOUS
031.8 DISEASES OTHER SPECIFIED
031.0 DISEASES PULMONARY
031.0 INTRACELLULARE (BATTEY BACILLUS) INFECTION
031.0 KANSASII INFECTION
031.1 MARINUM (M. BALNEI) INFECTION
031.1 ULCERANS INFECTION

0 MYCOBACTERIUM LEPRAE INFECTION SEE 'LEPROSY'
041.81 MYCOPLASMA INFECTION OR ORGANISM
483.0 MYCOPLASMA PNEUMONIA

MYCOSIS, MYCOTIC

117.9 UNSPECIFIED
111.9 CUTANEOUS NEC
202.1# FUNGOIDES M9700/3

5th Digit: 202.1

0. UNSPECIFIED SITE, EXTRANODAL AND SOLID ORGAN SITES
1. LYMPH NODES OF HEAD FACE NECK
2. LYMPH NODES INTRATHORACIC
3. LYMPH NODES ABDOMINAL
4. LYMPH NODES AXILLA AND UPPER LIMB
5. LYMPH NODES INGUINAL REGION AND LOWER LIMB
6. LYMPH NODES INTRAPELVIC
7. SPLEEN
8. LYMPH NODES MULTIPLE SITES

112.0 MOUTH
117.4 MYCETOMAS
118 OPPORTUNISTIC PATHOGENIC TO COMPROMISED HOSTS ONLY
117.9 PHARYNX
V75.4 SCREENING EXAM
111.9 SKIN NEC
112.0 STOMATITIS
117.9 TOENAIL
117.9 TONSIL
112.1 VAGINA
117.9 OTHER

379.43 MYDRIASIS PERSISTENT NOT DUE TO MYDRIATICS
742.59 MYELATELIA CONGENITAL
341.8 MYELINOSIS CENTRAL PONTINE
0 MYELITIS ACUTE SEE 'ENCEPHALITIS'
0 MYELITIS ASCENDING (TRANSVERSE) ABACTERIAL SEE 'ENCEPHALITIS'
756.89 MYELO-OSTEO-MUSCULODYSPLASIA HEREDITARIA

MYELOCELE

741.0# WITH HYDROCEPHALUS
741.9# WITHOUT HYDROCEPHALUS

5th Digit: 741.0, 9

0. REGION NOS
1. CERVICAL
2. DORSAL
3. LUMBAR

MYELOCYCSTOCELE

741.0# WITH HYDROCEPHALUS
741.9# WITHOUT HYDROCEPHALUS

5th Digit: 741.0, 9

0. REGION NOS
1. CERVICAL
2. DORSAL
3. LUMBAR

742.59 MYELODYSPLASIA CONGENITAL
238.7 MYELODYSPLASTIC SYNDROME
289.8 MYELOFIBROSIS
238.7 MYELOFIBROSIS WITH MYELOID METAPLASIA
V10.62 MYELOID LEUKEMIA HISTORY
288.0 MYELOKATHEXIS
214.9 MYELOLIPOMA SITE NOS
0 MYELOLIPOMA SITE SPECIFIED SEE 'BENIGN NEOPLASM', BY SITE M8870/0
203.0# MYELOMA M9730/3

5th Digit: 203.0

0. WITHOUT MENTION OF REMISSION
1. IN REMISSION

238.6 MYELOMA SOLITARY UNCERTAIN BEHAVIOR M9731/1
203.0# MYELOMATOSIS M9730/3

5th Digit: 203.0

0. WITHOUT MENTION OF REMISSION
1. IN REMISSION

IF MYELOPATHY IS NEOPLASTIC, CODE THE NEOPLASM FIRST WITH THE MYELOPATHY SECOND (336.3)

MYELOPATHY DISCOGENIC

722.70 INTERVERTEBRAL NOS
722.71 CERVICAL
722.72 DORSAL THORACIC
722.73 LUMBAR

MYELOPATHY NONDISCOGENIC

336.9 UNSPECIFIED
336.8 DRUG-INDUCED
336.3 NEOPLASTIC
336.8 RADIATION-INDUCED
336.1 SUBACUTE NECROTIC
336.8 OTHER SPECIFIED

MYELOPROLIFERATIVE

238.7 DISEASE OR SYNDROME (CHRONIC) SITE NOS M9960/1
0 DISEASE CHRONIC SITE SPECIFIED SEE 'NEOPLASM UNCERTAIN BEHAVIOR' BY SITE M9960/1

MYELOSCLEROSIS

238.7 WITH MYELOID METAPLASIA SITE NOS
0 WITH MYELOID METAPLASIA SITE SPECIFIED SEE 'NEOPLASM UNCERTAIN BEHAVIOR', BY SITE M9961/1

207.0# MYELOSIS ERYTHREMIC (ACUTE)

5th Digit: 207.0

0. WITHOUT MENTION OF REMISSION
1. WITH MENTION OF REMISSION

289.9 MYELOSUPPRESSION BONE MARROW DUE TO CHEMOTHERAPY

134.0 MYIASIS

MYOCARDIAL

429.1 ATROPHY
746.85 BRIDGE
861.01 CONTUSION
861.11 CONTUSION WITH OPEN WOUND INTO THORAX
277.3 DEGENERATION AMYLOID [425.7]
746.89 DEGENERATION CONGENITAL
429.1 DEGENERATION (FATTY) (MURAL) (MUSCULAR) WITH ARTERIOSCLEROSIS [440.9]
274.82 DEGENERATION GOUTY
402.## DEGENERATION HYPERTENSIVE

4th Digit: 402

0. MALIGNANT
1. BENIGN
9. UNSPECIFIED

5th Digit: 402

0. WITHOUT CHF
1. WITH CHF

M

MYOCARDIAL (continued)

404.## DEGENERATION HYPERTENSIVE WITH RENAL DISEASE

4th Digit: 404

0. MALIGNANT

1. BENIGN

9. UNSPECIFIED

5th Digit: 404

0. WITHOUT CHF OR RENAL FAILURE

1. WITH CHF

2. WITH RENAL FAILURE

3. WITH CHF AND RENAL FAILURE

093.82 DEGENERATION SYPHILITIC

429.1 DEGENERATION WITH ARTERIOSCLEROSIS [440.9]

0 DEGENERATION SEE ALSO 'CARDIOMYOPATHY'

0 DISEASE SEE 'CARDIOMYOPATHY'

V71.7 EVALUATION NO MI FOUND

428.9 FAILURE NOS

414.8 ISCHEMIA (CHRONIC)

411.89 ISCHEMIA ACUTE WITHOUT MI

411.81 ISCHEMIA ACUTE WITHOUT MI, WITH CORONARY (ARTERY) OCCLUSION

414.0# ISCHEMIA CHRONIC WITHOUT MI, WITH CORONARY (ARTERY) OCCLUSION DUE TO ATHEROSCLEROSIS

5th Digit: 414.0

0. UNSPECIFIED TYPE OF VESSEL, NATIVE OR GRAFT

1. NATIVE CORONARY VESSEL

2. AUTOLOGOUS VEIN BYPASS GRAFT

3. NONAUTOLOGOUS BIOLOGICAL BYPASS GRAFT

4. AUTOLOGOUS ARTERY BYPASS GRAFT (GASTROEPIPLOIC) (INTERNAL MAMMARY)

5. UNSPECIFIED TYPE OF BYPASS GRAFT

861.0# LACERATION

861.1# LACERATION WITH OPEN WOUND INTO THORAX

5th Digit: 861.0-1

2. WITHOUT PENETRATION OF HEART CHAMBERS

3. WITH PENETRATION OF HEART CHAMBERS

0 RUPTURE (NONTRAUMATIC) SEE 'MYOCARDIAL INFARCTION ACUTE'

861.03 RUPTURE TRAUMATIC

861.13 RUPTURE TRAUMATIC WITH OPEN WOUND INTO THORAX

ACUTE MYOCARDIAL INFARCTION - 410.## - THE FOLLOWING 5th DIGIT SUBCLASSIFICATION IS TO BE USED WITH CATEGORY 410.

0 - "EPISODE OF CARE UNSPECIFIED" - USE ONLY WHEN YOU HAVE INSUFFICIENT INFORMATION TO DETERMINE WHETHER EPISODE OF CARE IS INITIAL OR SUBSEQUENT.

1 - "INITIAL EPISODE OF CARE" - USE TO DESIGNATE THE ACUTE PHASE OF CARE, REGARDLESS OF THE LOCATION OF TREATMENT. THIS INCLUDES: 1) CASES ADMITTED TO INITIAL HOSPITAL 2) CASES TRANSFERRED FOR CARE OR TREATMENT OR BOTH 3) IF TRANSFERRED BACK TO INITIAL HOSPITAL DURING ACUTE PHASE OF CARE. EXAMPLE: ACUTE MI ADMITTED HOSPITAL II - 410.91, ACUTE MI FOR HEART CATHETER HOSPITAL II - 410.91, ACUTE MI RETURNED TO HOSPITAL I POST, HEART CATH DURING ACUTE PHASE OF CARE - 410.91, NOT DURING ACUTE PHASE - 410.92.

2 - "SUBSEQUENT EPISODE OF CARE" - USE TO DESIGNATE OBSERVATION, TREATMENT OR EVALUATION OF MI WITHIN 8 WEEKS OF ONSET, BUT FOLLOWING THE ACUTE PHASE, OR IN THE HEALING STATE WHERE THE EPISODE OF CARE MAY BE FOR RELATED OR UNRELATED CONDITION. EXAMPLE: PATIENT ADMITTED TO HOSPITAL 4 WEEKS POST ACUTE MI FOR (PTCA) - 410.92. PATIENT RETURNED TO HOSPITAL I AFTER (PTCA) ANGIOPLASTY WITH STABILIZATION OF HER MI. SHE HAS PICKED UP VIRUS INFECTION IN HOSPITAL II. DIAGNOSIS WOULD BE VIRUS INFECTION 079.99, ACUTE MI, SUBSEQUENT 410.92.

MYOCARDIAL INFARCTION ACUTE

410.9# UNSPECIFIED

410.1# ANTERIOR OTHER (CONTIGUOUS WITH SEPTUM)

410.1# ANTERIOR (WALL) (CONTIGUOUS WITH SEPTUM)

410.1# ANTEROAPICAL (CONTIGUOUS WITH SEPTUM)

410.0# ANTEROLATERAL

5th Digit: 410.0-1, 9

0. EPISODE UNSPECIFIED

1. INITIAL EPISODE

2. SUBSEQUENT EPISODE

MYOCARDIAL INFARCTION ACUTE (continued)

410.1# ANTEROSEPTAL (CONTIGUOUS WITH SEPTUM)

410.8# ATRIUM PAPILLARY OR SEPTUM ALONE

410.5# BASOLATERAL

410.4# DIAPHRAGMATIC

410.4# INFERIOR (WALL) (CONTIGUOUS WITH SEPTUM)

410.2# INFEROLATERAL

410.3# INFEROPOSTERIOR

410.5# LATERAL APICAL

410.5# LATERAL HIGH OR POSTERIOR

410.7# NON-Q WAVE

410.7# NONTRANSMURAL

410.6# POSTERIOR TRUE POSTERIOR (POSTEROBASAL)

410.5# POSTEROLATERAL

410.7# SUBENDOCARDIAL

5th Digit: 410.1-8

0. EPISODE UNSPECIFIED

1. INITIAL EPISODE

2. SUBSEQUENT EPISODE

MYOCARDIAL INFARCTION ASSOCIATED DIAGNOSES

412 DIAGNOSED ON EKG BUT PRESENTING NO SYMPTOMS

V71.7 EVALUATION NO MI FOUND

412 HISTORY

411.1 IMPENDING

412 OLD

411.0 POST MYOCARDIAL INFARCTION SYNDROME

IF THE DIAGNOSIS IS NOT SPECIFIED AS ACUTE ON THE RECORD, THE CODER IS REQUIRED TO SELECT THE CHRONIC OR NOS CODE. IF THE MEDICAL RECORD INDICATES THAT THE REASON THE PATIENT SOUGHT CARE WAS DUE TO AN EXACERBATION OF A CHRONIC CONDITION, CONSULT THE PHYSICIAN FOR FURTHER DOCUMENTATION.

MYOCARDITIS

429.0 UNSPECIFIED

422.90 ACUTE

422.92 ACUTE BACTERIAL

422.91 ACUTE IDIOPATHIC

422.90 ACUTE INTERSTITIAL

422.99 ACUTE OTHER SPECIFIED

429.0 ARTERIOSCLEROTIC [440.9]

429.0 CHRONIC INTERSTITIAL

425.4 CONSTRICTIVE

422.91 GIANT CELL (ACUTE) (SUBACUTE)

422.91 GRANULOMATOUS ACUTE (ISOLATED) (DIFFUSE)

0 HYPERTENSIVE SEE 'CARDIOMYOPATHY', HYPERTENSIVE

422.91 IDIOPATHIC GRANULOMATOUS

422.92 INFECTIVE

487.8 INFLUENZAL ACUTE [422.0]

422.99 MALIGNANT

036.43 MENINGOCOCCAL

422.90 NONRHEUMATIC, ACTIVE

422.90 PARENCHYMATOUS

422.92 PNEUMOCOCCAL [041.2]

391.2 RHEUMATIC ACUTE

398.0 RHEUMATIC CHRONIC

422.92 SEPTIC

422.92 STAPHYLOCOCCAL **[041.1#]**

5th Digit: 041.1

0. NOS

1. AUREUS

9. OTHER STAPH

391.2 STREPTOCOCCAL **[041.0#]**

5th Digit: 041.0

0. NOS

1. GROUP A

2. GROUP B

3. GROUP C

4. GROUP D (ENTEROCOCCUS)

5. GROUP G

9. OTHER STREP

MYOCARDITIS (continued)
422.92 SUPPURATIVE
422.93 TOXIC
422.91 VIRAL
074.23 VIRAL COXSACKIE
422.99 OTHER SPECIFIED ACUTE

MYOCARDITIS INFECTIOUS OR ASSOCIATED WITH OTHER DISEASES
074.23 ACUTE ASEPTIC (OF NEWBORN)
422.99 ACUTE OTHER
074.23 ASEPTIC NEWBORN
074.23 COXSACKIE
032.82 DIPHTHERIA
422.91 FIEDLER'S
422.91 GIANT CELL ACUTE
422.91 GRANULOMATOUS ISOLATED (DIFFUSE) ACUTE
422.91 IDIOPATHIC ACUTE, SUBACUTE
093.82 SYPHILIS
130.3 TOXOPLASMOSIS
017.9# TUBERCULOUS ACUTE [422.0]
5th Digit: 017.9
0. UNSPECIFIED
1. LAB NOT DONE
2. LABS PENDING
3. MICROSCOPY POSITIVE (IN SPUTUM)
4. CULTURE POSITIVE - MICROSCOPY NEGATIVE
5. CULTURE NEGATIVE - MICROSCOPY POSITIVE
6. CULTURE AND MICROSCOPY NEGATIVE CONFIRMED BY OTHER METHODS

333.2 MYOCLONUS
333.2 MYOCLONUS FAMILIAL ESSENTIAL
421.9 MYOENDOCARDITIS (ACUTE) (SUBACUTE)
229.9 MYOEPITHELIOMA SITE NOS
0 MYOEPITHELIOMA SITE SPECIFIED SEE 'BENIGN NEOPLASM', BY SITE M8982/0
724.2 MYOFASCIAL PAIN LOWER BACK (MYOFASCIITIS)
729.1 MYOFASCIAL PAIN SYNDROME (MYOFASCITIS)
729.1 MYOFASCITIS (ACUTE)
724.2 MYOFASCITIS LOWER BACK
728.2 MYOFIBROSIS
791.3 MYOGLOBINURIA (UNSPECIFIED)
351.8 MYOKYMIA FACIAL
215.# MYOMA M8895/0
4th Digit: 215
0. HEAD FACE NECK
2. UPPER LIMB SHOULDER
3. LOWER LIMB HIP
4. THORAX
5. ABDOMINAL HYPOCHONDRIUM
6. PELVIS BUTTOCK GROIN INGUINAL REGION PERINEUM
7. TRUNK NOS BACK NOS FLANK NOS
8. OTHER SPECIFIED SITES
9. SITE UNSPECIFIED

MYOMA UTERINE
218.9 UNSPECIFIED
218.1 INTRAMURAL
218.0 SUBMUCOUS
218.2 SUBSEROUS

MYOMETRITIS (SEE ALSO 'ENDOMETRITIS')
615.9 MYOMETRITIS
615.0 ACUTE
615.1 CHRONIC
670.0# MATERNAL DUE TO PREGNANCY
5th Digit: 670.0
0. UNSPECIFIED
2. DELIVERED WITH POSTPARTUM COMPLICATION
4. POSTPARTUM COMPLICATION

621.8 MYOMETRIUM ATROPHY
622.8 MYOMETRIUM ATROPHY CERVIX
040.0 MYONECROSIS, CLOSTRIDIAL

MYONEURAL
358.9 DISORDERS
358.8 DISORDERS OTHER NEC
358.2 DISORDERS TOXIC

MYOPATHY
359.9 NOS
255.4 ADDISONIAN [359.5]
277.3 AMYLOID [359.6]
359.0 BENIGN CONGENITAL
359.0 CENTRONUCLEAR
376.82 EXTRAOCULAR MUSCLES
253.2 HYPOPITUITARY [359.5]
244.# HYPOTHYROID [359.5]
4th Digit: 244
0. POSTSURGICAL
1. POSTABLATIVE (IRRADIATION)
2. IODINE INGESTION
3. PAS, PHENYLBUT, RESORCINOL
8. SECONDARY NEC
9. NOS
710.0 LUPUS [359.6]
359.0 MYOTUBULAR
359.1 OCULAR (HEREDITARY) (PROGRESSIVE)
446.0 POLYARTERITIS NODOSA [359.6]
714.0 RHEUMATOID [359.6]
135 SARCOID [359.6]
710.1 SCLERODERMA [359.6]
710.2 SJOGREN'S [359.6]
242.## THYROTOXIC [359.5]
4th Digit: 242
0. TOXIC DIFFUSE GOITER
1. TOXIC UNINODULAR GOITER
2. TOXIC MULTINODULAR GOITER
3. TOXIC NODULAR GOITER UNSPECIFIED
4. FROM ECTOPIC THYROID NODULE
8. OF OTHER SPECIFIED ORIGIN
9. WITHOUT GOITER OR OTHER CAUSE
5th Digit: 242
0. WITHOUT STORM
1. WITH STORM
359.4 TOXIC
255.0 WITH CUSHING'S SYNDROME [359.5]
244.# WITH MYXEDEMA [359.5]
4th Digit: 244
0. POSTSURGICAL
1. POSTABLATIVE (IRRADIATION)
2. IODINE INGESTION
3. PAS, PHENYLBUT, RESORCINOL
8. SECONDARY NEC
9. NOS
359.8 OTHER

MYOPERICARDITIS
420.90 ACUTE
423.8 CHRONIC
391.0 RHEUMATIC ACUTE
393 RHEUMATIC CHRONIC

367.1 MYOPIA
360.21 MYOPIA MALIGNANT
360.21 MYOPIA PROGRESSIVE HIGH (DEGENERATIVE)

M

171.# MYOSARCOMA M8895/3

4th Digit: 171

0. HEAD FACE NECK
2. UPPER LIMB LIMB SHOULDER
3. LOWER LIMB HIP
4. THORAX
5. ABDOMINAL HYPOCHONDRIUM
6. PELVIS BUTTOCK GROIN INGUINAL REGION PERINEUM
7. TRUNK NOS BACK NOS FLANK NOS
8. OTHER SPECIFIED SITES
9. SITE UNSPECIFIED

MYOSITIS

729.1 NOS
040.0 CLOSTRIDIAL
074.1 EPIDEMIC
728.0 INFECTIVE
728.81 INTERSTITIAL
376.12 ORBITAL
728.19 OSSIFICANS OTHER
728.11 OSSIFICANS PROGRESSIVE
728.12 OSSIFICANS TRAUMATIC
729.1 RHEUMATOID
095.6 SYPHILITIC
729.1 TRAUMATIC OLD
040.81 TROPICAL

728.2 MYOTATIC ATROPHY
359.2 MYOTONIA (ATROPHIC) CONGENITA
359.2 MYOTONIC DISORDERS
359.0 MYOTUBULAR MYOPATHY

MYRINGITIS

384.00 ACUTE
384.09 ACUTE OTHER SPECIFIED
384.01 BULLOSA HEMORRHAGIC ACUTE
384.1 CHRONIC
0 WITH OTITIS MEDIA SEE 'OTITIS MEDIA'

MYXEDEMA

244.9 NOS
244.# ADULT
244.# CEREBELLAR ATAXIA [334.4]
244.# CEREBRAL DEGENERATION [331.7]
243 CONGENITAL
244.# JUVENILE
293.0 MADNESS (ACUTE) **[244.#]**
244.# PRIMARY

4th Digit: 244

0. POSTSURGICAL
1. POSTABLATIVE (IRRADIATION)
2. IODINE INGESTION
3. PAS, PHENYLBUT, RESORCINOL
8. SECONDARY NEC
9. NOS

214.# MYXOLIPOMA M8852/0

4th Digit: 214

0. FACE SKIN AND SUBCUTANEOUS TISSUE
1. SKIN AND SUBCUTANEOUS TISSUE OTHER
2. INTRATHORACIC ORGANS
3. INTRA-ABDOMINAL ORGANS
4. SPERMATIC CORD
8. OTHER SPECIFIED SITES
9. UNSPECIFIED SITE

MYXOMA

215.# NOS M8840/0

4th Digit: 215

0. HEAD FACE NECK
2. UPPER LIMB SHOULDER
3. LOWER LIMB HIP
4. THORAX
5. ABDOMINAL HYPOCHONDRIUM
6. PELVIS BUTTOCK GROIN INGUINAL REGION PERINEUM
7. TRUNK NOS BACK NOS FLANK NOS
8. OTHER SPECIFIED SITES
9. SITE UNSPECIFIED

213.# ODONTOGENIC M9320/0

4th Digit: 213

0. SKULL FACE UPPER JAW
1. LOWER JAW (OR IF SITE UNSPECIFIED)

171.# MYXOSARCOMA M8840/3

4th Digit: 171

0. HEAD FACE NECK
2. UPPER LIMB SHOULDER
3. LOWER LIMB HIP
4. THORAX
5. ABDOMINAL HYPOCHONDRIUM
6. PELVIS BUTTOCK GROIN INGUINAL REGION PERINEUM
7. TRUNK NOS BACK NOS FLANK NOS
8. OTHER SPECIFIED SITES
9. SITE UNSPECIFIED

M

616.0 NABOTHIAN (GLAND) CYST OR FOLLICLE ECTROPION (NONOBSTETRICAL)
289.7 NADH [DPNH]-METHEMOGLOBIN-REDUCTASE DEFICIENCY CONGENITAL
287.1 NAEGELI'S DISEASE
136.2 NAEGLERIA MENINGOENCEPHALITIS
353.0 NAFFZIGER'S SYNDROME
756.0 NAGER-DE REYNIER SYNDROME (DYSOSTOSIS MANDIBULARIS)

NAIL
703.8 ATROPHY
757.5 ATROPHY CONGENITAL
883.0 AVULSION FINGER OR THUMB
883.1 AVULSION FINGER OR THUMB COMPLICATED
893.0 AVULSION TOE NAIL
893.1 AVULSION TOE NAIL COMPLICATED
307.9 BITING
757.5 DEFORMITY - CONGENITAL (FINGER OR TOE)
703.8 DEFORMITY - FINGER OR TOE
703.8 DEFORMITY - SPONGIFORM
703.8 DISCOLORATION
703.9 DISEASE UNSPECIFIED
703.8 DISEASE OTHER SPECIFIED NEC
703.8 HYPERTROPHY
681.9 INFECTION
681.02 INFECTION (PARONYCHIA OR ONYCHIA) FINGER
681.11 INFECTION (PARONYCHIA OR ONYCHIA) TOE
703.0 INGROWING WITH INFECTION
959.5 INJURY FINGER
959.7 INJURY TOE
756.89 PATELLA (HEREDITARY OSTEO-ONYCHODYSPLASIA)
703.8 THICKENING

066.1 NAIROBI SHEEP DISEASE
691.0 NAPKIN DERMATITIS (RASH)
301.81 NARCISSISTIC PERSONALITY
347 NARCOLEPSY
786.09 NARCOSIS CO 2 (RESPIRATORY)
763.5 NARCOSIS DUE TO DRUG (CORRECTLY ADMINISTERED) AFFECTING FETUS OR NEWBORN
763.5 NARCOTIC REACTION (INTOXICATION) MATERNAL DURING L&D AFFECTING FETUS OR NEWBORN
760.72 NARCOTIC TRANSMITTED VIA PLACENTA OR BREAST MILK AFFECTING FETUS OR NEWBORN
748.0 NARES ATRESIA (CONGENITAL)
748.0 NARES STENOSIS CONGENITAL
0 NASAL SEE 'NOSE, NASAL'

NASOLACRIMAL DUCT
743.65 ANOMALY OR ATRESIA CONGENITAL
375.56 OBSTRUCTION
743.65 OBSTRUCTION CONGENITAL
375.55 OBSTRUCTION NEONATAL
375.56 STENOSIS ACQUIRED

526.1 NASOPALATINE CYST

NASOPHARYNGEAL
478.29 ABSCESS
748.8 ATRESIA
472.2 ATROPHY
478.21 CELLULITIS
478.26 CYST
478.20 DISEASE
478.29 DISEASE OTHER SPECIFIED
478.25 EDEMA
959.09 INJURY
478.29 OBSTRUCTION
478.29 ULCER

NASOPHARYNGITIS
460 NOS
460 ACUTE [COMMON COLD]
460 ACUTE DUE TO RSV (RESPIRATORY SYNCYTIAL VIRUS) [079.6]
460 ACUTE INFECTIVE
472.2 CHRONIC
460 INFECTIVE
460 SUBACUTE
034.0 STREPTOCOCCAL
472.2 SUPPURATIVE (CHRONIC)
472.2 ULCERATIVE CHRONIC
472.1 WITH CHRONIC PHARYNGITIS

787.02 NAUSEA
787.01 NAUSEA WITH VOMITING
771.4 NAVEL CORD INFECTION PERINATAL
779.8 NAVEL DISEASE NEWBORN NEC
367.1 NEAR SIGHTEDNESS
780.2 NEAR-SYNCOPE
253.3 NEBECOURT'S SYNDROME
371.01 NEBULA CORNEA
743.43 NEBULA CORNEA CONGENITAL
743.42 NEBULA CORNEA CONGENITAL INTERFERING WITH VISION
126.1 NECATOR AMERICANUS INFECTION
126.9 NECATORIASIS

NECK
900.9 BLOOD VESSEL NOS INJURY
900.82 BLOOD VESSEL NEC INJURY - MULTIPLE
900.89 BLOOD VESSEL NEC INJURY - SPECIFIED NEC
719.88 CALCIFICATION (CERVICAL)
V48.1 DEFICIENCY
738.2 DEFORMITY ACQUIRED
744.9 DEFORMITY CONGENITAL
744.89 DEFORMITY CONGENITAL OTHER SPECIFIED
V48.7 DISFIGUREMENT
723.9 DISORDER (NECK REGION) (MUSCULOSKELETAL)
959.09 INJURY
925.2 INJURY (CRUSH)
910.8 INJURY OTHER AND UNSPECIFIED (SUPERFICIAL)
910.9 INJURY OTHER AND UNSPECIFIED (SUPERFICIAL) INFECTED
723.1 PAIN (NONDISCOGENIC)
V48.9 PROBLEM
V48.3 PROBLEM (MECHANICAL AND MOTOR)
V48.5 PROBLEM (SENSORY)
V48.8 PROBLEM (OTHER)
0 SEE ALSO 'CERVICAL'
847.0 SEPARATION (RUPTURE) (TEAR) (LACERATION)
723.5 SPASM
723.5 STIFF
847.0 STRAIN (SPRAIN) (AVULSION) (HEMARTHROSIS)
784.2 SWELLING MASS OR LUMP
784.9 SYMPTOM OTHER
744.5 WEBBING CONGENITAL

437.8 NECRENCEPHALUS
040.3 NECROBACILLOSIS
799.8 NECROBIOSIS
709.3 NECROBIOSIS LIPOIDICA
250.8# NECROBIOSIS LIPOIDICA DIABETICORUM [709.3]

5th Digit: 250.8

0. TYPE II, ADULT-ONSET, NON-INSULIN DEPENDENT (EVEN IF REQUIRING INSULIN), OR UNSPECIFIED; CONTROLLED

1. TYPE I, JUVENILE-ONSET OR INSULIN-DEPENDENT; CONTROLLED

2. TYPE II, ADULT-ONSET, NON-INSULIN DEPENDENT (EVEN IF REQUIRING INSULIN); UNCONTROLLED

3. TYPE I, JUVENILE-ONSET OR INSULIN-DEPENDENT; UNCONTROLLED

N

NECROSIS

785.4 NOS
255.8 ADRENAL (CAPSULE) (GLAND)
478.1 ANTRUM NASAL SINUS
441.9 AORTIC (HYALINE)
441.0# AORTIC DISSECTING CYSTIC MEDIAL
5th Digit: 441.0
0. SITE NOS
1. THORACIC
2. ABDOMINAL
3. THORACOABDOMINAL

441.5 AORTIC RUPTURED
446.0 ARTERITIS
447.5 ARTERY
733.40 ASEPTIC - BONE SITE NOS
733.42 ASEPTIC - FEMUR (HEAD AND NECK OF)
733.43 ASEPTIC - FEMUR (MEDIAL CONDYLE)
733.42 ASEPTIC - FEMUR (OTHER)
733.41 ASEPTIC - HUMERUS (HEAD OF)
733.44 ASEPTIC - TALUS
733.49 ASEPTIC - OTHER BONE SITE
0 AVASCULAR SEE 'NECROSIS', ASEPTIC, BY SITE
596.8 BLADDER (ASEPTIC) (SPHINCTER)
730.0# BONE ACUTE NOS
5th Digit: 730.0
0. SITE NOS
1. SHOULDER REGION
2. UPPER ARM (ELBOW) (HUMERUS)
3. FOREARM (RADIUS) (WRIST) (ULNA)
4. HAND (CARPAL) (METACARPAL) (FINGERS)
5. PELVIC REGION AND THIGH (HIP) (BUTTOCK) (FEMUR)
6. LOWER LEG (FIBULA) (KNEE) (PATELLA) (TIBIA)
7. ANKLE AND/OR FOOT (METATARSALS) (TOES) (TARSAL)
8. OTHER (HEAD) (NECK) (RIB) (SKULL) (TRUNK)
9. MULTIPLE

0 BONE ASEPTIC SEE 'NECROSIS', ASEPTIC
730.1# BONE DUE TO OSTEOMYELITIS CHRONIC (SEE ALSO 'OSTEOMYELITIS')
5th Digit: 730.1
0. SITE NOS
1. SHOULDER REGION
2. UPPER ARM (ELBOW) (HUMERUS)
3. FOREARM (RADIUS) (WRIST) (ULNA)
4. HAND (CARPAL) (METACARPAL) (FINGERS)
5. PELVIC REGION AND THIGH (HIP) (BUTTOCK) (FEMUR)
6. LOWER LEG (FIBULA) (KNEE) (PATELLA) (TIBIA)
7. ANKLE AND/OR FOOT (METATARSALS) (TOES) (TARSAL)
8. OTHER (HEAD) (NECK) (RIB) (SKULL) (TRUNK)
9. MULTIPLE

731.0 BONE DUE TO PAGET'S DISEASE
0 BONE DUE TO TUBERCULOSIS SEE 'TUBERCULOSIS', BONE
0 BONE EPIPHYSEAL ISCHEMIC SEE 'OSTEOCHONDROSIS'
478.1 BONE ETHMOID (NOSE)
733.40 BONE ISCHEMIC
526.4 BONE JAW
289.8 BONE MARROW
437.8 BRAIN
611.3 BREAST (ASEPTIC) (FAT) (SEGMENTAL)
519.1 BRONCHUS
437.8 CENTRAL NERVOUS SYSTEM NEC
437.8 CEREBELLAR
437.8 CEREBRAL NOS
742.4 CEREBRAL CONGENITAL
437.8 CEREBROSPINAL
371.40 CORNEA
0 DUE TO RADIATION / RADIUM SEE 'NECROSIS', BY SITE
0 DUE TO SWALLOWING CORROSIVE SUBSTANCE SEE 'BURN', BY SITE

NECROSIS (continued)

983.9 DUE TO POISONING BY PHOSPHORUS COMPOUNDS
0 DUE TO TUBERCULOSIS SEE 'TUBERCULOSIS'
385.24 EAR (OSSICLE)
0 EPIPHYSEAL ISCHEMIC SEE 'OSTEOCHONDROSIS'
530.89 ESOPHAGUS
478.1 ETHMOID (BONE)
374.50 EYELID
272.8 FATTY (GENERALIZED)
611.3 FATTY BREAST
569.89 FATTY INTESTINE
567.8 FATTY MESENTERY
567.8 FATTY OMENTUM
577.8 FATTY PANCREAS
567.8 FATTY PERITONEUM
709.3 FATTY SKIN (SUBCUTANEOUS)
778.1 FATTY SKIN (SUBCUTANEOUS) NEWBORN
733.42 FEMUR (ASEPTIC) (AVASCULAR)
733.42 FEMUR (ASEPTIC) (AVASCULAR) - HEAD
733.43 FEMUR (ASEPTIC) (AVASCULAR) - MEDIAL CONDYLE
733.42 FEMUR (ASEPTIC) (AVASCULAR) - NECK
575.0 GALLBLADDER (SEE ALSO 'CHOLECYSTITIS' ACUTE)
537.89 GASTRIC

646.6#: SPECIFY THE MATERNAL GENITAL NECROSIS WITH AN ADDITIONAL CODE.

646.6# GENITAL ORGAN OR TRACT MATERNAL COMPLICATING PREGNANCY
5th Digit: 646.6
0. EPISODE OF CARE UNSPECIFIED OR N/A
1. DELIVERED
2. DELIVERED WITH POSTPARTUM COMPLICATION
3 ANTEPARTUM COMPLICATION
4 POSTPARTUM COMPLICATION

478.79 GLOTTIS
0 HEART (MYOCARDIAL) (SUBENDOCARDIAL) SEE 'MYOCARDIAL INFARCTION ACUTE'
570 HEPATIC (SEE ALSO 'NECROSIS', LIVER)
733.42 HIP ASEPTIC (AVASCULAR) (SEE ALSO 'NECROSIS', FEMUR)
557.0 INTESTINE
785.4 ISCHEMIC (SEE ALSO 'GANGRENE')
583.9 KIDNEY NOS (BILATERAL)
584.9 KIDNEY ACUTE
583.6 KIDNEY CORTICAL
584.6 KIDNEY CORTICAL - ACUTE
760.1 KIDNEY CORTICAL - ACUTE AFFECTING FETUS OR NEWBORN
646.2# KIDNEY CORTICAL - ACUTE COMPLICATING PREGNANCY [584.6]
5th Digit: 646.2
0. EPISODE OF CARE UNSPECIFIED OR N/A
1. DELIVERED
2. DELIVERED WITH POSTPARTUM COMPLICATION
3 ANTEPARTUM COMPLICATION
4 POSTPARTUM COMPLICATION

639.3 KIDNEY CORTICAL - ACUTE FOLLOWING ABORTION
639.3 KIDNEY CORTICAL - ACUTE FOLLOWING ECTOPIC PREGNANCY
669.3# KIDNEY CORTICAL - ACUTE FOLLOWING LABOR AND DELIVERY
5th Digit: 669.3
0. EPISODE OF CARE UNSPECIFIED OR N/A
2. DELIVERED WITH POSTPARTUM COMPLICATION
4. POSTPARTUM COMPLICATION

639.3 KIDNEY CORTICAL - ACUTE FOLLOWING MOLAR PREGNANCY
0 KIDNEY CORTICAL - ACUTE WITH ABORTION SEE 'ABORTION', BY TYPE, WITH RENAL FAILURE
0 KIDNEY CORTICAL - ACUTE WITH ECTOPIC PREGNANCY SEE 'ECTOPIC PREGNANCY', BY SITE WITH COMPLICATION
0 KIDNEY CORTICAL - ACUTE WITH MOLAR PREGNANCY SEE 'MOLAR PREGNANCY', BY TYPE WITH COMPLICATION

NECROSIS (continued)

590.80 KIDNEY MEDULLARY (SEE ALSO 'PYELONEPHRITIS')
584.7 KIDNEY MEDULLARY - ACUTE RENAL FAILURE
583.7 KIDNEY MEDULLARY - IN GLOMERULONEPHRITIS NOS
584.5 KIDNEY TUBULAR
760.1 KIDNEY TUBULAR - AFFECTING FETUS OR NEWBORN
646.2# KIDNEY TUBULAR COMPLICATING PREGNANCY [584.5]

5th Digit: 646.2

- **0. EPISODE OF CARE UNSPECIFIED OR N/A**
- **1. DELIVERED**
- **2. DELIVERED WITH POSTPARTUM COMPLICATION**
- **3 ANTEPARTUM COMPLICATION**
- **4 POSTPARTUM COMPLICATION**

997.5 KIDNEY TUBULAR - DUE TO A PROCEDURE
639.3 KIDNEY TUBULAR - FOLLOWING ABORTION
639.3 KIDNEY TUBULAR - FOLLOWING ECTOPIC PREGNANCY
669.3# KIDNEY TUBULAR - FOLLOWING LABOR AND DELIVERY

5th Digit: 669.3

- **0. EPISODE OF CARE UNSPECIFIED OR N/A**
- **2. DELIVERED WITH POSTPARTUM COMPLICATION**
- **4. POSTPARTUM COMPLICATION**

639.3 KIDNEY TUBULAR - FOLLOWING MOLAR PREGNANCY
958.5 KIDNEY TUBULAR - TRAUMATIC
0 KIDNEY TUBULAR - WITH ABORTION SEE 'ABORTION', BY TYPE, WITH RENAL FAILURE
0 KIDNEY TUBULAR - WITH ECTOPIC PREGNANCY SEE 'ECTOPIC PREGNANCY', BY SITE, WITH COMPLICATION
0 KIDNEY TUBULAR - WITH MOLAR PREGNANCY SEE 'MOLAR PREGNANCY', BY TYPE, WITH COMPLICATION
478.79 LARYNX
570 LIVER (ACUTE) (CONGENITAL) (DIFFUSE) (MASSIVE) (SUBACUTE)
760.8 LIVER AFFFECTING FETUS OR NEWBORN
646.7# LIVER COMPLICATING PREGNANCY [570]

5th Digit: 646.7

- **0. EPISODE OF CARE UNSPECIFIED OR N/A**
- **1. DELIVERED**
- **3 ANTEPARTUM COMPLICATION**

639.8 LIVER FOLLOWING ABORTION
639.8 LIVER FOLLOWING ECTOPIC PREGNANCY
639.8 LIVER FOLLOWING MOLAR PREGNANCY
674.8# LIVER MATERNAL DUE TO PREGNANCY

5th Digit: 674.8

- **0. EPISODE OF CARE UNSPECIFIED OR N/A**
- **2. DELIVERED WITH POSTPARTUM COMPLICATION**
- **4. POSTPARTUM COMPLICATION**

639.8 LIVER POSTABORTAL
573.3 LIVER TOXIC (NONINFECTIOUS)
0 LIVER WITH ABORTION SEE 'ABORTION', BY TYPE, WITH OTHER SPECIFIED COMPLICATION
0 LIVER WITH ECTOPIC PREGNANCY SEE 'ECTOPIC PREGNANCY', BY SITE WITH COMPLICATION
0 LIVER WITH MOLAR PREGNANCY SEE 'MOLAR PREGNANCY', BY TYPE WITH COMPLICATION
513.0 LUNG
683 LYMPHATIC GLAND
611.3 MAMMARY GLAND
526.4 MANDIBLE
383.1 MASTOID (CHRONIC)
557.0 MESENTERY
567.8 MESENTERY FAT
0 MITRAL VALVE SEE 'MITRAL INSUFFICIENCY'
478.1 NASAL (SEPTUM)
478.1 NASAL SINUS (ANTRUM)
557.0 OMENTUM
567.8 OMENTUM FAT
557.0 OMENTUM WITH MESENTERIC INFARCTION

NECROSIS (continued)

376.10 ORBIT
385.24 OSSICLES, EAR (ASEPTIC)
614.2 OVARY (SEE ALSO 'SALPINGO-OOPHORITIS')
577.8 PANCREAS (ASEPTIC) (DUCT) (FAT)
577.0 PANCREAS ACUTE (ASEPTIC) (DUCT) (FAT)
577.0 PANCREAS INFECTIVE (ASEPTIC) (DUCT) (FAT)
590.80 PAPILLARY KIDNEY (SEE ALSO 'PYELONEPHRITIS')
557.0 PERITONEUM
567.8 PERITONEUM FAT
557.0 PERITONEUM WITH MESENTERIC INFARCTION
462 PHARYNX
288.0 PHARYNX IN GRANULOCYTOPENIA
253.2 PITUITARY (GLAND) (POSTPARTUM) (SHEEHAN)
656.7# PLACENTA AFFECTING MANAGEMENT OF MOTHER

5th Digit: 656.7

- **0. EPISODE OF CARE UNSPECIFIED OR N/A**
- **1. DELIVERED**
- **3 ANTEPARTUM COMPLICATION**

513.0 PNEUMONIA
513.0 PULMONARY
537.89 PYLORUS
0 RADIATION / RADIUM (DUE TO) SEE 'NECROSIS', BY SITE
0 RENAL SEE 'NECROSIS', KIDNEY
379.19 SCLERA
608.89 SCROTUM
709.8 SKIN OR SUBCUTANEOUS TISSUE
709.8 SKIN OR SUBCUTANEOUS TISSUE DUE TO BURN SEE 'BURN', BY SITE
785.4 SKIN OR SUBCUTANEOUS TISSUE GANGRENOUS
336.1 SPINAL CORD
730.18 SPINE, SPINAL (COLUMN) ACUTE
289.59 SPLEEN
537.89 STOMACH
528.1 STOMATITIS
709.3 SUBCUTANEOUS FAT
778.1 SUBCUTANEOUS FAT FETUS OR NEWBORN
255.8 SUPRARENAL (CAPSULE) (GLAND)
521.0 TOOTH
522.1 TOOTH PULP
608.89 TESTES
254.8 THYMUS (GLAND)
474.8 TONSIL
519.1 TRACHEA
0 TUBERCULOUS SEE 'TUBERCULOSIS'
997.5 TUBULAR (ACUTE) SPECIFIED AS DUE TO A PROCEDURE
762.6 UMBILICAL CORD AFFECTING FETUS OR NEWBORN
623.8 VAGINA
730.18 VERTEBRA (ACUTE) (LUMBAR)
015.0# VERTEBRAL COLUMN DUE TO TUBERCULOSIS **[730.8#]**

5th Digit: 015.0

- **0. NOS**
- **1. LAB NOT DONE**
- **2. LABS PENDING**
- **3. MICROSCOPY POSITIVE (IN SPUTUM)**
- **4. CULTURE POSITIVE - MICROSCOPY NEGATIVE**
- **5. CULTURE POSITIVE - MICROSCOPY POSITIVE**
- **6. CULTURE AND MICROSCOPY NEGATIVE - CONFIRMED BY OTHER METHODS**

5th Digit: 730.8

- **0. SITE NOS**
- **1. SHOULDER REGION**
- **2. UPPER ARM (ELBOW) (HUMERUS)**
- **3. FOREARM (RADIUS) (WRIST) (ULNA)**
- **4. HAND (CARPAL) (METACARPAL) (FINGERS)**
- **5. PELVIC REGION AND THIGH (HIP) (BUTTOCK) (FEMUR)**
- **6. LOWER LEG (FIBULA) (KNEE) (PATELLA) (TIBIA)**
- **7. ANKLE AND/OR FOOT (METATARSALS) (TOES) (TARSAL)**
- **8. OTHER (HEAD) (NECK) (RIB) (SKULL) (TRUNK)**
- **9. MULTIPLE**

0 X-RAY SEE 'NECROSIS', BY SITE

N

288.0 NECROTICANS AGRANULOCYTICA MUCOSITIS
777.5 NECROTIZING ENTEROCOLITIS IN FETUS OR NEWBORN
0 NECROTIZING FASCIITIS SEE 'FASCIITIS', NECROTIZING
584.7 NECROTIZING RENAL PAPILLITIS
446.4 NECROTIZING RESPIRATORY GRANULOMATOSIS
V15.42 NEGLECT HISTORY - ADULT
V15.42 NEGLECT HISTORY - CHILD OR NEWBORN
759.89 NEILL DINGWALL SYNDROME (MICROENCEPHALY AND DWARFISM)
359.0 NEMALINE BODY DISEASE
128.9 NEMATODE INFESTATION NEC CONJUNCTIVA
775.8 NEONATAL AMINO ACID DISORDER (METABOLIC), TRANSITORY
V23.5 NEONATAL DEATH HISTORY AFFECTING PREGNANCY SUPERVISION
776.8 NEONATAL HEMATOLOGICAL DISORDERS TRANSIENT OTHER SPECIFIED

NEONATAL JAUNDICE
774.2 ASSOCIATED WITH PRETERM DELIVERY
774.39 CONJUGATION OTHER
774.30 DELAYED CONJUGATION
774.4 DUE TO LIVER DAMAGE
774.6 FETAL
774.6 FETAL OTHER
774.0 FROM HEREDITARY ANEMIAS
774.5 FROM OTHER CAUSES
774.1 HEMOLYTIC

0 NEOPLASM BENIGN SEE 'BENIGN NEOPLASM', BY SITE
0 NEOPLASM IN SITU SEE 'CARCINOMA IN SITU', BY SITE
0 NEOPLASM MALIGNANT SEE 'CANCER' BY SITE
0 NEOPLASM METASTATIC SEE 'CANCER' BY SITE, METASTATIC.

NEOPLASM UNCERTAIN BEHAVIOR (QUICK REFERENCE)
235.# DIGESTIVE AND RESPIRATORY
4th Digit: 235
0. SALIVARY GLANDS, MAJOR
1. LIP, ORAL CAVITY, PHARYNX
2. STOMACH, INTESTINES, RECTUM
3. LIVER, BILIARY PASSAGES, GALLBLADDER
4. PERITONEUM, RETROPERITONEUM
5. OTHER AND UNSPECIFIED DIGESTIVE ORGANS
6. LARYNX
7. TRACHEA BRONCHUS LUNG
8. PLEURA, THYMUS, LUNG
9. OTHER AND UNSPECIFIED RESPIRATORY ORGANS
236.#(#) GENITOURINARY
4th or 4th and 5th Digit: 236
0. UTERUS
1. PLACENTA
2. OVARY
3. OTHER AND UNSPECIFIED FEMALE GENITAL ORGANS
4. TESTES
5. PROSTATE
6. OTHER AND UNSPECIFIED MALE GENITAL ORGANS
7. BLADDER
9#. OTHER AND UNSPECIFIED URINARY ORGANS
90. URINARY ORGAN, UNSPECIFIED
91. KIDNEY AND URETER
99. OTHER SPECIFIED

NEOPLASM UNCERTAIN BEHAVIOR (QUICK REFERENCE) (continued)
237.#(#) ENDOCRINE AND NERVOUS SYSTEM
4th or 4th and 5th Digit: 237
0. PITUITARY AND CRANIOPHARYNGEAL DUCT
1. PINEAL
2. ADRENAL, SUPRARENAL
3. PARAGANGLIA (AORTIC, CAROTID, COCCYGEAL, BODIES), GLOMUS JUGULARE
4. PARATHYROID, THYROID, OTHER AND UNSPECIFIED GLANDS
5. BRAIN AND SPINAL CORD
6. MENINGES
7#. NEUROFIBROMATOSIS
70. NOT OTHERWISE SPECIFIIED
71. TYPE 1
72. TYPE 2
9. CRANIAL NERVES, OTHER AND UNSPECIFIED PARTS OF THE NERVOUS SYSTEM
238.# OTHER AND UNSPECIFIED SITES
4th Digit: 238
0. BONE AND ARTICULAR CARTILAGE
1. CONNECTIVE AND OTHER SOFT TISSUE
2. SKIN
3. BREAST
4. POLYCYTHEMIA VERA
5. HISTIOCYTIC AND MAST CELLS
6. PLASMA CELLS
7. OTHER LYMPHATIC AND HEMOPOIETIC TISSUES
8. EYE, HEART, OTHER SPECIFIED
9. SITE UNSPECIFIED

0 BENIGN SEE 'BENIGN NEOPLASM', BY SITE •M8000/0
203.8# IMMUNOPROLIFERATIVE
5th Digit: 203.8
0. WITHOUT MENTION OF REMISSION
1. IN REMISSION

NEOPLASM UNCERTAIN BEHAVIOR: THE ULTIMATE BEHAVIOR OF THE NEOPLASM CANNOT BE DETERMINED AS TO WHETHER IT IS BENIGN OR MALIGNANT.

NEOPLASM UNCERTAIN BEHAVIOR
237.2 ADRENAL GLAND
235.3 AMPULLA OF VATER
235.5 ANAL CANAL
235.5 ANUS NOS
238.2 ANUS (SKIN) (MARGIN) (PERIANAL)
237.3 AORTIC BODY
235.1 ARYEPIGLOTTIC FOLD
235.6 ARYEPIGLOTTIC FOLD LARYNGEAL ASPECT
235.3 BILE DUCTS
235.3 BILIARY PASSAGES
236.7 BLADDER
238.0 BONE
237.5 BRAIN
238.3 BREAST SOFT TISSUE
235.7 BRONCHUS
237.3 CAROTID BODY
238.0 CARTILAGE ARTICULAR
237.5 CEREBELLOPONTINE ANGLE
237.6 CEREBRAL MENINGES
236.0 CERVIX STUMP
236.1 CHORIOADENOMA (DESTRUENS)
237.3 COCCYGEAL BODY
238.8 CONJUNCTIVA
238.1 CONNECTIVE
238.8 CORNEA
237.9 CRANIAL NERVE (CENTRAL)
237.0 CRANIOPHARYNGEAL DUCT
235.5 DIGESTIVE ORGANS UNSPECIFIED OTHER

NEOPLASM UNCERTAIN BEHAVIOR (continued)

238.8	EAR (EXTERNAL) (SKIN)
237.4	ENDOCRINE
235.6	EPIGLOTTIS
235.5	ESOPHAGUS
238.8	EYE
238.1	EYELID CARTILAGE
238.1	EYELID CONNECTIVE TISSUE
238.2	EYELID SKIN
235.3	GALLBLADDER
238.1	GANGLIA
236.3	GENITAL FEMALE ORGANS
236.6	GENITAL MALE ORGANS
235.1	GINGIVA
237.3	GLOMUS JUGULAR
238.8	HEART
238.7	HEMATOPOIETIC TISSUE
238.5	HISTIOCYTIC
235.1	HYPOPHARYNX
235.2	INTESTINES
236.91	KIDNEY
235.6	LARYNX
235.1	LIP
238.2	LIP (SKIN OF)
235.3	LIVER
235.7	LUNG
238.7	LYMPHATIC
238.5	MAST CELL
235.8	MEDIASTINUM
237.6	MENINGES
235.9	MIDDLE EAR
235.1	MOUTH
235.1	MOUTH GINGIVA
235.9	NASAL CAVITY
238.8	NASAL SKIN
235.1	NASOPHARYNX
238.1	NERVE - PARASYMPATHETIC, PERIPHERAL, SYMPATHETIC
237.9	NERVOUS SYSTEM OTHER AND UNSPECIFIED (CENTRAL)
237.7#	NEUROFIBROMATOSIS

5th Digit: 237.7

0. NOS OR MULTIPLE
1. TYPE I
2. TYPE II

235.1	ORAL CAVITY
235.1	OROPHARYNX
238.9	OTHER SITES AND TISSUES
236.2	OVARY
235.5	PANCREAS
237.3	PARAGANGLIA
237.4	PARATHYROID
235.0	PAROTID
238.8	PERICARDIUM
235.4	PERITONEUM
235.1	PHARYNX
237.1	PINEAL GLAND
237.0	PITUITARY
236.1	PLACENTA
238.6	PLASMA CELL
235.8	PLEURA
236.5	PROSTATE
235.2	RECTUM
235.9	RESPIRATORY ORGANS OTHER AND NOS
235.4	RETROPERITONEUM
235.1	SALIVARY GLAND (MINOR)
235.0	SALIVARY GLANDS MAJOR
235.9	SINUS (ACCESSORY)
238.2	SKIN
238.1	SOFT TISSUE SITE UNSPECIFIED
237.5	SPINAL CORD
237.6	SPINAL MENINGES
235.5	SPLEEN

NEOPLASM UNCERTAIN BEHAVIOR (continued)

235.2	STOMACH
235.0	SUBLINGUAL GLAND
235.0	SUBMANDIBULAR GLAND
237.2	SUPRARENAL GLAND
236.4	TESTIS
235.8	THYMUS
237.4	THYROID
235.1	TONGUE
235.7	TRACHEA
235.7	TRACHEOBRONCHIAL
236.91	URETER
236.90	URINARY ORGAN UNSPECIFIED
236.99	URINARY ORGAN OTHER
236.0	UTERUS
236.3	VAGINAL
236.2	VESICOVAGINAL
236.3	VESICOVAGINAL SEPTUM
235.6	VOCAL CORDS (TRUE) (FALSE)
235.0	WHARTON'S DUCT
237.3	ZUCKERKANDL'S ORGAN

NEOPLASM UNSPECIFIED NATURE: THE BEHAVIOR OR THE MORPHOLOGY IS UNSPECIFIED.

NEOPLASM UNSPECIFIED NATURE

239.0	ANUS
239.2	ANUS (MARGIN) (SKIN) (PERIANAL)
239.4	BLADDER
239.2	BONE
239.6	BRAIN
239.7	BRAIN (MENINGES)
239.3	BREAST
239.2	BREAST (SKIN OF)
239.9	CELLS SITE UNSPECIFIED
239.6	CEREBELLOPONTINE ANGLE
239.8	CONJUNCTIVA
239.2	CONNECTIVE TISSUE
239.8	CORNEA
239.7	CRANIAL NERVES
239.0	DIGESTIVE SYSTEM
239.7	ENDOCRINE
239.2	EYELID (SKIN OF)
239.5	GENITAL
239.2	GREAT VESSELS
239.1	LARYNX
239.0	LIP VERMILION BORDER
239.7	NERVOUS SYSTEM
239.1	NOSE
239.7	OPTIC NERVE
239.8	OTHER SPECIFIED SITES
239.8	PERICARDIUM
239.1	RESPIRATORY SYSTEM
239.2	SKIN
239.2	SOFT TISSUE
239.9	SITE UNSPECIFIED
239.0	TONGUE
239.1	TRACHEOBRONCHIAL
239.5	URINARY TRACT
239.5	VAGINA
239.5	VESICOVAGINAL SEPTUM
239.1	VOCAL CORDS (TRUE) (FALSE)
239.5	VULVA
239.0	WHARTON'S DUCT

239.# **NEOPLASM UNSPECIFIED NATURE**

4th Digit: 239

- **0. DIGESTIVE SYSTEM, ANAL**
- **1. RESPIRATORY SYSTEM**
- **2. BONE, SOFT TISSUE, SKIN, (ANAL SKIN MARGIN)**
- **3. BREAST**
- **4. BLADDER**
- **5. OTHER GENITOURINARY**
- **6. BRAIN**
- **7. ENDOCRINE GLANDS AND OTHER PARTS OF NERVOUS SYSTEM**
- **8. OTHER SPECIFIED SITES**
- **9. SITE UNSPECIFIED**

334.4 NEOPLASTIC CEREBELLAR ATAXIA

117.4 NEOTESTUDINA ROSATII INFECTION

364.42 NEOVASCULARIZATION OF IRIS OR CILIARY BODY

V45.89 NEPHRECTOMY STATUS

NEPHRITIS

583.# NOS

4th Digit: 583

- **0. PROLIFERATIVE**
- **1. MEMBRANOUS**
- **2. MEMBRANOPROLIFERATIVE, HYPOCOMPLEMENTEMIC PERSISTENT, LOBULAR, MESANGIOCAPILLARY, MIXED MEMBRANOUS AND PROLIFERATIVE**
- **4. RAPIDLY PROGRESSIVE, NECROTIZING**
- **6. WITH CORTICAL NECROSIS**
- **7. WITH MEDULLARY (PAPILLARY) NECROSIS**
- **9. UNSPECIFIED LESION IN KIDNEY**

580.# ACUTE

4th Digit: 580

- **0. PROLIFERATIVE OR POST STREPTOCOCCAL**
- **4. RAPIDLY PROGRESSIVE NECROTIZING, EXTRACAPILLARY WITH EPITHELIAL CRESCENTS**
- **9. UNSPECIFIED OR HEMORRHAGIC**

582.# CHRONIC

4th Digit: 582

- **0. PROLIFERATIVE**
- **1. MEMBRANOUS SCLEROSING, FOCAL, SEGMENTAL HYALINOSIS**
- **2. MEMBRANOPROLIFERATIVE, ENDOTHELIAL, HYPOCOMPLEMENTEMIC PERSISTENT, LOBULAR, MESANGIOCAPILLARY, MIXED MEMBRANOUS AND PROLIFERATIVE**
- **4. RAPIDLY PROGRESSIVE, NECROTIZING**
- **9. UNSPECIFIED OR HEMORRHAGIC**

581.# NEPHROTIC SYNDROME IN GLOMERULONEPHRITIS

4th Digit: 581

- **0. PROLIFERATIVE**
- **1. MEMBRANOUS, EPIMEMBRANOUS, IDIOPATHIC MEMBRANOUS, FOCAL, SCLEROSING, SEGMENTAL HYALINOSIS**
- **2. MEMBRANOPROLIFERATIVE, ENDOTHELIAL, HYPOCOMPLEMENTEMIC PERSISTENT, LOBULAR, MESANGIOCAPILLARY, MIXED MEMBRANOUS AND PROLIFERATIVE**
- **3. MINIMAL CHANGE, FOOT PROCESS DISEASE, LIPOID**
- **9. UNSPECIFIED**

NEPHRITIS DUE TO OTHER CAUSES

277.3 AMYLOID NOS [583.81]

277.3 AMYLOID CHRONIC [582.81]

277.3 AMYLOIDOSIS [583.81]

277.3 AMYLOIDOSIS CHRONIC [582.81]

583.89 ANALGESIC

403.90 ARTERIOLAR SEE 'HYPERTENSIVE RENAL DISEASE'

403.90 ARTERIOSCLEROTIC SEE 'HYPERTENSIVE RENAL DISEASE'

590.80 ASCENDING SEE ALSO 'PYELITIS'

582.9 ATROPHIC

NEPHRITIS DUE TO OTHER CAUSES (continued)

583.89 BASEMENT MEMBRANE NEC

446.21 BASEMENT MEMBRANE WITH PULMONARY HEMORRHAGE (GOODPASTURE'S SYNDROME) [583.81]

592.0 CALCULOUS, CALCULUS

403.90 CARDIAC, CARDIOVASCULAR SEE 'HYPERTENSIVE RENAL DISEASE'

587 CIRRHOTIC

580.9 CROUPOUS

250.4# DIABETIC (NEPHROPATHY) [583.81]

250.4# DIABETIC (NEPHROPATHY) WITH NEPHROTIC SYNDROME [581.81]

5th Digit: 250.4

- **0. TYPE II, ADULT-ONSET, NON-INSULIN DEPENDENT (EVEN IF REQUIRING INSULIN), OR UNSPECIFIED; CONTROLLED**
- **1. TYPE I, JUVENILE-ONSET OR INSULIN-DEPENDENT; CONTROLLED**
- **2. TYPE II, ADULT-ONSET, NON-INSULIN DEPENDENT (EVEN IF REQUIRING INSULIN); UNCONTROLLED**
- **3. TYPE I, JUVENILE-ONSET OR INSULIN-DEPENDENT; UNCONTROLLED**

032.89 DIPHTHERITIC [580.81]

421.0 ENDOCARDITIS BACTERIAL SUBACUTE (DUE TO) [580.81]

585 END STATE (CHRONIC) (TERMINAL)

581.1 EPIMEMBRANOUS

583.89 EXUDATIVE NOS

580.89 EXUDATIVE ACUTE

582.89 EXUDATIVE CHRONIC

581.89 EXUDATIVE WITH NEPHROTIC SYNDROME

098.19 GONOCOCCAL INFECTION (ACUTE) [583.81]

098.39 GONOCOCCAL INFECTION CHRONIC OR LASTING OVER TWO MONTHS [583.81]

274.10 GOUTY

274.11 GOUTY NEPHROLITHIASIS (URIC ACID STONES) [582.81]

070.9 HEPATIC INFECTIOUS [580.81]

759.89 HEREDITARY

588.8 HYPERCALCEMIC

403.## HYPERTENSIVE (CHRONIC) (INTERSTITIAL)

4th Digit: 403

- **0. MALIGNANT**
- **1. BENIGN**
- **9. UNSPECIFIED**

5th Digit: 403

- **0. WITHOUT RENAL FAILURE**
- **1. WITH RENAL FAILURE**

588.8 HYPOKALEMIC

583.89 IMMUNE COMPLEX NEC

590.80 INFECTIVE SEE ALSO 'PYELONEPHRITIS'

583.89 INTERSTITIAL (DIFFUSE) (FOCAL) NOS

580.89 INTERSTITIAL (DIFFUSE) (FOCAL) ACUTE

582.89 INTERSTITIAL (DIFFUSE) (FOCAL) CHRONIC

581.89 INTERSTITIAL (DIFFUSE) (FOCAL) WITH NEPHROTIC SYNDROME

984.9 DUE TO LEAD

984.9 LEAD (TOXIC)

583.2 LOBULAR (HYPOCOMPLEMENT) (MIXED)

710.0 LUPUS NOS [583.81]

710.0 LUPUS ACUTE [580.81]

710.0 LUPUS CHRONIC [582.81]

760.0 MATERNAL HYPERTENSION AFFECTING FETUS OR NEWBORN

760.1 MATERNAL RENAL DISEASE AFFECTING FETUS OR NEWBORN

642.1# MATERNAL WITH HYPERTENSION (COMPLICATING PREGNANCY)

5th Digit: 642.1

- **0. EPISODE OF CARE UNSPECIFIED OR N/A**
- **1. DELIVERED**
- **2. DELIVERED WITH POSTPARTUM COMPLICATION**
- **3. ANTEPARTUM COMPLICATION**
- **4. POSTPARTUM COMPLICATION**

NEPHRITIS DUE TO OTHER CAUSES (continued)

> *646.2#: SPECIFY THE MATERNAL NEPHRITIS WITH AN ADDITIONAL CODE.*

646.2# MATERNAL WITHOUT HYPERTENSION (COMPLICATING PREGNANCY)

5th Digit: 646.2
- **0. EPISODE OF CARE UNSPECIFIED OR N/A**
- **1. DELIVERED**
- **2. DELIVERED WITH POSTPARTUM COMPLICATION**
- **3. ANTEPARTUM COMPLICATION**
- **4. POSTPARTUM COMPLICATION**

072.79 MUMPS (DUE TO) [580.81]
581.89 PARENCHYMATOUS
753.12 POLYCYSTIC NOS
753.13 POLYCYSTIC ADULT TYPE
753.13 POLYCYSTIC AUTOSOMAL DOMINANT
753.14 POLYCYSTIC AUTOSOMAL RECESSIVE
753.14 POLYCYSTIC AUTOSOMAL CHILDHOOD TYPE (CPKD)
753.14 POLYCYSTIC AUTOSOMAL INFANTILE TYPE
590.80 PURULENT SEE ALSO 'PYELONEPHRITIS'
583.9 RENAL NECROSIS
583.6 RENAL NECROSIS CORTICAL
583.7 RENAL NECROSIS MEDULLARY (PAPILLARY)
593.9 SALT LOSING
584.9 SATURNINE
590.80 SEPTIC SEE ALSO 'PYELONEPHRITIS'
710.0 SLE (SYSTEMIC LUPUS ERYTHEMATOSUS) [583.81]
583.89 SPECIFIED PATHOLOGY NEC
580.89 SPECIFIED PATHOLOGY ACUTE
582.89 SPECIFIED PATHOLOGY CHRONIC
581.89 SPECIFIED PATHOLOGY WITH NEPHROTIC SYNDROME
V81.5 SCREENING
580.89 SPECIFIED PATHOLOGY ACUTE
590.80 STAPHYLOCOCCAL SEE ALSO 'PYELONEPHRITIS'
039.8 STREPTOTRICHOSIS [583.81]
581.9 SUBACUTE
590.80 SUPPURATIVE
095.4 SYPHILITIC (LATE)
095.5 SYPHILITIC CONGENITAL [583.81]
091.69 SYPHILITIC EARLY [583.81]
585 TERMINAL NEC (END-STAGE) (CHRONIC)
584.5 TOXIC SEE ALSO 'NEPHRITIS'
016.0# TUBERCULOSIS [583.81]

5th Digit: 016.0
- **0. NOS**
- **1. LAB NOT DONE**
- **2. LABS PENDING**
- **3. MICROSCOPY POSITIVE (IN SPUTUM)**
- **4. CULTURE POSITIVE - MICROSCOPY NEGATIVE**
- **5. CULTURE NEGATIVE - MICROSCOPY POSITIVE**
- **6. CULTURE AND MICROSCOPY NEGATIVE CONFIRMED BY OTHER METHODS**

002.0 TYPHOID WITH NEPHROTIC SYNDROME [581.81]
002.0 TYPHOID FEVER ACUTE [580.81]
580.9 WAR
581.9 WITH EDEMA
581.89 WITH GLOMERULONEPHRITIS

NEPHROBLASTOMA

189.0 SITE NOS
0 SITE SPECIFIED SEE 'CANCER' BY SITE M8960/3
189.0 EPITHELIAL SITE NOS
0 EPITHELIAL SITE SPECIFIED SEE 'CANCER' BY SITE M8961/3
189.0 MESENCHYMAL SITE NOS
0 MESENCHYMAL SITE SPECIFIED SEE 'CANCER' BY SITE M8962/3

275.49 NEPHROCALCINOSIS

592.0 NEPHROLITHIASIS
274.11 NEPHROLITHIASIS URIC ACID
236.99 NEPHROMA MESOBLASTIC SITE NOS
0 NEPHROMA MESOBLASTIC SITE SPECIFIED SEE 'NEOPLASM UNCERTAIN BEHAVIOR' BY SITE M8960/1
753.16 NEPHRONOPTHISIS
0 NEPHROPATHY SEE ALSO 'NEPHRITIS'
593.0 NEPHROPTOSIS

NEPHROSCLEROSIS

587 NEPHROSCLEROSIS NOS (SENILE)
274.10 GOUTY
403.## HYPERPLASTIC
403.## HYPERTENSIVE

4th Digit: 403
- **0. MALIGNANT**
- **1. BENIGN**
- **9. UNSPECIFIED**

5th Digit: 403
- **0. WITHOUT RENAL FAILURE**
- **1. WITH RENAL FAILURE**

584.# HYPERTENSIVE WITH ACUTE RENAL FAILURE (NON-HYPERTENSIVE) [**403.##**]

4th Digit: 584
- **5. WITH TUBULAR NECROSIS**
- **6. RENAL CORTICAL NECROSIS**
- **7. MEDULLARY (PAPILLARY) NECROSIS**
- **8. SPECIFIED PATHOLOGICAL LESION**
- **9. RENAL FAILURE UNSPECIFIED**

4th Digit: 403
- **0. MALIGNANT**
- **1. BENIGN**
- **9. UNSPECIFIED**

5th Digit: 403
- **0. WITHOUT RENAL FAILURE**
- **1. WITH RENAL FAILURE**

NEPHROSIS

581.9 NOS
250.4# DIABETIC [581.81]

5th Digit: 250.4
- **0. TYPE II, ADULT-ONSET, NON-INSULIN DEPENDENT (EVEN IF REQUIRING INSULIN), OR UNSPECIFIED; CONTROLLED**
- **1. TYPE I, JUVENILE-ONSET OR INSULIN-DEPENDENT; CONTROLLED**
- **2. TYPE II, ADULT-ONSET, NON-INSULIN DEPENDENT (EVEN IF REQUIRING INSULIN); UNCONTROLLED**
- **3. TYPE I, JUVENILE-ONSET OR INSULIN-DEPENDENT; UNCONTROLLED**

581.3 LIPOID
084.9 MALARIAL [573.2]
078.6 SYNDROME WITH EPIDEMIC FEVER

> *WHEN CODING AN INFECTION OF AN OSTOMY, USE AN ADDITIONAL CODE TO SPECIFY THE ORGANISM. SEE 'BACTERIAL INFECTION'*

NEPHROSTOMY

V55.6 CARE
V55.6 CATHETER ADJUSTMENT OR REPOSITIONING
V55.6 CATHETER REMOVAL OR REPLACEMENT
V55.6 CLOSURE
996.39 COMPLICATION DEVICE MECHANICAL
997.5 COMPLICATION STOMA
997.5 MALFUNCTION
V55.6 REMOVAL OR CHANGE
V44.6 STATUS
V55.6 TOILET STOMA

N

NEPHROTIC SYNDROME

581.# NEPHROTIC SYNDROME
4th Digit: 581
0. PROLIFERATIVE
1. MEMBRANOUS (SCLEROSING) (HYALINOSIS)
2. MEMBRANOPROLIFERATIVE (LOBULAR) (HYPOCOMPLEMENT)
3. MINIMAL CHANGE
9. UNSPECIFIED

277.3 AMYLOID [581.81]
250.4# DIABETIC [581.81]
5th Digit: 250.4
0. TYPE II, ADULT-ONSET, NON-INSULIN DEPENDENT (EVEN IF REQUIRING INSULIN), OR UNSPECIFIED; CONTROLLED
1. TYPE I, JUVENILE-ONSET OR INSULIN-DEPENDENT; CONTROLLED
2. TYPE II, ADULT-ONSET, NON-INSULIN DEPENDENT (EVEN IF REQUIRING INSULIN); UNCONTROLLED
3. TYPE I, JUVENILE-ONSET OR INSULIN-DEPENDENT; UNCONTROLLED

710.0 LUPUS (DUE TO) [581.81]
084.9 MALARIAL [581.81]
446.0 POLYARTERITIS (DUE TO) [581.81]
078.6 WITH EPIDEMIC HEMORRHAGIC FEVER
581.89 WITH GLOMERULONEPHRITIS AND NEPHRITIS (EXUDATIVE) (INTERSTITIAL) (DIFFUSE)

NERVE

742.8 AGENESIS CONGENITAL
355.9 DISORDER NEC
355.79 DISORDER- LOWER LIMB
354.8 DISORDER- UPPER LIMB
0 DIVISION SEE 'NERVE INJURY', BY SITE
996.2 GRAFT (PERIPHERAL) COMPLICATION (MECHANICAL)
996.63 GRAFT (PERIPHERAL) INFECTION OR INFLAMMATION
0 INJURY SEE 'NERVE INJURY'
0 LACERATION SEE 'NERVE INJURY' BY SPECIFIED SITE
0 PINCHED SEE 'NEUROPATHY', ENTRAPMENT
353.9 ROOT AND PLEXUS DISORDER (NONDISCOGENIC)
353.8 ROOT AND PLEXUS DISORDERS OTHER (NONDISCOGENIC)
794.10 STIMULATION ABNORMAL RESPONSE

NERVE INJURY

957.9 UNSPECIFIED NERVE
951.3 ABDUCENS
951.6 ACCESSORY
951.5 ACOUSTIC
955.0 AXILLARY
953.4 BRACHIAL PLEXUS
954.1 CELIAC GANGLION OR PLEXUS
953.0 CERVICAL ROOT
954.0 CERVICAL SYMPATHETIC
951.# CRANIAL
4th Digit: 951
0. OCULOMOTOR (3RD)
1. TROCHLEAR (4TH)
2. TRIGEMINAL (5TH)
3. ABDUCENS (6TH)
4. FACIAL (7TH)
5. ACOUSTIC (8TH)
6. ACCESSORY (11TH)
7. HYPOGLOSSAL (12TH)
8. OTHER: GLOSSOPHARYNGEAL (9TH), OLFACTORY (1ST), PNEUMOGASTRIC (10TH), VAGUS (10TH)
9. UNSPECIFIED

950.0 CRANIAL OPTIC (2ND NERVE)
956.4 CUTANEOUS SENSORY, LOWER LIMB
955.5 CUTANEOUS SENSORY, UPPER LIMB
955.6 DIGITAL
953.1 DORSAL ROOT

NERVE INJURY (continued)

951.5 EIGHTH CRANIAL
951.6 ELEVENTH CRANIAL
951.4 FACIAL
956.1 FEMORAL
951.2 FIFTH CRANIAL
951.8 FIRST CRANIAL
951.1 FOURTH CRANIAL
951.8 GLOSSOPHARYNGEAL
957.0 HEAD AND NECK SUPERFICIAL
951.7 HYPOGLOSSAL
954.1 INFERIOR MESENTERIC PLEXUS
907.9 LATE EFFECT - UNSPECIFIED NERVE
907.1 LATE EFFECT - CRANIAL
907.3 LATE EFFECT - NERVE ROOT(S)
907.5 LATE EFFECT - PELVIC GIRDLE AND LOWER LIMB PERIPHERAL
907.4 LATE EFFECT - SHOULDER GIRDLE AND UPPER LIMB PERIPHERAL
907.3 LATE EFFECT - SPINAL PLEXUS
907.3 LATE EFFECT - TRUNK NERVE
907.9 LATE EFFECT - OTHER SPECIFIED NERVE
953.2 LUMBAR ROOT
953.5 LUMBOSACRAL PLEXUS
955.1 MEDIAN
954.1 MESENTERIC PLEXUS INFERIOR
957.8 MULTIPLE NERVES NOS
953.8 MULTIPLE NERVE ROOT SITES
956.8 MULTIPLE NERVES OF PELVIC GIRDLE AND LOWER LIMB
955.8 MULTIPLE NERVES OF SHOULDER GIRDLE AND UPPER LIMB
955.4 MUSCULOCUTANEOUS
951.8 NINTH CRANIAL
951.0 OCULOMOTOR
951.8 OLFACTORY
950.# OPTIC NERVE AND PATHWAYS
4th Digit: 950
0. OPTIC NERVE INJURY (2ND CRANIAL NERVE)
1. OPTIC CHIASM
2. OPTIC PATHWAYS
3. VISUAL CORTEX
9. UNSPECIFIED

956.# PELVIC GIRDLE AND LOWER LIMB (PERIPHERAL NERVES)
4th Digit: 956
0. SCIATIC
1. FEMORAL
2. POSTERIOR TIBIAL
3. PERONEAL
4. CUTANEOUS SENSORY NERVE, LOWER LIMB
5. OTHER SPECIFIED
8. MULTIPLE
9. UNSPECIFIED

956.3 PERONEAL
951.8 PNEUMOGASTRIC
956.2 POSTERIOR TIBIAL
955.3 RADIAL
953.# ROOTS AND SPINAL PLEXUS INJURY
4th Digit: 953
0. CERVICAL ROOT
1. DORSAL ROOT
2. LUMBAR ROOT
3. SACRAL ROOT
4. BRACHIAL PLEXUS
5. LUMBOSACRAL PLEXUS
8. MULTIPLE SITES
9. UNSPECIFIED SITE

953.3 SACRAL ROOT
956.0 SCIATIC
950.0 SECOND CRANIAL
951.4 SEVENTH CRANIAL

NERVE INJURY (continued)

955.# SHOULDER GIRDLE AND UPPER LIMB (PERIPHERAL NERVES)

4th Digit: 955

0. AXILLARY
1. MEDIAN
2. ULNAR
3. RADIAL
4. MUSCULOCUTANEOUS
5. CUTANEOUS SENSORY NERVE, UPPER LIMB
6. DIGITAL
7. OTHER SPECIFIED
8. MULTIPLE
9. UNSPECIFIED

951.3 SIXTH CRANIAL
953.9 SPINAL ROOT
954.1 SPLANCHNIC
954.1 STELLATE GANGLION
951.8 TENTH CRANIAL
951.0 THIRD CRANIAL
956.2 TIBIAL POSTERIOR
951.2 TRIGEMINAL
951.1 TROCHLEAR
954.9 TRUNK - NOS
954.1 TRUNK - CELIAC GANGLION OR PLEXUS
954.0 TRUNK - CERVICAL SYMPATHETIC
954.1 TRUNK - INFERIOR MESENTERIC PLEXUS
954.1 TRUNK - SPLANCHNIC
954.1 TRUNK - STELLATE GANGLION
954.1 TRUNK - OTHER SYMPATHETIC
954.8 TRUNK - OTHER SPECIFIED
951.7 TWELFTH CRANIAL
955.2 ULNAR
951.8 VAGUS
951.8 OTHER SPECIFIED CRANIAL
956.5 OTHER SPECIFIED PELVIC GIRDLE AND LOWER LIMB
955.7 OTHER SPECIFIED SHOULDER GIRDLE AND UPPER LIMB
954.8 OTHER SPECIFIED TRUNK NERVES
957.1 OTHER SPECIFIED NERVES

799.2 NERVES

NERVOUS SYSTEM

742.8 ABSENCE (ATROPHY) CONGENITAL
742.9 ANOMALY
349.1 COMPLICATION FROM SURGICALLY IMPLANTED DEVICE - NONMECHANICAL
997.00 COMPLICATION POSTOPERATIVE IMMEDIATE NOS
997.01 COMPLICATION POSTOPERATIVE IMMEDIATE CENTRAL NERVOUS SYSTEM (ANOXIC BRAIN DAMAGE) (CEREBRAL HYPOXIA)
997.02 COMPLICATION POSTOPERATIVE IMMEDIATE CVA (STROKE) (BRAIN HEMORRHAGE)
997.09 COMPLICATION POSTOPERATIVE IMMEDIATE OTHER SPECIFIED
742.9 DEFORMITY CONGENITAL
349.89 DEGENERATION
V53.09 DEVICE (FITTING AND ADJUSTMENT) (REMOVAL) (REPLACEMENT)
996.63 DEVICE, IMPLANT OR GRAFT (INTERNAL PROSTHETIC) COMPLICATION - INFECTION OR INFLAMMATION
996.2 DEVICE, IMPLANT OR GRAFT COMPLICATION - MECHANICAL
996.75 DEVICE, IMPLANT OR GRAFT (INTERNAL PROSTHETIC) COMPLICATION - OTHER
349.9 DISORDER (CENTRAL) NEC
337.9 DISORDER - AUTONOMIC (PERIPHERAL)
352.9 DISORDER - CRANIAL
337.9 DISORDER - PARASYMPATHETIC
337.9 DISORDER - SYMPATHETIC
337.9 DISORDER - VEGETATIVE
V12.40 DISORDER HISTORY NOS
V12.49 DISORDER HISTORY OTHER
349.89 DISORDERS OTHER SPECIFED NEC
781.9 SYMPTOM OTHER SPECIFIED

799.2 NERVOUSNESS

757.1 NETHERTON'S SYNDROME (ICHTHYOSIFORM ERYTHRODERMA)

757.33 NETTLESHIP'S DISEASE CONGENITAL (URTICARIA PIGMENTOSA)

694.4 NEUMANN'S DISEASE (PEMPHIGUS VEGETANS)

NEURALGIA

0 SEE ALSO 'NEURITIS'
729.2 UNSPECIFIED (ACUTE) (OR RHEUMATIC)
352.4 ACCESSORY (NERVE)
388.5 ACOUSTIC (NERVE)
355.8 ANKLE
355.8 ANTERIOR CRURAL
787.99 ANUS OR RECTUM
723.4 ARM
388.5 AUDITORY (NERVE)
353.0 AXILLA
788.1 BLADDER
723.4 BRACHIAL
0 BRAIN SEE 'NEURALGIA' CRANIAL NERVE
625.9 BROAD LIGAMENT
0 CEREBRAL SEE 'NEURALGIA' CRANIAL NERVE
346.2# CILIARY

5th Digit: 346.2

0. WITHOUT MENTION INTRACTABLE MIGRAINE
1. WITH INTRACTABLE MIGRAINE

CRANIAL NERVE

352.9 NOS
352.0 FIRST
377.49 SECOND
378.51 THIRD PARTIAL
378.52 THIRD TOTAL
378.53 FOURTH
350.1 FIFTH OR TRIGEMINAL
378.54 SIXTH
351.9 SEVENTH NEC
388.5 EIGHTH
352.2 NINTH
352.3 TENTH
352.4 ELEVENTH
352.5 TWELFTH
352.6 MULTIPLE

NEURALGIA (continued)

388.71 EAR
352.1 EAR MIDDLE
351.8 FACIAL
354.9 FINGER
355.8 FLANK
355.8 FOOT
354.9 FOREARM
350.1 FOTHERGILL'S
053.12 FOTHERGILL'S POSTHERPETIC
352.1 GLOSSOPHARYNGEAL (NERVE)
355.8 GROIN
354.9 HAND
355.8 HEEL
346.2# HORTON'S

5th Digit: 346.2

0. WITHOUT MENTION INTRACTABLE MIGRAINE
1. WITH INTRACTABLE MIGRAINE

053.11 HUNT'S
352.5 HYPOGLOSSAL (NERVE)
355.8 ILIAC REGION
350.1 INFRAORBITAL
355.8 INGUINAL
353.8 INTERCOSTAL (NERVE)
053.19 INTERCOSTAL (NERVE) POSTHERPETIC
352.1 JAW
788.0 KIDNEY
355.8 KNEE
355.8 LOIN
0 MALARIAL SEE 'MALARIA'

N

NEURALGIA (continued)

385.89 MASTOID
352.1 MAXILLA
354.1 MEDIAN THENAR
355.6 METATARSAL
352.1 MIDDLE EAR
346.2# MIGRAINOUS
5th Digit: 346.2
0. WITHOUT MENTION INTRACTABLE MIGRAINE
1. WITH INTRACTABLE MIGRAINE

355.6 MORTON'S
0 NERVE CRANIAL SEE 'NEURALGIA' CRANIAL NERVE
0 NERVE OTHER SPECIFIED SEE NERVE BY SPECIFIC NAME, DISORDER
352.0 NOSE
784.0 OCCIPITAL
352.0 OLFACTORY (NERVE)
377.30 OPHTHALMIC
053.19 OPHTHALMIC POSTHERPETIC
377.30 OPTIC (NERVE)
607.9 PENIS
355.8 PERINEUM
511.0 PLEURA
053.19 POSTHERPETIC NEC
053.11 POSTHERPETIC GENICULATE GANGLION
053.19 POSTHERPETIC OPHTHALMIC
053.12 POSTHERPETIC TRIFACIAL
053.12 POSTHERPETIC TRIGEMINAL
355.8 PUBIC REGION
723.4 RADIAL (NERVE)
787.99 RECTUM
724.3 SACROILIAC JOINT
724.3 SCIATIC (NERVE)
608.9 SCROTUM
608.9 SEMINAL VESICLE
354.9 SHOULDER
337.0 SLUDER'S
608.9 SPERMATIC CORD
337.0 SPHENOPALATINE (GANGLION)
723.4 SUBSCAPULAR (NERVE)
723.4 SUPRASCAPULAR (NERVE)
608.89 TESTIS
354.1 THENAR (MEDIAN)
355.8 THIGH
352.5 TONGUE
350.1 TRIFACIAL
350.1 TRIGEMINAL (NERVE)
053.12 TRIGEMINAL (NERVE) POSTHERPETIC
388.71 TYMPANIC PLEXUS
723.4 ULNAR (NERVE)
352.3 VAGUS (NERVE)
354.9 WRIST
300.89 WRITERS'
333.84 WRITERS' ORGANIC

353.5 NEURALGIC AMYOTROPHY (NONDISCOGENIC)
300.5 NEURASTHENIA
780.79 NEURASTHENIA POSTFEBRILE
780.79 NEURASTHENIA POSTVIRAL

NEURILEMMOMA

225.1 ACOUSTIC (NERVE) BENIGN
192.0 ACOUSTIC (NERVE) MALIGNANT M9560/3
215.# BENIGN M9560/0
171.# MALIGNANT M9560/3
4th Digit: 171, 215
0. HEAD FACE NECK
2. UPPER LIMB SHOULDER
3. LOWER LIMB HIP
4. THORAX
5. ABDOMINAL HYPOCHONDRIUM
6. PELVIS BUTTOCK GROIN INGUINAL PERINEUM
7. TRUNK NOS BACK NOS FLANK NOS
8. OTHER SPECIFIED SITES
9. SITE NOS

171.9 NEURILEMMOSARCOMA SITE NOS
0 NEURILEMMOSARCOMA SITE SPECIFIED SEE 'CANCER' BY SITE SOFT TISSUE M9560/3
238.1 NEURINOMATOSIS SITE NOS
0 NEURINOMATOSIS SITE SPECIFIED SEE 'NEOPLASM UNCERTAIN BEHAVIOR' BY SITE M9560/1

NEURITIS

0 SEE ALSO 'NEURALGIA'
729.2 NOS
378.54 ABDUCENS NERVE
352.4 ACCESSORY NERVE
388.5 ACOUSTIC NERVE
094.86 ACOUSTIC SYPHILITIC
357.5 ALCOHOLIC
291.1 ALCOHOLIC WITH PSYCHOSIS (SEE ALSO 'PSYCHOSIS ALCOHOLIC')
277.3 AMYLOID [357.4]
355.8 ANTERIOR CRURAL
723.4 ARM
355.2 ASCENDING
0 ASSOCIATED WITH OTHER DISORDERS SEE 'NEURITIS ASSOCIATED WITH OTHER DISORDERS'
388.5 AUDITORY
353.0 AXILLARY NERVE (NONDISCOGENIC)
723.4 BRACHIAL NEC
722.0 BRACHIAL NEC DUE TO DISC DISPLACEMENT
723.4 CERVICAL
722.0 CERVICAL DUE TO DISPLACEMENT, PROLAPSE, PROTRUSION OR RUPTURE OF INTERVERTEBRAL DISC
353.8 CHEST WALL
353.8 COSTAL REGION (NONDISCOGENIC)
356.0 DEJERINE-SOTTAS
722.2 DISCOGENIC SYNDROME NOS
722.2 DUE TO DISPLACEMENT, PROLAPSE, PROTRUSION OR RUPTURE OF INTERVERTEBRAL DISC SITE NOS
388.5 EIGHTH NERVE
352.4 ELEVENTH NERVE
351.8 FACIAL NERVE
767.5 FACIAL NERVE NEWBORN
355.2 FEMORAL NERVE
350.1 FIFTH NERVE
352.0 FIRST NERVE
378.53 FOURTH NERVE
0 GENERAL SEE 'POLYNEUROPATHY'
351.1 GENICULATE GANGLION
053.11 GENICULATE GANGLION DUE TO HERPES
352.1 GLOSSOPHARYNGEAL
722.2 HNP (DUE TO) SITE NOS
722.0 HNP CERVICAL
722.10 HNP LUMBAR
722.11 HNP THORACIC
352.5 HYPOGLOSSAL (NERVE)
355.79 ILIOHYPOGASTRIC
355.8 ILIOINGUINAL
357.0 INFECTIOUS (MULTIPLE)
353.8 INTERCOSTAL
356.9 INTERSTITIAL HYPERTROPHIC PROGRESSIVE NEC
355.8 LEG
355.9 LIMB SITE UNSPECIFIED
355.8 LIMB LOWER, UNSPECIFIED
355.79 LIMB LOWER, OTHER SPECIFIED
354.9 LIMB UPPER, UNSPECIFIED
354.8 LIMB UPPER OTHER SPECIFIED
724.4 LUMBAR OR LUMBOSACRAL
722.10 LUMBAR OR LUMBOSACRAL DUE TO DISPLACEMENT, PROLAPSE, PROTRUSION OR RUPTURE OF INTERVERTEBRAL DISC
356.9 MULTIPLE (ACUTE) (INFECTIVE)
354.5 MULTIPLEX
354.1 MEDIAN NERVE
729.2 NERVE ROOT
352.1 NINTH NERVE

N

NEURITIS (continued)

378.52 OCULOMOTOR
352.0 OLFACTORY NERVE
377.30 OPHTHALMIC
053.19 OPHTHALMIC POSTHERPETIC
377.30 OPTIC
377.41 OPTIC (ISCHEMIC)
341.0 OPTIC IN MYELITIS
036.81 OPTIC MENINGOCCAL
377.30 OPTIC NERVE
377.33 OPTIC NUTRITIONAL
377.34 OPTIC TOXIC
355.8 PELVIC
0 PERIPHERAL (NERVE) SEE 'PERIPHERAL NEUROPATHY'
355.3 PERONEAL
352.3 PNEUMOGASTRIC
355.3 POPLITEAL LATERAL
355.4 POPLITEAL MEDIAN
052.7 POSTCHICKENPOX
053.19 POSTHERPETIC
356.9 PROGRESSIVE HYPERTROPHIC INTERSTITIAL NEC
723.4 RADIAL (NERVE)
377.32 RETROBULBAR
094.85 RETROBULBAR SYPHILITIC
729.2 RHEUMATIC (CHRONIC)
355.8 SACRAL
355.79 SAPHENOUS
355.0 SCIATIC MONONEURITIS
724.3 SCIATIC (NERVE) (SCIATICA)
722.10 SCIATIC (NERVE) (SCIATICA) DUE TO DISPLACEMENT, PROLAPSE, PROTRUSION OR RUPTURE OF INTERVERTEBRAL DISC
377.30 SECOND NERVE
999.5 SERUM
351.8 SEVENTH NERVE
767.5 SEVENTH NERVE NEWBORN
378.54 SIXTH NERVE
355.9 SPINAL (NERVE)
0 SPINAL ROOT SEE 'RADICULITIS'
723.4 SUBSCAPULAR (NERVE)
723.4 SUPRASCAPULAR (NERVE)
095.8 SYPHILITIC
352.3 TENTH NERVE
354.1 THENAR
378.52 THIRD NERVE
724.4 THORACIC OR THORACOLUMBAR
722.11 THORACIC OR THORACOLUMBAR DUE TO DISPLACEMENT, PROLAPSE, PROTRUSION OR RUPTURE OF INTERVERTEBRAL DISC
357.7 TOXIC
350.1 TRIGEMINAL
378.53 TROCHLEAR
352.5 TWELFTH NERVE
723.4 ULNAR (NERVE)
352.3 VAGUS (NERVE)
386.12 VESTIBULAR
0 SPECIFIED NERVE NEC SEE SPECIFIED NERVE BY SITE, DISORDER

NEURITIS ASSOCIATED WITH OTHER CONDITIONS

729.2 UNSPECIFIED (OR RHEUMATIC)
357.5 ALCOHOLIC
291.1 ALCOHOLIC WITH PSYCHOSIS (SEE ALSO 'PSYCHOSIS ALCOHOLIC')
277.3 AMYLOID (ANY SITE) [357.4]
265.0 BERIBERI (DUE TO) [357.4]

NEURITIS ASSOCIATED WITH OTHER CONDITIONS (continued)

250.6# DIABETIC [357.2]

5th Digit: 250.6

0. TYPE II, ADULT-ONSET, NON-INSULIN DEPENDENT (EVEN IF REQUIRING INSULIN), OR UNSPECIFIED; CONTROLLED
1. TYPE I, JUVENILE-ONSET OR INSULIN-DEPENDENT; CONTROLLED
2. TYPE II, ADULT-ONSET, NON-INSULIN DEPENDENT (EVEN IF REQUIRING INSULIN); UNCONTROLLED
3. TYPE I, JUVENILE-ONSET OR INSULIN-DEPENDENT; UNCONTROLLED

032.89 DIPHTHERITIC [357.4]
274.89 GOUTY [357.4]

646.4#: SPECIFY THE MATERNAL PERIPHERAL NEURITIS WITH AN ADDITIONAL CODE.

646.4# MATERNAL (PERIPHERAL) IN PREGNANCY

5th Digit: 646.4

0. EPISODE OF CARE UNSPECIFIED OR N/A
1. DELIVERED
2. DELIVERED WITH POSTPARTUM COMPLICATION
3. ANTEPARTUM COMPLICATION
4. POSTPARTUM COMPLICATION

265.0 MULTIPLEX ENDEMICA [357.4]
053.19 POSTHERPETIC
053.12 TRIFACIAL (POSTHERPETIC)

194.0 NEUROBLASTOMA SITE NOS
0 NEUROBLASTOMA SITE SPECIFIED SEE 'CANCER' BY SITE M9500/3

306.2 NEUROCIRCULATORY DISORDER PSYCHOGENIC
759.6 NEUROCUTANEOUS SYNDROME

229.9 NEUROCYTOMA SITE NOS
0 NEUROCYTOMA SITE SPECIFIED SEE 'BENIGN NEOPLASM', BY SITE M9506/0

691.8 NEURODERMATITIS
691.8 NEURODERMATITIS DIFFUSE OF BROCQ

199.1 NEUROEPITHELIOMA SITE NOS
0 NEUROEPITHELIOMA SITE SPECIFIED SEE 'CANCER' BY SITE M9503/3

CARCINOMAS AND NEOPLASMS SHOULD BE CODED BY SITE FIRST, NOT CELL TYPE. IF A SITE IS NOT SPECIFIED, THEN CODE BY CELL TYPE. CODE THE 'SITE NOS' ONLY IF NO SITE IS MENTIONED. WHEN NO SITE IS GIVEN, THE CODE REVERTS TO THE HISTOLOGICAL ORIGIN .

NEUROFIBROMA

215.# NOS M9540/0
215.# MELANOTIC M9541/0
215.# PLEXIFORM M9550/0

4th Digit: 215

0. HEAD FACE NECK
2. UPPER LIMB SHOULDER
3. LOWER LIMB HIP
4. THORAX
5. ABDOMINAL HYPOCHONDRIUM
6. PELVIS BUTTOCK GROIN INGUINAL REGION PERINEUM
7. TRUNK NOS BACK NOS FLANK NOS
8. OTHER SPECIFIED SITES
9. SITE NOS

NEUROFIBROMATOSIS

237.70 NOS M9540/1

171.# MALIGNANT M9540/3

4th Digit: 171

0. HEAD FACE NECK
2. UPPER LIMB SHOULDER
3. LOWER LIMB HIP
4. THORAX
5. ABDOMINAL HYPOCHONDRIUM
6. PELVIS BUTTOCK GROIN INGUINAL REGION PERINEUM
7. TRUNK NOS BACK NOS FLANK NOS
8. OTHER SPECIFIED SITES
9. SITE UNSPECIFIED

237.71 TYPE I [VON RECKLINGHAUSEN'S DISEASE]
237.72 TYPE II [ACOUSTIC NEUROFIBROMATOSIS]

171.# NEUROFIBROSARCOMA M9540/3

4th Digit: 171

0. HEAD FACE NECK
2. UPPER LIMB SHOULDER
3. LOWER LIMB HIP
4. THORAX
5. ABDOMINAL HYPOCHONDRIUM
6. PELVIS BUTTOCK GROIN INGUINAL REGION PERINEUM
7. TRUNK NOS BACK NOS FLANK NOS
8. OTHER SPECIFIED SITES
9. SITE UNSPECIFIED

596.54 NEUROGENIC BLADDER NOS
344.61 NEUROGENIC BLADDER WITH CAUDA EQUINA SYNDROME
0 NEUROGENIC BLADDER WITH INCONTINENCE SEE 'BLADDER DISORDERS WITH INCONTINENCE'
564.81 NEUROGENIC BOWEL
253.6 NEUROHYPOPHYSIS DISORDER NEC
333.92 NEUROLEPTIC MALIGNANT SYNDROME
781.8 NEUROLOGIC NEGLECT SYNDROME
V80.0 NEUROLOGICAL CONDITIONS SCREENING
781.9 NEUROLOGICAL DISORDER (SYMPTOM) (ILL DEFINED)

A NEUROMA IS A TUMOR OR GROWTH ON A NERVE, COMPOSED OF NERVE CELLS AND FIBERS.

NEUROMA

215.9 SITE NOS
0 SITE SPECIFIED SEE 'BENIGN NEOPLASM', BY SITE M9570/0
225.1 ACOUSTIC (8TH NERVE)
997.61 AMPUTATION STUMP
355.6 DIGITAL
355.6 MORTON'S
355.6 PLANTAR
355.8 SURGICAL - LOWER EXTREMITY (NONNEOPLASTIC)
354.9 SURGICAL - UPPER EXTREMITY (NONNEOPLASTIC)
355.8 TRAUMATIC OLD - LOWER EXTREMITY (NONNEOPLASTIC)
354.9 TRAUMATIC OLD - UPPER EXTREMITY (NONNEOPLASTIC)
0 TRAUMATIC OTHER SEE 'NERVE INJURY', BY SITE

358.9 NEUROMUSCULAR DISORDER NEC
359.1 NEUROMUSCULAR DISORDER - HEREDITARY NEC
358.8 NEUROMUSCULAR DISORDER - SPECIFIED NEC
358.2 NEUROMUSCULAR DISORDER - TOXIC
729.1 NEUROMYALGIA
341.0 NEUROMYELITIS OPTICA

216.# NEURONEVUS M8725/0

4th Digit: 216

0. LIP (SKIN OF)
1. EYELID INCLUDING CANTHUS
2. EAR (EXTERNAL) (AURICLE) (PINNA)
3. FACE (CHEEK) (NOSE) (EYEBROW) (TEMPLE)
4. SCALP NECK
5. TRUNK BACK EXCEPT SCROTUM
6. UPPER LIMB INCLUDING SHOULDER
7. LOWER LIMB INCLUDING HIP
8. OTHER SPECIFIED SITES
9. SKIN UNSPECIFIED

V53.02 NEUROPACEMAKER (BRAIN) (PERIPHERAL NERVE) (SPINAL CORD) FITTING AND ADJUSTMENT
V45.89 NEUROPACEMAKER STATUS

NEUROPATHY

355.9 NOS
357.5 ALCOHOLIC
291.1 ALCOHOLIC WITH PSYCHOSIS (SEE ALSO 'PSYCHOSIS ALCOHOLIC')
354.9 ARM NEC
353.0 AXILLARY NERVE
353.0 BRACHIAL PLEXUS
353.2 CERVICAL PLEXUS
357.8 CHRONIC PROGRESSIVE SEGMENTALLY DEMYELINATING
357.8 CHRONIC RELAPSING DEMYELINATING
356.2 CONGENITAL SENSORY
356.0 DEJERINE - SOTTAS
250.6# DIABETIC NOS [357.2]
250.6# DIABETIC PERIPHERAL AUTONOMIC [337.1]
250.6# DIABETIC POLYNEUROPATHY [357.2]

5th Digit: 250.6

0. TYPE II, ADULT-ONSET, NON-INSULIN DEPENDENT (EVEN IF REQUIRING INSULIN), OR UNSPECIFIED; CONTROLLED
1. TYPE I, JUVENILE-ONSET OR INSULIN-DEPENDENT; CONTROLLED
2. TYPE II, ADULT-ONSET, NON-INSULIN DEPENDENT (EVEN IF REQUIRING INSULIN); UNCONTROLLED
3. TYPE I, JUVENILE-ONSET OR INSULIN-DEPENDENT; UNCONTROLLED

032.89 DIPHTHERITIC [357.4]
355.9 ENTRAPMENT
355.79 ENTRAPMENT ILIOHYPOGASTRIC NERVE
355.79 ENTRAPMENT ILIOINGUINAL NERVE
355.1 ENTRAPMENT LATERAL CUTANEOUS NERVE OF THIGH
354.0 ENTRAPMENT MEDIAN
355.79 ENTRAPMENT OBTURATOR
355.3 ENTRAPMENT PERONEAL
355.5 ENTRAPMENT POSTERIOR TIBIAL
355.79 ENTRAPMENT SAPHENOUS
355.0 ENTRAPMENT SCIATIC
354.2 ENTRAPMENT ULNAR
351.9 FACIAL NERVE
356.9 HEREDITARY UNSPECIFIED
356.0 HEREDITARY PERIPHERAL
356.2 HEREDITARY SENSORY (RADICULAR)
356.# HYPERTROPHIC

4th Digit: 356

0. DEJERINE-SOTTAS
1. CHARCOT-MARIE-TOOTH
3. REFSUM
9. INTERSTITIAL

251.2 HYPOGLYCEMIA [357.4]
337.0 IDIOPATHIC PERIPHERAL AUTONOMIC
354.8 INTERCOSTAL
357.7 JAMAICAN (GINGER)
355.8 LEG NEC, LOWER EXTREMITY
353.1 LUMBAR PLEXUS
710.0 LUPUS (POLYNEUROPATHY) [357.1]

NEUROPATHY (continued)

354.1 MEDIAN
356.9 MULTIPLE NOS
356.1 MUSCULAR ATROPHY
357.3 NEOPLASTIC
377.3# OPTIC
5th Digit: 377.3
3. NUTRITIONAL
4. TOXIC
9. OTHER

377.41 OPTIC ISCHEMIA
265.2 PELLAGRA [357.4]
0 PERIPHERAL SEE 'NEUROPATHY PERIPHERAL'
355.6 PLANTAR NERVES
446.0 POLYARTERITIS NODOSA (POLYNEUROPATHY) [357.1]
277.1 PORPHYRIC [357.4]
356.9 PROGRESSIVE HYPERTROPHIC INTERSTITIAL
0 RADICULAR SEE 'RADICULITIS'
714.0 RHEUMATOID (POLYNEUROPATHY) [357.1]
135 SARCOID [357.4]
355.9 SPINAL NERVE
357.7 TOXIC
585 UREMIC (RENAL FAILURE) (CHRONIC) [357.4]
0 SEE ALSO 'NEURITIS'

NEUROPATHY PERIPHERAL

356.9 NOT OTHERWISE SPECIFIED
337.9 AUTONOMIC UNSPECIFIED
277.3 AUTONOMIC AMYLOIDOSIS [337.1]
274.89 AUTONOMIC GOUT [337.1]
242.9# AUTONOMIC HYPERTHYROIDISM [337.1]
5th Digit: 242.9
0. WITHOUT STORM
1. WITH STORM

337.0 AUTONOMIC IDIOPATHIC
357.6 DRUG INDUCED
356.0 HEREDITARY
356.2 HEREDITARY SENSORY
356.9 IDIOPATHIC
356.4 IDIOPATHIC PROGRESSIVE
356.8 IDIOPATHIC OTHER SPECIFIED
356.9 NERVE NOS
354.9 NERVE ARM NEC
907.4 NERVE INJURY LATE EFFECT (SHOULDER GIRDLE)
355.8 NERVE LEG, LOWER EXTREMITY
0 NERVE SEE 'POLYNEUROPATHY'
354.9 NERVE UPPER EXTREMITY
794.19 NERVOUS SYSTEM ABNORMAL FINDINGS FUNCTION STUDY

646.4#: SPECIFY THE MATERNAL PERIPHERAL NEURITIS WITH AN ADDITIONAL CODE.

646.4# NEURITIS (MATERNAL)
5th Digit: 646.4
0. EPISODE OF CARE UNSPECIFIED OR N/A
1. DELIVERED
2. DELIVERED WITH POSTPARTUM COMPLICATION
3. ANTEPARTUM COMPLICATION
4. POSTPARTUM COMPLICATION

0 SPINAL NERVE ROOT SEE 'RADICULITIS'
357.7 TOXIC INDUCED, (ARSENIC, LEAD, ORGANOPHOSPHATES)

0 NEUROPRAXIA SEE 'NERVE INJURY'
363.05 NEURORETINITIS

NEUROSIS, NEUROTIC

300.9 NOS
300.16 ACCIDENT
300.3 ANANCASTIC, ANANKASTIC
300.00 ANXIETY NOS
300.02 ANXIETY GENERALIZED
300.01 ANXIETY PANIC TYPE
300.5 ASTHENIC
306.53 BLADDER
306.2 CARDIAC (REFLEX)
306.2 CARDIOVASCULAR
627.2 CLIMACTERIC, NOS
306.4 COLON
300.16 COMPENSATORY
300.3 COMPULSIVE
300.11 CONVERSION
300.89 CRAFT
306.3 CUTANEOUS
300.6 DEPERSONALIZATION
300.4 DEPRESSIVE (REACTION) (TYPE)
300.89 DISORDER OTHER NEC
306.6 ENDOCRINE
300.89 ENVIRONMENTAL
300.5 FATIGUE
306.9 FUNCTIONAL
306.4 GASTRIC (GASTROINTESTINAL)
306.50 GENITOURINARY
306.2 HEART
V11.2 HISTORY
300.7 HYPOCHONDRIACAL
300.10 HYSTERICAL
300.11 HYSTERICAL CONVERSION TYPE
300.15 HYSTERICAL DISSOCIATIVE TYPE
300.3 IMPULSIVE
306.0 INCOORDINATION
306.1 INCOORDINATION LARYNX
306.1 INCOORDINATION VOCAL CORD
306.4 INTESTINE
306.1 LARYNX
300.11 LARYNX HYSTERICAL
306.1 LARYNX SENSORY
627.2 MENOPAUSE NOS
300.89 MIXED NEC
306.0 MUSCULOSKELETAL
300.3 OBSESSIONAL
300.3 OBSESSIONAL PHOBIA
300.3 OBSESSIVE COMPULSIVE
300.89 OCCUPATIONAL
306.7 OCULAR
307.0 ORAL
306.9 ORGAN
306.1 PHARYNX
300.20 PHOBIC
308.3 POSTTRAUMATIC (ACUTE) (SITUATIONAL)
309.81 POSTTRAUMATIC CHRONIC
300.89 PSYCHASTHENIC
300.16 RAILROAD
306.4 RECTUM
306.1 RESPIRATORY
306.4 RUMINATION
300.89 SENILE
302.70 SEXUAL
300.89 SITUATIONAL
300.9 STATE
300.6 STATE WITH DEPERSONALIZATION EPISODE
306.4 STOMACH
306.2 VASOMOTOR
306.4 VISCERAL
300.16 WAR
300.89 OTHER SPECIFIED TYPE

N

NEUROSYPHILIS:

WITH DEMENTIA [294.1]

094.9 NOS
094.3 ASYMPTOMATIC
090.40 CONGENITAL
094.1 GENERAL PARESIS
090.40 JUVENILE
094.1 PARETIC
094.0 TABETIC
094.89 OTHER

NEUTROPENIA

288.0 NOS
288.0 CHRONIC
288.0 CYCLIC
288.0 DRUG INDUCED
288.0 FEVER
288.0 GENETIC
288.0 IMMUNE
288.0 INFANTILE
288.0 MALIGNANT
288.0 PERIODIC
288.0 PERNICIOUS
038.9 SEPTIC [288.0]
288.0 SPLENIC
288.0 SPLENOMEGALY
288.0 TOXIC

NEUTROPENIA NEONATAL

776.7 ISOIMMUNE
776.7 MATERNAL TRANSFER
776.7 TRANSIENT

288.0 NEUTROPHIL ABSENCE
288.1 NEUTROPHIL, POLYMORPHONUCLEAR DISORDER (FUNCTIONAL)

NEVUS BENIGN

216.# NOS M8720/0
216.# ACHROMIC M8730/0
216.# AMELANOTIC M8730/0
228.00 ANGIOMATOUS M9120/0
216.# BALLOON CELL M8722/0
216.# BLUE M8780/0
216.# BLUE CELLULAR M8790/0
216.# BLUE GIANT M8790/0
216.# BLUE JADASSOHN'S M8780/0
228.00 CAPILLARY M9131/0
228.00 CAVERNOUS M9121/0
216.# CELLULAR M8720/0
216.# COMPOUND M8760/0
224.3 CONJUNCTIVA M8720/0
216.# DERMAL M8750/0
216.# DERMAL AND EPITHELIOID M8760/0
216.# EPITHELIOID AND SPINDLE CELL M8770/0
216.# GIANT PIGMENTED NEVUS M8761/0
216.# HAIRY M8720/0
216.# HALO M8723/0

4th Digit: 216

0. LIP (SKIN OF)
1. EYELID INCLUDING CANTHUS
2. EAR (EXTERNAL) (AURICLE) (PINNA)
3. FACE (CHEEK) (NOSE) (EYEBROW) (TEMPLE)
4. SCALP NECK
5. TRUNK BACK EXCEPT SCROTUM
6. UPPER LIMB INCLUDING SHOULDER
7. LOWER LIMB INCLUDING HIP
8. OTHER SPECIFIED SITES
9. SKIN UNSPECIFIED

NEVUS BENIGN (continued)

228.00 HEMANGIOMATOUS M9120/0
216.# INTRADERMAL M8750/0
216.# INTRAEPIDERMAL M8740/0
216.# INVOLUTIONAL M8724/0
216.# JUNCTIONAL M8740/0
216.# JUVENILE M8770/0
228.1 LYMPHATIC M9170/0
216.# MELANOTIC M8720/0
216.# NONPIGMENTED M8730/0
216.# NONVASCULAR M8720/0
216.# PAPILLARIS M8720/0
216.# PAPILLOMATOSUS M8720/0
216.# PILOSUS M8720/0
216.# PIGMENTED M8720/0
216.# SPINDLE CELL AND EPITHELIOID M8770/0
216.# SYRINGOCYSTADENOMATOUS PAPILLIFEROUS M8406/0

4th Digit: 216

0. LIP (SKIN OF)
1. EYELID INCLUDING CANTHUS
2. EAR (EXTERNAL) (AURICLE) (PINNA)
3. FACE (CHEEK) (NOSE) (EYEBROW) (TEMPLE)
4. SCALP NECK
5. TRUNK BACK EXCEPT SCROTUM
6. UPPER LIMB INCLUDING SHOULDER
7. LOWER LIMB INCLUDING HIP
8. OTHER SPECIFIED SITES
9. SKIN UNSPECIFIED

173.# NEVUS BLUE MALIGNANT OR OTHER M8780/3

4th Digit: 173

0. LIP
1. EYELID
2. EAR (AURICLE) (AURICULAR) CANAL (EXTERNAL) (ACOUSTIC) MEATUS PINNA
3. UNSPECIFIED PART FACE CHEEK (EXTERNAL) CHIN EYEBROW FOREHEAD NOSE (EXT) TEMPLE
4. SCALP AND NECK
5. TRUNK AXILLA BREAST (OR MASTECTOMY SITE) BUTTOCK GROIN PERIANAL SKIN PERINEUM UMBILICUS
6. UPPER LIMB SHOULDER
7. LOWER LIMB HIP
8. OTHER SPECIFIED SKIN SITE CONTIGUOUS OR OVERLAPPING UNDETERMINED POINT OF ORIGIN
9. SITE UNSPECIFIED

NEVUS - OTHER

702.8 ACANTHOTIC
709.09 ANEMIC, ANEMICUS
448.1 ARANEUS
709.09 AVASCULOSUS
757.33 COMEDONICUS
757.32 FLAMMEUS
759.89 FLAMMEUS OSTEOHYPERTROPHIC
238.2 GIANT PIGMENTED SITE NOS M8761/1
0 JUNCTIONAL IN MALIGNANT MELANOMA SEE 'MELANOMA BY SITE' M8740/3
224.0 MAGNOCELLULAR SITE NOS M8726/0
759.5 MULTIPLEX
448.1 NONNEOPLASTIC
648.9# NON-NEOPLASTIC MATERNAL CURRENT (CO-EXISTENT) IN PREGNANCY [448.1]

5th Digit: 648.9

0. EPISODE OF NOS OR N/A
1. DELIVERED
2. DELIVERED WITH POSTPARTUM COMPLICATION
3. ANTEPARTUM COMPLICATION
4. POSTPARTUM COMPLICATION

750.26 ORAL MUCOSA, WHITE SPONGE
757.33 PIGMENTED SYSTEMATICUS
757.32 PORTWINE CONGENITAL

N

NEVUS - OTHER (continued)
757.32 SANGUINEOUS
702.8 SEBACEOUS, SENILE
448.1 SENILE
448.1 SPIDER
448.1 STELLAR
757.32 STRAWBERRY
757.33 UNIUS LATERIS
757.32 UNNA'S
757.32 VASCULAR
757.33 VERRUCOUS

0 NEWBORN DELIVERY OUTCOME, SEE 'OUTCOME OF DELIVERY'

0 NEWBORN EVALUATION FOR SUSPECTED CONDITION NOT FOUND SEE 'OBSERVATION NEWBORN/INFANT SUSPECTED CONDITION (UNDIAGNOSED) (UNPROVEN) NOT FOUND'

077.8 NEWCASTLE CONJUNCTIVITIS
279.13 NEZELOF'S SYNDROME (PURE ALYMPHOCYTOSIS)
099.4# NGU
5th Digit: 099.4
0. UNSPECIFIED
1. CHLAMYDIA TRACHOMATIS
9. OTHER SPECIFIED ORGANISM

265.2 NIACIN DEFICIENCY
099.1 NICOLAS (-DURAND) -FAVRE DISEASE (CLIMATIC BUBO)
265.2 NICOTINAMIDE DEFICIENCY
265.2 NICOTINIC ACID DEFICIENCY

0 NIDDM (NON INSULIN DEPENDENT DIABETES MELLITUS) SEE 'DIABETES'

272.7 NIEMANN PICK CEREBRAL DEGENERATION [330.2]
272.7 NIEMANN PICK DISEASE OR SYNDROME (LIPID HISTIOCYTOSIS)

NIGHT BLINDNESS
368.60 NOS
368.63 ABNORMAL DARK ADAPTATION CURVE
368.62 ACQUIRED
368.61 CONGENITAL
368.63 DUE TO DELAYED ADAPTATION OF CONES OR RODS
264.5 DUE TO VITAMIN A DEFICIENCY
368.69 OTHER

729.82 NIGHT CRAMPS (LIMB)
780.8 NIGHT SWEATS
307.47 NIGHTMARES
352.2 NINTH CRANIAL NERVE ATROPHY
352.2 NINTH CRANIAL NERVE DISORDER NEC
951.8 NINTH CRANIAL NERVE INJURY

NIPPLE
757.6 ABSENCE CONGENITAL
757.6 ACCESSORY CONGENITAL
675.8# AND BREAST INFECTION OTHER SPECIFIED MATERNAL DUE TO PREGNANCY
675.9# AND BREAST INFECTION MATERNAL DUE TO PREGNANCY
5th Digit: 675.8, 9
0. EPISODE OF CARE UNSPECIFIED OR N/A
1. DELIVERED
2. DELIVERED WITH POSTPARTUM COMPLICATION
3. ANTEPARTUM COMPLICATION
4. POSTPARTUM COMPLICATION

611.79 DISCHARGE NONPUERPERAL
611.9 DISORDER
611.2 FISSURE
676.1# FISSURE (LACTATING) DUE TO PREGNANCY
5th Digit: 676.1
0. EPISODE OF CARE UNSPECIFIED OR N/A
1. DELIVERED
2. DELIVERED WITH POSTPARTUM COMPLICATION
3. ANTEPARTUM COMPLICATION
4. POSTPARTUM COMPLICATION

NIPPLE (continued)
611.0 INFLAMMATION NONPUERPERAL
675.0# INFLAMMATION DUE TO PREGNANCY
5th Digit: 675.0
0. EPISODE OF CARE UNSPECIFIED OR N/A
1. DELIVERED
2. DELIVERED WITH POSTPARTUM COMPLICATION
3. ANTEPARTUM COMPLICATION
4. POSTPARTUM COMPLICATION

611.79 INVERSION (RETRACTION) NONPUERPERAL
757.6 INVERSION (RETRACTION) CONGENITAL
676.0# INVERSION (RETRACTION) DUE TO PREGNANCY
5th Digit: 676.0
0. EPISODE OF CARE UNSPECIFIED OR N/A
1. DELIVERED
2. DELIVERED WITH POSTPARTUM COMPLICATION
3. ANTEPARTUM COMPLICATION
4. POSTPARTUM COMPLICATION

757.6 SUPERNUMERARY CONGENITAL

437.5 NISHIMOTO (-TAKEUCHI) DISEASE
458.2 NITRITOID CRISIS - ADVERSE EFFECT (POSTOPERATIVE) (PROPERLY TAKEN)
961.1 NITRITOID CRISIS - POISONING (OVERDOSE) (IMPROPERLY TAKEN)
790.6 NITROGEN DERIVATIVES, BLOOD ABNORMAL FINDINGS
270.9 NITROGEN METABOLISM DISORDER
104.0 NJOVERA
333.92 NMS (NEUROLEPTIC MALIGNANT SYNDROME)
799.9 NO DIAGNOSIS FOR CAUSE OF DEATH
0 NOCARDIOSIS SEE 'ACTINOMYCOSIS'
788.43 NOCTURIA
788.36 NOCTURNAL ENURESIS
788.43 NOCTURNAL FREQUENCY (MICTURITION)
427.60 NODAL PREMATURE CONTRACTION
371.46 NODULAR DEGENERATION CORNEA
728.79 NODULAR FASCIITIS
202.0# NODULAR LYMPHOMA M9690\3
5th Digit: 202.0
0. UNSPECIFIED SITE, EXTRANODAL AND SOLID ORGAN SITES
1. LYMPH NODES OF HEAD FACE NECK
2. LYMPH NODES INTRATHORACIC
3. LYMPH NODES ABDOMINAL
4. LYMPH NODES AXILLA AND UPPER LIMB
5. LYMPH NODES INGUINAL REGION AND LOWER LIMB
6. LYMPH NODES INTRAPELVIC
7. SPLEEN
8. LYMPH NODES MULTIPLE SITES

NODULE, NODE
039.9 ACTINOMYCOTIC (SEE ALSO 'ACTINOMYCOSIS')
0 ARTHRITIC SEE 'ARTHRITIS OSTEOARTHRITIS (DEGNERATIVE)'
782.2 CUTANEOUS
715.04 HAYGARTH'S
715.04 HEBERDEN'S
102.7 JUXTA-ARTICULAR
095.7 JUXTA-ARTICULAR - SYPHILITIC
102.7 JUXTA-ARTICULAR - YAWS
478.79 LARYNX
518.89 LUNG, SOLITARY
492.8 LUNG, SOLITARY EMPHYSEMATOUS
051.1 MILKERS'
421.0 OSLER'S
600 PROSTATE
729.89 RHEUMATIC
0 RHEUMATOID SEE 'RHEUMATOID ARTHRITIS'

N

NODULE, NODE (continued)

0 SCHMORL'S SEE 'SCHMORL'S NODES'
608.4 SCROTUM (INFLAMMATORY)
478.5 SINGERS'
782.2 SKIN
518.89 SOLITARY, LUNG
492.8 SOLITARY, LUNG EMPHYSEMATOUS
782.2 SUBCUTANEOUS
241.0 THYROID (GLAND) (NONTOXIC) (UNINODULAR)
242.1# THYROID (GLAND) (NONTOXIC) (UNINODULAR) WITH HYPERTHYROIDISM
242.1# THYROID (GLAND) (NONTOXIC) (UNINODULAR) WITH THYROTOXICOSIS
242.1# THYROID (GLAND) (UNINODULAR) TOXIC
242.1# THYROID (GLAND) (UNINODULAR) TOXIC WITH HYPERTHYROIDISM

5th Digit: 242.1

0. WITHOUT MENTION OF THYROTOXIC CRISIS OR STORM
1. WITH MENTION OF THYROTOXIC CRISIS OR STORM

0 TUBERCULOUS SEE 'TUBERCULOSIS', LYMPH NODES
478.5 VOCAL CORDS

388.10 NOISE EFFECTS (INNER EAR)
388.12 NOISE INDUCED HEARING LOSS
V15.81 NONCOMPLIANCE WITH MEDICAL TREATMENT (HISTORY)
998.83 NON-HEALING SURGICAL WOUND
V72.85 NONSTRESS TEST (FOR PREGNANCY)
234.9 NONINFILTRATING INTRACYSTIC CARCINOMA SITE NOS
0 NONINFILTRATING INTRACYSTIC CARCINOMA SITE SPECIFIED SEE 'CA IN SITU' BY SITE M8504/2
757.0 NONNE-MILROY-MEIGE DISEASE OR SYNDROME (CHRONIC HEREDITARY EDEMA)
300.16 NONSENSE SYNDROME
733.82 NONUNION FRACTURE
759.89 NOONAN'S SYNDROME
259.3 NOREPINEPHRINE ECTOPIC SECRETION
289.8 NORMOBLASTOSIS
743.8 NORRIE'S DISEASE (CONGENITAL PROGRESSIVE OCULOACOUSTICOCEREBRAL DEGENERATION)
116.0 NORTH AMERICAN BLASTOMYCOSIS
082.2 NORTH ASIAN TICK FEVER
008.63 NORWALK VIRUS ENTERITIS

NOSE, NASAL

738.0 ABSENCE
748.1 ABSENCE CONGENITAL
748.1 ACCESSORY CONGENITAL
478.1 ADHESIONS
748.1 ANOMALIES OTHER CONGENITAL
738.0 ATRESIA
748.0 ATRESIA CONGENITAL
754.0 BENT CONGENITAL
784.7 BLEED
738.0 BONES OVERDEVELOPMENT
748.1 CLEFT CONGENITAL
478.1 CONGESTION
795.3 CULTURE POSITIVE
738.0 DEFORMITY
748.1 DEFORMITY CONGENITAL
754.0 DEVIATION NASAL SEPTUM CONGENITAL
478.1 DISCHARGE
478.1 DISEASE
478.1 DISORDER

NOSE, NASAL (continued)

478.1 HYPERPLASIA (LYMPHOID) (POLYPOID)
959.09 INJURY
910.8 INJURY OTHER AND UNSPECIFIED (SUPERFICIAL)
910.9 INJURY OTHER AND UNSPECIFIED (SUPERFICIAL) INFECTED
748.1 NOTCHING OF TIP CONGENITAL
478.1 OBSTRUCTION
375.56 OBSTRUCTION DUCT
375.55 OBSTRUCTION DUCT NEONATAL
478.1 OCCLUSION
748.0 OCCLUSION CONGENITAL
471.9 POLYP
212.0 POLYP ADENOMATOUS
478.1 REDNESS
470 SEPTUM - DEVIATED
754.0 SEPTUM - DEVIATED CONGENITAL
478.1 SEPTUM - NECROSIS
478.1 SEPTUM - PERFORATION
748.1 SEPTUM - PERFORATION CONGENITAL
095.8 SEPTUM - PERFORATION SYPHILTIC
478.1 SEPTUM - SPUR
478.1 SEPTUM - ULCER (ABSCESS) (NECROSIS)
456.8 SEPTUM - VARICES
456.8 SEPTUM - VARICOSE ULCER
478.1 SINUS CYST (MUCOCELE) (RHINOLITH)
748.1 SINUS DEFORMITY CONGENITAL
0 SINUS OBSTRUCTION SEE 'SINUSITIS'
748.1 SINUS PERFORATION CONGENITAL
754.0 SQUASHED CONGENITAL
478.1 STUFFY
478.1 SYNECHIA
726.91 SPUR BONE
478.1 SPUR (SEPTUM)
478.0 TURBINATE HYPERTROPHY

378.52 NOTHNAGEL'S OPHTHALMOPLEGIA-CEREBELLAR ATAXIA SYNDROME
443.89 NOTHNAGEL'S VASOMOTOR ACROPARESTHESIA SYNDROME
760.70 NOXIOUS SUBSTANCE TRANSMITTED VIA PLACENTA OR BREAST MILK AFFECTING FETUS OR NEWBORN - NOS
760.75 NOXIOUS SUBSTANCE (COCAINE) TRANSMITTED VIA PLACENTA OR BREAST MILK AFFECTING FETUS OR NEWBORN
760.79 NOXIOUS SUBSTANCE TRANSMITTED VIA PLACENTA OR BREAST MILK AFFECTING FETUS OR NEWBORN - OTHER SPECIFIED
781.6 NUCHAL RIGIDITY
366.16 NUCLEAR SCLEROSIS SENILE CATARACT
352.6 NUCLEUS AMBIGUOUS-HYPOGLOSSAL SYNDROME
782.0 NUMBNESS
832.01 NURSEMAID'S ELBOW
831.0# NURSEMAID'S SHOULDER

5th Digit: 831.0

0. NOS
1. ANTERIOR DISLOCATION
2. POSTERIOR DISLOCATION
3. INFERIOR DISLOCATION
4. ACROMIOCLAVICULAR (JOINT)
9. OTHER

573.8 NUTMEG LIVER
783.9 NUTRITION PROBLEM

NUTRITIONAL DEFICIENCY

269.9 UNSPECIFIED
261 ATROPHY
269.8 DEFICIENCY OTHER
783.4 DEFICIENCY WITH FAILURE TO THRIVE

NUTRITIONAL DEFICIENCY (continued)

V77.9 DISEASE SCREENING
269.9 DISORDER
760.4 DISORDERS MATERNAL AFFECTING FETUS OR NEWBORN
783.3 FEEDING PROBLEMS
779.3 FEEDING PROBLEMS IN NEWBORN
V12.1 HISTORY
261 MARASMUS
648.9# MATERNAL CURRENT (CO-EXISTENT) IN PREGNANCY

5th Digit: 648.9

0. EPISODE OF CARE NOS OR N/A
1. DELIVERED
2. DELIVERED WITH POSTPARTUM COMPLICATION
3. ANTEPARTUM COMPLICATION
4. POSTPARTUM COMPLICATION

281.2 MEGALOBLASTIC ANEMIA (OF INFANCY)

368.60 NYCTALOPIA
788.43 NYCTURIA
302.89 NYMPHOMANIA

NYSTAGMUS

379.50 NOS
386.11 BENIGN POSITIONAL
386.2 CENTRAL POSITIONAL
379.51 CONGENITAL
379.53 DEPRIVATION (VISUAL DEPRIVATION)
379.55 DISSOCIATED
379.52 LATENT
379.54 VESTIBULAR (DISORDER OF VESTIBULAR SYSTEM)
379.56 OTHER FORMS

066.3 O'NYONG NYONG FEVER (VIRAL)
0 OA (OSTEOARTHRITIS) SEE 'OSTEOARTHRITIS'
270.2 OASTHOUSE URINE DISEASE
162.9 OAT CELL CARCINOMA SITE NOS
0 OAT CELL CARCINOMA SITE SPECIFIED SEE 'CANCER' BY SITE M8042/3
756.0 OAV SYNDROME (OCULOAURICULOVERTEBRAL DYSPLASIA)

OBESITY

278.00 NOS
255.8 ADRENAL
V65.3 DIETARY COUNSELING AND SURVEILLANCE
253.8 DUE TO ADIPOSOGENITAL DYSTROPHY
259.9 DUE TO ENDOCRINE DISTURBANCE
783.6 DUE TO EXCESSIVE EATING
278.00 DUE TO HYPERALIMENTATION
259.9 DUE TO HORMONE DISTURBANCE
259.9 DUE TO INFANTILISM DISTURBANCE
259.9 ENDOCRINE IN ORIGIN
278.00 METABOLIC
278.01 MORBID
783.6 POLYPHAGIC (HYPERALIMENTATION) (OVEREATING)
V77.8 SCREENING
0 SEE ALSO 'WEIGHT', GAIN

OBLIQUE LIE

652.3# NOS
660.0# NOS OBSTRUCTING LABOR [652.3#]

5th Digit: 652.3, 660.0
0. EPISODE OF CARE UNSPECIFIED OR N/A
1. DELIVERED
3. ANTEPARTUM COMPLICATION

761.7 AFFECTING FETUS OR NEWBORN BEFORE L&D
652.6# WITH MULTIPLE GESTATION
660.0# WITH MULTIPLE GESTATION OBSTRUCTING LABOR [652.6#]

5th Digit: 652.6, 660.0
0. EPISODE OF CARE UNSPECIFIED OR N/A
1. DELIVERED
3. ANTEPARTUM COMPLICATION

599.84 OBLITERATION URETHRA
447.1 OBLITERATIVE VASCULAR DISEASE
291.2 OBS ALCOHOLIC (SEE ALSO 'PSYCHOSIS ALCOHOLIC')
294.9 OBS (CHRONIC)

V71 - V71.9 ARE ALWAYS SEQUENCED FIRST--THEY DESCRIBE THE EVALUATION AND OBSERVATION FOR SUSPECTED INJURY OR ILLNESS. EXAMPLE: EVALUATION OF A PATIENT IN A MOTOR VEHICLE ACCIDENT WITH NO APPARENT INJURY.

OBSERVATION FOR SUSPECTED CONDITION (UNDIAGNOSED) (UNPROVEN) NOT FOUND

V71.9 UNSPECIFIED
V71.6 ABUSE - CHILD OR ADULT
V71.3 ACCIDENT AT WORK
V71.4 ACCIDENT NEC
V71.8 ACUTE ABDOMEN
V71.01 ANTISOCIAL BEHAVIOR - ADULT
V71.02 ANTISOCIAL BEHAVIOR - CHILD OR ADOLESCENT
V71.6 ASSAULT WITH NO NEED FOR MEDICAL TREATMENT
V71.1 CANCER
V71.7 CARDIOVASCULAR DISEASE
V71.4 CONCUSSION - ACCIDENTAL
V71.6 CONCUSSION - INFLICTED
V71.3 CONCUSSION - WORK RELATED
V71.8 CVA (CEREBROVASCULAR ACCIDENT)
V71.8 FOREIGN BODY INGESTION
V71.01 GANG ACTIVITY - ADULT WITHOUT MANIFEST PSYCHIATRIC DISORDER
V71.02 GANG ACTIVITY - CHILD OR ADOLESCENT WITHOUT MANIFEST PSYCHIATRIC DISORDER

OBSERVATION FOR SUSPECTED CONDITION (UNDIAGNOSED) (UNPROVEN) NOT FOUND (continued)

V71.8 HEMORRHAGE (NON TRAUMATIC) (POST OP)
V71.09 MENTAL CONDITION
V71.4 MVA (MOTOR VEHICLE ACCIDENT) WITH NO APPARENT INJURY
V71.7 MYOCARDIAL INFARCTION

NEWBORN (28 DAYS OR LESS)

V29.9 UNSPECIFIED
V29.8 CARDIOVASCULAR DISEASE
V29.8 CONGENITAL ABNORMALITY
V29.3 GENETIC CONDITION
V29.8 INGESTION FOREIGN OBJECT
V29.0 INFECTIOUS DISEASE
V29.8 INJURY
V29.3 METABOLIC CONDITION
V29.8 NEOPLASM
V29.1 NEUROLOGICAL DISEASE
V29.8 POISONING
V29.2 RESPIRATORY CONDITION
V29.8 SPECIFIED NEC

OBSERVATION FOR SUSPECTED CONDITION (UNDIAGNOSED) (UNPROVEN) NOT FOUND (continued)

V71.02 PSYCHIATRIC DISORDER - ADOLESCENT OR CHILD WITH ANTISOCIAL BEHAVIOR (GANG ACTIVITY)
V71.01 PSYCHIATRIC DISORDER - ADULT WITH ANTISOCIAL BEHAVIOR (GANG ACTIVITY)
V71.09 PSYCHIATRIC DISORDER OTHER
V71.5 RAPE (ALLEGED)
V71.8 RUPTURE OF MEMBRANES PREMATURE
V71.5 SEDUCTION (ALLEGED)
V71.8 SEPSIS
V71.8 STROKE
V71.8 SUICIDE ATTEMPT (ALLEGED)
V71.2 TUBERCULOSIS
V71.4 OTHER ACCIDENT
V71.6 OTHER INFLICTED INJURY
V71.8 OTHER SPECIFIED SUSPECTED CONDITIONS

301.4 OBSESSIONAL PERSONALITY
300.3 OBSESSIVE COMPULSIVE NEUROSIS (DISORDER) (SYNDROME)
301.4 OBSESSIVE COMPULSIVE PERSONALITY

648.##: USE AN ADDITIONAL CODE TO IDENTIFY THE SPECIFIC MATERNAL BACK DISORDER OR NUTRITIONAL DEFIECIENCY.

OBSTETRICAL

648.7# BONE DISORDER MATERNAL CURRENT (CO-EXISTENT) (BACK PELVIS LOWER LIMBS)

5th Digit: 648.7
0. EPISODE OF CARE UNSPECIFIED OR N/A
1. DELIVERED
2. DELIVERED WITH POSTPARTUM COMPLICATION
3. ANTEPARTUM COMPLICATION
4. POSTPARTUM COMPLICATION

V13.2 DISORDER HISTORY (NONGRAVID)
V23.4 HISTORY POOR AFFECTING PREGNANCY SUPERVISION
648.9# NUTRITIONAL DEFICIENCIES MATERNAL CURRENT (CO-EXISTENT)
669.4# SURGERY OR MEDICAL PROCEDURES COMPLICATION, OTHER
665.9# TRAUMA
665.8# TRAUMA OTHER SPECIFIED

5th Digit: 648.9, 665.8-9, 669.4
0. EPISODE OF CARE UNSPECIFIED OR N/A
1. DELIVERED
2. DELIVERED WITH POSTPARTUM COMPLICATION
3. ANTEPARTUM COMPLICATION
4. POSTPARTUM COMPLICATION

564.0 OBSTIPATION
306.4 OBSTIPATION PSYCHOGENIC [564.0]
0 OBSTRUCTION SEE ANATOMICAL SITE, OBSTRUCTION
593.89 OBSTRUCTIVE NEPHROPATHY
599.6 OBSTRUCTIVE UROPATHY
553.8 OBTURATOR HERNIA
355.79 OBTURATOR MONONEUROPATHY
355.79 OBTURATOR NERVE COMPRESSION (ENTRAPMENT)
355.79 OBTURATOR NERVE DISORDER (LESION)
959.09 OCCIPITAL INJURY
784.0 OCCIPITAL NEURALGIA
739.0 OCCIPITOCERVICAL REGION SEGMENTAL OR SOMATIC DYSFUNCTION
0 OCCLUSION ARTERIES EXTREMITIES SEE 'ARTERY, ARTERIAL', OCCLUSION
0 OCCLUSION SEE ANATOMICAL SITE, OCCLUSION
792.1 OCCULT BLOOD IN STOOL
727.2 OCCUPATIONAL BURSITIS
300.89 OCCUPATIONAL DISORDER PSYCHOGENIC
V70.5 OCCUPATIONAL EXAM (HEALTH)
V57.21 OCCUPATIONAL THERAPY
270.2 OCHRONOSIS AMINO ACID METABOLISM AROMATIC DISTURBANCES
270.2 OCHRONOSIS ARTHRITIS [713.0]

OCULAR

0 OCULAR SEE ALSO EYE
360.32 FISTULA (CAUSING HYPOTONY) (POSTINFLAMMATORY) (POST OP) (POSTTRAUMATIC)
365.04 HYPERTENSION
871.1 LACERATION WITH PROLAPSE OF INTRAOCULAR TISSUE
871.0 LACERATION WITHOUT PROLAPSE
996.69 LENS PROSTHESIS COMPLICATION - INFECTION OR INFLAMMATION
996.53 LENS PROSTHESIS COMPLICATION - MECHANICAL
996.79 LENS PROSTHESIS COMPLICATION - OTHER
378.87 MOTION DISTURBANCE
306.7 MOTION DISTURBANCE PSYCHOGENIC
743.69 MUSCLE ABSENCE (CONGENITAL)
378.60 MUSCLE DEFORMITY ACQUIRED
743.9 MUSCLE DEFORMITY (CONGENITAL)
378.9 MUSCLE DISEASE
359.1 MUSCULAR DYSTROPHY
378.71 RETRACTION SYNDROME

364.24 OCULOCUTANEOUS SYNDROME
378.87 OCULOGYRIC CRISIS
306.7 OCULOGYRIC CRISIS PSYCHOGENIC

OCULOMOTOR

344.89 ALTERNATING PARALYSIS
794.14 FUNCTION STUDY ABNORMAL
378.51 NERVE DISORDER (ATROPHY) (PALSY) - PARTIAL
378.52 NERVE DISORDER (ATROPHY) (PALSY) - TOTAL
951.0 NERVE INJURY
344.89 NERVE PARALYSIS
378.81 SYNDROME

359.1 OCULOPHARYNGEAL MUSCULAR DYSTROPHY

099.3 OCULOURETHROARTICULAR SYNDROME
099.3 OCULOURETHROARTICULAR SYNDROME WITH ARTHROPATHY [711.1#]

5th Digit: 711.1
0. SITE NOS
1. SHOULDER REGION
2. UPPER ARM (ELBOW) (HUMERUS)
3. FOREARM (RADIUS) (WRIST) (ULNA)
4. HAND (CARPAL) (METACARPAL) (FINGERS)
5. PELVIC REGION AND THIGH (HIP) (BUTTOCK) (FEMUR)
6. LOWER LEG (FIBULA) (KNEE) (PATELLA) (TIBIA)
7. ANKLE AND/OR FOOT (METATARSALS) (TOES) (TARSALS)
8. OTHER (HEAD) (NECK) (RIB) (SKULL) (TRUNK) (VERTEBRAE)
9. MULTIPLE

099.3 OCULOURETHROARTICULAR SYNDROME WITH CONJUNCTIVITIS [372.33]
732.1 ODELBERG'S DISEASE (JUVENILE OSTEOCHONDROSIS)
213.# ODONTOAMELOBLASTOMA M9311/0

4th Digit: 213
0. SKULL FACE UPPER JAW
1. LOWER JAW (OR IF SITE UNSPECIFIED)

521.0 ODONTOCLASIA
520.5 ODONTOGENESIS IMPERFECTA

ODONTOGENIC

526.0 CYST
213.# CYST CALCIFYING M9301/0
238.0 TUMOR M9270/1
213.# TUMOR ADENOMATOID M9300/0
213.# TUMOR BENIGN M9270/0
213.# TUMOR EPITHELIAL M9340/0
170.# TUMOR MALIGNANT M9270/3
213.# TUMOR SQUAMOUS M9312/0

4th Digit: 170, 213
0. SKULL FACE UPPER JAW
1. LOWER JAW (OR IF SITE UNSPECIFIED)

ODONTOMA

213.# UNSPECIFIED M9280/0
213.# COMPLEX M9282/0
213.# COMPOUND M9281/0

4th Digit: 213
0. SKULL FACE UPPER JAW
1. LOWER JAW (OR IF SITE UNSPECIFIED)

170.# ODONTOSARCOMA AMELOBLASTIC M9290/3

4th Digit: 213
0. SKULL FACE UPPER JAW
1. LOWER JAW (OR IF SITE UNSPECIFIED)

787.2 ODYNOPHAGIA
127.7 OESOPHAGOSTOMUM APIOSTOMUM AND RELATED SPECIES INFECTION
134.0 OESTRUS OVIS INFESTATION
560.89 OGILVIE'S SYNDROME (SYMPATHICOTONIC COLON OBSTRUCTION)
0 OGILVIE'S SYNDROME SEE 'OBSTRUCTION', BOWEL
368.61 OGUCHI'S (RETINA) DISEASE
021.9 OHARA'S DISEASE (SEE ALSO 'TULAREMIA')
797 OLD AGE (CAUSE OF MORBIDITY AND MORTALITY)
726.33 OLECRANON BURSITIS

OLFACTORY

352.0 NERVE ATROPHY
352.0 NERVE DISORDERS
951.8 NERVE INJURY
352.0 NERVE NEURITIS
160.0 NEUROGENIC TUMOR SITE NOS
0 NEUROGENIC TUMOR SITE SPECIFIED SEE 'CANCER' BY SITE M9520/3

285.9 OLIGOCYTHEMIA

191.9 OLIGODENDROBLASTOMA SITE NOS

0 OLIGODENDROBLASTOMA SITE SPECIFIED SEE 'CANCER' BY SITE M9460/3

OLIGODENDROGLIOMA

191.9 SITE NOS

0 SITE SPECIFIED SEE 'CANCER' BY SITE M9450/3

191.9 ANAPLASTIC TYPE SITE NOS

0 ANAPLASTIC TYPE SITE SPECIFIED SEE 'CANCER' BY SITE M9451/3

520.0 OLIGODONTIA

658.0# OLIGOHYDRAMNIOS

5th Digit: 658.0

0. EPISODE OF CARE UNSPECIFIED OR N/A
1. DELIVERED
3. ANTEPARTUM COMPLICATION

761.2 OLIGOHYDRAMNIOS AFFECTING FETUS OR NEWBORN

658.1# OLIGOHYDRAMNIOS DUE TO PREMATURE RUPTURE OF MEMBRANES

5th Digit: 658.1

0. EPISODE OF CARE UNSPECIFIED OR N/A
1. DELIVERED
3. ANTEPARTUM COMPLICATION

705.0 OLIGOHYDROSIS

626.1 OLIGOMENORRHEA

606.1 OLIGOSPERMIA

788.5 OLIGURIA

639.3 OLIGURIA POST (ABORTIVE) (ECTOPIC) (MOLAR) PREGNANCY

997.5 OLIGURIA POSTOPERATIVE

333.0 OLIVOPONTOCEREBELLAR ATROPHY OR DEGENERATION

756.4 OLLIER'S DISEASE CONGENITAL (CHONDRODYSPLASIA)

771.4 OMPHALITIS NEWBORN

771.3 OMPHALITIS TETANUS

756.79 OMPHALOCELE

751.0 OMPHALOMESENTERIC DUCT PERSISTENT (CONGENITAL)

125.3 ONCHOCERCA VOLVULUS INFECTION

125.3 ONCHOCERCIASIS

125.3 ONCHOCERCIASIS EYELID [373.6]

125.3 ONCHOCERCOSIS

295.4# ONEIROPHRENIA ACUTE EPISODE

5th Digit: 295.4

0. UNSPECIFIED
1. SUBCHRONIC
2. CHRONIC
3. SUBCHRONIC WITH ACUTE EXACERBATION
4. CHRONIC WITH ACUTE
5. IN REMISSION

703.8 ONYCHAUXIS

757.5 ONYCHAUXIS CONGENITAL

ONYCHIA

681.02 FINGER

681.11 TOE

112.3 CANDIDAL DIGIT NOS [681.9]

112.3 CANDIDAL FINGER [681.02]

112.3 CANDIDAL TOE [681.11]

110.1 DERMATOPHYTIC

110.1 TINEA DIGIT NOS [681.9]

110.1 TINEA FINGER [681.02]

110.1 TINEA TOE [681.11]

703.0 ONYCHOCRYPTOSIS

703.8 ONYCHOGRYPOSIS

703.8 ONYCHOLYSIS

110.1 ONYCHOMYCOSIS (FINGER) (TOE)

110.1 ONYCHOMYCOSIS BLASTOMYCOSIS

112.3 ONYCHOMYCOSIS CANDIDAL

V45.89 OOPHORECTOMY STATUS

OOPHORITIS

614.2 NOS

614.0 ACUTE

614.1 CHRONIC

072.79 MUMPS

016.6# TUBERCULOUS

5th Digit: 016.6

0. UNSPECIFIED
1. LAB NOT DONE
2. LABS PENDING
3. MICROSCOPY POSITIVE (IN SPUTUM)
4. CULTURE POSITIVE - MICROSCOPY NEGATIVE
5. CULTURE NEGATIVE - MICROSCOPY POSITIVE
6. CULTURE AND MICROSCOPY NEGATIVE CONFIRMED BY OTHER METHODS

524.2 OPEN BITE (ANTERIOR) (POSTERIOR)

> *WHEN AN OPEN WOUND OR LACERATION IS ACCOMPANIED BY CELLULITIS, TWO CODES ARE NEEDED, THE CODE FOR THE **COMPLICATED** OPEN WOUND OR LACERATION AND A CODE FOR THE CELLULITIS. SEQUENCING DEPENDS ON WHICH DIAGNOSIS REQUIRED THE MAJOR WORK AND EFFORT.*

OPEN WOUND

0 SEE ALSO 'LACERATION', BY SITE

879.8 NOS

879.9 NOS COMPLICATED

879.2 ABDOMEN WALL ANTERIOR

879.3 ABDOMEN WALL ANTERIOR COMPLICATED

879.4 ABDOMEN WALL LATERAL

879.5 ABDOMEN WALL LATERAL COMPLICATED

873.62 ALVEOLAR (GUM)

873.72 ALVEOLAR (GUM) COMPLICATED

891.0 ANKLE

891.1 ANKLE COMPLICATED

891.2 ANKLE WITH TENDON INVOLVEMENT

879.6 ANUS

879.7 ANUS COMPLICATED

863.89 ANUS (SPHINCTER) INTERNAL

565.0 ANUS NONTRAUMATIC NONPUERPERAL

884.0 ARM NOS

884.1 ARM NOS COMPLICATED

884.2 ARM NOS WITH TENDON INVOLVEMENT

0 ARM LOWER SEE 'OPEN WOUND' FOREARM

884.0 ARM MULTIPLE SITES

884.1 ARM MULTIPLE SITES COMPLICATED

884.0 ARM MULTIPLE SITES OF ONE UPPER LIMB

884.2 ARM MULTIPLE SITES WITH TENDON INVOLVEMENT

880.03 ARM UPPER

880.13 ARM UPPER COMPLICATED

880.23 ARM UPPER WITH TENDON INVOLVEMENT

0 ARTERY SEE SPECIFIC ARTERY

872.02 AUDITORY CANAL

872.12 AUDITORY CANAL COMPLICATED

872.01 AURICLE (PINNA)

872.11 AURICLE (PINNA) COMPLICATED

880.02 AXILLA

880.12 AXILLA COMPLICATED

880.22 AXILLA WITH TENDON INVOLVEMENT

WHEN AN OPEN WOUND OR LACERATION IS ACCOMPANIED BY CELLULITIS, TWO CODES ARE NEEDED, THE CODE FOR THE __COMPLICATED__ OPEN WOUND OR LACERATION AND A CODE FOR THE CELLULITIS. SEQUENCING DEPENDS ON WHICH DIAGNOSIS REQUIRED THE MAJOR WORK AND EFFORT.

OPEN WOUND (continued)

880.09 AXILLA WITH OTHER SITES OF UPPER ARM
880.19 AXILLA WITH OTHER SITES OF UPPER ARM COMPLICATED
880.29 AXILLA WITH OTHER SITES OF UPPER ARM WITH TENDON INVOLVEMENT

876.0 BACK
876.1 BACK COMPLICATED

0 BLOOD VESSEL SEE 'BLOOD VESSEL INJURY', BY SITE

879.0 BREAST
879.1 BREAST COMPLICATED

0 BROW SEE 'OPEN WOUND', EYEBROW

873.61 BUCCAL MUCOSA
873.71 BUCCAL MUCOSA COMPLICATED

877.0 BUTTOCK
877.1 BUTTOCK COMPLICATED

891.0 CALF
891.1 CALF COMPLICATED
891.2 CALF WITH TENDON INVOLVEMENT

870.8 CANALICULUS LACRIMALIS
870.2 CANALICULUS LACRIMALIS WITH LACERATION OF EYELID

870.8 CANTHUS, EYE

873.41 CHEEK EXTERNAL
873.51 CHEEK EXTERNAL COMPLICATED

873.61 CHEEK INTERNAL
873.71 CHEEK INTERNAL COMPLICATED

875.0 CHEST WALL
875.1 CHEST WALL COMPLICATED

873.44 CHIN
873.54 CHIN COMPLICATED

363.63 CHOROID

878.8 CLITORIS
878.9 CLITORIS COMPLICATED

872.64 COCHLEA
872.74 COCHLEA COMPLICATED

871.9 CONJUNCTIVA (ALONE)
0 CORNEA SEE 'OPEN WOUND', EYEBALL

875.0 COSTAL REGION
875.1 COSTAL REGION COMPLICATED

0 DESCEMET'S MEMBRANE SEE 'OPEN WOUND', EYEBALL

872.8 EAR
872.9 EAR COMPLICATED

872.01 EAR AURICLE (PINNA)
872.11 EAR AURICLE (PINNA) COMPLICATED

872.02 EAR CANAL
872.12 EAR CANAL COMPLICATED

872.61 EAR DRUM
872.71 EAR DRUM COMPLICATED

872.00 EAR EXTERNAL NOS
872.10 EAR EXTERNAL NOS COMPLICATED

872.62 EAR OSSICLES (INCUS) (MALLEUS) (STAPES)
872.72 EAR OSSICLES (INCUS) (MALLEUS) (STAPES) COMPLICATED

872.69 EAR OTHER AND MULTIPLE SITES
872.79 EAR OTHER AND MULTIPLE SITES COMPLICATED

OPEN WOUND (continued)

881.01 ELBOW
881.11 ELBOW COMPLICATED
881.21 ELBOW WITH TENDON INVOLVEMENT

878.2 EPIDIDYMIS
878.3 EPIDIDYMIS COMPLICATED

879.2 EPIGASTRIC REGION
879.3 EPIGASTRIC REGION COMPLICATED

874.01 EPIGLOTTIS
874.11 EPIGLOTTIS COMPLICATED

874.4 ESOPHAGUS CERVICAL
874.5 ESOPHAGUS CERVICAL COMPLICATED

872.63 EUSTACHIAN TUBE
872.73 EUSTACHIAN TUBE COMPLICATED

871.4 EYE
870.9 EYE (OCULAR ADNEXA)
870.8 EYE (OCULAR ADNEXA) OTHER SPECIFIED
870.3 EYE (ORBIT) PENETRATING
0 EYE WITH FOREIGN BODY SEE 'FOREIGN BODY', EYE

871.9 EYEBALL NOS
871.7 EYEBALL PENETRATING NOS
871.2 EYEBALL WITH PARTIAL LOSS OF INTRAOCULAR TISSUE
0 EYEBALL WITH FOREIGN BODY SEE 'FOREIGN BODY', EYE
871.1 EYEBALL WITH PROLAPSE OF INTRAOCULAR TISSUE
871.0 EYEBALL WITHOUT PROLAPSE OF INTRAOCULAR TISSUE

873.42 EYEBROW
873.52 EYEBROW COMPLICATED

A COMPLICATED LACERATION OR OPEN WOUND IS DEFINED AS THAT WHICH IS INFECTED, CONTAINS A FOREIGN BODY, OR IS GROSSLY CONTAMINATED.

870.0 EYELID AND PERIOCULAR AREA
870.1 EYELID FULL THICKNESS
870.2 EYELID INVOLVING LACRIMAL PASSAGES

873.40 FACE
873.50 FACE COMPLICATED

873.49 FACE OTHER AND MULTIPLE SITES
873.59 FACE OTHER AND MULTIPLE SITES COMPLICATED

883.0 FINGER (NAIL)
883.1 FINGER (NAIL) COMPLICATED
883.2 FINGER (NAIL) WITH TENDON INVOLVEMENT

879.4 FLANK
879.5 FLANK COMPLICATED

892.0 FOOT
892.1 FOOT COMPLICATED
892.2 FOOT WITH TENDON INVOLVEMENT

881.00 FOREARM
881.10 FOREARM COMPLICATED
881.20 FOREARM WITH TENDON INVOLVEMENT

873.42 FOREHEAD
873.52 FOREHEAD COMPLICATED

878.8 GENITALIA
878.9 GENITALIA COMPLICATED

873.62 GINGIVA
873.72 GINGIVA COMPLICATED

0 GLOBE SEE 'OPEN WOUND', EYEBALL

879.4 GROIN
879.5 GROIN COMPLICATED

873.62 GUM
873.72 GUM COMPLICATED

882.0 HAND
882.1 HAND COMPLICATED
882.2 HAND WITH TENDON INVOLVEMENT

O

WHEN AN OPEN WOUND OR LACERATION IS ACCOMPANIED BY CELLULITIS, TWO CODES ARE NEEDED, THE CODE FOR THE __COMPLICATED__ OPEN WOUND OR LACERATION AND A CODE FOR THE CELLULITIS. SEQUENCING DEPENDS ON WHICH DIAGNOSIS REQUIRED THE MAJOR WORK AND EFFORT.

OPEN WOUND (continued)

873.8 HEAD
873.9 HEAD COMPLICATED

0 HEEL SEE 'OPEN WOUND', FOOT

890.0 HIP
890.1 HIP COMPLICATED
890.2 HIP WITH TENDON INVOLVEMENT

878.6 HYMEN
878.7 HYMEN COMPLICATED

879.4 HYPOCHONDRIUM
879.5 HYPOCHONDRIUM COMPLICATED

879.2 HYPOGASTRIC REGION
879.3 HYPOGASTRIC REGION COMPLICATED

879.4 ILIAC REGION
879.5 ILIAC REGION COMPLICATED

879.4 INGUINAL REGION
879.5 INGUINAL REGION COMPLICATED

892.0 INSTEP
892.1 INSTEP COMPLICATED
892.2 INSTEP WITH TENDON INVOLVEMENT

0 INTERNAL ORGAN SEE SPECIFIC ORGAN

876.0 INTERSCAPULAR REGION
876.1 INTERSCAPULAR REGION COMPLICATED

0 IRIS SEE 'OPEN WOUND', EYEBALL

873.44 JAW
873.54 JAW COMPLICATED

891.0 KNEE
891.1 KNEE COMPLICATED
891.2 KNEE WITH TENDON INVOLVEMENT

878.4 LABIA
878.5 LABIA COMPLICATED

A COMPLICATED LACERATION OR OPEN WOUND IS DEFINED AS THAT WHICH IS INFECTED, CONTAINS A FOREIGN BODY, OR IS GROSSLY CONTAMINATED.

870.8 LACRIMAL APPARATUS, GLAND OR SAC
870.2 LACRIMAL APPARATUS, GLAND OR SAC WITH LACERATION OF EYELID

874.## LARYNX
4th Digit: 874
0. UNSPECIFIED
1. COMPLICATED
5th Digit: 874
0. LARYNX WITH TRACHEA
1. LARYNX

906.1 LATE EFFECT EXTREMITIES
906.0 LATE EFFECT HEAD, NECK OR TRUNK
905.8 LATE EFFECT WITH TENDON INVOLVEMENT

891.0 LEG NOS OR LOWER
891.1 LEG NOS OR LOWER COMPLICATED
891.2 LEG NOS OR LOWER WITH TENDON INVOLVEMENT

890.0 LEG UPPER
890.1 LEG UPPER COMPLICATED
890.2 LEG UPPER WITH TENDON INVOLVEMENT

OPEN WOUND (continued)

OPEN WOUND INCLUDES LACERATION, PUNCTURE WOUND, ANIMAL BITES, FOREIGN BODY, OR AVULSION.

894.0 LIMB LOWER NOS OR MULTIPLE SITES
894.1 LIMB LOWER NOS OR MULTIPLE SITES COMPLICATED
894.2 LIMB LOWER NOS OR MULTIPLE SITES WITH TENDON INVOLVEMENT

884.0 LIMB UPPER NOS OR MULTIPLE SITES
884.1 LIMB UPPER NOS OR MULTIPLE SITES COMPLICATED
884.2 LIMB UPPER NOS OR MULTIPLE SITES WITH TENDON INVOLVEMENT

873.43 LIP
873.53 LIP COMPLICATED

876.0 LOIN
876.1 LOIN COMPLICATED

876.0 LUMBAR REGION
876.1 LUMBAR REGION COMPLICATED

873.41 MALAR
873.51 MALAR COMPLICATED

873.44 MANDIBLE
873.54 MANDIBLE COMPLICATED

873.49 MASTOID
873.59 MASTOID COMPLICATED

875.0 MIDTHORACIC REGION
875.1 MIDTHORACIC REGION COMPLICATED

873.60 MOUTH
873.70 MOUTH COMPLICATED

873.64 MOUTH FLOOR
873.74 MOUTH FLOOR COMPLICATED

873.69 MOUTH OTHER AND MULTIPLE SITES
873.79 MOUTH OTHER AND MULTIPLE SITES COMPLICATED

879.8 MULTIPLE
879.9 MULTIPLE COMPLICATED

894.0 MULTIPLE LOWER LIMB
894.1 MULTIPLE LOWER LIMB COMPLICATED
894.2 MULTIPLE LOWER LIMB WITH TENDON INVOLVEMENT

884.0 MULTIPLE UPPER LIMB
884.1 MULTIPLE UPPER LIMB COMPLICATED
884.2 MULTIPLE UPPER LIMB WITH TENDON INVOLVEMENT

0 NAIL SEE 'OPEN WOUND', FINGER, THUMB OR TOE

0 NASAL SEE 'OPEN WOUND', NOSE

873.22 NASOPHARYNX
873.32 NASOPHARYNX COMPLICATED

874.8 NECK
874.9 NECK COMPLICATED

874.8 NECK NAPE
874.9 NECK NAPE COMPLICATED

874.8 NECK OTHER AND UNSPECIFIED
874.9 NECK OTHER AND UNSPECIFIED COMPLICATED

0 NERVE SEE 'LACERATION', NERVE BY SITE

998.83 NON-HEALING SURGICAL

873.20 NOSE
873.30 NOSE COMPLICATED

873.22 NOSE CAVITY
873.32 NOSE CAVITY COMPLICATED

873.29 NOSE MULTIPLE SITES
873.39 NOSE MULTIPLE SITES COMPLICATED

873.21 NOSE SEPTUM
873.31 NOSE SEPTUM COMPLICATED

*WHEN AN OPEN WOUND OR LACERATION IS ACCOMPANIED BY CELLULITIS, TWO CODES ARE NEEDED, THE CODE FOR THE **COMPLICATED** OPEN WOUND OR LACERATION AND A CODE FOR THE CELLULITIS. SEQUENCING DEPENDS ON WHICH DIAGNOSIS REQUIRED THE MAJOR WORK AND EFFORT.*

OPEN WOUND (continued)

873.23 NOSE SINUS
873.33 NOSE SINUS COMPLICATED

0 OCCIPITAL REGION SEE 'OPEN WOUND', SCALP

870.9 OCULAR ADNEXA
870.8 OCULAR ADNEXA OTHER SPECIFIED

870.8 ORBIT
870.3 ORBIT PENETRATING
870.4 ORBIT PENETRATING WITH FOREIGN BODY
870.9 ORBITAL REGION

0 ORGAN INTERNAL SEE SPECIFIC ORGAN

872.62 OSSICLES EAR
872.72 OSSICLES EAR COMPLICATED

873.65 PALATE
873.75 PALATE COMPLICATED

0 PALM SEE 'OPEN WOUND', HAND

874.2 PARATHYROID GLAND
874.3 PARATHYROID GLAND COMPLICATED

0 PARIETAL REGION SEE 'OPEN WOUND', SCALP

879.6 PELVIC REGION
879.7 PELVIC REGION COMPLICATED

878.0 PENIS
878.1 PENIS COMPLICATED

879.6 PERINEUM
879.7 PERINEUM COMPLICATED

870.8 PERIOCULAR AREA
870.0 PERIOCULAR AREA WITH LACERATION OF SKIN

874.4 PHARYNX
874.5 PHARYNX COMPLICATED

872.01 PINNA
872.11 PINNA COMPLICATED

891.0 POPLITEAL
891.1 POPLITEAL COMPLICATED
891.2 POPLITEAL WITH TENDON INVOLVEMENT

0 PREPUCE SEE 'OPEN WOUND', PENIS

879.2 PUBIC REGION
879.3 PUBIC REGION COMPLICATED

878.8 PUDENDA
878.9 PUDENDA COMPLICATED

878.8 RECTOVAGINAL SEPTUM
878.9 RECTOVAGINAL SEPTUM COMPLICATED

877.0 SACRAL REGION
877.1 SACRAL REGION COMPLICATED

0 SACROILIAC REGION SEE 'OPEN WOUND', SACRAL REGION

873.69 SALIVARY (DUCTS) (GLAND)
873.79 SALIVARY (DUCTS) (GLAND) COMPLICATED

873.0 SCALP
873.1 SCALP COMPLICATED

880.01 SCAPULAR
880.11 SCAPULAR COMPLICATED
880.21 SCAPULAR WITH TENDON INVOLVEMENT

871.9 SCLERA

OPEN WOUND (continued)

878.2 SCROTUM
878.3 SCROTUM COMPLICATED

891.0 SHIN
891.1 SHIN COMPLICATED
891.2 SHIN WITH TENDON INVOLVEMENT

880.00 SHOULDER
880.10 SHOULDER COMPLICATED
880.20 SHOULDER WITH TENDON INVOLVEMENT

880.09 SHOULDER AND ARM MULTIPLE SITES
880.19 SHOULDER AND ARM MULTIPLE SITES COMPLICATED
880.29 SHOULDER AND ARM MULTIPLE SITES WITH TENDON INVOLVEMENT

879.8 SKIN NOS
879.9 SKIN NOS COMPLICATED

0 SPERMATIC CORD (SCROTAL) SEE 'OPEN WOUND', SCROTUM

0 SPINAL CORD SEE 'SPINAL CORD INJURY', BY SITE

875.0 STERNAL REGION
875.1 STERNAL REGION COMPLICATED

0 SUBMAXILLARY REGION SEE 'OPEN WOUND', JAW
0 SUBMENTAL REGION SEE 'OPEN WOUND', JAW

0 SUBUNGUAL SEE 'OPEN WOUND', FINGER, THUMB OR TOE

874.8 SUPRACLAVICULAR REGION
874.9 SUPRACLAVICULAR REGION COMPLICATED

0 SUPRAORBITAL SEE 'OPEN WOUND', FOREHEAD

873.49 TEMPLE
873.59 TEMPLE COMPLICATED

0 TEMPORAL REGION SEE 'OPEN WOUND', TEMPLE

0 TENDON SEE 'LACERATION', TENDON BY SITE

878.2 TESTIS
878.3 TESTIS COMPLICATED

890.0 THIGH
890.1 THIGH COMPLICATED
890.2 THIGH WITH TENDON INVOLVEMENT

875.0 THORAX EXTERNAL
875.1 THORAX EXTERNAL COMPLICATED

874.8 THROAT
874.9 THROAT COMPLICATED

883.0 THUMB (NAIL)
883.1 THUMB (NAIL) COMPLICATED
883.2 THUMB (NAIL) WITH TENDON INVOLVEMENT

874.2 THYROID GLAND
874.3 THYROID GLAND COMPLICATED

893.0 TOE (NAIL)
893.1 TOE (NAIL) COMPLICATED
893.2 TOE (NAIL) WITH TENDON INVOLVEMENT

873.64 TONGUE
873.74 TONGUE COMPLICATED

873.64 TONGUE AND FLOOR OF MOUTH
873.74 TONGUE AND FLOOR OF MOUTH COMPLICATED

874.## TRACHEA

4th Digit: 874
- **0. UNSPECIFIED**
- **1. COMPLICATED**

5th Digit: 874
- **0. TRACHEA WITH LARYNX**
- **2. TRACHEA**

O

WHEN AN OPEN WOUND OR LACERATION IS ACCOMPANIED BY CELLULITIS, TWO CODES ARE NEEDED, THE CODE FOR THE ***COMPLICATED*** *OPEN WOUND OR LACERATION AND A CODE FOR THE CELLULITIS. SEQUENCING DEPENDS ON WHICH DIAGNOSIS REQUIRED THE MAJOR WORK AND EFFORT.*

OPEN WOUND (continued)

879.6 TRUNK
879.7 TRUNK COMPLICATED

878.2 TUNICA VAGINALIS
878.3 TUNICA VAGINALIS COMPLICATED

872.61 TYMPANIC MEMBRANE
872.71 TYMPANIC MEMBRANE COMPLICATED

879.2 UMBILICAL REGION
879.3 UMBILICAL REGION COMPLICATED

873.69 UVULA
873.79 UVULA COMPLICATED

878.6 VAGINA
878.7 VAGINA COMPLICATED

871.2 VITREOUS (HUMOR)

878.4 VULVA
878.5 VULVA COMPLICATED

881.02 WRIST
881.12 WRIST COMPLICATED
881.22 WRIST WITH TENDON INVOLVEMENT

709.01 OPHIASIS
771.6 OPHTHALMIA NEONATORUM
098.40 OPHTHALMIA NEONATORUM GONOCOCCAL
360.14 OPHTHALMIA NODOSA
370.31 OPHTHALMIA PHLYCTENULAR
377.30 OPHTHALMIC NEURITIS

OPHTHALMOPLEGIA

378.9 NOS
378.52 CEREBELLAR ATAXIA SYNDROME
242.## EXOPHTHALMIC [376.22]

4th Digit: 242
- **0. DIFFUSE**
- **1. UNINODULAR**
- **2. MULTINODULAR**
- **3. NODULAR UNSPECIFIED**
- **4. ECTOPIC THYROID NODULE**
- **8. OTHER SPECIFIED**
- **9. NOS**

5th Digit: 242
- **0. WITHOUT MENTION OF THYROTOXIC CRISIS OR STORM**
- **1. WITH MENTION OF THYROTOXIC CRISIS OR STORM**

378.55 EXTERNAL
378.86 INTERNUCLEAR
378.72 PROGRESSIVE EXTERNAL
333.0 PROGRESSIVE SUPRANUCLEAR
378.56 TOTAL
367.52 TOTAL OR COMPLETE (INTERNAL)

763.5 OPIATE REACTION (INTOXICATION) MATERNAL DURING L&D AFFECTING FETUS OR NEWBORN
305.5# OPIOID ABUSE (NONDEPENDENT)
304.0# OPIOID ADDICTION (DEPENDENT)
304.7# OPIOID ADDICTION MIXED WITH ANY OTHER DRUG DEPENDENCE

5th Digit: 304.0, 7, 305.5
- **0. NOS**
- **1. CONTINUOUS**
- **2. EPISODIC**
- **3. IN REMISSION**

524.00 OPISTHOGNATHISM
121.0 OPISTHORCHIASIS
289.51 OPITZ'S DISEASE (CONGESTIVE SPLENOMEGALY)

305.5# OPIUM ABUSE (NONDEPENDENT)
304.0# OPIUM ADDICTION (DEPENDENT)
304.7# OPIUM ADDICTION MIXED WITH ANY OTHER DRUG DEPENDENCE

5th Digit: 304.0, 7, 305.5
- **0. UNSPECIFIED**
- **1. CONTINUOUS**
- **2. EPISODIC**
- **3. IN REMISSION**

358.8 OPPENHEIM'S DISEASE (MYONEURAL DISORDER)
250.8# OPPENHEIM-URBACH DISEASE OR SYNDROME (NECROBIOSIS LIPOIDICA DIABETICORUM) [709.3]

5th Digit: 250.8
- **0. TYPE II, ADULT-ONSET, NON-INSULIN DEPENDENT (EVEN IF REQUIRING INSULIN), OR UNSPECIFIED; CONTROLLED**
- **1. TYPE I, JUVENILE-ONSET OR INSULIN-DEPENDENT; CONTROLLED**
- **2. TYPE II, ADULT-ONSET, NON-INSULIN DEPENDENT (EVEN IF REQUIRING INSULIN); UNCONTROLLED**
- **3. TYPE I, JUVENILE-ONSET OR INSULIN-DEPENDENT; UNCONTROLLED**

313.81 OPPOSITIONAL DISORDER (EMOTIONAL DISTURBANCES OF CHILDHOOD OR ADOLESCENCE)

379.59 OPSOCLONUS

OPTIC ATROPHY

377.10 NOS
377.16 HEREDITARY
377.15 PARTIAL
377.12 POSTINFLAMMATORY
377.11 PRIMARY
094.84 SYPHILITIC
090.49 SYPHILITIC CONGENITAL
094.0 SYPHILITIC TABES DORSALIS
377.13 WITH RETINAL DYSTROPHIES

OPTIC CHIASM

377.54 DISORDERS WITH INFLAMMATORY DISORDERS
377.52 DISORDERS WITH NEOPLASMS NEC
377.51 DISORDERS WITH PITUITARY NEOPLASMS AND DISORDERS
377.53 DISORDERS WITH VASCULAR DISORDERS
950.1 INJURY

OPTIC DISC

743.57 ANOMALIES SPECIFIED CONGENITAL
377.14 ATROPHY (CUPPING) GLAUCOMATOUS
377.23 COLOBOMA
743.57 COLOBOMA CONGENITAL
377.22 CRATER-LIKE HOLES
377.15 PALLOR (TEMPORAL)

OPTIC NERVE

377.9 AND VISUAL PATHWAYS DISORDER
377.10 ATROPHY - NOS
377.14 ATROPHY - GLAUCOMATOUS
377.16 ATROPHY - HEREDITARY
377.15 ATROPHY - PARTIAL
377.12 ATROPHY - POSTINFLAMMATORY
377.11 ATROPHY - PRIMARY
094.84 ATROPHY - SYPHILITIC
090.49 ATROPHY - SYPHILITIC CONGENITAL
094.0 ATROPHY - SYPHILITIC TABES DORSALIS
377.13 ATROPHY - WITH RETINAL DYSTROPHIES
377.49 COMPRESSION

OPTIC NERVE (continued)
377.49 DISORDER - NEC
377.41 DISORDER - ISCHEMIC
377.33 DISORDER - NUTRITIONAL
377.34 DISORDER - TOXIC
377.42 HEMORRHAGE SHEATHS
950.0 INJURY
950.9 INJURY UNSPECIFIED
950.9 TRAUMATIC BLINDNESS

OPTIC NEURITIS
377.30 NOS
341.0 IN MYELITIS
377.41 ISCHEMIC
036.81 MENINGOCOCCAL
377.33 NUTRITIONAL
377.32 RETROBULBAR ACUTE
094.85 RETROBULBAR SYPHILITIC
377.34 TOXIC
377.39 OTHER

377.31 OPTIC PAPILLITIS
950.2 OPTIC PATHWAYS INJURY
377.63 OPTIC RADIATION DISORDER
377.63 OPTIC TRACTS DISORDER
379.57 OPTOKINETIC RESPONSE ABNORMAL

ORAL
528.3 ABSCESS
528.9 DISEASE (SOFT TISSUE)
528.9 DISEASE (SOFT TISSUE) OTHER SPECIFIED
759.89 FACIAL-DIGITAL SYNDROME
528.3 FISTULA
528.7 HYPERPLASIA - EPITHELIAL
523.8 HYPERPLASIA - GUM
528.9 HYPERPLASIA - IRRITATIVE
529.8 HYPERPLASIA - TONGUE
528.9 HYPERPLASIA - SOFT TISSUE NEC (INFLAMMATORY) (IRRITATIVE) (MUCOSA)
528.7 LEUKOEDEMA

ORBIT, ORBITAL
743.66 ANOMALIES (SPECIFIED) CONGENITAL
376.45 ATROPHY
376.40 DEFORMITY
376.44 DEFORMITY ASSOCIATED WITH CRANIOFACIAL DEFORMITIES
376.47 DEFORMITY DUE TO TRAUMA OR SURGERY
376.43 DEFORMITY LOCAL DUE TO BONE DISEASE
376.9 DISORDER
376.89 DISORDERS OTHER
376.46 ENLARGEMENT
376.42 EXOSTOSIS
376.41 HYPERTELORISM
996.69 IMPLANT COMPLICATION - INFECTION OR INFLAMMATION
996.59 IMPLANT COMPLICATION - MECHANICAL
996.79 IMPLANT COMPLICATION - OTHER
376.00 INFLAMMATION ACUTE
376.10 INFLAMMATION CHRONIC
376.13 PARASITIC INFESTATION
376.11 PSEUDOTUMOR (INFLAMMATORY)

ORCHITIS
604.90 NOS
072.0 MUMPS
098.13 GONOCOCCAL ACUTE
098.33 GONOCOCCAL CHRONIC
<u>032.89</u> <u>DIPHTHERITIC</u> [604.91]
<u>125.9</u> <u>FILARIAL</u> [604.91]
604.99 OTHER
<u>095.8</u> <u>SYPHILITIC</u> [604.91]

ORCHITIS (continued)
016.5# TUBERCULOUS
5th Digit: 016.5
0. UNSPECIFIED
1. LAB NOT DONE
2. LABS PENDING
3. MICROSCOPY POSITIVE (IN SPUTUM)
4. CULTURE POSITIVE - MICROSCOPY NEGATIVE
5. CULTURE NEGATIVE - MICROSCOPY POSITIVE
6. CULTURE AND MICROSCOPY NEGATIVE CONFIRMED BY OTHER METHODS
604.0 WITH ABSCESS
0 WITH ABSCESS OF KNOWN ORGANISM SEE 'ABSCESS', TESTIS

759.89 ORDIGITOFACIAL SYNDROME
051.2 ORF

744.05 ORGAN OF CORTI ANOMALY (CONGENITAL)

ORGANIC
293.83 AFFECTIVE SYNDROME NEC
292.84 AFFECTIVE SYNDROME DRUG INDUCED
293.83 AFFECTIVE SYNDROME TRANSIENT DEPRESSIVE TYPE
293.84 ANXIETY SYNDROME

BRAIN SYNDROME
310.9 NOS
294.9 CHRONIC
291.2 CHRONIC ALCOHOLIC (SEE ALSO 'PSYCHOSIS ALCOHOLIC')
294.8 DUE TO DIALYSIS
293.9 DUE TO DIALYSIS TRANSIENT
265.2 DUE TO NICOTINE ACID DEFICIENCY
310.2 DUE TO TRAUMA (POSTCONCUSSIONAL)
294.8 <u>EPILEPTIC</u> [<u>**345.##**</u>]
4th Digit: 345
0. GENERALIZED NONCONVULSIVE
1. GENERALIZED CONVULSIVE
4. PARTIAL, WITH IMPAIRMENT OF CONSCIOUSNESS
5. PARTIAL, WITHOUT IMPAIRMENT OF CONSCIOUSNESS
6. INFANTILE SPASMS
7. EPILEPSIA PARTIALIS CONTINUA
8. OTHER FORMS
9. UNSPECIFIED, NOS
5th Digit: 345
0. WITHOUT MENTION OF INTRACTABLE EPILEPSY
1. WITH INTRACTABLE EPILEPSY
294.8 <u>EPILEPTIC GRAND MAL STATUS</u> [<u>345.3</u>]
294.8 <u>EPILEPTIC PETIT MAL STATUS</u> [<u>345.2</u>]
294.8 OTHER SPECIFIED

DELUSIONAL SYNDROME
293.81 NOS
291.5 ALCOHOL INDUCED (SEE ALSO 'PSYCHOSIS ALCOHOLIC')
292.11 DRUG INDUCED (SEE ALSO 'PSYCHOSIS DRUG INDUCED')
290.42 DUE TO OR ASSOCIATED WITH <u>ARTERIOSCLEROSIS</u> [<u>437.0</u>]
290.12 DUE TO OR ASSOCIATED WITH PRESENILE BRAIN DISEASE
290.20 DUE TO OR ASSOCIATED WITH SENILITY

DEPRESSIVE SYNDROME
293.83 NOS
292.84 DRUG INDUCED
290.43 DUE TO OR ASSOCIATED WITH <u>ARTERIOSCLEROSIS</u> [<u>437.0</u>]
290.13 DUE TO OR ASSOCIATED WITH PRESENILE BRAIN DISEASE
290.21 DUE TO OR ASSOCIATED WITH SENILITY

ORGANIC (continued)

293.82 HALLUCINOSIS SYNDROME
292.84 HALLUCINOSIS SYNDROME DRUG INDUCED
310.1 PERSONALITY SYNDROME
292.89 PERSONALITY SYNDROME DRUG INDUCED
293.9 PSYCHOSIS DUE TO OR ASSOCIATED WITH PHYSICAL CONDITION
293.81 PSYCHOSIS DUE TO OR ASSOCIATED WITH PHYSICAL CONDITION WITH DELUSIONS
293.82 PSYCHOSIS DUE TO OR ASSOCIATED WITH PHYSICAL CONDITION WITH HALLUCINATIONS
310.1 PSYCHOSYNDROME OF NONPSYCHOTIC SEVERITY
293.84 PSYCHOTIC TRANSIENT STATE - ANXIETY TYPE

302.73 ORGASM INHIBITED FEMALE PSYCHOSEXUAL
302.74 ORGASM INHIBITED MALE PSYCHOSEXUAL

121.1 ORIENTAL LIVER FLUKE DISEASE
121.2 ORIENTAL LUNG FLUKE DISEASE
085.1 ORIENTAL SORE

593.4 ORMOND'S DISEASE OR SYNDROME
270.6 ORNITHINE METABOLISM DISORDERS

ORNITHOSIS

073.9 NOS
073.7 ENCEPHALITIS [323.0]
073.0 LOBULAR PNEUMONITIS
073.0 PNEUMONIA
073.8 WITH UNSPECIFIED COMPLICATION
073.7 WITH OTHER SPECIFIED COMPLICATIONS

066.3 OROPOUCHE FEVER (VIRAL)
088.0 OROYA FEVER

V53.4 ORTHODONTIC DEVICES FITTING AND ADJUSTMENT
V58.5 ORTHODONTICS AFTERCARE

ORTHOPEDIC

V54.9 AFTERCARE
V54.8 AFTERCARE OTHER
V54.0 AFTERCARE REMOVAL OF ANY INTERNAL FIXATION
996.67 DEVICE (INTERNAL) COMPLICATION - INFECTION OR INFLAMMATION (PIN) (ROD) (SCREW)
996.4 DEVICE (INTERNAL) COMPLICATION -MECHANICAL
996.78 DEVICE (INTERNAL) COMPLICATION - OTHER
V53.7 DEVICE FITTING AND ADJUSTMENT (BRACE) (CAST) (CORSET) (SHOES)
V52.0 PROSTHESIS FITTING (REMOVAL) - ARM
V52.1 PROSTHESIS FITTING (REMOVAL) - LEG
V52.8 PROSTHESIS FITTING (REMOVAL) - OTHER

786.02 ORTHOPNEA
V57.4 ORTHOPTIC TRAINING
333.0 ORTHOSTATIC HYPOTENSIVE-DYSAUTONOMIC DYSKINETIC SYNDROME
V57.81 ORTHOTIC TRAINING

0 OS CALCIS SEE 'CALCANEUS'

732.4 OSGOOD SCHLATTER DISEASE (TIBIA TUBERCLE)

421.0 OSLER'S NODE
238.4 OSLER (-VAQUEZ) DISEASE (POLYCYTHEMIA VERA) M9950/1
448.0 OSLER-WEBER-RENDU SYNDROME (FAMILIAL HEMORRHAGIC TELANGIECTASIA)

744.03 OSSEOUS MEATUS (EAR) ABSENCE OR ATRESIA

724.8 OSSIFICATION POSTERIOR LONGITUDINAL LIGAMENT

723.7 OSSIFICATION POSTERIOR LONGITUDINAL LIGAMENT CERVICAL REGION

OSTEITIS (SEE ALSO 'OSTEOMYELITIS')

730.2# NOS

5th Digit: 730.2

0. SITE UNSPECIFIED
1. SHOULDER REGION
2. UPPER ARM (ELBOW) (HUMERUS)
3. FOREARM (RADIUS) (WRIST) (ULNA)
4. HAND (CARPAL) (METACARPAL) (FINGERS)
5. PELVIC REGION AND THIGH (HIP) (BUTTOCK) (FEMUR)
6. LOWER LEG (FIBULA) (KNEE) (PATELLA) (TIBIA)
7. ANKLE AND/OR FOOT (METATARSALS) (TOES) (TARSALS)
8. OTHER (HEAD) (NECK) (RIB) (SKULL) (TRUNK) (VERTEBRAE)
9. MULTIPLE

733.5 CONDENSANS
731.1 DEFORMANS NEOPLASTIC (MALIGNANT) [**170.#**]

4th Digit: 170

0. SKULL AND FACE
1. MANDIBLE
2. VERTEBRAL COLUMN
3. RIBS STERNUM CLAVICLE
4. SCAPULA LONG BONES UPPER LIMB
5. SHORT BONES UPPER LIMB
6. PELVIC BONES SACRUM COCCYX
7. LONG BONES LOWER LIMB
8. SHORT BONES LOWER LIMB
9. SITE UNSPECIFIED

731.0 DEFORMANS WITHOUT MENTION OF BONE TUMOR
250.8# DIABETIC [731.8]

5th Digit: 250.8

0. TYPE II, ADULT-ONSET, NON-INSULIN DEPENDENT (EVEN IF REQUIRING INSULIN), OR UNSPECIFIED; CONTROLLED
1. TYPE I, JUVENILE-ONSET OR INSULIN-DEPENDENT; CONTROLLED
2. TYPE II, ADULT-ONSET, NON-INSULIN DEPENDENT (EVEN IF REQUIRING INSULIN); UNCONTROLLED
3. TYPE I, JUVENILE-ONSET OR INSULIN-DEPENDENT; UNCONTROLLED

102.6 DUE TO YAWS
252.0 FIBROSA CYSTICA
756.59 FIBROSA DISSEMINATA

OSTEOARTHRITIS IS THE MOST COMMON TYPE OF ARTHRITIS, SOMETIMES REFERRED TO AS DEGENERATIVE JOINT DISEASE. CLASSIFICATION IS GENERALLY CODED TO LOCALIZED (PRIMARY OR SECONDARY), OR GENERALIZED.

OSTEOARTHRITIS

715.9# NOS

5th Digit: 715.9

0. SITE UNSPECIFIED
1. SHOULDER REGION
2. UPPER ARM (ELBOW) (HUMERUS)
3. FOREARM (RADIUS) (WRIST) (ULNA)
4. HAND (CARPAL) (METACARPAL) (FINGERS)
5. PELVIC REGION AND THIGH (HIP) (BUTTOCK) (FEMUR)
6. LOWER LEG (FIBULA) (KNEE) (PATELLA) (TIBIA)
7. ANKLE AND/OR FOOT (METATARSALS) (TOES)(TARSALS)
8. OTHER (HEAD) (NECK) (RIB) (SKULL) (TRUNK) (VERTEBRAE)

715.0# GENERALIZED

5th Digit: 715.0

0. SITE UNSPECIFIED
4. HAND (CARPAL) (METACARPAL) (FINGERS)
9. MULTIPLE

OSTEOARTHRITIS (continued)

715.3# LOCALIZED
715.1# LOCALIZED PRIMARY (BY JOINT)
715.2# LOCALIZED SECONDARY (BY JOINT)

5th Digit: 715.1-3

- **0. SITE UNSPECIFIED**
- **1. SHOULDER REGION**
- **2. UPPER ARM (ELBOW) (HUMERUS)**
- **3. FOREARM (RADIUS) (WRIST) (ULNA)**
- **4. HAND (CARPAL) (METACARPAL) (FINGERS)**
- **5. PELVIC REGION AND THIGH (HIP) (BUTTOCK) (FEMUR)**
- **6. LOWER LEG (FIBULA) (KNEE) (PATELLA) (TIBIA)**
- **7. ANKLE AND/OR FOOT (METATARSALS) (TOES)(TARSALS)**
- **8. OTHER (HEAD) (NECK) (RIB) (SKULL) (TRUNK) (VERTEBRAE)**

715.8# MULTIPLE SITES (BY JOINT) (NOT SPECIFIED AS GENERALIZED)

5th Digit: 715.8

- **0. SITE UNSPECIFIED**
- **9. MULTIPLE**

OSTEOARTHRITIS OF SPINE

-WITH OSTEOPOROSIS [733.0#]

721.0 CERVICAL
721.1 CERVICAL WITH MYELOPATHY (CORD COMPRESSION)
721.3 LUMBAR
721.42 LUMBAR WITH MYELOPATHY (CORD COMPRESSION)
721.3 LUMBOSACRAL
721.42 LUMBOSACRAL WITH MYELOPATHY (CORD COMPRESSION)
721.90 SPINE
721.91 SPINE WITH MYELOPATHY (CORD COMPRESSION)
721.2 THORACIC
721.41 THORACIC WITH MYELOPATHY (CORD COMPRESSION)
721.7 TRAUMATIC

WITH OSTEOPOROSIS [733.0#]

5th Digit: 733.0

- **0. UNSPECIFIED**
- **1. SENILE**
- **2. IDIOPATHIC**
- **3. DISUSE**
- **9. DRUG INDUCED**

0 OSTEOARTHROPATHY SEE 'OSTEOARTHRITIS'
731.2 OSTEOARTHROPATHY HYPERTROPHIC PULMONARY
0 OSTEOARTHROSIS SEE 'OSTEOARTHRITIS'
213.# OSTEOBLASTOMA M9200/0

4th Digit: 213

- **0. SKULL FACE UPPER JAW**
- **1. LOWER JAW**
- **2. SPINE**
- **3. RIB STERNUM CLAVICLE**
- **4. UPPER LIMB LONG BONES SCAPULA**
- **5. UPPER LIMB SHORT BONES**
- **6. PELVIS SACRUM COCCYX**
- **7. LOWER LIMB LONG BONE**
- **8. LOWER LIMB SHORT BONE**
- **9. SITE UNSPECIFIED**

OSTEOCHONDRITIS

732.9 NOS
732.7 DISSECANS
732.6 JUVENILE

277.5 OSTEOCHONDRODYSTROPHY

213.# OSTEOCHONDROMA M9210/1

4th Digit: 213

- **0. SKULL FACE UPPER JAW**
- **1. LOWER JAW**
- **2. SPINE**
- **3. RIB STERNUM CLAVICLE**
- **4. UPPER LIMB LONG BONES SCAPULA**
- **5. UPPER LIMB SHORT BONES**
- **6. PELVIS SACRUM COCCYX**
- **7. LOWER LIMB LONG BONE**
- **8. LOWER LIMB SHORT BONE**
- **9. SITE UNSPECIFIED**

238.0 OSTEOCHONDROMATOSIS SITE NOS
0 OSTEOCHONDROMATOSIS SITE SPECIFIED SEE 'NEOPLASM UNCERTAIN BEHAVIOR', BY SITE M9210/1

732.9 OSTEOCHONDROPATHY NOS

OSTEOCHONDROSIS

732.9 NOS
732.6 SITE NOS JUVENILE
732.# SPECIFIED SITE (JUVENILE)

4th Digit: 732

- **0. SPINE**
- **1. HIP AND PELVIS**
- **3. UPPER EXTREMITY**
- **4. LOWER EXTREMITY EXCLUDING FOOT**
- **5. FOOT**
- **6. OTHER**

737.0 SPINE ADOLESCENT POSTURAL KYPHOSIS
732.8 SPINE ADULT
732.0 SPINE JUVENILE
090.0 SYPHILITIC

757.39 OSTEODERMOPATHIC HYPEROSTOSIS SYNDROME

OSTEODYSTROPHY

588.0 AZOTEMIC
756.50 CONGENITAL
756.59 CONGENITAL OTHER
588.0 RENAL

252.0 OSTEOFIBROCYSTIC DISEASE
756.51 OSTEOGENESIS IMPERFECTA
213.# OSTEOID OSTEOMA M9191/0
213.# OSTEOMA M9180/0

4th Digit: 213

- **0. SKULL FACE UPPER JAW**
- **1. LOWER JAW**
- **2. SPINE**
- **3. RIB STERNUM CLAVICLE**
- **4. UPPER LIMB LONG BONES SCAPULA**
- **5. UPPER LIMB SHORT BONES**
- **6. PELVIS SACRUM COCCYX**
- **7. LOWER LIMB LONG BONE**
- **8. LOWER LIMB SHORT BONE**
- **9. SITE UNSPECIFIED**

268.2 OSTEOMALACIA VITAMIN D DEFICIENCY
275.3 OSTEOMALACIA VITAMIN D RESISTANT

O

OSTEOMYELITIS

730.2# NOS

730.0# ACUTE

730.1# CHRONIC

5th Digit: 730.0-2

- **0. SITE UNSPECIFIED**
- **1. SHOULDER REGION**
- **2. UPPER ARM (ELBOW) (HUMERUS)**
- **3. FOREARM (RADIUS) (WRIST) (ULNA)**
- **4. HAND (CARPAL) (METACARPAL) (FINGERS)**
- **5. PELVIC REGION AND THIGH (HIP) (BUTTOCK) (FEMUR)**
- **6. LOWER LEG (FIBULA) (KNEE) (PATELLA) (TIBIA)**
- **7. ANKLE AND/OR FOOT (METATARSALS) (TOES) (TARSALS)**
- **8. OTHER (HEAD) (NECK) (RIB) (SKULL) (TRUNK) (VERTEBRAE)**
- **9. MULTIPLE**

250.8# DIABETIC [731.8] **[730.0#]**

5th Digit: 250.8

- **0. TYPE II, ADULT-ONSET, NON-INSULIN DEPENDENT (EVEN IF REQUIRING INSULIN), OR UNSPECIFIED; CONTROLLED**
- **1. TYPE I, JUVENILE-ONSET OR INSULIN-DEPENDENT; CONTROLLED**
- **2. TYPE II, ADULT-ONSET, NON-INSULIN DEPENDENT (EVEN IF REQUIRING INSULIN); UNCONTROLLED**
- **3. TYPE I, JUVENILE-ONSET OR INSULIN-DEPENDENT; UNCONTROLLED**

5th Digit: 730.0

- **0. SITE UNSPECIFIED**
- **1. SHOULDER REGION**
- **2. UPPER ARM (ELBOW) (HUMERUS)**
- **3. FOREARM (RADIUS) (WRIST) (ULNA)**
- **4. HAND (CARPAL) (METACARPAL) (FINGERS)**
- **5. PELVIC REGION AND THIGH (HIP) (BUTTOCK) (FEMUR)**
- **6. LOWER LEG (FIBULA) (KNEE) (PATELLA) (TIBIA)**
- **7. ANKLE AND/OR FOOT (METATARSALS) (TOES) (TARSALS)**
- **8. OTHER (HEAD) (NECK) (RIB) (SKULL) (TRUNK) (VERTEBRAE)**
- **9. MULTIPLE**

526.4 JAW (ACUTE) (CHRONIC) (NEONATAL) (SUPPURATIVE)

0 OLD SEE 'OSTEOMYELITIS', CHRONIC

376.03 ORBITAL

383.20 PETROUS

383.21 PETROUS ACUTE

383.22 PETROUS CHRONIC

003.24 SALMONELLA

0 SCLEROSING OF GARRE SEE 'OSTEOMYELITIS', CHRONIC

095.5 SYPHILITIC

OSTEOMYELITIS (continued)

015.## TUBERCULOUS [730.8#]

4th Digit: 015

- **0. VERTEBRAL COLUMN**
- **1. HIP**
- **2. KNEE**
- **5. LIMB BONES**
- **6. MASTOID**
- **7. OTHER SPECIFIED BONE**
- **8. OTHER SPECIFIED JOINT**
- **9. UNSPECIFIED BONES AND JOINT**

5th Digit: 015

- **0. UNSPECIFIED**
- **1. LAB NOT DONE**
- **2. LABS PENDING**
- **3. MICROSCOPY POSITIVE (IN SPUTUM)**
- **4. CULTURE POSITIVE - MICROSCOPY NEGATIVE**
- **5. CULTURE NEGATIVE - MICROSCOPY POSITIVE**
- **6. CULTURE AND MICROSCOPY NEGATIVE CONFIRMED BY OTHER METHODS**

5th Digit: 730.8

- **0. SITE UNSPECIFIED**
- **1. SHOULDER REGION**
- **2. UPPER ARM (ELBOW) (HUMERUS)**
- **3. FOREARM (RADIUS) (WRIST) (ULNA)**
- **4. HAND (CARPAL) (METACARPAL) (FINGERS)**
- **5. PELVIC REGION AND THIGH (HIP) (BUTTOCK) (FEMUR)**
- **6. LOWER LEG (FIBULA) (KNEE) (PATELLA) (TIBIA)**
- **7. ANKLE AND/OR FOOT (METATARSALS) (TOES) (TARSALS)**
- **8. OTHER (HEAD) (NECK) (RIB) (SKULL) (TRUNK) (VERTEBRAE)**
- **9. MULTIPLE**

002.0 TYPHOID [730.8#]

5th Digit: 730.8

- **0. SITE UNSPECIFIED**
- **1. SHOULDER REGION**
- **2. UPPER ARM (ELBOW) (HUMERUS)**
- **3. FOREARM (RADIUS) (WRIST) (ULNA)**
- **4. HAND (CARPAL) (METACARPAL) (FINGERS)**
- **5. PELVIC REGION AND THIGH (HIP) (BUTTOCK) (FEMUR)**
- **6. LOWER LEG (FIBULA) (KNEE) (PATELLA) (TIBIA)**
- **7. ANKLE AND/OR FOOT (METATARSALS) (TOES) (TARSALS)**
- **8. OTHER (HEAD) (NECK) (RIB) (SKULL) (TRUNK) (VERTEBRAE)**
- **9. MULTIPLE**

045.## OSTEOPATHY DUE TO POLIOMYELITIS [730.7#]

4th Digit: 045

- **0. ACUTE BULBAR PARALYTIC**
- **1. ACUTE WITH OTHER PARALYSIS**
- **2. ACUTE NON PARALYTIC**
- **9. ACUTE UNSPECIFIED**

5th Digit: 045

- **0. POLIOVIRUS UNSPECIFIED**
- **1. POLIOVIRUS TYPE I**
- **2. POLIOVIRUS TYPE II**
- **3. POLIOVIRUS TYPE III**

5th Digit: 730.7

- **0. SITE UNSPECIFIED**
- **1. SHOULDER REGION**
- **2. UPPER ARM (ELBOW) (HUMERUS)**
- **3. FOREARM (RADIUS) (WRIST) (ULNA)**
- **4. HAND (CARPAL) (METACARPAL) (FINGERS)**
- **5. PELVIC REGION AND THIGH (HIP) (BUTTOCK) (FEMUR) AND THIGH**
- **6. LOWER LEG (FIBULA) (KNEE) (PATELLA) (TIBIA)**
- **7. ANKLE AND/OR FOOT (METATARSALS) (TOES) (TARSALS)**
- **8. OTHER (HEAD) (NECK) (RIB) (SKULL) (TRUNK) (VERTEBRAE)**
- **9. MULTIPLE**

0	OSTEOPATHY SEE ALSO 'OSTEITIS'
733.90	OSTEOPENIA
756.52	OSTEOPETROSIS
0	OSTEOPHYTE SEE 'EXOSTOSIS'
756.53	OSTEOPOIKILOSIS

OSTEOPOROSIS

733.00	NOS
733.03	DISUSE
733.09	DRUG INDUCED
733.02	IDIOPATHIC
268.2	OSTEOMALACIA SYNDROME
733.01	POSTMENOPAUSAL
733.01	SENILE
733.00	VERTEBRA

756.51	OSTEOPSATHYROSIS CONGENITAL

OSTEOSARCOMA

170.#	NOS M9180/3
170.#	CHONDROBLASTIC M9181/3
170.#	FIBROBLASTIC M9182/3
170.#	IN PAGET'S DISEASE OF BONE M9184/3
170.#	JUXTACORTICAL M9190/3
170.#	TELANGIECTATIC M9183/3

4th Digit: 170

0. SKULL AND FACE
1. MANDIBLE
2. VERTEBRAL COLUMN
3. RIBS STERNUM CLAVICLE
4. SCAPULA LONG BONES UPPER LIMB
5. SHORT BONES UPPER LIMB
6. PELVIC BONES SACRUM COCCYX
7. LONG BONES LOWER LIMB
8. SHORT BONES LOWER LIMB
9. SITE UNSPECIFIED

756.52	OSTEOSCLEROSIS CONGENITAL
756.89	OSTERREICHER-TURNER (HEREDITARY OSTEO-ONYCHODYSPLASIA)
745.61	OSTIUM PRIMUM DEFECT CONGENITAL
745.5	OSTIUM SECUNDUM (PATENT) (PERSISTENT) CONGENITAL

> *WHEN CODING AN INFECTION OF AN OSTOMY, USE AN ADDITIONAL CODE TO SPECIFY THE ORGANISM. SEE 'BACTERIAL INFECTION'*

OSTOMY

V55.9	CARE (CLOSURE) (TOILET) (ATTENTION) (REMOVAL OR REPLACEMENT)
V55.4	CARE (CLOSURE) (TOILET) (ATTENTION) (REMOVAL OR REPLACEMENT) OTHER DIGESTIVE
V55.6	CARE (CLOSURE) (TOILET) (ATTENTION) (REMOVAL OR REPLACEMENT) OTHER URINARY
V55.8	CARE (CLOSURE) (TOILET) (ATTENTION) (REMOVAL OR REPLACEMENT) OTHER SPECIFIED SITE
V44.9	STATUS UNSPECIFIED OSTOMY
V44.4	STATUS OTHER G.I. TRACT
V44.6	STATUS OTHER URINARY
V44.8	STATUS OTHER OSTOMY
0	SEE ALSO CECOSTOMY, COLOSTOMY, CYSTOSTOMY, ENTEROSTOMY, GASTROSTOMY, ILEOSTOMY, JEJUNOSTOMY, NEPHROSTOMY, TRACHEOSTOMY, URETEROSTOMY, URETHROSTOMY

757.7	OSTOMYLOSIS ACROMEGLIOID
756.59	OSTRUM-FURST SYNDROME
V57.21	OT (OCCUPATIONAL THERAPY)
388.70	OTALGIA
388.11	OTIC BLAST INJURY

OTITIS

NOS

382.9	NOS (ACUTE)
382.4	PURULENT
381.4	SECRETORY (SEROUS)
382.4	SUPPURATIVE
381.4	WITH EFFUSION

CHRONIC

382.9	NOS
381.20	MUCOID, MUCOUS
382.3	PURULENT
381.3	SECRETORY
381.10	SEROUS
382.3	SUPPURATIVE
381.3	WITH EFFUSION

OTITIS (continued)

136.8	DIFFUSE PARASITIC
0	EXTERNA SEE 'OTITIS EXTERNA'
0	INSIDIOSA SEE 'OTOSCLEROSIS'
0	INTERNA SEE 'LABYRINTHITIS'
0	MEDIA SEE 'OTITIS MEDIA'

OTITIS EXTERNA

380.10	NOS
380.22	ACTINIC
380.10	ACUTE
380.10	ACUTE INFECTIVE
117.3	ASPERGILLOSIS [380.15]
112.82	CANDIDA
380.22	CHEMICAL
380.21	CHOLESTEATOMA
380.23	CHRONIC
380.16	CHRONIC INFECTIVE
380.22	CONTACT
111.3	DERMATOMYCOTIC (TINEA) (RINGWORM) [380.15]
110.8	DERMATOPHYTOSIS [380.15]
380.22	ECZEMATOID
035	ERYSIPELAS [380.13]
680.0	FURUNCULAR [380.13]
054.73	HERPES SIMPLEX
053.71	HERPES ZOSTER
684	IMPETIGO [380.13]
380.14	MALIGNANT
380.15	MYCOTIC
111.9	OTOMYCOSIS [380.15]
380.22	REACTIVE
690.10	SEBORRHEIC DERMATITIS NOS [380.13]
690.11	SEBORRHEIC DERMATITIS CAPITIS [380.13]
690.12	SEBORRHEIC DERMATITIS INFANTILE [380.13]
690.18	SEBORRHEIC DERMATITIS OTHER [380.13]
380.12	SWIMMER'S EAR
111.8	TROPICAL [380.15]
380.22	OTHER ACUTE
380.23	OTHER CHRONIC
380.16	OTHER CHRONIC INFECTIVE

> *MANY CARRIERS REQUIRE VERIFICATION OF THE PRESENCE OF EFFUSION (A DICTATED EXPLANATION BY THE PHYSICIAN) FOR ANY PE TUBES PLACED FOR CHRONIC NONSUPPURATIVE OTITIS MEDIA. (381.3).*

OTITIS MEDIA

NOS

382.9	NOS
993.0	DUE TO BAROTRAUMA
909.4	DUE TO BAROTRAUMA - LATE EFFECT
381.4	NONSUPPURATIVE (ALLERGIC) (EXUDATIVE) (TRANSUDATIVE) (SECRETORY) (MUCOID) (CATARRHAL)
381.4	NONSUPPURATIVE (ALLERGIC) (EXUDATIVE) (TRANSUDATIVE) (SECRETORY) (MUCOID) (CATARRHAL) WITH EFFUSION
055.2	POSTMEASLES
381.4	SEROUS (MUCOID) (CATARRHAL)
382.4	SUPPURATIVE

OTITIS MEDIA (continued)

ACUTE

382.9 NOS
381.00 NOS WITH EFFUSION
0 ADHESIVE SEE 'ADHESION, ADHESIVE', OTITIS
381.04 ALLERGIC
381.00 EXUDATIVE
487.8 INFLUENZAL [382.02]
055.2 MEASLES (DUE TO)
381.02 MUCOID
381.05 MUCOID ALLERGIC
381.03 SANGUINOUS
381.06 SANGUINOUS ALLERGIC
034.1 SCARLET FEVER (DUE TO) [382.02]
381.01 SEROUS
381.04 SEROUS ALLERGIC
382.00 SUPPURATIVE
382.01 SUPPURATIVE WITH SPONTANEOUS RUPTURE OF EAR DRUM

CHRONIC

382.9 NOS
381.3 ALLERGIC
112.82 CANDIDAL
381.20 MUCOID
381.29 MUCOSANGUINOUS
381.3 NONSUPPURATIVE (ALLERGIC) (EXUDATIVE) (TRANSUDATIVE) (SECRETORY) (MUCOID) (CATARRHAL)
381.3 NONSUPPURATIVE (ALLERGIC) (EXUDATIVE) (TRANSUDATIVE) (SECRETORY) (MUCOID) (CATARRHAL) WITH EFFUSION
381.19 SEROSANGUINOUS
381.10 SEROUS SIMPLE
382.3 SUPPURATIVE
382.1 SUPPURATIVE TUBOTYMPANIC WITH ANTERIOR PERFORATION OF EAR DRUM
382.2 SUPPURATIVE WITH POSTERIOR OR SUPERIOR MARGINAL PERFORATION EAR DRUM
017.4# TUBERCULOUS CHRONIC

5th Digit: 017.4

0. UNSPECIFIED
1. LAB NOT DONE
2. LABS PENDING
3. MICROSCOPY POSITIVE (IN SPUTUM)
4. CULTURE POSITIVE - MICROSCOPY NEGATIVE
5. CULTURE NEGATIVE - MICROSCOPY POSITIVE
6. CULTURE AND MICROSCOPY NEGATIVE CONFIRMED BY OTHER METHODS

385.03 TYMPANOSCLEROSIS (DUE TO)

386.8 OTOCONIA
388.71 OTOGENIC PAIN
386.19 OTOLITH SYNDROME
111.8 OTOMYCOSIS [380.15]
117.3 OTOMYCOSIS ASPERGILLUS [380.15]
112.82 OTOMYCOSIS CANDIDA
759.89 OTOPALATATODIGITAL SYNDROME
388.69 OTORRHAGIA
388.60 OTORRHEA
388.61 OTORRHEA CEREBROSPINAL FLUID

OTOSCLEROSIS

387.9 OTOSCLEROSIS
387.2 COCHLEAR
387.2 OTIC CAPSULE
387.0 OVAL WINDOW
387.1 OVAL WINDOW OBLITERATIVE
387.2 ROUND WINDOW
387.8 OTHER

715.35 OTTO'S DISEASE

OUTCOME OF DELIVERY

V30.# SINGLE LIVEBORN (CODE ON INFANT'S RECORD)
V27.0 SINGLE LIVEBORN (CODE ON MOTHER'S RECORD)
V27.1 SINGLE STILLBORN (CODE ON MOTHER'S RECORD)
V31.# TWIN MATE, LIVEBORN (CODE ON INFANT'S RECORD)
V27.2 TWIN MATE, LIVEBORN (CODE ON MOTHER'S RECORD)
V27.3 TWIN MATE,ONE LIVEBORN ONE STILLBORN (CODE ON MOTHER'S RECORD)
V32.# TWIN MATE, STILLBORN (CODE ON INFANT'S RECORD)
V27.4 TWIN MATE, STILLBORN (CODE ON MOTHER'S RECORD)
V33.# TWIN, UNSPECIFIED (CODE ON INFANT'S RECORD)
V34.# OTHER MULTIPLE, MATES ALL LIVEBORN (CODE ON INFANT'S RECORD)
V27.5 OTHER MULTIPLE, MATES ALL LIVEBORN (CODE ON MOTHER'S RECORD)
V35.# OTHER MULTIPLE, MATES ALL STILLBORN (CODE ON INFANT'S RECORD)
V27.7 OTHER MULTIPLE, MATES ALL STILLBORN (CODE ON MOTHER'S RECORD)
V36.# OTHER MULTIPLE, MATES LIVEBORN AND STILLBORN (CODE ON INFANT'S RECORD)
V27.6 OTHER MULTIPLE, MATES LIVEBORN AND STILLBORN (CODE ON MOTHER'S RECORD)
V37.# OTHER MULTIPLE, UNSPECIFIED (CODE ON INFANT'S RECORD)
V39.# UNSPECIFIED (SINGLE OR MULTIPLE) (CODE ON INFANT'S RECORD)
V27.9 UNSPECIFIED (SINGLE OR MULTIPLE) (CODE ON MOTHER'S RECORD)

4th Digit: V30 - V39

0. BORN IN HOSPITAL
1. BORN BEFORE ADMISSION TO HOSPITAL
2. BORN OUTSIDE HOSPITAL AND NOT HOSPITALIZED

5th Digit: V30.0 - V39.0

USE ONLY WITH 4th Digit 0., BORN IN HOSPITAL
0. DELIVERED WITHOUT MENTION OF CESAREAN SECTION
1. DELIVERED BY CESAREAN SECTION

353.0 OUTLET COMPRESSION SYNDROME (THORACIC)
653.3# OUTLET CONTRACTION PELVIS
660.1# OUTLET CONTRACTION PELVIS OBSTRUCTING LABOR [653.3#]

5th Digit: 653.3, 660.1

0. EPISODE OF CARE UNSPECIFIED OR N/A
1. DELIVERED
3. ANTEPARTUM CONDITION OR COMPLICATION

OUT-TOEING (DUE TO)

754.62 CALCANEOVALGUS
755.63 FEMORAL RETROVERSION
754.61 FLATFEET
755.69 TIBIA TORSION, EXTERNAL

282.1 OVALOCYTOSIS CONGENITAL
282.1 OVALOCYTOSIS HEREDITARY
0 OVARIAN SEE 'OVARY, OVARIAN'

OVARY, OVARIAN

620.8 ABSENCE
752.0 ABSENCE CONGENITAL
752.0 ACCESSORY CONGENITAL
614.6 ADHESION
752.0 ADHESION CONGENITAL (TO CECUM, KIDNEY, OMENTUM)
620.4 AND FALLOPIAN TUBE PROLAPSE OR HERNIA
902.81 ARTERY INJURY
908.4 ARTERY INJURY LATE EFFECT
902.81 ARTERY LACERATION (RUPTURE) (HEMATOMA) (AVULSION) (ANEURYSM) TRAUMATIC
908.4 ARTERY LACERATION LATE EFFECT
620.3 ATROPHY (SENILE)

O

OVARY, OVARIAN (continued)
620.8 CALCIFICATION
0 CYST SEE 'CYST', OVARY
220 CYSTADENOMA
620.2 CYSTOMA SIMPLE
620.9 DISEASE - NEC (NONINFLAMMATORY)
620.2 DISEASE - CYSTIC
256.4 DISEASE - POLYCYSTIC
620.8 DISEASE - SPECIFIED NEC
614.9 DISORDER INFLAMMATORY - NOS
614.8 DISORDER INFLAMMATORY - OTHER
620.9 DISORDER NONINFLAMMATORY - NOS
620.8 DISORDER NONINFLAMMATORY - OTHER
620.4 DISPLACEMENT
752.0 DISPLACEMENT - CONGENITAL
256.9 DYSFUNCTION
256.2 DYSFUNCTION POSTIRRADIATION
256.8 DYSFUNCTION OTHER
758.6 DYSGENESIS
752.0 ECTOPIC CONGENITAL
256.3 FAILURE
256.2 FAILURE IATROGENIC (POST IRRADIATION) (POSTSURGICAL)
256.2 FAILURE POSTABLATIVE
256.3 FAILURE PRIMARY
256.1 HYPERFUNCTION OTHER
620.8 HYPERPLASIA
256.1 HYPERSTIMULATION
620.8 INFARCTION
867.6 INJURY TRAUMATIC
867.7 INJURY TRAUMATIC WITH OPEN WOUND INTO CAVITY
908.2 INJURY LATE EFFECT
256.1 OVERSTIMULATION
620.5 PEDICLE TORSION
633.2 PREGNANCY
633.2 PREGNANCY WITH COMPLICATION DURING TREATMENT [639.#]
639.# PREGNANCY WITH COMPLICATION FOLLOWING TREATMENT
4th Digit: 639
0. GENITAL TRACT AND PELVIC INFECTION
1. DELAYED OR EXCESSIVE HEMORRHAGE
2. DAMAGE TO PELVIC ORGANS AND TISSUE
3. RENAL FAILURE
4. METABOLIC DISORDERS
5. SHOCK
6. EMBOLISM
8. OTHER SPECIFIED COMPLICATION
9. UNSPECIFIED COMPLICATION
620.4 PROLAPSE (HERNIA)
V50.42 REMOVAL PROPHYLACTIC
620.8 RUPTURE (NONPREGNANT)
620.8 RUPTURE WITH HEMOPERITONEUM (NON TRAUMATIC) [568.81]
620.3 SENILE INVOLUTION
752.0 STREAK CONGENITAL

OVARY, OVARIAN (continued)
620.5 TORSION
902.82 VEIN INJURY
908.4 VEIN INJURY LATE EFFECT
902.82 VEIN LACERATION (RUPTURE) (HEMATOMA) (AVULSION)
908.4 VEIN LACERATION LATE EFFECT
593.4 VEIN SYNDROME

314.01 OVERACTIVITY NOS (ADULT) (CHILD)
313.0 OVERANXIOUS DISORDER OF CHILDHOOD AND ADOLESCENCE

OVERBITE
524.2 DEEP (EXCESSIVE)
524.2 EXCESSIVE
524.2 HORIZONTAL (EXCESSIVE)
524.2 VERTICAL (EXCESSIVE)

977.9 OVERDOSE DRUG UNSPECIFIED
0 OVERDOSE SEE APPENDIX B, DRUGS AND CHEMICALS

OVEREATING
783.6 NOS (UNSPECIFIED CAUSE)
307.51 NON-ORGANIC
278.00 WITH OBESITY

524.2 OVERJET

OVERLOAD
276.6 FLUID
276.7 POTASSIUM
276.0 SODIUM

255.3 OVERPRODUCTION ACTH
255.0 OVERPRODUCTION CORTISOL
253.0 OVERPRODUCTION GROWTH HORMONE
242.8# OVERPRODUCTION TSH
5th Digit: 242.8
0. WITHOUT THYROTOXIC CRISIS OR STORM
1. WITH MENTION OF THROTOXIC CRISIS OR STORM

747.21 OVERRIDING AORTA CONGENITAL
780.79 OVERSTRAINED
0 OVERUSE SYNDROME SEE 'BURSITIS OCCUPATIONAL'
278.00 OVERWEIGHT
780.79 OVERWORK

620.8 OVIDUCT ABSENCE OR ATRESIA
752.19 OVIDUCT ABSENCE OR ATRESIA CONGENITAL
620.3 OVIDUCT ATROPHY (SENILE) ACQUIRED
619.2 OVIDUCT FISTULA EXTERNAL
628.2 OVIDUCT OCCLUSION
752.19 OVIDUCT OCCLUSION CONGENITAL

626.5 OVULATION BLEEDING
625.2 OVULATION PAIN

286.3 OWREN'S (CONGENITAL) DISEASE OR SYNDROME (SEE ALSO 'COAGULATION DEFECT')

758.6 OX SYNDROME
271.8 OXALOSIS CARBOHYDRATE TRANSPORT DISORDERS
756.0 OXYCEPHALY
790.91 OXYGEN SATURATION ABNORMAL FINDING
127.4 OXYURIASIS
127.4 OXYURIS VERMICULARIS INFECTION
472.0 OZENA

756.59 PAAS' DISEASE

PACEMAKER (CARDIAC)

V53.31 BATTERY REPLACEMENT
V53.39 CAROTID SINUS FITTING AND ADJUSTMENT
996.61 COMPLICATION - INFECTION OR INFLAMMATION
996.01 COMPLICATION - MECHANICAL (BREAKDOWN) (PERFORATION) (DISPLACED)
996.72 COMPLICATION - OTHER
V53.31 FITTING AND ADJUSTMENT
V45.01 IN SITU STATUS
996.01 MALFUNCTION (BREAKDOWN) (PERFORATION) (DISPLACED)
V53.31 REPROGRAMMING
V45.01 STATUS POSTSURGICAL (IN SITU)
429.4 SYNDROME

427.61 PAC'S (PREMATURE ATRIAL CONTRACTIONS)
322.9 PACHYMENINGITIS
757.5 PACHYONYCHIA CONGENITAL
216.# PACINIAN TUMOR M9507/0

4th Digit: 216

0. LIP (SKIN OF)
1. EYELID INCLUDING CANTHUS
2. EAR (EXTERNAL) (AURICLE) (PINNA)
3. FACE (CHEEK) (NOSE) (EYEBROW) (TEMPLE)
4. SCALP NECK
5. TRUNK BACK EXCEPT SCROTUM
6. UPPER LIMB INCLUDING SHOULDER
7. LOWER LIMB INCLUDING HIP
8. OTHER SPECIFIED SITES
9. SKIN UNSPECIFIED

PAGET'S DISEASE

731.0 BONE (OSTEITIS DEFORMANS)
174.# BREAST INFILTRATING DUCT CARCINOMA M8541/3
174.# BREAST SOFT/CONNECTIVE TISSUE M8540/3

4th Digit: 174

0. NIPPLE AND AREOLA
1. CENTRAL PORTION
2. UPPER INNER QUADRANT
3. LOWER INNER QUADRANT
4. UPPER OUTER QUADRANT
5. LOWER OUTER QUADRANT
6. AXILLARY TAIL
8. MASTECTOMY SITE, INNER LOWER MIDLINE OUTER UPPER ECTOPIC SITES, SITES CONTIGUOUS OVERLAPPING SITES UNDETERMINED
9. BREAST (FEMALE) SITE UNSPECIFIED

199.1 EXTRA MAMMARY (EXCEPT PAGET'S DISEASE OF BONE) SITE NOS
0 EXTRA MAMMARY (EXCEPT PAGET'S DISEASE OF BONE) SITE SPECIFIED SEE 'CANCER' BY SITE M8542/3

453.8 PAGET-SCHROETTER SYNDROME (INTERMITTENT VENOUS CLAUDICATION)

VAGUE AND ILL DEFINED SIGNS AND SYMPTOMS SHOULD BE CODED ONLY IF A DEFINITIVE DIAGNOSIS IS NOT ESTABLISHED. THEY ARE HOWEVER, VALUABLE AS ADDITIONAL CODES IN AN ACCURATE ACCOUNTING OF THE PATIENT ENCOUNTER.

PAIN

789.0# ABDOMINAL (REBOUND TENDERNESS)

5th Digit: 789.0

0. UNSPECIFIED SITE
1. UPPER RIGHT QUADRANT
2. UPPER LEFT QUADRANT
3. LOWER RIGHT QUADRANT
4. LOWER LEFT QUADRANT
5. PERIUMBILIC
6. EPIGASTRIC
7. GENERALIZED
9. OTHER SPECIFIED SITE (MULTIPLE)

PAIN (continued)

789.09 ABDOMINAL PAIN OTHER SPECIFIED SITE-MULTIPLE
719.47 ANKLE JOINT
307.89 ANKLE PSYCHOGENIC
729.5 ARCH FOOT
729.5 ARM
724.5 BACK (POSTURAL)
724.2 BACK LOW
307.89 BACK PSYCHOGENIC
788.9 BLADDER
611.71 BREAST
307.89 BREAST PSYCHOGENIC
786.52 BREATHING
337.0 CAROTID ARTERY
723.3 CERVICAL - BRACHIAL (SYNDROME)
786.50 CHEST (SEE ALSO 'CHEST PAIN')
786.52 CHEST WALL ANTERIOR
724.79 COCCYX
625.0 COITUS FEMALE
302.76 COITUS FEMALE PSYCHOGENIC
608.89 COITUS MALE
302.76 COITUS MALE PSYCHOGENIC
786.52 DIAPHRAGM
388.70 EAR
388.72 EAR REFERRED
719.42 ELBOW
307.89 ELBOW PSYCHOGENIC
789.06 EPIGASTRIC
379.91 EYE
784.0 FACE
350.2 FACE ATYPICAL
351.8 FACE NEUROGENIC
719.44 FINGER JOINTS
729.5 FINGER SOFT TISSUE
789.09 FLANK
729.5 FOOT ARCH
719.47 FOOT JOINT
729.5 FOOT SOFT TISSUE
729.5 FOOT AND/OR TOES
307.89 FOOT PSYCHOGENIC
729.5 FOREARM
780.9 GENERALIZED
608.9 GENITAL MALE
307.89 GENITAL MALE PSYCHOGENIC
529.6 GLOTTIC (TONGUE)
789.09 GROIN
781.9 GROWING
719.44 HAND JOINTS
307.89 HAND PSYCHOGENIC
729.5 HAND SOFT TISSUE
784.0 HEAD
719.45 HIP
307.89 HIP PSYCHOGENIC
526.9 JAW
307.89 JAW PSYCHOGENIC
719.40 JOINT
307.89 JOINT PSYCHOGENIC
788.0 KIDNEY
719.46 KNEE
307.89 KNEE PSYCHOGENIC
729.5 LEG
729.5 LIMB
724.2 LUMBAR
526.9 MAXILLA
719.49 MULTIPLE SITES (JOINT)
307.89 MULTIPLE SITES PSYCHOGENIC
729.1 MUSCLE
786.59 MUSCLE - INTERCOSTAL
729.1 MYOFASCIAL
723.1 NECK (NONDISCOGENIC)
729.2 NERVE
729.1 NEUROMUSCULAR
478.1 NOSE

PAIN (continued)

379.91 ORBITAL
719.48 OTHER JOINTS
388.71 OTOGENIC
719.45 PELVIC BONE STRUCTURES
307.89 PELVIC BONE STRUCTURES PSYCHOGENIC
625.9 PELVIC FEMALE (ORGANIC)
307.89 PELVIC FEMALE PSYCHOGENIC
789.09 PELVIC MALE
307.89 PELVIC MALE PSYCHOGENIC
789.05 PERIUMBILIC
786.52 PLEURITIC (CHEST)
786.51 PRECORDIAL (CHEST)
996.7 PROSTHETIC COMPLICATION INTERNAL (DEVICE) (IMPLANT) (GRAFT)
307.80 PSYCHOGENIC SITE UNSPECIFIED
307.89 PSYCHOGENIC OTHER SPECIFIED SITES
569.42 RECTUM
786.52 RESPIRATION
729.1 RHEUMATIC MUSCULAR
786.50 RIB
724.6 SACROILIAC
709.2 SCAR
724.3 SCIATIC
719.41 SHOULDER
307.89 SHOULDER PSYCHOGENIC
478.1 SINUS
306.3 SKIN PSYCHOGENIC
729.2 SPINAL ROOT SEE ALSO 'RADICULITIS'
536.8 STOMACH
998.89 SUTURES (WIRE)
0 SYNDROME SEE 'PAIN' BY SPECIFIED SITE
348.8 THALAMIC
724.1 THORACIC SPINE (NONVERTEBRAL) (NONDISCOGENIC)
784.1 THROAT
524.6# TMJ

5th Digit: 524.6

0. UNSPECIFIED
1. ADHESIONS AND ANKYLOSIS
2. ARTHRALGIA
3. ARTICULAR DISC DISORDER (REDUCING OR NON REDUCING)
9. OTHER SPECIFIED JOINT DISORDER

729.5 TOE SOFT TISSUE
525.9 TOOTH
789.05 UMBILICAL
788.1 URINATION
724.5 VERTEBROGENIC
998.89 WIRE SUTURES
719.43 WRIST
307.89 WRIST PSYCHOGENIC

162.3 PAINFUL APICOCOSTAL VERTEBRAL SYNDROME M8010/3
726.19 PAINFUL ARC SYNDROME
287.2 PAINFUL BRUISING SYNDROME
266.2 PAINFUL FEET SYNDROME
709.2 PAINFUL SCAR
788.1 PAINFUL URINATION
0 PAINT GUN INJURY SEE 'OPEN WOUND', BY SITE, COMPLICATED
528.9 PALATE (SOFT) DISEASE (HYPERPLASIA)
959.09 PALATE INJURY

719.3# PALINDROMIC RHEUMATISM

5th Digit: 719.3

0. SITE UNSPECIFIED
1. SHOULDER REGION
2. UPPER ARM (ELBOW) (HUMERUS)
3. FOREARM (RADIUS) (WRIST) (ULNA)
4. HAND (CARPAL) (METACARPAL) (FINGERS)
5. PELVIC REGION AND THIGH (HIP) (BUTTOCK) (FEMUR)
6. LOWER LEG (FIBULA) (KNEE) (PATELLA) (TIBIA)
7. ANKLE AND/OR FOOT (METATARSALS) (TOES) (TARSALS)
8. OTHER
9. MULTIPLE

362.63 PALISADE DEGENERATION RETINA

WHEN USING CODE V66.7, CODE THE TERMINAL ILLNESS FIRST.

V66.7 PALLIATIVE CARE FOR END-OF-LIFE, HOSPICE OR TERMINAL CARE
782.61 PALLOR SKIN

PALMAR

903.4 ARTERY INJURY
908.3 ARTERY INJURY LATE EFFECT
903.4 ARTERY LACERATION (RUPTURE) (HEMATOMA) (AVULSION) (ANEURYSM) TRAUMATIC
908.3 ARTERY LACERATION LATE EFFECT
726.4 BURSITIS
757.2 CREASES ABNORMAL CONGENITAL
695.0 ERYTHEMA
728.6 FASCIA CONTRACTURE

785.1 PALPITATIONS
335.20 PALSY ATROPHIC DIFFUSE
333.0 PALSY PROGRESSIVE SUPRANUCLEAR
335.23 PALSY PSEUDOBULBAR
356.8 PALSY SUPRANUCLEAR NEC
333.0 PALSY SUPRANUCLEAR PROGRESSIVE
201.9# PALTAUF-STERNBERG DISEASE

5th Digit: 201.9

0. UNSPECIFIED SITE, EXTRANODAL AND SOLID ORGAN SITES
1. LYMPH NODES OF HEAD FACE NECK
2. LYMPH NODES INTRATHORACIC
3. LYMPH NODES ABDOMINAL
4. LYMPH NODES AXILLA AND UPPER LIMB
5. LYMPH NODES INGUINAL REGION AND LOWER LIMB
6. LYMPH NODES INTRAPELVIC
7. SPLEEN
8. LYMPH NODES MULTIPLE SITES

446.0 PANARTERITIS NODOSA
446.0 PANARTERITIS NODOSA POLYNEUROPATHY [357.1]
162.3 PANCOAST'S SYNDROME (CARCINOMA, PULMONARY APEX) M8010/3
556.6 PANCOLITIS

PANCREAS, PANCREATIC

577.0 ABSCESS
577.8 ABSENCE (POSTOPERATIVE) (POSTTRAUMATIC)
751.7 ABSENCE CONGENITAL
751.7 ACCESSORY CONGENITAL
751.7 AGENESIS
751.7 ANNULAR CONGENITAL
577.8 ATROPHY
577.8 CALCIFICATION
577.2 CYST OR PSEUDOCYST

PANCREAS, PANCREATIC (continued)

577.9 DISEASE
577.2 DISEASE - CYSTIC
751.7 DISEASE - CYSTIC CONGENITAL
277.00 DISEASE - FIBROCYSTIC
277.01 DISEASE - FIBROCYSTIC WITH MECONIUM ILEUS
251.9 DISORDER OF INTERNAL SECRETION (NON-DIABETIC)
251.8 DISORDER OF INTERNAL SECRETION (NON-DIABETIC) OTHER
V59.8 DONOR NON-AUTOGENOUS
577.8 DUCT CALCULUS
577.8 DUCT OBSTRUCTION
751.7 ECTOPIC
277.0# FIBROCYSTIC DISEASE

5th Digit: 277.0

0. WITHOUT MENTION OF MECONIUM ILEUS
1. WITH MECONIUM ILEUS

577.8 FIBROSIS (ATROPHY) (CALCULUS) (CIRRHOSIS)
794.9 FUNCTION STUDY ABNORMAL
751.7 HETEROTOPIA CONGENITAL
751.7 HYPOPLASIA CONGENITAL
863.8# INJURY
863.9# INJURY WITH OPEN WOUND INTO CAVITY

5th Digit: 863.8-9

1. HEAD
2. BODY
3. TAIL
4. MULTIPLE AND UNSPECIFIED SITES

908.1 INJURY LATE EFFECT
251.5 ISLET ALPHA CELLS HYPERPLASIA WITH GASTRIN EXCESS
251.1 ISLET BETA CELLS HYPERPLASIA
251.9 ISLET CELL HYPERPLASIA
211.7 ISLET CELL TUMOR
577.8 NECROSIS NOS (ASEPTIC) (FAT)
577.0 NECROSIS ACUTE OR INFECTIVE
577.8 OTHER SPECIFIED DISEASES
442.84 PANCREATICODUODENAL ARTERY (ANEURYSM) (A-V FISTULA) (CIRSOID) (FALSE) (VARICOSE)
794.9 RADIOISOTOPE STUDY ABNORMAL
794.9 SCAN ABNORMAL
579.4 STEATORRHEA
996.86 TRANSPLANT REJECTION (FAILURE)
V42.83 TRANSPLANT STATUS

0 PANCREATIC SEE 'PANCREAS, PANCREATIC'

PANCREATITIS

577.0 NOS
577.0 ACUTE
577.0 APOPLECTIC
577.0 CALCEREOUS
577.1 CHRONIC (INFECTIOUS) (INTERSTITIAL)
577.0 GANGRENOUS
577.0 HEMORRHAGIC
072.3 MUMPS
577.1 PAINLESS
577.0 RECURRENT ACUTE
577.1 RECURRENT CHRONIC
577.1 RELAPSING
577.0 SUBACUTE
577.0 SUPPURATIVE

577.8 PANCREATOLITHIASIS
284.8 PANCYTOPENIA
284.0 PANCYTOPENIA CONGENITAL
046.2 PANENCEPHALITIS SCLEROSING SUBACUTE
253.7 PANHYPOPITUITARISM IATROGENIC
253.2 PANHYPOPITUITARISM (POSTPARTUM) (SYNDROME)

300.01 PANIC ATTACK (NEUROTIC)
0 PANIC ATTACK (TRANSIENT) DUE TO GROSS STRESS REACTION (ACUTE) SEE 'STRESS REACTION', ACUTE
300.01 PANIC DISORDER
300.21 PANIC DISORDER WITH AGORAPHOBIA

238.7 PANMYELOSIS ACUTE SITE NOS
0 PANMYELOSIS ACUTE SITE SPECIFIED SEE 'NEOPLASM UNCERTAIN BEHAVIOR' BY SITE M9951/1
732.3 PANNER'S DISEASE (OSTEOCHONDROSIS)

PANNICULITIS

729.30 NOS
724.8 BACK
729.31 KNEE
723.6 NECK
729.30 NODULAR, NONSUPPURATIVE
729.39 OTHER SITE
724.8 SACRAL

076.1 PANNUS TRACHOMATOUS

360.02 PANOPHTHALMITIS
461.8 PANSINUSITIS
360.12 PANUVEITIS

PAP SMEAR

795.0 CERVIX ABNORMAL (DYSKARYOTIC)
622.1 CIN I
622.1 CIN II
233.1 CIN III (SEVERE)
0 FOLLOWUP TO PREVIOUS TREATMENT OF A DISORDER WITHOUT RECURRENCE SEE 'FOLLOWUP EXAM'
V72.3 ROUTINE WITH GYN EXAM
V76.2 ROUTINE WITHOUT GYN EXAM
V71.1 SUSPECTED NEOPLASM (UNPROVEN) (UNDIAGNOSED)
795.1 OTHER SITE ABNORMAL

PAPILLARY CARCINOMA

199.1 SITE NOS
0 SITE SPECIFIED SEE 'CANCER' BY SITE M8050/3
234.9 IN SITU SITE NOS
0 IN SITU SITE SPECIFIED SEE 'CA IN SITU' BY SITE M8050/2
183.0 SEROUS SURFACE SITE NOS
0 SEROUS SURFACE SITE SPECIFIED SEE 'CANCER' BY SITE M8461/3
199.1 SQUAMOUS CELL SITE NOS
0 SQUAMOUS CELL SITE SPECIFIED SEE 'CANCER' BY SITE M8052/3
199.1 TRANSITIONAL CELL SITE NOS
0 TRANSITIONAL CELL SITE SPECIFIED SEE 'CANCER' BY SITE M8130/3

216.# PAPILLARY HYDROADENOMA M8405/0

4th Digit: 216

0. LIP (SKIN OF)
1. EYELID INCLUDING CANTHUS
2. EAR (EXTERNAL) (AURICLE) (PINNA)
3. FACE (CHEEK) (NOSE) (EYEBROW) (TEMPLE)
4. SCALP NECK
5. TRUNK BACK EXCEPT SCROTUM
6. UPPER LIMB INCLUDING SHOULDER
7. LOWER LIMB INCLUDING HIP
8. OTHER SPECIFIED SITES
9. SKIN UNSPECIFIED

PAPILLARY MUSCLE

429.81 ATROPHY
429.81 DEGENERATION
429.81 DYSFUNCTION (DISORDER)
429.81 INCOMPETENCE
429.81 INCOORDINATION
410.8# INFARCTION ACUTE

5th Digit: 410.8

0. EPISODE UNSPECIFIED
1. INITIAL EPISODE
2. SUBSEQUENT EPISODE

PAPILLARY MUSCLE (continued)

429.6 RUPTURE

410.8# RUPTURE (DYSFUNCTION) (POST INFARCTION) ACUTE, < 8 WEEKS

5th Digit: 410.8

0. EPISODE UNSPECIFIED

1. INITIAL EPISODE

2. SUBSEQUENT EPISODE

429.79 RUPTURE (DYSFUNCTION) (POST INFARCTION) > 8 WEEKS [414.8]

429.81 SCARRING

429.81 SYNDROME

410.8# SYNDROME WITH MYOCARDIAL INFARCTION

5th Digit: 410.8

0. EPISODE UNSPECIFIED

1. INITIAL EPISODE

2. SUBSEQUENT EPISODE

216.# PAPILLARY SYRINGADENOMA M8406/0

4th Digit: 216

0. LIP (SKIN OF)

1. EYELID INCLUDING CANTHUS

2. EAR (EXTERNAL) (AURICLE) (PINNA)

3. FACE (CHEEK) (NOSE) (EYEBROW) (TEMPLE)

4. SCALP NECK

5. TRUNK BACK EXCEPT SCROTUM

6. UPPER LIMB INCLUDING SHOULDER

7. LOWER LIMB INCLUDING HIP

8. OTHER SPECIFIED SITES

9. SKIN UNSPECIFIED

PAPILLEDEMA

377.00 NOS

377.02 WITH DECREASED OCULAR PRESSURE

377.01 WITH INCREASED INTRACRANIAL PRESSURE

377.03 WITH RETINAL DISORDER

377.31 PAPILLITIS OPTIC

PAPILLOMA

229.9 SITE NOS (EXCEPT PAPILLOMA OF URINARY BLADDER)

0 SITE SPECIFIED SEE 'BENIGN NEOPLASM', BY SITE (EXCEPT PAPILLOMA OF URINARY BLADDER) M8050/0

078.11 ACUMINATUM (MALE) (FEMALE)

217 BREAST LACTIFEROUS DUCT (SOLITARY) SITE NOS

0 BREAST LACTIFEROUS DUCT (SOLITARY) SITE SPECIFIED SEE 'BENIGN NEOPLASM', BREAST

225.0 CHOROID PLEXUS SITE NOS M9390/0

0 CHOROID PLEXUS SITE SPECIFIED SEE 'BENIGN NEOPLASM', BY SITE

191.5 CHOROID PLEXUS MALIGNANT SITE NOS

0 CHOROID PLEXUS MALIGNANT SITE SPECIFIED SEE 'CANCER' BY SITE M9390/3

229.9 INTRADUCTAL SITE NOS

0 INTRADUCTAL SITE SPECIFIED SEE 'BENIGN NEOPLASM', BY SITE M8503/0

229.9 INVERTED SITE NOS

0 INVERTED SITE SPECIFIED SEE 'BENIGN NEOPLASM', BY SITE M8053/0

212.0 SCHNEIDERIAN SITE NOS

0 SCHNEIDERIAN SITE SPECIFIED SEE 'BENIGN NEOPLASM', BY SITE M8121/0

220 SEROUS SURFACE SITE NOS

0 SEROUS SURFACE - BENIGN SITE SPECIFIED SEE 'BENIGN NEOPLASM' BY SITE M8461/0

236.2 SEROUS SURFACE - BORDERLINE MALIGNANCY SITE NOS

0 SEROUS SURFACE - BORDERLINE MALIGNANCY SITE SPECIFIED SEE 'NEOPLASM UNCERTAIN BEHAVIOR', BY SITE M8461/1

229.9 SQUAMOUS CELL SITE NOS

0 SQUAMOUS CELL SITE SPECIFIED SEE 'BENIGN NEOPLASM', BY SITE M8052/0

PAPILLOMA (continued)

229.9 TRANSITIONAL CELL SITE NOS

0 TRANSITIONAL CELL SITE SPECIFIED SEE 'BENIGN NEOPLASM', BY SITE M8120/0

238.1 TRANSITIONAL CELL - INVERTED TYPE SITE NOS

0 TRANSITIONAL CELL - INVERTED TYPE SITE SPECIFIED SEE 'NEOPLASM UNCERTAIN BEHAVIOR', BY SITE M8121/1

238.9 UROTHELIAL SITE NOS

0 UROTHELIAL SITE SPECIFIED SEE 'NEOPLASM UNCERTAIN BEHAVIOR' BY SITE M8120/1

229.9 VERRUCOUS SITE NOS

0 VERRUCOUS SITE SPECIFIED SEE 'BENIGN NEOPLASM', BY SITE M8051/0

0 VERRUCOUS CARCINOMA SITE SPECIFIED SEE 'CANCER', BY SITE M8051/3

238.9 VILLOUS SITE NOS

0 VILLOUS SITE SPECIFIED SEE 'NEOPLASM UNCERTAIN BEHAVIOR' BY SITE M8261/1

PAPILLOMATOSIS

229.9 SITE NOS

0 SITE SPECIFIED SEE 'BENIGN NEOPLASM', BY SITE M8060/0

229.9 INTRADUCTAL SITE NOS

0 INTRADUCTAL SITE SPECIFIED SEE 'BENIGN NEOPLASM', BY SITE M8505/0

217 SUBAREOLAR DUCT SITE NOS

0 SUBAREOLAR DUCT SITE SPECIFIED SEE 'BENIGN NEOPLASM', BY SITE M8506/0

079.4 PAPILLOMAVIRUS INFECTION

078.1# PAPILLOMAVIRUS WART

5th Digit: 078.1

0. UNSPECIFIED, CONDYLOMA NOS, VERRUCA NOS, VERRUCA VULGARIS, WARTS (INFECTIOUS)

1. CONDYLOMA ACUMINATUM

9. OTHER SPECIFIED VIRAL, GENITAL NOS, VERRUCA: PLANA, PLANTARIS

759.89 PAPILLON-LEAGE AND PSAUME (ORODIGITOFACIAL DYSOSTOSIS)

709.8 PAPULAR ERUPTION

747.42 PAPVR (PARTIAL ANOMALOUS PULMONARY VENOUS RETURN)

772.0 PARABIOTIC (TRANSFUSION) SYNDROME-DONOR (TWIN)

776.4 PARABIOTIC (TRANSFUSION) SYNDROME-RECIPIENT (TWIN)

746.5 PARACHUTE DEFORMITY MITRAL VALVE CONGENITAL

116.1 PARACOCCIDIOIDOMYCOSIS PULMONARY

116.1 PARACOCCIDIOIDOMYCOSIS VISCERAL

374.43 PARADOXICAL FACIAL MOVEMENTS

PARAGANGLIOMA

237.3 SITE NOS

0 SITE SPECIFIED SEE 'NEOPLASM UNCERTAIN BEHAVIOR', BY SITE M8680/1

237.3 EXTRA ADRENAL SITE NOS

0 EXTRA ADRENAL SITE SPECIFIED SEE 'NEOPLASM UNCERTAIN BEHAVIOR', BY SITE M8693/1

194.6 EXTRA ADRENAL - MALIGNANT SITE NOS

0 EXTRA ADRENAL - MALIGNANT SITE SPECIFIED SEE 'CANCER' BY SITE M8693/3

194.6 MALIGNANT SITE NOS

0 MALIGNANT SITE SPECIFIED SEE 'CANCER' BY SITE M8680/3

237.3 PARASYMPATHETIC SITE NOS

0 PARASYMPATHETIC SITE SPECIFIED SEE 'NEOPLASM UNCERTAIN BEHAVIOR' BY SITE M8682/1

237.3 SYMPATHETIC SITE NOS

0 SYMPATHETIC SITE SPECIFIED SEE 'NEOPLASM UNCERTAIN BEHAVIOR' BY SITE M8681/1

781.1 PARAGEUSIA
121.2 PARAGONIMIASIS
121.2 PARAGONIMUS INFECTION
286.3 PARAHEMOPHILIA
079.89 PARAINFLUENZA VIRUS INFECTION
690.8 PARAKERATOSIS
696.2 PARAKERATOSIS VARIEGATA

PARALYSIS, PARALYTIC

344.9 UNSPECIFIED
355.9 ABDOMEN (MUSCLES)
355.9 ABDUCTOR
352.4 ACCESSORY NERVE
344.9 ACQUIRED (OLD) (CAUSE OTHER OR UNSPECIFIED)
332.0 AGITANS (SYNDROME)
344.89 ALTERNATING
355.8 ANKLE
569.49 ANUS (SPHINCTER)
344.4# ARM (MONOPLEGIA)

5th Digit: 344.4
- **0. UNSPECIFIED SIDE**
- **1. DOMINANT SIDE**
- **2. NONDOMINANT SIDE**

344.2 ARMS BOTH (DIPLEGIA)
358.0 ASTHENIC BULBAR
355.9 ATROPHY
344.89 BABINSKI-NAGEOTTE'S
355.9 BACK (MUSCLES)
344.89 BENEDIKT'S
767.7 BIRTH INJURY
0 BLADDER SEE 'BLADDER DISORDERS', PARALYSIS
767.6 BRACHIAL PLEXUS (BIRTH TRAUMA)
353.0 BRACHIAL PLEXUS (NONDISCOGENIC)
437.8 BRAIN (CORTICAL)
344.89 BROWN-SEQUARD'S
335.22 BULBAR (CHRONIC) (PROGRESSIVE)
428.9 CARDIAC
0 CEREBRAL SPASTIC INFANTILE SEE 'CEREBRAL PALSY'
437.8 CEREBROCEREBELLAR
337.0 CERVICAL SYMPATHETIC
344.89 CESTAN-CHENAIS
378.81 CONJUGATE CORTICAL (NUCLEAR) (SUPRANUCLEAR)
378.83 CONVERGENCE
767.7 CRANIAL NERVE DUE TO BIRTH TRAUMA
344.89 CROSSED LEG
519.4 DIAPHRAGM
564.89 DIGESTIVE ORGANS NEC
344.2 DIPLEGIA
781.4 EXTREMITY TRANSIENT
367.51 EYE (INTRINSIC)
378.51 EYE (OBLIQUE)
359.3 FAMILIAL PERIODIC
354.9 FINGER NEC
094.1 GENERAL (OF THE INSANE) (PROGRESSIVE)
353.4 GLUTEAL (NONDISCOGENIC)
354.9 HAND
349.89 HEMIFACIAL PROGRESSIVE
342.## HEMIPLEGIA

4th Digit: 342
- **0. FLACCID**
- **1. SPASTIC**
- **8. OTHER SPECIFIED**
- **9. UNSPECIFIED**

5th Digit: 342
- **0. UNSPECIFIED SIDE**
- **1. DOMINANT SIDE**
- **2. NONDOMINANT SIDE**

359.3 HYPOKALEMIC FAMILIAL PERIODIC
300.11 HYSTERICAL (CONVERSION)

PARALYSIS, PARALYTIC (continued)

560.1 ILEUS
564.89 INTESTINAL
767.0 INTRACRANIAL (BIRTH TRAUMA)
364.8 IRIS
344.89 JACKSON'S
478.30 LARYNX
478.34 LARYNX BILATERAL COMPLETE
478.33 LARYNX BILATERAL PARTIAL
478.32 LARYNX UNILATERAL COMPLETE
478.31 LARYNX UNILATERAL PARTIAL
438.50 LATE EFFECT CEREBROVASCULAR DISEASE -CAUDA EQUINA SYNDROME [344.60]
438.50 LATE EFFECT CEREBROVASCULAR DISEASE - CAUDA EQUINA SYNDROME WITH NEUROGENIC BLADDER [344.61]
438.2# LATE EFFECT CEREBROVASCULAR DISEASE - HEMIPLEGIA OR HEMIPARESIS

5th Digit: 438.2
- **0. UNSPECIFIED SIDE**
- **1. DOMINANT SIDE**
- **2. NONDOMINANT SIDE**

438.53 LATE EFFECT CEREBROVASCULAR DISEASE - LOCKED IN STATE [344.81]
438.4# LATE EFFECT CEREBROVASCULAR DISEASE - MONOPLEGIA LOWER LIMB
438.3# LATE EFFECT CEREBROVASCULAR DISEASE - MONOPLEGIA UPPER LIMB

5th Digit: 438.3-4
- **0. UNSPECIFIED SIDE**
- **1. DOMINANT SIDE**
- **2. NONDOMINANT SIDE**

438.5# LATE EFFECT CEREBROVASCULAR DISEASE - OTHER PARALYTIC SYNDROME

5th Digit: 438.5
- **0. UNSPECIFIED SIDE**
- **1. DOMINANT SIDE**
- **2. NONDOMINANT SIDE**
- **3. BILATERAL**

438.53 LATE EFFECT CEREBROVASCULAR DISEASE - QUADRIPLEGIA [**344.0#**]

5th Digit: 344.0
- **0. UNSPECIFIED**
- **1. C1 - C4, COMPLETE**
- **2. C1 - C4, INCOMPLETE**
- **3. C5 - C7, COMPLETE**
- **4. C5 - C7, INCOMPLETE**
- **9. OTHER QUADRIPLEGIA**

984.9 LEAD TOXICITY
781.4 LIMB TRANSIENT
344.81 LOCKED IN STATE
344.1 LOWER EXTREMITIES (PARAPLEGIA)
344.3# LOWER LIMB MONOPLEGIA (OLD)

5th Digit: 344.3
- **0. UNSPECIFIED SIDE**
- **1. DOMINANT SIDE**
- **2. NONDOMINANT SIDE**

354.1 MEDIAN NERVE
344.89 MEDULLARY (TEGMENTAL)
344.89 MESENCEPHALIC
344.89 MESENCEPHALIC TEGMENTAL
344.89 MILLARD-GUBLER-FOVILLE
344.5 MONOPLEGIA UNSPECIFIED
344.3# MONOPLEGIA LOWER LIMB (OLD)
344.4# MONOPLEGIA UPPER LIMB (OLD)

5th Digit: 344.3-4
- **0. UNSPECIFIED SIDE**
- **1. DOMINANT SIDE**
- **2. NONDOMINANT SIDE**

359.9 MUSCLE
344.89 NUCLEAR ASSOCIATED

PARALYSIS, PARALYTIC (continued)

378.9 OCULAR NOS
352.6 OCULOFACIAL (CONGENITAL)
344.89 OCULOMOTOR ALTERNATING
767.7 PERIPHERAL NERVE DUE TO BIRTH TRAUMA
354.8 PHRENIC NERVE
767.7 PHRENIC NERVE DUE TO BIRTH TRAUMA
344.89 POSTEPILEPTIC (TRANSITORY)
094.1 PROGRESSIVE (GENERAL)
335.23 PSEUDOBULBAR
306.0 PSYCHOGENIC
379.49 PUPILLARY
355.8 QUADRICEPS
344.0# QUADRIPLEGIA

5th Digit: 344.0

- **0. UNSPECIFIED**
- **1. C1 - C4, COMPLETE**
- **2. C1 - C4, INCOMPLETE**
- **3. C5 - C7, COMPLETE**
- **4. C5 - C7, INCOMPLETE**
- **9. OTHER QUADRIPLEGIA**

354.3 RADIAL NERVE
767.6 RADIAL NERVE (BIRTH TRAUMA)
344.89 RESPIRATORY CENTER NEC
770.8 RESPIRATORY NEWBORN
344.9 SENILE
355.9 SERRATUS (ANTERIOR)
354.9 SHOULDER
344.9 SPASTIC
344.89 SPINAL CORD LATE EFFECT NEC
352.4 STERNOMASTOID
536.3 STOMACH
354.8 SUBSCAPULARIS
334.9 SUPERIOR NUCLEAR NEC
344.89 SUPRANUCLEAR
333.0 SUPRANUCLEAR PROGRESSIVE
344.89 SYNDROME ACQUIRED SPECIFIED NEC
094.89 SYPHILITIC
989.5 TICK
344.89 TODD'S
529.8 TONGUE
781.4 TRANSIENT EXTREMITY
781.4 TRANSIENT LIMB
352.4 TRAPEZIUS
354.9 TRICEPS
350.9 TRIGEMINAL NERVE
378.53 TROCHLEAR NERVE
354.2 ULNAR NERVE
344.2 UPPER EXTREMITIES (DIPLEGIA)
344.4# UPPER LIMB MONOPLEGIA (OLD)

5th Digit: 344.4

- **0. UNSPECIFIED SIDE**
- **1. DOMINANT SIDE**
- **2. NONDOMINANT SIDE**

352.3 VAGUS NERVE
0 VESICAL SEE 'BLADDER DISORDERS', PARALYSIS
344.89 WEBER'S

PARAMETRITIS

614.3 ACUTE
614.4 CHRONIC OR UNSPECIFIED
639.0 FOLLOWING ECTOPIC MOLAR OR ABORTED PREGNANCY
016.7# TUBERCULOUS

5th Digit: 016.7

- **0. UNSPECIFIED**
- **1. LAB NOT DONE**
- **2. LABS PENDING**
- **3. MICROSCOPY POSITIVE (IN SPUTUM)**
- **4. CULTURE POSITIVE - MICROSCOPY NEGATIVE**
- **5. CULTURE NEGATIVE - MICROSCOPY POSITIVE**
- **6. CULTURE AND MICROSCOPY NEGATIVE CONFIRMED BY OTHER METHODS**

614.4 PARAMETRIUM ABSCESS CHRONIC OR UNSPECIFIED
629.9 PARAMETRIUM DISEASE
359.2 PARAMYOTONIA CONGENITA
0 PARANEOPLASTIC SYNDROME SEE SPECIFIC DISORDER

PARANOIA

297.1 PARANOIA
291.5 ALCOHOLIC
292.11 DRUG INDUCED
297.8 QUERULANS
293.81 TRANSIENT ORGANIC

PARANOID

297.9 DISORDER
297.3 DISORDER SHARED (INDUCED)
301.0 PERSONALITY
297.9 REACTION
298.3 REACTION ACUTE (PSYCHOTIC)
295.3# SCHIZOPHRENIC

5th Digit: 295.3

- **0. UNSPECIFIED**
- **1. SUBCHRONIC**
- **2. CHRONIC**
- **3. SUBCHRONIC WITH ACUTE EXACERBRATION**
- **4. CHRONIC WITH ACUTE**
- **5. IN REMISSION**

PARANOID STATES (DELUSIONAL DISORDERS)

297.9 NOS
291.5 ALCOHOLIC
292.11 INDUCED BY DRUGS
297.2 INVOLUTIONAL
297.1 PARANOID (CHRONIC)
297.2 PARAPHRENIA
297.3 SHARED DELUSION
297.0 SIMPLE
297.8 OTHER SPECIFIED

784.3 PARAPHASIA
302.9 PARAPHILIA
605 PARAPHIMOSIS
297.2 PARAPHRENIA

344.1 PARAPLEGIA ACQUIRED (OLD) (CAUSE OTHER OR UNSPECIFIED)
343.0 PARAPLEGIA CONGENITAL
334.1 PARAPLEGIA HEREDITARY SPASTIC
438.53 PARAPLEGIA LATE EFFECT OF CEREBROVASCULAR DISEASE [344.1]
728.10 PARAPLEGIC CALCIFICATION (MASSIVE)

273.1 PARAPROTEINEMIA
696.2 PARAPSORIASIS
696.2 PARAPSORIASIS LICHENOIDES CHRONICA
057.8 PARASCARLATINA

PARASITIC DISEASE

136.9 NOS
123.9 CEREBRAL NEC
V12.00 HISTORY NOS
V18.8 HISTORY FAMILY
V12.09 HISTORY OTHER SPECIFIED
129 INTESTINAL NOS
139.8 LATE EFFECT

647.8#: USE AN ADDITIONAL CODE TO IDENTIFY THE MATERNAL PARASITIC DISEASE.

647.8# MATERNAL CURRENT (CO-EXISTENT) IN PREGNANCY

5th Digit: 647.8

- **0. EPISODE OF CARE UNSPECIFIED OR N/A**
- **1. DELIVERED**
- **2. DELIVERED WITH POSTPARTUM COMPLICATION**
- **3. ANTEPARTUM COMPLICATION**
- **4. POSTPARTUM COMPLICATION**

PARASITIC DISEASE (continued)

112.0 MOUTH
V75.8 SCREENING EXAM PARASITIC INFECTIONS OTHER SPECIFIED
134.9 SKIN NEC
112.0 TONGUE
136.8 OTHER SPECIFIED

300.29 PARASITOPHOBIA

780.59 PARASOMNIA
307.47 PARASOMNIA NONORGANIC
752.69 PARASPADIAS CONGENITAL
351.8 PARASPASM FACIALIS
337.9 PARASYMPATHETIC NERVOUS SYSTEM DISORDER NEC

PARATHYROID

759.2 GLAND ABSENT (CONGENITAL)
252.8 GLAND CYST
252.9 GLAND DISORDER
252.8 GLAND DISORDER SPECIFIED NEC
252.8 GLAND HEMORRHAGE (INFARCT)
252.8 HEMORRHAGE
252.0 HYPERPLASIA (GLAND)
959.09 INJURY (GLAND)
252.1 TETANY

252.1 PARATHYROIDITIS AUTOIMMUNE
077.0 PARATRACHOMA

PARATYPHOID FEVER

002.9 NOS
002.1 A
002.2 B
002.3 C

753.8 PARAURETHRAL DUCT ABSENCE
051.9 PARAVACCINIA
570 PARENCHYMATOUS LIVER DEGENERATION
V61.3 PARENT PROBLEM (AGED) (IN-LAW)
0 PARESIS SEE 'PARALYSIS'
782.0 PARESTHESIA SKIN
378.81 PARINAUD'S SYNDROME (PARALYSIS OF CONJUGATE UPWARD GAZE)
372.02 PARINAUD'S SYNDROME - OCULOGLANDULAR
759.6 PARKES WEBER AND DIMITRI SYNDROME (ENCEPHALOCUTANEOUS ANGIOMATOSIS)
0 PARKINSON'S (PARKINSONIAN) DISEASE OR SYNDROME SEE 'PARKINSONISM'

PARKINSONISM

332.0 NOS
332.1 DRUG INDUCED
332.0 IDIOPATHIC
333.4 IN HUNTINGDON'S DISEASE
332.0 IN PROGRESSIVE SUPRANUCLEAR OPHTHALMOGPLEGIA
333.0 IN SHY-DRAGER SYNDROME
332.0 PRIMARY
332.1 SECONDARY
094.82 SYPHILITIC
333.0 WITH ORTHOSTATIC HYPOTENSION

523.9 PARODONTAL DISEASE
681.02 PARONYCHIA FINGER
681.11 PARONYCHIA TOE
0 PARONYCHIA SEE ALSO 'ONYCHIA'
781.1 PAROSMIA
527.8 PAROTID DUCT ATRESIA
750.23 PAROTID DUCT ATRESIA CONGENITAL
527.8 PAROTID DUCT OBSTRUCTION
750.21 PAROTID GLAND ABSENCE (CONGENITAL)
527.0 PAROTID GLAND ATROPHY

PAROTITIS

527.2 NOS
527.2 ALLERGIC
072.9 EPIDEMIC
072.9 INFECTIOUS
072.9 MUMPS
527.2 SURGICAL (POSTOPERATIVE) (NOT MUMPS)
527.2 TOXIC

PAROXYSMAL

427.0 ATRIAL TACHYCARDIA
333.5 CHOREOATHETOSIS
780.39 DISORDER (ATTACK), MIXED
427.2 TACHYCARDIA
316 TACHYCARDIA PSYCHOGENIC
427.1 TACHYCARDIA VENTRICULAR

090.0 PARROT'S DISEASE (SYPHILITIC OSTEOCHONDRITIS)
0 PARROT FEVER SEE 'ORNITHOSIS'
242.0# PARRY'S DISEASE OR SYNDROME (EXOPHTHALMIC GOITER)

5th Digit: 242.0

0. WITHOUT MENTION OF THYROTOXIC CRISIS OR STORM

1. WITH MENTION OF THYROTOXIC CRISIS OR STORM

349.89 PARRY-ROMBERG SYNDROME
242.0# PARSON'S DISEASE (EXOPHTHALMIC GOITER)

5th Digit: 242.0

0. WITHOUT MENTION OF THYROTOXIC CRISIS OR STORM

1. WITH MENTION OF THYROTOXIC CRISIS OR STORM

353.5 PARSONAGE-ALDREN-TURNER SYNDROME
353.5 PARSONAGE-TURNER SYNDROME
363.21 PARS PLANITIS
353.5 PARSONAGE ALDREN TURNER SYNDROME (NONDISCOGENIC)
790.92 PARTIAL THROMBOPLASTIN TIME (PTT) ABNORMAL
553.1 PARUMBILICAL HERNIA
551.1 PARUMBILICAL HERNIA GANGRENOUS
552.1 PARUMBILICAL HERNIA INCARCERATED
301.84 PASSIVE AGGRESSIVE PERSONALITY
301.6 PASSIVE DEPENDENT PERSONALITY DISORDER
301.6 PASSIVE PERSONALITY
0 PASTEURELLA PESTIS SEE 'PLAGUE'
027.2 PASTEURELLA PSEUDOTUBERCULOSIS INFECTION
027.2 PASTEURELLA SEPTICA (CAT BITE) (DOG BITE)
0 PASTEURELLA TULAREMSIS SEE 'TULAREMIA'
027.2 PASTEURELLOSIS
427.0 PAT PAROXYSMAL ATRIAL TACHYCARDIA
316 PAT PSYCHOGENIC [427.0]
758.1 PATAU'S SYNDROME (TRISOMY D1)

PATELLA, PATELLAR

755.64 ABSENCE CONGENITAL
755.64 BIPARTITE
717.7 CHONDROMALACIA
755.64 RUDIMENTARY CONGENITAL
717.89 SLIPPING
844.8 SPRAIN
717.89 SPRAIN - OLD
726.64 TEDINITIS
727.66 TENDON RUPTURE NONTRAUMATIC
844.8 TENDON RUPTURE TRAUMATIC

726.69 PATELLOFEMORAL STRESS SYNDROME

747.0 PATENT DUCTUS ARTERIOSUS
747.0 PATENT DUCTUS BOTALLI
745.5 PATENT FORAMEN BOTALLI
745.5 PATENT FORAMEN OVALE CONGENITAL
753.7 PATENT URACHUS CONGENITAL
V70.4 PATERNITY TESTING
280.8 PATERSON (-BROWN) (-KELLY) SYNDROME (SIDEROPENIC DYSPHAGIA)
V72.6 PATHOLOGY
301.9 PATHOLOGICAL PERSONALITY (DISORDER)
302.9 PATHOLOGICAL SEXUALITY
V64.2 PATIENT DECISION - PROCEDURE (SURGICAL) NOT CARRIED OUT
V62.6 PATIENT DECISION - PROCEDURE (SURGICAL) NOT CARRIED OUT FOR REASONS OF CONSCIENCE OR RELIGION
0 PATIENT SEE 'PERSON'
362.61 PAVING STONE DEGENERATION (RETINAL)
593.6 PAVY'S DISEASE
111.2 PAXTON'S DISEASE (WHITE PIEDRA)
569.89 PAYR'S SPLENIC FLEXURE SYNDROME
0 PCL (POSTERIOR CRUCIATE LIGAMENT) SEE 'POSTERIOR', CRUCIATE
996.69 PE TUBE COMPLICATION - INFECTION OR INFLAMMATION
996.59 PE TUBE COMPLICATION - MALFUNCTION
996.79 PE TUBE COMPLICATION - OTHER COMPLICATION
V53.09 PE TUBE REMOVAL
0 PEARL-WORKERS DISEASE SEE 'OSTEOMYELITIS', CHRONIC
447.8 PECTORAL GIRDLE SYNDROME
447.8 PECTORALIS MINOR SYNDROME

PECTUS

738.3 CARINATUM ACQUIRED
754.82 CARINATUM CONGENITAL
738.3 EXCAVATUM ACQUIRED
754.81 EXCAVATUM CONGENITAL
738.3 RECURVATUM ACQUIRED
754.81 RECURVATUM CONGENITAL

PEDICULOSIS

132.9 NOS
132.0 CAPITIS (HEAD LOUSE)
132.1 CORPORIS (BODY LOUSE)
V01.8 EXPOSURE
132.0 EYELID [373.6]
132.3 MIXED INFESTATION
132.2 PUBIS (PUBIC LOUSE)

302.2 PEDOPHILIA
302.2 PEDOPHILIC HOMOSEXUAL
0 PEG TUBE SEE 'GASTROSTOMY'
0 PEL-EBSTEIN SEE 'HODGKIN'S DISEASE'
288.2 PELGER HUET SYNDROME (HEREDITARY HYPOSEGMENTATION)
287.0 PELIOSIS RHEUMATICA
330.0 PELIZAEUS MERZBACHER DISEASE
330.0 PELIZAEUS MERZBACHER DISEASE WITH DEMENTIA [294.1]
265.2 PELLAGRA
265.2 PELLAGRA (ALCOHOLIC)
270.0 PELLAGRA CEREBELLAR ATAXIA-RENAL AMINOACIDURIA SYNDROME
265.2 PELLAGRA POLYNEUROPATHY [357.4]
726.62 PELLEGRINI STIEDA SYNDROME (CALCIFICATION KNEE JOINT)
265.2 PELLAGROID SYNDROME
259.8 PELLIZZI'S SYNDROME (PINEAL)

0 PELVIC SEE 'PELVIS, PELVIC'

PELVIS, PELVIC

902.9 BLOOD VESSEL INJURY - NOS
902.87 BLOOD VESSEL INJURY - MULTIPLE
902.89 BLOOD VESSEL INJURY - SPECIFIED NEC
763.1 BONY AFFECTING FETUS OR NEWBORN
653.0# BONY COMPLICATING PREGNANCY, L&D
660.1# BONY OBSTRUCTING LABOR **[653.0#]**

5th Digit: 653.0, 660.1
0. EPISODE OF CARE UNSPECIFIED OR N/A
1. DELIVERED
3. ANTEPARTUM COMPLICATION

614.4 CELLULITIS FEMALE
614.3 CELLULITIS FEMALE - ACUTE
614.4 CELLULITIS FEMALE - CHRONIC
639.0 CELLULITIS FEMALE - FOLLOWING ABORTION OR ECTOPIC / MOLAR PREGNANCY
016.7# CELLULITIS FEMALE - TUBERCULOUS

5th Digit: 016.7
0. UNSPECIFIED
1. LAB NOT DONE
2. LABS PENDING
3. MICROSCOPY POSITIVE (IN SPUTUM)
4. CULTURE POSITIVE - MICROSCOPY NEGATIVE
5. CULTURE NEGATIVE - MICROSCOPY POSITIVE
6. CULTURE AND MICROSCOPY NEGATIVE CONFIRMED BY OTHER METHODS

567.2 CELLULITIS MALE
625.5 CONGESTION (-FIBROSIS) SYNDROME
763.1 CONTRACTED AFFECTING FETUS OR NEWBORN
653.1# CONTRACTED - NOS COMPLICATING PREGNANCY CHILDBIRTH OR PUERPERIUM
660.1# CONTRACTED - NOS OBSTRUCTING LABOR **[653.1#]**
653.2# CONTRACTED - INLET COMPLICATING PREGNANCY CHILDBIRTH OR PUERPERIUM
660.1# CONTRACTED - INLET OBSTRUCTING LABOR **[653.2#]**
653.8# CONTRACTED - MIDPLANE (MIDPELVIC) COMPLICATING PREGNANCY CHILDBIRTH OR PUERPERIUM
660.1# CONTRACTED - MIDPLANE (MIDPELVIC) OBSTRUCTING LABOR **[653.8#]**
653.3# CONTRACTED - OUTLET COMPLICATING PREGNANCY CHILDBIRTH OR PUERPERIUM
660.1# CONTRACTED - OUTLET OBSTRUCTING LABOR **[653.3#]**

5th Digit: 653.1-3, 8, 660.1
0. EPISODE OF CARE UNSPECIFIED OR N/A
1. DELIVERED
3. ANTEPARTUM COMPLICATION

738.6 DEFORMITY ACQUIRED
763.1 DEFORMITY AFFECTING FETUS OR NEWBORN
755.60 DEFORMITY CONGENITAL
614.9 DISEASE FEMALE NEC
614.8 DISEASE FEMALE SPECIFIED NEC
653.0# DISPROPORTION IN PREGNANCY (PELVIC DEFORMITY UNSPECIFIED)
660.1# DISPROPORTION OBSTRUCTING LABOR (BONY PELVIC DEFORMITY UNSPECIFIED) **[653.0#]**

5th Digit: 653.0, 660.1
0. EPISODE OF CARE UNSPECIFIED OR N/A
1. DELIVERED
3. ANTEPARTUM COMPLICATION

V72.3 EXAM ANNUAL (PERIODIC)
654.4# FLOOR REPAIR (PREVIOUS) COMPLICATING PREGNANCY CHILDBIRTH OR PUREPERIUM
660.2# FLOOR REPAIR (PREVIOUS) OBSTRUCTING LABOR **[654.4#]**

5th Digit: 654.4
0. EPISODE OF CARE UNSPECIFIED OR N/A
1. DELIVERED
2. DELIVERED WITH POSTPARTUM COMPLICATION
3. ANTEPARTUM COMPLICATION
4. POSTPARTUM COMPLICATION

5th Digit: 660.2
0. EPISODE OF CARE UNSPECIFIED OR N/A
1. DELIVERED
3. ANTEPARTUM COMPLICATION

PELVIS, PELVIC (continued)

614.9 INFECTION FEMALE NOS
614.9 INFLAMMATORY DISEASE FEMALE - NOS
614.3 INFLAMMATORY DISEASE FEMALE - ACUTE
614.4 INFLAMMATORY DISEASE FEMALE - CHRONIC
760.8 INFLAMMATORY DISEASE MATERNAL - AFFECTING FETUS OR NEWBORN
670.0# INFLAMMATORY DISEASE MATERNAL DUE TO PREGNANCY NOS - MAJOR PUERPERAL [614.9]
670.0# INFLAMMATORY DISEASE MATERNAL DUE TO PREGNANCY ACUTE - MAJOR PUERPERAL [614.3]
670.0# INFLAMMATORY DISEASE MATERNAL DUE TO PREGNANCY CHRONIC - MAJOR PUERPERAL [614.4]

5th Digit: 670.0
0. EPISODE OF CARE UNSPECIFIED OR N/A
2. DELIVERED WITH POSTPARTUM COMPLICATION
4. POSTPARTUM COMPLICATION

639.0 INFLAMMATORY DISEASE MATERNAL - FOLLOWING ABORTION OR ECTOPIC / MOLAR PREGNANCY
0 INFLAMMATORY DISEASE MATERNAL - IN ABORTION SEE 'ABORTION', BY TYPE WITH SHOCK
646.6# INFLAMMATORY DISEASE MATERNAL NOS -MINOR COMPLICATING PREGNANCY [614.9]
646.6# INFLAMMATORY DISEASE MATERNAL ACUTE -MINOR COMPLICATING PREGNANCY [614.3]
646.6# INFLAMMATORY DISEASE MATERNAL CHRONIC -MINOR COMPLICATING PREGNANCY [614.4]

5th Digit: 646.6
0. EPISODE OF CARE UNSPECIFIED OR N/A
1. DELIVERED
2. DELIVERED WITH POSTPARTUM COMPLICATION
3. ANTEPARTUM COMPLICATION
4. POSTPARTUM COMPLICATION

016.7# INFLAMMATORY DISEASE TUBERCULOUS

5th Digit: 016.7
0. UNSPECIFIED
1. LAB NOT DONE
2. LABS PENDING
3. MICROSCOPY POSITIVE (IN SPUTUM)
4. CULTURE POSITIVE - MICROSCOPY NEGATIVE
5. CULTURE NEGATIVE - MICROSCOPY POSITIVE
6. CULTURE AND MICROSCOPY NEGATIVE CONFIRMED BY OTHER METHODS

614.8 INFLAMMATORY DISEASE - OTHER SPECIFIED
719.85 JOINT CALCIFICATION (PELVIC REGION)
718.15 JOINT LOOSE BODY (PELVIC REGION)
789.39 MASS
738.6 OBLIQUITY
629.9 ORGAN DISEASE FEMALE - NOS
629.8 ORGAN DISEASE FEMALE - OTHER SPECIFIED NEC
867.8 ORGAN INJURY TRAUMATIC
867.9 ORGAN INJURY TRAUMATIC WITH OPEN WOUND INTO CAVITY
908.2 ORGAN INJURY LATE EFFECT
763.89 ORGAN OR SOFT TISSUE ABNORMALITY AFFECTING FETUS OR NEWBORN
654.9# ORGAN OR SOFT TISSUE ABNORMALITY COMPLICATING PREGNANCY
660.2# ORGAN OR SOFT TISSUE ABNORMALITY OBSTRUCTING LABOR [654.9#]

5th Digit: 654.9
0. EPISODE OF CARE UNSPECIFIED OR N/A
1. DELIVERED
2. DELIVERED WITH POSTPARTUM COMPLICATION
3. ANTEPARTUM COMPLICATION
4. POSTPARTUM COMPLICATION

5th Digit: 660.2
0. EPISODE OF CARE UNSPECIFIED OR N/A
1. DELIVERED
3. ANTEPARTUM COMPLICATION

PELVIS, PELVIC (continued)

625.9 PAIN FEMALE
789.09 PAIN MALE
568.0 PERITONEAL ADHESIONS
560.81 PERITONEAL ADHESIONS WITH INTESTINAL OBSTRUCTION
614.6 PERITONEAL ADHESIONS - FEMALE
614.6 PERITONEAL ADHESIONS - FEMALE POSTOPERATIVE (POSTINFECTION)
614.7 PERITONITIS CHRONIC FEMALE
567.2 PERITONITIS CHRONIC MALE
016.7# PERITONITIS FEMALE TUBERCULOUS

5th Digit: 016.7
0. UNSPECIFIED
1. LAB NOT DONE
2. LABS PENDING
3. MICROSCOPY POSITIVE (IN SPUTUM)
4. CULTURE POSITIVE - MICROSCOPY NEGATIVE
5. CULTURE NEGATIVE - MICROSCOPY POSITIVE
6. CULTURE AND MICROSCOPY NEGATIVE CONFIRMED BY OTHER METHODS

639.0 PERITONITIS FOLLOWING ABORTION OR ECTOPIC / MOLAR PREGNANCY
739.5 REGION SEGMENTAL OR SOMATIC DYSFUNCTION
654.4# RIGID FLOOR COMPLICATING PREGNANCY CHILDBIRTH OR PUREPERIUM
660.2# RIGID FLOOR OBSTRUCTING LABOR [654.4#]

5th Digit: 654.4
0. EPISODE OF CARE UNSPECIFIED OR N/A
1. DELIVERED
2. DELIVERED WITH POSTPARTUM COMPLICATION
3. ANTEPARTUM COMPLICATION
4. POSTPARTUM COMPLICATION

5th Digit: 660.2
0. EPISODE OF CARE UNSPECIFIED OR N/A
1. DELIVERED
3. ANTEPARTUM COMPLICATION

848.5 SEPARATION (RUPTURE) (TEAR) (LACERATION)
848.5 STRAIN (SPRAIN) (AVULSION) (HEMARTHROSIS)
789.9 SYMPTOM OTHER
789.69 TENDERNESS
456.5 VARICES

PEMPHIGOID

694.5 NOS
694.60 BENIGN MUCOUS MEMBRANE
694.61 BENIGN MUCOUS MEMBRANE WITH OCULAR INVOLVEMENT
694.5 BULLOUS
694.60 CICATRICIAL
694.61 CICATRICIAL WITH OCULAR INVOLVEMENT
694.2 JUVENILE
694.60 MUCOSYNECHIAL ATROPHIC BULLOUS DERMATITIS
694.61 MUCOSYNECHIAL ATROPHIC BULLOUS DERMATITIS WITH OCULAR INVOLVEMENT

PEMPHIGUS

694.4 NOS
694.5 BENIGN
694.4 BRAZILIAN
694.0 CIRCINATUS
694.61 CONJUNCTIVA
694.4 ERYTHEMATOSUS
694.4 FOLIACEUS
694.4 FRAMBESIODES
785.4 GANGRENOUS SEE ALSO 'GANGRENE'
694.4 MALIGNANT
684 NEONATORUM
694.61 OCULAR
694.4 PAPILLARIS
694.4 SEBORRHEIC
694.4 SOUTH AMERICAN
694.4 VEGETANS
694.4 VULGARIS

243 PENDRED'S SYNDROME (FAMILIAL GOITER WITH DEAF-MUTISM)

701.9 PENDULOUS ABDOMEN

345.5# PENFIELD'S SYNDROME (SEE ALSO 'EPILEPSY')

5th Digit: 345.5

0. WITHOUT MENTION OF INTRACTABLE EPILEPSY

1. WITH INTRACTABLE EPILEPSY

V14.0 PENICILLIN ALLERGY (HISTORY)

V09.0 PENICILLIN RESISTANT INFECTION (SEE 'DRUG RESISTANCE')

0 PENILE SEE 'PENIS, PENILE'

PENIS, PENILE

607.89 ABSENCE
752.69 ABSENCE CONGENITAL
752.69 ACCESSORY (CONGENITAL)
752.69 AGENESIS (CONGENITAL)
752.69 ATRESIA (CONGENITAL)
607.89 ATROPHY
607.2 BOIL (ABSCESS) (CARBUNCLE)
607.89 CALCIFICATION
607.2 CELLULITIS
752.69 CLEFT (CONGENITAL)
752.69 CLOSURE IMPERFECT (CONGENITAL)
752.65 CONCEALED (CONGENITAL)
752.69 CURVATURE (LATERAL) (CONGENITAL)
788.7 DISCHARGE
607.9 DISORDER
607.2 DISORDER INFLAMMATORY
607.89 DISORDER OTHER SPECIFIED
752.69 DOUBLE (CONGENITAL)
752.69 ELONGATION FRENULUM (CONGENITAL)
607.82 EMBOLISM (HEMATOMA) (HEMORRHAGE) NONTRAUMATIC
607.83 EDEMA
607.89 FIBROSIS
607.89 GANGRENE NONINFECTIVE
752.69 GLANS DIVISION (CONGENITAL)
752.65 HIDDEN (CONGENITAL)
752.69 HOODED (CONGENITAL)
607.89 HYPERTROPHY
752.69 HYPOPLASIA CONGENITAL
959.1 INJURY OTHER AND NOS
911.8 INJURY OTHER AND NOS SUPERFICIAL
911.9 INJURY OTHER AND NOS SUPERFICIAL INFECTED
607.0 LEUKOPLAKIA KRAUROSIS
752.69 MALPOSITION CONGENITAL
752.64 MICROPENIS (CONGENITAL)
607.81 OSSIFICATION
607.9 PAIN
307.89 PAIN PSYCHOGENIC
607.89 PHAGEDENA
605 PHIMOSIS
996.65 PROSTHESIS (IMPLANT) COMPLICATION - INFECTION OR INFLAMMATION
996.39 PROSTHESIS (IMPLANT) COMPLICATION - MECHANICAL
996.76 PROSTHESIS (IMPLANT) COMPLICATION - OTHER
607.82 THROMBOSIS
607.89 TORSION
752.69 TORSION CONGENITAL
607.89 ULCER (CHRONIC)
607.82 VASCULAR DISORDERS
752.69 OTHER SPECIFIED ANOMALY CONGENITAL

758.81 PENTA X SYNDROME

282.2 PENTOSE PHOSPHATE PATHWAY DISORDER WITH ANEMIA

271.8 PENTOSURIA ESSENTIAL BENIGN

536.8 PEPTIC DISORDER ACID

536.9 PEPTIC DISORDER FUNCTIONAL - NEC

533.## PEPTIC ULCER (SYNDROME)

533.## PEPTIC ULCER DUE TO HELICOBACTER PYLORI INFECTION [041.86]

4th Digit: 533

0. ACUTE WITH HEMORRHAGE

1. ACUTE WITH PERFORATION

2. ACUTE WITH HEMORRHAGE AND PERFORATION

3. ACUTE

4. CHRONIC OR UNSPECIFIED WITH HEMORRHAGE

5. CHRONIC OR UNSPECIFIED WITH PERFORATION

6. CHRONIC OR UNSPECIFIED WITH HEMORRHAGE AND PERFORATION

7. CHRONIC

9. UNSPECIFIED AS ACUTE OR CHRONIC

5th Digit: 533

0. WITHOUT OBSTRUCTION

1. OBSTRUCTED

V12.71 PEPTIC ULCER HISTORY

041.84 PEPTOCOCCUS INFECTION

041.84 PEPTOSTREPTOCOCCUS INFECTION

447.8 PERABDUCTION SYNDROME

V45.82 PERCUTANEOUS TRANSLUMINAL CORONARY ANGIOPLASTY (PTCA) STATUS

V65.2 PEREGRINATING PATIENT

PERFORATION

473.0 ANTRUM (SINUS)
540.0 APPENDIX
540.1 APPENDIX WITH PERITONEAL ABSCESS
745.5 ATRIAL SEPTUM, MULTIPLE
384.22 ATTIC EAR
384.81 ATTIC EAR HEALED
576.3 BILE DUCT
575.4 BILE DUCT CYSTIC
867.0 BLADDER
639.2 BLADDER FOLLOWING ABORTION, ECTOPIC OR MOLAR PREGNANCY
596.6 BLADDER NONTRAUMATIC (URINARY)
665.5# BLADDER OBSTETRICAL TRAUMA

5th Digit: 665.5

0. EPISODE OF CARE UNSPECIFIED OR N/A

1. DELIVERED

4. POSTPARTUM COMPLICATION

867.0 BLADDER TRAUMATIC
0 BLADDER WITH ABORTION SEE 'ABORTION', BY TYPE, WITH DAMAGE TO PELVIC ORGANS OR TISSUE
0 BLADDER WITH ECTOPIC PREGNANCY SEE 'ECTOPIC PREGNANCY', BY SITE WITH COMPLICATION
0 BLADDER WITH MOLAR PREGNANCY SEE 'MOLAR PREGNANCY', BY TYPE WITH COMPLICATION
569.83 BOWEL
777.6 BOWEL FETUS OR NEWBORN
639.2 BOWEL FOLLOWING ABORTION, ECTOPIC OR MOLAR PREGNANCY
665.5# BOWEL OBSTETRICAL TRAUMA

5th Digit: 665.5

0. EPISODE OF CARE UNSPECIFIED OR N/A

1. DELIVERED

4. POSTPARTUM COMPLICATION

0 BOWEL WITH ABORTION SEE 'ABORTION', BY TYPE, WITH DAMAGE TO PELVIC ORGANS OR TISSUE
0 BOWEL WITH ECTOPIC PREGNANCY SEE 'ECTOPIC PREGNANCY', BY SITE WITH COMPLICATION
0 BOWEL WITH MOLAR PREGNANCY SEE 'MOLAR PREGNANCY', BY TYPE WITH COMPLICATION

PERFORATION (continued)

639.2 BROAD LIGAMENT FOLLOWING ABORTION, ECTOPIC OR MOLAR PREGNANCY

665.6# BROAD LIGAMENT OBSTETRICAL TRAUMA

5th Digit: 665.6

0. EPISODE OF CARE UNSPECIFIED OR N/A
1. DELIVERED
4. POSTPARTUM COMPLICATION

0 BROAD LIGAMENT WITH ABORTION SEE 'ABORTION', BY TYPE, WITH DAMAGE TO PELVIC ORGANS OR TISSUE

0 BROAD LIGAMENT WITH ECTOPIC PREGNANCY SEE 'ECTOPIC PREGNANCY', BY SITE WITH COMPLICATION

0 BROAD LIGAMENT WITH MOLAR PREGNANCY SEE 'MOLAR PREGNANCY', BY TYPE WITH COMPLICATION

0 BY DEVICE, IMPLANT OR GRAFT SEE 'COMPLICATION OF A DEVICE, IMPLANT OR GRAFT - MECHANICAL'

998.4 BY FOREIGN BODY LEFT ACCIDENTALLY IN OPERATION WOUND

998.2 BY INSTRUMENT (ANY) DURING A PROCEDURE, ACCIDENTAL

540.0 CECUM

540.1 CECUM WITH PERITONEAL ABSCESS

867.4 CERVIX

639.2 CERVIX FOLLOWING ABORTION, ECTOPIC OR MOLAR PREGNANCY

665.3# CERVIX OBSTETRICAL TRAUMA

5th Digit: 665.3

0. EPISODE OF CARE UNSPECIFIED OR N/A
1. DELIVERED
4. POSTPARTUM COMPLICATION

0 CERVIX WITH ABORTION SEE 'ABORTION', BY TYPE, WITH DAMAGE TO PELVIC ORGANS OR TISSUE

0 CERVIX WITH ECTOPIC PREGNANCY SEE 'ECTOPIC PREGNANCY', BY SITE WITH COMPLICATION

0 CERVIX WITH MOLAR PREGNANCY SEE 'MOLAR PREGNANCY', BY TYPE WITH COMPLICATION

569.83 COLON

576.3 COMMON DUCT (BILE)

370.00 CORNEA NOS

370.06 CORNEA DUE TO ULCERATION

575.4 CYSTIC DUCT

0 DIVERTICULUM SEE ANATOMICAL SITE

0 DUODENUM ULCER SEE 'ULCER', DUODENUM WITH PERFORATION

0 EAR DRUM SEE 'PERFORATION' TYMPANIC MEMBRANE

0 ENTERITIS SEE 'ENTERITIS'

530.4 ESOPHAGUS

473.2 ETHMOID SINUS

0 EYE TRAUMATIC SEE 'EYE INJURIES'

0 FOREIGN BODY - EXTERNAL SITE SEE 'LACERATION', COMPLICATED

0 FOREIGN BODY - INTERNAL SITE, BY INGESTED OBJECT SEE 'FOREIGN BODY'

473.1 FRONTAL SINUS

575.4 GALLBLADDER

0 GASTRIC ULCER SEE 'ULCER', GASTRIC WITH PERFORATION

0 HEART VALVE SEE 'ENDOCARDITIS'

569.83 ILEUM

665.5# ILEUM OBSTETRICAL TRAUMA

5th Digit: 665.5

0. EPISODE OF CARE UNSPECIFIED OR N/A
1. DELIVERED
4. POSTPARTUM COMPLICATION

777.6 ILEUM PERINATAL

0 INSTRUMENTAL EXTERNAL SEE 'LACERATION'

665.9# INSTRUMENTAL PREGNANT UTERUS COMPLICATING DELIVERY

5th Digit: 665.9

0. EPISODE OF CARE UNSPECIFIED OR N/A
1. DELIVERED
2. DELIVERED WITH POSTPARTUM COMPLICATION
3. ANTEPARTUM COMPLICATION
4. POSTPARTUM COMPLICATION

PERFORATION (continued)

998.2 INSTRUMENTAL SURGICAL ACCIDENTAL

569.83 INTESTINE

665.5# INTESTINE OBSTETRICAL TRAUMA

5th Digit: 665.5

0. EPISODE OF CARE UNSPECIFIED OR N/A
1. DELIVERED
4. POSTPARTUM COMPLICATION

777.6 INTESTINE PERINATAL

0 INTESTINE WITH ABORTION SEE 'ABORTION', BY TYPE, WITH DAMAGE TO PELVIC ORGANS OR TISSUE

0 INTESTINE WITH ECTOPIC PREGNANCY SEE 'ECTOPIC PREGNANCY', BY SITE WITH COMPLICATION

0 INTESTINE WITH MOLAR PREGNANCY SEE 'MOLAR PREGNANCY', BY TYPE WITH COMPLICATION

569.83 INTESTINE ULCERATIVE NEC

569.83 JEJUNUM

665.5# JEJUNUM OBSTETRICAL TRAUMA

5th Digit: 665.5

0. EPISODE OF CARE UNSPECIFIED OR N/A
1. DELIVERED
4. POSTPARTUM COMPLICATION

777.6 JEJUNUM PERINATAL

0 JEJUNUM ULCER SEE 'ULCER', GASTROJEJUNAL WITH PERFORATION

383.89 MASTOID (ANTRUM) (CELL)

473.0 MAXILLARY SINUS

0 MEMBRANA TYMPANI SEE 'PERFORATION' TYMPANIC MEMBRANE

478.1 NASAL SEPTUM

748.1 NASAL SEPTUM CONGENITAL

095.8 NASAL SEPTUM SYPHILITIC

473.9 NASAL SINUS NOS

748.1 NASAL SINUS CONGENITAL

0 ORGAN INTERNAL TRAUMATIC SEE ANATOMICAL SITE

526.89 PALATE (HARD)

095.8 PALATE (HARD OR SOFT) SYPHILITIC

528.9 PALATE (SOFT)

526.89 PALATINE VAULT

095.8 PALATINE VAULT SYPHILITIC

090.5 PALATINE VAULT SYPHILITIC CONGENITAL

664.1# PELVIC FLOOR OBSTETRICAL TRAUMA

5th Digit: 664.1

0. EPISODE OF CARE UNSPECIFIED OR N/A
1. DELIVERED
4. POSTPARTUM COMPLICATION

0 PELVIC FLOOR WITH ABORTION SEE 'ABORTION', BY TYPE, WITH DAMAGE TO PELVIC ORGANS OR TISSUE

0 PELVIC FLOOR WITH ECTOPIC PREGNANCY SEE 'ECTOPIC PREGNANCY', BY SITE WITH COMPLICATION

0 PELVIC FLOOR WITH MOLAR PREGNANCY SEE 'MOLAR PREGNANCY', BY TYPE WITH COMPLICATION

639.2 PELVIC ORGAN FOLLOWING ABORTION, ECTOPIC OR MOLAR PREGNANCY

665.5# PELVIC ORGAN OBSTETRICAL TRAUMA

5th Digit: 665.5

0. EPISODE OF CARE UNSPECIFIED OR N/A
1. DELIVERED
4. POSTPARTUM COMPLICATION

0 PELVIC ORGAN WITH ABORTION SEE 'ABORTION', BY TYPE, WITH DAMAGE TO PELVIC ORGANS OR TISSUE

0 PELVIC ORGAN WITH ECTOPIC PREGNANCY SEE 'ECTOPIC PREGNANCY', BY SITE WITH COMPLICATION

0 PELVIC ORGAN WITH MOLAR PREGNANCY SEE 'MOLAR PREGNANCY', BY TYPE WITH COMPLICATION

879.6 PERINEUM

0 PERIURETHRAL TISSUE WITH ABORTION SEE 'ABORTION', BY TYPE, WITH DAMAGE TO PELVIC ORGANS OR TISSUE

0 PERIURETHRAL TISSUE WITH ECTOPIC PREGNANCY SEE 'ECTOPIC PREGNANCY', BY SITE WITH COMPLICATION

0 PERIURETHRAL TISSUE WITH MOLAR PREGNANCY SEE 'MOLAR PREGNANCY', BY TYPE WITH COMPLICATION

478.29 PHARYNX

PERFORATION (continued)

0 PYLORIC ULCER SEE 'ULCER', STOMACH WITH PERFORATION
569.49 RECTUM
569.83 SIGMOID
473.9 SINUS NOS
473.3 SPHENOIDAL SINUS
0 STOMACH DUE TO ULCER SEE 'ULCER', STOMACH WITH PERFORATION
998.2 SURGICAL (ACCIDENTAL) (DUE TO INSTRUMENT)
384.20 TYMPANIC MEMBRANE (POSTTRAUMATIC) (PERSISTENT) - NOS
384.22 TYMPANIC MEMBRANE (POSTTRAUMATIC) (PERSISTENT) - ATTIC
384.21 TYMPANIC MEMBRANE (POSTTRAUMATIC) (PERSISTENT) - CENTRAL
384.81 TYMPANIC MEMBRANE (POSTTRAUMATIC) (PERSISTENT) - HEALED
384.24 TYMPANIC MEMBRANE (POSTTRAUMATIC) (PERSISTENT) - MULTIPLE
384.22 TYMPANIC MEMBRANE (POSTTRAUMATIC) (PERSISTENT) - PARS FLACCIDA
384.23 TYMPANIC MEMBRANE (POSTTRAUMATIC) (PERSISTENT) - OTHER MARGINAL
0 TYMPANIC MEMBRANE (POSTTRAUMATIC) (PERSISTENT) - WITH OTITIS MEDIA SEE 'OTITIS MEDIA'
384.25 TYMPANIC MEMBRANE (POSTTRAUMATIC) (PERSISTENT) - TOTAL
872.61 TYMPANIC MEMBRANE - TRAUMATIC
002.0 TYPHOID, GASTROINTESTINAL
0 ULCER SEE 'ULCER', BY SITE WITH PERFORATION
593.89 URETER
639.2 URETHRA FOLLOWING ABORTION, ECTOPIC OR MOLAR PREGNANCY
665.5# URETHRA OBSTETRICAL TRAUMA

5th Digit: 665.5

0. EPISODE OF CARE UNSPECIFIED OR N/A
1. DELIVERED
4. POSTPARTUM COMPLICATION

0 URETHRA WITH ABORTION SEE 'ABORTION', BY TYPE, WITH DAMAGE TO PELVIC ORGANS OR TISSUE
0 URETHRA WITH ECTOPIC PREGNANCY SEE 'ECTOPIC PREGNANCY', BY SITE WITH COMPLICATION
0 URETHRA WITH MOLAR PREGNANCY SEE 'MOLAR PREGNANCY', BY TYPE WITH COMPLICATION
867.4 UTERUS
996.32 UTERUS BY INTRAUTERINE CONTRACEPTIVE DEVICE
639.2 UTERUS FOLLOWING ABORTION, ECTOPIC OR MOLAR PREGNANCY
665.5# UTERUS OBSTETRICAL TRAUMA

5th Digit: 665.5

0. EPISODE OF CARE UNSPECIFIED OR N/A
1. DELIVERED
4. POSTPARTUM COMPLICATION

0 UTERUS WITH ABORTION SEE 'ABORTION', BY TYPE, WITH DAMAGE TO PELVIC ORGANS OR TISSUE
0 UTERUS WITH ECTOPIC PREGNANCY SEE 'ECTOPIC PREGNANCY', BY SITE WITH COMPLICATION
0 UTERUS WITH MOLAR PREGNANCY SEE 'MOLAR PREGNANCY', BY TYPE WITH COMPLICATION
763.89 UTERUS WITH OBSTETRICAL TRAUMA AFFECTING FETUS OR NEWBORN
528.9 UVULA
095.8 UVULA SYPHILITIC
665.4# VAGINA COMPLICATING DELIVERY NOS
665.4# VAGINA COMPLICATING DELIVERY WITH HIGH VAGINAL WALL OR SULCUS LACERATION

5th Digit: 665.4

0. EPISODE OF CARE UNSPECIFIED OR N/A
1. DELIVERED
4. POSTPARTUM COMPLICATION

PERFORATION (continued)

664.## VAGINA COMPLICATING DELIVERY WITH PERINEAL LACERATION

4th Digit: 664

0. FRIST DEGREE
1. SECOND DEGREE
2. THIRD DEGREE
3. FOURTH DEGREE
4. UNSPECIFIED

5th Digit: 664

0. EPISODE OF CARE UNSPECIFIED OR N/A
1. DELIVERED
4. POSTPARTUM COMPLICATION

639.2 VAGINA FOLLOWING ABORTION, ECTOPIC OR MOLAR PREGNANCY
623.4 VAGINA NONPUERPERAL, NONTRAUMATIC
623.4 VAGINA OLD OR POSTPARTAL
0 VAGINA WITH ABORTION SEE 'ABORTION', BY TYPE, WITH DAMAGE TO PELVIC ORGANS OR TISSUE
0 VAGINA WITH ECTOPIC PREGNANCY SEE 'ECTOPIC PREGNANCY', BY SITE WITH COMPLICATION
0 VAGINA WITH MOLAR PREGNANCY SEE 'MOLAR PREGNANCY', BY TYPE WITH COMPLICATION
799.8 VISCUS NEC
868.00 VISCUS NEC TRAUMATIC
868.10 VISCUS NEC TRAUMATIC WITH OPEN WOUND INTO CAVITY

698.0 PERIANAL ITCH
522.9 PERIAPICAL TISSUES DISEASE NEC
446.0 PERIARTERITIS NODOSA
446.0 PERIARTERITIS NODOSA POLYNEUROPATHY [357.1]
726.2 PERIARTHRITIS SHOULDER
726.4 PERIARTHRITIS WRIST
0 PERICARDIAL SEE 'PERICARDIUM, PERICARDIAL'

PERICARDITIS

423.9 NOS
420.90 ACUTE
420.99 ACUTE BACTERIAL
420.90 ACUTE INFECTIVE
391.0 ACUTE RHEUMATIC
392.0 ACUTE RHEUMATIC WITH CHOREA
420.99 ACUTE SEPTIC
423.1 ADHESIVE
420.99 BACTERIAL (ACUTE)
420.91 BENIGN (ACUTE)
423.8 CHOLESTEROL (CHRONIC)
423.8 CHRONIC
393 CHRONIC RHEUMATIC
423.2 CONSTRICTIVE
098.83 GONOCOCCAL
420.90 HEMORRHAGIC (ACUTE)
420.91 IDIOPATHIC (ACUTE)
036.41 MENINGOCOCCAL
420.90 NEOPLASTIC (ACUTE)
423.1 OBLITERATIVE

998.59: POSTOPERATIVE PERICARDITIS, USE AN ADDITIONAL CODE TO IDENTIFY THE SPECIFIC TYPE OF PERICARDITIS.

998.59 POSTOPERATIVE
420.99 PURULENT (ACUTE)
391.0 RHEUMATIC (ACUTE)
392.0 RHEUMATIC (ACUTE) WITH CHOREA
393 RHEUMATIC OR INACTIVE CHRONIC WITH CHOREA
420.90 SICCA (ACUTE)
420.99 SUPPURATIVE (ACUTE)
420.91 VIRAL ACUTE

PERICARDITIS OTHER

039.8 ACTINOMYCOTIC (ACUTE) [420.0]
006.8 AMEBIC (ACUTE) [420.0]
074.21 COXSACKIE
411.0 DRESSLER'S
115.93 HISTOPLASMA
115.03 HISTOPLASMA CAPSULATUM
115.13 HISTOPLASMA DUBOISII
039.8 NOCARDIA (DUE TO) (ACUTE) [420.0]
423.1 OBLITERANS OBLITERATING (PLASTIC)
420.99 PNEUMOCOCCAL (ACUTE) [041.2]

> *998.59: POSTOPERATIVE PERICARDITIS, USE AN ADDITIONAL CODE TO IDENTIFY THE SPECIFIC TYPE OF PERICARDITIS.*

998.59 POSTOPERATIVE
420.99 STAPHYLOCOCCAL (ACUTE) [041.1#]
5th Digit: 041.1
0. NOS
1. AUREUS
9. OTHER STAPH

420.99 STREPTOCOCCAL (ACUTE) [041.0#]
5th Digit: 041.0
0. NOS
1. GROUP A
2. GROUP B
3. GROUP C
4. GROUP D (ENTEROCOCCUS)
5. GROUP G
9. OTHER STREP

093.81 SYPHILIS
017.9# TB [420.0]
5th Digit: 017.9
0. UNSPECIFIED
1. LAB NOT DONE
2. LABS PENDING
3. MICROSCOPY POSITIVE (IN SPUTUM)
4. CULTURE POSITIVE - MICROSCOPY NEGATIVE
5. CULTURE NEGATIVE - MICROSCOPY POSITIVE
6. CULTURE AND MICROSCOPY NEGATIVE CONFIRMED BY OTHER METHODS

585 UREMIC (RENAL FAILURE) (CHRONIC) [420.0]

PERICARDIUM, PERICARDIAL

746.89 ABSENCE (CONGENITAL)
423.1 ADHERENT
423.1 ADHESION (NONRHEUMATIC)
423.8 CALCIFICATION
746.89 DEFECT CONGENITAL
423.9 DISEASE
423.8 DISEASE SPECIFIED TYPE NEC
0 DISEASE RHEUMATIC SEE 'RHEUMATIC'
423.8 DIVERTICULUM
746.89 DIVERTICULUM CONGENITAL
423.9 EFFUSION
420.90 EFFUSION ACUTE
391.0 EFFUSION ACUTE RHEUMATIC
393 EFFUSION CHRONIC RHUEMATIC
423.1 FIBROSIS
423.8 FISTULA
423.1 MILK SPOTS
423.1 SOLDIERS' PATCHES

523.3 PERICEMENTITIS ACUTE
523.4 PERICEMENTITIS CHRONIC

0 PERICHOLECYSITIS SEE 'CHOLECYSITIS'

PERICHONDRITIS

380.00 AURICLE
380.01 AURICLE ACUTE
380.02 AURICLE CHRONIC
478.71 LARYNX

PERICHONDRITIS (continued)

380.00 PINNA
380.01 PINNA ACUTE
380.02 PINNA CHRONIC

569.89 PERICOLITIS INTESTINE

523.3 PERICORONITIS ACUTE
523.4 PERICORONITIS CHRONIC

375.32 PERIDACRYOCYSTITIS ACUTE
610.4 PERIDUCTAL MASTITIS
421.9 PERIENDOCARDITIS (ACUTE) (SUBACUTE)
704.8 PERIFOLLICULITIS
704.8 PERIFOLLICULITIS CAPITIS ABSCEDENS ET SUFFODIENS
704.8 PERIFOLLICULITIS SCALP

099.56 PERIHEPATITIS CHLAMYDIAL

PERIMETRITIS

615.9 PERIMETRITIS
615.0 ACUTE
615.1 CHRONIC
670.0# MATERNAL DUE TO PREGNANCY
5th Digit: 670.0
0. UNSPECIFIED
2. DELIVERED WITH POSTPARTUM COMPLICATION
4. POSTPARTUM COMPLICATION

> *FURTHER SPECIFY THESE PERINATAL DISEASES OR DISORDERS WITH AN ADDITIONAL CODE(S) FOR THE SPECIFIC CONDITION.*

PERINATAL

779.9 CONDITION
779.8 CONDITIONS OTHER SPECIFIED
777.9 DIGESTIVE SYSTEM DISORDER
775.9 ENDOCRINE AND METABOLIC DISORDERS
776.9 HEMATOLOGICAL DISORDERS
771.8 INFECTION OTHER
778.9 INTEGUMENTARY AND TEMPERATURE REGULATION DISORDERS
0 JAUNDICE SEE 'JAUNDICE NEONATAL'
V13.7 PROBLEM HISTORY

0 PERINEAL SEE 'PERINEUM, PERINEAL'
590.2 PERINEPHRIC ABSCESS

PERINEUM, PERINEAL

624.9 DISEASE FEMALE
624.8 DISEASE FEMALE - OTHER SPECIFIED NEC
616.9 DISEASE FEMALE - INFLAMMATORY
616.8 DISEASE FEMALE - INFLAMMATORY OTHER SPECIFIED NEC
682.2 DISEASE MALE - INFLAMMATORY
654.8# FIBROSIS (RIGID) COMPLICATING CHILDBIRTH
660.2# FIBROSIS OBSTRUCTING LABOR [654.8#]
5th Digit: 654.8
0. EPISODE OF CARE UNSPECIFIED OR N/A
1. DELIVERED
2. DELIVERED WITH POSTPARTUM COMPLICATION
3. ANTEPARTUM COMPLICATION
4. POSTPARTUM COMPLICATION
5th Digit: 660.2
0. EPISODE OF CARE UNSPECIFIED OR N/A
1. DELIVERED
3. ANTEPARTUM COMPLICATION

785.4 GANGRENE
959.1 INJURY
911.8 INJURY OTHER AND NOS SUPERFICIAL
911.9 INJURY OTHER AND NOS SUPERFICIAL INFECTED

PERINEUM, PERINEAL (continued)

664.4# LACERATION OBSTETRICAL
664.0# LACERATION OBSTETRICAL - 1ST DEGREE
664.1# LACERATION OBSTETRICAL - 2ND DEGREE
664.2# LACERATION OBSTETRICAL - 3RD DEGREE
664.3# LACERATION OBSTETRICAL - 4TH DEGREE

5th Digit: 664.0-4
0. EPISODE OF CARE UNSPECIFIED OR N/A
1. DELIVERED
4. POSTPARTUM COMPLICATION

879.6 LACERATION TRAUMATIC
654.8# SURGERY PREVIOUS COMPLICATING PREGNANCY CHILDBIRTH OR PUREPERIUM
660.2# SURGERY PREVIOUS OBSTRUCTING LABOR [654.8#]

5th Digit: 654.8
0. EPISODE OF CARE UNSPECIFIED OR N/A
1. DELIVERED
2. DELIVERED WITH POSTPARTUM COMPLICATION
3. ANTEPARTUM COMPLICATION
4. POSTPARTUM COMPLICATION

5th Digit: 660.2
0. EPISODE OF CARE UNSPECIFIED OR N/A
1. DELIVERED
3. ANTEPARTUM COMPLICATION

664.9# TRAUMA - NOS DURING DELIVERY
0 TRAUMA - LACERATION DURING DELIVERY SEE 'PERINEUM, PERINEAL' LACERATION
664.8# TRAUMA - OTHER SPECIFIED DURING DELIVERY

5th Digit: 664.8-9
0. EPISODE OF CARE UNSPECIFIED OR N/A
1. DELIVERED
4. POSTPARTUM COMPLICATION

380.02 PERIOCHONDRITIS AURICLE CHRONIC
380.02 PERIOCHONDRITIS PINNA CHRONIC

277.3 PERIODIC FAMILIAL (REIMANN'S) DISEASE NEC
359.3 PERIODIC FAMILIAL PARALYSIS
277.3 PERIODIC SYNDROME

523.3 PERIODONTAL ABSCESS
522.8 PERIODONTAL CYST
523.9 PERIODONTAL DISEASE NEC
523.8 PERIODONTAL DISEASE SPECIFIED NEC
523.8 PERIODONTAL OCCLUSION, TRAUMATIC

PERIODONTITIS

523.4 NOS
523.3 ACUTE
522.4 ACUTE APICAL (PULPAL)
522.6 APICAL CHRONIC
523.4 CHRONIC
522.6 CHRONIC APICAL

523.5 PERIODONTOSIS
733.90 PERIOSTEAL DISORDER NOS

PERIOSTITIS

730.3# NOS

5th Digit: 730.3
0. SITE UNSPECIFIED
1. SHOULDER REGION
2. UPPER ARM (ELBOW) (HUMERUS)
3. FOREARM (RADIUS) (WRIST) (ULNA)
4. HAND (CARPAL) (METACARPAL) (FINGERS)
5. PELVIC REGION AND THIGH (HIP) (BUTTOCK) (FEMUR)
6. LOWER LEG (FIBULA) (KNEE) (PATELLA) (TIBIA)
7. ANKLE AND/OR FOOT (METATARSALS) (TOES) (TARSALS)
8. OTHER (HEAD) (NECK) (RIB) (SKULL) (TRUNK) (VERTEBRAE)
9. MULTIPLE

526.5 ALVEOLODENTAL
102.6 DUE TO YAWS

PERIOSTITIS (continued)

526.4 JAW
376.02 ORBITAL
095.5 SYPHILITIC
091.61 SYPHILITIC SECONDARY
0 WITH OSTEOMYELITIS SEE 'OSTEOMYELITIS'

0 PERIOSTOSIS SEE 'PERIOSTITIS'

0 PERIPHERAL ARTERY OCCLUSION SEE 'ARTERY, ARTERIAL', OCCLUSION

V53.02 PERIPHERAL NERVE NEUROPACEMAKER (FITTING AND ADJUSTMENT) (REMOVAL) (REPLACEMENT)

PERIPHERAL NEUROPATHY

356.9 NOT OTHERWISE SPECIFIED
337.9 AUTONOMIC UNSPECIFIED
277.3 AUTONOMIC AMYLOIDOSIS [337.1]
274.89 AUTONOMIC GOUT [337.1]
242.9# AUTONOMIC HYPERTHYROIDISM [337.1]

5th Digit: 242.9
0. WITHOUT STORM
1. WITH STORM

337.0 AUTONOMIC IDIOPATHIC
357.6 DRUG INDUCED NEUROPATHY
356.0 HEREDITARY
356.2 HEREDITARY SENSORY
356.9 IDIOPATHIC
356.4 IDIOPATHIC PROGRESSIVE
356.8 IDIOPATHIC OTHER SPECIFIED
356.9 NERVE NOS
354.9 NERVE ARM NEC
907.4 NERVE INJURY LATE EFFECT (SHOULDER GIRDLE)
355.8 NERVE LEG, LOWER EXTREMITY
0 NERVE SEE 'POLYNEUROPATHY'
354.9 NERVE UPPER EXTREMITY
794.19 NERVOUS SYSTEM ABNORMAL FINDINGS FUNCTION STUDY
0 SPINAL NERVE ROOT SEE 'RADICULITIS'
357.7 TOXIC INDUCED, (ARSENIC, LEAD, ORGANOPHOSPHATES)

V42.82 PERIPHERAL STEM CELLS TRANSPLANT STATUS

YOU SHOULD NOT ASSUME A CAUSE AND EFFECT RELATIONSHIP BETWEEN DIABETES AND PERIPHERAL VASCULAR DISEASE. UNLESS THE PHYSICIAN STATES THAT THE PERIPHERAL VASCULAR DISEASE IS DIABETIC OR DUE TO DIABETES, CODE THE CONDITIONS SEPARATELY OR ASK THE PHYSICIAN TO DOCUMENT THE DIAGNOSIS CLEARLY.

PERIPHERAL VASCULAR

747.6# ANOMALIES (CONGENITAL) (ABERRANT) (ABSENCE) (AGENESIS) (ACCESSORY) (ANEURYSM) (ATRESIA) (DEFORMITY) (HYPOPLASIA) (MALPOSITION)

5th Digit: 747.6
0. UNSPECIFIED SITE
1. GASTROINTESTINAL VESSEL
2. RENAL VESSEL
3. UPPER LIMB VESSEL
4. LOWER LIMB VESSEL
9. OTHER SPECIFIED SITE PERIPHERAL VASCULAR

443.9 DISEASE NOS
250.7# DISEASE DIABETIC [443.81]

5th Digit: 250.7
0. TYPE II, ADULT-ONSET, NON-INSULIN DEPENDENT (EVEN IF REQUIRING INSULIN), OR UNSPECIFIED; CONTROLLED
1. TYPE I, JUVENILE-ONSET OR INSULIN-DEPENDENT; CONTROLLED
2. TYPE II, ADULT-ONSET, NON-INSULIN DEPENDENT (EVEN IF REQUIRING INSULIN); UNCONTROLLED
3. TYPE I, JUVENILE-ONSET OR INSULIN-DEPENDENT; UNCONTROLLED

PERIPHERAL VASCULAR (continued)

648.9#: USE AN ADDITIONAL CODE TO IDENTIFY THE PERIPHERAL VASCULAR DISEASE.

648.9# DISEASE MATERNAL CURRENT (CO-EXISTENT) IN PREGNANCY
5th Digit: 648.9
0. EPISODE OF NOS OR N/A
1. DELIVERED
2. DELIVERED WITH POSTPARTUM COMPLICATION
3. ANTEPARTUM COMPLICATION
4. POSTPARTUM COMPLICATION
443.89 DISEASE SPECIFIED TYPE NEC

590.2 PERIRENAL ABSCESS
569.89 PERISIGMOIDITIS INTESTINE
289.59 PERISPLENITIS
787.4 PERISTALSIS VISIBLE
787.4 PERISTALSIS REVERSE(D)
0 PERITONEAL SEE 'PERITONEUM, PERITONEAL'

PERITONEUM, PERITONEAL
568.0 ADHESIONS
751.4 ADHESIONS CONGENITAL
614.6 ADHESIONS FEMALE
614.6 ADHESIONS FEMALE PELVIC
614.6 ADHESIONS FEMALE POSTOPERATIVE (POSTINFECTION)
568.0 ADHESIONS MALE
614.6 ADHESIONS PELVIC POSTOPERATIVE (POSTINFECTION)
568.0 ADHESIONS POSTOPERATIVE (POSTINFECTION)
568.89 CYST
0 DIALYSIS SEE 'DIALYSIS' PERITONEAL
568.9 DISORDER
629.9 DISORDER PELVIC FEMALE - NOS
629.8 DISORDER PELVIC FEMALE - OTHER SPECIFIED
568.82 EFFUSION (CHRONIC) NONASCITES
792.9 FLUID ABNORMAL
568.89 GRANULOMA
868.03 INJURY
868.03 INJURY - TRAUMATIC
868.13 INJURY - TRAUMATIC WITH OPEN WOUND INTO CAVITY
908.1 INJURY - LATE EFFECT
0 PREGNANCY SEE 'ECTOPIC PREGNANCY (RUPTURED) (UNRUPTURED)'
761.4 PREGNANCY AFFECTING FETUS OR NEWBORN

WHEN CODING AN INFECTION, USE AN ADDITIONAL CODE, [041.#], TO IDENTIFY THE ORGANISM. SEE 'BACTERIAL INFECTION'.

PERITONITIS
567.9 NOS
567.2 ACUTE
567.2 ACUTE GENERALIZED
567.2 ACUTE OTHER SUPPURATIVE
540.0 APPENDICITIS ACUTE (WITH)
540.1 APPENDICITIS WITH PERITONEAL ABSCESS
998.7 ASEPTIC (ACUTE REACTION TO FOREIGN SUBSTANCE ACCIDENTALLY LEFT DURING A PROCEDURE)
567.2 BACTERIAL
277.3 BENIGN PAROXYSMAL
567.8 BILE
567.8 DUE TO TALC
998.7 CHEMICAL - ACUTE REACTION TO FOREIGN SUBSTANCE ACCIDENTALLY LEFT DURING A PROCEDURE
567.8 CHEMICAL - TALC
099.56 CHLAMYDIAL
567.8 CHRONIC PROLIFERATIVE
777.6 CONGENITAL NEC

PERITONITIS (continued)
567.2 DIAPHRAGMATIC (SUBPHRENIC)
567.2 DIFFUSE NEC
032.83 DIPHTHERIA
567.2 DUE TO STAPHYLOCOCCAL **[041.1#]**
5th Digit: 041.1
0. NOS
1. AUREUS
9. OTHER STAPH
567.2 DUE TO STREPTOCOCCAL **[041.0#]**
5th Digit: 041.0
0. NOS
1. GROUP A
2. GROUP B
3. GROUP C
4. GROUP D (ENTEROCOCCUS)
5. GROUP G
9. OTHER STREP
567.8 FAT NECROSIS
098.86 GONOCOCCAL
777.6 MECONIUM
567.8 MESENTERIC SAPONIFICATION
0 OBSTETRICAL SEE 'PERITONITIS OBSTETRICAL'
567.8 OTHER SPECIFIED
577.8 PANCREATIC
614.5 PELVIC ACUTE OR UNSPECIFIED (FEMALE)
614.7 PELVIC CHRONIC FEMALE
016.7# PELVIC FEMALE TUBERCULOUS
5th Digit: 016.7
0. UNSPECIFIED
1. LAB NOT DONE
2. LABS PENDING
3. MICROSCOPY POSITIVE (IN SPUTUM)
4. CULTURE POSITIVE - MICROSCOPY NEGATIVE
5. CULTURE NEGATIVE - MICROSCOPY POSITIVE
6. CULTURE AND MICROSCOPY NEGATIVE CONFIRMED BY OTHER METHODS
567.2 PELVIC MALE
277.3 PERIODIC FAMILIAL
567.1 PNEUMOCOCCAL
998.7 POSTOPERATIVE DUE TO FOREIGN SUBSTANCE ACCIDENTALLY LEFT
998.59 POSTOPERATIVE INFECTIVE [567.2]
567.2 SUBPHRENIC
567.2 SUPPURATIVE
095.2 SYPHILITIC
090.0 SYPHILITIC CONGENITAL [567.0]
014.0# TUBERCULOUS
5th Digit: 014.0
0. NOS
1. LAB NOT PENDING
2. LABS PENDING
3. MICROSCOPY POSITIVE (IN SPUTUM)
4. CULTURE POSITIVE - MICROSCOPY NEGATIVE
5. CULTURE NEGATIVE - MICROSCOPY POSITIVE
6. CULTURE AND MICROSCOPY NEGATIVE CONFIRMED BY OTHER METHODS
567.8 URINE

PERITONITIS OBSTETRICAL
639.0 FOLLOWING ABORTION
639.0 FOLLOWING ECTOPIC OR MOLAR PREGNANCY
638.0# IN ABORTION FAILED ATTEMPTED
636.0# IN ABORTION ILLEGALLY INDUCED
635.0# IN ABORTION LEGALLY INDUCED
634.0# IN ABORTION SPONTANEOUS
635.0# IN ABORTION THERAPEUTIC
637.0# IN ABORTION UNSPECIFIED
5th Digit: 634.0, 635.0, 636.0, 637.0, 638.0
0. NOS
1. INCOMPLETE
2. COMPLETE

PERITONITIS OBSTETRICAL (continued)
670.0# PELVIC MATERNAL DUE TO PREGNANCY
5th Digit: 670.0
0. UNSPECIFIED
2. DELIVERED WITH POSTPARTUM COMPLICATION
4. POSTPARTUM COMPLICATION

475 PERITONSILLAR ABSCESS
475 PERITONSILLAR CELLULITIS

614.6 PERITUBAL ADHESIONS
614.6 PERITUBAL ADHESIONS POSTOPERATIVE (POSTINFECTION)

593.89 PERIURETERITIS
593.4 PERIURETHRAL FIBROSIS SYNDROME
639.2 PERIURETHRAL INJURY FOLLOWING ABORTION, ECTOPIC OR MOLAR PREGNANCY

362.18 PERIVASCULITIS RETINAL

686.8 PERLECHE
112.0 PERLECHE MONILIAL
266.0 PERLECHE RIBOFLAVIN DEFICIENCY

281.0 PERNICIOUS ANEMIA
281.0 PERNICIOUS ANEMIA CONGENITAL

991.5 PERNIOSIS ERYTHEMA
909.4 PERNIOSIS ERYTHEMA LATE EFFECT

PERONEAL
356.1 MUSCULAR ATROPHY
355.3 NERVE DISORDER
956.3 NERVE INJURY
355.3 NEURITIS (COMMON)
726.79 TENDINITIS
727.09 TENDONS DISLOCATING

719.65 PERRIN-FERRATON DISEASE (SNAPPING HIP)
V62.4 PERSECUTION SOCIAL
751.5 PERSISTENT CLOACA CONGENITAL
747.89 PERSISTENT FETAL CIRCULATION SYNDROME
654.8# PERSISTENT HYMEN COMPLICATING CHILDBIRTH
660.2# PERSISTENT HYMEN OBSTRUCTING LABOR [654.8#]
5th Digit: 654.8
0. EPISODE OF CARE UNSPECIFIED OR N/A
1. DELIVERED
2. DELIVERED WITH POSTPARTUM COMPLICATION
3. ANTEPARTUM COMPLICATION
4. POSTPARTUM COMPLICATION

5th Digit: 660.2
0. EPISODE OF CARE UNSPECIFIED OR N/A
1. DELIVERED
3. ANTEPARTUM COMPLICATION

757.4 PERSISTENT LANUGO CONGENITAL
763.1 PERSISTENT OCCIPITOPOSTERIOR POSITION AFFECTING FETUS OR NEWBORN
747.89 PERSISTENT PULMONARY HYPERTENSION CONGENITAL
745.0 PERSISTENT TRUNCUS ARTERIOSUS CONGENITAL HISTORY
780.03 PERSISTENT VEGETATIVE STATE
743.51 PERSISTENT VITREOUS HYPERPLASIA CONGENITAL

V60.3 PERSON LIVING ALONE
V60.6 PERSON LIVING IN RESIDENTIAL INSTITUTION
V60.4 PERSON UNABLE TO CARE FOR SELF

0 PERSONAL HISTORY SEE 'HISTORY'
310.1 PERSONALITY CHANGE

WHEN CODING A PERSONALITY DISORDER, USE AN ADDITIONAL CODE FOR ANY ASSOCIATED NEUROSIS, PSYCHOSIS OR PHYSICAL CONDITION.

PERSONALITY DISORDER
301.9 NOS
301.10 AFFECTIVE
301.3 AGGRESSIVE
301.7 AMORAL
301.4 ANANCASTIC
301.7 ANTISOCIAL
301.7 ASOCIAL
301.6 ASTHENIC
301.82 AVOIDANT
301.83 BORDERLINE
301.4 COMPULSIVE
301.13 CYCLOID (CYCLOTHYMIC)
301.6 DEPENDENT
301.12 DEPRESSIVE CHRONIC
292.89 DRUG INDUCED [304.##]
4th Digit: 304
0. OPIOID
1. BARBITURATE, SEDATIVES, AND TRANQUILIZERS WITH A SIMILAR EFFECT
2. COCAINE
3. CANNABIS
4. AMPHETAMINE TYPE
5. HALLUCINOGENIC
6. OTHER SPECIFIED
7. MIXED WITH OPIOID
8. MIXED
9. NOS
5th Digit: 304
0. UNSPECIFIED
1. CONTINUOUS
2. EPISODIC
3. IN REMISSION

300.14 DUAL
301.7 DYSSOCIAL
301.89 ECCENTRIC
301.59 EMOTIONALLY UNSTABLE
301.3 EPILEPTOID
301.3 EXPLOSIVE
301.0 FANATIC
301.50 HISTRIONIC
301.11 HYPERTHYMIC
301.11 HYPOMANIC CHRONIC
301.50 HYSTERICAL
301.89 IMMATURE
301.6 INADEQUATE
301.21 INTROVERTED
301.59 LABILE
301.89 MASOCHISTIC
300.14 MULTIPLE
301.51 MUNCHAUSEN
301.81 NARCISSISTIC
300.5 NEURASTHENIA
301.4 OBSESSIONAL
301.0 PARANOID
301.6 PASSIVE
301.84 PASSIVE AGGRESSIVE
301.6 PASSIVE DEPENDENT
301.9 PATHOLOGICAL
301.9 PATTERN DISTURBANCE
301.59 PSYCHO-INFANTILE
301.9 PSYCHOPATHIC
0 PSYCHOTIC SEE 'PSYCHOSIS'
301.20 SCHIZOID
301.21 SCHIZOID INTROVERTED
0 SCHIZOPHRENIC SEE ALSO 'SCHIZOPHRENIA'
301.22 SCHIZOTYPAL

PERSONALITY DISORDER (continued)
301.59 SEDUCTIVE
301.7 SOCIOPATHIC
301.9 TRAIT DISTURBANCE
301.4 TYPE A

732.1 PERTHES' DISEASE (CAPITAL FEMORAL OSTEOCHONDROSIS)

PERTUSSIS
033.0 BORDETALLA
033.1 BORDETALLA PARAPERTUSSIS
V01.8 EXPOSURE
V74.8 SCREENING EXAM
V03.6 VACCINATION (SINGLE)

299.8# PERVASIVE DEVELOPMENTAL DISORDER - CHILDHOOD ONSET
5th Digit: 299.8
0. CURRENT OR ACTIVE STATE
1. RESIDUAL STATE

PES
726.61 ANSERINUS TENDINITIS
754.71 CAVUS
736.79 PLANOVALGUS (ACQUIRED)
754.69 PLANOVALGUS (CONGENITAL)
734 PLANUS (ACQUIRED) FLAT FOOT
754.61 PLANUS (CONGENITAL)
736.79 TALIPES DEFORMITY ACQUIRED NEC
754.50 VARUS CONGENITAL
736.79 OTHER ACQUIRED NEC

020.8 PESTIS MINOR

782.7 PETECHIAE
772.6 PETECHIAE FETUS OR NEWBORN
743.44 PETERS' ANOMALY
710.3 PETGES-CLEJAT SYNDROME (POIKILODERMATOMYOSITIS)
345.0# PETIT MAL
5th Digit: 345.0
0. WITHOUT MENTION OF INTRACTABLE EPILEPSY
1. WITH INTRACTABLE EPILEPSY

345.2 PETIT MAL STATUS

0 PETIT'S DISEASE SEE 'HERNIA' LUMBAR
117.6 PETRIELLIDOSIS

383.20 PETROSITIS
383.21 PETROSITIS ACUTE
383.22 PETROSITIS CHRONIC

759.6 PEUTZ-JEGHERS SYNDROME
607.81 PEYRONIES DISEASE

075 PFEIFFER'S DISEASE (INFECTIOUS MONONUCLEOSIS)
755.55 PFEIFFER SYNDROME (ACROCEPHALOSYNDACTYLY)

117.8 PHAEHYPHOMYCOSIS INFECTION

785.4 PHAGEDENA
440.24 PHAGEDENA ARTERIOSCLEROTIC ISCHEMIC GANGRENE (SENILE)
440.3# PHAGEDENA DUE TO BYPASS GRAFT ARTERIOSCLEROSIS [785.4]
5th Digit: 440.3
0. UNSPECIFIED GRAFT
1. AUTOLOGOUS VEIN BYPASS GRAFT
2. NONAUTOLOGOUS BIOLOGICAL BYPASS GRAFT

686.09 PHAGEDENA GEOMETRIC
099.8 PHAGEDENIC BUBO NEC

996.53 PHAKIA DISLOCATED
996.69 PHAKIA INFECTION OR INFLAMMATION
996.79 PHAKIA OTHER COMPLICATION

0 PHALANGES SEE 'FINGER' OR 'THUMB' OR 'TOE'
353.6 PHANTOM LIMB (SYNDROME) (NONDISCOGENIC)
0 PHARYNGEAL SEE 'PHARYNX, PHARYNGEAL'

PHARYNGITIS
462 ACUTE
462 ACUTE GANGRENOUS
462 ACUTE INFECTIVE
462 ACUTE PHLEGMONOUS
462 ACUTE PNEUMOCOCCAL
462 ACUTE STAPHYLOCOCCAL
462 ACUTE SUPPURATIVE
472.1 ATROPHIC
099.51 CHLAMYDIAL
472.1 CHRONIC
472.1 CHRONIC GRANULAR
074.0 COXSACKIE VIRUS
098.6 GONOCOCCAL
054.79 HERPES SIMPLEX
472.1 HYPERTROPHIC
487.1 INFLUENZAL
074.8 LYMPHONODULAR ACUTE
075 MONONUCLEOSIS
034.0 STREPTOCOCCAL
462 ULCERATIVE
074.0 VESICULAR
462 VIRAL

077.2 PHARYNGOCONJUNCTIVAL FEVER
077.2 PHARYNGOCONJUNCTIVITIS VIRAL
530.6 PHARYNGOESOPHAGEAL DIVERTICULUM (ESOPHAGEAL)
465.8 PHARYNGOTRACHEITIS ACUTE
478.9 PHARYNGOTRACHEITIS CHRONIC

PHARYNX, PHARYNGEAL
478.29 ABSCESS
478.22 ABSCESS PARAPHARYNGEAL
478.24 ABSCESS RETROPHARYNGEAL
750.29 ANOMALY OTHER SPECIFIED (CONGENITAL)
478.29 ATROPHY
925.2 CRUSH INJURY
478.26 CYST
478.20 DISEASE
478.29 DISEASE OTHER NEC
750.27 DIVERTICULUM CONGENITAL
478.25 EDEMA
478.29 HYPERPLASIA (LYMPHOID)
750.29 IMPERFORATE CONGENITAL
959.09 INJURY
478.29 OBSTRUCTION
474.00 POSTERIOR LYMPHOID TISSUE INFECTION
750.27 POUCH CONGENITAL
279.11 POUCH SYNDROME
478.29 ULCER

304.4# PHENMETRAZINE DEPENDENCE
5th Digit: 304.4
0. UNSPECIFIED
1. CONTINUOUS
2. EPISODIC
3. IN REMISSION

270.1 PHENYLKETONURIA (PKU)
V77.3 PHENYLKETONURIA SCREENING (PKU)
270.1 PHENYLPYRUVIC OLIGOPHRENIA AMINO ACID DISORDER (METABOLIC)

PHEOCHROMOCYTOMA
227.0 SITE NOS
0 SITE SPECIFIED SEE 'BENIGN NEOPLASM', BY SITE M8700/0
194.0 MALIGNANT SITE NOS
0 MALIGNANT SITE SPECIFIED SEE 'CANCER' BY SITE M8700/3
255.6 SYNDROME

117.8 PHIALOPHORA GOUGEROTII INFECTION
117.8 PHIALOPHORA JEANSELMEI INFECTION
117.2 PHIALOPHORA VERRUCOSA INFECTION

605 PHIMOSIS
605 PHIMOSIS CONGENITAL
747.6# PHLEBECTASIA CONGENITAL PERIPHERAL VASCULAR
5th Digit: 747.6
0. PERIPHERAL VASCULAR UNSPECIFIED SITE
1. GASTROINTESTINAL VESSEL
2. RENAL VESSEL
3. UPPER LIMB VESSEL
4. LOWER LIMB VESSEL
9. OTHER SPECIFIED SITE PERIPHERAL VASCULAR

454.9 PHLEBECTASIA PERIPHERAL VASCULAR SEE ALSO 'VARICOSE VEINS' LOWER EXTREMITIES
0 PHLEBECTASIA OTHER SITES SEE 'VARICES' BY SPECIFIED SITE

PHLEBITIS
451.9 PHLEBITIS SITE NOS
451.82 ANTECUBITAL VEIN
451.83 ARM DEEP
451.82 ARM SUPERFICIAL
451.84 ARM NEC
451.89 AXILLARY VEIN
451.82 BASILIC VEIN
451.83 BRACHIAL VEIN
451.82 CEPHALIC VEIN
997.2 DURING OR RESULTING FROM A PROCEDURE
451.11 FEMORAL VEIN (DEEP) (SUPERFICIAL)
451.19 FEMOROPOPLITEAL VEIN
999.2 FOLLOWING INFUSION PERFUSION OR TRANSFUSION
274.89 GOUTY [451.9]
451.89 HEPATIC VEIN
451.81 ILIAC VEIN
451.11 ILIOFEMORAL
326 INTRACRANIAL LATE EFFECT
325 INTRACRANIAL SINUS
451.89 JUGULAR VEIN
451.2 LEG
451.2 LOWER EXTREMITIES
451.19 LOWER EXTREMITIES DEEP VESSELS OTHER SPECIFIED

648.9#: USE AN ADDITIONAL CODE TO IDENTIFY THE SPECIFIC PHLEBITIS.

648.9# MATERNAL CURRENT (CO-EXISTENT) IN PREGNANCY
671.9# MATERNAL DUE TO PREGNANCY
5th Digit: 648.9, 671.9
0. EPISODE OF CARE UNSPECIFIED OR N/A
1. DELIVERED
2. DELIVERED WITH POSTPARTUM COMPLICATION
3. ANTEPARTUM COMPLICATION
4. POSTPARTUM COMPLICATION

451.19 POPLITEAL VEIN
572.1 PORTAL VEIN
997.2 POSTOPERATIVE
451.83 RADIAL VEIN
362.18 RETINAL
451.0 SAPHENOUS VEIN (GREATER) (LESSER)
451.89 SUBCLAVIAN VEIN
451.19 TIBIAL VEIN
451.83 ULNAR VEIN
451.84 UPPER EXTREMITIES
451.83 UPPER EXTREMITIES DEEP VESSELS
451.82 UPPER EXTREMITIES SUPERFICIAL VESSELS

459.89 PHLEBOSCLEROSIS

PHLEBOTHROMBOSIS (DEEP-VEIN) COMPLICATING PREGNANCY OR THE PUERPERIUM
671.3# MATERNAL DUE TO PREGNANCY ANTEPARTUM
5th Digit: 671.3
0. EPISODE OF CARE NOS OR N/A
1. DELIVERED
3. ANTEPARTUM COMPLICATION

671.4# MATERNAL DUE TO PREGNANCY POSTPARTUM
5th Digit: 671.4
0. UNSPECIFIED
2. DELIVERED, WTIH POSTPARTUM COMPLICATION
4. POSTPARTUM CONDITION OR COMPLICATION

066.0 PHLEBOTOMUS FEVER
475 PHLEGMONOUS ANGINA
370.31 PHLYCTENULOSIS

PHOBIA
300.20 NOS
300.29 ACROPHOBIA
300.22 AGORAPHOBIA
300.21 AGORAPHOBIA WITH PANIC ATTACKS
300.29 ANIMAL
300.29 CLAUSTROPHOBIA
300.29 CROWDS
300.23 EATING IN PUBLIC
300.3 OBSESSIONAL (ANY)
300.21 OPEN SPACES WITH PANIC ATTACKS
300.29 PARASITES
300.23 PUBLIC-SPEAKING
300.23 SOCIAL
300.21 STREETS WITH PANIC ATTACKS
300.21 TRAVEL WITH PANIC ATTACKS
300.23 WASHING IN PUBLIC
300.29 OTHER SIMPLE

610.1 PHOCAS' DISEASE

PHOCOMELIA
755.4 NOS
755.32 LOWER LIMB
755.33 LOWER LIMB COMPLETE
755.35 LOWER LIMB DISTAL
755.34 LOWER LIMB PROXIMAL
755.22 UPPER LIMB
755.23 UPPER LIMB COMPLETE
755.25 UPPER LIMB DISTAL
755.24 UPPER LIMB PROXIMAL

PHONOCARDIOGRAM
794.39 ABNORMAL
V71.7 FOR SUSPECTED DISEASE
V72.81 PREOPERATIVE
V72.85 ROUTINE

275.3 PHOSPHATE ABNORMAL FINDINGS
588.0 PHOSPHATE LOSING TUBULAR DISORDERS
275.3 PHOSPHATE METABOLISM DISORDER

271.2 PHOSPHOFRUCTOKINASE DEFICIENCY
271.0 PHOSPHOGLUMOTASE DEFICIENCY
271.0 PHOSPHOHEXOSISOMERASE DEFICIENCY

275.3 PHOSPHORUS ABNORMAL FINDINGS
275.3 PHOSPHORUS METABOLISM DISORDER

692.72 PHOTOALLERGIC RESPONSE (ACUTE)
031.9 PHOTOCHROMOGENIC DISEASE (ACID-FAST BACILLI) - NONPULMONARY
031.0 PHOTOCHROMOGENIC DISEASE (ACID-FAST BACILLI) - PULMONARY

692.72 PHOTODERMATITIS SUN
692.82 PHOTODERMATITIS LIGHT OTHER

370.24 PHOTOKERATITIS

368.13 PHOTOPHOBIA
368.15 PHOTOPSIA
363.31 PHOTORETINITIS
363.31 PHOTORETINOPATHY
692.72 PHOTOSENSITIVITY SUNLIGHT
692.82 PHOTOSENSITIVITY LIGHT OTHER
692.72 PHOTOSENSITIZATION SUNLIGHT
692.82 PHOTOSENSITIZATION LIGHT OTHER
692.72 PHOTOTOXIC RESPONSE (ACUTE)
990 PHOTOTHERAPY COMPLICATION
530.89 PHRENIC AMPULLA
354.8 PHRENIC NERVE NEURITIS (DISORDER)
767.7 PHRENIC NERVE PARALYSIS NEWBORN (BIRTH TRAUMA)
017.3# PHTHISICAL CORNEA [371.05]

5th Digit: 017.3

0. UNSPECIFIED
1. LAB NOT DONE
2. LABS PENDING
3. MICROSCOPY POSITIVE (IN SPUTUM)
4. CULTURE POSITIVE - MICROSCOPY NEGATIVE
5. CULTURE NEGATIVE - MICROSCOPY POSITIVE
6. CULTURE AND MICROSCOPY NEGATIVE CONFIRMED BY OTHER METHODS

360.41 PHTHISIS BULBI
132.2 PHTHIRUS PUBIS (PUBIC LOUSE)
127.7 PHYSALOPTERIASIS INFECTION
306.9 PHYSICAL DISORDER PSYCHOGENIC
0 PHYSICAL EXAM SEE 'EXAM'
V57.1 PHYSICAL THERAPY THERAPEUTIC AND REMEDIAL EXERCISES (EXCEPT BREATHING)
935.2 PHYTOBEZOAR GASTRIC
936 PHYTOBEZOAR INTESTINE
102.1 PIANOMA SEE ALSO 'YAWS'
307.52 PICA
300.11 PICA HYSTERICAL

PICK'S DISEASE

331.1 NOS
331.1 NOS WITH DEMENTIA [294.1]
331.1 BRAIN
331.1 BRAIN WITH DEMENTIA [294.1]
331.1 CEREBRAL ATROPHY
331.1 CEREBRAL ATROPHY WITH DEMENTIA [294.1]
423.2 HEART (AND LIVER) (SYNDROME)
272.7 LIPID HISTIOCYTOSIS
423.2 PERICARDIUM (SYNDROME)

701.8 PICK-HERXHEIMER SYNDROME (DIFFUSE IDIOPATHIC CUTANEOUS ATROPHY)
278.8 PICKWICKIAN SYNDROME (CARDIOPULMONARY OBESITY)

PID (PELVIC INFLAMMATORY DISEASE)

614.9 NOS
614.3 ACUTE
614.4 CHRONIC
760.8 MATERNAL - AFFECTING FETUS OR NEWBORN
639.0 MATERNAL - FOLLOWING ABORTION OR ECTOPIC/MOLAR PREGNANCY
0 MATERNAL - IN ABORTION SEE 'ABORTION' BY TYPE WITH SHOCK
670.0# MATERNAL NOS - MAJOR PUERPERAL [614.9]
670.0# MATERNAL ACUTE - MAJOR PUERPERAL [614.3]
670.0# MATERNAL CHRONIC - MAJOR PUERPERAL [614.4]

5th Digit: 670.0

0. EPISODE OF CARE UNSPECIFIED OR N/A
2. DELIVERED WITH POSTPARTUM COMPLICATION
4. POSTPARTUM COMPLICATION

PID (PELVIC INFLAMMATORY DISEASE) (continued)

646.6# MATERNAL NOS - MINOR COMPLICATING PREGNANCY [614.9]
646.6# MATERNAL ACUTE - MINOR COMPLICATING PREGNANCY [614.3]
646.6# MATERNAL CHRONIC - MINOR COMPLICATING PREGNANCY [614.4]

5th Digit: 646.6

0. EPISODE OF CARE UNSPECIFIED OR N/A
1. DELIVERED
2. DELIVERED WITH POSTPARTUM COMPLICATION
3. ANTEPARTUM COMPLICATION
4. POSTPARTUM COMPLICATION

016.7# TUBERCULOUS

5th Digit: 016.7

0. UNSPECIFIED
1. LAB NOT DONE
2. LABS PENDING
3. MICROSCOPY POSITIVE (IN SPUTUM)
4. CULTURE POSITIVE - MICROSCOPY NEGATIVE
5. CULTURE NEGATIVE - MICROSCOPY POSITIVE
6. CULTURE AND MICROSCOPY NEGATIVE CONFIRMED BY OTHER METHODS

614.8 OTHER SPECIFIED

518.3 PIE SYNDROME (PULMONARY INFILTRATION WITH EOSINOPHILIA)
709.09 PIEBALDISM
111.3 PIEDRAIA HORTAI INFECTION
731.2 PIERRE MARIE-BAMBERGER SYNDROME (HYPERTROPHIC PULMONARY OSTEOARTHROPATHY)
258.1 PIERRE MAURIAC'S SYNDROME (DIABETES-DWARFISM-OBESITY)
756.0 PIERRE ROBIN SYNDROME
732.1 PIERSON'S DISEASE (OSTEOCHONDROSIS)
754.82 PIGEON CHEST (BREAST) CONGENITAL
495.2 PIGEON FANCIERS' (BREEDERS') DISEASE
735.8 PIGEON TOE
364.53 PIGMENT DISPERSION SYNDROME, IRIS
333.0 PIGMENTARY PALLIDAL ATROPHY OR DEGENERATION BASAL GANGLIA

PIGMENTATION (ABNORMAL)

709.00 ANOMALY NEC
0 ANOMALY SEE 'DYSCHROMIA'
709.09 ARSENICAL DUE TO DRUG OR CORRECT SUBSTANCE PROPERLY ADMINISTERED
743.53 CHOROID DISORDER, CONGENITAL
372.55 CONJUNCTIVA
371.10 CORNEA - NOS
371.11 CORNEA - ANTERIOR
371.13 CORNEA - POSTERIOR
371.12 CORNEA - STROMAL
374.52 EYELIDS ACQUIRED
757.33 EYELIDS CONGENITAL
743.57 OPTIC PAPILLA CONGENITAL
362.74 RETINA ACQUIRED
743.53 RETINA CONGENITAL

216.# PIGMENTED NEVUS M8720/0

4th Digit: 216

0. LIP (SKIN OF)
1. EYELID INCLUDING CANTHUS
2. EAR (EXTERNAL) (AURICLE) (PINNA)
3. FACE (CHEEK) (NOSE) (EYEBROW) (TEMPLE)
4. SCALP NECK
5. TRUNK BACK EXCEPT SCROTUM
6. UPPER LIMB INCLUDING SHOULDER
7. LOWER LIMB INCLUDING HIP
8. OTHER SPECIFIED SITES
9. SKIN UNSPECIFIED

757.4 PILI ANNULATI TORTI (CONGENITAL)
704.8 PILI INCARNATI
216.# PILOMATRIXOMA M8110/0
4th Digit: 216
0. LIP (SKIN OF)
1. EYELID INCLUDING CANTHUS
2. EAR (EXTERNAL) (AURICLE) (PINNA)
3. FACE (CHEEK) (NOSE) (EYEBROW) (TEMPLE)
4. SCALP NECK
5. TRUNK BACK EXCEPT SCROTUM
6. UPPER LIMB INCLUDING SHOULDER
7. LOWER LIMB INCLUDING HIP
8. OTHER SPECIFIED SITES
9. SKIN UNSPECIFIED

PILONIDAL
685.1 CYST (SINUS) (FISTULA)
685.0 CYST WITH ABSCESS
685.1 FISTULA (SINUS)
685.0 FISTULA (SINUS) WITH ABSCESS

V54.0 PIN REMOVAL (ORTHOPEDIC)
0 PINCHED NERVE SEE 'NEUROPATHY', ENTRAPMENT
259.8 PINEAL CALCIFICATION
259.8 PINEAL GLAND DISEASE (DYSFUNCTION)
259.8 PINEAL SYNDROME
237.1 PINEALOMA SITE NOS
0 PINEALOMA SITE SPECIFIED SEE 'NEOPLASM UNCERTAIN BEHAVIOR' BY SITE M9360/1
194.8 PINEOBLASTOMA SITE NOS
0 PINEOBLASTOMA SITE SPECIFIED SEE 'CANCER' BY SITE M9362/3
237.1 PINEOCYTOMA SITE NOS
0 PINEOCYTOMA SITE SPECIFIED SEE 'NEOPLASM UNCERTAIN BEHAVIOR' BY SITE M9361/1
372.51 PINGUECULA
985.0 PINK DISEASE
492.8 PINK PUFFER SYNDROME
697.1 PINKUS' DISEASE (LICHEN NITIDUS)

PINNA
738.7 ACQUIRED DEFORMITIES (CAULIFLOWER EAR)
380.32 ACQUIRED DEFORMITIES NONINFECTIONS
274.81 DISORDER GOUTY
380.30 DISORDER NONINFECTIOUS
380.39 DISORDER NONINFECTIOUS OTHER SPECIFIED
380.31 HEMATOMA OF AURICLE
380.11 INFECTION ACUTE

622.4 PINPOINT OS (UTERI) SEE ALSO 'CERVIX' STRICTURE

PINTA
103.9 NOS
103.0 CHANCRE (PRIMARY)
103.1 ERYTHEMATOUS PLAQUES
103.1 HYPERKERATOSIS
103.1 INTERMEDIATE LESIONS
103.2 LATE LESIONS
103.3 MIXED LESIONS
103.0 PAPULE (PRIMARY)
103.0 PRIMARY LESIONS

103.0 PINTID OF PINTA
127.4 PINWORM INFECTION
270.7 PIPECOLIC ACIDEMIA
733.5 PIRIFORM SCLEROSIS OF ILIUM
355.0 PIRIFORMIS SYNDROME
066.8 PIRY FEVER

PITUITARY
253.2 CACHEXIA
253.9 DISEASE (GLAND)
253.7 DISORDER IATROGENIC
253.9 DISORDER THALAMIC
253.7 DISORDER THALAMIC - IATROGENIC
253.7 DISORDER THALAMIC - POSTABLATIVE
253.4 DISORDER THALAMIC ANTERIOR NEC
253.4 DISORDERS OTHER (ANTERIOR)
253.3 DWARFISM
253.9 DYSFUNCTION
259.3 ECTOPIC SECRETION (POSTERIOR)
253.8 EMBOLISM
759.2 GLAND ABSENCE (CONGENITAL)
253.4 HORMONE DEFICIENCY ANTERIOR
253.1 HYPERFUNCTION
253.2 HYPOFUNCTION
253.2 INSUFFICIENCY
253.7 INSUFFICIENCY IATROGENIC
253.2 NECROSIS POSTPARTUM
495.8 SNUFF-TAKERS' DISEASE
253.0 SYNDROME

PITYRIASIS
696.5 NOS
696.5 ALBA (STREPTOGENES)
690.11 CAPITIS
696.3 CIRCINATA (ET MACULATA)
695.89 HEBRA
696.2 LICHENOIDES ET VARIOLIFORMIS
696.8 LIKE DISORDER NEC
111.1 NIGRA
696.3 ROSEA
696.4 RUBRA PILARIS
690.18 SICCA
690.8 SIMPLEX
111.0 VERSICOLOR

066.3 PIXUNA FEVER (VIRAL)
270.1 PKU (PHENYLKETONURIA)
V77.3 PKU SCREENING

FETAL OR NEWBORN CODES (760-779), SOMETIMES REQUIRE AN ADDITIONAL CODE TO FURTHER SPECIFY THE CAUSE OF THE CONDITION, THE INFECTING ORGANISM, OR COMPLICATING DIAGNOSES. WHENEVER APPROPRIATE, DESCRIBE THE PATIENT'S MEDICAL SITUATION AS CLEARLY AND CONCISELY AS POSSIBLE USING MULTIPLE CODES.

PLACENTA, PLACENTAL
656.9# UNSPECIFIED PROBLEM AFFECTING MANAGEMENT OF MOTHER
5th Digit: 656.9
0. EPISODE OF CARE UNSPECIFIED OR N/A
1. DELIVERED
3. ANTEPARTUM COMPLICATION

762.2 ABNORMAL - AFFECTING FETUS OR NEWBORN
762.1 ABNORMAL - AFFECTING FETUS OR NEWBORN WITH HEMORRHAGE
656.7# ABNORMAL - AFFECTING MANAGEMENT OF MOTHER
641.8# ABNORMAL - WITH HEMORRHAGE AFFECTING MANAGEMENT OF MOTHER
5th Digit: 641.8, 656.7
0. EPISODE OF CARE UNSPECIFIED OR N/A
1. DELIVERED
3. ANTEPARTUM COMPLICATION

793.9 ABNORMAL FINDING (X-RAY) (ULTRASOUND) (THERMOGRAPHY)
794.9 ABNORMAL FINDING (RADIOISOTOPE LOCALIZATION)
641.2# ABRUPTIO OR ABLATIO
5th Digit: 641.2
0. EPISODE OF CARE UNSPECIFIED OR N/A
1. DELIVERED
3. ANTEPARTUM COMPLICATION

PLACENTA, PLACENTAL (continued)

762.1 ABRUPTIO OR ABLATIO AFFECTING FETUS OR NEWBORN
0 ACCRETA SEE 'PLACENTA, PLACENTAL' RETAINED
0 ADHERENT SEE 'PLACENTA, PLACENTAL' RETAINED
0 BIPARTITA SEE 'PLACENTA, PLACENTAL' ABNORMAL
762.1 DAMAGE DUE TO AMNIOCENTESIS, C-SECTION, OR SURGICAL INDUCTION - AFFECTING FETUS OR NEWBORN
762.2 DISEASE AFFECTING FETUS OR NEWBORN
656.7# DISEASE AFFECTING MANAGEMENT OF MOTHER

5th Digit: 656.7
0. EPISODE OF CARE UNSPECIFIED OR N/A
1. DELIVERED
3. ANTEPARTUM COMPLICATION

762.2 DYSFUNCTION SYNDROME
794.9 FUNCTION STUDY ABNORMAL
762.2 INFARCT AFFECTING FETUS OR NEWBORN
656.7# INFARCT AFFECTING MANAGEMENT OF MOTHER

5th Digit: 656.7
0. EPISODE OF CARE UNSPECIFIED OR N/A
1. DELIVERED
3. ANTEPARTUM COMPLICATION

762.2 INSUFFICIENCY AFFECTING FETUS OR NEWBORN
656.5# INSUFFICIENCY AFFECTING MANAGEMENT OF MOTHER

5th Digit: 656.5
0. EPISODE OF CARE UNSPECIFIED OR N/A
1. DELIVERED
3. ANTEPARTUM COMPLICATION

762.2 INSUFFICIENCY SYNDROME
0 LOW IMPLANTATION SEE 'PLACENTA, PLACENTAL' PREVIA
0 LOW LYING SEE 'PLACENTA, PLACENTAL' PREVIA
762.1 MALFORMATION AFFECTING FETUS OR NEWBORN
656.7# MALFORMATION AFFECTING MANAGEMENT OF MOTHER
641.8# MALFORMATION WITH HEMORRHAGE AFFECTING MANAGEMENT OF MOTHER

5th Digit: 641.8, 656.7
0. EPISODE OF CARE UNSPECIFIED OR N/A
1. DELIVERED
3. ANTEPARTUM COMPLICATION

0 MALPOSITION SEE 'PLACENTA, PLACENTAL' PREVIA
658.4# PLACENTITIS

5th Digit: 658.4
0. EPISODE OF CARE UNSPECIFIED OR N/A
1. DELIVERED
3. ANTEPARTUM COMPLICATION

762.7 PLACENTITIS AFFECTING FETUS OR NEWBORN
674.4# POLYP MATERNAL DUE TO PREGNANCY

5th Digit: 674.4
0. UNSPECIFIED
2. DELIVERED WITH POSTPARTUM COMPLICATION
4. POSTPARTUM COMPLICATION

0 PREMATURE SEPARATION SEE 'PLACENTA, PLACENTAL' ABRUPTIO
762.0 PREVIA AFFECTING FETUS OR NEWBORN
641.0# PREVIA (DURING PREGNANCY) (BEFORE LABOR)
641.1# PREVIA WITH HEMORRHAGE

5th Digit: 641.0-1
0. EPISODE OF CARE UNSPECIFIED OR N/A
1. DELIVERED
3. ANTEPARTUM COMPLICATION

794.9 RADIOISOTOPE STUDY ABNORMAL
667.0# RETAINED
667.1# RETAINED FRAGMENTS
666.0# RETAINED WITH POSTPARTUM HEMORRHAGE
666.2# RETAINED WITH POSTPARTUM HEMORRHAGE SECOND STAGE
667.1# RETAINED PRODUCTS OF CONCEPTUS

5th Digit: 666.0, 2, 667.0-1
0. NOS
2. DELIVERED WITH POSTPARTUM COMPLICATION
4. POSTPARTUM COMPLICATION

095.8 SYPHILITIC

PLACENTA, PLACENTAL (continued)

762.3 TRANSFUSION SYNDROMES AFFECTING FETUS OR NEWBORN
762.3 TRANSFUSION SYNDROMES AFFECTING FETUS OR NEWBORN - WITH FETAL BLOOD LOSS [772.0]
762.3 TRANSFUSION SYNDROMES AFFECTING FETUS OR NEWBORN - WITH POLYCYTHEMIA NEONATORUM [776.4]
656.7# VARICES
656.8# OTHER SPECIFIED PROBLEMS AFFECTING MANAGEMENT OF MOTHER

5th Digit: 656.7-8
0. EPISODE OF CARE UNSPECIFIED OR N/A
1. DELIVERED
3. ANTEPARTUM COMPLICATION

658.4# PLACENTITIS

5th Digit: 658.4
0. EPISODE OF CARE UNSPECIFIED OR N/A
1. DELIVERED
3. ANTEPARTUM COMPLICATION

762.7 PLACENTITIS AFFECTING FETUS OR NEWBORN
754.0 PLAGIOCEPHALY

PLAGUE

020.9 NOS
020.8 ABORTIVE
020.8 AMBULATORY
020.0 BUBONIC
020.1 CELLULOCUTANEOUS
020.5 PNEUMONIA
020.3 PNEUMONIA PRIMARY
020.4 PNEUMONIA SECONDARY
V74.8 SCREENING EXAM
020.2 SEPSIS
V03.3 VACCINATION
020.8 OTHER SPECIFIED TYPES

736.79 PLANOVALGUS DEFORMITY (ACQUIRED)
754.69 PLANOVALGUS DEFORMITY CONGENITAL

PLANTAR

904.6 ARTERY INJURY (DEEP VESSELS)
908.3 ARTERY INJURY (DEEP VESSELS) - LATE EFFECT
904.6 BLOOD VESSEL LACERATION DEEP VESSELS (RUPTURE) (HEMATOMA) (AVULSION) (ANEURYSM) TRAUMATIC
908.3 BLOOD VESSEL LACERATION DEEP VESSELS LATE EFFECT
728.71 FASCIITIS (SYNDROME) (TRAUMATIC)
355.6 NERVE DISORDER
956.5 NERVE INJURY
907.5 NERVE INJURY - LATE EFFECT
355.6 NERVE LESION
904.6 VEIN INJURY (DEEP VESSELS)
908.3 VEIN INJURY (DEEP VESSELS) - LATE EFFECT
078.19 WARTS

PLASMA CELL

610.4 MASTITIS
203.0# MYELOMA

5th Digit: 203.0
0. WITHOUT MENTION OF REMISSION
1. IN REMISSION

0 MYELOMA SITE SPECIFIED SEE 'CANCER' BY SITE M9730/3
229.9 TUMOR BENIGN SITE NOS
0 TUMOR BENIGN SITE SPECIFIED SEE 'BENIGN NEOPLASM', BY SITE M9731/0
203.8# TUMOR MALIGNANT SITE NOS

5th Digit: 203.8
0. WITHOUT MENTION OF REMISSION
1. IN REMISSION

0 TUMOR MALIGNANT SITE SPECIFIED SEE 'CANCER' BY SITE M7931/3
238.6 TUMOR UNCERTAIN BEHAVIOR UNSPECIFIED

286.2 PLASMA THROMBOPLASTIN ANTECEDENT (PTA) DEFICIENCY
286.1 PLASMA THROMBOPLASTIN COMPONENT DEFICIENCY
203.1# PLASMACYTIC LEUKEMIA M9830/3
5th Digit: 203.1
0. WITHOUT MENTION OF REMISSION
1. IN REMISSION

238.6 PLASMACYTOMA SITE NOS
0 PLASMACYTOMA SITE SPECIFIED SEE 'NEOPLASM UNCERTAIN BEHAVIOR' BY SITE M9731/1
0 PLASMACYTOMA BENIGN SITE SPECIFIED SEE 'BENIGN NEOPLASM', BY SITE M9731/0
203.8# PLASMACYTOMA MALIGNANT SITE NOS M9731/3
5th Digit: 203.8
0. WITHOUT MENTION OF REMISSION
1. IN REMISSION

288.8 PLASMACYTOSIS
V50.1 PLASTIC SURGERY (ELECTIVE) (FOR UNACCEPTABLE COSMETIC APPEARANCE)
V51 PLASTIC SURGERY REVISION OF OLD INJURY
V54.0 PLATE REMOVAL (ORTHOPEDIC)
287.1 PLATELET DEFECT
286.9 PLATELET STICKY SYNDROME
756.0 PLATYBASIA
756.19 PLATYSPONDYLIA SUPERNUMERARY VERTEBRA
199.1 PLEOMORPHIC CARCINOMA SITE NOS
0 PLEOMORPHIC CARCINOMA SITE SPECIFIED SEE 'CANCER' BY SITE M8022/3
782.62 PLETHORA
776.4 PLETHORA NEWBORN

PLEURA, PLEURAL

511.0 ADHESION
511.0 CALCIFICATION
786.52 CHEST PAIN
511.0 DISEASE (CAVITY) (SEE ALSO 'PLEURISY')
511.9 EFFUSION - UNSPECIFIED
511.9 EFFUSION - FETUS OR NEWBORN
197.2 EFFUSION - MALIGNANT
511.9 EFFUSION - PLEURISY NOS
997.3 EFFUSION - POST OP
511.1 EFFUSION - <u>PNEUMOCOCCAL</u> <u>[041.2]</u>
511.1 EFFUSION - <u>STAPHYLOCOCCAL</u> **<u>[041.1#]</u>**
5th Digit: 041.1
0. UNSPECIFIED
1. AUREUS
9. OHER

511.1 EFFUSION - <u>STREPTOCOCCAL</u> **<u>[041.0#]</u>**
5th Digit: 041.0
0. NOS
1. GROUP A
2. GROUP B
3. GROUP C
4. GROUP D (ENTEROCOCCUS)
5. GROUP G
9. OTHER STREP

862.39 EFFUSION - TRAUMATIC WITH OPEN WOUND
862.29 EFFUSION - TRAUMATIC WITHOUT OPEN WOUND
012.0# EFFUSION - TUBERCULOUS
010.1# EFFUSION - TUBERCULOUS PRIMARY PROGRESSIVE
5th Digit: 010.1, 012.0
0. UNSPECIFIED
1. LAB NOT DONE
2. LABS PENDING
3. MICROSCOPY POSITIVE (IN SPUTUM)
4. CULTURE POSITIVE - MICROSCOPY NEGATIVE
5. CULTURE NEGATIVE - MICROSCOPY POSITIVE
6. CULTURE AND MICROSCOPY NEGATIVE CONFIRMED BY OTHER METHODS

PLEURA, PLEURAL (continued)

511.0 FIBRIN DEPOSIT
511.0 FIBROSIS
792.9 FLUID ABNORMAL
748.8 FOLDS ANOMALY CONGENITAL
786.7 FRICTION RUB
862.29 INJURY
862.39 INJURY WITH OPEN WOUND
908.0 INJURY LATE EFFECT
748.8 SACS AND PERICARDIAL SACS ABNORMAL COMMUNICATION
511.0 THICKENING

PLEURISY

511.0 UNSPECIFIED
511.9 UNSPECIFIED WITH EFFUSION
511.0 ACUTE
511.0 ACUTE (STERILE) DIAPHRAGMATIC
511.0 ACUTE (STERILE) FIBRINOUS
511.0 ACUTE (STERILE) INTERLOBULAR
511.0 BACTERIAL
511.1 BACTERIAL WITH EFFUSION
511.8 ENCYSTED
511.9 EXUDATIVE
511.8 HEMORRHAGIC
487.1 INFLUENZAL
511.1 OTHER SPECIFIED WITH EFFUSION
511.1 <u>PNEUMOCOCCAL</u> WITH EFFUSION <u>[041.2]</u>
511.9 SEROUS
511.1 <u>STAPHYLOCOCCAL</u> WITH EFFUSION **<u>[041.1#]</u>**
5th Digit: 041.1
0. NOS
1. AUREUS
9. OTHER STAPH

511.1 <u>STREPTOCOCCAL</u> WITH EFFUSION **<u>[041.0#]</u>**
5th Digit: 041.0
0. NOS
1. GROUP A
2. GROUP B
3. GROUP C
4. GROUP D (ENTEROCOCCUS)
5. GROUP G
9. OTHER STREP

510.9 SUPPURATIVE (SEPTIC) (PURULENT) (FIBRINOPURULENT)
012.0# TUBERCULOUS
010.1# TUBERCULOUS PRIMARY PROGRESSIVE
5th Digit: 010.1, 012.0
0. UNSPECIFIED
1. LAB NOT DONE
2. LABS PENDING
3. MICROSCOPY POSITIVE (IN SPUTUM)
4. CULTURE POSITIVE - MICROSCOPY NEGATIVE
5. CULTURE NEGATIVE - MICROSCOPY POSITIVE
6. CULTURE AND MICROSCOPY NEGATIVE CONFIRMED BY OTHER METHODS

485 PLEUROBRONCHOPNEUMONIA
786.52 PLEURODYNIA
074.1 PLEURODYNIA EPIDEMIC
573.8 PLEUROHEPATITIS
420.90 PLEUROPERICARDITIS ACUTE
041.81 PLEUROPNEUMONIA LIKE ORGANISM (PPLO) (INFECTING ORGANISM)
727.89 PLICA SYNOVIUM
474.8 PLICA TONSIL
335.24 PLS
984.9 PLUMBISM

242.3# PLUMMER'S DISEASE (TOXIC NODULAR GOITER)
5th Digit: 242.3
0. WITHOUT STORM
1. WITH STORM

280.8 PLUMMER-VINSON SYNDROME (SIDEROPENIC DYSPHAGIA)
260 PLURICARENTIAL (PLURIDEFICIENCY) OF INFANCY SYNDROME
258.8 PLURIGLANDULAR ATROPHY
258.8 PLURIGLANDULAR (COMPENSATORY) SYNDROME
625.4 PMS
786.09 PND PAROXYSMAL NOCTURUAL DYSPNEA
958.0 PNEUMATHEMIA
908.6 PNEUMATHEMIA LATE EFFECT
348.8 PNEUMATOCELE INTRACRANIAL
518.89 PNEUMATOCELE LUNG
492.0 PNEUMATOCELE TENSION
599.84 PNEUMATURIA
348.8 PNEUMOCEPHALUS
0 PNEUMOCOCCAL ARTHRITIS SEE 'ARTHRITIS OTHER SPECIFIED' PYOGENIC
038.2 PNEUMOCOCCAL SEPSIS
038.2 PNEUMOCOCCEMIA
V01.8 PNEUMOCOCCUS EXPOSURE
041.2 PNEUMOCOCCUS INFECTION OR ORGANISM

PNEUMOCONIOSIS

505 NOS
503 ALUMINUM
501 ASBESTOS
495.1 BAGASSE
503 BAUXITE
503 BERYLLIUM
500 COAL WORKERS'
504 COTTON DUST
506.9 FUMES VAPORS (FROM SILO)
503 GRAPHITE HARD METAL
503 INORGANIC DUST OTHER
502 MICA TALC
504 ORGANIC DUST NEC
502 SILICA OR SILICATES OTHER DUE TO

136.3 PNEUMOCYSTOSIS
793.0 PNEUMOENCEPHALOGRAM ABNORMAL
352.3 PNEUMOGASTRIC NERVE ATROPHY
352.3 PNEUMOGASTRIC NERVE DISORDER
951.8 PNEUMOGASTRIC NERVE INJURY
511.8 PNEUMOHEMOTHORAX
860.4 PNEUMOHEMOTHORAX TRAUMATIC
860.5 PNEUMOHEMOTHORAX TRAUMATIC WITH OPEN WOUND
423.9 PNEUMOHYDROPERICARDIUM
518.1 PNEUMOMEDIASTINUM
770.2 PNEUMOMEDIASTINUM PERINATAL PERIOD
117.9 PNEUMOMYCOSIS

IF THE PHYSICIAN HAS NOT SPECIFIED WHETHER THE ORGANISM CAUSING THE PNEUMONIA IS BACTERIAL OR VIRAL, CODE 486; 'PNEUMONIA UNSPECIFIED. A MORE SPECIFIC CODE CAN BE ASSIGNED ONLY IF A THOROUGH REVIEW OF THE MEDICAL RECORD SUBSTANTIATES A MORE SPECIFIC DIAGNOSIS.

PNEUMONIA

486 UNSPECIFIED
480.0 ADENOVIRAL
518.3 ALLERGIC
482.81 ANAEROBIC

PNEUMONIA (continued)

WHEN BOTH ASPIRATION PNEUMONIA 507.0 AND BACTERIAL PNEUMONIA 480-483 ARE DOCUMENTED ON THE SAME ENCOUNTER, BOTH CONDITIONS SHOULD BE CODED. SEQUENCING DEPENDS ON THE REASON FOR ENCOUNTER.

ASPIRATION

507.0 NOS
770.1 FETAL
507.0 FOOD REGURGITATED
506.0 FUMES OR VAPORS (CHEMICAL) (ACUTE)
507.0 GASTRIC SECRETIONS
516.8 LIPOID ENDOGENOUS
507.1 LIPOID EXOGENOUS
770.1 NEWBORN

***668.0#:** WHEN CODING A MATERNAL ASPIRATION PNEUMONIA/PNEUMONITIS USE AN ADDITIONAL CODE TO SHOW THE TYPE OF ASPIRATION.*

668.0# OBSTETRICAL MATERNAL (MOTHER'S RECORD)
5th Digit: 668.0
0. EPISODE OF CARE NOS OR N/A
1. DELIVERED
2. DELIVERED WITH POSTPARTUM COMPLICATION
3. ANTEPARTUM COMPLICATION
4. POSTPARTUM COMPLICATION

507.1 OILS OR ESSENCES
997.3 POSTOPERATIVE
507.0 VOMITUS
507.8 OTHER SOLIDS OR LIQUIDS

PNEUMONIA (continued)

482.9 BACTERIAL
482.89 BACTERIAL SPECIFIED NEC
482.83 BACTERIUM ANITRATUM
482.81 BACTEROIDES (MELANINOGENICUS)
485 BROCHOPNEUMONIA (CONFLUENT) (CROUPOUS) (DIFFUSE) (DISSEMINATED) (LOBAR) (HEMORRHAGIC) (TERMINAL)
482.81 BUTYRIVIBRIO (FIBRIOSOLVENS)
112.4 CANDIDIASIS
466.19 CAPILLARY
483.1 CHLAMYDIAL
482.81 CLOSTRIDIUM (HAEMOLYTICUM) (NOVYI)
481 COMMUNITY ACQUIRED
481 DIPLOCOCCAL
483.0 EATON'S AGENT
482.82 ESCHERICHIA COLI (E. COLI)
482.81 EUBACTERIUM
482.0 FRIEDLANDER'S BACILLUS
482.81 FUSOBACTERIUM (NUCLEATUM)
513.0 GANGRENOUS
482.81 GRAM-NEGATIVE ANAEROBIC
482.83 GRAM-NEGATIVE BACTERIA NEC
482.2 HEMOPHILUS INFLUENZA
482.83 HERELLEA
514 HYPOSTATIC
770.0 INFECTIVE ACQUIRED PRENATALLY
487.0 INFLUENZA
516.8 INTERSTITIAL (DESQUAMATIVE) (LYMPHOID)
482.0 KLEBSIELLA PNEUMONIAE
482.84 LEGIONNAIRES'
481 LOBAR
485 LOBULAR
038.8 METASTATIC NEC [484.8]
483.8 MICROORGANISM OTHER SPECIFIED
483.0 MYCOPLASMA PNEUMONIAE
513.0 NECROTIC
486 OBSTRUCTIVE (BRONCHOGENIC NEOPLASM)

PNEUMONIA (continued)

480.2 PARAINFLUENZA
514 PASSIVE
482.81 PEPTOCOCCUS
482.81 PEPTOSTREPTOCOCCUS
483.0 PLEUROPNEUMONIA-LIKE ORGANISM (PPLO)
481 PNEUMOCOCCAL
V03.82 PNEUMOCOCCAL VACCINATION
997.3 POST OP
483.0 PPLO
770.0 PRENATALLY ACQUIRED INFECTIVE
486 PRIMARY ATYPICAL
482.81 PROPIONIBACTERIUM
482.83 PROTEUS
482.1 PSEUDOMONAS
480.1 RESPIRATORY SYNCYTIAL VIRUS
997.3 RESULTING FROM A PROCEDURE
485 SEGMENTAL
482.83 SERRATIA (MARCESCENS)
482.4# STAPHYLOCOCCAL

5th Digit: 482.4
0. NOS
1. AUREUS
9. OTHER STAPH

482.3# STREPTOCOCCAL
482.3# STREPTOCOCCAL BETAHEMOLYTIC

5th Digit: 482.3
0. NOS
1. GROUP A
2. GROUP B
9. OTHER STREPTOCOCCUS

481 STREPTOCOCCUS PNEUMONIAE
V03.82 STREPTOCOCCUS PNEUMONIAE VACCINATION
958.8 TRAUMATIC
908.6 TRAUMATIC LATE EFFECT
V03.82 VACCINATION
052.1 VARICELLA
482.81 VEILLONELLA
480.8 VIRAL NEC
480.9 VIRAL
482.89 OTHER SPECIFIED BACTERIA
483.8 OTHER SPECIFIED ORGANISM

THE CODE IN THE LEFT MARGIN ALWAYS SEQUENCES FIRST. THE ADDITIONAL CODE IN BRACKETS TO THE RIGHT OF THE DESCRIPTION IS SEQUENCED SECONDARILY. UNDERLINING SHOWS THE CODE NUMBER THAT CORRESPONDS TO THE UNDERLINED VERBAL DESCRIPTION. UNDERLINING NEVER IMPLIES CORRECT SEQUENCING.

PNEUMONIA - OTHER

039.1 ACTINOMYCOTIC
022.1 ANTHRAX [484.5]
117.3 ASPERGILLA [484.6]
482.89 BACTERIA NEC [041.89]
112.4 CANDIDIASIS LUNG
466.19 CAPILLARY (BRONCHIOLITIS) (WITH BRONCHOSPASM OR OBSTRUCTION)
483.1 CHLAMYDIAL (PNEUMONIAE) (TRACHOMATIS)
073.0 CHLAMYDIAL PSITTACI
078.5 CMV [484.1]
114.# COCCIDIOIDOMYCOSIS

4th Digit: 114
0. ACUTE (PRIMARY)
4. CHRONIC (SECONDARY)
5. UNSPECIFIED

770.0 CONGENITAL
078.5 CYTOMEGALIC INCLUSION [484.1]
506.0 DUE TO FUMES AND VAPORS
518.3 EOSINOPHILIC

PNEUMONIA - OTHER (continued)

117.9 FUNGUS [484.7]
513.0 GANGRENOUS
487.0 GRIPPAL
083.0 HIBERNO-VERNAL [484.8]
115.95 HISTOPLASMOSIS
115.05 HISTOPLASMOSIS CAPSULATUM
115.15 HISTOPLASMOSIS DUBOISII
514 HYPOSTATIC
136.9 INFECTIOUS DISEASES [484.8]
516.8 INTERSTITIAL (DESQUAMATIVE) (LYMPHOID)
516.8 LIPOID ENDOGENOUS
507.1 LIPOID EXOGENOUS
038.8 METASTATIC DUE TO BLOOD BOURNE BACTERIA [484.8]
038.8 METASTATIC DUE TO SEPSIS [484.8]
484.7 MYCOTIC (OTHER) (SYSTEMIC)
039.1 NOCARDIA
486 ORGANISM UNSPECIFIED
073.0 ORNITHOSIS
483.8 OTHER SPECIFIED ORGANISM
514 PASSIVE
033.# PERTUSSIS [484.3]

5th Digit: 033
0. B. PERTUSSIS
1. B. PARAPERTUSSIS
8. B. BRONCHISEPTICA
9. UNSPECIFIED ORGANISM

136.3 PNEUMOCYSTIS CARINII
055.1 POSTMEASLES
083.0 Q FEVER [484.8]
390 RHEUMATIC [517.1]
083.9 RICKETTSIA [484.8]
771.0 RUBELLA PNEUMONITIS CONGENITAL
003.22 SALMONELLA
104.8 SPIROCHETAL [484.8]
130.4 TOXOPLASMOSIS
958.8 TRAUMATIC
011.6# TUBERCULOUS

5th Digit: 011.6
0. UNSPECIFIED
1. LAB NOT DONE
2. LABS PENDING
3. MICROSCOPY POSITIVE (IN SPUTUM)
4. CULTURE POSITIVE - MICROSCOPY NEGATIVE
5. CULTURE NEGATIVE - MICROSCOPY POSITIVE
6. CULTURE AND MICROSCOPY NEGATIVE CONFIRMED BY OTHER METHODS

021.2 TULAREMIA
483.1 TWAR AGENT
002.# TYPHOID [484.8]

4th Digit: 002
0. PARATYPHOID FEVER
1. PARATYPHOID FEVER A
2. PARATYPHOID FEVER B
3. PARATYPHOID FEVER C
9. PARATYPHOID FEVER UNSPECIFIED

052.1 VARICELLA
033.# WHOOPING COUGH [484.3]

5th Digit: 033
0. B. PERTUSSIS
1. B. PARAPERTUSSIS
8. B. BRONCHISEPTICA
9. UNSPECIFIED ORGANISM

PNEUMONITIS

486 NOS
495.9 ALLERGIC
495.8 ALLERGIC OTHER SPECIFIED

ASPIRATION

507.0 NOS
770.1 FETAL
507.0 FOOD REGURGITATED
506.0 FUMES OR VAPORS (CHEMICAL) (ACUTE)
507.0 GASTRIC SECRETIONS
516.8 LIPOID ENDOGENOUS
507.1 LIPOID EXOGENOUS
770.1 NEWBORN

> ***668.0#:*** *WHEN CODING A MATERNAL ASPIRATION PNEUMONIA/PNEUMONITIS USE AN ADDITIONAL CODE TO SHOW THE TYPE OF ASPIRATION.*

668.0# OBSTETRICAL MATERNAL (MOTHER'S RECORD)
5th Digit: 668.0
0. EPISODE OF CARE NOS OR N/A
1. DELIVERED
2. DELIVERED WITH POSTPARTUM COMPLICATION
3. ANTEPARTUM COMPLICATION
4. POSTPARTUM COMPLICATION

507.1 OILS OR ESSENCES
997.3 POSTOPERATIVE
771.0 RUBELLA CONGENITAL
507.0 VOMITUS
507.8 OTHER SOLIDS OR LIQUIDS

PNEUMONITIS (continued)

506.0 CHEMICAL (OR FUMES)
495.9 HYPERSENSITIVITY
770.1 MECONIUM FETUS OR NEWBORN
508.0 RADIATION
0 SEE ALSO 'PNEUMONIA'
495.7 VENTILATION

516.9 PNEUMONOPATHY ALVEOLAR AND PARIETOALVEOLAR
504 PNEUMONOPATHY - INHALATION OTHER DUST
527.8 PNEUMOPAROTID
420.90 PNEUMOPERICARDITIS ACUTE
770.2 PNEUMOPERICARDIUM PERINATAL PERIOD
568.89 PNEUMOPERITONEUM
770.2 PNEUMOPERITONEUM FETUS OR NEWBORN
420.99 PNEUMOPYOPERICARDIUM
503 PNEUMOSIDEROSIS (OCCUPATIONAL)

PNEUMOTHORAX

512.1 ACCIDENTAL DURING A PROCEDURE
770.2 CONGENITAL
512.1 DUE TO OPERATIVE PROCEDURE
512.1 IATROGENIC
770.2 PERINATAL PERIOD
512.1 POSTOPERATIVE
512.8 SPONTANEOUS
512.8 SPONTANEOUS ACUTE OR CHRONIC
512.1 TENSION IATROGENIC
512.1 TENSION POSTOPERATIVE
512.0 TENSION SPONTANEOUS
860.0 TENSION TRAUMATIC
860.1 TENSION TRAUMATIC WITH OPEN WOUND INTO THORAX
908.0 TENSION TRAUMATIC LATE EFFECT
860.0 TRAUMATIC
860.4 TRAUMATIC WITH HEMOTHORAX
860.1 TRAUMATIC WITH OPEN WOUND INTO THORAX
908.0 TRAUMATIC LATE EFFECT

PNEUMOTHORAX (continued)

011.7# TUBERCULOUS
5th Digit: 011.7
0. UNSPECIFIED
1. LAB NOT DONE
2. LABS PENDING
3. MICROSCOPY POSITIVE (IN SPUTUM)
4. CULTURE POSITIVE - MICROSCOPY NEGATIVE
5. CULTURE NEGATIVE - MICROSCOPY POSITIVE
6. CULTURE AND MICROSCOPY NEGATIVE CONFIRMED BY OTHER METHODS

132.2 PHTHIRUS PUBIS
790.91 PO2 OXYGEN RATIO ABNORMAL
790.0 POIKILOCYTOSIS
790.0 POIKILOCYTOSIS ABNORMAL FINDINGS
709.09 POIKILODERMA
757.33 POIKILODERMA CONGENITAL
710.3 POIKILODERMATOMYOSITIS
744.29 POINTED EAR CONGENITAL
692.6 POISON IVY DERMATITIS
692.6 POISON OAK DERMATITIS
692.6 POISON SUMAC DERMATITIS
692.6 POISON VINE DERMATITIS

> *POISONING - MEDICINAL: CONDITIONS CAUSED BY MEDICINAL SUBSTANCES ARE CLASSIFIED AS A POISONING WHEN THE SUBSTANCE INVOLVED IS IMPROPERLY TAKEN. CODE THE POISONING FROM THE SECTION BELOW FIRST, THEN THE MANIFESTATION, WITH AN ADDITIONAL 'E-CODE' TO FURTHER CLASSIFY THE POISONING. (SEE APPENDIX 'A', 'POISONING').*

POISONING - MEDICINAL

0 SEE ALSO APPENDIX B, DRUG AND CHEMICALS INDEX
977.9 UNSPECIFIED DRUG OR MEDICINAL SUBSTANCES
965.#(#) ANALGESICS, ANTIPYRETICS, AND ANTIRHEUMATICS
4th or 4th and 5th Digit: 965
0#. OPIATES AND RELATED NARCOTICS
00.OPIUM (ALKALOIDS) UNSPECIFIED
01. HEROIN
02. METHADONE
09. OTHER (CODEINE) (MEPERIDINE) (MORPHINE)
1. SALICYLATES
4. AROMATIC ANALGESICS, NEC
5. PYRAZOLE DERIVATIVES
6#. ANTIRHEUMATICS (ANTIPHLOGISTICS)
61. PROPIONIC ACID DERIVATIVES
69. OTHER ANTIRHEUMATICS
7. OTHER NON-NARCOTIC ANALGESICS
8. OTHER SPECIFIED ANALGESICS AND ANTIPYRETICS
9. UNSPECIFIED ANALGESIC AND ANTIPYRETIC

960.# ANTIBIOTICS
4th Digit: 960
0. PENICILLINS
1. ANTIFUNGAL ANTIBIOTICS
2. CHLORAMPHENICOL GROUP
3. ERYTHROMYCIN AND OTHER MACROLIDES
4. TETRACYCLINE GROUP
5. CEPHALOSPORIN GROUP
6. ANTIMYCOBACTERIAL GROUP
7. ANTINEOPLASTIC ANTIBIOTICS
8. OTHER SPECIFIED ANTIBIOTICS
9. UNSPECIFIED ANTIBIOTICS

POISONING - MEDICINAL (continued)

961.# OTHER ANTI-INFECTIVES

4th Digit: 961

- **0. SULFONAMIDES**
- **1. ARSENICAL ANTI-INFECTIVES**
- **2. HEAVY METAL ANTI-INFECTIVES**
- **3. QUINOLINE AND HYDROXYQUINOLINE DERIVATIVES**
- **4. ANTIMALARIALS AND DRUGS ACTING ON OTHER BLOOD PROTOZOA**
- **5. OTHER ANTIPROTOZOAL DRUGS**
- **6. ANTHELMINTICS**
- **7. ANTIVIRAL DRUGS**
- **8. OTHER ANTIMYCOBACTERIAL DRUGS**
- **9. OTHER AND UNSPECIFIED ANTI-INFECTIVES**

966.# ANTICONVULSANTS AND ANTI-PARKINSONISM DRUGS

4th Digit: 966

- **0. OXAZOLIDINE DERIVATIVES**
- **1. HYDANTOIN DERIVATIVES**
- **2. SUCCINIMIDES**
- **3. OTHER AND UNSPECIFIED ANTICONVULSANTS**
- **4. ANTI-PARKINSONISM DRUGS**

971.# AUTONOMIC NERVOUS SYSTEM DRUGS - (PRIMARILY AFFECTING)

4th Digit: 971

- **0. PARASYMPATHOMIMETICS (CHOLINERGICS)**
- **1. PARASYMPATHOLYTICS (ANTICHOLINERGICS AND ANTIMUSCARINICS) AND SPASMOLYTICS**
- **2. SYMPATHOMIMETICS (ADRENERGICS)**
- **3. SYMPATHOLYTICS (ANTIADRENERGICS)**
- **9. UNSPECIFIED DRUG PRIMARILY AFFECTING AUTONOMIC NERVOUS SYSTEM**

964.# BLOOD CONSTITUENT AGENTS (PRIMARILY AFFECTING)

4th Digit: 964

- **0. IRON AND ITS COMPOUNDS**
- **1. LIVER PREPARATIONS AND OTHER ANTIANEMIC AGENTS**
- **2. ANTICOAGULANTS**
- **3. VITAMIN K (PHYTONADIONE)**
- **4. FIBRINOLYSIS-AFFECTING DRUGS**
- **5. ANTICOAGULANT ANTAGONISTS AND OTHER COAGULANTS**
- **6. GAMMA GLOBULIN**
- **7. NATURAL BLOOD AND BLOOD PRODUCTS**
- **8. OTHER SPECIFIED AGENTS AFFECTING BLOOD CONSTITUENTS**
- **9. UNSPECIFIED AGENTS AFFECTING BLOOD CONSTITUENTS**

972.# CARDIOVASCULAR SYSTEM DRUGS - (PRIMARILY AFFECTING)

4th Digit: 972

- **0. CARDIAC RHYTHM REGULATORS**
- **1. CARDIOTONIC GLYCOSIDES AND DRUGS OF SIMILAR ACTION**
- **2. ANTILIPEMIC AND ANTIARTERIOSCLEROTIC DRUGS**
- **3. GANGLION-BLOCKING AGENTS**
- **4. CORONARY VASODILATORS**
- **5. OTHER VASODILATORS**
- **6. OTHER ANTIHYPERTENSIVE AGENTS**
- **7. ANTIVARICOSE DRUGS, INCLUDING SCLEROSING AGENTS**
- **8. CAPILLARY-ACTIVE DRUGS**
- **9. OTHER AND NOS AGENTS PRIMARILY AFFECTING THE CARDIOVASCULAR SYSTEM**

POISONING - MEDICINAL (continued)

973.# GASTROINTESTINAL SYSTEM DRUGS (PRIMARILY AFFECTING)

4th Digit: 973

- **0. ANTACIDS AND ANTIGASTRIC SECRETION DRUGS**
- **1. IRRITANT CATHARTICS**
- **2. EMOLLIENT CATHARTICS**
- **3. OTHER CATHARTICS, INCLUDING INTESTINAL ATONIA DRUGS**
- **4. DIGESTANTS**
- **5. ANTIDIARRHEAL DRUGS**
- **6. EMETICS**
- **8. OTHER SPECIFIED AGENTS**
- **9. UNSPECIFIED AGENT AFFECTING THE GASTROINTESTINAL SYSTEM**

962.# HORMONES AND SYNTHETIC SUBSTITUTES

4th Digit: 962

- **0. ADRENAL CORTICAL STEROIDS**
- **1. ANDROGENS AND ANABOLIC CONGENERS**
- **2. OVARIAN HORMONES AND SYNTHETIC SUBSTITUTES**
- **3. INSULINS AND ANTIDIABETIC AGENTS**
- **4. ANTERIOR PITUITARY HORMONES**
- **5. POSTERIOR PITUITARY HORMONES**
- **6. PARATHYROID AND PARATHYROID DERIVATIVES**
- **7. THYROID AND THYROID DERIVATIVES**
- **8. ANTITHYROID AGENTS**
- **9. OTHER AND UNSPECIFIED HORMONES AND SYNTHETIC SUBSTITUTES**

967.# SEDATIVES AND HYPNOTICS

4th Digit: 967

- **0. BARBITURATES**
- **1. CHLORAL HYDRATE GROUP**
- **2. PARALDEHYDE**
- **3. BROMINE COMPOUNDS**
- **4. METHAQUALONE COMPOUNDS**
- **5. GLUTETHIMIDE GROUP**
- **6. MIXED SEDATIVES, NEC**
- **8. OTHER SEDATIVES AND HYPNOTICS**
- **9. UNSPECIFIED SEDATIVE OR HYPNOTIC**

968.# OTHER DEPRESSANTS AND ANESTHETICS (CENTRAL NERVOUS SYSTEM)

4th Digit: 968

- **0. CNS MUSCLE TONE DEPRESSANTS**
- **1. HALOTHANE**
- **2. OTHER GASEOUS ANESTHETICS**
- **3. INTRAVENOUS ANESTHETICS**
- **4. OTHER AND UNSPECIFIED GENERAL ANESTHETICS**
- **5. SURFACE (TOPICAL) AND INFILTRATION ANESTHETICS**
- **6. PERIPHERAL NERVE- AND PLEXUS-BLOCKING ANESTHETICS**
- **7. SPINAL ANESTHETICS**
- **9. OTHER AND UNSPECIFIED LOCAL ANESTHETICS**

969.# PSYCHOTROPIC AGENTS

4th Digit: 969

- **0. ANTIDEPRESSANTS**
- **1. PHENOTHIAZINE-BASED TRANQUILIZERS**
- **2. BUTYROPHENONE-BASED TRANQUILIZERS**
- **3. OTHER ANTIPSYCHOTICS, NEUROLEPTICS, AND MAJOR TRANQUILIZERS**
- **4. BENZODIAZEPINE-BASED TRANQUILIZERS**
- **5. OTHER TRANQUILIZERS**
- **6. PSYCHODYSLEPTICS, (HALLUCINOGENS)**
- **7. PSYCHOSTIMULANTS**
- **8. OTHER SPECIFIED PSYCHOTROPIC AGENTS**
- **9. UNSPECIFIED PSYCHOTROPIC AGENT**

POISONING - MEDICINAL (continued)

976.# SKIN AND MUCOUS MEMBRANE, OPHTHALMOLOGICAL, OTORHINOLARYNGOLOGICAL, AND DENTAL DRUGS - (PRIMARILY AFFECTING)

4th Digit: 976

- **0. LOCAL ANTI-INFECTIVES AND ANTI-INFLAMMATORY DRUGS**
- **1. ANTIPRURITICS**
- **2. LOCAL ASTRINGENTS AND LOCAL DETERGENTS**
- **3. EMOLLIENTS, DEMULCENTS, AND PROTECTANTS**
- **4. KERATOLYTICS, KERATOPLASTICS, OTHER HAIR TREATMENT DRUGS AND PREPARATIONS**
- **5. EYE ANTI-INFECTIVES AND OTHER EYE DRUGS**
- **6. ANTI-INFECTIVES AND OTHER DRUGS AND PREPARATIONS FOR EAR, NOSE, AND THROAT**
- **7. DENTAL DRUGS TOPICALLY APPLIED**
- **8. OTHER AGENTS PRIMARILY AFFECTING SKIN AND MUCOUS MEMBRANE**
- **9. UNSPECIFIED AGENT PRIMARILY AFFECTING SKIN AND MUCOUS MEMBRANE**

975.# SMOOTH MUSCLES, SKELETAL MUSCLES, RESPIRATORY SYSTEM DRUGS (PRIMARILY ACTING ON)

4th Digit: 975

- **0. OXYTOCIC AGENTS**
- **1. SMOOTH MUSCLE RELAXANTS**
- **2. SKELETAL MUSCLE RELAXANTS**
- **3. OTHER AND UNSPECIFIED DRUGS ACTING ON MUSCLES**
- **4. ANTITUSSIVES**
- **5. EXPECTORANTS**
- **6. ANTI-COMMON COLD DRUGS**
- **7. ANTIASTHMATICS**
- **8. OTHER AND UNSPECIFIED RESPIRATORY DRUGS**

970.# STIMULANTS (CENTRAL NERVOUS SYSTEM)

4th Digit: 970

- **0. ANALEPTICS**
- **1. OPIATE ANTAGONISTS**
- **8. OTHER SPECIFIED CNS STIMULANTS**
- **9. UNSPECIFIED CNS STIMULANTS**

963.# SYSTEMIC AGENTS (PRIMARILY)

4th Digit: 963

- **0. ANTIALLERGIC AND ANTIEMETIC DRUGS**
- **1. ANTINEOPLASTIC AND IMMUNOSUPPRESSIVE DRUGS**
- **2. ACIDIFYING AGENTS**
- **3. ALKALIZING AGENTS**
- **4. ENZYMES NEC**
- **5. VITAMINS NEC. (A) (D)**
- **8. OTHER SPECIFIED SYSTEMIC AGENTS**
- **9. UNSPECIFIED SYSTEMIC AGENTS**

978.# VACCINES BACTERIAL

4th Digit: 978

- **0. BCG**
- **1. TYPHOID AND PARATYPHOID**
- **2. CHOLERA**
- **3. PLAGUE**
- **4. TETANUS**
- **5. DIPHTHERIA**
- **6. PERTUSSIS VACCINE COMBINATIONS WITH A PERTUSSIS COMPONENT**
- **8. OTHER AND UNSPECIFIED BACTERIAL VACCINE**
- **9. MIXED BACTERIAL VACCINES EXCEPT COMBINATIONS WITH PERTUSSIS COMPONENT**

POISONING - MEDICINAL (continued)

979.# OTHER VACCINES AND BIOLOGICAL SUBSTANCES

4th Digit: 979

- **0. SMALLPOX VACCINE**
- **1. RABIES VACCINE**
- **2. TYPHUS VACCINE**
- **3. YELLOW FEVER VACCINE**
- **4. MEASLES VACCINE**
- **5. POLIOMYELITIS VACCINE**
- **6. OTHER AND UNSPECIFIED VIRAL AND RICKETTSIAL VACCINES**
- **7. MIXED VIRAL-RICKETTSIAL AND BACTERIAL VACCINES, EXCEPT COMBINATIONS WITH A PERTUSSIS COMPONENT**
- **9. OTHER AND UNSPECIFIED VACCINES AND BIOLOGICAL SUBSTANCES**

974.# WATER, MINERAL, AND URIC ACID METABOLISM DRUGS

4th Digit: 974

- **0. MERCURIAL DIURETICS**
- **1. PURINE DERIVATIVE DIURETICS**
- **2. CARBONIC ACID ANHYDRASE INHIBITORS**
- **3. SALURETICS**
- **4. OTHER DIURETICS**
- **5. ELECTROLYTIC, CALORIC, AND WATER-BALANCE AGENTS**
- **6. OTHER MINERAL SALTS, NEC**
- **7. URIC ACID METABOLISM DRUGS**

977.# OTHER DRUGS AND MEDICINAL SUBSTANCES

4th Digit: 977

- **0. DIETETICS**
- **1. LIPOTROPICS**
- **2. ANTIDOTES AND CHELATING AGENTS, NEC**
- **3. ALCOHOL DETERRENTS**
- **4. PHARMACEUTICAL EXCIPIENTS**
- **8. OTHER SPECIFIED DRUGS AND MEDICINALS**
- **9. UNSPECIFIED DRUG OR MEDICINAL SUBSTANCE**

POISONING - NONMEDICINAL

989.9 UNSPECIFIED SUBSTANCE CHIEFLY NONMEDICINAL AS TO SOURCE
796.0 ABNORMAL
790.3 ABNORMAL FINDINGS (NONSPECIFIC) (ALCOHOL ONLY)
982.8 ACETONE (SOLVENT)
989.7 AFLATOXIN AND OTHER MYCOTOXIN [FOOD CONTAMINANTS]
980.9 ALCOHOL
980.2 ALCOHOL (RUBBING)
980.8 ALCOHOL OTHER SPECIFIED
989.2 ALDRIN
985.4 ANTIMONY AND ITS COMPOUNDS
985.1 ARSENIC AND ITS COMPOUNDS
989.81 ASBESTOS
982.0 BENZENE AND HOMOLOGUES (SOLVENT)
981 BENZINE
988.2 BERRIES AND OTHER PLANTS
985.3 BERYLLIUM AND ITS COMPOUNDS
985.8 BRASS FUMES
987.5 BROMOBENZYL CYANIDE
987.0 BUTANE
985.5 CADMIUM AND ITS COMPOUNDS
989.3 CARBAMATE
989.3 CARBARYL
983.0 CARBOLIC ACID OR PHENOL
982.2 CARBON BISULFIDE (SOLVENT)
982.2 CARBON DISULFIDE (SOLVENT)
986 CARBON MONOXIDE FROM ANY SOURCE
982.1 CARBON TETRACHLORIDE (SOLVENT)
983.9 CAUSTIC

POISONING - NONMEDICINAL (continued)

989.2 CHLORDANE
989.9 CHLORINATED HYDROCARBON
987.6 CHLORINE GAS
987.5 CHLOROACETOPHENONE
985.6 CHROMIUM
985.8 COPPER SALTS
983.0 CRESOL
989.2 DDT
989.6 DETERGENTS
987.4 DICHLOROMONOFLUOROMETHANE
989.3 DICHLORVOS
989.2 DIELDRIN
980.2 DIMETHYL CARBINOL
796.0 DRUGS (HEAVY METALS) ABNORMAL
981 ETHER PETROLEUM

> ***980.0 ETHYL ALCOHOL:*** *USE AN ADDITIONAL CODE TO IDENTIFY ASSOCIATED DRUNKENNESS. SEE 'DRUNKENNESS.'*

980.0 ETHYL ALCOHOL
987.5 ETHYLIODOACETATE
988.0 FISH AND SHELLFISH
987.4 FREON
980.3 FUSEL OIL
987.9 GAS FUME OR VAPOR
981 GASOLINE
987.1 HYDROCARBON GAS OTHER
983.1 HYDROCHLORIC ACID (LIQUID)
987.7 HYDROCYANIC ACID (GAS) (FUMES) (VAPORS)
989.4 INSECTICIDE MIXTURES
985.8 IRON COMPOUNDS
980.2 ISOPROPANOL
981 KEROSENE
909.1 LATE EFFECT NONMEDICAL SUBSTANCES
989.82 LATEX
984.1 LEAD (TETRAETHYL)
984.1 LEAD ACETATE
984.9 LEAD COMPOUND
984.8 LEAD COMPOUNDS OTHER
984.0 LEAD DIOXIDE
984.0 LEAD SALTS
983.2 LYE
989.3 MALATHION
985.2 MANGANESE AND ITS COMPOUNDS
985.0 MERCURY AND ITS COMPOUNDS
985.9 METAL
980.1 METHANOL
988.1 MUSHROOMS
981 NAPTHA PETROLEUM
985.8 NICKEL COMPOUNDS
983.1 NITRIC ACID
987.2 NITROGEN DIOXIDE
982.4 NITROGLYCOL (SOLVENT)
987.2 NITROUS FUMES
988.8 NOXIOUS SUBSTANCES EATEN AS FOOD OTHER SPECIFIED
989.3 ORGANOPHOSPHATE AND CARBAMATE
981 PARAFFIN WAX
989.3 PARATHION
989.4 PESTICIDES NEC OTHER
981 PETROLEUM (SPIRIT)
989.3 PHORATE
989.3 PHOSDRIN
987.8 PHOSGENE
987.8 POLYESTER FUMES
989.0 POTASSIUM CYANIDE
983.2 POTASSIUM HYDROXIDE
987.0 PROPANE

POISONING - NONMEDICINAL (continued)

> ***989.83 SILICONE:*** *FOR SILICONE USED IN MEDICAL DEVICES, IMPLANTS AND GRAFTS SEE 'COMPLICATION OF A DEVICE, IMPLANT OR GRAFT.'*

989.83 SILICONE
989.6 SOAPS AND DETERGENTS
989.0 SODIUM CYANIDE
983.2 SODIUM HYDROXIDE
982.8 SOLVENT (NONPETROLEUM BASED) OTHER
989.1 STRYCHNINE AND SALTS
987.3 SULFUR DIOXIDE
983.1 SULFURIC ACID
987.5 TEAR GAS
982.3 TETRACHLOROETHYLENE (SOLVENT)
989.84 TOBACCO
982.3 TRICHLOROETHYLENE (SOLVENT)
989.5 VENOM
989.89 OTHER SUBSTANCES CHIEFLY NONMEDICINAL AS TO SOURCE

0 POISONING SEE ALSO APPENDIX B, DRUG AND CHEMICALS INDEX

0 POLIO SEE 'POLIOMYELITIS'
045.0# POLIOENCEPHALITIS BULBAR ACUTE, PARALYTIC
045.0# POLIOENCEPHALOMYELITIS BULBAR ACUTE ANTERIOR, PARALYTIC

5th Digit: 045.0

0. UNSPECIFIED
1. TYPE I
2. TYPE II
3. TYPE III

POLIOMYELITIS

045.9# ACUTE UNSPECIFIED
045.2# ACUTE ANTERIOR NONPARALYTIC
045.1# ACUTE ATROPHIC
045.2# ACUTE EPIDEMIC NONPARALYTIC
045.1# ACUTE EPIDEMIC PARALYTIC
045.1# ACUTE INFANTILE PARALYTIC
138 ACUTE LATE EFFECTS
045.2# ACUTE NONPARALYTIC
045.1# ACUTE PARALYTIC
045.1# ACUTE SPINAL PARALYTIC
045.0# BULBAR ACUTE ANTERIOR PARALYTIC
045.0# BULBAR ACUTE ANTERIOR POLIOENCEPHALOMYELITIS PARALYTIC
045.0# BULBAR ACUTE INFANTILE PARALYTIC
045.0# BULBAR ACUTE PARALYTIC
045.0# BULBAR ACUTE POLIOENCEPHALITIS PARALYTIC
045.1# OTHER PARALYSIS ACUTE

5th Digit: 045.0-2, 9

0. UNSPECIFIED
1. TYPE I
2. TYPE II
3. TYPE III

V01.2 EXPOSURE
V12.02 HISTORY
V73.0 SCREENING EXAM
V04.0 VACCINATION

704.3 POLIOSIS
704.3 POLIOSIS CIRCUMSCRIPTA ACQUIRED
V62.4 POLITICAL DISCRIMINATION CAUSING ENCOUNTER
788.41 POLLAKIURIA
705.83 POLLITZER'S DISEASE (HIDRADENITIS SUPPURATIVA)
729.9 POLYALGIA

POLYARTERITIS

446.0 NODOSA
446.0 NODOSA MYOPATHY [359.6]
446.0 NODOSA WITH DEMENTIA [294.1]
648.9# MATERNAL CURRENT (CO-EXISTENT) IN PREGNANCY [446.0]

5th Digit: 648.9

- **0. EPISODE OF NOS OR N/A**
- **1. DELIVERED**
- **2. DELIVERED WITH POSTPARTUM COMPLICATION**
- **3. ANTEPARTUM COMPLICATION**
- **4. POSTPARTUM COMPLICATION**

POLYARTHRITIS

716.5# NOS

5th Digit: 716.5

- **0. SITE NOS**
- **1. SHOULDER REGION**
- **2. UPPER ARM (ELBOW) (HUMERUS)**
- **3. FOREARM (RADIUS) (WRIST) (ULNA)**
- **4. HAND (CARPAL) (METACARPAL) (FINGERS)**
- **5. PELVIC REGION (HIP) (BUTTOCK) (FEMUR)**
- **6. LOWER LEG (FIBULA) (KNEE) (PATELLA) (TIBIA)**
- **7. ANKLE AND/OR FOOT (METATARSALS) (TOES) (TARSALS)**
- **8. OTHER (HEAD) (NECK) (RIB) (SKULL) (TRUNK) (VERTEBRAE)**
- **9. MULTIPLE**

714.0 ATROPHIC
714.9 INFLAMMATORY
714.89 INFLAMMATORY NEC
714.31 JUVENILE ACUTE
714.30 JUVENILE CHRONIC

260 POLYCARENTIAL OF INFANCY SYNDROME
733.99 POLYCHONDRITIS RELAPSING

POLYCYSTIC DISEASE

759.89 NOS (CONGENITAL)
753.12 KIDNEY (CONGENITAL)
753.13 KIDNEY (CONGENITAL) - ADULT TYPE (APKD)
753.13 KIDNEY (CONGENITAL) - AUTOSOMAL DOMINANT
753.14 KIDNEY (CONGENITAL) - AUTOSOMAL RECESSIVE
753.14 KIDNEY (CONGENITAL) - CHILDHOOD TYPE (INFANTILE) (CPKD)
V18.61 KIDNEY FAMILY HISTORY
751.62 LIVER CONGENITAL
518.89 LUNG (PULMONARY)
748.4 LUNG (PULMONARY) - CONGENITAL
256.4 OVARIES
759.0 SPLEEN

POLYCYTHEMIA

790.0 NOS
289.0 ACQUIRED
289.0 BENIGN
289.6 BENIGN FAMILIAL
776.4 DUE TO DONOR TWIN TRANSFUSION
289.0 DUE TO FALL IN PLASMA VOLUME
289.0 DUE TO HIGH ALTITUDE
776.4 DUE TO MATERNAL TWIN TRANSFUSION
289.0 EMOTIONAL
289.6 ERYTHROCYTOSIS BENIGN FAMILIAL
289.0 ERYTHROPOEITIN INDUCED
289.0 ERYTHROPOIETIN
289.6 FAMILIAL
289.0 HEMOGLOBIN
289.0 HIGH OXYGEN AFFINITY
289.0 HYPOXEMIC
238.4 PRIMARY
776.4 NEONATORUM
762.3 NEONATORUM PLACENTAL TRANSFUSION [776.4]
289.0 NEPHROGENOUS

POLYCYTHEMIA (continued)

289.0 RELATIVE
776.4 SECONDARY
289.0 SECONDARY (ACQUIRED)
289.0 SPURIOUS
289.0 STRESS
238.4 VERA SITE NOS
0 VERA SITE SPECIFIED SEE 'NEOPLASM UNCERTAIN BEHAVIOR' BY SITE M9950/1

POLYDACTYLY

755.00 DIGITS
755.01 FINGERS
755.02 TOES

783.5 POLYDIPSIA

199.1 POLYEMBRYOMA SITE NOS
0 POLYEMBRYOMA SITE SPECIFIED SEE 'CANCER' BY SITE M9072/3

258.9 POLYGLANDULAR DYSFUNCTION (ENDOCRINE)
258.8 POLYGLANDULAR DYSFUNCTION OR SYNDROME OTHER SPECIFIED (ENDOCRINE)

199.1 POLYGONAL CELL CARCINOMA SITE NOS
0 POLYGONAL CELL CARCINOMA SITE SPECIFIED SEE 'CANCER' BY SITE M8034/3

657.0# POLYHYDRAMNIOS

5th Digit: 657.0

- **0. EPISODE OF CARE UNSPECIFIED OR N/A**
- **1. DELIVERED**
- **3. ANTEPARTUM COMPLICATION**

761.3 POLYHYDRAMNIOS AFFECTING FETUS OR NEWBORN

626.2 POLYMENORRHEA
692.72 POLYMORPHOUS LIGHT ERUPTION (ACUTE)
725 POLYMYALGIA RHEUMATICA

POLYMYOSITIS

710.4 POLYMYOSITIS
728.19 POLYMYOSITIS OSSIFICANS
710.3 SKIN INVOLVEMENT
710.4 WITH LUNG INVOLVEMENT [517.8]

357.0 POLYNEURITIS ACUTE INFECTIVE
291.1 POLYNEURITIS ALCOHOLIC PSYCHOSIS
291.5 POLYNEURITIS ALCOHOLIC PSYCHOSIS WITH DELUSIONS
291.3 POLYNEURITIS ALCOHOLIC PSYCHOSIS WITH HALLUCINATIONS
352.6 POLYNEURITIS CRANIALIS
357.8 POLYNEURITIS DEMYELINATING CHRONIC INFLAMMATORY
357.0 POLYNEURITIS POSTINFECTIOUS
0 POLYNEURITIS SEE ALSO 'NEUROPATHY'

POLYNEUROPATHY

357.9 NOS
357.5 ALCOHOLIC
277.3 AMYLOID [357.4]
265.0 BERIBERI [357.4]
266.2 DEFICIENCY OF B- COMPLEX [357.4]
266.9 DEFICIENCY OF VITAMIN B [357.4]
266.1 DEFICIENCY OF VITAMIN B6 [357.4]
269.2 DEFICIENCY VITAMIN [357.4]
357.8 DEMYELINATING CHRONIC PROGRESSIVE (RELAPSING)

POLYNEUROPATHY (continued)

250.6#	DIABETIC [357.2]
250.6#	DIABETIC PERIPHERAL AUTONOMIC [337.1]
	5th Digit: 250.6
	0. TYPE II, ADULT-ONSET, NON-INSULIN DEPENDENT (EVEN IF REQUIRING INSULIN), OR UNSPECIFIED; CONTROLLED
	1. TYPE I, JUVENILE-ONSET OR INSULIN-DEPENDENT; CONTROLLED
	2. TYPE II, ADULT-ONSET, NON-INSULIN DEPENDENT (EVEN IF REQUIRING INSULIN); UNCONTROLLED
	3. TYPE I, JUVENILE-ONSET OR INSULIN-DEPENDENT; UNCONTROLLED
357.6	DUE TO DRUGS
710.0	DUE TO LUPUS ERYTHEMATOUS [357.1]
356.0	HEREDITARY
356.4	IDIOPATHIC PROGRESSIVE
269.2	IN AVITAMINOSIS [357.4]
269.1	IN AVITAMINOSIS SPECIFIED NEC [357.4]
710.9	IN COLLAGEN VASCULAR DISEASE [357.1]
199.1	MALIGNANT (NEOPLASTIC) [357.3]
072.72	MUMPS
265.2	PELLAGRA [357.4]
277.1	PORPHYRIA [357.4]
053.13	POSTHERPETIC
724.4	RADICULAR THORACIC NEC
714.0	RHEUMATOID ARTHRITIS [357.1]
353.1	SACRAL PLEXUS
135	SARCOIDOSIS [357.4]
355.0	SCIATIC
356.2	SENSORY (HEREDITARY)
355.9	SPINAL NERVE NEC
729.2	SPINAL NERVE ROOT
0	SPINAL NERVE ROOT SEE 'RADICULITIS'
357.7	TOXIC
350.8	TRIGEMINAL SENSORY
354.2	ULNAR NERVE
354.9	UPPER EXTREMITY NEC
585	UREMIC [357.4]
266.2	VITAMIN B12 [357.4]
281.0	VITAMIN B12 WITH ANEMIA (PERNICIOUS) [357.4]
357.8	OTHER SPECIFIED
0	SEE ALSO 'NEUROPATHY'

368.15	POLYOPIA REFRACTIVE
752.8	POLYORCHISM CONGENITAL
756.54	POLYOSTOTIC FIBROUS DYSPLASIA BONE
744.1	POLYOTIA CONGENITAL

POLYPS OF SITES NOT LISTED BELOW SHOULD BE CODED TO DISEASE OF THE SPECIFIED ANATOMICAL SITE.

POLYP

471.8	ACCESSORY SINUS
212.0	ACCESSORY SINUS ADENOMATOUS
199.1	ADENOCARCINOMA SITE NOS
0	ADENOCARCINOMA SITE SPECIFIED SEE 'CANCER' BY SITE M8210/3
471.0	ADENOID
212.0	ADENOID ADENOMATOUS
0	ADENOMATOUS UNSPECIFIED SEE 'BENIGN NEOPLASM', BY SITE M8210/0
211.4	ANAL (CANAL) ADENOMATOUS
569.0	ANAL (CANAL) NONADENOMATOUS
471.8	ANTRUM
212.0	ANTRUM ADENOMATOUS
624.6	BARTHOLIN'S GLAND
620.8	BROAD LIGAMENT OR FALLOPIAN TUBE (NONPREGNANT)

POLYP (continued)

211.3	CECUM
622.7	CERVIX
219.0	CERVIX ADENOMATOUS
622.7	CERVIX MUCOUS
0	CERVIX (MATERNAL) SEE CERVIX ABNORMALITY MATERNAL
471.0	CHOANAL
212.0	CHOANAL ADENOMATOUS
575.6	CHOLESTEROL
624.6	CLITORIS
211.3	COLON ADENOMATOUS M/8210/0
569.89	COLON NONADENOMATOUS
211.4	COLON, RECTOSIGMOID JUNCTION ADENOMATOUS
621.0	CORPUS UTERI
575.6	CYSTIC DUCT
522.0	DENTAL PULP
385.30	EAR (MIDDLE)
621.0	ENDOMETRIUM
471.8	ETHMOID SINUS
212.0	ETHMOID SINUS ADENOMATOUS
620.8	FALLOPIAN TUBE
624.8	FEMALE GENITAL ORGANS NEC
471.8	FRONTAL SINUS
212.0	FRONTAL SINUS ADENOMATOUS
575.6	GALLBLADDER
624.8	GENITAL ORGANS (FEMALE) NEC
523.8	GINGIVAL
523.8	GUM
211.3	ILEUM
624.6	LABIA AND VULVA
478.4	LARYNX
212.1	LARYNX ADENOMATOUS
471.8	MAXILLARY SINUS
212.0	MAXILLARY SINUS ADENOMATOUS
229.9	MULTIPLE ADENOMATOUS SITE NOS
0	MULTIPLE ADENOMATOUS SITE SPECIFIED SEE 'BENIGN NEOPLASM', BY SITE M8221/0
621.0	MYOMETRIUM
212.0	NARES ADENOMATOUS
471.9	NARES ANTERIOR
471.0	NARES POSTERIOR
471.9	NASAL (MUCOUS)
212.0	NASAL (MUCOUS) ADENOMATOUS
471.0	NASAL CAVITY
212.0	NASAL CAVITY ADENOMATOUS
471.9	NASAL SEPTUM
212.0	NASAL SEPTUM ADENOMATOUS
471.0	NASAL CHOANAL
212.0	NASAL CHOANAL ADENOMATOUS
471.0	NASOPHARYNGEAL
212.0	NASOPHARYNGEAL ADENOMATOUS
0	NEOPLASTIC SEE 'BENIGN NEOPLASM', BY SITE M/8210/0
620.8	OVIDUCT
620.8	PARATUBAL
478.29	PHARYNX
750.29	PHARYNX CONGENITAL
674.4#	PLACENTAL MATERNAL DUE TO PREGNANCY
	5th Digit: 674.4
	0. UNSPECIFIED
	2. DELIVERED WITH POSTPARTUM COMPLICATION
	4. POSTPARTUM COMPLICATION
600	PROSTATE
624.6	PUDENDAL
569.0	RECTAL
211.4	RECTAL ADENOMATOUS
569.0	RECTAL NONADENOMATOUS
211.4	RECTOSIGMOID ADENOMATOUS
471.8	SINUS NOS
471.8	SPHENOIDAL SINUS
212.0	SPHENOIDAL SINUS ADENOMATOUS
211.1	STOMACH M8210/0

POLYP (continued)

471.8 TURBINATE (MUCOUS MEMBRANE)
212.0 TURBINATE (MUCOUS MEMBRANE) ADENOMATOUS
593.89 URETER
599.3 URETHRA
621.0 UTERINE
620.8 UTERINE LIGAMENT
620.8 UTERINE TUBE
763.89 UTERUS BODY (CORPUS) (MUCOUS) AFFECTING FETUS OR NEWBORN
654.1# UTERUS BODY (CORPUS) (MUCOUS) IN PREGNANCY
660.2# UTERUS BODY (CORPUS) (MUCOUS) OBSTRUCTING LABOR **[654.1#]**

5th Digit: 654.1
- **0. EPISODE OF CARE UNSPECIFIED OR N/A**
- **1. DELIVERED**
- **2. DELIVERED WITH POSTPARTUM COMPLICATION**
- **3. ANTEPARTUM COMPLICATION**

5th Digit: 660.2
- **0. EPISODE OF CARE UNSPECIFIED OR N/A**
- **1. DELIVERED**
- **3. ANTEPARTUM COMPLICATION**

623.7 VAGINA
478.4 VOCAL CORD
212.1 VOCAL CORD ADENOMATOUS
624.6 VULVA

783.6 POLYPHAGIA ORGANIC
471.1 POLYPOID SINUS DEGENERATION
357.0 POLYRADICULITIS (ACUTE)
278.00 POLYSARCIA
759.0 POLYSPLENIA SYNDROME
704.1 POLYTRICHIA
788.42 POLYURIA

271.0 POMPE'S DISEASE (GLYCOGENOSIS II)
705.81 POMPHOLYX

015.9# PONCET'S DISEASE (TUBERCULOUS RHEUMATISM) (SEE ALSO 'TUBERCULOSIS')

5th Digit: 015.9
- **0. UNSPECIFIED**
- **1. LAB NOT DONE**
- **2. LABS PENDING**
- **3. MICROSCOPY POSITIVE (IN SPUTUM)**
- **4. CULTURE POSITIVE - MICROSCOPY NEGATIVE**
- **5. CULTURE NEGATIVE - MICROSCOPY POSITIVE**
- **6. CULTURE AND MICROSCOPY NEGATIVE CONFIRMED BY OTHER METHODS**

433.8# PONTINE ARTERY OCCLUSION OR SYNDROME
433.8# PONTINE ARTERY THROMBOSIS (EMBOLISM) (DEFORMANS)

5th Digit: 433.8
- **0. WITHOUT CEREBRAL INFARCTION**
- **1. WITH CEREBRAL INFARCTION**

431 PONTINE HEMORRHAGE (CEREBRAL)
674.0# PONTINE HEMORRHAGE MATERNAL DUE TO PREGNANCY

5th Digit: 674.0
- **0. EPISODE OF CARE UNSPECIFIED OR N/A**
- **1. DELIVERED**
- **2. DELIVERED WITH POSTPARTUM COMPLICATION**
- **3. ANTEPARTUM COMPLICATION**
- **4. POSTPARTUM COMPLICATION**

INJURY OF A BLOOD VESSEL CAN BE A LACERATION, A-V FISTULA, ANEURYSM, OR HEMATOMA. USE THE "INJURY" CODE FOUND BY ANATOMICAL SITE (THE NAME OF THE BLOOD VESSEL).

POPLITEAL

442.3 ARTERY ANEURYSM
440.2# ARTERY ARTERIOSCLEROSIS

5th Digit: 440.2
- **0. UNSPECIFIED**
- **1. WITH INTERMITTENT CLAUDICATION**
- **2. WITH REST PAIN, OR REST PAIN AND (INTERMITTENT CLAUDICATION)**
- **3. WITH ULCERATION, OR ULCERATION AND (INTERMITTENT CLAUDICATION) (REST PAIN)**
- **4. WITH ISCHEMIC GANGRENE, OR ISCHEMIC GANGRENE AND (INTERMITTENT CLAUDICATION) (REST PAIN) (ULCERATION)**
- **9. OTHER ATHEROSCLEROSIS EXTREMITIES**

440.3# ARTERY BYPASS GRAFT ARTERIOSCLEROSIS

5th Digit: 440.3
- **0. UNSPECIFIED GRAFT**
- **1. AUTOLOGOUS VEIN BYPASS GRAFT**
- **2. NONAUTOLOGOUS BIOLOGICAL BYPASS GRAFT**

904.41 ARTERY INJURY
908.3 ARTERY INJURY LATE EFFECT
447.8 ENTRAPMENT (SYNDROME)
904.42 VEIN INJURY
908.3 VEIN INJURY LATE EFFECT
904.40 VESSEL INJURY VESSEL UNSPECIFIED
908.3 VESSEL INJURY LATE EFFECT
756.89 WEB SYNDROME

POPLITEAL NERVE

355.3 DISORDER LATERAL
355.4 DISORDER MEDIAL
355.3 NEURITIS LATERAL
355.4 NEURITIS MEDIAL

348.0 PORENCEPHALY
742.4 PORENCEPHALY CONGENITAL

123.0 PORK TAPEWORM (ADULT) (INFECTION)
757.39 POROTERATOSIS

277.1 PORPHYRIA
277.1 PORPHYRIA POLYNEUROPATHY [357.4]

277.1 PORPHYRIN METABOLISM DISORDER
277.1 PORPHYRINURIA

PORTAL

571.5 CIRRHOSIS
571.5 CIRRHOSIS WITH ESOPHAGEAL VARICES **[456.2#]**

5th Digit: 456.2
- **0. WITH BLEEDING**
- **1. WITHOUT BLEEDING**

572.3 HYPERTENSION
572.3 HYPERTENSION WITH ESOPHAGEAL VARICES **[456.2#]**

5th Digit: 456.2
- **0. WITH BLEEDING**
- **1. WITHOUT BLEEDING**

452 OBSTRUCTION
572.2 SYSTEMIC ENCEPHALOPATHY
572.1 THROMBOPHLEBITIS
747.49 VEIN ABSENCE (ATRESIA)
452 VEIN EMBOLISM
902.33 VEIN INJURY
908.4 VEIN INJURY LATE EFFECT
452 VEIN OBSTRUCTION
572.1 VEIN PHLEBITIS
452 VEIN THROMBOSIS
093.89 VEIN THROMBOSIS DUE TO SYPHILIS
572.1 VEIN THROMBOSIS INFECTIONAL OR SEPTIC
572.1 VEIN THROMBOPHLEBITIS

757.32 PORTWINE STAIN CONGENITAL

114.9 POSADAS-WERNICKE DISEASE
V46.8 POSSUM DEPENDENCE

627.4 POSTARTIFICIAL MENOPAUSE SYNDROME
429.4 POSTCARDIOTOMY SYNDROME
576.0 POSTCHOLECYSTECTOMY SYNDROME
626.7 POSTCOITAL BLEEDING
429.4 POSTCOMMISSUROTOMY SYNDROME
310.2 POSTCONCUSSION SYNDROME (POSTCONTUSIONAL SYNDROME) (MENTAL DISORDER)

310.8 POSTENCEPHALITIS SYNDROME (MENTAL DISORDER)

372.64 POSTENUCLEATION CONTRACTION EYE SOCKET

POSTERIOR

723.2 CERVICAL SYMPATHETIC SYNDROME
433.8# COMMUNICATING ARTERY OBSTRUCTION (THROMBOSIS)
5th Digit: 433.8
0. WITHOUT CEREBRAL INFARCTION
1. WITH CEREBRAL INFARCTION

844.2 CRUCIATE LIGAMENT SPRAIN, STRAIN ACUTE
717.84 CRUCIATE LIGAMENT SPRAIN, STRAIN OLD
348.4 FOSSA COMPRESSION SYNDROME
436 INFERIOR CEREBELLAR ARTERY SYNDROME
524.2 LINGUAL OCCLUSION MANDIBULAR TEETH
743.54 SEGMENT CONGENITAL FOLDS AND CYSTS
904.53 TIBIAL ARTERY INJURY
908.3 TIBIAL ARTERY INJURY LATE EFFECT
355.5 TIBIAL NERVE COMPRESSION
956.2 TIBIAL NERVE INJURY
907.5 TIBIAL NERVE INJURY LATE EFFECT
904.54 TIBIAL VEIN INJURY
908.3 TIBIAL VEIN INJURY LATE EFFECT

564.2 POSTGASTRECTOMY SYNDROME (DUMPING) (POSTGASTRIC SURGERY)

780.79 POSTHEPATITIS SYNDROME
053.11 POSTHERPETIC (NEURALGIA) GENICULATE GANGLION (SYNDROME)
053.19 POSTHERPETIC (NEURALGIA) INTERCOSTAL (ZOSTER) OPHTHALMICA (SYNDROME)
053.12 POSTHERPETIC TRIGEMINAL NEURALGIA

411.0 POSTINFARCTION SYNDROME
780.79 POSTINFLUENZA (ASTHENIA) SYNDROME
990 POSTIRRADIATION SYNDROME

POSTLAMINECTOMY SYNDROME IS THE CONTINUOUS PROGRESSION OF SCAR TISSUE FORMATION AT THE LAMINECTOMY SITE. THIS CONDITION IS MARKED BY CONSTANT PAIN DUE TO THE SCAR TISSUE AND IS A BASICALLY UNTREATABLE CONDITION. ASSIGN A CODE FROM THIS SECTION WHEN THE PHYSICIAN STATES THAT THE PAIN IS DUE TO SCAR TISSUE.

POSTLAMINECTOMY SYNDROME

722.80 NOS
722.81 CERVICAL
722.83 LUMBAR
722.82 THORACIC

310.0 POSTLEUKOTOMY SYNDROME (STATE)
310.0 POSTLOBOTOMY SYNDROME

457.0 POSTMASTECTOMY LYMPHEDEMA SYNDROME
766.2 POSTMATURE SYNDROME (OF NEWBORN)

627.1 POSTMENOPAUSAL BLEEDING
627.9 POSTMENOPAUSAL DISORDER UNSPECIFIED
627.8 POSTMENOPAUSAL DISORDER OTHER SPECIFIED NEC
V07.4 POSTMENOPAUSAL HORMONE REPLACEMENT THERAPY (PROPHYLACTIC)

411.0 POSTMYOCARDIAL INFARCTION SYNDROME
473.9 POSTNASAL DRIP

579.2 POSTOPERATIVE BLIND LOOP SYNDROME
998.9 POSTOPERATIVE COMPLICATION OR SYNDROME NOS (SEE ALSO 'COMPLICATION')
998.89 POSTOPERATIVE COMPLICATION SPECIFIED NEC (SEE ALSO 'COMPLICATION')
0 POSTOPERATIVE STATUS SEE 'STATUS'

POSTPARTUM

V24.0 CARE IMMEDIATELY AFTER DELIVERY (ROUTINE)
V24.1 CARE LACTATING MOTHER
V24.2 CARE ROUTINE FOLLOW-UP
648.4# BLUES
648.4# DEPRESSION - NOS [311]
648.4# DEPRESSION - PSYCHOTIC - RECURRENT [**296.3#**]
648.4# DEPRESSION - PSYCHOTIC - SINGLE EPISODE [**296.2#**]
5th Digit: 648.4
0. EPISODE OF CARE NOS
1. DELIVERED WITH OR WITHOUT MENTION OF ANTEPARTUM CONDITION
2. DELIVERED WITH MENTION OF POSTPARTUM COMPLICATION
3. ANTEPARTUM CONDITION
4. POSTPARTUM COMPLICATION

5th Digit: 296.2-3
0. UNSPECIFIED
1. MILD
2. MODERATE
3. SEVERE WITHOUT MENTION OF PSYCHOTIC BEHAVIOR
4. SEVERE SPECIFIED AS WITH PSYCHOTIC BEHAVIOR
5. IN PARTIAL OR UNSPECIFIED REMISSION

253.2 PANHYPOPITUITARY SYNDROME

999.8 POSTPERFUSION SYNDROME NEC
996.85 POSTPERFUSION BONE MARROW SYNDROME NEC
429.4 POSTPERICARDIOTOMY SYNDROME
459.1 POSTPHLEBITIS SYNDROME
648.9# POSTPHLEBITIS SYNDROME MATERNAL CURRENT (CO-EXISTENT) IN PREGNANCY [459.1]
5th Digit: 648.9
0. EPISODE OF NOS OR N/A
1. DELIVERED
2. DELIVERED WITH POSTPARTUM COMPLICATION
3. ANTEPARTUM COMPLICATION
4. POSTPARTUM COMPLICATION

138 POST POLIO SYNDROME
138 POSTPOLIOMYELITIS SYNDROME

V58.49 POSTSURGICAL AFTERCARE NEC
244.0 POSTSURGICAL HYPOTHYROIDISM
V45.89 POSTSURGICAL STATUS NEC

766.2 POST TERM INFANT
645.0# POST TERM PREGNANCY
5th Digit: 645.0
0. EPISODE OF CARE UNSPECIFIED OR N/A
1. DELIVERED
3. ANTEPARTUM COMPLICATION

998.11 POST TONSILLECTOMY HEMORRHAGE

287.4 POSTTRANSFUSION PURPURA
310.2 POSTTRAUMATIC BRAIN SYNDROME NONPSYCHOTIC

POSTTRAUMATIC STRESS SYNDROME

309.81 STRESS SYNDROME - UNSPECIFIED
308.3 ACUTE
308.3 BRIEF
309.81 CHRONIC
309.81 PROLONGED

337.2# POSTTRAUMATIC SYMPATHETIC DYSTROPHY
5th Digit: 337.2
0. UNSPECIFIED
1. UPPER LIMB
2. LOWER LIMB
9. OTHER SPECIFIED SITE

958.3 POSTTRAUMATIC WOUND INFECTION
908.6 POSTTRAUMATIC WOUND INFECTION LATE EFFECT
781.9 POSTURE ABNORMAL
564.2 POSTVAGOTOMY SYNDROME
429.4 POSTVALVULOTOMY SYNDROME
780.79 POSTVIRAL SYNDROME (ASTHENIA) (MALAISE OR FATIGUE)
514 POTAIN'S DISEASE (PULMONARY EDEMA)
536.1 POTAIN'S SYNDROME (GASTRECTASIS WITH DYSPEPSIA)

POTASSIUM
276.8 DEFICIENCY (HYPOKALEMIA)
269.3 DEFICIENCY NUTRITIONAL
276.7 ELEVATED, EXCESS (HYPERKALEMIA)
276.7 INTOXICATION SYNDROME

POTT'S DISEASE (TUBERCULOSIS OF THE SPINE)
015.0# NOS [730.88]
015.0# OSTEOMYELITIS [730.88]
015.0# PARAPLEGIA [730.88]
015.0# SPINAL CURVATURE [737.43]
015.0# SPONDYLITIS [720.81]
5th Digit: 015.0
0. UNSPECIFIED
1. LAB NOT DONE
2. LABS PENDING
3. MICROSCOPY POSITIVE (IN SPUTUM)
4. CULTURE POSITIVE - MICROSCOPY NEGATIVE
5. CULTURE NEGATIVE - MICROSCOPY POSITIVE
6. CULTURE AND MICROSCOPY NEGATIVE CONFIRMED BY OTHER METHODS

440.24 POTT'S ISCHEMIC GANGRENE
753.0 POTTER'S DISEASE OR SYNDROME
754.0 POTTER'S FACIES
714.2 POULET'S DISEASE
V60.2 POVERTY
063.8 POWASSAN ENCEPHALITIS
795.5 PPD POSITIVE (WITHOUT ACTIVE TB)
041.81 PPLO INFECTION
V03.82 PPV VACCINATION
759.81 PRADER (-LABHART) -WILLI (-FANCONI) SYNDROME
744.1 PREAURICULAR APPENDAGE CONGENITAL
744.47 PREAURICULAR CYST CONGENITAL
744.46 PREAURICULAR SINUS OR FISTULA CONGENITAL
0 PRECANCEROUS MELANOSIS SEE 'CA IN SITU' SKIN BY SITE M8741/2
433.9# PRECEREBRAL ARTERY EMBOLISM, THROMBOSIS, OBSTRUCTION OR OCCLUSION
433.3# PRECEREBRAL ARTERY EMBOLISM, THROMBOSIS, OBSTRUCTION OR OCCLUSION MULTIPLE AND BILATERAL
433.8# PRECEREBRAL ARTERY EMBOLISM, THROMBOSIS, OBSTRUCTION OR OCCLUSION OTHER SPECIFIED
5th Digit: 433.3, 8-9
0. WITHOUT CEREBRAL INFARCTION
1. WITH CEREBRAL INFARCTION

763.6 PRECIPITATE DELIVERY AFFECTING FETUS OR NEWBORN
661.3# PRECIPITATE LABOR
5th Digit: 661.3
0. EPISODE OF CARE UNSPECIFIED OR N/A
1. DELIVERED
3. ANTEPARTUM COMPLICATION

PRECOCIOUS PUBERTY
259.1 NOS
255.2 CORTICAL HYPERFUNCTION (ADRENAL)
256.1 OVARIAN HYPERFUNCTION
256.0 OVARIAN HYPERFUNCTION ESTROGEN (HYPERESTROGENISM)
259.8 PINEAL TUMOR
257.0 TESTICULAR HYPERFUNCTION

786.51 PRECORDIAL CHEST PAIN
785.3 PRECORDIAL FRICTION
790.2 PREDIABETES
775.8 PREDIABETES COMPLICATING FETUS OR NEWBORN
648.8# PREDIABETES IN PREGNANCY
5th Digit: 648.8
0. EPISODE OF CARE UNSPECIFIED OR N/A
1. DELIVERED
2. DELIVERED WITH POSTPARTUM COMPLICATION
3. ANTEPARTUM COMPLICATION
4. POSTPARTUM COMPLICATION

PRE-ECLAMPSIA
642.4# NOS
760.0 AFFECTING FETUS OR NEWBORN
642.4# MILD
642.7# OR ECLAMPSIA WITH PRE-EXISTING HYPERTENSION
642.5# SEVERE
5th Digit: 642.4-5, 7
0. EPISODE OF CARE UNSPECIFIED OR N/A
1. DELIVERED
2. DELIVERED WITH POSTPARTUM COMPLICATION
3. ANTEPARTUM COMPLICATION
4. POSTPARTUM COMPLICATION

V70.5 PREEMPLOYMENT EXAM (HEALTH)
365.00 PREGLAUCOMA

PREGNANCY
V72.4 EXAM (UNCONFIRMED PREGNANCY)
0 COMPLICATIONS SEE ALSO 'LABOR AND DELIVERY COMPLICATIONS' (FOR COMPLICATIONS OF L AND D)
0 COMPLICATIONS SEE ALSO 'PREGNANCY COMPLICATIONS'
646.9# COMPLICATION UNSPECIFIED
5th Digit: 646.9
0. EPISODE OF CARE UNSPECIFIED OR N/A
1. DELIVERED
3. ANTEPARTUM COMPLICATION

761.9 COMPLICATION UNSPECIFIED AFFECTING FETUS OR NEWBORN

646.8#: SPECIFY THE MATERNAL COMPLICATION WITH AN ADDITIONAL CODE.

646.8# COMPLICATION OTHER SPECIFIED
5th Digit: 646.8
0. EPISODE OF CARE UNSPECIFIED OR N/A
1. DELIVERED
2. DELIVERED WITH POSTPARTUM COMPLICATION
3. ANTEPARTUM COMPLICATION
4. POSTPARTUM COMPLICATION

761.8 COMPLICATION OTHER SPECIFIED AFFECTING FETUS OR NEWBORN
300.11 FALSE
V22.2 INCIDENTAL FINDING
677 LATE EFFECT
645.0# POST TERM
5th Digit: 645.0
0. EPISODE OF CARE UNSPECIFIED OR N/A
1. DELIVERED
3. ANTEPARTUM COMPLICATION

779.6 TERMINATION CAUSING FETAL DEATH

PREGNANCY COMPLICATIONS

ABNORMALITIES OF PELVIC ORGANS OR TISSUE: COMPLICATING PREGNANCY, (CHILDBIRTH) (PUERPERIUM)

654.4# BLADDER DILATATION
660.2# BLADDER DILATATION OBSTRUCTING LABOR **[654.4#]**
654.5# CERVICAL INCOMPETENCE
660.2# CERVICAL INCOMPETENCE OBSTRUCTING LABOR **[654.5#]**
654.6# CERVICAL POLYP
660.2# CERVICAL POLYP OBSTRUCTING LABOR **[654.6#]**
654.6# CERVICAL STENOSIS
660.2# CERVICAL STENOSIS OBSTRUCTING LABOR **[654.6#]**
654.6# CERVIX ABNORMALITY
660.2# CERVIX ABNORMALITY OBSTRUCTING LABOR **[654.6#]**
654.6# CERVIX CICATRIX
660.2# CERVIX CICATRIX OBSTRUCTING LABOR **[654.6#]**
654.6# CERVIX RIGID
660.2# CERVIX RIGID OBSTRUCTING LABOR **[654.6#]**
654.6# CERVIX TUMOR
660.2# CERVIX TUMOR OBSTRUCTING LABOR **[654.6#]**
654.2# CESAREAN SECTION (PREVIOUS)
660.2# CESAREAN SECTION (PREVIOUS) OBSTRUCTING LABOR **[654.2#]**
654.4# CYSTOCELE
660.2# CYSTOCELE OBSTRUCTING LABOR **[654.4#]**
654.4# KIDNEY ECTOPIC
660.2# KIDNEY ECTOPIC OBSTRUCTING LABOR **[654.4#]**
654.6# LOCKED TWINS
660.5# LOCKED TWINS OBSTRUCTING LABOR **[654.6#]**
654.9# OTHER AND UNSPECIFIED ABNORMALITY
660.2# OTHER AND UNSPECIFIED ABNORMALITY OBSTRUCTING LABOR **[654.9#]**
654.4# PENDULOUS ABDOMEN
660.2# PENDULOUS ABDOMEN OBSTRUCTING LABOR **[654.4#]**
654.8# PERINEAL FIBROSIS
660.2# PERINEAL FIBROSIS OBSTRUCTING LABOR **[654.8#]**
654.8# PERINEUM RIGID
660.2# PERINEUM RIGID OBSTRUCTING LABOR **[654.8#]**

5th Digit: 654.2, 4-6, 8-9

0. EPISODE OF CARE UNSPECIFIED OR N/A
1. DELIVERED
2. DELIVERED WITH POSTPARTUM COMPLICATION
3. ANTEPARTUM COMPLICATION
4. POSTPARTUM COMPLICATION

5th Digit: 660.2

0. EPISODE OF CARE UNSPECIFIED OR N/A
1. DELIVERED
3. ANTEPARTUM COMPLICATION

PREGNANCY COMPLICATIONS

ABNORMALITIES OF PELVIC ORGANS OR TISSUE: COMPLICATING PREGNANCY, (CHILDBIRTH) (PUERPERIUM) (continued)

654.8# PERSISTENT HYMEN
660.2# PERSISTENT HYMEN OBSTRUCTING LABOR **[654.8#]**
654.2# PREVIOUS C SECTION
660.2# PREVIOUS C SECTION OBSTRUCTING LABOR **[654.2#]**
654.4# RECTOCELE
660.2# RECTOCELE OBSTRUCTING LABOR **[654.4#]**
654.7# SEPTATE VAGINA
660.2# SEPTATE VAGINA OBSTRUCTING LABOR **[654.7#]**
654.5# SHIRODKAR SUTURE
660.2# SHIRODKAR SUTURE OBSTRUCTING LABOR **[654.5#]**
654.0# UTERINE ABNORMALITY CONGENITAL
660.2# UTERINE ABNORMALITY CONGENITAL OBSTRUCTING LABOR **[654.0#]**
654.0# UTERINE BICORNIS
660.2# UTERINE BICORNIS OBSTRUCTING LABOR **[654.0#]**
654.1# UTERINE FIBROID
660.2# UTERINE FIBROID OBSTRUCTING LABOR **[654.1#]**
654.4# UTERINE SACCULATION
660.2# UTERINE SACCULATION OBSTRUCTING LABOR **[654.4#]**
654.4# UTERUS PROLAPSE
660.2# UTERUS PROLAPSE OBSTRUCTING LABOR **[654.4#]**
654.3# UTERUS RETROVERTED (INCARCERATED)
660.2# UTERUS RETROVERTED (INCARCERATED) OBSTRUCTING LABOR **[654.3#]**
654.7# VAGINA ABNORMALITY
660.2# VAGINA ABNORMALITY OBSTRUCTING LABOR **[654.7#]**
654.7# VAGINAL PROLAPSE
660.2# VAGINAL PROLAPSE OBSTRUCTING LABOR **[654.7#]**
654.7# VAGINAL STENOSIS
660.2# VAGINAL STENOSIS OBSTRUCTING LABOR **[654.7#]**
654.7# VAGINAL TUMOR
660.2# VAGINAL TUMOR OBSTRUCTING LABOR **[654.7#]**
654.8# VULVA ABNORMALITY
660.2# VULVA ABNORMALITY OBSTRUCTING LABOR **[654.8#]**
654.8# VULVA TUMOR
660.2# VULVA TUMOR OBSTRUCTING LABOR **[654.8#]**
671.1# VULVA VARICOSE VEINS
660.2# VULVA VARICOSE VEINS OBSTRUCTING LABOR **[671.1#]**

5th Digit: 654.0-5, 7-8, 671.1

0. EPISODE OF CARE UNSPECIFIED OR N/A
1. DELIVERED
2. DELIVERED WITH POSTPARTUM COMPLICATION
3. ANTEPARTUM COMPLICATION
4. POSTPARTUM COMPLICATION

5th Digit: 660.2

0. EPISODE OF CARE UNSPECIFIED OR N/A
1. DELIVERED
3. ANTEPARTUM COMPLICATION

PREGNANCY COMPLICATIONS

DELIVERY PROBLEMS:

MALPRESENTATION/MALPOSITION

652.2# BREECH DELIVERY
660.0# BREECH DELIVERY OBSTRUCTING LABOR [652.2#]
652.1# BREECH OR MALPRESENTATION CONVERTED TO CEPHALIC
660.0# BREECH OR MALPRESENTATION CONVERTED TO CEPHALIC OBSTRUCTING LABOR [652.1#]
652.2# BREECH PRESENTATION WITHOUT VERSION
660.0# BREECH PRESENTATION OBSTRUCTING LABOR [652.2#]
652.6# BREECH PRESENTATION WITH MULTIPLE GESTATION
660.0# BREECH PRESENTATION WITH MULTIPLE GESTATION OBSTRUCTING LABOR [652.6#]
652.4# BROW PRESENTATION
660.0# BROW PRESENTATION OBSTRUCTING LABOR [652.4#]
652.2# BUTTOCKS PRESENTATION
660.0# BUTTOCKS PRESENTATION OBSTRUCTING LABOR [652.2#]
652.1# CEPHALIC VERSION
660.0# CEPHALIC VERSION OBSTRUCTING LABOR [652.1#]
652.4# CHIN PRESENTATION
660.0# CHIN PRESENTATION OBSTRUCTING LABOR [652.4#]
652.2# COMPLETE BREECH PRESENTATION
660.0# COMPLETE BREECH PRESENTATION OBSTRUCTING LABOR [652.2#]
652.8# COMPOUND PRESENTATION
660.0# COMPOUND PRESENTATION OBSTRUCTING LABOR [652.8#]
652.6# COMPOUND PRESENTATION WITH MULTIPLE GESTATION
660.0# COMPOUND PRESENTATION WITH MULTIPLE GESTATION OBSTRUCTING LABOR [652.6#]
652.4# EXTENDED HEAD PRESENTATION
660.0# EXTENDED HEAD PRESENTATION OBSTRUCTING LABOR [652.4#]
652.4# FACE PRESENTATION
660.0# FACE PRESENTATION OBSTRUCTING LABOR [652.4#]
652.8# FACE TO PUBES PRESENTATION
660.0# FACE TO PUBES PRESENTATION OBSTRUCTING LABOR [652.8#]
652.8# FOOTLING PRESENTATION
660.0# FOOTLING PRESENTATION OBSTRUCTING LABOR [652.8#]
652.2# FRANK BREECH PRESENTATION
660.0# FRANK BREECH PRESENTATION OBSTRUCTING LABOR [652.2#]
652.5# HIGH HEAD AT TERM
660.0# HIGH HEAD AT TERM OBSTRUCTING LABOR [652.5#]
652.8# INCOMPLETE BREECH PRESENTATION
660.0# INCOMPLETE BREECH PRESENTATION OBSTRUCTING LABOR [652.8#]
652.6# LOCKED TWINS
660.0# LOCKED TWINS OBSTRUCTING LABOR [652.6#]
652.9# MALPRESENTATION NOS
660.0# MALPRESENTATION NOS OBSTRUCTING LABOR [652.9#]
652.3# OBLIQUE LIE
660.0# OBLIQUE LIE OBSTRUCTING LABOR [652.3#]
652.7# PROLAPSE ARM
660.0# PROLAPSE ARM OBSTRUCTING LABOR [652.7#]
652.8# PROLAPSE FOOT
660.0# PROLAPSE FOOT OBSTRUCTING LABOR [652.8#]
652.8# PROLAPSE LEG
660.0# PROLAPSE LEG OBSTRUCTING LABOR [652.8#]
660.3# TRANSVERSE ARREST AND PERSISTENT OCCIPITOPOSTERIOR POSITION
652.3# TRANSVERSE LIE
660.0# TRANSVERSE LIE OBSTRUCTING LABOR [652.3#]
652.0# UNSTABLE LIE
660.0# UNSTABLE LIE OBSTRUCTING LABOR [652.0#]

5th Digit: 652.0-9, 660.0, 3

0. EPISODE OF CARE UNSPECIFIED OR N/A
1. DELIVERED
3. ANTEPARTUM COMPLICATION

DISPROPORTION

653.4# CEPHALOPELVIC DISPROPORTION
660.1# CEPHALOPELVIC DISPROPORTION OBSTRUCTING LABOR [653.4#]
653.9# DISPROPORTION NOS
660.1# DISPROPORTION NOS OBSTRUCTING LABOR [653.9#]
653.7# CONJOINED TWINS
660.1# CONJOINED TWINS OBSTRUCTING LABOR [653.7#]
653.7# FETAL ASCITES
660.1# FETAL ASCITES OBSTRUCTING LABOR [653.7#]
653.7# FETAL HYDROPS
660.1# FETAL HYDROPS OBSTRUCTING LABOR [653.7#]
656.6# FETAL "LARGE FOR DATES" AFFECTING MANAGEMENT OF MOTHER
653.5# FETAL "LARGE FOR DATES" CAUSING DISPROPORTION
660.1# FETAL "LARGE FOR DATES" (EXCEPTIONALLY LARGE) OBSTRUCTING LABOR [653.5#]
653.7# FETAL MYELOMENINGOCELE
660.1# FETAL MYELOMENINGOCELE OBSTRUCTING LABOR [653.7#]
653.7# FETAL SACRAL TERATOMA
660.1# FETAL SACRAL TERATOMA OBSTRUCTING LABOR [653.7#]
653.7# FETAL TUMOR
660.1# FETAL TUMOR OBSTRUCTING LABOR [653.7#]
653.4# FETOPELVIC DISPROPORTION
660.1# FETOPELVIC DISPROPORTION OBSTRUCTING LABOR [653.4#]
653.7# FETUS ABNORMALITY (OTHER)
660.1# FETUS ABNORMALITY (OTHER) OBSTRUCTING LABOR [653.7#]
655.0# FETUS HYDROCEPHALIC (KNOWN/SUSPECTED) AFFECTING MANAGEMENT OF MOTHER
653.6# FETUS HYDROCEPHALIC CAUSING DISPROPORTION
660.1# FETUS HYDROCEPHALIC OBSTRUCTING LABOR [653.6#]
653.2# INLET CONTRACTION (PELVIS)
660.1# INLET CONTRACTION (PELVIS) OBSTRUCTING LABOR [653.2#]
653.3# OUTLET CONTRACTION PELVIS
660.1# OUTLET CONTRACTION PELVIS OBSTRUCTING LABOR [653.3#]
653.0# PELVIC DEFORMITY NOS
660.1# PELVIC DEFORMITY NOS OBSTRUCTING LABOR [653.0#]
653.1# PELVIS CONTRACTED
660.1# PELVIS CONTRACTED OBSTRUCTING LABOR [653.1#]
653.8# SHOULDER DYSTOCIA, CAUSING DISPROPORTION
660.1# SHOULDER DYSTOCIA, CAUSING DISPROPORTION OBSTRUCTING LABOR [653.8#]
660.4# SHOULDER GIRDLE DYSTOCIA OBSTRUCTING LABOR
653.8# OTHER DISPROPORTION
660.1# OTHER DISPROPORTION OBSTRUCTING LABOR [653.8#]

5th Digit: 653.0-9, 655.0, 656.6, 660.1, 660.4

0. EPISODE OF CARE UNSPECIFIED OR N/A
1. DELIVERED
3. ANTEPARTUM COMPLICATION

PREGNANCY COMPLICATIONS

LABOR PROBLEMS

669.9# COMPLICATION NOS
- 5th Digit: 669.9
  - 0. EPISODE OF CARE UNSPECIFIED OR N/A
  - 1. DELIVERED
  - 2. DELIVERED WITH POSTPARTUM COMPLICATION
  - 3. ANTEPARTUM COMPLICATION
  - 4. POSTPARTUM COMPLICATION

659.3# BACTEREMIA DURING LABOR
660.6# FAILED TRIAL
- 5th Digit: 659.3, 660.6
  - 0. EPISODE OF CARE UNSPECIFIED OR N/A
  - 1. DELIVERED
  - 3. ANTEPARTUM COMPLICATION

644.1# FALSE > 37 WEEKS
644.0# FALSE> 22 AND < 37 WEEKS
- 5th Digit: 644.0-1
  - 0. EPISODE OF CARE UNSPECIFIED OR N/A
  - 3. ANTEPARTUM COMPLICATION

660.8# OBSTRUCTED BY OTHER CAUSES
661.3# PRECIPITATE
- 5th Digit: 661.3, 660.8
  - 0. EPISODE OF CARE UNSPECIFIED OR N/A
  - 1. DELIVERED
  - 3. ANTEPARTUM COMPLICATION

644.2# PREMATURE WITH ONSET OF DELIVERY < 37 WEEKS
- 5th Digit: 644.2
  - 0. EPISODE OF CARE UNSPECIFIED OR N/A
  - 1. DELIVERED

644.0# PREMATURE WITHOUT DELIVERY > 22 AND < 37 WEEKS
- 5th Digit: 644.0
  - 0. EPISODE OF CARE UNSPECIFIED OR N/A
  - 3. ANTEPARTUM COMPLICATION

662.1# PROLONGED
662.0# PROLONGED FIRST STAGE
662.2# PROLONGED SECOND STAGE
659.2# PYREXIA OR FEVER DURING LABOR
- 5th Digit: 659.2, 662.0-2
  - 0. EPISODE OF CARE UNSPECIFIED OR N/A
  - 1. DELIVERED
  - 3. ANTEPARTUM COMPLICATION

669.1# SHOCK DURING LABOR AND DELIVERY
- 5th Digit: 669.1
  - 0. EPISODE OF CARE UNSPECIFIED OR N/A
  - 1. DELIVERED
  - 2. DELIVERED WITH POSTPARTUM COMPLICATION
  - 3. ANTEPARTUM COMPLICATION
  - 4. POSTPARTUM COMPLICATION

644.1# THREATENED > 37 WEEKS
644.0# THREATENED > 22 AND < 37 WEEKS
- 5th Digit: 644.0-1
  - 0. EPISODE OF CARE UNSPECIFIED OR N/A
  - 3. ANTEPARTUM COMPLICATION

663.0# UMBILICAL CORD PROLAPSE
665.0# UTERUS RUPTURE BEFORE ONSET OF LABOR
- 5th Digit: 665.0, 663.0
  - 0. EPISODE OF CARE UNSPECIFIED OR N/A
  - 1. DELIVERED
  - 3. ANTEPARTUM COMPLICATION

PREGNANCY COMPLICATIONS

LABOR PROBLEMS (continued)

665.1# UTERUS RUPTURE UNSPECIFIED
665.1# UTERUS RUPTURE DURING LABOR
- 5th Digit: 665.1
  - 0. EPISODE OF CARE UNSPECIFIED OR N/A
  - 1. DELIVERED

669.8# COMPLICATION OTHER
- 5th Digit: 669.8
  - 0. EPISODE OF CARE UNSPECIFIED OR N/A
  - 1. DELIVERED
  - 2. DELIVERED WITH POSTPARTUM COMPLICATION
  - 3. ANTEPARTUM COMPLICATION
  - 4. POSTPARTUM COMPLICATION

PREGNANCY COMPLICATIONS

MATERNAL CONDITIONS

*WHEN CODING A MATERNAL CONDITION USING A CODE LISTED BELOW IN THE CATEGORIES OF **646.##**, **647.##** OR **648.##**, USE AN ADDITIONAL CODE TO IDENTIFY THE SPECIFIC CONDITION.*

646.9# UNSPECIFIED

ELDERLY MULTIGRAVIDA: SECOND OR MORE PREGNANCY IN A WOMAN WHO WILL BE 35 YEARS OF AGE OR OLDER AT EXPECTED DATE OF DELIVERY.

659.6# AGE ADVANCED - ELDERLY MULTIGRAVIDA

ELDERLY PRIMIGRAVIDA: FIRST PREGNANCY IN A WOMAN WHO WILL BE 35 YEARS OF AGE OR OLDER AT EXPECTED DATE OF DELIVERY.

659.5# AGE ADVANCED - ELDERLY PRIMIGRAVIDA

YOUNG MATERNAL AGE: PREGNANCY IN FEMALE WHO IS LESS THAN 16 YEARS OLD AT EXPECTED DATE OF DELIVERY.

659.8# AGE YOUNG MATERNAL COMPLICATING LABOR AND DELIVERY
- 5th Digit: 646.9, 659.5-6, 8
  - 0. EPISODE OF CARE UNSPECIFIED OR N/A
  - 1. DELIVERED
  - 3. ANTEPARTUM COMPLICATION

647.6# AIDS CURRENT (CO-EXISTENT) [042]
648.2# ANEMIA CURRENT (CO-EXISTENT)
647.8# BACTEREMIA CURRENT (CO-EXISTENT)
646.5# BACTERIURIA ASYMPTOMATIC
654.4# BLADDER DILATATION
648.7# BONE AND JOINT DISORDER BACK PELVIS AND LOWER LIMBS CURRENT (CO-EXISTENT)
648.6# CARDIOVASCULAR DISEASE OTHER SPECIFIED CURRENT (CO-EXISTENT)
648.5# CARDIOVASCULAR DISORDER CONGENITAL CURRENT (CO-EXISTENT)
648.0# DIABETES CURRENT (CO-EXISTENT)
648.8# DIABETES GESTATIONAL
669.0# DISTRESS (L AND D)
0 ECLAMPSIA SEE 'ECLAMPSIA'
646.1# EDEMA WITHOUT MENTION OF HYPERTENSION
648.3# DRUG DEPENDENCE CURRENT (CO-EXISTENT)
647.1# GONORRHEA CURRENT (CO-EXISTENT)
- 5th Digit: 646.1, 5, 647.1, 6, 8, 648.0, 2-3, 5-8, 654.4, 669.0
  - 0. EPISODE OF CARE UNSPECIFIED OR N/A
  - 1. DELIVERED
  - 2. DELIVERED WITH POSTPARTUM COMPLICATION
  - 3. ANTEPARTUM COMPLICATION
  - 4. POSTPARTUM COMPLICATION

WHEN CODING A MATERNAL CONDITION USING A CODE LISTED BELOW IN THE CATEGORIES OF 646.##, 647.## OR 648.##, USE AN ADDITIONAL CODE TO IDENTIFY THE SPECIFIC CONDITION.

640.9# HEMORRHAGE ANTEPARTUM (< 22 WEEKS)
641.9# HEMORRHAGE ANTEPARTUM NOS
641.3# HEMORRHAGE ANTEPARTUM ASSOCIATED WITH COAGULATION DEFECTS
641.8# HEMORRHAGE ANTEPARTUM OTHER

5th Digit: 640.9, 641.3, 8-9
- **0. EPISODE OF CARE NOS OR N/A**
- **1. DELIVERED**
- **3. ANTEPARTUM COMPLICATION**

648.9# HEMORRHOIDS CURRENT (CO-EXISTENT)
671.8# HEMORRHOIDS DUE TO PREGNANCY

5th Digit: 648.9, 671.8
- **0. EPISODE OF CARE UNSPECIFIED OR N/A**
- **1. DELIVERED**
- **2. DELIVERED WITH POSTPARTUM COMPLICATION**
- **3. ANTEPARTUM COMPLICATION**
- **4. POSTPARTUM COMPLICATION**

646.7# HEPATITIS

5th Digit: 646.7
- **0. EPISODE OF CARE UNSPECIFIED OR N/A**
- **1. DELIVERED**
- **3. ANTEPARTUM COMPLICATION**

WHEN CODING A MATERNAL CONDITION USING A CODE LISTED BELOW IN THE CATEGORIES OF 646.##, 647.## OR 648.##, USE AN ADDITIONAL CODE TO IDENTIFY THE SPECIFIC CONDITION.

647.6# HEPATITIS VIRAL CURRENT (CO-EXISTENT)
647.6# HIV ASYMPTOMATIC CURRENT (CO-EXISTENT) [V08]
647.6# HIV SYMPTOMATIC CURRENT (CO-EXISTENT) [042]
0 HYPERTENSION SEE 'HYPERTENSION COMPLICATING PREGNANCY'
648.0# HYPOGLYCEMIC REACTION DIABETIC (DIETARY) CURRENT (CO-EXISTENT) [251.2]
648.8# HYPOGLYCEMIC REACTION GESTATIONAL DIABETES (DIETARY) [251.2]
669.2# HYPOTENSION SYNDROME
646.6# INFECTION GENITOURINARY
647.9# INFECTION OR INFESTATION - NOS CURRENT (CO-EXISTENT)
647.8# INFECTION OR INFESTATION - OTHER SPECIFIED CURRENT (CO-EXISTENT)

5th Digit: 646.6, 647.6, 8-9, 648.0, 8
- **0. EPISODE OF CARE UNSPECIFIED OR N/A**
- **1. DELIVERED**
- **2. DELIVERED WITH POSTPARTUM COMPLICATION**
- **3. ANTEPARTUM COMPLICATION**
- **4. POSTPARTUM COMPLICATION**

670.0# INFECTION MAJOR PUERPERAL, ENDOMETRITIS DUE TO PREGNANCY
670.0# INFECTION MAJOR PUERPERAL, PELVIC CELLULITIS DUE TO PREGNANCY
670.0# INFECTION MAJOR PUERPERAL, PELVIC SEPSIS DUE TO PREGNANCY
670.0# INFECTION MAJOR PUERPERAL, PERITONITIS DUE TO PREGNANCY
670.0# INFECTION MAJOR PUERPERAL, PYEMIA DUE TO PREGNANCY
670.0# INFECTION MAJOR PUERPERAL, SALPINGITIS DUE TO PREGNANCY

5th Digit: 670.0
- **0. EPISODE OF CARE UNSPECIFIED OR N/A**
- **2. DELIVERED WITH POSTPARTUM COMPLICATION**
- **4. POSTPARTUM COMPLICATION**

PREGNANCY COMPLICATIONS

MATERNAL CONDITIONS (continued)

WHEN CODING A MATERNAL CONDITION USING A CODE LISTED BELOW IN THE CATEGORIES OF 646.##, 647.## OR 648.##, USE AN ADDITIONAL CODE TO IDENTIFY THE SPECIFIC CONDITION.

647.6# INFECTION VIRAL CURRENT (CO-EXISTENT)
648.9# INJURY-TRAUMA NON-OBSTETRICAL CURRENT (CO-EXISTENT)

5th Digit: 647.6, 648.9
- **0. EPISODE OF CARE UNSPECIFIED OR N/A**
- **1. DELIVERED**
- **2. DELIVERED WITH POSTPARTUM COMPLICATION**
- **3. ANTEPARTUM COMPLICATION**
- **4. POSTPARTUM COMPLICATION**

646.7# LIVER DISORDER

5th Digit: 646.7
- **0. EPISODE OF CARE UNSPECIFIED OR N/A**
- **1. DELIVERED**
- **3. ANTEPARTUM COMPLICATION**

648.9# LYMPHATIC DISORDER CURRENT (CO-EXISTENT)
648.4# MENTAL DISORDER CURRENT (CO-EXISTENT)

5th Digit: 648.4, 9
- **0. EPISODE OF CARE UNSPECIFIED OR N/A**
- **1. DELIVERED**
- **2. DELIVERED WITH POSTPARTUM COMPLICATION**
- **3. ANTEPARTUM COMPLICATION**
- **4. POSTPARTUM COMPLICATION**

ELDERLY MULTIGRAVIDA: SECOND OR MORE PREGNANCY IN A WOMAN WHO WILL BE 35 YEARS OF AGE OR OLDER AT EXPECTED DATE OF DELIVERY.

659.6# MULTIGRAVIDA ELDERLY

5th Digit: 659.6
- **0. EPISODE OF CARE UNSPECIFIED OR N/A**
- **1. DELIVERED**
- **3. ANTEPARTUM COMPLICATION**

646.4# NEURITIS PERIPHERAL
648.9# NUTRITIONAL DEFICIENCIES CURRENT (CO-EXISTENT)
646.1# OBESITY SYNDROME
648.9# PHLEBITIS (ANY TYPE) CURRENT (CO-EXISTENT)

5th Digit: 646.1, 4, 648.9
- **0. EPISODE OF CARE UNSPECIFIED OR N/A**
- **1. DELIVERED**
- **2. DELIVERED WITH POSTPARTUM COMPLICATION**
- **3. ANTEPARTUM COMPLICATION**
- **4. POSTPARTUM COMPLICATION**

671.3# PHLEBITIS DEEP (VEIN) DUE TO PREGNANCY

5th Digit: 671.3
- **0. EPISODE OF CARE NOS OR N/A**
- **1. DELIVERED**
- **3. ANTEPARTUM COMPLICATION**

671.9# PHLEBITIS DUE TO PREGNANCY
671.2# PHLEBITIS SUPERFICIAL (VEIN) DUE TO PREGNANCY
671.5# PHLEBITIS OTHER DUE TO PREGNANCY
648.9# PHLEBOTHROMBOSIS CURRENT (CO-EXISTENT)

5th Digit: 648.9, 671.2, 5, 9
- **0. EPISODE OF CARE UNSPECIFIED OR N/A**
- **1. DELIVERED**
- **2. DELIVERED WITH POSTPARTUM COMPLICATION**
- **3. ANTEPARTUM COMPLICATION**
- **4. POSTPARTUM COMPLICATION**

671.3# PHLEBOTHROMBOSIS DEEP-VEIN ANTEPARTUM DUE TO PREGNANCY

5th Digit: 671.3
- **0. EPISODE OF CARE NOS OR N/A**
- **1. DELIVERED**
- **3. ANTEPARTUM COMPLICATION**

PREGNANCY COMPLICATIONS

MATERNAL CONDITIONS (continued)

*WHEN CODING A MATERNAL CONDITION USING A CODE LISTED BELOW IN THE CATEGORIES OF **646.##, 647.##** OR **648.##**, USE AN ADDITIONAL CODE TO IDENTIFY THE SPECIFIC CONDITION.*

671.4# PHLEBOTHROMBOSIS DEEP-VEIN POSTPARTUM DUE TO PREGNANCY

5th Digit: 671.4

0. UNSPECIFIED
2. DELIVERED, WITH POSTPARTUM COMPLICATION
4. POSTPARTUM CONDITION OR COMPLICATION

642.4# PRE-ECLAMPSIA (NOS) (MILD)
642.5# PRE-ECLAMPSIA SEVERE
642.7# PRE-ECLAMPSIA WITH PRE-EXISTING HYPERTENSION

5th Digit: 642.4-5, 7

0. EPISODE OF CARE UNSPECIFIED OR N/A
1. DELIVERED
2. DELIVERED WITH POSTPARTUM COMPLICATION
3. ANTEPARTUM COMPLICATION
4. POSTPARTUM COMPLICATION

ELDERLY PRIMIGRAVIDA: FIRST PREGNANCY IN A WOMAN WHO WILL BE 35 YEARS OF AGE OR OLDER AT EXPECTED DATE OF DELIVERY.

659.5# PRIMIGRAVIDA ELDERLY

5th Digit: 659.5

0. EPISODE OF CARE UNSPECIFIED OR N/A
1. DELIVERED
3. ANTEPARTUM COMPLICATION

646.8# PRURITUS (PUPP)

5th Digit: 646.8

0. EPISODE OF CARE UNSPECIFIED OR N/A
1. DELIVERED
2. DELIVERED WITH POSTPARTUM COMPLICATION
3. ANTEPARTUM COMPLICATION
4. POSTPARTUM COMPLICATION

659.2# PYREXIA OR FEVER DURING LABOR

5th Digit: 659.2

0. EPISODE OF CARE UNSPECIFIED OR N/A
1. DELIVERED
3. ANTEPARTUM COMPLICATION

646.2# RENAL DISEASE WITHOUT MENTION OF HYPERTENSION
647.5# RUBELLA CURRENT (CO-EXISTENT)
647.0# SYPHILIS CURRENT (CO-EXISTENT)
648.9# THROMBOSIS (ANY TYPE) CURRENT (CO-EXISTENT)
671.3# THROMBOSIS DEEP (VEIN) DUE TO PREGNANCY
671.9# THROMBOSIS DUE TO PREGNANCY
671.2# THROMBOSIS SUPERFICIAL (VEIN) DUE TO PREGNANCY
671.5# THROMBOSIS OTHER DUE TO PREGNANCY
648.1# THYROID DYSFUNCTION CURRENT (CO-EXISTENT)
647.3# TUBERCULOSIS CURRENT (CO-EXISTENT)
646.2# UREMIA
646.8# UTERINE IRRITABILITY COMPLICATING PREGNANCY
648.9# VARICOSE VEINS ANY SITE CURRENT (CO-EXISTENT)
671.0# VARICOSE VEINS DUE TO PREGNANCY
671.1# VARICOSE VEINS VULVA AND PERINEUM DUE TO PREGNANCY
648.9# VASCULAR DISORDER CURRENT (CO-EXISTENT)
647.6# VIRAL DISEASE CURRENT (CO-EXISTENT)

5th Digit: 646.2, 8, 647.0, 3, 5, 6, 648.1, 9, 671.0-3, 5, 9

0. EPISODE OF CARE UNSPECIFIED OR N/A
1. DELIVERED
2. DELIVERED WITH POSTPARTUM COMPLICATION
3. ANTEPARTUM COMPLICATION
4. POSTPARTUM COMPLICATION

PREGNANCY COMPLICATIONS

MATERNAL CONDITIONS (continued)

*WHEN CODING A MATERNAL CONDITION USING A CODE LISTED BELOW IN THE CATEGORIES OF **646.##, 647.##** OR **648.##**, USE AN ADDITIONAL CODE TO IDENTIFY THE SPECIFIC CONDITION.*

646.1# WEIGHT GAIN EXCESSIVE
648.9# OTHER CURRENT (CO-EXISTENT) CONDITION (DISEASE)
646.8# OTHER SPECIFIED COMPLICATION ARISING DURING PREGNANCY
647.8# OTHER SPECIFIED INFECTIOUS AND PARASITIC DISEASE CURRENT (CO-EXISTENT)
647.2# OTHER SPECIFIED VENEREAL DISEASE CURRENT (CO-EXISTENT)
647.6# OTHER SPECIFIED VIRAL DISEASE CURRENT (CO-EXISTENT)

5th Digit: 646.1, 8, 647.2, 6, 8, 648.9

0. EPISODE OF CARE UNSPECIFIED OR N/A
1. DELIVERED
2. DELIVERED WITH POSTPARTUM COMPLICATION
3. ANTEPARTUM COMPLICATION
4. POSTPARTUM COMPLICATION

PREGNANCY COMPLICATIONS

MATERNAL DISORDERS AFFECTING FETUS OR NEWBORN

IN ORDER TO USE THE FOLLOWING CODES, THE MEDICAL RECORD MUST SPECIFY THAT THE MATERNAL CONDITION IS A CAUSE OF MORBIDITY OR MORTALITY IN THE FETUS OR NEWBORN. THE MERE FACT THAT THE CONDITION EXISTED IN THE MOTHER OR COMPLICATED THE PREGNANCY DOES NOT WARRANT THE USE OF THESE CODES ON THE NEWBORN'S RECORD. REMEMBER, CODES 760-763 APPLY ONLY TO THE INFANT AND ARE NEVER ASSIGNED TO THE MOTHER'S RECORD. CONVERSELY, NEVER CODE THE MOTHER'S CONDITION WITH THESE FETAL/NEWBORN CODES.

762.9 UNSPECIFIED ABNORMALITIES OF CHORION AND AMNION
761.9 UNSPECIFIED COMPLICATIONS - DUE TO CURRENT PREGNANCY
760.9 UNSPECIFIED CONDITIONS - UNRELATED TO CURRENT PREGNANCY
762.6 UNSPECIFIED CONDITIONS OF UMBILICAL CORD
763.9 UNSPECIFIED DISORDER - DUE TO LABOR AND DELIVERY
761.4 ABDOMINAL PREGNANCY
763.1 ABNORMALITY BONY
763.89 ABNORMALITY SOFT TISSUES
761.8 ABORTION SPONTANEOUS
762.1 ABRUPTIO PLACENTAE
760.79 ADRENOGENITAL IATROGENIC SYNDROME AFFECTING FETUS OR NEWBORN
760.71 ALCOHOL TRANSMITTED VIA PLACENTA OR BREAST MILK
762.1 AMNIOCENTESIS DAMAGE TO PLACENTA
762.8 AMNION ADHESION TO FETUS
762.7 AMNIONITIS
763.5 ANALGESICS ADMINISTERED DURING LABOR AND DELIVERY
763.5 ANESTHETICS ADMINISTERED DURING LABOR AND DELIVERY
760.74 ANTIBIOTICS (ANTI-INFECTIVES) TRANSMITTED VIA PLACENTA OR BREAST MILK
760.1 BACTERIURIA
763.1 BLADDER DILATATION
762.1 BLOOD LOSS MATERNAL
763.0 BREECH DELIVERY AND EXTRACTION
761.7 BREECH MALPRESENTATION BEFORE LABOR AND DELIVERY

PREGNANCY COMPLICATIONS

MATERNAL DISORDERS AFFECTING FETUS OR NEWBORN (continued)

IN ORDER TO USE THE FOLLOWING CODES, THE MEDICAL RECORD MUST SPECIFY THAT THE MATERNAL CONDITION IS A CAUSE OF MORBIDITY OR MORTALITY IN THE FETUS OR NEWBORN. THE MERE FACT THAT THE CONDITION EXISTED IN THE MOTHER OR COMPLICATED THE PREGNANCY DOES NOT WARRANT THE USE OF THESE CODES ON THE NEWBORN'S RECORD. REMEMBER, CODES 760-763 APPLY ONLY TO THE INFANT AND ARE NEVER ASSIGNED TO THE MOTHER'S RECORD. CONVERSELY, NEVER CODE THE MOTHER'S CONDITION WITH THESE FETAL/NEWBORN CODES.

760.8	CERVICITIS
763.89	CERVIX ABNORMALITY
761.0	CERVIX INCOMPETENT
763.89	CERVIX SCAR
763.1	CERVIX SCAR OBSTRUCTING LABOR
763.89	CERVIX STENOSIS/STRICTURE
763.1	CERVIX STENOSIS/STRICTURE OBSTRUCTING LABOR
763.4	CESAREAN DELIVERY
763.89	CESAREAN SCAR PREVIOUS
762.1	CESAREAN SECTION DAMAGE (SEPARATION) (HEMORRHAGE) TO PLACENTA
762.7	CHORIOAMNIONITIS
762.9	CHORION AND AMNION ABNORMALITY
762.8	CHORION AND AMNION ABNORMALITIES OTHER SPECIFIED
760.3	CIRCULATORY DISEASE MATERNAL CHRONIC
763.89	CLEIDOTOMY FETAL
760.75	COCAINE TRANSMITTED VIA PLACENTA OR BREAST MILK
763.7	CONTRACTION RING
760.75	CRACK (COCAINE) TRANSMITTED VIA PLACENTA OR BREAST MILK
763.89	CRANIOCLASIS, FETAL
763.89	CRANIOTOMY, FETAL
763.89	CYSTOCELE
763.1	CYSTOCELE OBSTRUCTING LABOR
761.6	DEATH (MATERNAL)
763.89	DELAYED BIRTH OR DELIVERY NEC
763.89	DELAYED BIRTH OR DELIVERY SECOND TWIN, TRIPLET ETC.
763.0	DELIVERY AND EXTRACTION
763.6	DELIVERY RAPID SECOND STAGE
760.76	DES (DIETHYLSTILBESTROL) TRANSMITTED VIA PLACENTA OR BREAST MILK
763.89	DESTRUCTIVE OPERATION OR PROCEDURE ON LIVE FETUS TO FACILITATE DELIVERY
775.0	DIABETES CAUSING FETAL HYPOGLYCEMIA
760.76	DIETHYLSTILBESTROL (DES) TRANSMITTED VIA PLACENTA OR BREAST MILK
763.5	DRUG REACTION MATERNAL
761.4	ECTOPIC PREGNANCY
763.89	ENDOCERVICAL OS STENOSIS/STRICTURE
763.1	ENDOCERVICAL OS STENOSIS/STRICTURE OBSTRUCTING LABOR
760.8	ENDOMETRITIS
763.89	EXHAUSTION MATERNAL
761.7	EXTERNAL VERSION MALPRESENTATION BEFORE LABOR AND DELIVERY
763.89	EXTRACTION FETAL MANUAL OR WITH HOOK
762.3	FETAL BLOOD LOSS DUE TO PLACENTAL TRANSFUSION [772.0]
763.89	FORCED BIRTH
763.2	FORCEPS DELIVERY
760.73	HALLUCINOGENIC TRANSMITTED VIA PLACENTA OR BREAST MILK
762.1	HEMORRHAGE COMPLICATING PREGNANCY, ANTEPARTUM
763.89	HEMORRHAGE DUE TO COAGULATION DEFECT
760.8	HEPATITIS MATERNAL
761.3	HYDRAMNIOS ACUTE (CHRONIC)
760.0	HYPERTENSIVE DISORDERS MATERNAL

MATERNAL DISORDERS AFFECTING FETUS OR NEWBORN (continued)

760.79	IMMUNE SERA TRANSMITTED VIA PLACENTA OR BREAST MILK
763.89	INDUCTION OF LABOR (MEDICAL)
760.8	INFECTION GENITAL TRACT OTHER LOCALIZED MATERNAL
760.2	INFECTION MATERNAL NOT MANIFESTED IN FETUS OR NEWBORN
760.1	INFECTION URINARY TRACT
760.2	INFLUENZA
763.89	INJURY DUE TO OBSTETRICAL TRAUMA
760.5	INJURY MATERNAL
761.4	INTRAPERITONEAL PREGNANCY
760.1	KIDNEY NECROSIS
760.8	LIVER NECROSIS
761.7	MALPRESENTATION/MALPOSITION BEFORE LABOR
763.1	MALPRESENTATION/MALPOSITION DURING LABOR
761.6	MATERNAL DEATH
760.79	MEDICINAL AGENTS NEC TRANSMITTED VIA PLACENTA OR BREAST MILK
762.7	MEMBRANITIS
763.89	MULTIPARITY
761.5	MULTIPLE PREGNANCY
763.5	NARCOSIS DUE TO DRUG (CORRECTLY ADMINISTERED)
763.5	NARCOTIC REACTION (INTOXICATION) MATERNAL DURING L&D
760.72	NARCOTIC TRANSMITTED VIA PLACENTA OR BREAST MILK
760.70	NOXIOUS SUBSTANCE UNSPECIFIED TRANSMITTED VIA PLACENTA OR BREAST MILK
760.79	NOXIOUS SUBSTANCE OTHER SPECIFIED TRANSMITTED VIA PLACENTA OR BREAST MILK
760.4	NUTRITIONAL DEFICIENCY DISORDERS MATERNAL
761.7	OBLIQUE LIE BEFORE LABOR AND DELIVERY
761.2	OLIGOHYDRAMNIOS
763.5	OPIATE REACTION (INTOXICATION) MATERNAL DURING L&D
763.89	OS UTERI STRICTURE
763.1	OS UTERI STRICTURE OBSTRUCTING LABOR
763.89	OVARIAN CYST
763.1	OVARIAN CYST OBSTRUCTING LABOR
763.1	PELVIS BONY
763.1	PELVIS CONTRACTED
763.89	PELVIS CYST
763.1	PELVIS CYST OBSTRUCTING LABOR
763.89	PELVIS DEFORMITY
760.8	PELVIS INFLAMMATORY DISEASE
763.89	PELVIS ORGANS OR SOFT TISSUE ABNORMALITY
763.89	PELVIS ORGANS SURGERY PREVIOUS
763.1	PELVIS ROBERT'S
763.89	PENDULOUS ABDOMEN
761.4	PERITONEAL PREGNANCY
763.1	PERSISTENT OCCIPITOPOSTERIOR POSITION
762.1	PLACENTA DAMAGE
762.2	PLACENTA INFARCTION
762.0	PLACENTA PREVIA
762.3	PLACENTA TRANSFUSION SYNDROMES
762.7	PLACENTITIS
762.3	POLYCYTHEMIA NEONATORUM PLACENTAL TRANSFUSION [776.4]
761.3	POLYHYDRAMNIOS
763.6	PRECIPITATE DELIVERY
760.0	PRE-ECLAMPSIA
761.1	PREMATURE RUPTURE OF MEMBRANES
760.3	RESPIRATORY DISEASE MATERNAL CHRONIC
762.1	RUPTURE MARGINAL SINUS
760.8	SALPINGITIS
763.1	SHOULDER DYSTOCIA
763.1	SHOULDER PRESENTATION
763.1	SPONDYLOLISTHESIS
763.1	SPONDYLOLYSIS
760.6	SURGERY MATERNAL
762.1	SURGICAL INDUCTION WITH DAMAGE TO PLACENTA

PREGNANCY COMPLICATIONS

MATERNAL DISORDERS AFFECTING FETUS OR NEWBORN (continued)

IN ORDER TO USE THE FOLLOWING CODES, THE MEDICAL RECORD MUST SPECIFY THAT THE MATERNAL CONDITION IS A CAUSE OF MORBIDITY OR MORTALITY IN THE FETUS OR NEWBORN. THE MERE FACT THAT THE CONDITION EXISTED IN THE MOTHER OR COMPLICATED THE PREGNANCY DOES NOT WARRANT THE USE OF THESE CODES ON THE NEWBORN'S RECORD. REMEMBER, CODES 760-763 APPLY ONLY TO THE INFANT AND ARE NEVER ASSIGNED TO THE MOTHER'S RECORD. CONVERSELY, NEVER CODE THE MOTHER'S CONDITION WITH THESE FETAL/NEWBORN CODES.

760.70 TOXIC SUBSTANCE NOS TRANSMITTED VIA PLACENTA OR BREAST MILK
760.79 TOXIC SUBSTANCE NEC TRANSMITTED VIA PLACENTA OR BREAST MILK
763.5 TRANQUILIZER REACTION (MATERNAL)
761.7 TRANSVERSE LIE BEFORE LABOR AND DELIVERY
763.1 TRANSVERSE LIE-PRESENTATION DURING LABOR AND DELIVERY
761.5 TRIPLET PREGNANCY
761.4 TUBAL PREGNANCY
761.5 TWIN PREGNANCY
762.5 UMBILICAL CORD ENTANGLEMENT (CORD AROUND NECK, KNOT, TORSION)
762.4 UMBILICAL CORD PROLAPSE (PRESENTATION)
762.6 UMBILICAL CORD OTHER AND UNSPECIFIED CONDITIONS
761.7 UNSTABLE LIE BEFORE LABOR AND DELIVERY
760.1 URINARY TRACT DISEASES MATERNAL
763.89 UTERUS ABNORMALITY
763.89 UTERUS ABSCESS (TO ABDOMINAL WALL)
763.89 UTERUS ADHESION
763.89 UTERUS BICORNIS/DOUBLE
763.89 UTERUS BODY POLYP (CORPUS) (MUCOUS)
763.7 UTERUS CONTRACTIONS ABNORMAL
763.7 UTERUS HYPERTONIC/HYPOTONIC
763.7 UTERUS INERTIA-DYSFUNCTION
763.89 UTERUS PERFORATION WITH OBSTETRICAL TRAUMA
763.1 UTERUS PROLAPSE
763.89 UTERUS RUPTURE
763.1 UTERUS SACCULATION
763.89 UTERUS SHAPE ABNORMALITY
763.89 UTERUS SURGERY PREVIOUS
763.89 UTERUS VERSION
763.3 VACUUM EXTRACTOR DELIVERY
763.3 VACUUM RUPTURE
763.89 VAGINA ABNORMALITY
763.89 VAGINA STENOSIS/STRICTURE
763.1 VAGINA STENOSIS/STRICTURE OBSTRUCTING LABOR
760.8 VAGINITIS
763.89 VULVA ABNORMALITY
762.8 OTHER SPECIFIED ABNORMALITIES OF CHORION AND AMNION
761.8 OTHER SPECIFIED COMPLICATIONS - DUE TO CURRENT PREGNANCY
760.8 OTHER SPECIFIED CONDITIONS - UNRELATED TO CURRENT PREGNANCY
762.6 OTHER SPECIFIED CONDITIONS OF UMBILICAL CORD
763.89 OTHER SPECIFIED DISORDER - DUE TO LABOR AND DELIVERY

PREGNANCY SUPERVISION

V22.0 NORMAL - FIRST
V22.1 NORMAL - OTHER THAN FIRST
V23.9 HIGH RISK
V23.2 HIGH RISK - ABORTION HISTORY

ELDERLY MULTIGRAVIDA: SECOND OR MORE PREGNANCY IN A WOMAN WHO WILL BE 35 YEARS OF AGE OR OLDER AT EXPECTED DATE OF DELIVERY.

V23.82 HIGH RISK - ELDERLY MULTIGRAVIDA

PREGNANCY SUPERVISION (continued)

ELDERLY PRIMIGRAVIDA: FIRST PREGNANCY IN A WOMAN WHO WILL BE 35 YEARS OF AGE OR OLDER AT EXPECTED DATE OF DELIVERY.

V23.81 HIGH RISK - ELDERLY PRIMIGRAVIDA
V23.3 HIGH RISK - GRAND MULTIPARITY
V23.1 HIGH RISK - HYDATIDIFORM MOLE HISTORY
V23.0 HIGH RISK - INFERTILITY HISTORY
V23.89 HIGH RISK - MENTAL DISORDER HISTORY
V23.5 HIGH RISK - NEONATAL DEATH HISTORY
V23.4 HIGH RISK - POOR OBSTETRICAL HISTORY
V23.7 HIGH RISK - PRENATAL CARE POOR OR NONE
V23.5 HIGH RISK - STILLBIRTH HISTORY
V23.1 HIGH RISK - TROPHOBLASTIC DISEASE HISTORY
V23.1 HIGH RISK - VESICULAR MOLE HISTORY

YOUNG MULTIGRAVIDA: SECOND OR MORE PREGNANCY IN A FEMALE WHO IS LESS THAN 16 YEARS OLD AT EXPECTED DATE OF DELIVERY.

V23.84 HIGH RISK - YOUNG MULTIGRAVIDA

YOUNG PRIMIGRAVIDA: FIRST PREGNANCY IN A FEMALE WHO IS LESS THAN 16 YEARS OLD AT EXPECTED DATE OF DELIVERY.

V23.83 HIGH RISK - YOUNG PRIMIGRAVIDA
V23.89 HIGH RISK - OTHER SPECIFIED

V22.2 PREGNANT STATE (INCIDENTAL FINDING)

411.1 PREINFARCTION ANGINA
411.1 PREINFARCTION SYNDROME

733.09 PREISER'S DISEASE (OSTEOPOROSIS)
238.7 PRELEUKEMIC SYNDROME
754.32 PRELUXATION OF HIP
524.04 PREMAXILLAR RETRUSION (DEVELOPMENTAL)

PREMATURE

427.61 ATRIAL CONTRACTIONS
427.60 BEATS
756.0 CLOSURE CRANIAL SUTURES
644.2# DELIVERY <37 WEEKS
5th Digit: 644.2
0. EPISODE OF CARE UNSPECIFIED OR N/A
1. DELIVERED

302.75 EJACULATION (PSYCHOSEXUAL)
704.3 GREY HAIR
0 INFANT SEE 'PREMATURE INFANT'
427.60 JUNCTIONAL CONTRACTIONS
644.0# LABOR FALSE >22 AND <37 WEEKS
644.1# LABOR FALSE >37 WEEKS
644.0# LABOR THREATENED >22 AND <37 WEEKS
644.1# LABOR THREATENED >37 WEEKS
5th Digit: 644.0-1
0. EPISODE OF CARE UNSPECIFIED OR N/A
3. ANTEPARTUM COMPLICATION

644.2# LABOR WITH DELIVERY <37 WEEKS
5th Digit: 644.2
0. EPISODE OF CARE UNSPECIFIED OR N/A
1. DELIVERED

761.1 RUPTURE OF MEMBRANES - AFFECTING FETUS
V71.8 RUPTURE OF MEMBRANES - EVALUATION, NOT FOUND
658.1# RUPTURE OF MEMBRANES OBSTETRICAL
5th Digit: 658.1
0. EPISODE OF CARE UNSPECIFIED OR N/A
1. DELIVERED
3. ANTEPARTUM COMPLICATION

259.8 SENILITY SYNDROME
427.69 VENTRICULAR CONTRACTIONS

765.##: USE AN ADDITIONAL CODE IF NECESSARY, TO FURTHER SPECIFY THE CONDITION OF THE PREMATURE INFANT.

PREMATURE INFANT
765.10 >28 WEEKS AND/OR WEIGHT UNSPECIFIED
765.14 >28 WEEKS AND/OR 1000-1249 GRAMS
765.15 >28 WEEKS AND/OR 1250-1499 GRAMS
765.16 >28 WEEKS AND/OR 1500-1749 GRAMS
765.17 >28 WEEKS AND/OR 1750-1999 GRAMS
765.18 >28 WEEKS AND/OR 2000-2499 GRAMS
765.19 >28 WEEKS AND/OR 2500 GRAMS AND OVER

PREMATURE INFANT EXTREME
765.00 <28 WEEKS AND/OR WEIGHT UNSPECIFIED
765.01 <28 WEEKS AND/OR LESS THAN 500 GRAMS
765.02 <28 WEEKS AND/OR 500-749 GRAMS
765.03 <28 WEEKS AND/OR 750-999 GRAMS

627.0 PREMENOPAUSAL MENORRHAGIA
625.4 PREMENSTRUAL (TENSION) SYNDROME

PRENATAL CARE
V23.7 POOR (INSUFFICIENT) OR NONE
V22.0 NORMAL (FIRST)
V22.1 NORMAL (OTHER THAN FIRST)

V72.#, 'PREOPERATIVE EXAMINATION' IDENTIFIES THE TYPE OF EXAM DONE RATHER THAN THE TYPE OF SURGERY TO BE PERFORMED. THE PREOPERATIVE EXAMINATION CODES SHOULD BE LISTED FIRST FOLLOWED BY THE CODE FOR THE CONDITION NECESSITATING THE SURGERY.

PREOPERATIVE EXAMINATION
V72.84 UNSPECIFIED OR GENERAL
V72.81 CARDIOVASCULAR
V72.82 RESPIRATORY
V72.83 OTHER SPECIFIED

726.65 PREPATELLAR BURSITIS
362.56 PRERETINAL FIBROSIS
388.01 PRESBYACUSIS
605 PREPUCE ADHERENT
530.89 PRESBYESOPHAGUS
310.1 PRESBYOPHRENIA ORGANIC
367.4 PRESBYOPIA
V70.5 PRESCHOOL CHILDREN HEALTH EXAM
V25.01 PRESCRIPTION ORAL CONTRACEPTIVES
V68.1 PRESCRIPTION REPEAT ISSUE
0 PRESENTATION (ABNORMAL) SEE 'MALPOSITION/MALPRESENTATION'
756.11 PRESPONDYLOLISTHESIS (LUMBOSACRAL) CONGENITAL
996.59 PRESSURE EQUALIZATION (PE) TUBE COMPLICATION - MALFUNCTION
996.69 PRESSURE EQUALIZATION (PE) TUBE COMPLICATION - INFECTION OR INFLAMMATION
996.79 PRESSURE EQUALIZATION (PE) TUBE COMPLICATION - OTHER COMPLICATION
365.00 PRESSURE INTRAOCULAR INCREASED (GLAUCOMA SUSPECT)
780.2 PRESYNCOPE
100.89 PRETIBIAL FEVER
536.9 PRE ULCER SYNDROME
607.3 PRIAPISM
782.0 PRICKLING SENSATION SKIN

770.4 PRIMARY ATELECTASIS
334.2 PRIMARY CEREBELLAR DEGENERATION
335.24 PRIMARY LATERAL SCLEROSIS
661.0# PRIMARY UTERINE INERTIA

ELDERLY PRIMIGRAVIDA: FIRST PREGNANCY IN A WOMAN WHO WILL BE 35 YEARS OF AGE OR OLDER AT EXPECTED DATE OF DELIVERY.

659.5# PRIMIGRAVIDA ELDERLY
5th Digit: 659.5, 661.0
0. EPISODE OF CARE UNSPECIFIED OR N/A
1. DELIVERED
3. ANTEPARTUM COMPLICATION

436 PRIND
759.5 PRINGLE'S DISEASE (TUBEROUS SCLEROSIS)
786.52 PRINZMETAL-MASSUMI ANTERIOR CHEST WALL SYNDROME
V70.5 PRISONER HEALTH EXAM
286.3 PROACCELERIN DEFICIENCY

PROBLEM HEAD, NECK, TRUNK, LIMB
V48.9 HEAD NOS
V48.9 NECK NOS
V48.9 TRUNK NOS
V49.9 LIMB NOS

V48.0 HEAD DEFICIENCY
V48.1 NECK DEFICIENCY
V48.1 TRUNK DEFICIENCY
V49.0 LIMB DEFICIENCY

V48.6 HEAD DISFIGUREMENT
V48.7 NECK DISFIGUREMENT
V48.7 TRUNK DISFIGUREMENT
V49.4 LIMB DISFIGUREMENT

V48.2 HEAD MECHANICAL AND MOTOR
V48.3 NECK MECHANICAL AND MOTOR
V48.3 TRUNK MECHANICAL AND MOTOR
V49.1 LIMB MECHANICAL
V49.2 LIMB MOTOR

V48.4 HEAD SENSORY
V48.5 NECK SENSORY
V48.5 TRUNK SENSORY
V49.3 LIMB SENSORY

V48.8 HEAD OTHER
V48.8 NECK OTHER
V48.8 TRUNK OTHER
V49.5 LIMB OTHER
V49.8 LIMB OTHER SPECIFIED AFFECTING HEALTH STATUS

PROBLEM LIFESTYLE
V69.9 PROBLEM NOS
V69.1 DIET AND EATING HABITS INAPPROPRIATE
V69.3 GAMBLING AND BETTING
V69.0 PHYSICAL EXERCISE (LACK OF)
V69.8 SELF-DAMAGING BEHAVIOR
V69.2 SEXUAL BEHAVIOR HIGH RISK
V69.8 OTHER LIFESTYLE PROBLEMS

PROBLEM MENTAL BEHAVIORAL
V40.9 BEHAVIORAL
V40.1 COMMUNICATION
V40.0 LEARNING
V40.9 MENTAL
V40.1 SPEECH
V40.3 OTHER SPECIFIED BEHAVIORAL
V40.2 OTHER SPECIFIED MENTAL

PROBLEM SOCIAL

V62.4 ACCULTURATION
V61.29 ADOPTED CHILD
V61.3 AGED PARENTS OR IN-LAWS
V61.49 CARE OF SICK OR HANDICAPPED FAMILY MEMBER
V61.29 CONCERNING ADOPTED OR FOSTER CHILD OTHER (REASON FOR ENCOUNTER)
V62.3 EDUCATIONAL CIRCUMSTANCES (REASON FOR ENCOUNTER)
V61.41 FAMILY ALCOHOLISM (REASON FOR ENCOUNTER)
V61.9 FAMILY CIRCUMSTANCE UNSPECIFIED (REASON FOR ENCOUNTER)
V61.8 FAMILY MEMBERS NEC (REASON FOR ENCOUNTER)
V61.29 FOSTER CHILD (REASON FOR ENCOUNTER)
V61.6 ILLEGITIMACY TO FAMILY
V62.81 INTERPERSONAL NEC
V62.5 LEGAL
V62.89 LIFE CIRCUMSTANCE
V61.10 MARITAL
V61.5 MULTIPARITY IN FAMILY
V62.2 OCCUPATIONAL OTHER CIRCUMSTANCES OR MALADJUSTMENT
V61.20 PARENT-CHILD RELATIONSHIP
V61.10 PARTNER
V62.89 PHASE OF LIFE
V62.9 PSYCHOSOCIAL
V62.81 RELATIONAL
V62.6 RELIGIOUS REGARDING MEDICAL CARE
V62.89 RELIGIOUS OTHER THAN MEDICAL CARE
V61.8 SIBLING RELATIONAL
V62.0 UNEMPLOYMENT (AS CAUSE OF)
V61.7 UNWANTED PREGNANCY IN FAMILY
V62.1 WORK ENVIRONMENT (ADVERSE EFFECTS OF)

PROBLEM WITH

V40.1 COMMUNICATION
V41.3 EAR (OTHER SPECIFIED)
V41.1 EYE
V48.9 HEAD
V48.0 HEAD DEFICIENCY
V48.6 HEAD DISFIGUREMENT
V48.2 HEAD MECHANICAL AND MOTOR
V48.4 HEAD SENSORY
V48.8 HEAD OTHER
V41.2 HEARING
V47.0 INTERNAL ORGANS DEFICIENCY
V47.1 INTERNAL ORGANS MECHANICAL AND MOTOR
V40.0 LEARNING

V49.9 LIMB
V49.0 LIMB DEFICIENCY
V49.4 LIMB DISFIGUREMENT
V49.1 LIMB MECHANICAL
V49.2 LIMB MOTOR
V49.3 LIMB SENSORY
V49.5 LIMB OTHER
V49.8 LIMB OTHER SPECIFIED

V41.6 MASTICATION

V48.9 NECK
V48.1 NECK DEFICIENCY
V48.7 NECK DISFIGUREMENT
V48.3 NECK MECHANICAL AND MOTOR
V48.5 NECK SENSORY
V48.8 NECK OTHER

V41.7 SEXUAL FUNCTION
V41.0 SIGHT
V41.5 SMELL
V41.9 SPECIAL FUNCTIONS
V41.8 SPECIAL FUNCTIONS OTHER SPECIFIED
V40.1 SPEECH
V41.6 SWALLOWING
V41.5 TASTE

PROBLEM WITH (continued)

V48.9 TRUNK
V48.1 TRUNK DEFICIENCY
V48.7 TRUNK DISFIGUREMENT
V48.3 TRUNK MECHANICAL AND MOTOR
V48.8 TRUNK OTHER
V48.5 TRUNK SENSORY

V41.4 VOICE (WITH PRODUCTION)

PROBLEM WITH INTERNAL ORGANS

V47.3 DIGESTIVE
V47.2 EXERCISE INTOLERANCE CARDIOVASCULAR (RESPIRATORY) AT REST
V47.5 GENITAL
V47.9 INTERNAL ORGAN NOS
V47.0 INTERNAL ORGANS DEFICIENCY
V47.1 INTERNAL ORGANS MECHANICAL AND MOTOR
V47.4 URINARY NEC

PROBLEM WITH SPECIAL SENSES AND FUNCTION

V41.9 SPECIAL FUNCTIONS NOS
V41.3 EAR OTHER SPECIFIED
V41.1 EYE OTHER SPECIFIED
V41.2 HEARING
V41.6 MASTICATION
V41.7 SEXUAL FUNCTION
V41.0 SIGHT
V41.5 SMELL
V41.6 SWALLOWING
V41.5 TASTE
V41.4 VOICE (WITH PRODUCTION)
V41.8 OTHER SPECIFIED SPECIAL FUNCTIONS

PROCEDURE (SURGICAL) NOT DONE

V64.3 NEC
V64.1 DUE TO CONTRAINDICATION
V64.4 LAPAROSCOPIC CONVERTED TO OPEN PROCEDURE
V64.2 PATIENT DECISION
V64.6 PATIENT DECISION FOR REASONS OF CONSCIENCE OR RELIGION
V64.3 OTHER REASONS NEC

569.1 PROCIDENTIA ANUS RECTUM (SPHINCTER)
537.89 PROCIDENTIA STOMACH
286.3 PROCONVERTIN DEFICIENCY CONGENITAL

V26.4 PROCREATIVE COUNSELING
V26.9 PROCREATIVE MANAGEMENT NOS
V26.8 PROCREATIVE MANAGEMENT SPECIFIED NEC

PROCTALGIA

569.42 PROCTALGIA
564.6 FUGAX
564.6 SPASMODIC
307.89 SPASMODIC PSYCHOGENIC

569.49 PROCTITIS
555.1 PROCTITIS GRANULOMATOUS
556.2 PROCTITIS ULCERATIVE (CHRONIC)

556.2 PROCTOCOLITIS IDIOPATHIC

556.3 PROCTOSIGMOIDITIS ULCERATIVE
729.9 PROFICHET'S SYNDROME
259.8 PROGERIA (SYNDROME)
524.10 PROGNATHISM

PROGRESSIVE

335.22 BULBAR PALSY
046.3 MULTIFOCAL LEUKOENCEPHALOPATHY
335.21 MUSCULAR ATROPHY
335.0 MUSCULAR ATROPHY OF INFANCY
333.2 MYOCLONIC EPILEPSY
333.0 PALLIDAL DEGENERATION
709.09 PIGMENTARY DERMATOSIS

PROGRESSIVE (continued)

288.1 SEPTIC GRANULOMATOSIS
333.0 SUPRANUCLEAR OPHTHALMOPLEGIA
333.0 SUPRANUCLEAR PALSY

PROLACTIN

253.4 DEFICIENCY
253.1 EXCESS

PROLAPSE

569.1 ANAL
756.71 BLADDER (MUCOSA) CONGENITAL (FEMALE) (MALE)
618.0 BLADDER FEMALE
618.0 BLADDER FEMALE WITH STRESS INCONTINENCE [625.6]
618.0 BLADDER FEMALE WITH OTHER URINARY INCONTINENCE [788.3#]

5th Digit: 788.3
- 0. UNSPECIFIED
- 1. URGE INCONTINENCE
- 3. MIXED URGE AND STRESS (MALE) (FEMALE)
- 4 WITHOUT SENSORY AWARENESS
- 5. POST-VOID DRIBBLING
- 6. NOCTURNAL ENURESIS
- 7. CONTINUOUS LEAKAGE
- 9. OTHER

596.8 BLADDER MALE
569.69 CECOSTOMY
569.69 COLOSTOMY
372.73 CONJUNCTIVA
537.89 DUODENAL
569.69 ENTEROSTOMY
996.59 EYE IMPLANT (ORBITAL)
537.89 GASTRIC (MUCOSA)
618.9 GENITAL FEMALE
618.9 GENITAL FEMALE WITH STRESS INCONTINENCE [625.6]
618.9 GENITAL FEMALE WITH OTHER URINARY INCONTINENCE [788.3#]

5th Digit: 788.3
- 0. UNSPECIFIED
- 1. URGE INCONTINENCE
- 3. MIXED URGE AND STRESS
- 4 WITHOUT SENSORY AWARENESS
- 5. POST-VOID DRIBBLING
- 6. NOCTURNAL ENURESIS
- 7. CONTINUOUS LEAKAGE
- 9. OTHER

618.8 GENITAL OTHER SPECIFIED FEMALE
618.8 GENITAL OTHER SPECIFIED FEMALE WITH STRESS INCONTINENCE [625.6]
618.8 GENITAL OTHER SPECIFIED FEMALE WITH OTHER URINARY INCONTINENCE [788.3#]

5th Digit: 788.3
- 0. UNSPECIFIED
- 1. URGE INCONTINENCE
- 3. MIXED URGE AND STRESS
- 4 WITHOUT SENSORY AWARENESS
- 5. POST-VOID DRIBBLING
- 6. NOCTURNAL ENURESIS
- 7. CONTINUOUS LEAKAGE
- 9. OTHER

360.81 GLOBE
569.69 ILEOSTOMY
569.89 INTESTINE
364.8 IRIS
871.1 IRIS (TRAUMATIC) (ACUTE)
569.69 JEJUNOSTOMY
996.53 LENS IMPLANT (OCULAR)
424.0 MITRAL VALVE
620.4 OVARY AND FALLOPIAN TUBE
618.8 PELVIC FLOOR FEMALE
618.8 PELVIC FLOOR FEMALE WITH STRESS INCONTINENCE [625.6]

PROLAPSE (continued)

618.8 PELVIC FLOOR FEMALE WITH OTHER URINARY INCONTINENCE [788.3#]

5th Digit: 788.3
- 0. UNSPECIFIED
- 1. URGE INCONTINENCE
- 3. MIXED URGE AND STRESS
- 4 WITHOUT SENSORY AWARENESS
- 5. POST-VOID DRIBBLING
- 6. NOCTURNAL ENURESIS
- 7. CONTINUOUS LEAKAGE
- 9. OTHER

618.8 PERINEUM FEMALE
618.8 PERINEUM FEMALE WITH STRESS INCONTINENCE [625.6]
618.8 PERINEUM FEMALE WITH OTHER URINARY INCONTINENCE [788.3#]

5th Digit: 788.3
- 0. UNSPECIFIED
- 1. URGE INCONTINENCE
- 3. MIXED URGE AND STRESS
- 4 WITHOUT SENSORY AWARENESS
- 5. POST-VOID DRIBBLING
- 6. NOCTURNAL ENURESIS
- 7. CONTINUOUS LEAKAGE
- 9. OTHER

569.1 RECTAL
593.89 URETER
599.5 URETHRA
618.1 UTERUS
618.1 UTERUS FIRST DEGREE
618.1 UTERUS SECOND DEGREE
618.1 UTERUS THIRD DEGREE
618.4 UTERUS AND VAGINA
618.3 UTERUS AND VAGINA COMPLETE
618.2 UTERUS AND VAGINA INCOMPLETE
618.0 VAGINA (WITHOUT UTERINE PROLAPSE)
618.5 VAGINA AFTER HYSTERECTOMY

PROLAPSE COMPLICATING PREGNANCY

652.7# ARM
660.0# ARM OBSTRUCTING LABOR [652.7#]
652.6# ARM WITH MULTIPLE GESTATION
660.0# ARM WITH MULTIPLE GESTATION OBSTRUCTING LABOR [652.6#]

5th Digit: 652.6-7, 660.0
- 0. EPISODE OF CARE UNSPECIFIED OR N/A
- 1. DELIVERED
- 3. ANTEPARTUM COMPLICATION

762.4 CORD AFFECTING FETUS OR NEWBORN
652.8# FOOT
660.0# FOOT OBSTRUCTING LABOR [652.8#]
652.8# LEG
660.0# LEG OBSTRUCTING LABOR [652.8#]
663.0# UMBILICAL CORD

5th Digit: 652.8, 660.0, 663.0
- 0. EPISODE OF CARE UNSPECIFIED OR N/A
- 1. DELIVERED
- 3. ANTEPARTUM COMPLICATION

654.4# UTERUS COMPLICATING PREGNANCY
660.2# UTERUS OBSTRUCTING LABOR [654.4#]
654.4# VAGINAL (PUERPERAL)
660.2# VAGINAL (PUERPERAL) OBSTRUCTING LABOR [654.4#]

5th Digit: 654.4
- 0. EPISODE OF CARE UNSPECIFIED OR N/A
- 1. DELIVERED
- 2. DELIVERED WITH POSTPARTUM COMPLICATION
- 3. ANTEPARTUM COMPLICATION
- 4. POSTPARTUM COMPLICATION

5th Digit: 660.2
- 0. EPISODE OF CARE UNSPECIFIED OR N/A
- 1. DELIVERED
- 3. ANTEPARTUM COMPLICATION

728.79 PROLIFERATIVE FIBROMATOSIS (SARCOMATOUS)
270.8 PROLINE METABOLISM DISORDERS
270.8 PROLINEMIA
270.8 PROLINURIA
766.2 PROLONGED GESTATION SYNDROME
736.79 PRONATION ANKLE (FOOT)
755.67 PRONATION ANKLE FOOT CONGENITAL

PROPHYLACTIC

V07.39 ANTIBIOTIC ADMINISTRATION
V07.2 ANTIVENIN ADMINISTRATION
V50.41 BREAST REMOVAL
V50.41 BREAST REMOVAL DUE TO FAMILY HISTORY CANCER BREAST [V16.3]
V07.39 CHEMOTHERAPEUTIC AGENT ADMINISTRATION NEC
V07.31 FLUORIDE ADMINISTRATION
V07.2 GAMMA GLOBULIN ADMINISTRATION
V07.4 HORMONE REPLACEMENT THERAPY POSTMENOPAUSAL
0 IMMUNIZATION SEE 'VACCINATION'
V07.0 ISOLATION
V07.9 MEASURE
V50.42 OVARY REMOVAL
V50.42 OVARY REMOVAL DUE TO FAMILY HISTORY OF OVARIAN CANCER [V16.41]
V50.49 ORGAN REMOVAL OTHER SPECIFIED
V07.2 RHOGAM ADMINISTRATION
V07.2 TETANUS ANTITOXIN ADMINISTRATION
V07.8 TOXOXIFEN ADMINISTRATION DUE TO FAMILY HISTORY CANCER BREAST [V16.3]
0 VACCINATION OR INOCULATION SEE 'VACCINATION'
V07.8 OTHER SPECIFIED MEASURE

041.84 PROPIONIBACTERIUM INFECTION
376.30 PROPTOSIS OCULAR
V62.5 PROSECUTION PROBLEM (REASON FOR ENCOUNTER)
079.81 PROSPECT HILL VIRUS

PROSTATE

601.2 ABSCESS
602.8 ABSENCE
752.8 ABSENCE CONGENITAL
600 ADENOFIBROMATOUS HYPERTROPHY
600 ADENOFIBROMATOUS HYPERTROPHY WITH INCONTINENCE **[788.3#]**

5th Digit: 788.3

0. UNSPECIFIED
1. URGE INCONTINENCE
2. STRESS, MALE
3. MIXED URGE AND STRESS
4 WITHOUT SENSORY AWARENESS
5. POST-VOID DRIBBLING
6. NOCTURNAL ENURESIS
7. CONTINUOUS LEAKAGE
9. OTHER

752.8 APLASIA CONGENITAL
602.2 ATROPHY
600 BENIGN ADENOMA
600 BENIGN ADENOMA WITH INCONTINENCE **[788.3#]**
600 BENIGN HYPERTROPHY
600 BENIGN HYPERTROPHY WITH INCONTINENCE **[788.3#]**
222.2 BENIGN NEOPLASM
222.2 BENIGN NEOPLASM WITH INCONTINENCE **[788.3#]**

5th Digit: 788.3

0. UNSPECIFIED
1. URGE INCONTINENCE
2. STRESS, MALE
3. MIXED URGE AND STRESS
4 WITHOUT SENSORY AWARENESS
5. POST-VOID DRIBBLING
6. NOCTURNAL ENURESIS
7. CONTINUOUS LEAKAGE
9. OTHER

PROSTATE (continued)

602.0 CALCULUS
V76.44 CANCER SCREENING
602.1 CONGESTION OR HEMORRHAGE
602.9 DISORDER
602.8 DISORDER SPECIFIED TYPE NEC
602.8 DYSPLASIA
600 ENLARGEMENT
600 FIBROADENOMA
600 FIBROADENOMA WITH INCONTINENCE **[788.3#]**
600 HYPERPLASIA
600 HYPERPLASIA WITH INCONTINENCE **[788.3#]**
867.6 INJURY
867.7 INJURY WITH OPEN WOUND INTO CAVITY
908.2 INJURY LATE EFFECT
600 MEDIAN BAR
600 MEDIAN BAR WITH INCONTINENCE **[788.3#]**
600 MYOMA
600 MYOMA WITH INCONTINENCE **[788.3#]**
600 NODULE
600 NODULE WITH INCONTINENCE **[788.3#]**
600 OBSTRUCTION
600 OBSTRUCTION WITH INCONTINENCE **[788.3#]**

5th Digit: 788.3

0. UNSPECIFIED
1. URGE INCONTINENCE
2. STRESS, MALE
3. MIXED URGE AND STRESS
4 WITHOUT SENSORY AWARENESS
5. POST-VOID DRIBBLING
6. NOCTURNAL ENURESIS
7. CONTINUOUS LEAKAGE
9. OTHER

790.93 PSA ELEVATED
790.93 SPECIFIC ANTIGEN (PSA) ELEVATED
016.5# TB [608.81]

5th Digit: 016.5

0. UNSPECIFIED
1. LAB NOT DONE
2. LABS PENDING
3. MICROSCOPY POSITIVE (IN SPUTUM)
4. CULTURE POSITIVE - MICROSCOPY NEGATIVE
5. CULTURE NEGATIVE - MICROSCOPY POSITIVE
6. CULTURE AND MICROSCOPY NEGATIVE CONFIRMED BY OTHER METHODS

596.0 VALVE OBSTRUCTION (PROSTATIC) (URINARY)
602.8 OTHER SPECIFIED DISORDER NEC

PROSTATITIS

601.9 NOS
601.0 ACUTE
039.8 ACTINOMYCOTIC [601.4]
116.0 BLASTOMYCOTIC [601.4]
601.8 CAVITARY
099.54 CHLAMYDIAL
601.1 CHRONIC
601.8 DIVERTICULAR
098.12 GONOCOCCAL ACUTE
098.32 GONOCOCCAL CHRONIC
601.8 GRANULOMATOUS
112.2 MONILIAL
095.8 SYPHILITIC [601.4]
131.03 TRICHOMONAL

601.3 PROSTATOCYSTITIS

PROSTHESIS (FITTING AND ADJUSTMENT) (REMOVAL)

V52.9 NOS
V52.0 ARM
V52.4 BREAST
V52.3 DENTURES
V52.2 EYE
V52.1 LEG
V52.8 OTHER SPECIFIED

PROSTHESIS (STATUS)

V43.5 BLADDER
V43.82 BREAST
V45.83 BREAST REMOVAL
0 COMPLICATION SEE 'COMPLICATION'
V43.0 EYE GLOBE
V43.1 EYE LENS
V43.2 HEART
V43.3 HEART VALVE
V43.4 HEART VESSEL
V43.89 INTESTINE
V43.60 JOINT
V43.66 JOINT ANKLE
V43.62 JOINT ELBOW
V43.69 JOINT FINGER
V43.64 JOINT HIP
V43.65 JOINT KNEE
V43.61 JOINT SHOULDER
V43.63 JOINT WRIST
V43.69 JOINT OTHER
V43.89 KIDNEY
V43.81 LARYNX
V43.7 LIMB
V43.89 LIVER
V43.89 LUNG
V43.89 ORGAN OTHER
V43.89 PANCREAS
V43.83 SKIN ARTIFICIAL
V43.89 TISSUE OTHER
V43.89 OTHER ORGAN OR TISSUE

V70.5 PROSTITUTES HEALTH EXAM

PROSTRATION

780.79 NOS
992.5 HEAT
992.4 HEAT - SALT DEPLETION
992.4 HEAT - SALT AND WATER DEPLETION
992.3 HEAT - WATER DEPLETION
300.5 NERVOUS
779.8 NEWBORN
797 SENILE

368.51 PROTAN DEFECT
368.51 PROTANOMALY
368.51 PROTANOPIA

273.9 PROTEIN PLASMA METABOLISM DISORDER
273.8 PROTEIN PLASMA METABOLISM ABNORMALITY SPECIFIED NEC
790.99 PROTEIN SERUM NEC ABNORMAL FINDINGS
273.8 PROTEIN TRANSPORT ABNORMALITY

790.99 PROTEINEMIA
272.8 PROTEINOSIS LIPID

PROTEINURIA

791.0 NOS
791.0 BENCE-JONES

PROTEINURIA (continued)

646.2# MATERNAL (GESTATIONAL) COMPLICATING PREGNANCY WITHOUT MENTION OF HYPERTENSION

5th Digit: 646.2

0. EPISODE OF CARE UNSPECIFIED OR N/A
1. DELIVERED
2. DELIVERED WITH POSTPARTUM COMPLICATION
3. ANTEPARTUM COMPLICATION
4. POSTPARTUM COMPLICATION

593.6 ORTHOSTATIC
593.6 POSTURAL BENIGN

041.6 PROTEUS MIRABILIS MORGANII INFECTION OR ORGANISM
008.3 PROTEUS MIRABILIS MORGANII GASTROENTERITIS
757.39 PROTEUS SYNDROME (DERMAL HYPOPLASIA)

PROTHROMBIN

286.3 DEFICIENCY CONGENITAL
286.7 DEFICIENCY DUE TO LIVER DISEASE
286.7 TIME INCREASED DUE TO LIVER DISEASE
790.92 TIME (PROLONGED)

790.92 PROTIME ABNORMAL
286.7 PROTIME TIME INCREASED DUE TO LIVER DISEASE

277.1 PROTOCOPROPORPHYRIA
277.1 PROTOPORPHYRIA

136.8 PROTOZOAL DISEASE OTHER SPECIFIED NEC
007.9 PROTOZOAL INTESTINAL DISEASE
007.8 PROTOZOAL INTESTINAL DISEASES OTHER SPECIFIED

701.5 PROUD FLESH
756.71 PRUNE BELLY SYNDROME

PRURIGO

698.2 NOS
691.8 ASTHMA SYNDROME
691.8 BESNIER'S (INFANTILE ECZEMA)
691.8 ECZEMATODES ALLERGICUM
692.72 ESTIVALIS
698.2 HEBRA'S
692.72 HUTCHINSON'S
698.2 MITIS
698.3 NODULARIS
698.2 PRURIGO
698.2 SIMPLEX

PRURITUS

698.9 NOS
698.0 ANI
698.9 EAR
379.99 EYE
698.1 GENITAL ORGANS
698.8 HIEMALIS

646.8#: SPECIFY THE MATERNAL PRURITUS WITH AN ADDITIONAL CODE.

646.8# MATERNAL COMPLICATING PREGNANCY

5th Digit: 646.8

0. EPISODE OF CARE UNSPECIFIED OR N/A
1. DELIVERED
2. DELIVERED WITH POSTPARTUM COMPLICATION
3. ANTEPARTUM COMPLICATION
4. POSTPARTUM COMPLICATION

306.3 PSYCHOGENIC
698.1 SCROTUM
306.3 SCROTUM PSYCHOGENIC
698.8 SENILIS
698.8 UREMIC
698.1 VULVA

790.93 PSA ELEVATED ABNORMAL FINDINGS

0 PSEUDOANEURYSM SEE 'ANEURYSM'

733.82 PSEUDARTHROSIS
V45.4 PSEUDARTHROSIS FOLLOWING FUSION (STATUS)

335.23 PSEUDOBULBAR PALSY
727.89 PSEUDOBURSA

701.8 PSEUDOCANTHOSIS NIGRICANS
354.0 PSEUDOCARPAL TUNNEL SYNDROME (SUBLIMIS)
289.8 PSEUDOCHOLINESTERASE DEFICIENCY
705.89 PSEUDOCHROMIDROSIS
051.1 PSEUDOCOWPOX
732.1 PSEUDOCOXALGIA
300.11 PSEUDOCYESIS
577.2 PSEUDOCYST PANCREAS
361.19 PSEUDOCYST RETINA

518.89 PSEUDOEMPHYSEMA
265.1 PSEUDOENCEPHALITIS SUPERIOR (ACUTE) HEMORRHAGIC

268.2 PSEUDOFRACTURE (IDIOPATHIC) (MULTIPLE) (SPONTANEOUS)(SYMMETRICAL)
025 PSEUDOGLANDERS
360.44 PSEUDOGLIOMA
0 PSEUDOGOUT SEE 'CHONDROCALCINOSIS'

780.1 PSEUDOHALLUCINATION
782.0 PSEUDOHEMIANESTHESIA
272.7 PSEUDO-HURLER'S (MUCOLIPIDOSIS III)

PSEUDOHEMOPHILIA
287.8 HEREDITARY CAPILLARY FRAGILITY
287.8 TYPE A
286.4 TYPE B
287.8 VASCULAR

PSEUDOHERMAPHRODITISM
255.2 ADRENAL FEMALE
752.7 CONGENITAL
255.2 FEMALE (ADRENOCORTICAL)
257.8 MALE (GONADAL)
257.8 MALE WITH TESTICULAR FEMINIZATION
256.4 STEIN LEVENTHAL (POLYCYSTIC OVARY)
255.2 VIRILISM-HIRSUTISM SYNDROME

348.2 PSEUDOHYDROCEPHALUS
275.49 PSEUDOHYPOPARATHYROIDISM

285.8 PSEUDOLEUKEMIA INFANTILE

101 PSEUDOMEMBRANOUS ANGINA
008.45 PSEUDOMEMBRANOUS COLITIS
777.5 PSEUDOMEMBRANOUS ENTEROCOLITIS IN NEWBORN

349.2 PSEUDOMENINGOCELE, ACQUIRED (SPINAL)
626.8 PSEUDOMENSTRUATION

PSEUDOMONAS
008.42 GASTROENTERITIS
041.7 INFECTION
024 INFECTION MALLEI
025 INFECTION PSEUDOMALLEI
038.43 INFECTION WITH SEPSIS

197.6 PSEUDOMYXOMA PERITONEI SITE NOS
0 PSEUDOMYXOMA PERITONEI SITE SPECIFIED SEE 'CANCER' BY SITE M8480/6

377.24 PSEUDONEURITIS (OPTIC NERVE) (PAPILLA)

564.89 PSEUDOOBSTRUCTION (INTESTINE)

377.24 PSEUDOPAPILLEDEMA
358.0 PSEUDOPARALYTICA SYNDROME
704.09 PSEUDOPELADE
V43.1 PSEUDOPHAKIA

556.4 PSEUDOPOLYPOSIS COLON
348.0 PSEUDOPORENCEPHALY
275.49 PSEUDOPSEUDOHYPOPARATHYROIDISM
372.52 PSEUDOPTERYGIUM
374.34 PSEUDOPTOSIS

362.65 PSEUDORETINITIS PIGMENTOSA
057.8 PSEUDORUBELLA

PSEUDOSARCOMATOUS
199.1 CARCINOMA SITE NOS
0 CARCINOMA SITE SPECIFIED SEE 'CANCER' BY SITE M8033/3
728.79 FIBROMATOSIS (PROLIFERATIVE) (SUBCUTANEOUS)

057.8 PSEUDOSCARLATINA

046.1 PSEUDOSCLEROSIS (JAKOB'S) (SPASTIC) BRAIN
046.1 PSEUDOSCLEROSIS (JAKOB'S) (SPASTIC) BRAIN WITH DEMENTIA [294.1]

799.8 PSEUDOTABES

780.39 PSEUDOTETANUS (SEE ALSO 'CONVULSIONS')
348.2 PSEUDOTUMOR CEREBRI
376.11 PSEUDOTUMOR ORBIT (INFLAMMATORY)
759.89 PSEUDO-TURNER'S SYNDROME

305.3# PSILOCYBIN ABUSE (NONDEPENDENT)
304.5# PSILOCYBIN ADDICTION (DEPENDENT)
5th Digit: 304.5, 305.3
0. UNSPECIFIED
1. CONTINUOUS
2. EPISODIC
3. IN REMISSION

073.9 PSITTACOSIS
726.5 PSOAS TENDINITIS

PSORIASIS
696.1 NOS
696.0 ARTHRITIC
696.0 ARTHROPATHIC
528.6 BUCCAL
528.6 MOUTH
691.0 NAPKIN ERUPTION
316 PSYCHOGENIC [696.1]
696.8 OTHER SPECIFIED

136.4 PSOROSPERMIASIS

300.89 PSYCHASTHENIA
300.89 PSYCHASTHENIC NEUROSIS

V70.1 PSYCHIATRIC EXAM GENERAL REQUESTED BY AUTHORITY
V70.2 PSYCHIATRIC EXAM GENERAL OTHER AND UNSPECIFIED

316 PSYCHOGENIC CAUSE OF (OR ASSOCIATED WITH) OTHER ORGANIC DISEASE
300.9 PSYCHOGENIC DISORDER (NEUROTIC) NEC
307.80 PSYCHOGENIC PAIN SITE UNSPECIFIED
316 PSYCHOGENIC PIELINOSIS
298.8 PSYCHOGENIC STUPOR
298.2 PSYCHOGENIC TWILIGHT STATE

301.59 PSYCHOINFANTILE PERSONALITY
V15.4# PSYCHOLOGICAL TRAUMA HISTORY
5th Digit: V15.4
1. PHYSICAL ABUSE, RAPE
2. EMOTIONAL ABUSE, NEGLECT
9. OTHER

300.11 PSYCHOMOTOR DISORDER NEC - HYSTERICAL
307.9 PSYCHOMOTOR DISORDER NEC - PSYCHOGENIC

300.9 PSYCHONEUROSIS
301.89 PSYCHONEUROTIC PERSONALITY

PSYCHO-ORGANIC SYNDROME

293.9 NOS
293.0 ACUTE
293.84 ANXIETY TYPE
293.83 DEPRESSIVE TYPE
293.82 HALLUCINATORY TYPE
310.1 NONPSYCHOTIC SEVERITY
310.8 NONPSYCHOTIC SEVERITY, SPECIFIED FOCAL (PARTIAL)
293.81 PARANOID TYPE
293.1 SUBACUTE
293.89 OTHER SPECIFIED

301.9 PSYCHOPATHIC PERSONALITY DISORDER
306.9 PSYCHOPHYSIOLOGIC DISORDER

PSYCHOSEXUAL DYSFUNCTION

302.70 NOS
302.72 FRIGIDITY
302.85 IDENTITY DISORDER ADULT
302.6 IDENTITY DISORDER CHILDHOOD
302.72 IMPOTENCE
302.79 SEXUAL AVERSION
306.51 VAGINISMUS
302.76 WITH DYSPAREUNIA FUNCTIONAL
302.73 WITH INHIBITED FEMALE ORGASM
302.74 WITH INHIBITED MALE ORGASM
302.71 WITH INHIBITED SEXUAL DESIRE
302.72 WITH INHIBITED SEXUAL EXCITEMENT
302.75 WITH PREMATURE EJACULATION
302.79 OTHER SPECIFIED

PSYCHOSIS

298.9 NOS
296.90 AFFECTIVE
295.4# CONFUSIONAL TYPE ACUTE EPISODE

5th Digit: 295.4

0. NOS
1. SUBCHRONIC
2. CHRONIC
3 SUBCHRONIC WITH ACUTE EXACERBATION
4. CHRONIC WITH ACUTE
5. IN REMISSION

296.90 MELANCHOLIC

> ***PSYCHOSIS ALCOHOLIC, 291.#(#),** REQUIRES TWO CODES: CODE THE PSYCHOSIS FIRST WITH AN ADDITIONAL CODE FOR THE DEPENDENCE / NON DEPENDENCE. SEE 'ALCOHOL ABUSE', (DEPENDENT) (NON DEPENDENT).*

PSYCHOSIS ALCOHOLIC

291.9 NOS
291.0 ACUTE WITH DELIRIUM
291.3 ACUTE WITH HALLUCINATION
291.1 AMNESTIC SYNDROME
291.0 DELIRIUM (TREMENS)
291.5 DELUSIONS
291.2 DEMENTIA NOS
291.3 HALLUCINOSIS
291.4 INTOXICATION PATHOLOGIC (IDIOSYNCRATIC)
291.5 JEALOUSY
291.1 KORSAKOFF'S
291.2 ORGANIC BRAIN SYNDROME
291.5 PARANOID
291.1 POLYNEURITIC
291.5 POLYNEURITIC WITH DELUSIONS
291.3 POLYNEURITIC WITH HALLUCINATIONS
291.1 WITH AMNESIA PERSISTING
291.89 WITH ANXIETY
291.89 WITH MOOD DISTURBANCE
291.89 WITH SEXUAL DYSFUNCTION
291.89 WITH SLEEP DISTURBANCE
291.0 WITHDRAWAL DELIRIUM
291.3 WITHDRAWAL HALLUCINOSIS
291.81 WITHDRAWAL SYNDROME

PSYCHOSIS ARTERIOSCLEROTIC

290.40 NOS [437.0]
290.41 ACUTE [437.0]
290.41 WITH CONFUSIONAL STATE [437.0]
290.41 WITH DELIRIUM [437.0]
290.42 WITH DELUSION [437.0]
290.43 WITH DEPRESSION [437.0]
290.42 PARANOID OR DELUSIONAL [437.0]
290.40 UNCOMPLICATED [437.0]

PSYCHOSIS CHILDHOOD

299.90 ACTIVE STATE
299.91 RESIDUAL STATE
299.80 ATYPICAL ACTIVE STATE
299.81 ATYPICAL RESIDUAL STATE
299.00 AUTISTIC ACTIVE STATE
299.01 AUTISTIC RESIDUAL STATE
299.80 BORDERLINE ACTIVE STATE
299.81 BORDERLINE RESIDUAL STATE
299.10 DISINTEGRATIVE ACTIVE STATE
299.11 DISINTEGRATIVE RESIDUAL STATE
299.00 INFANTILE ACTIVE STATE
299.01 INFANTILE RESIDUAL STATE

> ***PSYCHOSIS DRUG INDUCED, 292.#(#),** REQUIRES TWO CODES: CODE THE PSYCHOSIS FIRST WITH AN ADDITIONAL CODE FOR THE DEPENDENCE / NON DEPENDENCE. SEE 'DRUG ABUSE', (DEPENDENT) (NON DEPENDENT).*

PSYCHOSIS DRUG INDUCED

292.9 NOS
292.11 DELUSIONAL
292.12 DRUG WITH HALLUCINATION
292.12 HALLUCINATORY
292.2 PATHOLOGICAL DRUG INTOXICATION (BRIEF)
292.83 WITH AMNESTIC SYNDROME
292.89 WITH ANXIETY
292.81 WITH DELERIUM
292.82 WITH DEMENTIA
292.89 WITH MOOD DISTURBANCE
292.84 WITH ORGANIC AFFECTIVE SYNDROME (DEPRESSIVE STATE)
292.89 WITH SEXUAL DYSFUNCTION
292.89 WITH SLEEP DISTURBANCE
292.0 WITHDRAWL
292.89 OTHER

PSYCHOSIS NON ORGANIC (STRESS INDUCED)

298.9 NOS
298.9 ATYPICAL
298.8 BRIEF REACTIVE
298.0 DEPRESSIVE TYPE
298.1 EXCITATIVE TYPE
298.1 HYSTERICAL (ACUTE)
298.8 HYSTERICAL BRIEF REACTIVE
298.8 INCIPIENT
298.8 INVOLUTIONAL
298.9 NONORGANIC
297.9 PARANOID
298.3 PARANOID (ACUTE) (PSYCHOGENIC)
297.1 PARANOID (CHRONIC)
298.4 PARANOID (CHRONIC) PSYCHOGENIC
298.3 PARANOID PSYCHOGENIC (PROTRACTED)
298.8 PSYCHOGENIC
298.8 REACTIVE BRIEF HYSTERICAL
298.2 REACTIVE CONFUSION
298.0 REACTIVE DEPRESSIVE
298.4 REACTIVE PARANOID, PROTRACTED

PSYCHOSIS ORGANIC

294.9 NOS
291.2 ALCOHOLIC
293.9 INFECTIVE
294.8 MIXED PARANOID AND AFFECTIVE STATES
293.9 POSTTRAUMATIC

PSYCHOSIS ORGANIC TRANSIENT

293.9 NOS
293.84 ANXIETY TYPE
293.0 ASSOCIATED WITH ENDOCRINE, METABOLIC, OR CEREBROVASCULAR DISORDER ACUTE
293.1 ASSOCIATED WITH ENDOCRINE OR METABOLIC DISORDER SUBACUTE
293.9 ASSOCIATED WITH PHYSICAL CONDITION
293.81 ASSOCIATED WITH PHYSICAL CONDITION WITH DELUSIONS
293.82 ASSOCIATED WITH PHYSICAL CONDITION WITH HALLUCINATIONS
293.0 DELIRIUM ACUTE
293.1 DELIRIUM SUBACUTE
293.81 DELUSIONAL SYNDROME
293.83 DEPRESSIVE TYPE
293.82 HALLUCINOSIS SYNDROME
293.0 INFECTIVE ACUTE
293.1 INFECTIVE SUBACUTE
293.0 ORGANIC REACTION ACUTE
293.1 ORGANIC REACTION SUBACUTE
293.81 PARANOID TYPE
293.0 POSTTRAUMATIC ACUTE
293.1 POSTTRAUMATIC SUBACUTE
293.89 OTHER SPECIFIED TYPE

PSYCHOSIS ORGANIC - OTHER

330.1 CEREBRAL LIPIDOSIS WITH DEMENTIA [294.1]
046.1 DUE TO JAKOB CREUTZFELDT DISEASE OR SYNDROME WITH DEMENTIA [294.1]
294.8 EPILEPTIC [**345.##**]

4th Digit: 345

0. GENERALIZED NONCONVULSIVE
1. GENERALIZED CONVULSIVE
4. PARTIAL, WITH IMPAIRMENT OF CONSCIOUSNESS
5. PARTIAL, WITHOUT IMPAIRMENT OF CONSCIOUSNESS
6. INFANTILE SPASMS
7. EPILEPSIA PARTIALIS CONTINUA
8. OTHER FORMS
9. UNSPECIFIED, NOS

5th Digit: 345

0. WITHOUT MENTION OF INTRACTABLE EPILEPSY
1. WITH INTRACTABLE EPILEPSY

294.8 EPILEPTIC GRAND MAL STATUS [345.3]
345.3 EPILEPTIC GRAND MAL STATUS WITH DEMENTIA [294.1]
294.8 EPILEPTIC PETIT MAL STATUS [345.2]
345.2 EPILEPTIC PETIT MAL STATUS WITH DEMENTIA [294.1]
345.## EPILEPTIC WITH DEMENTIA [294.1]

4th Digit: 345

0. GENERALIZED NONCONVULSIVE
1. GENERALIZED CONVULSIVE
4. PARTIAL, WITH IMPAIRMENT OF CONSCIOUSNESS
5. PARTIAL, WITHOUT IMPAIRMENT OF CONSCIOUSNESS
6. INFANTILE SPASMS
7. EPILEPSIA PARTIALIS CONTINUA
8. OTHER FORMS
9. UNSPECIFIED, NOS

5th Digit: 345

0. WITHOUT MENTION OF INTRACTABLE EPILEPSY
1. WITH INTRACTABLE EPILEPSY

PSYCHOSIS ORGANIC - OTHER (continued)

275.1 HEPATOLENTICULAR DEGENERATION WITH DEMENTIA [294.1]
333.4 HUNTINGTON'S CHOREA WITH DEMENTIA [294.1]
046.1 JAKOB CREUTZFELDT (PRESENILE) WITH DEMENTIA [294.1]
0 MANIC DEPRESSIVE SEE 'MANIC DEPRESSIVE PSYCHOSIS'
340 MULTIPLE SCLEROSIS WITH DEMENTIA [294.1]
294.9 ORGANIC BRAIN SYNDROME CHRONIC
446.0 POLYARTERITIS NODOSA WITH DEMENTIA [294.1]
094.1 SYPHILITIC WITH DEMENTIA [294.1]

> ***290 .#(#) PSYCHOSIS: CODE FIRST ANY ASSOCIATED NEUROLOGICAL CONDITION.***

PSYCHOSIS PRESENILE

290.10 UNCOMPLICATED
290.12 PARANOID
295.7# SCHIZO-AFFECTIVE

5th Digit: 295.7

0. UNSPECIFIED
1. SUBCHRONIC
2. CHRONIC
3. SUBCHRONIC WITH ACUTE EXACERBATION
4. CHRONIC WITH ACUTE
5. IN REMISSION

290.11 WITH DELIRIUM
290.12 WITH DELUSIONS
290.13 WITH DEPRESSIVE FEATURES

> ***290 .#(#) PSYCHOSIS: CODE FIRST ANY ASSOCIATED NEUROLOGICAL CONDITION.***

PSYCHOSIS SENILE

290.20 NOS
290.20 DELUSIONAL
290.20 PARANOID
290.8 PRESBYOPHRENIC
094.1 SYPHILITIC [294.1]
290.3 WITH DELERIUM
290.21 WITH DEPRESSION

> *SPECIFY THE MATERNAL PSYCHOSIS WITH AN ADDITIONAL CODE. SEE 'PSYCHOSIS'.*

PSYCHOSIS WITH PREGNANCY

648.4# NOS
648.4# MAJOR DEPRESSIVE - RECURRENT [**296.3#**]
648.4# MAJOR DEPRESSIVE - SINGLE EPISODE [**296.2#**]

5th Digit: 648.4

0. EPISODE OF CARE UNSPECIFIED OR N/A
1. DELIVERED
2. DELIVERED WITH POSTPARTUM COMPLICATION
3. ANTEPARTUM COMPLICATION
4. POSTPARTUM COMPLICATION

5th Digit: 296.2-3

0. UNSPECIFIED
1. MILD
2. MODERATE
3. SEVERE WITHOUT MENTION OF PSYCHOTIC BEHAVIOR
4. SEVERE SPECIFIED AS WITH PSYCHOTIC BEHAVIOR
5. IN PARTIAL OR UNSPECIFIED REMISSION

306.9 PSYCHOSOMATIC DISORDER
306.9 PSYCHOSOMATIC REACTION
V67.3 PSYCHOTHERAPY AND OTHER TREATMENT FOLLOWUP EXAM
V66.3 PSYCHOTHERAPY CONVALESCENCE

V57.1 PT (PHYSICAL THERAPY)
790.92 PT PROLONGED
286.7 PT PROLONGED DUE TO LIVER DISEASE
286.2 PTA DEFICIENCY
286.1 PTC DEFICIENCY
V45.82 PTCA STATUS (PERCUTANEOUS TRANSLUMINAL CORONARY ANGIOPLASTY)

PTERYGIUM
372.40 NOS
372.43 CENTRAL
744.5 COLLI CONGENITAL
372.44 DOUBLE
372.42 PERIPHERAL PROGRESSIVE
372.41 PERIPHERAL STATIONARY
372.52 PSEUDOPTERYGIUM
372.45 RECURRENT

758.6 PTERYGOLYMPHANGIECTASIA SYNDROME
0 PTHIRUS SEE 'PEDICULOSIS'

PTOSIS
611.8 BREAST
270.2 EPICANTHUS SYNDROME
569.89 INTESTINE

PTOSIS OF THE EYE
374.30 NOS
743.61 CONGENITAL
374.33 MECHANICAL
374.32 MYOGENIC
374.31 PARALYTIC
374.34 PSEUDOPTOSIS

790.92 PTT PROLONGED
286.7 PTT PROLONGED DUE TO LIVER DISEASE
848.8 PUBALGIA

PUBERTY
259.9 ABNORMAL
626.3 BLEEDING
259.0 DELAYED
259.1 PRECOCIOUS - NOS
255.2 PRECOCIOUS - CORTICAL HYPERFUNCTION (ADRENAL)
256.1 PRECOCIOUS - OVARIAN HYPERFUNCTION
256.0 PRECOCIOUS - OVARIAN HYPERFUNCTION ESTROGEN (HYPERESTROGENISM)
259.8 PRECOCIOUS - PINEAL TUMOR
257.0 PRECOCIOUS - TESTICULAR HYPERFUNCTION
259.1 PREMATURE - NOS
255.2 PREMATURE - CORTICAL HYPERFUNCTION (ADRENAL)
259.8 PREMATURE - PINEAL TUMOR
253.1 PREMATURE - PITUITARY (ANTERIOR) HYPERFUNCTION
V21.1 STATE

665.6# PUBIC BONE SEPARATION (OBSTETRICAL)
5th Digit: 665.6
0. EPISODE OF CARE UNSPECIFIED OR N/A
1. DELIVERED
4. POSTPARTUM COMPLICATION

132.2 PUBIC LICE
739.5 PUBIC REGION SEGMENTAL OR SOMATIC DYSFUNCTION
848.5 PUBIC SYMPHYSIS SEPARATION
553.8 PUDENDAL HERNIA
099.2 PUDENDAL ULCER
528.5 PUENTE'S (SIMPLE GLANDULAR CHEILITIS)
672.0# PUERPERAL FEVER
670.0# PUERPERAL FEVER SEPTIC
4th Digit: 670.0, 672.0
0. UNSPECIFIED
2. DELIVERED WITH POSTPARTUM COMPLICATION
4. POSTPARTUM COMPLICATION

PULMONARY
235.7 ADENOMATOUS TUMOR SITE NOS
0 ADENOMATOUS TUMOR SITE SPECIFIED SEE 'NEOPLASM UNCERTAIN BEHAVIOR', BY SITE M8250/1
516.2 ALVEOLAR MICROLITHIASIS
516.0 ALVEOLAR PROTEINOSIS
416.0 ARTERIOSCLEROSIS SYNDROME
747.3 ARTERY - ABSENCE CONGENITAL
747.3 ARTERY - AGENESIS CONGENITAL
417.1 ARTERY - ANEURYSM
747.3 ARTERY - ANOMALY CONGENITAL
417.8 ARTERY - ARTERITIS
747.3 ARTERY - ATRESIA CONGENITAL
747.3 ARTERY - COARCTATION CONGENITAL
417.9 ARTERY - DISEASE
417.8 ARTERY - ENDARTERITIS
747.3 ARTERY - HYPOPLASIA CONGENITAL
415.19 ARTERY - INFARCTION
415.11 ARTERY - INFARCTION IATROGENIC
415.11 ARTERY - INFARCTION POSTOPERATIVE
901.41 ARTERY - INJURY
908.4 ARTERY - INJURY LATE EFFECT
901.41 ARTERY - LACERATION (RUPTURE) (HEMATOMA) (AVULSION)
908.4 ARTERY - LACERATION LATE EFFECT
417.8 ARTERY - RUPTURE
417.8 ARTERY - STENOSIS (STRICTURE) ACQUIRED
747.3 ARTERY - STENOSIS CONGENITAL
417.8 ARTERY - STRICTURE
668.0# ASPIRATION FOLLOWING ANESTHESIA OR OTHER SEDATION IN L AND D
5th Digit: 668.0
0. EPISODE OF CARE UNSPECIFIED OR N/A
1 DELIVERED
2. DELIVERED WITH POSTPARTUM COMPLICATION
3. ANTEPARTUM COMPLICATION
4. POSTPARTUM COMPLICATION

417.9 BLOOD VESSEL - CIRCULATION DISEASE
901.40 BLOOD VESSEL - INJURY
908.4 BLOOD VESSEL - INJURY OR LACERATION LATE EFFECT
901.40 BLOOD VESSEL - LACERATION (RUPTURE) (HEMATOMA) (AVULSION) (ANEURYSM) TRAUMATIC
417.8 BLOOD VESSEL - RUPTURE
518.0 COLLAPSE
770.5 COLLAPSE PERINATAL
514 CONGESTION
861.21 CONTUSION
861.31 CONTUSION WITH OPEN WOUND INTO THORAX
908.0 CONTUSION LATE EFFECT
417.9 DISEASE CIRCULATION
416.9 DISEASE HEART
416.0 DISEASE HYPERTENSIVE VASCULAR (CARDIOVASCULAR)
496 DISEASE OBSTRUCTIVE CHRONIC (SEE ALSO 'COPD')
424.3 DISEASE VALVE
508.0 DISORDER DUE TO RADIATION ACUTE
508.1 DISORDER DUE TO RADIATION CHRONIC
508.8 DISORDER DUE TO OTHER EXTERNAL AGENTS
508.9 DISORDER DUE TO UNSPECIFIED EXTERNAL AGENTS
0 EDEMA SEE 'PULMONARY EDEMA'
V12.51 EMBOLISM HISTORY
415.11 EMBOLISM - IATROGENIC
673.2# EMBOLISM MATERNAL DUE TO PREGNANCY
5th Digit: 673.2
0. EPISODE OF CARE UNSPECIFIED OR N/A
1. DELIVERED
2. DELIVERED WITH POSTPARTUM COMPLICATION
3. ANTEPARTUM COMPLICATION
4. POSTPARTUM COMPLICATION

415.19 EMBOLISM - OTHER AND UNSPECIFIED
415.11 EMBOLISM - POSTOPERATIVE

PULMONARY (continued)

417.8	ENDARTERITIS
515	FIBROSIS - CHRONIC OR UNSPECIFIED
506.4	FIBROSIS - DUE TO FUMES AND VAPORS
508.1	FIBROSIS - DUE TO RADIATION
508.0	FIBROSIS - DUE TO RADIATION ACUTE
508.1	FIBROSIS - DUE TO RADIATION CHRONIC
508.8	FIBROSIS - DUE TO OTHER EXTERNAL AGENTS
508.9	FIBROSIS - DUE TO UNSPECIFIED EXTERNAL AGENTS
516.3	FIBROSIS - IDIOPATHIC (INTERSTITIAL) (DIFFUSE)
770.7	FIBROSIS - INTERSTITIAL OF PREMATURITY
710.1	FIBROSIS - SCLEROSIS DUE TO SCLERODERMA [517.8]
V71.8	FUNCTION STUDIES TO EVALUATE RESPIRATORY DISEASE OR INSUFFICIENCY
794.2	FUNCTION STUDY ABNORMAL
416.8	HEART DISEASE CHRONIC OTHER
770.3	HEMORRHAGE PERINATAL
747.89	HYPERTENSION PERSISTENT CONGENITAL
416.0	HYPERTENSION PRIMARY CHRONIC
416.8	HYPERTENSION SECONDARY CHRONIC
731.2	HYPERTROPHIC OSTEOARTHROPATHY
769	HYPOPERFUSION SYNDROME (IDIOPATHIC)
770.4	IMMATURITY
424.3	INCOMPETENCE
415.19	INFARCTION
415.11	INFARCTION IATROGENIC
415.11	INFARCTION POSTOPERATIVE
518.3	INFILTRATE
793.1	INFILTRATE X-RAY FINDING
861.20	INJURY NOS
861.30	INJURY NOS WITH OPEN WOUND INTO THORAX
908.0	INJURY NOS LATE EFFECT
518.82	INSUFFICIENCY ACUTE
0	INSUFFICIENCY VALVE SEE 'PULMONARY', VALVLE INSUFFICIENCY
861.22	LACERATION
861.32	LACERATION WITH OPEN WOUND INTO THORAX
908.0	LACERATION LATE EFFECT
518.89	NODULE
731.2	OSTEOARTHROPATHY HYPERTROPHIC
V81.4	PERFUSION SCREENING
424.3	REGURGITATION SEE ALSO 'PULMONARY' VALVE INSUFFICIENCY
446.21	RENAL (HEMORRHAGIC) SYNDROME
746.01	VALVE - ABSENCE (CONGENITAL)
746.00	VALVE - ANOMALY (CONGENITAL)
746.01	VALVE - ATRESIA (CONGENITAL)

PULMONIC INCOMPETENCE AND PULMONIC REGURGITATION ARE SYNONYMS FOR PULMONIC INSUFFICIENCY.

424.3	VALVE INSUFFICIENCY
421.0	VALVE INSUFFICIENCY - BACTERIAL (ACUTE) (CHRONIC)
746.09	VALVE INSUFFICIENCY - CONGENITAL
397.1	VALVE INSUFFICIENCY - RHEUMATIC
093.24	VALVE INSUFFICIENCY - SYPHILITIC
424.3	VALVE OBSTRUCTION (SEE ALSO 'ENDOCARDITIS', PULMONARY)
424.3	VALVE STENOSIS
421.0	VALVE STENOSIS - BACTERIAL (ACUTE) (CHRONIC)
746.02	VALVE STENOSIS - CONGENITAL
746.83	VALVE STENOSIS - CONGENITAL INFUNDIBULAR
746.83	VALVE STENOSIS - CONGENITAL SUBPULMONARY
397.1	VALVE STENOSIS - RHEUMATIC
093.24	VALVE STENOSIS - SYPHILITIC
424.3	VALVE STENOSIS - WITH INSUFFICIENCY
421.0	VALVE STENOSIS - WITH INSUFFICIENCY BACTERIAL (ACUTE) (CHRONIC)
397.1	VALVE STENOSIS - WITH INSUFFICIENCY RHEUMATIC
093.24	VALVE STENOSIS - WITH INSUFFICIENCY SYPHILITIC

PULMONARY (continued)

747.49	VEIN - ABSENCE OR ATRESIA (CONGENITAL)
747.42	VEIN - ANOMALOUS RETURN (CONNECTION) (PARTIAL)
747.40	VEIN - ANOMALY CONGENITAL
901.42	VEIN - AVULSION (ANEURYSM) TRAUMATIC
415.19	VEIN - INFARCTION
415.11	VEIN - INFARCTION IATROGENIC
415.11	VEIN - INFARCTION POSTOPERATIVE
901.42	VEIN - INJURY
901.42	VEIN - LACERATION (RUPTURE) (HEMATOMA)
908.4	VEIN - LATE EFFECT OF AVULSION, INJURY OR LACERATION
747.49	VEIN - OBSTRUCTION
747.42	VEIN - RETURN PARTIAL ANOMALOUS CONNECTION (RETURN)
747.41	VEIN - RETURN TOTAL ANOMALOUS CONNECTION (RETURN)
417.8	VEIN - STRICTURE
747.49	VEIN - TRANSPOSITION

PULMONARY EDEMA

514	NOS
518.4	ACUTE
507.0	ACUTE ASPIRATION
428.1	ACUTE CARDIOGENIC
506.1	ACUTE CHEMICAL OR FUMES
518.4	ACUTE DUE TO PNEUMONIA
518.4	ACUTE POSTOPERATIVE
428.0	ACUTE WITH CHF (RIGHT HEART FAILURE)
402.91	ACUTE WITH HYPERTENSIVE HEART FAILURE
402.11	ACUTE WITH HYPERTENSIVE HEART FAILURE BENIGN
402.01	ACUTE WITH HYPERTENSIVE HEART FAILURE MALIGNANT
428.1	ACUTE WITH LEFT HEART FAILURE
518.5	ADULT RESPIRATORY DISTRESS SYNDROME ASSOCIATED WITH SHOCK
507.0	ASSOCIATED WITH ASPIRATION PNEUMONIA [518.82]
514	ASSOCIATED WITH HYPOSTATIC PNEUMONIA
518.82	ASSOCIATED WITH OTHER CONDITIONS
518.81	ASSOCIATED WITH RESPIRATORY FAILURE - ACUTE IN OTHER CONDITIONS
518.84	ASSOCIATED WITH RESPIRATORY FAILURE - ACUTE AND CHRONIC IN OTHER CONDITIONS
518.83	ASSOCIATED WITH RESPIRATORY FAILURE - CHRONIC IN OTHER CONDITIONS
514	CHRONIC
518.4	DUE TO ARDS [518.82]
518.4	DUE TO ARDS DRUG OVERDOSE
518.5	DUE TO ARDS POST OP WITH SHOCK
518.5	DUE TO ARDS TRAUMATIC [518.4]
508.1	DUE TO RADIATION CHRONIC
508.0	DUE TO RADIATION PNEUMONITIS
508.8	DUE TO OTHER EXTERNAL AGENTS
508.9	DUE TO UNSPECIFIED EXTERNAL AGENTS
518.4	DUE TO RENAL FAILURE [585]
518.4	DUE TO SEPSIS [038.39]
518.4	DUE TO SEPSIS (GRAM NEGATIVE) [785.59]
518.5	DUE TO SHOCK LUNG
518.5	DUE TO SHOCK TRAUMATIC
518.5	FOLLOWING TRAUMA AND SURGERY
518.4	POSTOPERATIVE ACUTE
518.4	POSTOPERATIVE ACUTE DUE TO FLUID OVERLOAD [276.6]
391.8	RHEUMATIC ACUTE
398.91	RHEUMATIC CHRONIC
392.0	RHEUMATIC WITH CHOREA
428.1	WITH HEART DISEASE OR FAILURE, LEFT
428.0	WITH HEART DISEASE OR FAILURE, RIGHT
428.0	WITH HEART DISEASE OR FAILURE, COMBINED

522.9	PULP (DENTAL) DISEASE NOS
0	PULP (DENTAL) SEE ALSO 'TOOTH PULP AND PERIAPICAL DISORDERS'
522.1	PULP GANGRENE
522.0	PULPITIS (TOOTH)

785.0 PULSE RAPID
427.89 PULSE SLOW
785.9 PULSE WEAK
446.7 PULSELESS DISEASE OR SYNDROME
375.52 PUNCTA LACRIMALIA OCCLUSION
0 PUNCTURE WOUND SEE 'OPEN WOUND'

PUPIL
743.46 ATRESIA CONGENITAL
364.75 DEFORMED
379.43 DILATATION
379.40 DYSFUNCTION
379.49 DYSFUNCTION HIPPUS
379.46 DYSFUNCTION TONIC
364.75 ECTOPIC
364.76 FIXED
364.75 RUPTURE SPHINCTER

PUPILLARY
364.74 MEMBRANE
743.46 MEMBRANE PERSISTENT
364.74 OCCLUSION
379.49 PARALYSIS
379.46 REACTION (MYOTONIC) (TONIC)
364.74 SECLUSION

646.8# PUPP COMPLICATING PREGNANCY
5th Digit: 646.8
0. EPISODE OF CARE UNSPECIFIED OR N/A
1. DELIVERED
2. DELIVERED WITH POSTPARTUM COMPLICATION
3. ANTEPARTUM COMPLICATION
4. POSTPARTUM COMPLICATION

277.2 PURINE AMINO ACID DISORDER (METABOLISM) NEC

PURPURA
287.2 NOS
287.0 ABDOMINAL
287.0 ALLERGIC
287.0 ANAPHYLACTOID
709.1 ANNULARIS TELANGIECTODES
287.2 AUTOERYTHROCYTE SENSITIZATION
287.0 AUTOIMMUNE
287.0 BACTERIAL
273.2 CRYOGLOBULINEMIC
287.2 DEVIL'S PINCHES
287.1 DUE TO QUALITATIVE PLATELET DEFECTS
286.6 FIBRINOLYTIC
286.6 FULMINANS
287.3 HEMORRHAGIC
287.0 HENOCH'S
287.0 HENOCH SCHONLEIN
273.0 HYPERGAMMAGLOBULINEMIC
287.3 IDIOPATHIC
287.2 NONTHROMBOCYTOPENIC
287.0 NONTHROMBOCYTOPENIC HEMORRHAGIC
287.0 NONTHROMBOCYTOPENIC IDIOPATHIC
709.09 PIGMENTARIA
287.4 POSTTRANSFUSION
287.2 RED CELL MEMBRANE SENSITIVITY
287.0 RHEUMATICA
287.2 SENILE
287.2 SIMPLEX
287.1 THROMBASTHENIA
287.1 THROMBOCYTASTHENIA
287.1 THROMBOCYTOPATHY
287.3 THROMBOCYTOPENIC CONGENITAL OR HEREDITARY
666.3# THROMBOCYTOPENIC (PUERPERIUM) (POSTPARTUM)
5th Digit: 666.3
0. UNSPECIFIED
2. DELIVERED WITH POSTPARTUM COMPLICATION
4. POSTPARTUM COMPLICATION

PURPURA (continued)
446.6 THROMBOCYTOPENIC THROMBOTIC
287.1 THROMBOPATHY
287.0 TOXIC
050.0 VARIOLOSA
287.0 VASCULAR
287.0 VISCERAL SYMPTOMS

792.1 PUS IN STOOL
599.0 PUS IN URINE
022.0 PUSTULE MALIGNANT
686.9 PUSTULE SKIN/SUBCUTANEOUS (NONMALIGNANT)
281.0 PUTNAM'S DISEASE OR SYNDROME (SUBACUTE COMBINED SCLEROSIS WITH PERNICIOUS ANEMIA) [336.2]

427.69 PVC'S

593.89 PYELECTASIA
0 PYELITIS SEE 'PYELONEPHRITIS'
593.89 PYELOCALIECTASIS

PYELONEPHRITIS
590.80 NOS
590.10 ACUTE
590.11 ACUTE WITH RENAL MEDULLARY NECROSIS
112.2 CANDIDAL
590.00 CHRONIC
590.00 CHRONIC WITH VESICOURETERAL REFLUX [**593.7#**]
5th Digit: 593.7
0. UNSPECIFIED
1. WITH REFLUX NEPHROPATHY, UNILATERAL
2. WITH REFLUX NEPHROPATHY, BILATERAL
3. WITH REFLUX NEPHROPATHY UNSPECIFIED

590.01 CHRONIC WITH RENAL MEDULLARY NECROSIS
590.01 CHRONIC WITH RENAL MEDULLARY NECROSIS WITH VESICOURETERAL REFLUX [**593.7#**]
5th Digit: 593.7
0. UNSPECIFIED
1. WITH REFLUX NEPHROPATHY, UNILATERAL
2. WITH REFLUX NEPHROPATHY, BILATERAL
3. WITH REFLUX NEPHROPATHY UNSPECIFIED

646.6#: SPECIFY THE MATERNAL PYELONEPHRITIS WITH AN ADDITIONAL CODE.

646.6# MATERNAL COMPLICATING PREGNANCY
5th Digit: 646.6
0. EPISODE OF CARE NOS OR N/A
1. DELIVERED
2. DELIVERED WITH POSTPARTUM COMPLICATION
3. ANTEPARTUM COMPLICATION
4. POSTPARTUM COMPLICATION

016.0# TUBERCULOUS [590.81]
5th Digit: 016.0
0. NOS
1. LAB NOT DONE
2. LABS PENDING
3. MICROSCOPY POSITIVE (IN SPUTUM)
4. CULTURE POSITIVE - MICROSCOPY NEGATIVE
5. CULTURE NEGATIVE - MICROSCOPY POSITIVE
6. CULTURE AND MICROSCOPY NEGATIVE CONFIRMED BY OTHER METHODS

590.3 PYELOURETERITIS CYSTICA

PYEMIA
771.8 NEWBORN
0 OBSTRUCTIVE SEE 'SEPSIS'
572.1 PORTAL (VEIN)
999.3 POSTVACCINAL
0 SEE 'SEPSIS'

759.4 PYGOPAGUS

345.0# PYKNO EPILEPSY PYKNOLEPSY (IDIOPATHIC)

5th Digit: 345.0

0. WITHOUT MENTION OF INTRACTABLE EPILEPSY

1. WITH INTRACTABLE EPILEPSY

756.89 PYLE (-COHN) DISEASE (CRANIOMETAPHYSEAL DYSPLASIA)

572.1 PYLEPHLEBITIS SUPPURATIVE

572.1 PYLETHROMBOPHLEBITIS

PYLORIC

537.0 CONSTRICTION

537.0 OBSTRUCTION OR OCCLUSION

537.0 STENOSIS HYPERTROPHIC

537.0 STENOSIS HYPERTROPHIC NONINFANTILE

537.0 STRICTURE

PYLORIC STENOSIS CONGENITAL OR INFANTILE

750.5 CONSTRICTION

750.5 HYPERTROPHY

750.5 SPASM

750.5 STENOSIS

750.5 STENOSIS HYPERTROPHIC

750.5 STRICTURE

537.89 PYLORODUODENAL SYNDROME

537.81 PYLOROSPASM

750.5 PYLOROSPASM CONGENITAL

686.0# PYODERMA, PYODERMATITIS

5th Digit: 686.0

0. UNPECIFIED

1. GANGRENOSUM

9. OTHER PYODERMA

686.1 PYOGENIC GRANULOMA

528.9 PYOGENIC GRANULOMA OF ORAL MUCOSA

615.9 PYOMETRA UTERUS - NOS

615.0 PYOMETRA UTERUS - ACUTE

615.1 PYOMETRA UTERUS - CHRONIC

510.9 PYOPNEUMOTHORAX

614.2 PYOSALPINX

510.9 PYOTHORAX

333.90 PYRAMIDAL TRACT DISEASE

332.0 PYRAMIDOPALLIDONIGRAL SYNDROME

117.4 PYRENOCHAETA ROMEROI INFECTION

780.6 PYREXIA

659.2# PYREXIA MATERNAL DURING LABOR

5th Digit: 659.2

0. EPISODE OF CARE UNSPECIFIED OR N/A

1. DELIVERED

3. ANTEPARTUM COMPLICATION

778.4 PYREXIA NEWBORN ENVIRONMENTALLY INDUCED

672.0# PYREXIA PUERPERAL

670.0# PYREXIA PUERPERAL SEPTIC

4th Digit: 670.0, 672.0

0. UNSPECIFIED

2. DELIVERED WITH POSTPARTUM COMPLICATION

4. POSTPARTUM COMPLICATION

0 PYREXIA SEE ALSO 'FEVER'

266.1 PYRIDOXINE DEFICIENCY (PYRIDOXAL, PYRIDOXAMINE)

355.0 PYRIFORMIS SYNDROME

277.2 PYRIMIDINE AMINO ACID DISORDER (METABOLISM) NEC

312.33 PYROMANIA

787.1 PYROSIS

277.1 PYRROLOPORPHYRIA

791.9 PYURIA (BACTERIAL)

083.0 Q FEVER
794.31 Q-T INTERVAL PROLONGATION SYNDROME
368.46 QUADRANT ANOPSIA
890.2 QUADRICEPS TENDON LACERATION
891.2 QUADRICEPS TENDON LACERATION (KNEE)
727.65 QUADRICEPS TENDON RUPTURE
843.8 QUADRICEPS TENDON RUPTURE - HIP AND THIGH (TRAUMATIC)
844.8 QUADRICEPS TENDON RUPTURE - KNEE AND LEG (TRAUMATIC)
0 QUADRIPARESIS SEE 'QUADRIPLEGIA'

QUADRIPLEGIA

344.0# ACQUIRED (LONG STANDING) ANY CAUSE
5th Digit: 344.0
0. UNSPECIFIED
1. C1 - C4, COMPLETE
2. C1 - C4, INCOMPLETE
3. C5 - C7, COMPLETE
4. C5 - C7, INCOMPLETE
9. OTHER QUADRIPLEGIA

434.1# CEREBRAL EMBOLIC (CURRENT)
5th Digit: 434.1
0. WITHOUT CEREBRAL INFARCTION
1. WITH CEREBRAL INFARCTION

437.8 CEREBRAL INJURY
767.0 CEREBRAL INJURY BIRTH TRAUMA (NEWBORN)
434.0# CEREBRAL THROMBOTIC
5th Digit: 434.0
0. WITHOUT CEREBRAL INFARCTION
1. WITH CEREBRAL INFARCTION

438.53 LATE EFFECT OF CEREBROVASCULAR DISEASE **[344.0#]**
5th Digit: 344.0
0. UNSPECIFIED
1. C1 - C4, COMPLETE
2. C1 - C4, INCOMPLETE
3. C5 - C7, COMPLETE
4. C5 - C7, INCOMPLETE
9. OTHER QUADRIPLEGIA

344.81 LOCKED IN STATE
344.0# SPINAL ACQUIRED (LONG STANDING)
5th Digit: 344.0
0. UNSPECIFIED
1. C1 - C4, COMPLETE
2. C1 - C4, INCOMPLETE
3. C5 - C7, COMPLETE
4. C5 - C7, INCOMPLETE
9. OTHER QUADRIPLEGIA

767.4 SPINAL INJURY BIRTH TRAUMA (NEWBORN)
0 SPINAL INJURY CURRENT SEE 'SPINAL CORD INJURY'

651.2# QUADRUPLET GESTATION
651.5# QUADRUPLET WITH ONE OR MORE LOSSES
5th Digit: 651.2, 5
0. EPISODE OF CARE NOS OR N/A
1. DELIVERED
3. ANTEPARTUM COMPLICATION

301.3 QUARRELSOMENESS
082.3 QUEENSLAND TICK TYPHUS
727.04 QUERVAIN'S TENDON SHEATH
245.1 QUERVAIN'S THYROID (SUBACUTE GRANULOMATOUS THYROIDITIS)
233.5 QUEYRAT'S ERYTHROPLASIA SITE NOS
0 QUEYRAT'S ERYTHROPLASIA SITE SPECIFIED SEE 'CA IN SITU' BY SITE M8080/2
0 QUINCKE'S SEE 'ANGIONEUROTIC EDEMA'
704.09 QUINQUAUD DISEASE (ACNE DECALVANS)
083.1 QUINTAN FEVER

0 RABBIT FEVER SEE 'TULAREMIA'

RABIES

071 RABIES
V01.5 EXPOSURE
V04.5 VACCINATION

RACHISCHISIS

741.0# WITH HYDROCEPHALUS
741.9# WITHOUT HYDROCEPHALUS
5th Digit: 741.0,9
0. REGION NOS
1. CERVICAL
2. DORSAL
3. LUMBAR

442.0 ARTERY ANEURYSM (RUPTURED) (CIRSOID) (VARIX) (FALSE)
440.2# ARTERY ARTERIOSCLEROSIS (DEGENERATION)
5th Digit: 440.2
0. UNSPECIFIED
1. WITH INTERMITTENT CLAUDICATION
2. WITH REST PAIN, OR REST PAIN AND (INTERMITTENT CLAUDICATION)
3. WITH ULCERATION, OR ULCERATION AND (INTERMITTENT CLAUDICATION) (REST PAIN)
4. WITH ISCHEMIC GANGRENE, OR ISCHEMIC GANGRENE AND (INTERMITTENT CLAUDICATION) (REST PAIN) (ULCERATION)
9. OTHER ATHEROSCLEROSIS EXTREMITIES

444.21 ARTERY (EMBOLISM)(THROMBOSIS) (OCCLUSION) (INFARCTION)
440.3# ARTERY BYPASS GRAFT ARTERIOSCLEROSIS
5th Digit: 440.3
0. UNSPECIFIED GRAFT
1. AUTOLOGOUS VEIN BYPASS GRAFT
2. NONAUTOLOGOUS BIOLOGICAL BYPASS GRAFT

903.2 ARTERY INJURY
908.3 ARTERY INJURY LATE EFFECT
903.2 BLOOD VESSELS INJURY
908.3 BLOOD VESSELS INJURY LATE EFFECT
903.2 BLOOD VESSELS LACERATION (RUPTURE) (HEMATOMA)
908.3 BLOOD VESSELS LACERATION LATE EFFECT
354.3 NERVE DISORDER (PALSY) (LESION)
955.3 NERVE INJURY
907.4 NERVE INJURY LATE EFFECT
723.4 NERVE NEURITIS
354.3 NERVE PALSY ACUTE
354.3 NERVE PARALYSIS
767.6 NERVE PARALYSIS BIRTH TRAUMA
727.04 STYLOID TENOSYNOVITIS
903.2 VEIN INJURY
908.3 VEIN INJURY LATE EFFECT
451.83 VEIN PHLEBITIS

RADIATION

0 BURN SEE 'BURN', BY SITE
595.82 CYSTITIS
692.82 DERMATITIS (SEE ALSO 'DERMATITIS')
558.1 ENTEROCOLITIS
V82.5 EXPOSURE SCREENING
508.1 FIBROSIS PULMONARY
909.2 LATE EFFECT
990 SICKNESS
990 THERAPY COMPLICATION

RADICULAR SYNDROME

729.2 NOS
724.4 LOWER LIMBS
723.4 UPPER LIMBS
767.4 UPPER LIMBS NEWBORN

RADICULITIS
729.2 RADICULITIS
723.4 ACCESSORY NERVE
724.4 ANTERIOR CRURAL
723.4 BRACHIAL (NONDISCOGENIC)
723.4 CERVICAL
723.4 CERVICAL (NONDISCOGENIC)
724.4 LEG
724.4 LUMBAR
724.4 THORACIC

357.0 RADICULOMYELITIS (ACUTE)
0 RADICULOPATHY SEE 'RADICULITIS'

990 RADIOACTIVE FALLOUT
909.2 RADIOACTIVE FALLOUT LATE EFFECT
0 RADIOACTIVE IODINE THERAPY CODE THE UNDERLYING DISEASE
V82.5 RADIOACTIVE SUBSTANCE INGESTION SCREENING

0 RADIOCARPAL JOINT SEE 'DISLOCATION', WRIST
842.02 RADIOCARPAL SEPARATION (RUPTURE) (TEAR) (LACERATION)
842.02 RADIOCARPAL STRAIN (SPRAIN) (AVULSION) (HEMARTHROSIS)

692.82 RADIODERMATITIS

841.2 RADIOHUMERAL SEPARATION (RUPTURE) (TEAR) (LACERATION)
841.2 RADIOHUMERAL STRAIN (SPRAIN) (AVULSION) (HEMARTHROSIS)

794.19 RADIOISOTOPE SCAN ABNORMAL

RADIOLOGICAL EXAM
793.# ABNORMAL FINDINGS (NONSPECIFIC)
4th Digit: 793
0. SKULL AND HEAD
1. LUNG FIELD
2. OTHER INTRATHORACIC ORGAN
3. BILIARY TRACT
4. GASTROINTESTINAL TRACT
5. GENITOURINARY ORGANS
6. ABDOMINAL AREA INCLUDING RETROPERITONEUM
7. MUSCULOSKELETAL SYSTEM
8. BREAST
9. OTHER
V72.5 EXAM NEC
V71.2 EXAM FOR TB

IF ENOUNTER IS FOR RADIOTHERAPY SEQUENCE THE RADIOTHERAPY FIRST, WITH AN ADDITIONAL CODE FOR THE CANCER.

RADIOTHERAPY
V58.1 ADMISSION
990 COMPLICATION
V66.1 CONVALESCENCE
V67.1 FOLLOWUP EXAM
V58.0 ENCOUNTER
V58.0 MAINTENANCE
V58.0 SESSION
0 SESSION FOR RADIOACTIVE IMPLANT CODE THE CANCER BY SITE
0 SESSION FOR RADIOACTIVE IODINE THERAPY CODE THE UNDERLYING DISEASE

755.53 RADIOULNAR SYNOSTOSIS

755.26 RADIUS AGENESIS (CONGENITAL)
755.21 RADIUS AGENESIS (CONGENITAL) - WITH ABSENCE COMPLETE DISTAL ELEMENTS
755.26 RADIUS AGENESIS - WITH ABSENCE INCOMPLETE DISTAL ELEMENTS
755.25 RADIUS AND ULNA ABSENCE CONGENITAL
736.00 RADIUS DEFORMITY
755.50 RADIUS DEFORMITY CONGENITAL

446.7 RAEDER-HARBITZ PULSELESS DISEASE OR SYNDROME

022.1 RAG SORTER'S DISEASE

786.7 RALES

334.2 RAMSAY HUNT'S DYSSYNERGIA CEREBELLARIS MYOCLONICA SYNDROME
053.11 RAMSAY HUNT'S HERPETIC GENICULATE GANGLIONITIS SYNDROME

0 RAMUS SEE ALSO 'MANDIBLE, MANDIBULAR'

0 RANGE OF MOTION (JOINT) LIMITATION SEE 'STIFF, STIFFNESS', JOINT'
527.6 RANULA
750.26 RANULA CONGENITAL

0 RAPE - CODE SPECIFIED INJURY(IES)
V71.5 RAPE EXAM FOR ALLEGED RAPE
0 RAPE IN AN ABUSIVE RELATIONSHIP SEE 'ABUSE', CHILD OR 'ABUSE', ADULT

V21.0 RAPID GROWTH IN CHILDHOOD
307.45 RAPID TIME ZONE CHANGE SYNDROME
078.89 RASH ECHO 9 VIRUS
782.1 RASH NONSPECIFIC

026.9 RAT BITE FEVER
026.0 RAT BITE FEVER DUE TO SPIRILLUM MINOR (S. MINUS)
026.1 RAT BITE FEVER DUE TO STREPTOBACILLUS MONILIFORMIS

989.5 RATTLESNAKE BITE
995.0 RATTLESNAKE BITE WITH ANAPHYLAXIS [989.5]

433.8# RAYMOND (-CESTAN) SYNDROME
5th Digit: 433.8
0. WITHOUT CEREBRAL INFARCTION
1. WITH CEREBRAL INFARCTION

443.0 RAYNAUD'S SYNDROME / PHENOMENON (PAROXYSMAL DIGITAL CYANOSIS)
648.9# RAYNAUD'S SYNDROME / PHENOMENOM (PAROXYSMAL DIGITAL CYANOSIS) MATERNAL CURRENT (CO-EXISTENT) IN PREGNANCY [443.0]
5th Digit: 648.9
0. EPISODE OF NOS OR N/A
1. DELIVERED
2. DELIVERED WITH POSTPARTUM COMPLICATION
3. ANTEPARTUM COMPLICATION
4. POSTPARTUM COMPLICATION

443.0 RAYNAUD'S SYNDROME (PAROXYSMAL DIGITAL CYANOSIS) WITH GANGRENE [785.4]

769 RDS NEWBORN (RESPIRATORY DISTRESS SYNDROME)

493.90 REACTIVE AIRWAY DISEASE (SEE ALSO 'ASTHMA')
313.89 REACTIVE ATTACHMENT DISORDER (INFANCY OR EARLY CHILDHOOD)
300.4 REACTIVE DEPRESSION (NEUROTIC)

READING DISORDER
315.00 NOS
315.01 ALEXIA
315.02 DEVELOPMENTAL DYSLEXIA
315.09 SPELLING
315.09 OTHER SPECIFIED

789.6# REBOUND TENDERNESS
5th Digit: 789.6
0. UNSPECIFIED SITE
1. UPPER RIGHT QUADRANT
2. UPPER LEFT QUADRANT
3. LOWER RIGHT QUADRANT
4. LOWER LEFT QUADRANT
5. PERIUMBILIC
6. EPIGASTRIC
7. GENERALIZED
9. OTHER SPECIFIED SITE (MULTIPLE)

524.06 RECESSION CHIN
0 RECKLINGHAUSEN'S DISEASE SEE 'VON RECKLINGHAUSEN'S'
610.1 RECLUS' DISEASE (CYSTIC)
081.1 RECRUDESCENT TYPHUS
0 RECTAL SEE 'RECTUM, RECTAL'

RECTOCELE
618.# FEMALE
618.# FEMALE WITH STRESS INCONTINENCE [625.6]
618.# FEMALE WITH OTHER URINARY INCONTINENCE **[788.3#]**

4th Digit: 618
0. WITHOUT UTERINE PROLAPSE
2. WITH INCOMPLETE UTERINE PROLAPSE
3. WITH COMPLETE UTERINE PROLAPSE
4. UTERINE PROLAPSE UNSPECIFIED

5th Digit: 788.3
0. UNSPECIFIED
1. URGE INCONTINENCE
3. MIXED URGE AND STRESS
4 WITHOUT SENSORY AWARENESS
5. POST-VOID DRIBBLING
6. NOCTURNAL ENURESIS
7. CONTINUOUS LEAKAGE
9. OTHER

654.4# COMPLICATING PREGNANCY
660.2# OBSTRUCTING LABOR **[654.4#]**

5th Digit: 654.4
0. EPISODE OF CARE NOS OR N/A
1. DELIVERED
2. DELIVERED WITH POSTPARTUM COMPLICATION
3. ANTEPARTUM COMPLICATION
4. POSTPARTUM COMPLICATION

5th Digit: 660.2
0. EPISODE OF CARE NOS OR N/A
1. DELIVERED
3. ANTEPARTUM COMPLICATION

0 GRAVID SEE 'UTERUS, UTERINE DISORDERS COMPLICATING PREGNANCY', ABNORMALITY IN SHAPE OR POSITION
569.49 MALE

562.10 RECTOSIGMOID DIVERTICULA
751.5 RECTOSIGMOID DIVERTICULA CONGENITAL
569.89 RECTOSIGMOID LESION
560.9 RECTOSIGMOID OBSTRUCTION (SEE ALSO 'INTESTINE, INTESTINAL' OBSTRUCTION)
211.4 RECTOSIGMOID POLYP ADENOMATOUS
569.89 RECTOSIGMOIDITIS
556.3 RECTOSIGMOIDITIS ULCERATIVE (CHRONIC)
752.49 RECTOVAGINAL FISTULA CONGENITAL

RECTUM, RECTAL
569.49 ABSENCE
751.2 ABSENCE CONGENITAL
751.2 ATRESIA CONGENITAL
569.3 BLEEDING
569.49 CRYPT
569.49 DISEASE NEC
306.4 DISORDER PSYCHOGENIC
562.10 DIVERTICULA
569.49 ECTROPION
565.1 FISTULA
569.49 GRANULOMA (RUPTURE) (PAPILLARY HYPERTROPHY)
751.2 IMPERFORATE CONGENITAL
569.49 INFECTION
569.49 INFLAMMATION

RECTUM, RECTAL (continued)
863.45 INJURY
863.55 INJURY - WITH OPEN WOUND
908.1 INJURY - LATE EFFECT
863.46 INJURY - MULTIPLE SITES
863.56 INJURY - MULTIPLE SITES WITH OPEN WOUND
863.49 INJURY - OTHER
863.59 INJURY - OTHER WITH OPEN WOUND INTO CAVITY
564.89 IRRITABILTY
569.49 LESION
787.99 MASS
787.99 NEURALGIA
569.49 OBSTRUCTION
569.42 PAIN
211.4 POLYP ADENOMATOUS
569.0 POLYP NONADENOMATOUS
569.1 PROLAPSE (SPHINCTER)
455.9 SKIN TAGS (HEMORRHOIDAL)
787.99 SPHINCTER IMPAIRMENT
564.89 STASIS
569.2 STRICTURE / STENOSIS
751.2 STRICTURE - CONGENITAL
947.3 STRICTURE - DUE TO CHEMICAL BURN
569.2 STRICTURE - DUE TO RADIATION BURN
098.7 STRICTURE - GONOCOCCAL
099.1 STRICTURE - INFLAMMATORY
095.8 STRICTURE - SYPHILITIC
787.99 SWELLING
455.9 TAG (HEMORRHOIDAL)
787.99 TENESMUS
564.89 TIGHTNESS
569.41 ULCER

087.9 RECURRENT FEVER (RELAPSING)
352.3 RECURRENT LARYNGEAL NERVE DISORDER
790.0 RED BLOOD CELL ABNORMAL MORPHOLOGY OR VOLUME
284.9 RED BLOOD CELL (IDIOPATHIC) ABSENCE
284.0 RED BLOOD CELL ABSENCE CONGENITAL
790.0 RED BLOOD CELLS VOLUME ABNORMAL TEST RESULTS
133.8 RED BUG BITE
284.8 RED CELL APLASIA ACQUIRED (SECONDARY)
284.0 RED CELL APLASIA CONGENITAL (PRIMARY)
V68.81 REFERRAL OF PATIENT WITHOUT EXAMINATION OR TREATMENT
796.1 REFLEX ABNORMAL (DISORDER)
337.2# REFLEX SYMPATHETIC DYSTROPHY

5th Digit: 337.2
0. UNSPECIFIED
1. UPPER LIMB
2. LOWER LIMB
9. OTHER SPECIFIED SITE

REFRACTIVE
367.81 CHANGE TRANSIENT
368.15 DIPLOPIA
367.9 DISORDER (SEE ALSO SPECIFIC DISORDER)
367.89 DISORDER DRUG INDUCED OR TOXIC
367.89 DISORDER OTHER SPECIFIED
368.15 POLYOPIA

356.3 REFSUM'S DISEASE OR SYNDROME (HEREDOPATHIA ATACTICA POLYNEURITIFORMIS)
356.3 REFSUM'S RETINAL DYSTROPHY [362.72]
V70.5 REFUGEES HEALTH EXAM
V15.81 REFUSAL OF TREATMENT AGAINST MEDICAL ADVICE
V62.6 REFUSAL OF TREATMENT RELIGION BASED
V64.2 REFUSAL OF TREATMENT (SURGERY) (PROCEDURE) PATIENT'S DECISION

REGIONAL ENTERITIS

555.9 NOS
555.1 LARGE INTESTINE
555.0 SMALL INTESTINE
555.2 SMALL INTESTINE WITH LARGE INTESTINE

520.4 REGIONAL ODONTODYSPLASIA
779.3 REGURGITATION OF FOOD NEONATAL
307.53 REGURGITATION PSYCHOGENIC ORIGIN OF FOOD WITH RESWALLOWING

WHEN A CODE FROM V57.# REHABILITATION IS ASSIGNED AS THE PRINCIPAL DIAGNOSIS, A SECONDARY CODE (S) SHOULD BE ASSIGNED TO IDENTIFY AND EXPLAIN THE CONDITION(S) REQUIRING THE REHABILITATION SERVICES.

V57.4 ORTHOPTIC TRAINING DUE TO FRACTURE FEMUR CLOSED INTRACAPSULAR [820.00]

REHABILITATION

V57.9 NOS
V57.0 BREATHING EXERCISES
V57.81 GAIT OR ORTHOTIC TRAINING
V57.89 MULTIPLE TYPES
V57.21 OCCUPATIONAL THERAPY
V57.4 ORTHOPTIC TRAINING
V57.1 PHYSICAL THERAPY
V57.9 PROCEDURE
V57.89 PROCEDURE (OTHER)
V57.3 SPEECH THERAPY
V57.22 VOCATIONAL THERAPY
V57.89 OTHER

536.8 REICHMANN'S DISEASE OR SYNDROME (GASTROSUCCORRHEA)
245.3 REIDEL'S THYROIDITIS
257.2 REIFENSTEIN'S SYNDROME (HEREDITARY FAMILIAL HYPOGONADISM, MALE)
337.9 REILLY'S PHENOMENON OR SYNDROME
277.3 REIMANN'S (PERIODIC) DISEASE

REITER'S

099.3 DISEASE OR SYNDROME
099.3 DISEASE OR SYNDROME WITH ARTHROPATHY [711.1#]

5th Digit: 711.1

0. SITE NOS
1. SHOULDER REGION
2. UPPER ARM (ELBOW) (HUMERUS)
3. FOREARM (RADIUS) (WRIST) (ULNA)
4. HAND (CARPAL) (METACARPAL) (FINGERS)
5. PELVIC REGION AND THIGH (HIP) (BUTTOCK) (FEMUR)
6. LOWER LEG (FIBULA) (KNEE) (PATELLA) (TIBIA)
7. ANKLE AND/OR FOOT (METATARSALS) (TOES) (TARSALS)
8. OTHER (HEAD) (NECK) (RIB) (SKULL) (TRUNK) (VERTEBRAE)
9. MULTIPLE

099.3 DISEASE OR SYNDROME WITH CONJUNCTIVITIS [372.33]
655.4# DISEASE MATERNAL (WITH KNOWN / SUSPECTED DAMAGE TO FETUS)

5th Digit: 655.4

0. EPISODE OF CARE NOS OR N/A
1. DELIVERED
3. ANTEPARTUM COMPLICATION

647.2# DISEASE MATERNAL CURRENT (CO-EXISTENT) IN PREGNANCY

5th Digit: 647.2

0. EPISODE OF CARE NOS OR N/A
1. DELIVERED
2. DELIVERED WITH POSTPARTUM COMPLICATION
3. ANTEPARTUM COMPLICATION
4. POSTPARTUM COMPLICATION

RELAPSING FEVER

087.9 NOS
087.0 LOUSE BORNE
087.1 TICK BORNE

313.3 RELATIONSHIP PROBLEM (EMOTIONAL DISTURBANCE OF CHILDHOOD OR ADOLESCENCE)
0 RELATIONSHIP PROBLEM WITH CONDUCT DISORDER SEE 'CONDUCT DISORDER'

RELAXATION

596.59 BLADDER
0 BLADDER WITH INCONTINENCE SEE 'BLADDER DISORDERS WITH INCONTINENCE'
530.89 CARDIOESOPHAGEAL
519.4 DIAPHRAGMATIC
734 FOOT (ARCH)
618.8 PELVIC FLOOR
618.8 PELVIS
618.8 PERINEUM
599.84 URETHRA
618.8 UTERUS (VAGINA)
596.59 VESICAL
0 VESICAL WITH INCONTINENCE SEE 'BLADDER DISORDERS WITH INCONTINENCE'

V62.4 RELIGIOUS DISCRIMINATION CAUSING ENCOUNTER
V62.6 RELIGIOUS PROBLEM REGARDING MEDICAL CARE
V62.89 RELIGIOUS PROBLEM OTHER THAN MEDICAL CARE

RENAL

590.2 ABSCESS
753.0 AGENESIS CONGENITAL
593.7# AGENESIS CONGENITAL WITH VESICOURETERAL REFLUX [753.0]

5th Digit: 593.7

0. UNSPECIFIED
1. WITH REFLUX NEPHROPATHY, UNILATERAL
2. WITH REFLUX NEPHROPATHY, BILATERAL
3. WITH REFLUX NEPHROPATHY UNSPECIFIED

747.62 ANOMALY PERIPHERAL VASCULAR (ABERRANT) (ABSENCE) (AGENESIS) (ACCESSORY) (ANEURYSM) (ATRESIA) (DEFORMITY) (HYPOPLASIA) (MALPOSITION)
0 ARTERY DISORDER SEE 'RENAL ARTERY'
587 ATROPHY
583.89 BASEMENT MEMBRANE DISEASE NEC
593.89 CALCIFICATION
592.0 CALCULUS
274.11 CALCULUS - URIC ACID
189.0 CELL CARCINOMA SITE NOS
0 CELL CARCINOMA SITE SPECIFIED SEE 'CANCER' BY SITE M8312/3
587 CIRRHOSIS
788.0 COLIC
866.01 CONTUSION
866.11 CONTUSION WITH OPEN WOUND INTO CAVITY
908.1 CONTUSION LATE EFFECT
593.81 CRISIS
593.2 CYST
591 CYST - CALYCEAL OR PYELOGENIC
753.10 CYST CONGENITAL
753.11 CYST CONGENITAL - SINGLE OR SOLITARY
753.19 CYST CONGENITAL - MULTICYSTIC
V45.1 DIALYSIS STATUS

RENAL (continued)

593.9 DISEASE NOS
277.3 DISEASE AMYLOIDOSIS [583.81]
0 DISEASE CHRONIC SEE 'NEPHRITIS', CHRONIC
753.10 DISEASE CYSTIC CONGENITAL
250.4# DISEASE DIABETIC [583.81]
5th Digit: 250.4
0. TYPE II, ADULT-ONSET, NON-INSULIN DEPENDENT (EVEN IF REQUIRING INSULIN), OR UNSPECIFIED; CONTROLLED
1. TYPE I, JUVENILE-ONSET OR INSULIN-DEPENDENT; CONTROLLED
2. TYPE II, ADULT-ONSET, NON-INSULIN DEPENDENT (EVEN IF REQUIRING INSULIN); UNCONTROLLED
3. TYPE I, JUVENILE-ONSET OR INSULIN-DEPENDENT; UNCONTROLLED

585 DISEASE END STAGE
593.9 DISEASE FUNCTIONAL
098.19 DISEASE GONOCOCCAL [583.81]
274.10 DISEASE GOUTY
403.## DISEASE HYPERTENSIVE
4th Digit: 403
0. MALIGNANT
1. BENIGN
9. NOS
5th Digit: 403
0. WITHOUT RENAL FAILURE
1. WITH RENAL FAILURE

710.0 DISEASE LUPUS (SYSTEMIC LUPUS ERYTHEMATOSUS (DUE TO) [583.81]
760.1 DISEASE MATERNAL AFFECTING FETUS OR NEWBORN

646.2#: SPECIFY THE MATERNAL RENAL DISEASE WITH AN ADDITIONAL CODE.

646.2# DISEASE MATERNAL COMPLICATING PREGNANCY
5th Digit: 646.2
0. EPISODE OF CARE NOS OR N/A
1. DELIVERED
2. DELIVERED WITH POSTPARTUM COMPLICATION
3. ANTEPARTUM COMPLICATION
4. POSTPARTUM COMPLICATION

0 DISEASE MATERNAL HYPERTENSIVE SEE 'ECLAMPSIA' OR 'PRE-ECLAMPSIA'
588.0 DISEASE PHOSPHATE-LOSING (TUBULAR)
753.12 DISEASE POLYCYSTIC (CONGENITAL)
753.13 DISEASE POLYCYSTIC (CONGENITAL) - ADULT TYPE (APKD)
753.13 DISEASE POLYCYSTIC (CONGENITAL) - AUTOSOMAL DOMINANT
753.14 DISEASE POLYCYSTIC (CONGENITAL) - AUTOSOMAL RECESSIVE
753.14 DISEASE POLYCYSTIC (CONGENITAL) - CHILDHOOD TYPE (INFANTILE) (CPKD)
0 DISEASE SEE ALSO 'NEPHRITIS'
095.4 DISEASE SYPHILITIC
016.0# DISEASE TUBERCULOUS [583.81]
5th Digit: 016.0
0. NOS
1. LAB NOT DONE
2. LABS PENDING
3. MICROSCOPY POSITIVE (IN SPUTUM)
4. CULTURE POSITIVE - MICROSCOPY NEGATIVE
5. CULTURE NEGATIVE - MICROSCOPY POSITIVE
6. CULTURE AND MICROSCOPY NEGATIVE CONFIRMED BY OTHER METHODS

584.5 DISEASE TUBULAR
581.9 DISEASE WITH EDEMA
588.9 DISORDER IMPAIRED FUNCTION
588.8 DISORDER OTHER SPECIFIED
593.89 DIVERTICULUM
588.0 DWARFISM
753.15 DYSPLASIA

RENAL (continued)

593.7# DYSPLASIA WITH VESICOURETERAL REFLUX [753.15]
5th Digit: 593.7
0. UNSPECIFIED
1. WITH REFLUX NEPHROPATHY, UNILATERAL
2. WITH REFLUX NEPHROPATHY, BILATERAL
3. WITH REFLUX NEPHROPATHY UNSPECIFIED

0 FAILURE SEE 'RENAL FAILURE'
593.81 EMBOLISM
753.19 FIBROCYSTIC DISEASE
587 FIBROSIS
588.9 FUNCTION IMPAIRED (DISORDER NOS) (DUE TO)
588.8 FUNCTION IMPAIRED (DISORDER) SPECIFIED NEC
794.4 FUNCTION TEST ABNORMAL
250.4# GLOMERULOHYALINOSIS - DIABETIC SYNDROME [583.81]
5th Digit: 250.4
0. TYPE II, ADULT-ONSET, NON-INSULIN DEPENDENT (EVEN IF REQUIRING INSULIN), OR UNSPECIFIED; CONTROLLED
1. TYPE I, JUVENILE-ONSET OR INSULIN-DEPENDENT; CONTROLLED
2. TYPE II, ADULT-ONSET, NON-INSULIN DEPENDENT (EVEN IF REQUIRING INSULIN); UNCONTROLLED
3. TYPE I, JUVENILE-ONSET OR INSULIN-DEPENDENT; UNCONTROLLED

593.81 HEMORRHAGE
753.0 HYPOPLASIA
588.0 INFANTILISM
593.81 INFARCTION
866.## INJURY
4th Digit: 866
0. CLOSED
1. WITH OPEN WOUND INTO CAVITY
5th Digit: 866
0. INJURY NOS
1. CONTUSION/HEMATOMA
2. LACERATION
3. RUPTURE

908.1 INJURY LATE EFFECT
593.9 INSUFFICIENCY
866.02 LACERATION
866.12 LACERATION WITH OPEN WOUND INTO CAVITY
908.1 LACERATION LATE EFFECT
592.0 LITHIASIS
593.9 MASS
593.89 OBSTRUCTION
588.0 OSTEODYSTROPHY
788.0 PAIN
593.89 POLYP
588.0 RICKETS
587 SCLEROSIS
0 SCLEROSIS HYPERTENSIVE SEE 'HYPERTENSIVE', RENAL DISEASE
593.81 THROMBOSIS
588.8 TRANSPORT DISORDER NEC
270.0 TRANSPORT AMINO ACID DISORDER NEC (METABOLISM)
588.8 TUBULAR ACIDOSIS (LIGHTWOOD'S)
0 VEIN DISORDER SEE 'RENAL VEIN (VESSEL)'
0 SEE ALSO 'KIDNEY'

RENAL ARTERY

747.62 ANOMALIES MULTIPLE CONGENITAL
747.62 ANOMALY PERIPHERAL VASCULAR (ABERRANT) (ABSENCE) (AGENESIS) (ACCESSORY) (ANEURYSM) (DEFORMITY) (HYPOPLASIA) (MALPOSITION)
442.1 ANEURYSM (A-V FISTULA) (CIRSOID) (FALSE) (VARICOSE) (RUPTURED)
440.1 ARTERIOSCLEROSIS (DEGENERATION) (DEFORMANS) (ARTERITIS)
593.81 EMBOLISM

RENAL ARTERY (continued)

593.81 HEMORRHAGE
447.3 HYPERPLASIA
593.81 INFARCTION (HEMORRHAGE)
902.41 INJURY
908.4 INJURY LATE EFFECT
593.81 ISCHEMIA
902.41 LACERATION (RUPTURE) (HEMATOMA) (AVULSION) (ANEURYSM) TRAUMATIC
908.4 LACERATION LATE EFFECT
593.81 OCCLUSION
440.1 STENOSIS
440.1 STRICTURE
593.81 THROMBOSIS

WHEN YOU HAVE A PATIENT WITH BOTH RENAL FAILURE AND HYPERTENSION, ICD 9-CM DOES PRESUME A CAUSE AND EFFECT RELATIONSHIP AND YOU SHOULD ASSIGN CODES FROM 403.##, (HYPERTENSIVE RENAL DISEASE). HOWEVER, IF YOU HAVE ACUTE RENAL FAILURE NOT DUE TO HYPERTENSION ALONG WITH HYPERTENSIVE RENAL DISEASE, TWO CODES ARE REQUIRED. ONE IS FOR THE ACUTE RENAL FAILURE (584.#), AND ONE IS AN ADDITIONAL CODE FOR THE HYPERTENSIVE RENAL DISEASE (403.##).

RENAL FAILURE

586 NOS
584.# ACUTE
4th Digit: 584
5. WITH ACUTE TUBULAR NECROSIS
6. WITH CORTICAL NECROSIS
7. WITH MEDULLARY (PAPILLARY) NECROSIS
8. WITH OTHER SPECIFIED PATHOLOGICAL LESION IN KIDNEY
9. RENAL FAILURE UNSPECIFIED

669.3# ACUTE FOLLOWING L AND D
5th Digit: 669.3
0. NOS
2. DELIVERED WITH POSTPARTUM COMPLICATION
4. POSTPARTUM COMPLICATION

584.# ACUTE WITH HYPERTENSION [401.#]
4th Digit: 584
5. WITH ACUTE TUBULAR NECROSIS
6. WITH CORTICAL NECROSIS
7. WITH MEDULLARY NECROSIS
8. WITH OTHER SPECIFIED PATHOLOGICAL LESION IN KIDNEY
9. RENAL FAILURE UNSPECIFIED
4th Digit: 401
0. MALIGNANT, ACCELERATED
1. BENIGN
9. NOS

584.# ACUTE NON-HYPERTENSIVE WITH HYPERTENSIVE RENAL DISEASE [403.##]
4th Digit: 584
5. WITH ACUTE TUBULAR NECROSIS
6. WITH CORTICAL NECROSIS
7. WITH MEDULLARY NECROSIS
8. WITH OTHER SPECIFIED PATHOLOGICAL LESION IN KIDNEY
9. RENAL FAILURE UNSPECIFIED
4th Digit: 403
0. MALIGNANT
1. BENIGN
9. UNSPECIFIED
5th Digit: 403
0. WITHOUT CHRONIC RENAL FAILURE
1. WITH CHRONIC RENAL FAILURE

585 CHRONIC
585 CHRONIC WITH NEUROPATHY [357.4]
585 CHRONIC WITH PERICARDITIS [420.0]
585 CHRONIC WITH POLYNEUROPATHY [357.4]

RENAL FAILURE (continued)

958.5 CRUSH INJURY (FOLLOWING)
908.6 CRUSH INJURY (FOLLOWING) LATE EFFECT
997.5 DUE TO PROCEDURE

HYPERTENSIVE

404.93 AND CHF WITH HYPERTENSIVE HEART AND RENAL DISEASE
404.13 AND CHF WITH HYPERTENSIVE HEART AND RENAL DISEASE - BENIGN
404.03 AND CHF WITH HYPERTENSIVE HEART AND RENAL DISEASE - MALIGNANT
0 ASSOCIATED WITH ABORTION SEE 'ABORTION'
403.91 CHRONIC WITH RENAL HYPERTENSIVE DISEASE
403.11 CHRONIC WITH RENAL HYPERTENSIVE DISEASE - BENIGN
403.01 CHRONIC WITH RENAL HYPERTENSIVE DISEASE - MALIGNANT
404.92 HEART AND RENAL DISEASE
404.12 HEART AND RENAL DISEASE - BENIGN
404.02 HEART AND RENAL DISEASE - MALIGNANT

RENAL FAILURE (continued)

584.7 NECROTIZING RENAL PAPILLITIS
639.3 POST (ABORTIVE) (ECTOPIC) (MOLAR) PREGNANCY
997.5 POST OP
639.3 SHUTDOWN POST (ABORTIVE) (ECTOPIC) (MOLAR) PREGNANCY
958.5 TRAUMATIC
908.6 TRAUMATIC LATE EFFECT

RENAL VEIN (VESSEL)

747.62 ANOMALY PERIPHERAL VASCULAR (ABERRANT) (ABSENCE) (AGENESIS) (ACCESSORY) (ANEURYSM) (DEFORMITY) (HYPOPLASIA) (MALPOSITION)
902.42 VEIN INJURY
908.4 VEIN INJURY LATE EFFECT
902.42 VEIN LACERATION (RUPTURE) (HEMATOMA) (AVULSION) (ANEURYSM) TRAUMATIC
908.4 VEIN LACERATION LATE EFFECT
453.3 VEIN THROMBOSIS (EMBOLISM)
902.40 VESSEL INJURY - NOS
902.49 VESSEL INJURY - SPECIFIED NEC
908.4 VESSEL INJURY - LATE EFFECT
902.40 VESSEL NOS LACERATION (RUPTURE) (HEMATOMA) (AVULSION) (ANEURYSM) TRAUMATIC
908.4 VESSEL NOS LACERATION LATE EFFECT

448.0 RENDU-OSLER-WEBER DISEASE OR SYNDROME (FAMILIAL HEMORRHAGIC TELANGIECTASIA)

648.9# RENDU-OSLER-WEBER DISEASE OR SYNDROME (FAMILIAL HEMORRHAGIC TELANGIECTASIA) MATERNAL CURRENT (CO-EXISTENT) IN PREGNANCY [448.0]
5th Digit: 648.9
0. EPISODE OF NOS OR N/A
1. DELIVERED
2. DELIVERED WITH POSTPARTUM COMPLICATION
3. ANTEPARTUM COMPLICATION
4. POSTPARTUM COMPLICATION

790.99 RENIN ELEVATED

753.0 RENOFACIAL SYNDROME (CONGENITAL BILIARY FIBROANGIOMATOSIS)

253.8 RENON-DELILLE SYNDROME

403.## RENOVASCULAR DISEASE (ARTERIOSCLEROTIC) DUE TO HYPERTENSION

4th Digit: 403
- **0. MALIGNANT**
- **1. BENIGN**
- **9. NOS**

5th Digit: 403
- **0. WITHOUT RENAL FAILURE**
- **1. WITH RENAL FAILURE**

405.91 RENOVASCULAR DISEASE WITH SECONDARY HYPERTENSION - UNSPECIFIED

405.11 RENOVASCULAR DISEASE WITH SECONDARY HYPERTENSION - BENIGN

405.01 RENOVASCULAR DISEASE WITH SECONDARY HYPERTENSION - MALIGNANT

727.2 REPETITIVE USE SYNDROME BURSITIS

REPLACEMENT STATUS

V43.5 BLADDER (ARTIFICIAL) (PROSTHESIS)
V43.4 BLOOD VESSEL (ARTIFICIAL) (PROSTHESIS)
V43.82 BREAST (ARTIFICIAL) (PROSTHESIS)
V43.0 EYE GLOBE (ARTIFICIAL) (PROSTHESIS)
V43.2 HEART (ARTIFICIAL) (PROSTHESIS)
V43.3 HEART VALVE (ARTIFICIAL) (PROSTHESIS)
V43.89 INTESTINE (ARTIFICIAL) (PROSTHESIS)
V43.60 JOINT
V43.66 JOINT ANKLE
V43.69 JOINT FINGER
V43.62 JOINT ELBOW
V43.64 JOINT HIP
V43.65 JOINT KNEE
V43.61 JOINT SHOULDER
V43.63 JOINT WRIST
V43.69 JOINT OTHER
V43.89 KIDNEY (ARTIFICIAL) (PROSTHESIS)
V43.81 LARYNX (ARTIFICIAL) (PROSTHESIS)
V43.1 LENS (ARTIFICIAL) (PROTHESIS)
V43.7 LIMB (ARTIFICIAL) (PROSTHESIS)
V43.89 LIVER (ARTIFICIAL) (PROSTHESIS)
V43.89 LUNG (ARTIFICIAL) (PROSTHESIS)
V43.89 ORGAN OTHER (ARTIFICIAL) (PROSTHESIS)
V43.89 PANCREAS (ARTIFICIAL) (PROSTHESIS)
V43.83 SKIN ARTIFICIAL
V43.89 TISSUE OTHER (ARTIFICIAL) (PROSTHESIS)
V43.89 OTHER ORGAN OR TISSUE (ARTIFICIAL) (PROSTHESIS)

0 RESISTANCE TO DRUGS BY MICROORGANISMS SEE 'DRUG RESISTANCE'

RESPIRATION, RESPIRATORY

786.00 ABNORMALITY
748.9 ANOMALY (SYSTEM) UNSPECIFIED CONGENITAL
748.8 ANOMALY (SYSTEM) OTHER SPECIFIED CONGENITAL
799.1 ARREST
799.1 ARREST CAUSE UNCERTAIN

DISORDER

519.9 UNSPECIFIED
770.9 UNSPECIFIED FETUS AND NEWBORN
465.9 ACUTE (UPPER) NEC
519.9 CHRONIC
770.7 CHRONIC ARISING IN PERINATAL PERIOD
760.3 CHRONIC MATERNAL AFFECTING FETUS OR NEWBORN
508.9 DUE TO ASPIRATION OF LIQUIDS OR SOLIDS
506.9 DUE TO FUMES AND VAPORS
506.3 DUE TO FUMES AND VAPORS - ACUTE / SUBACUTE
506.4 DUE TO FUMES AND VAPORS - CHRONIC
508.0 DUE TO RADIATION ACUTE
508.1 DUE TO RADIATION CHRONIC
508.8 DUE TO OTHER EXTERNAL AGENTS
508.9 DUE TO UNSPECIFIED EXTERNAL AGENTS
0 FAILURE SEE 'RESPIRATORY', FAILURE
V12.6 HISTORY

RESPIRATION, RESPIRATORY (continued)

DISORDER

306.1 PSYCHOGENIC
V81.3 SCREENING (FOR CHRONIC BRONCHITIS AND EMPHYSEMA)
V81.4 SCREENING (FOR OTHER RESPIRATORY DISEASES)
519.8 SPECIFIED NEC

DISTRESS

786.09 NOS
518.82 ACUTE
518.82 ACUTE NEC
770.8 NEWBORN
770.8 PERINATAL PERIOD
518.5 SYNDROME ADULT (FOLLOWING SHOCK, SURGERY OR TRAUMA)
518.82 SYNDROME ADULT (FOLLOWING SHOCK, SURGERY OR TRAUMA) SPECIFIED NEC
769 SYNDROME NEWBORN

FAILURE

518.81 NOS
518.81 ACUTE
518.84 ACUTE AND CHRONIC (ACUTE ON CHRONIC)
518.83 CHRONIC
518.5 DUE TO (TRAUMA SURGERY SHOCK)
770.8 NEWBORN
770.8 PERINATAL

INFECTION, UPPER

465.9 ACUTE
487.1 ACUTE INFLUENZAL
465.0 ACUTE LARYNGOPHARYNGITIS
465.8 ACUTE (MULTIPLE SITES)
034.0 ACUTE STREPTOCOCCAL
519.8 CHRONIC

INSUFFICIENCY

786.09 NOS
518.82 ACUTE
518.82 NEC

RESPIRATION, RESPIRATORY (continued)

786.09 KUSSMAUL (AIR HUNGER)
786.09 NARCOSIS CO 2 (CARBON DIOXIDE)
519.8 OBSTRUCTION (AIRWAY) NEC
496 OBSTRUCTION (CHRONIC) COPD
934.9 OBSTRUCTION DUE TO FOREIGN BODY
748.8 OBSTRUCTION UPPER CONGENITAL
748.9 ORGAN ABSENCE CONGENITAL
786.52 PAINFUL
344.89 PARALYSIS (SYSTEM)
786.06 RAPID
786.9 SYMPTOMS (SYSTEM)
079.6 SYNCYTIAL VIRUS
466.11 SYNCYTIAL VIRUS BRONCHIOLITIS
460 SYNCYTIAL VIRUS COMMON COLD-LIKE [079.6]
460 SYNCYTIAL VIRUS NASOPHARYNGITIS ACUTE [079.6]
480.1 SYNCYTIAL VIRUS PNEUMONIA (BRONCHOPNEUMONIA)
466.0 SYNCYTIAL VIRUS TRACHEOBRONCHITIS [079.6]
519.9 SYSTEM DISORDER NOS
519.8 SYSTEM DISORDER NEC
306.1 SYSTEM DISORDER PSYCHOGENIC
478.9 TRACT UPPER ATROPHY

V46.1 RESPIRATOR DEPENDENCE

0 RESPIRATORY SEE 'RESPIRATION, RESPIRATORY'

333.99 RESTLESS LEGS (SYNDROME)

799.2 RESTLESSNESS

V60.1 RESTRICTION OF SPACE (INADEQUATE HOUSING)

667.0# RETAINED PLACENTA
666.0# RETAINED PLACENTA WITH POSTPARTUM HEMORRHAGE
666.2# RETAINED PLACENTA WITH POSTPARTUM HEMORRHAGE SECOND STAGE
667.1# RETAINED PRODUCTS OF CONCEPTUS

5th Digit: 666.0, 2, 667.0-1
0. NOS
2. DELIVERED WITH POSTPARTUM COMPLICATION
4. POSTPARTUM COMPLICATION

0 RETARDATION DEVELOPMENTAL LANGUAGE OR LEARNING SKILLS - SEE 'DEVELOPMENTAL DISORDER'
0 RETARDATION FETAL GROWTH SEE 'FETAL - INFANT'S RECORD', GROWTH RETARDATION

RETARDATION MENTAL
319 UNSPECIFIED
317 MILD IQ 50-70
318.0 MODERATE IQ 35-49
318.1 SEVERE IQ 20-34
318.2 PROFOUND
V18.4 FAMILY HISTORY
V79.2 SCREENING

783.4 RETARDATION PHYSICAL
276.2 RETENTION CARBON DIOXIDE
788.2# RETENTION URINE

5th Digit: 788.2
0. UNSPECIFIED
1. INCOMPLETE BLADDER EMPTYING
9. OTHER SPECIFIED RETENTION

997.5 RETENTION URINE POSTOPERATIVE
362.64 RETICULAR DEGENERATION SENILE
701.8 RETICULATA ATROPHIC
790.99 RETICULOCYTOSIS
0 RETICULOENDOTHELIAL CYTOMYCOSIS SEE 'HISTOPLASMOSIS'
289.9 RETICULOENDOTHELIAL HYPERPLASIA (CELL)
202.5# RETICULOENDOTHELIOSIS INFANTILE ACUTE M9722/3
202.3# RETICULOENDOTHELIOSIS MALIGNANT M9720/3
200.8# RETICULOLYMPHOSARCOMA (DIFFUSE) M9613/3

5th Digit: 200.8, 202.3, 5
0. UNSPECIFIED SITE, EXTRANODAL AND SOLID ORGAN SITES
1. LYMPH NODES OF HEAD FACE NECK
2. LYMPH NODES INTRATHORACIC
3. LYMPH NODES ABDOMINAL
4. LYMPH NODES AXILLA AND UPPER LIMB
5. LYMPH NODES INGUINAL REGION AND LOWER LIMB
6. LYMPH NODES INTRAPELVIC
7. SPLEEN
8. LYMPH NODES MULTIPLE SITES

RETICULOSARCOMA
200.0# NOS M9640/3
202.0# FOLLICULAR OR NODULAR M9642/3

5th Digit: 200.0, 202.0
0. UNSPECIFIED SITE, EXTRANODAL AND SOLID ORGAN SITES
1. LYMPH NODES OF HEAD FACE NECK
2. LYMPH NODES INTRATHORACIC
3. LYMPH NODES ABDOMINAL
4. LYMPH NODES AXILLA AND UPPER LIMB
5. LYMPH NODES INGUINAL REGION AND LOWER LIMB
6. LYMPH NODES INTRAPELVIC
7. SPLEEN
8. LYMPH NODES MULTIPLE SITES

V10.71 HISTORY (NOT IN REMISSION)

RETICULOSARCOMA (continued)
200.0# NODULAR M9642/3
200.0# PLEOMORPHIC CELL TYPE M9641/3

5th Digit: 200.0
0. UNSPECIFIED SITE, EXTRANODAL AND SOLID ORGAN SITES
1. LYMPH NODES OF HEAD FACE NECK
2. LYMPH NODES INTRATHORACIC
3. LYMPH NODES ABDOMINAL
4. LYMPH NODES AXILLA AND UPPER LIMB
5. LYMPH NODES INGUINAL REGION AND LOWER LIMB
6. LYMPH NODES INTRAPELVIC
7. SPLEEN
8. LYMPH NODES MULTIPLE SITES

202.3# RETICULOSIS MALIGNANT M9720/3
202.5# RETICULOSIS OF INFANCY ACUTE M9722/3

5th Digit: 202.3, 5
0. UNSPECIFIED SITE, EXTRANODAL AND SOLID ORGAN SITES
1. LYMPH NODES OF HEAD FACE NECK
2. LYMPH NODES INTRATHORACIC
3. LYMPH NODES ABDOMINAL
4. LYMPH NODES AXILLA AND UPPER LIMB
5. LYMPH NODES INGUINAL REGION AND LOWER LIMB
6. LYMPH NODES INTRAPELVIC
7. SPLEEN
8. LYMPH NODES MULTIPLE SITES

RETINA, RETINAL
0 ABLATIO SEE 'RETINAL DETACHMENT'
794.11 ABNORMAL FUNCTION STUDIES
743.58 ANEURYSM CONGENITAL
0 ARTERITIS SEE 'RETINAL ARTERITIS (VARICES)'
0 ATROPHY SEE 'RETINAL DEGENERATION'
0 ATROPHY HEREDITARY SEE 'RETINAL DYSTROPHY'
361.30 BREAK NOS
743.56 CHANGES OTHER CONGENITAL
368.34 CORRESPONDENCE ABNORMAL WITH BINOCULAR VISION DISORDER
362.83 COTTON WOOL SPOTS
361.13 CYST PRIMARY
361.14 CYST SECONDARY
362.89 DEGENERATION (SEE ALSO 'RETINAL DEGENERATION')
361.9 DETACHMENT (SEE ALSO 'RETINAL DETACHMENT')
361.04 DIALYSIS (JUVENILE) WITH DETACHMENT
362.9 DISORDER
362.89 DISORDER SPECIFIED NEC
0 DYSTROPHY SEE 'RETINAL DYSTROPHY'
362.83 EDEMA (LOCALIZED) (MACULAR) (PERIPHERAL)
362.53 EDEMA (LOCALIZED) (MACULAR) (PERIPHERAL) CYSTOID
362.82 EXUDATES AND DEPOSITS
228.03 HEMANGIOMA
362.81 HEMORRHAGE (PERIRETINAL) (DEEP) (SUBRETINAL)
362.84 INFARCTION
921.3 INJURY CONTUSION
362.84 ISCHEMIA
362.13 LIGHT REFLEX INCREASED
362.14 MICROANEURYSMS
362.33 MICROEMBOLISMS
362.16 NEOVASCULARIZATION
362.85 NERVE FIBER BUNDLE DEFECTS

361.32 OPERCULUM
361.01 OPERCULUM WITH DETACHMENT

362.42 PIGMENT EPITHELIUM DETACHMENT EXUDATIVE
362.43 PIGMENT EPITHELIUM DETACHMENT HEMORRHAGIC
362.42 PIGMENT EPITHELIUM DETACHMENT SEROUS
361.19 PSEUDOCYST

RETINA, RETINAL (continued)

361.30 RUPTURE
0 RUPTURE WITH DETACHMENT SEE 'RETINAL DETACHMENT'
363.30 SCAR
363.35 SCAR DISSEMINATED
363.33 SCAR OF POSTERIOR POLE
363.34 SCAR PERIPHERAL
363.31 SCAR SOLAR
362.17 SCLEROSIS (SENILE) (VASCULAR)
362.40 SEPARATION LAYER UNSPECIFIED
362.13 SILVER WIRE ARTERIES
362.89 TESSELLATED FUNDUS (TIGROID)
362.30 VASCULAR OCCLUSION
362.13 VASCULAR SHEATHING
362.35 VEIN CENTRAL OCCLUSION
362.35 VEIN CENTRAL OCCLUSION CAUSING GLAUCOMA [365.63]
362.37 VEIN ENGORGEMENT
362.37 VEIN OCCLUSION PARTIAL OR INCIPIENT
362.36 VEIN OCCLUSION TRIBUTARY OR BRANCH
362.17 VESSEL TORTUOUS ACQUIRED
743.58 VESSEL TORTUOUS CONGENITAL

RETINAL ARTERITIS (VARICES)

362.18 ARTERITIS
362.18 ENDARTERITIS
362.14 MICROANEURYSMS
362.16 NEOVASCULARIZATION
362.18 PERIVASCULITIS
362.18 PHLEBITIS
362.15 TELANGIECTASIA
362.17 VARICES
362.18 VASCULITIS

RETINAL ARTERY OCCLUSION (OBSTRUCTION)

362.30 NOS
362.32 BRANCH
362.31 CENTRAL
362.33 PARTIAL
362.34 TRANSIENT
362.32 TRIBUTARY

RETINAL DEFECT

361.30 WITHOUT DETACHMENT
361.32 HORSESHOE TEAR WITHOUT DETACHMENT
361.33 MULTIPLE WITHOUT DETACHMENT
361.31 ROUND HOLE WITHOUT DETACHMENT
0 WITH DETACHMENT SEE 'RETINAL DETACHMENT'

RETINAL DEGENERATION

0 HEREDITARY SEE 'RETINAL DYSTROPHY', HEREDITARY
362.63 LATTICE (PALISADE)
362.62 MICROCYSTOID
362.61 PAVING STONE
362.60 PERIPHERAL
362.65 SECONDARY PIGMENTARY
362.66 SECONDARY VITREORETINAL
362.64 SENILE (RETICULAR)
0 WITH RETINAL DEFECT SEE 'RETINAL DETACHMENT'

RETINAL DETACHMENT

361.9 NOS
361.06 OLD DELIMITED
361.06 OLD PARTIAL
361.07 OLD TOTAL OR SUBTOTAL
361.00 PARTIAL RETINAL DEFECT
361.01 PARTIAL WITH SINGLE DEFECT
361.02 PARTIAL WITH MULTIPLE DEFECTS
361.03 PARTIAL WITH GIANT TEAR
362.42 PIGMENT EPITHELIUM SEROUS
362.43 PIGMENT EPITHELIUM HEMORRHAGIC

RETINAL DETACHMENT (continued)

361.04 RECENT WITH RETINAL DIALYSIS
361.05 RECENT TOTAL OR SUBTOTAL
361.2 SEROUS
362.41 SEROUS WITH CENTRAL SEROUS RETINOPATHY
361.81 TRACTION
361.81 TRACTION WITH VITREORETINAL ORGANIZATION
361.2 WITHOUT RETINAL DEFECT
361.89 OTHER FORM

RETINAL DYSTROPHY

272.5 BASSEN KORNZWEIG [362.72]
330.1 CEREBRORETINAL [362.71]
362.70 HEREDITARY
362.74 HEREDITARY - ALBIPUNCTATE
362.77 HEREDITARY - DRUSEN
362.76 HEREDITARY - FUNDUS FLAVIMACULATUS
362.77 HEREDITARY - HYALINE
362.74 HEREDITARY - PIGMENTARY
362.76 HEREDITARY - PRIMARILY INVOLVING RETINAL PIGMENT EPITHELIUM
362.77 HEREDITARY - PRIMARILY OF BRUCH'S MEMBRANE
362.75 HEREDITARY - PROGRESSIVE CONE (-ROD)
362.77 HEREDITARY - PSEUDOINFLAMMATORY FOVEAL
362.75 HEREDITARY - STARGARDT'S DISEASE
362.76 HEREDITARY - VITELLIFORM
362.73 HEREDITARY - VITREORETINAL
356.3 REFSUM'S DISEASE [362.72]
272.7 SYSTEMIC LIPIDOSES (DUE TO) [362.71]

RETINAL TEAR

361.30 NOS
361.00 NOS WITH DETACHMENT
361.03 GIANT
361.32 HORSESHOE
361.33 MULTIPLE
361.02 MULTIPLE WITH DETACHMENT
361.06 OLD PARTIAL
361.07 OLD TOTAL
361.31 ROUND HOLE WITHOUT DETACHMENT
361.05 TOTAL
361.07 TOTAL OLD
0 WITH DETACHMENT SEE RETINAL DETACHMENT

RETINAL VEIN OCCLUSION (OBSTRUCTION)

362.30 NOS
362.36 BRANCH
362.35 CENTRAL (TOTAL)
362.37 INCIPIENT
362.37 PARTIAL
362.36 TRIBUTARY

RETINITIS

363.20 NOS
363.10 DISSEMINATED
363.14 DISSEMINATED METASTATIC
363.00 FOCAL
363.05 FOCAL JUXTAPAPILLARY (AND RETINOCHOROIDITIS)
363.06 FOCAL MACULAR OR PARAMACULAR (AND RETINOCHOROIDITIS)
363.07 FOCAL OTHER POSTERIOR POLE (AND RETINOCHOROIDITIS)
363.08 FOCAL PERIPHERAL POLE (AND RETINOCHOROIDITIS)
115.92 HISTOPLASMA
115.02 HISTOPLASMA CAPSULATUM
115.12 HISTOPLASMA DUBOISII
362.74 PIGMENTOSA HEREDITARY
362.29 PROLIFERANS
0 SEE ALSO 'CHORIORETINITIS'
094.84 SYPHILITIC

RETINOBLASTOMA
190.5 SITE NOS
0 SITE SPECIFIED SEE 'CANCER' BY SITE M9510/3
190.5 DIFFERENTIATED TYPE SITE NOS
0 DIFFERENTIATED TYPE SITE SPECIFIED SEE 'CANCER' BY SITE M9511/3
190.5 UNDIFFERENTIATED TYPE SITE NOS
0 UNDIFFERENTIATED TYPE SITE SPECIFIED SEE 'CANCER' BY SITE M9512/3

0 RETINOCHORIORETINITIS SEE 'RETINITIS'

RETINOCHOROIDITIS
363.10 DISSEMINATED NOS
363.15 DISSEMINATED EPITHELIOPATHY (PIGMENTARY)
130.2 DUE TO ACQUIRED TOXOPLASMOSIS
363.00 FOCAL
094.83 SYPHILITIC

RETINOPATHY
440.8 ARTERIOSCLEROTIC [362.13]
362.10 BACKGROUND
362.41 CENTRAL SEROUS
250.5# DIABETIC BACKGROUND OR UNSPECIFIED [362.01]
250.5# DIABETIC PROLIFERATIVE [362.02]
5th Digit: 250.5
0. TYPE II, ADULT-ONSET, NON-INSULIN DEPENDENT (EVEN IF REQUIRING INSULIN), OR UNSPECIFIED; CONTROLLED
1. TYPE I, JUVENILE-ONSET OR INSULIN-DEPENDENT; CONTROLLED
2. TYPE II, ADULT-ONSET, NON-INSULIN DEPENDENT (EVEN IF REQUIRING INSULIN); UNCONTROLLED
3. TYPE I, JUVENILE-ONSET OR INSULIN-DEPENDENT; UNCONTROLLED
362.12 EXUDATIVE
362.11 HYPERTENSIVE
362.14 MICROANEURYSMS
362.21 OF PREMATURITY
362.17 OTHER INTRARETINAL MICROVASCULAR ABNORMALITIES
362.29 PROLIFERATIVE (OTHER) (NONDIABETIC)
282.60 PROLIFERATIVE DUE TO SICKLE CELL ANEMIA [362.29]
363.31 SOLAR
362.13 VASCULAR (CHANGES)

RETINOSCHISIS
361.10 NOS
361.12 BULLOUS
361.11 FLAT
362.73 JUVENILE HEREDITARY

752.52 RETRACTILE TESTIS (CONGENITAL)
378.71 RETRACTION SYNDROME (DUANE'S)
094.85 RETROBULBAR NEURITIS SYPHILITIC
753.4 RETROCAVAL URETER CONGENITAL
524.10 RETROGNATHISM
362.21 RETROLENTAL FIBROPLASIA

RETROPERITONEAL
568.89 CYST
593.4 FIBROSIS IDIOPATHIC (SYNDROME)
568.81 HEMOPERITONEUM NONTRAUMATIC
553.8 HERNIA
551.8 HERNIA GANGRENOUS
552.8 HERNIA INCARCERATED
868.04 HERNIATION TRAUMATIC
868.14 HERNIATION TRAUMATIC WITH OPEN WOUND INTO CAVITY
908.1 HERNIATION TRAUMATIC LATE EFFECT
868.04 INJURY
868.14 INJURY WITH OPEN WOUND INTO CAVITY
908.1 INJURY LATE EFFECT
789.39 MASS
789.09 PAIN
789.69 TENDERNESS

621.6 RETROVERTED UTERUS
654.3# RETROVERTED UTERUS (INCARCERATED) COMPLICATING CHILDBIRTH
5th Digit: 654.3
0. EPISODE OF CARE NOS OR N/A
1. DELIVERED
2. DELIVERED WITH POSTPARTUM COMPLICATION
3. ANTEPARTUM COMPLICATION
4. POSTPARTUM COMPLICATION

AIDS, ARC AND SYMPTOMATIC HIV INFECTIONS ALL CODE TO 042. THIS CODE SHOULD BE SEQUENCED AS THE PRINCIPAL DIAGNOSIS WITH AN ADDITIONAL CODE FOR ANY MANIFESTATION. EXCEPTION: IF THE ENCOUNTER IS FOR AN UNRELATED CONDITION SUCH AS A TRAUMA, SEQUENCE THE TRAUMA AS THE PRINCIPAL DIAGNOSIS, FOLLOWED BY THE 042 WITH ADDITIONAL CODES FOR THE MANIFESTATIONS.

RETROVIRUS
079.50 UNSPECIFIED
042 HIV 1 (HUMAN IMMUNODEFICIENCY VIRUS, TYPE 1)
079.53 HIV 2 (HUMAN IMMUNODEFICIENCY VIRUS, TYPE 2)
079.51 HTLV 1 (HUMAN T-CELL LYMPHOTROPHIC VIRUS TYPE 1)
079.52 HTLV 2 (HUMAN T-CELL LYMPHOTROPHIC VIRUS TYPE 2)
042 HTLV 3 (HUMAN T-CELL LYMPHOTROPHIC VIRUS TYPE 3)
042 LAV (LYMPHADENOPATHY-ASSOCIATED VIRUS)
079.59 OTHER SPECIFIED RETROVIRUS

524.04 RETRUSION PREMAXILLA (DEVELOPMENTAL)
330.8 RETT'S SYNDROME
331.81 REYE'S SYNDROME
253.2 REYE-SHEEHAN SYNDROME (POSTPARTUM PITUITARY NECROSIS)

RH INCOMPATIBILITY
773.0 CAUSING HEMOLYTIC DISEASE (FETUS) (NEWBORN)
773.0 FETUS OR NEWBORN
999.7 INFUSION OR TRANSFUSION REACTION
656.1# MATERNAL AFFECTING MANAGEMENT OF MOTHER
5th Digit: 656.1
0. EPISODE OF CARE NOS OR N/A
1. DELIVERED
3. ANTEPARTUM COMPLICATION

728.89 RHABDOMYOLYSIS IDIOPATHIC

RHABDOMYOMA
215.# NOS M8900/0
215.# ADULT M8904/0
215.# FETAL M8903/0
4th Digit: 215
0. HEAD FACE NECK
2. UPPER LIMB SHOULDER
3. LOWER LIMB HIP
4. THORAX
5. ABDOMINAL HYPOCHONDRIUM
6. PELVIS BUTTOCK GROIN INGUINAL REGION PERINEUM
7. TRUNK NOS BACK NOS FLANK NOS
8. OTHER SPECIFIED SITES
9. SITE UNSPECIFIED

RHABDOMYOSARCOMA
171.# NOS M8900/0
171.# ALVEOLAR M8920/3
171.# EMBRYONAL M8910/3
171.# MIXED TYPE M8902/3
171.# PLEOMORPHIC M8901/3
4th Digit: 171
0. HEAD FACE NECK
2. UPPER LIMB SHOULDER
3. LOWER LIMB HIP
4. THORAX
5. ABDOMINAL HYPOCHONDRIUM
6. PELVIS BUTTOCK GROIN INGUINAL REGION PERINEUM
7. TRUNK NOS BACK NOS FLANK NOS
8. OTHER SPECIFIED SITES
9. SITE NOS

0 RHEGMATOGENOUS RETINAL DETACHMENT SEE 'RETINAL DETACHMENT'

RHEUMATIC
396.9 AORTIC AND MITRAL VALVE DISEASE NOS
395.1 AORTIC INSUFFICIENCY
396.3 AORTIC INSUFFICIENCY AND MITRAL INSUFFICIENCY
395.0 AORTIC STENOSIS
395.2 AORTIC STENOSIS WITH INSUFFICIENCY
396.2 AORTIC STENOSIS AND MITRAL INSUFFICIENCY
396.0 AORTIC STENOSIS AND MITRAL STENOSIS
395.9 AORTIC VALVE DISEASE CHRONIC
V82.2 DISORDER SCREENING
396.8 OTHER AORTIC STENOSIS AND/OR INSUFFICIENCY WITH MITRAL STENOSIS AND/OR INSUFFICIENCY
394.1 MITRAL INSUFFICIENCY
396.3 MITRAL INSUFFICIENCY AND AORTIC INSUFFICIENCY
394.0 MITRAL STENOSIS
396.1 MITRAL STENOSIS AND AORTIC INSUFFICIENCY
394.2 MITRAL STENOSIS WITH INSUFFICIENCY
394.9 MITRAL VALVE DISEASE OTHER AND UNSPECIFIED
729.1 MYOSITIS
396.8 OTHER MITRAL STENOSIS AND/OR INSUFFICIENCY WITH AORTIC STENOSIS AND/OR INSUFFICIENCY
397.0 TRICUSPID DISEASE
397.0 TRICUSPID INSUFFICIENCY
397.0 TRICUSPID STENOSIS

RHEUMATIC ACUTE
390 ARTHRITIS
391.9 CARDITIS
392.9 CHOREA
392.0 CHOREA WITH HEART INVOLVEMENT
391.8 DISEASE ACTIVE WITH OTHER OR MULTIPLE TYPES OF HEART INVOLVEMENT
391.1 ENDOCARDITIS
390 FEVER (WITHOUT MENTION OF HEART INVOLVEMENT)
391.9 HEART DISEASE
391.8 HEART DISEASE OTHER (WITH OTHER OR MULTIPLE)
391.2 MYOCARDITIS
391.8 PANCARDITIS
391.0 PERICARDITIS

RHEUMATIC CHRONIC
398.90 CARDITIS
398.91 CHF
397.9 ENDOCARDITIS
398.90 HEART DISEASE
398.99 HEART DISEASE OTHER
398.91 LEFT VENTRICULAR FAILURE
393 MEDIASTINOPERICARDITIS
398.0 MYOCARDITIS
393 MYOPERICARDITIS
393 PERICARDITIS
397.1 PULMONIC INSUFFICIENCY (REGURGITATION)
397.1 PULMONIC STENOSIS
V82.2 SCREENING

729.0 RHEUMATISM

RHEUMATOID
714.2 CARDITIS
714.81 LUNG
714.0 MYOPATHY [359.6]

RHEUMATOID ARTHRITIS
714.0 ADULT
714.30 JUVENILE CHRONIC OR UNSPECIFIED
714.33 JUVENILE MONOARTICULAR
714.32 JUVENILE PAUCIARTICULAR
714.31 JUVENILE POLYARTICULAR ACUTE
V82.1 SCREENING
720.0 SPINE
714.2 WITH VISCERAL OR SYSTEMIC INVOLVEMENT

RHINITIS
472.0 NOS
460 ACUTE
460 ACUTE INFECTIVE
477.9 ALLERGIC
477.8 ALLERGIC DUE TO ANIMAL (DANDER) (HAIR) (EPIDERMIS)
477.8 ALLERGIC DUE TO DUST MITES
477.0 ALLERGIC DUE TO POLLEN
477.8 ALLERGIC DUE TO OTHER ALLERGEN
493.9# ALLERGIC WITH ASTHMA
493.0# ALLERGIC WITH ASTHMA WITH STATED CAUSE
5th Digit: 493.0, 9
1. WITHOUT STATUS
2. WITH STATUS
472.0 ATROPHIC
472.0 CHRONIC
472.0 CHRONIC ATROPHIC
472.0 CHRONIC GRANULOMATOUS
472.0 HYPERTROPHIC
472.0 OBSTRUCTIVE
472.0 ULCERATIVE
477.9 VASOMOTOR
491.21 WITH ACUTE BRONCHITIS
491.20 WITH CHRONIC BRONCHITIS
491.21 WITH CHRONIC BRONCHITIS WITH EXACERBATION

478.1 RHINOLITH SINUS (NASAL)
460 RHINOPHARYNGITIS ACUTE
472.2 RHINOPHARYNGITIS CHRONIC
102.5 RHINOPHARYNGITIS MUTILANS (DESTRUCTIVE ULCERATING)
695.3 RHINOPHYMA

RHINORRHEA
349.81 CEREBROSPINAL FLUID
478.1 RHINORRHEA
0 SEE 'RHINITIS'

040.1 RHINOSCLEROMA
117.0 RHINOSPORIDIOSIS
117.0 RHINOSPORIDIUM SEEBERI INFECTION
079.3 RHINOVIRUS (INFECTION) (INFECTING AGENT)
117.7 RHIZOPUS INFECTION
086.4 RHODESIAN SLEEPING SICKNESS
V07.2 RHOGAM ADMINISTRATION (PROPHYLACTIC)
701.8 RHYTIDOSIS FAVALIS
701.8 RHYTIDS

RIB
748.3 ABSENCE
756.3 ABSENCE CONGENITAL
756.3 ACCESSORY
739.8 CAGE SEGMENTAL OR SOMATIC DYSFUNCTION
719.88 CALCIFICATION
738.3 DEFORMITY ACQUIRED
756.3 EXTRA
756.3 FUSION CONGENITAL
848.3 SEPARATION (RUPTURE) (TEAR) (LACERATION)
733.99 SLIPPED
848.3 STRAIN (SPRAIN) (AVULSION) (HEMARTHROSIS)
756.3 SUPERNUMERARY CONGENITAL
353.0 SYNDROME CERVICAL

266.0 RIBOFLAVIN DEFICIENCY

718.1# RICE BODIES (OLD)
5th Digit: 718.1
0. SITE NOS
1. SHOULDER REGION
2. UPPER ARM (ELBOW) (HUMERUS)
3. FOREARM (RADIUS) (WRIST) (ULNA)
4. HAND (CARPAL) (METACARPAL) (FINGERS)
5. PELVIC REGION AND THIGH (HIP) (BUTTOCK) (FEMUR)
7. ANKLE AND/OR FOOT (METATARSALS) (TOES) (TARSALS)
8. OTHER SPECIFIED SITES
9. MULTIPLE

717.6 RICE BODIES (OLD) - KNEE (JOINT)
724.9 RICE BODIES (OLD) - VERTEBRAL FACET

RICKETS
268.0 ACTIVE
268.0 ACUTE
268.0 ADOLESCENT
268.0 ADULT
579.0 CELIAC (DISEASE)
268.0 CHEST WALL
268.0 CONGENITAL
268.0 CURRENT
756.4 FETAL
267 HEMORRHAGIC
270.0 HYPOPHOSPHATEMIC WITH NEPHROTIC-GLYCOSURIC DWARFISM
268.0 INFANTILE
268.0 INTESTINAL
588.0 KIDNEY
268.1 LATE EFFECT
588.0 RENAL
267 SCURVY
275.3 VITAMIN D-RESISTANT

RICKETTSIAL, RICKETTSIOSIS
083.9 DISEASE NOS
083.8 DISEASE OTHER SPECIFIED TYPE
083.2 POX
083.0 Q FEVER
V75.0 SCREENING EXAM

TICK-BORNE
082.9 NOS
082.1 BOUTONNEUSE FEVER
082.2 NORTH ASIAN FEVER
082.3 QUEENSLAND FEVER
082.0 SPOTTED FEVER
082.8 OTHER SPECIFIED

RICKETTSIAL, RICKETTSIOSIS (continued)
083.1 TRENCH FEVER
083.2 VESICULAR

368.16 RIDDOCH'S SYNDROME (VISUAL DISORIENTATION)
733.99 RIDER'S BONE CALCIFICATION
744.29 RIDGE EAR CONGENITAL
428.1 RIDLEY'S SYNDROME
245.3 RIEDEL'S DISEASE (LIGNEOUS THYROIDITIS)
751.69 RIEDEL'S LOBE LIVER
743.44 RIEGER'S ANOMALY OR SYNDROME (MESODERMAL DYSGENESIS, ANTERIOR OCULAR SEGMENT)
709.09 RIEHL'S MELANOSIS
282.4 RIETTI-GREPPI-MICHELI SYNDROME (THALASSEMIA MINOR)
066.3 RIFT VALLEY FEVER (VIRAL)
529.0 RIGA (-FEDE) DISEASE (CACHECTIC APHTHAE)
523.4 RIGGS' DISEASE (COMPOUND PERIODONTITIS)

426.4 RIGHT BUNDLE BRANCH BLOCK
428.0 RIGHT HEART FAILURE (SECONDARY TO LEFT HEART FAILURE)
518.0 RIGHT MIDDLE LOBE SYNDROME
428.0 RIGHT VENTRICULAR FAILURE
429.3 RIGHT VENTRICULAR HYPERTROPHY
0 RIGHT VENTRICULAR OBSTRUCTION SYNDROME SEE 'CHF (CONGESTIVE HEART FAILURE)'

789.4# RIGIDITY ABDOMEN
5th Digit: 789.4
0. UNSPECIFIED SITE
1. UPPER RIGHT QUADRANT
2. UPPER LEFT QUADRANT
3. LOWER RIGHT QUADRANT
4. LOWER LEFT QUADRANT
5. PERIUMBILIC
6. EPIGASTRIC
7. GENERALIZED
9. OTHER SPECIFIED SITE (MULTIPLE)

742.8 RILEY-DAY SYNDROME (FAMILIAL DYSAUTONOMIA)
661.4# RING CONTRACTION COMPLICATING DELIVERY
5th Digit: 661.4
0. EPISODE OF CARE NOS OR N/A
1. DELIVERED
3. ANTEPARTUM COMPLICATION

110.9 RINGWORM
0 RINGWORM SEE 'TINEA'

695.1 RITTER LYELL SYNDROME (SSSS)
695.81 RITTER'S DISEASE
039.3 RIVALTA'S DISEASE (CERVICOFACIAL ACTINOMYCOSIS)
755.69 ROBERT'S PELVIS
763.1 ROBERT'S PELVIS AFFECTING FETUS
653.0# ROBERT'S PELVIS WITH DISPROPORTION
660.1# ROBERT'S PELVIS WITH DISPROPORTION CAUSING OBSTRUCTION **[653.0#]**
5th Digit: 653.0, 660.1
0. EPISODE OF CARE NOS OR N/A
1. DELIVERED
3. ANTEPARTUM COMPLICATION

756.0 ROBIN'S SYNDROME
125.3 ROBLES' DISEASE (ONCHOCERCIASIS) [360.13]

0 ROCHALIMEA SEE 'RICKETSIOSIS'
082.0 ROCKY MOUNTAIN SPOTTED FEVER
370.07 RODENT ULCER CORNEA
0 RODENT ULCER SKIN SEE 'CANCER', SKIN

745.4 ROGER'S DISEASE (CONGENITAL INTERVENTRICULAR SEPTAL DEFECT)

570 ROKITANSKY'S DISEASE (SEE ALSO 'NECROSIS', LIVER)
752.49 ROKITANSKY-KUSTER-HAUSER SYNDROME (CONGENITAL ABSENCE, VAGINA)

794.31 ROMANO-WARD SYNDROME (PROLONGED Q-T INTERVAL)
720.1 ROMANUS LESION
349.89 ROMBERG'S DISEASE OR SYNDROME

ROSACEA
695.3 NOS
695.3 ACNE
695.3 CONJUNCTIVITIS [372.31]
695.3 KERATITIS [370.49]

516.0 ROSEN-CASTLEMAN-LIEBOW SYNDROME (PULMONARY PROTEINOSIS)
286.2 ROSENTHAL'S DISEASE (FACTOR XI DEFICIENCY)
057.8 ROSEOLA (INFANTUM)

066.3 ROSS RIVER FEVER (VIRAL)
536.8 ROSSBACH'S DISEASE (HYPERCHLORHYDRIA)
306.4 ROSSBACH'S DISEASE (HYPERCHLORHYDRIA) - PSYCHOGENIC

ROTATOR CUFF

727.61 CAPSULE RUPTURE NONTRAUMATIC
840.4 CAPSULE RUPTURE TRAUMATIC
727.61 RUPTURE COMPLETE NONTRAUMATIC
840.4 RUPTURE TRAUMATIC
840.4 SEPARATION (RUPTURE) (TEAR) (LACERATION)
840.4 SPRAIN
840.4 STRAIN (SPRAIN) (AVULSION) (HEMARTHROSIS)
726.10 SYNDROME NOS
726.10 TEAR DEGENERATIVE
727.61 TEAR NONTRAUMATIC
840.4 TEAR TRAUMATIC

008.61 ROTAVIRUS ENTERITIS
355.1 ROTH (-BERNHARDT) DISEASE OR SYNDROME
757.33 ROTHMUND'S SYNDROME (CONGENITAL POIKILODERMA)
277.4 ROTOR'S SYNDROME (IDIOPATHIC HYPERBILIRUBINEMIA)
752.8 ROUND LIGAMENT ABSENCE (APLASIA) (CONGENITAL)
867.6 ROUND LIGAMENT INJURY TRAUMATIC
867.7 ROUND LIGAMENT INJURY TRAUMATIC WITH OPEN WOUND
646.8# ROUND LIGAMENT SYNDROME COMPLICATING PREGNANCY [625.9]

5th Digit: 646.8

- **0. EPISODE OF CARE NOS OR N/A**
- **1. DELIVERED**
- **2. DELIVERED WITH POSTPARTUM COMPLICATION**
- **3. ANTEPARTUM COMPLICATION**
- **4. POSTPARTUM COMPLICATION**

127.0 ROUNDWORM INFECTION
334.3 ROUSSY-LEVY SYNDROME
757.39 ROY (-JUTRAS) SYNDROME (ACROPACHYDERMA)

RSV (RESPIRATORY SYNCYTIAL VIRUS)

079.6 NOS
466.11 BRONCHIOLITIS
460 COMMON COLD-LIKE [079.6]
460 NASOPHARYNGITIS ACUTE [079.6]
480.1 PNEUMONIA (BRONCHOPNEUMONIA)
466.0 TRACHEOBRONCHITIS [079.6]

751.2 RS WADE SYNDROME

RUBELLA

056.9 RUBELLA
056.71 ARTHRITIS
771.0 CONGENITAL OR PERINATAL
056.01 ENCEPHALITIS
V01.4 EXPOSURE
V73.3 SCREENING EXAM
056.79 SPECIFIED COMPLICATION OTHER
771.0 SYNDROME (CONGENITAL)
V04.3 VACCINATION ALONE
056.09 WITH NEUROLOGICAL COMPLICATION OTHER
056.8 WITH NOS COMPLICATION
056.00 WITH NOS NEUROLOGICAL COMPLICATION (RUBEOLA MOBILLI)

RUBELLA COMPLICATING PREGNANCY

655.3# MATERNAL AFFECTING FETUS

5th Digit: 655.3

- **0. EPISODE OF CARE NOS OR N/A**
- **1. DELIVERED**
- **3. ANTEPARTUM COMPLICATION**

RUBELLA COMPLICATING PREGNANCY (continued)

647.5#: USE AN ADDITIONAL CODE TO IDENTIFY THE MATERNAL RUBELLA.

647.5# MATERNAL CURRENT (COEXISTENT)

5th Digit: 647.5

- **0. EPISODE OF CARE NOS OR N/A**
- **1. DELIVERED**
- **2. DELIVERED WITH POSTPARTUM COMPLICATION**
- **3. ANTEPARTUM COMPLICATION**
- **4. POSTPARTUM COMPLICATION**

0 RUBEOLA SEE 'MEASLES'
364.42 RUBEOSIS IRIDIS
759.89 RUBINSTEIN-TAYBI'S SYNDROME (BRACHYDACTYLIA, SHORT STATURE AND MENTAL RETARDATION)
759.89 RUD'S SYNDROME (MENTAL DEFICIENCY, EPILEPSY AND INFANTILISM)
755.22 RUDIMENTARY ARM
272.7 RUITER-POMPEN (-WYERS) SYNDROME (ANGIOKERATOMA CORPORIS DIFFUSUM)

RUMINATION

300.3 NEUROTIC
300.3 OBSESSIONAL
307.53 PSYCHOGENIC

281.0 RUNEBERG'S DISEASE (PROGRESSIVE PERNICIOUS ANEMIA)
766.2 RUNGE'S SYNDROME (POSTMATURITY)
726.69 RUNNER'S KNEE

RUPTURE

845.09 ACHILLES TENDON (TRAUMATIC)
441.5 AORTA NOS
441.1 AORTA ASCENDING
093.0 AORTA SYPHILITIC
441.1 AORTIC ARCH

447.2 ARTERY
0 ARTERY TRAUMATIC SEE SPECIFIC ARTERY, INJURY
840.8 BICEPS LONG HEAD (TRAUMATIC)
576.3 BILE DUCT
459.0 BLOOD VESSEL
363.63 CHOROID

0 COLLATERAL LIGAMENTS SEE 'SPRAIN'

384.20 EAR DRUM (POST TRAUMA POST INFECTIVE)
872.61 EAR DRUM TRAUMATIC
872.71 EAR DRUM TRAUMATIC COMPLICATED

862.22 ESOPHAGUS TRAUMATIC
862.32 ESOPHAGUS TRAUMATIC WITH OPEN WOUND INTO CAVITY

871.1 EYE WITH EXPOSURE OF INTRAOCULAR TISSUE
871.2 EYE WITH PARTIAL LOSS OF INTRAOCULAR TISSUE
620.8 FALLOPIAN TUBE HYDATID OF MORGAGNI CONGENITAL
575.4 GALLBLADDER
537.89 GASTRIC OR DUODENAL
623.8 HYMEN

0 INTERNAL ORGAN TRAUMATIC SEE SPECIFIC ORGAN, INJURY
0 JOINT SEE 'SPRAIN'
866.03 KIDNEY
866.13 KIDNEY WITH OPEN WOUND INTO CAVITY

0 LIGAMENTS OF JOINT NONTRAUMATIC SEE 'ARTICULAR CARTILAGE DERANGEMENT'
0 LIGAMENTS OF JOINT TRAUMATIC SEE 'SPRAIN'
762.1 MARGINAL SINUS AFFECTING FETUS OR NEWBORN
761.1 MEMBRANES PREMATURE AFFECTING FETUS (SEE ALSO 'RUPTURE OBSTETRICAL', MEMBRANES)

RUPTURE (continued)

728.83 MUSCLE NONTRAUMATIC
0 MUSCLE NEC TRAUMATIC SEE 'SPRAIN' BY SITE
0 MUSCLE TRAUMATIC WITH OPEN WOUND SEE 'LACERATION' BY SITE
840.4 MUSCULOTENDINOUS CUFF (NONTRAUMATIC) (SHOULDER)
0 MYOCARDIUM (NONTRAUMATIC) SEE 'MYOCARDIAL INFARCTION ACUTE'
861.03 MYOCARDIUM TRAUMATIC
861.13 MYOCARDIUM TRAUMATIC WITH OPEN WOUND INTO THORAX
620.8 OVARY OR FALLOPIAN TUBE (NONPREGNANT)
620.8 OVARY WITH HEMOPERITONEUM (NON TRAUMATIC) [568.81]
620.8 OVIDUCT
577.8 PANCREAS
844.8 PATELLAR TENDON (TRAUMATIC)
624.8 PERINEUM
417.8 PULMONARY VESSEL
844.8 QUADRICEPS (TRAUMATIC)
843.8 QUADRICEPS TENDON - HIP AND THIGH (TRAUMATIC)
844.8 QUADRICEPS TENDON - KNEE AND LEG (TRAUMATIC)
569.49 RECTAL SPHINCTER

767.4 SPINE OR SPINAL CORD BIRTH TRAUMA

865.04 SPLEEN
767.8 SPLEEN BIRTH TRAUMA
865.14 SPLEEN WITH OPEN WOUND INTO CAVITY

767.8 STOMACH (BIRTH TRAUMA)
0 TENDON NONTRAUMATIC SEE 'TENDON', RUPTURE
0 TENDON TRAUMATIC SEE 'SPRAIN'
457.8 THORACIC DUCT
599.84 URETHRA
0 UTERUS OBSTETRICAL SEE 'RUPTURE OBSTETRICAL'
0 VEIN TRAUMATIC SEE SPECIFIC VEIN, INJURY

RUPTURE OBSTETRICAL

658.3# MEMBRANES ARTIFICIAL WITH DELAYED DELIVERY
V71.8 MEMBRANES EVALUATION, NOT FOUND
658.1# MEMBRANES PREMATURE
658.2# MEMBRANES SPONTANEOUS WITH DELAYED DELIVERY

5th Digit: 658.1-3
0. EPISODE OF CARE NOS OR N/A
1. DELIVERED
3. ANTEPARTUM COMPLICATION

665.1# UTERUS NOS
665.1# UTERUS DURING LABOR

5th Digit: 665.1
0. EPISODE OF CARE NOS OR N/A
1. DELIVERED

665.0# UTERUS BEFORE ONSET OF LABOR

5th Digit: 665.0
0. EPISODE OF CARE NOS OR N/A
1. DELIVERED
3. ANTEPARTUM COMPLICATION

759.89 RUSSELL (-SILVER) SYNDROME (CONGENITAL HEMIHYPERTROPHY AND SHORT STATURE)
063.0 RUSSIAN SPRING SUMMER (TAIGA) ENCEPHALITIS
0 RUST'S DISEASE SEE 'TUBERCULOSIS', SPONDYLOPATHY
203.0# RUSTITSKII'S MULTIPLE MYELOMA M9730/3

5th Digit: 203.0
0. WITHOUT MENTION OF REMISSION
1. IN REMISSION

751.3 RUYSCH'S DISEASE CONGENITAL
426.0 RYTAND-LIPSITCH SYNDROME (COMPLETE ATRIOVENTRICULAR BLOCK)

379.57 SACCADIC EYE MOVEMENTS DEFICIENCY
330.1 SACH'S (-TAY) DISEASE
270.7 SACCHAROPINURIA
756.15 SACRALIZATION-SCOLIOSIS-SCIATICA SYNDROME
0 SACRAL SEE 'SACRUM, SACRAL'
739.4 SACROCOCCYGEAL REGION SEGMENTAL OR SOMATIC DYSFUNCTION

SACROILIAC
755.69 DEFORMITY CONGENITAL
755.69 FUSION CONGENITAL
724.6 JOINT DISORDER NEC (NONVERTEBRAL) (NONDISCOGENIC)
846.1 LIGAMENT SEPARATION (RUPTURE) (TEAR) (LACERATION)
846.1 LIGAMENT STRAIN (SPRAIN) (AVULSION) (HEMARTHROSIS)
739.4 REGION SEGMENTAL OR SOMATIC DYSFUNCTION
846.9 REGION SEPARATION (RUPTURE) (TEAR) (LACERATION) UNSPECIFIED SITE
846.8 REGION SEPARATION (RUPTURE) (TEAR) (LACERATION) OTHER SPECIFIED SITES
846.9 REGION STRAIN (SPRAIN) (AVULSION) (HEMARTHROSIS) UNSPECIFIED SITE
846.8 REGION STRAIN (SPRAIN) (AVULSION) (HEMARTHROSIS) OTHER SPECIFIED SITES
724.6 SYNDROME

720.2 SACROILIITIS
846.2 SACROSPINATUS SEPARATION (RUPTURE) (TEAR) (LACERATION)
846.2 SACROSPINATUS STRAIN (SPRAIN) (AVULSION) (HEMARTHROSIS)
846.3 SACROTUBEROUS SEPARATION (RUPTURE) (TEAR) (LACERATION)
846.3 SACROTUBEROUS STRAIN (SPRAIN) (AVULSION) (HEMARTHROSIS)

SACRUM, SACRAL
756.13 ABSENCE CONGENITAL
724.6 ANKYLOSIS (NONVERTEBRAL) (NONDISCOGENIC)
724.6 DISORDER
724.6 INSTABILITY (NONVERTEBRAL) (NONDISCOGENIC)
953.3 NERVE ROOT INJURY
739.4 REGION SEGMENTAL OR SOMATIC DYSFUNCTION
847.3 SEPARATION (RUPTURE) (TEAR) (LACERATION)
847.3 STRAIN (SPRAIN) (AVULSION) (HEMARTHROSIS)

309.1 SAD (SEASONAL AFFECTIVE DISORDER)
302.84 SADISM SEXUAL
370.04 SAEMISCH'S ULCER
379.46 SAENGER'S SYNDROME
0 SAH SEE 'SUBARACHNOID', HEMORRHAGE
692.74 SAILORS' SKIN
117.7 SAKSENAEA INFECTION
345.6# SALAAM ATTACKS

5th Digit: 345.6

0. WITHOUT MENTION OF INTRACTABLE EPILEPSY
1. WITH INTRACTABLE EPILEPSY

781.0 SALAAM TIC
792.4 SALIVA ABNORMAL

SALIVARY DUCT
527.8 ATRESIA
750.23 ATRESIA CONGENITAL
527.0 ATROPHY
527.9 DISEASE NEC
750.23 IMPERFORATE CONGENITAL
078.5 INCLUSION DISEASE
034.0 INCLUSION STREPTOCOCCAL
959.09 INJURY

SALIVARY DUCT (continued)
527.8 OBSTRUCTION
527.5 OBSTRUCTION WITH CALCULUS
527.8 STENOSIS
527.8 STRICTURE
078.5 VIRUS DISEASE

SALIVARY GLAND
527.3 ABSCESS
750.21 ABSENCE CONGENITAL
750.22 ACCESSORY CONGENITAL
527.8 ATRESIA
750.23 ATRESIA CONGENITAL
527.0 ATROPHY
527.9 DISEASE NEC
527.7 DISTURBANCE SALIVARY SECRETION
527.4 FISTULA
750.24 FISTULA CONGENITAL
527.1 HYPERPLASIA
527.1 HYPERTROPHY
078.5 INCLUSION DISEASE
034.0 INCLUSION STREPTOCOCCAL
959.09 INJURY
527.8 LYMPHOEPITHELIAL LESION BENIGN
527.6 MUCOCELE
078.5 VIRUS DISEASE

527.5 SALIVARY SYSTEM CALCULUS

SALMONELLA
003.23 ARTHRITIS
V02.3 CARRIER
003.0 GASTROENTERITIS
003.9 INFECTION
003.20 INFECTION LOCALIZED
003.29 INFECTIONS LOCALIZED OTHER
003.8 INFECTIONS OTHER SPECIFIED
003.21 MENINGITIS
003.24 OSTEOMYELITIS
003.22 PNEUMONIA
003.1 SEPSIS

SALPINGITIS
614.2 NOS
614.0 ACUTE
614.0 ACUTE AND OOPHORITIS
760.8 AFFECTING FETUS OR NEWBORN
614.1 CHRONIC
614.1 CHRONIC AND OOPHORITIS
614.1 FOLLICULARIS
639.0 FOLLOWING ABORTION OR ECTOPIC/MOLAR PREGNANCY
098.17 GONOCOCCAL ACUTE
098.37 GONOCOCCAL CHRONIC
614.1 ISTHMICA NODOSA
670.0# MATERNAL DUE TO PREGNANCY

5th Digit: 670.0

0. NOS
2. DELIVERED WITH POSTPARTUM COMPLICATION
4. POSTPARTUM COMPLICATION

016.6# TUBERCULOUS

5th Digit: 016.6

0. NOS
1. LAB NOT DONE
2. LABS PENDING
3. MICROSCOPY POSITIVE (IN SPUTUM)
4. CULTURE POSITIVE - MICROSCOPY NEGATIVE
5. CULTURE NEGATIVE - MICROSCOPY POSITIVE
6. CULTURE AND MICROSCOPY NEGATIVE CONFIRMED BY OTHER METHODS

S

SALPINGO-OOPHORITIS
614.2 NOS
614.0 ACUTE
614.1 CHRONIC

620.4 SALPINGOCELE

992.8 SALT DEPLETION SYNDROME DUE TO HEAT
992.4 SALT DEPLETION SYNDROME DUE TO HEAT CAUSING HEAT EXHAUSTION OR PROSTRATION
593.9 SALT LOSING (DEPLETION) SYNDROME
371.46 SALZMANN'S NODULAR DYSTROPHY
114.# SAN JOAQUIN VALLEY FEVER
4th Digit: 114
0. ACUTE (PRIMARY)
4. CHRONIC (SECONDARY)
5. UNSPECIFIED

134.1 SAND FLEA INFESTATION
297.1 SANDER'S DISEASE (PARANOIA)
066.0 SANDFLY FEVER
330.1 SANDHOFF'S DISEASE
126.9 SANDWORM DISEASE
277.5 SANFILIPPO'S SYNDROME
334.2 SANGER BROWN CEREBELLA DEGENERATION

082.0 SAO PAULO FEVER

SAPHENOUS
904.7 ARTERY INJURY
908.3 ARTERY INJURY LATE EFFECT
355.79 MONONEUROPATHY
355.79 NERVE COMPRESSION (ENTRAPMENT)
355.79 NERVE DISORDER (LESION) (NEURITIS)
904.3 VEIN (GREATER) (LESSER) INJURY
908.3 VEIN (GREATER) (LESSER) INJURY LATE EFFECT
904.3 VEIN (GREATER) (LESSER) LACERATION
908.3 VEIN (GREATER) (LESSER) LACERATION LATE EFFECT
451.0 VEIN PHLEBITIS

136.5 SARCOCYSTIS LINDEMANNI INFECTION

SARCOID, SARCOIDOSIS
135 ANY SITE OR UNSPECIFIED
135 MENINGITIS [321.4]
135 MYOPATHY [359.6]
135 POLYNEUROPATHY [357.4]
V82.8 SARCOID TEST
V82.8 SCREENING EXAM
135 WITH LUNG INVOLVEMENT [517.8]

SARCOMA
171.9 SITE NOS
0 SITE SPECIFIED SEE 'CANCER' BY SITE SOFT TISSUE M8800/3
171.# ALVEOLAR SOFT PART M9581/3
4th Digit: 171
0. HEAD FACE NECK
2. UPPER LIMB SHOULDER
3. LOWER LIMB HIP
4. THORAX
5. ABDOMINAL HYPOCHONDRIUM
6. PELVIS BUTTOCK GROIN INGUINAL REGION PERINEUM
7. TRUNK NOS BACK NOS FLANK NOS
8. OTHER SPECIFIED SITES
9. SITE NOS

191.6 CEREBELLAR SITE NOS
0 CEREBELLAR SITE SPECIFIED SEE 'CANCER' BY SITE M9480/3

SARCOMA (continued)
171.# CLEAR CELL OF TENDONS AND APONEUROSES M9044/3
171.# EMBRYONAL M8991/3
4th Digit: 171
0. HEAD FACE NECK
2. UPPER LIMB SHOULDER
3. LOWER LIMB HIP
4. THORAX
5. ABDOMINAL HYPOCHONDRIUM
6. PELVIS BUTTOCK GROIN INGUINAL REGION PERINEUM
7. TRUNK NOS BACK NOS FLANK NOS
8. OTHER SPECIFIED SITES
9. SITE NOS

182.1 ENDOMETRIAL ISTHMUS M8930/3
182.0 ENDOMETRIAL STROMA UTERINE BODY, NOS M8930/3
171.# EPITHELIOID CELL M8804/3
4th Digit: 171
0. HEAD FACE NECK
2. UPPER LIMB SHOULDER
3. LOWER LIMB HIP
4. THORAX
5. ABDOMINAL HYPOCHONDRIUM
6. PELVIS BUTTOCK GROIN INGUINAL REGION PERINEUM
7. TRUNK NOS BACK NOS FLANK NOS
8. OTHER SPECIFIED SITES
9. SITE NOS

170.# EWING'S M9260/3
4th Digit: 170
0. SKULL AND FACE
1. MANDIBLE
2. VERTEBRAL COLUMN
3. RIBS STERNUM CLAVICLE
4. SCAPULA LONG BONES UPPER LIMB
5. SHORT BONES UPPER LIMB
6. PELVIC BONES SACRUM COCCYX
7. LONG BONES LOWER LIMB
8. SHORT BONES LOWER LIMB
9. SITE NOS

171.# GIANT CELL (EXCEPT OF BONE)
4th Digit: 171
0. HEAD FACE NECK
2. UPPER LIMB SHOULDER
3. LOWER LIMB HIP
4. THORAX
5. ABDOMINAL HYPOCHONDRIUM
6. PELVIS BUTTOCK GROIN INGUINAL REGION PERINEUM
7. TRUNK NOS BACK NOS FLANK NOS
8. OTHER SPECIFIED SITES
9. SITE NOS

176.# KAPOSI'S M9140/3
4th Digit: 176
0. SKIN
1. SOFT TISSUE
2. SOFT PALATE
3. GASTROINTESTINAL
4. LUNG
5. LYMPH NODES
8. OTHER SPECIFIED SITES (EXTERNAL GENITALIA) (SCROTUM) (VULVA)
9. SITE UNSPECIFIED

155.0 KUPFFER CELL SITE NOS
0 MAST CELL SEE 'CANCER' BY SITE M9740/3
191.9 MONSTROCELLULAR SITE NOS
0 MONSTROCELLULAR SITE SPECIFIED SEE 'CANCER' BY SITE M9481/3

SARCOMA (continued)

205.3# MYELOID M9930/3

5th Digit: 205.3

0. WITHOUT MENTION OF REMISSION

1. IN REMISSION

200.0# RETICULUM CELL NOS M9640/3

200.0# RETICULUM CELL PLEOMORPHIC CELL TYPE M9641/3

5th Digit: 200.0

0. UNSPECIFIED SITE, EXTRANODAL AND SOLID ORGAN SITES

1. LYMPH NODES OF HEAD FACE NECK

2. LYMPH NODES INTRATHORACIC

3. LYMPH NODES ABDOMINAL

4. LYMPH NODES AXILLA AND UPPER LIMB

5. LYMPH NODES INGUINAL REGION AND LOWER LIMB

6. LYMPH NODES INTRAPELVIC

7. SPLEEN

8. LYMPH NODES MULTIPLE SITES

171.# SMALL CELL M8803/3

171.# SPINDLE CELL M8801/3

171.# SYNOVIAL M9040/3

171.# SYNOVIAL BIPHASIC TYPE M9043/3

171.# SYNOVIAL EPITHELIOID CELL TYPE M9042/3

171.# SYNOVIAL SPINDLE CELL M9041/3

4th Digit: 171

0. HEAD FACE NECK

2. UPPER LIMB SHOULDER

3. LOWER LIMB HIP

4. THORAX

5. ABDOMINAL HYPOCHONDRIUM

6. PELVIS BUTTOCK GROIN INGUINAL REGION PERINEUM

7. TRUNK NOS BACK NOS FLANK NOS

8. OTHER SPECIFIED SITES

9. SITE NOS

SARCOMATOSIS

171.# NOS M8800/9

4th Digit: 171

0. HEAD FACE NECK

2. UPPER LIMB SHOULDER

3. LOWER LIMB HIP

4. THORAX

5. ABDOMINAL HYPOCHONDRIUM

6. PELVIS BUTTOCK GROIN INGUINAL REGION PERINEUM

7. TRUNK NOS BACK NOS FLANK NOS

8. OTHER SPECIFIED SITES

9. SITE NOS

192.1 MENINGEAL SITE NOS

0 MENINGEAL SITE SPECIFIED SEE 'CANCER' BY SITE M9539/3

133.0 SARCOPTES SCABIEI INFESTATION

133.0 SARCOPTIC ITCH SCABIES

270.8 SARCOSINEMIA

136.5 SARCOSPORIDIOSIS

354.3 SATURDAY NIGHT SYNDROME

302.89 SATYRIASIS

695.89 SAVILL'S DISEASE (EPIDEMIC EXFOLIATIVE DERMATITIS)

SAWYER JONES SYNDROME

492.8 NOS

491.21 WITH ACUTE BRONCHITIS

491.20 WITH CHRONIC BRONCHITIS

491.21 WITH CHRONIC BRONCHITIS WITH EXACERBATION

421.0 SBE

133.0 SCABIES (NORWEGIAN)

253.0 SCAGLIETTI-DAGNINI SYNDROME (ACROMEGALIC MACROSPONDYLITIS)

0 SCALD INJURY SEE 'BURN', BY SITE

695.1 SCALDED SKIN SYNDROME STAPHYLOCOCCAL (SSSS)

353.0 SCALENUS ANTICUS SYNDROME (NONDISCOGENIC)

SCALP INJURY

959.09 NOS

767.1 BIRTH TRAUMA

910.8 OTHER AND UNSPECIFIED (SUPERFICIAL)

910.9 OTHER AND UNSPECIFIED (SUPERFICIAL) INFECTED

767.8 SCALPEL WOUND (BIRTH TRAUMA)

SCAPULAR

755.59 ABSENCE CONGENITAL

755.52 ELEVATION CONGENITAL

959.2 INJURY UNSPECIFIED (SCAPULAR REGION)

912.8 REGION INJURY OTHER AND UNSPECIFIED SUPERFICIAL

912.9 REGION INJURY OTHER AND UNSPECIFIED SUPERFICIAL (INFECTED)

354.8 SCAPULOCOSTAL SYNDROME

726.2 SCAPULOHUMERAL FIBROSITIS

726.2 SCAPULOHUMERAL IMPINGEMENT

359.1 SCAPULOHUMERAL MYOPATHY

359.1 SCAPULOPERONEAL SYNDROME

723.4 SCAPULOVERTEBRAL SYNDROME

SCAR

709.2 NOS

654.6# CERVIX COMPLICATING PREGNANCY

660.2# CERVIX OBSTRUCTING LABOR [654.6#]

5th Digit: 654.6

0. EPISODE OF CARE NOS OR N/A

1. DELIVERED

2. DELIVERED WITH POSTPARTUM COMPLICATION

3. ANTEPARTUM COMPLICATION

4. POSTPARTUM COMPLICATION

5th Digit: 660.2

0. EPISODE OF CARE NOS OR N/A

1. DELIVERED

3. ANTEPARTUM COMPLICATION

763.1 CERVIX OBSTRUCTING LABOR AFFECTING FETUS OR NEWBORN

654.2# CESAREAN PREVIOUS

660.2# CESAREAN PREVIOUS OBSTRUCTING LABOR [654.2#]

5th Digit: 654.2

0. EPISODE OF CARE NOS OR N/A

1. DELIVERED

2. DELIVERED WITH POSTPARTUM COMPLICATION

3. ANTEPARTUM COMPLICATION

4. POSTPARTUM COMPLICATION

5th Digit: 660.2

0. EPISODE OF CARE NOS OR N/A

1. DELIVERED

3. ANTEPARTUM COMPLICATION

763.89 CESAREAN PREVIOUS COMPLICATING PREGNANCY AFFECTING FETUS OR NEWBORN

701.4 CHELOID

363.3# CHORIORETINAL

5th Digit: 363.3

0. NOS

2 MACULAR

3. POSTERIOR POLE NEC

4. PERIPHERAL

5. DISSEMINATED

0 CHOROID SEE 'SCAR', CHORIORETINAL

423.9 COMPRESSION PERICARDIAL

757.39 CONGENITAL NOS

372.64 CONJUNCTIVA (POST ENUCLEATION)

S

SCAR (continued)

371.00 CORNEA
264.6 CORNEA DUE TO VITAMIN A DEFICIENCY
264.6 CORNEA XEROPHTHALMIC
537.3 DUODENAL (BULB) (CAP)
571.9 HEPATIC POSTNECROTIC
701.4 KELOID
624.4 LABIA
571.9 LIVER POSTNECROTIC
518.89 LUNG (BASE)
363.32 MACULA
363.35 MACULA DISSEMINATED
363.34 MACULA PERIPHERAL
728.89 MUSCLE
412 MYOCARDIUM POST MI
709.2 PAINFUL
429.81 PAPILLARY MUSCLE
423.9 PERICARDIAL COMPRESSION
363.33 POSTERIOR POLE RETINA
571.9 POSTNECROTIC HEPATIC
571.9 POSTNECROTIC LIVER
V15.4# PSYCHOLOGICAL HISTORY

5th Digit: V15.4

1. PHYSICAL ABUSE, RAPE
2. EMOTIONAL ABUSE, NEGLECT
9. OTHER

363.30 RETINA
363.35 RETINA DISSEMINATED
363.32 RETINA OTHER MACULAR
363.33 RETINA OTHER POSTERIOR POLE
363.34 RETINA PERIPHERAL
363.31 RETINA SOLAR
0 REVISION USING PLASTIC SURGERY (OF OLD INJURY) - CODE 'SCAR' BY SITE
709.2 SKIN (ADHERENT) (ATROPHIC) (FIBROSIS)
709.2 SKIN CAUSING DISFIGUREMENT
701.4 SKIN KELOID
478.9 TRACHEA
621.8 UTERINE NEC
654.9# UTERINE COMPLICATING PREGNANCY AND CHILDBIRTH

5th Digit: 654.9

0. EPISODE OF CARE NOS OR N/A
1. DELIVERED
2. DELIVERED WITH POSTPARTUM COMPLICATION
3. ANTEPARTUM COMPLICATION
4. POSTPARTUM COMPLICATION

763.89 UTERINE COMPLICATING PREGNANCY AFFECTING FETUS OR NEWBORN
0 UTERINE FROM PREVIOUS CESAREAN DELIVERY SEE 'SCAR', CESAREAN PREVIOUS
624.4 VULVA (OLD)

134.1 SCARABIASIS
034.1 SCARLATINAL ANGINA
695.0 SCARLATINIFORM ERYTHEMA

034.1 SCARLET FEVER
034.1 SCARLET FEVER OTITIS MEDIA [382.02]

709.09 SCHAMBERG'S DISEASE (PROGRESSIVE PIGMENTARY DERMATOSIS)
530.3 SCHATZKI'S RING
750.3 SCHATZKI'S RING CONGENITAL
135 SCHAUMANN'S SYNDROME (SARCOIDOSIS)

277.5 SCHEIE'S SYNDROME (MUCOPOLYSACCHARIDOSIS IS)
117.1 SCHENCK'S DISEASE (SPOROTRICHOSIS)
732.0 SCHEUERMANN'S DISEASE (OSTEOCHONDROSIS)
755.59 SCHEUTHAUER-MARIE-SAINTON SYNDROME (CLEIDOCRANIALIS DYSOSTOSIS)

V74.3 SCHICK SCREENING EXAM
341.1 SCHILDER'S DISEASE
610.1 SCHIMMELBUSCH'S DISEASE (HYPERPLASIA)
759.6 SCHIRMER'S SYNDROME (ENCEPHALOCUTANEOUS ANGIOMATOSIS)
756.79 SCHISTOCELIA

SCHISTOSOMA, SCHISTOSOMIASIS

120.9 INFECTION
120.2 ASIATIC
120.0 BLADDER
120.8 BOVIS INFECTION
120.3 CERCARIAE INFECTION
120.8 CHESTERMANI
120.1 COLON
120.3 CUTANEOUS
120.3 DERMATITIS
120.2 EASTERN
120.0 GENITOURINARY TRACT
120.0 HAEMATOBIUM
120.8 INTERCALATUM
120.1 INTESTINAL
120.2 JAPONICUM
120.2 KATAYAMA
120.2 LUNG
120.1 MANSONI
120.8 MATTHEII
120.2 ORIENTAL
120.2 PULMONARY
V75.5 SCREENING EXAM
120.8 SPINDALE INFECTION
120.0 VESICAL
120.8 OTHER SPECIFIED

742.4 SCHIZENCEPHALY
0 SCHIZO-AFFECTIVE DISORDER SEE 'SCHIZOPHRENIA'

313.22 SCHIZOID DISORDER CHILDHOOD / ADOLESCENCE
301.20 SCHIZOID PERSONALITY DISORDER
301.21 SCHIZOID PERSONALITY DISORDER - INTROVERTED
301.22 SCHIZOID PERSONALITY DISORDER - SCHIZOTYPAL
0 SCHIZOMYCETOMA (ACTINOMYCOTIC) SEE 'ACTINOMYCOSIS'

SCHIZOPHRENIA

295.9# NOS
295.8# ATYPICAL
295.2# CATALEPSY
295.2# CATATONIC
295.8# CENESTHOPATHIC
299.90 CHILDHOOD TYPE NOS, ACTIVE STATE
299.91 CHILDHOOD TYPE NOS, RESIDUAL STATE
295.6# CHRONIC UNDIFFERENTIATED
295.7# CYCLIC NOS
295.4# CYCLIC ACUTE
295.1# DISORGANIZED TYPE
295.4# EPISODE ACUTE
295.2# FLEXIBILITAS CEREA
295.1# HEBEPHRENIC
V11.0 HISTORY
295.5# LATENT (BORDERLINE) (INCIPIENT) (PREPSYCHOTIC)

5th Digit: 295.1-2, 4-9

0. NOS
1. SUBCHRONIC
2. CHRONIC
3. SUBCHRONIC WITH ACUTE EXACERBATION
4. CHRONIC WITH ACUTE
5. IN REMISSION

SCHIZOPHRENIA (continued)

SPECIFY THE MATERNAL SCHIZOPHRENIA WITH AN ADDITIONAL CODE. SEE 'SCHIZOPHRENIA'.

648.4# MATERNAL CURRENT (CO-EXISTENT) IN PREGNANCY
5th Digit: 648.4
0. EPISODE OF CARE NOS OR N/A
1. DELIVERED
2. DELIVERED WITH POSTPARTUM COMPLICATION
3. ANTEPARTUM COMPLICATION
4. POSTPARTUM COMPLICATION

295.9# MIXED
295.7# MIXED WITH AFFECTIVE PSYCHOSIS
295.3# PARANOID
295.3# PARAPHRENIC
295.5# PRODROMAL
295.5# PSEUDONEUROTIC
295.5# PSEUDOPSYCHOPATHIC
295.9# REACTION
295.6# RESIDUAL
295.6# RESTZUSTAND
295.7# SCHIZO AFFECTIVE
5th Digit: 295.3, 5-7, 9
0. NOS
1. SUBCHRONIC
2. CHRONIC
3. SUBCHRONIC WITH ACUTE EXACERBATION
4. CHRONIC WITH ACUTE
5. IN REMISSION

301.20 SCHIZOID PERSONALITY
295.4# SCHIZOPHRENIA CYCLIC ACUTE
295.9# SCHIZOPHRENIC REACTION ACUTE
295.8# SCHIZOPHRENIC UNDIFFERENTIATED ACUTE
295.9# SCHIZOPHRENIFORM PSYCHOSIS ACUTE
295.7# SCHIZOPHRENIFORM PSYCHOSIS, AFFECTIVE TYPE
295.4# SCHIZOPHRENIFORM PSYCHOSIS, CONFUSIONAL TYPE
295.4# SCHIZOPHRENIFORM SCHIZOPHRENIC EPISODE (ATTACK)
295.0# SIMPLE
299.90 SYNDROME OF CHILDHOOD, ACTIVE STATE
299.91 SYNDROME OF CHILDHOOD, RESIDUAL STATE
295.9# UNDIFFERENTIATED
295.8# UNDIFFERENTIATED ACUTE
5th Digit: 295.0, 4, 7-9
0. NOS
1. SUBCHRONIC
2. CHRONIC
3. SUBCHRONIC WITH ACUTE EXACERBATION
4. CHRONIC WITH ACUTE
5. IN REMISSION

SCHIZOPHRENIA CHILDHOOD TYPE
299.90 ACTIVE STATE (SYNDROME)
299.80 ATYPICAL ACTIVE STATE
299.81 ATYPICAL RESIDUAL STATE
299.01 AUTISTIC ACTIVE STATE
299.00 AUTISTIC RESIDUAL STATE
299.10 DISINTEGRATIVE ACTIVE STATE
299.11 DISINTEGRATIVE RESIDUAL STATE
299.91 RESIDUAL STATE (SYNDROME)

301.22 SCHIZOTYPAL PERSONALITY DISORDER
732.4 SCHLATTER-OSGOOD DISEASE
732.4 SCHLATTER'S TIBIA (TUBERCLE)
352.6 SCHMIDT'S SYNDROME (SPHALLO-PHARYNGO-LARYNGEAL HEMIPLEGIA)
258.1 SCHMIDT'S SYNDROME (THYROID-ADRENOCORTICAL INSUFFICIENCY)
352.6 SCHMIDT'S SYNDROME (VAGOACCESSORY)

SCHMORL'S NODES
722.30 NOS
722.32 LUMBAR
722.31 THORACIC
722.39 OTHER

047.9 SCHNEIDER'S SYNDROME
160.0 SCHNEIDERIAN CARCINOMA SITE NOS
0 SCHNEIDERIAN CARCINOMA SITE SPECIFIED SEE 'CANCER' BY SITE M8121/3
259.2 SCHOLTE'S SYNDROME (MALIGNANT CARCINOID)
330.0 SCHOLZ'S (-BIELSCHOWSKY-HENNEBERG) DISEASE OR SYNDROME
287.0 SCHONLEIN (-HENOCH) DISEASE (PURPURA RHEUMATICA)
V70.5 SCHOOL EXAM (HEALTH)
002.9 SCHOTTMULLER'S DISEASE (SEE ALSO 'PARATYPHOID FEVER')
255.3 SCHROEDER'S SYNDROME (ENDOCRINE-HYPERTENSIVE)
277.8 SCHULLER-CHRISTIAN DISEASE OR SYNDROME (CHRONIC HISTIOCYTOSIS X)
288.0 SCHULTZ'S DISEASE OR SYNDROME (AGRANULOCYTOSIS)
V74.8 SCHULTZ CHARLTON SCREENING EXAM
333.6 SCHWALBE ZIEHEN OPPENHEIM DISEASE
0 SCHWANNOMA BENIGN SEE 'BENIGN NEOPLASM', BY SITE M9560/0
0 SCHWANNOMA MALIGNANT SEE 'CANCER' BY SITE M9560/3
756.89 SCHWARTZ (-JAMPEL) SYNDROME
253.6 SCHWARTZ-BARTTER SYNDROME (INAPPROPRIATE SECRETION OF ANTIDIURETIC HORMONE)
701.3 SCHWENINGER-BUZZI DISEASE (MACULAR ATROPHY)

SCIATIC
0 HERNIA SEE 'HERNIA', SCIATIC
355.0 NERVE DISORDER
355.0 NERVE ENTRAPMENT
956.0 NERVE INJURY
355.0 NERVE LESION
724.3 NERVE NEURALGIA (SCIATICA UNSPECIFIED)
724.3 NERVE NEURITIS

SCIATICA
722.10 DISCOGENIC
722.73 DISCOGENIC WITH MYELOPATHY
355.0 DUE TO SPECIFIED LESION
724.3 NONVERTEBRAL (NONDISCOGENIC)

794.19 SCIATIPHOTOGRAPHY ABNORMAL
747.49 SCIMITAR SYNDROME (ANOMALOUS VENOUS DRAINAGE, RIGHT LUNG TO INFERIOR VENA CAVA)
368.12 SCINTILLATING SCOTOMA
199.1 SCIRRHOUS ADENOCARCINOMA SITE NOS
0 SCIRRHOUS ADENOCARCINOMA SITE SPECIFIED SEE 'CANCER' BY SITE M8141/3

SCLERA, SCLERAL
379.09 ABSCESS
743.47 ANOMALIES SPECIFIED CONGENITAL
743.47 BLUE (CONGENITAL)
379.16 CALCIFICATION
379.16 DISORDERS DEGENERATIVE OTHER
379.19 DISORDERS OTHER
379.11 ECTASIA
379.11 STAPHYLOMA
379.14 STAPHYLOMA - ANTERIOR LOCALIZED
379.13 STAPHYLOMA - EQUATORIAL
379.12 STAPHYLOMA - POSTICUM
379.15 STAPHYLOMA - RING

778.1 SCLEREMA NEONATORUM

SCLERITIS

379.00 NOS
379.02 AND EPISCLERITIS NODULAR
379.01 AND EPISCLERITIS PERIODICA FUGAX
379.03 ANTERIOR
379.06 BRAWNY
379.05 CORNEAL INVOLVEMENT
379.01 PERIODICA FUGAX
379.07 POSTERIOR
095.0 SYPHILITIC

S

256.4 SCLEROCYSTIC OVARY SYNDROME
701.0 SCLERODACTYLIA

SCLERODERMA

710.1 NOS
701.0 CIRCUMSCRIBED
701.0 CIRCUMSCRIBED OR LOCALIZED
710.1 MYOPATHY [359.6]
710.1 WITH LUNG INVOLVEMENT [517.2]

379.04 SCLEROMALACIA PERFORANS
379.05 SCLEROPERIKERATITIS
193 SCLEROSING CARCINOMA (NONENCAPSULATED) SITE NOS
0 SCLEROSING CARCINOMA (NONENCAPSULATED) SITE SPECIFIED SEE 'CANCER' BY SITE M8350/3

SCLEROSIS

255.8 ADRENAL (GLAND)
331.0 ALZHEIMER'S
0 ALZHEIMER'S WITH DEMENTIA SEE 'ALZHEIMER'S', DEMENTIA
335.20 AMYOTROPHIC (LATERAL)
424.1 ANNULARIS FIBROSI AORTIC
424.0 ANNULARIS FIBROSI MITRAL
440.0 AORTA, AORTIC
424.1 AORTIC VALVE SEE ALSO 'ENDOCARDITIS AORTIC'
340 ASCENDING MULTIPLE
341.1 BALO'S (CONCENTRIC)
733.99 BONE (LOCALIZED) NEC
0 BRAIN SEE 'BRAIN', SCLEROSIS
340 BULBAR PROGRESSIVE
426.50 BUNDLE OF HIS NOS
426.3 BUNDLE OF HIS LEFT
426.4 BUNDLE OF HIS RIGHT
404.90 CARDIORENAL
429.2 CARDIOVASCULAR
404.90 CARDIOVASCULAR RENAL
330.0 CENTROLOBAR FAMILIAL
340 CEREBROSPINAL (DISSEMINATED) (MULTIPLE)
437.0 CEREBROVASCULAR
363.40 CHOROID
363.56 CHOROID DIFFUSE
341.1 CONCENTRIC BALOS
370.54 CORNEA
0 CORONARY SEE 'ARTERIOSCLEROSIS, ARTERIOSCLEROTIC', CORONARY
624.8 CORPUS CAVERNOSUM FEMALE
607.89 CORPUS CAVERNOSUM MALE
424.1 DEWITZKY'S AORTIC
424.0 DEWITZKY'S MITRAL
341.1 DIFFUSE NEC
0 DISEASE HEART SEE 'ARTERIOSCLEROSIS, ARTERIOSCLEROTIC', CORONARY
340 DISSEMINATED
340 DORSAL
621.8 ENDOMETRIUM
333.90 EXTRAPYRAMIDAL
366.16 EYE NUCLEAR (SENILE)
334.0 FRIEDREICH'S (SPINAL CORD)
608.89 FUNICULAR (SPERMATIC CORD)

SCLEROSIS (continued)

535.4# GASTRITIS

5th Digit: 535.4

0. WITHOUT HEMORRHAGE
1. WITH HEMORRHAGE

457.8 GLAND (LYMPHATIC)
571.9 HEPATIC
334.2 HEREDITARY CEREBELLAR
334.0 HEREDITARY SPINAL
730.1# IDIOPATHIC CORTICAL (GARRE'S)

5th Digit: 730.1

0. SITE NOS
1. SHOULDER REGION
2. UPPER ARM (ELBOW) (HUMERUS)
3. FOREARM (RADIUS) (WRIST) (ULNA)
4. HAND (CARPAL) (METACARPAL) (FINGERS)
5. PELVIC REGION AND THIGH (HIP) (BUTTOCK) (FEMUR)
6. LOWER LEG (FIBULA) (KNEE) (PATELLA) (TIBIA)
7. ANKLE AND/OR FOOT (METATARSALS) (TOES)
8. OTHER (HEAD) (NECK) (RIB) (SKULL) (VERTEBRAE)
9. MULTIPLE

733.5 ILIUM PIRIFORM
340 INSULAR
251.8 INSULAR PANCREAS
251.8 ISLANDS OF LANGERHANS
478.79 LARYNX
571.9 LIVER
515 LUNG NOS
383.1 MASTOID
440.20 MONCKEBERG'S (MEDIAL) SEE ALSO 'ARTERIOSCLEROSIS, ARTERIOSCLEROTIC', EXTREMITIES
340 MULTIPLE (BRAIN STEM) (CEREBRAL) (GENERALIZED) (SPINAL CORD)
366.16 NUCLEAR (SENILE) EYE
620.8 OVARY
577.8 PANCREAS
607.89 PENIS
440.20 PERIPHERAL ARTERIES NEC
733.5 PIRIFORM OF ILIUM
340 PLAQUES
258.8 PLURIGLANDULAR
258.8 POLYGLANDULAR
094.0 POSTERIOR (SPINAL CORD) (SYPHILITIC)
607.89 PREPUCE
335.24 PRIMARY LATERAL
710.1 PROGRESSIVE SYSTEMIC
515 PULMONARY
416.0 PULMONARY ARTERY
424.3 PULMONARY VALVE
587 RENAL
362.17 RETINA (SENILE) (VASCULAR)
395.9 RHEUMATIC AORTIC VALVE
394.9 RHEUMATIC MITRAL VALVE
341.1 SCHILDER'S

SPINAL

336.8 NOS (CORD) (GENERAL) (PROGRESSIVE) (TRANSVERSE)
357.0 ASCENDING
340 DISSEMINATED
334.0 HEREDITARY (FRIEDREICH'S) (MIXED)
335.24 LATERAL
340 MULTIPLE
094.0 POSTERIOR (SYPHILITIC)

SCLEROSIS (continued)

537.89 STOMACH
425.3 SUBENDOCARDIAL CONGENITAL
710.1 SYSTEMIC PROGRESSIVE
710.1 SYSTEMIC PROGRESSIVE WITH LUNG INVOLVEMENT [517.2]

SCLEROSIS (continued)
759.5 TUBEROUS (BRAIN)
385.00 TYMPANIC MEMBRANE SEE ALSO 'TYMPANOSCLEROSIS'
459.89 VEIN

379.07 SCLEROTENONITIS

SCOLIOSIS
737.30 NOS
737.30 AND KYPHOSCOLIOSIS IDIOPATHIC
737.43 ASSOCIATED WITH OTHER CONDITIONS
356.1 CHARCOT MARIE TOOTH [737.43]
737.33 DUE TO RADIATION
737.31 INFANTILE IDIOPATHIC (RESOLVING)
277.5 MUCOPOLYSACCHARIDOSIS [737.43]
237.7# NEUROFIBROMATOSIS [737.43]
5th Digit: 237.7
0. UNSPECIFIED
1. TYPE I
2. TYPE II
733.0# OSTEOPOROSIS [737.43]
5th Digit: 733.0
0. UNSPECIFIED
1. SENILE
2. IDIOPATHIC
3. DISUSE
9. OTHER
252.0 OTEITIS FIBROSA CYSTICA [737.43]
045.## POLIOMYELITIS ACUTE [737.43]
4th Dgit: 045
0. ACUTE BULBAR PARALYTIC
1. ACUTE WITH OTHER PARALYSIS
2. ACUTE NON PARALYTIC
9. ACUTE UNSPECIFIED
5th Digit: 045
0. NOS
1. TYPE I
2. TYPE II
3. TYPE III
138 POLIOMYELITIS LATE EFFECT [737.43]
754.2 POSTURAL CONGENITAL
737.32 PROGRESSIVE INFANTILE IDIOPATHIC
737.34 THORACOGENIC
737.39 OTHER
237.7# VON RECKLINGHAUSEN'S DISEASE [737.43]
5th Digit: 237.7
0. NOS OR MULTIPLE
1. TYPE I
2. TYPE II

SCOTOMA
368.44 NOS
368.43 ARCUATE
368.43 BJERRUM
368.42 BLIND SPOT AREA
368.41 CENTRAL
368.41 CENTROCECAL
368.42 PARACECAL
368.41 PARACENTRAL
368.12 SCINTILLATING
368.43 SEIDEL

SCREENING
V82.9 UNSPECIFIED CONDITION
V79.1 ALCOHOLISM
V28.1 ALPHA FETOPROTEIN LEVELS IN AMNIOTIC FLUID
V78.0 ANEMIA
V78.1 ANEMIA DEFICIENCY UNSPECIFIED
V28.9 ANTENATAL
V28.8 ANTENATAL OTHER SPECIFIED
V73.5 ARTHROPOD BORNE VIRAL
V81.4 ASTHMA

SCREENING (continued)
V74.9 BACTERIAL AND SPIROCHETAL
V74.8 BACTERIAL SPIROCHETAL DISEASES OTHER SPECIFIED
V81.5 BACTERIURIA ASYMPTOMATIC
V28.2 BASED ON AMNIOCENTESIS OTHER
V78.9 BLOOD DISORDERS
V78.8 BLOOD DISORDERS OTHER SPECIFIED
V78.9 BLOOD FORMING ORGANS DISORDER
V78.8 BLOOD FORMING ORGANS DISORDER OTHER SPECIFIED
V81.3 BRONCHITIS (CHRONIC)
V74.8 BRUCELLOSIS
V76.9 CANCER NOS
V76.3 CANCER BLADDER
V76.10 CANCER BREAST UNSPECIFIED
V76.11 CANCER BREAST MAMMOGRAM FOR HIGH RISK PATIENT
V76.12 CANCER BREAST MAMMOGRAM NEC
V76.19 CANCER BREAST SPECIFIED TYPE NEC
V76.2 CANCER CERVIX
V76.42 CANCER ORAL CAVITY
V76.44 CANCER PROSTATE
V76.41 CANCER RECTAL
V76.0 CANCER RESPIRATORY ORGANS
V76.43 CANCER SKIN
V76.45 CANCER TESTIS
V76.49 CANCER OTHER SITES
V76.8 OTHER NEOPLASMS (BENIGN) (TUMORS)
V81.2 CARDIOVASCULAR CONDITIONS
V80.2 CATARACT
V75.3 CHAGAS' DISEASE
V82.5 CHEMICAL POISONING AND OTHER CONTAMINATION
V73.98 CHLAMYDIA
V73.88 CHLAMYDIA OTHER SPECIFIED
V74.0 CHOLERA
V77.9 CHOLESTEROL
V28.0 CHROMOSOMAL ANOMALIES BY AMNIOCENTESIS
V82.4 CHROMOSOMAL ANOMALIES MATERNAL POSTNATAL
V82.3 CONGENITAL HIP DISLOCATION
V74.4 CONJUNCTIVITIS (BACTERIAL)
V77.6 CYSTIC FIBROSIS
V73.5 DENGUE FEVER
V79.0 DEPRESSION
V79.9 DEVELOPMENTAL HANDICAPS
V79.8 DEVELOPMENTAL HANDICAPS (OTHER)
V79.3 DEVELOPMENTAL HANDICAPS IN EARLY CHILDHOOD
V77.1 DIABETES MELLITUS
V74.3 DIPHTHERIA
V70.3 DRUG ADMINISTRATIVE
V70.4 DRUG MEDICOLEGAL
V80.3 EAR DISEASES
V81.3 EMPHYSEMA
V73.5 ENCEPHALITIS (MOSQUITO BORNE)
V73.5 ENCEPHALITIS (TICK BORNE)
V77.9 ENDOCRINE DISORDER
V80.2 EYE ANOMALY CONGENITAL
V80.2 EYE CONDITIONS OTHER
V28.4 FETAL GROWTH RETARDATION USING ULTRASONICS
V75.6 FILARIASIS
V77.4 GALACTOSEMIA
V81.6 GENITOURINARY CONDITIONS OTHER AND UNSPECIFIED
V80.1 GLAUCOMA
V77.5 GOUT
V82.5 HEAVY METAL POISONING
V75.7 HELMINTHIASIS INTESTINAL
V78.3 HEMOGLOBINOPATHIES OTHER
V73.5 HEMORRHAGIC FEVER
V73.89 HIV
V81.1 HYPERTENSION
V77.9 IMMUNITY DISORDERS
V75.9 INFECTIOUS DISEASE
V78.0 IRON DEFICIENCY ANEMIA
V81.0 ISCHEMIC HEART DISEASE
V28.5 ISOIMMUNIZATION ANTENATAL

S

SCREENING (continued)

V75.2	LEISHMANIASIS
V74.2	LEPROSY
V74.8	LEPTOSPIROSIS
V80.2	MACULAR SENILE LESIONS
V75.1	MALARIA
V28.3	MALFORMATION USING ULTRASONICS ANTENATAL
V77.2	MALNUTRITION
V76.11	MAMMOGRAM FOR HIGH RISK PATIENT
V76.12	MAMMOGRAM NEC
V73.2	MEASLES
V79.9	MENTAL DISORDERS
V79.8	MENTAL DISORDERS OTHER
V79.2	MENTAL RETARDATION
V77.7	METABOLISM (OTHER INBORN ERRORS)
V77.6	MUCOVISCIDOSIS
V82.6	MULTIPHASIC
V75.4	MYCOTIC INFECTIONS
V76.8	NEOPLASMS OTHER (BENIGN) (TUMORS)
V80.0	NEUROLOGICAL CONDITIONS
V77.8	OBESITY
V75.8	PARASITIC INFECTIONS OTHER
V77.3	PHENYLKETONURIA
V74.8	PLAGUE
V82.5	POISONING FROM CONTAMINATED WATER SUPPLY
V73.0	POLIOMYELITIS
V82.5	RADIATION EXPOSURE
V82.5	RADIOACTIVE SUBSTANCE INGESTION
V81.4	RESPIRATORY CONDITIONS
V82.2	RHEUMATIC DISORDERS
V82.1	RHEUMATOID ARTHRITIS
V75.0	RICKETTSIAL DISEASES
V73.3	RUBELLA
V75.5	SCHISTOSOMIASIS
V78.2	SICKLE CELL DISEASE OR TRAIT
V82.0	SKIN CONDITIONS
V75.3	SLEEPING SICKNESS
V73.1	SMALLPOX
V28.6	STREPTOCOCCUS B ANTENATAL
V74.5	SYPHILIS
V74.8	TETANUS
V77.0	THYROID DISORDERS
V73.6	TRACHOMA
V74.1	TUBERCULOSIS
V74.5	VENEREAL DISEASE
V73.99	VIRAL DISEASE UNSPECIFIED
V73.89	VIRAL DISEASE OTHER SPECIFIED
V82.5	WATER SUPPLY CONTAMINATION
V74.8	WHOOPING COUGH
V74.6	YAWS
V73.4	YELLOW FEVER
V82.8	OTHER SPECIFIED CONDITIONS

V54.0	SCREW REMOVAL (ORTHOPEDIC)
017.2#	SCROFULA
017.0#	SCROFULODERMA

5th Digit: 017.0, 2

- **0. NOS**
- **1. LAB NOT DONE**
- **2. LABS PENDING**
- **3. MICROSCOPY POSITIVE (IN SPUTUM)**
- **4. CULTURE POSITIVE - MICROSCOPY NEGATIVE**
- **5. CULTURE NEGATIVE - MICROSCOPY POSITIVE**
- **6. CULTURE AND MICROSCOPY NEGATIVE CONFIRMED BY OTHER METHODS**

SCROTUM, SCROTAL

608.4	ABSCESS (CELLULITIS) (BOIL) (CARBUNCLE)
752.8	ABSENCE CONGENITAL
608.89	ATROPHY (FIBROSIS) (HYPERTROPHY) (ULCER)
608.4	CELLULITIS
608.9	DISORDER NOS

SCROTUM, SCROTAL (continued)

608.83	HEMORRHAGE (THROMBOSIS) (HEMATOMA) NONTRAUMATIC
878.2	INJURY TRAUMATIC
878.3	INJURY TRAUMATIC WITH OPEN WOUND
911.8	INJURY OTHER AND UNSPECIFIED SUPERFICIAL
911.9	INJURY OTHER AND UNSPECIFIED SUPERFICIAL (INFECTED)
608.4	NODULE INFLAMMATORY
456.4	VARICES

081.2	SCRUB TYPHUS
267	SCURVY (VITAMIN C DEFICIENCY)
272.7	SEA-BLUE HISTIOCYTE SYNDROME
275.49	SEABRIGHT-BANTAM SYNDROME (PSEUDOHYPOPARATHYROIDISM)
994.6	SEASICKNESS
909.4	SEASICKNESS LATE EFFECT
989.5	SEA SNAKE BITE
<u>995.0</u>	SEA SNAKE BITE WITH <u>ANAPHYLAXIS</u> [989.5]
309.1	SEASONAL AFFECTIVE DISORDER (SAD)

SEBACEOUS

706.2	CYST
610.8	CYST BREAST
374.84	CYST EYELID
629.8	CYST GENITAL ORGANS NEC - FEMALE
608.89	CYST GENITAL ORGANS NEC - MALE
706.2	CYST SCROTUM
706.9	GLAND DISEASE NEC

SEBORRHEA, SEBORRHEIC

706.3	NOS
690.11	CAPITIS
695.4	CONGESTIVA
706.3	CORPORIS
690.10	DERMATITIS NOS
690.12	DERMATITIS INFANTILE
690.18	DERMATITIS OTHER
690.18	ECZEMA
690.12	ECZEMA INFANTILE
702.1#	KERATOSIS

5th Digit: 702.1

- **1. INFLAMED**
- **9. OTHER**

705.89	NIGRICANS
690.18	SICCA
702.1#	WART

5th Digit: 702.1

- **1. INFLAMED**
- **9. OTHER**

759.89	SECKEL'S SYNDROME
377.10	SECOND CRANIAL NERVE ATROPHY
377.49	SECOND CRANIAL NERVE DISORDER OTHER NEC
426.13	SECOND DEGREE HEART BLOCK AV OTHER
664.1#	SECOND DEGREE LACERATION (PERINEAL)

5th Digit: 664.1

- **0. EPISODE OF CARE NOS OR N/A**
- **1. DELIVERED**
- **4. POSTPARTUM COMPLICATION**

362.65	SECONDARY PIGMENTARY RETINAL DEGENERATION
661.1#	SECONDARY UTERINE INERTIA

5th Digit: 661.1

- **0. EPISODE OF CARE NOS OR N/A**
- **1. DELIVERED**
- **3. ANTEPARTUM COMPLICATION**

362.66	SECONDARY VITREORETINAL DEGENERATION

782.3 SECRETAN'S DISEASE OR SYNDROME (POSTTRAUMATIC EDEMA)
710.2 SECRETOINHIBITOR SYNDROME (KERATOCONJUNCTIVITIS SICCA)

668.##: USE AN ADDITIONAL CODE TO FURTHER SPECIFY THE COMPLICATION OF ANESTHESIA OR OTHER SEDATION.

SEDATION COMPLICATING L & D
668.9# COMPLICATION NOS
668.1# CARDIAC COMPLICATIONS
668.2# CENTRAL NERVOUS SYSTEM COMPLICATIONS
668.0# PULMONARY COMPLICATIONS
668.8# OTHER SPECIFIED COMPLICATIONS
5th Digit: 668.0-9
0. EPISODE OF CARE NOS OR N/A
1. DELIVERED
2. DELIVERED WITH POSTPARTUM COMPLICATION
3. ANTEPARTUM COMPLICATION
4. POSTPARTUM COMPLICATION

304.1# SEDATIVE ADDICTION NEC (DEPENDENT)
305.4# SEDATIVE HYPNOTIC ABUSE NONDEPENDENT
5th Digit: 304.1, 305.4
0. NOS
1. CONTINUOUS
2. EPISODIC
3. IN REMISSION

790.1 SED RATE ELEVATED
790.1 SEDIMENTATION RATE ELEVATED
301.59 SEDUCTIVE PERSONALITY DISORDER
757.1 SEELIGMANN'S SYNDROME (ICHTHYOSIS CONGENITA)
0 SEGMENTAL DYSFUNCTION SEE 'SOMATIC DYSFUNCTION'

SEIZURE
780.39 NOS
780.39 CONVULSIVE
780.39 DISORDER
0 EPILEPTIC SEE 'SEIZURE EPILEPTIC'
780.39 EPILEPTIFORM, EPILEPTOID
780.31 FEBRILE
780.39 INFANTILE
779.0 NEWBORN
780.39 RECURRENT
780.39 REPETITIVE
780.39 UNKNOWN ETIOLOGY

SEIZURE EPILEPTIC
345.9# NOS
345.5# FOCAL (MOTOR)
345.0# GENERALIZED PETIT MAL NONCONVULSIVE
345.1# GENERALIZED GRAND MAL CONVULSIVE
345.2 PETIT MAL STATUS
345.3 GRAND MAL STATUS
345.4# PARTIAL WITH IMPAIRMENT OF CONSCIOUSNESS
345.5# PARTIAL WITHOUT IMPAIRMENT OF CONSCIOUSNESS
345.6# INFANTILE SPASMS
345.7# EPILEPSIA PARTIALIS CONTINUA
345.8# OTHER
5th Digit: 345.0-1, 4-9
0. WITHOUT MENTION OF INTRACTABLE EPILEPSY
1. WITH INTRACTABLE EPILEPSY

V69.8 SELF-DAMAGING BEHAVIOR PROBLEM
792.2 SEMEN ABNORMAL
780.09 SEMICOMA
780.09 SEMICONSCIOUSNESS

SEMILUNAR CARTILAGE
717.89 CALCIFICATION
717.5 DERANGEMENT (KNEE) OLD
717.5 DISEASE CYSTIC
836.2 TEAR (KNEE) ACUTE

SEMINAL VESICLE
608.0 ABSCESS (CELLULITIS)
608.89 ABSENCE
752.8 ABSENCE CONGENITAL
608.89 ATROPHY (FIBROSIS) (HYPERTROPHY) (ULCER)
608.9 DISORDER
608.83 HEMORRHAGE (THROMBOSIS) (HEMATOMA) NONTRAUMATIC
867.6 INJURY (TRAUMATIC)
867.7 INJURY WITH OPEN WOUND INTO CAVITY
908.2 INJURY LATE EFFECT

SEMINAL VESICULITIS
608.0 SEMINAL VESICULITIS
098.14 GONOCOCCAL ACUTE
098.34 GONOCOCCAL CHRONIC

257.2 SEMIFEROUS TUBULE FAILURE (ADULT)

SEMINOMA
186.9 SITE NOS
0 SITE SPECIFIED SEE 'CANCER' BY SITE M9061/3
186.9 ANAPLASTIC TYPE SITE NOS
0 ANAPLASTIC TYPE SITE SPECIFIED SEE 'CANCER' BY SITE M9062/3
186.9 SPERMATOCYTIC SITE NOS
0 SPERMATOCYTIC SITE SPECIFIED SEE 'CANCER' BY SITE M9063/3

694.4 SENEAR-USHER DISEASE OR SYNDROME (PEMPHIGUS ERYTHEMATOSUS)
797 SENESCENCE CAUSE OF MORBIDITY AND MORTALITY

SENILE
797 ASTHENIA CAUSE OF MORBIDITY AND MORTALITY
797 ATROPHY
701.8 ATROPHY SKIN
701.3 ATROPHY SKIN DEGENERATIVE
371.41 CORNEAL CHANGES
797 DEBILITY CAUSE OF MORBIDITY AND MORTALITY
331.2 DEGENERATION OF BRAIN
701.3 DEGENERATIVE ATROPHY
694.5 DERMATITIS HERPETIFORMIS
709.3 DERMATOSIS
797 EXHAUSTION CAUSE OF MORBIDITY AND MORTALITY
362.52 MACULAR DEGENERATION DISCIFORM
362.64 RETICULAR DEGENERATION
702.0 WART

SENILE PSYCHOSIS (DEMENTIA)
290.0 UNCOMPLICATED
290.20 DELUSIONAL
290.3 WITH DELIRIUM
290.20 WITH DELUSION
290.21 WITH DEPRESSIVE FEATURES

702.0 SENILIS KERATOSIS
259.8 SENILISM SYNDROME
310.1 SENILITY ORGANIC NONPSYCHOTIC
797 SENILITY WITHOUT PSYCHOSIS CAUSE OF MORBIDITY AND MORTALITY
782.0 SENSATION DISTURBANCE SKIN

S

S

297.8 SENSITIVER BEZIEHUNGSWAHN
313.21 SENSITIVITY REACTION OF CHILDHOOD AND ADOLESCENCE

SENSORY
780.39 AND MOTOR ATTACK
781.8 EXTINCTION
781.8 NEGLECT
V48.4 PROBLEM - HEAD
V48.5 PROBLEM - NECK
V48.5 PROBLEM - TRUNK

079.81 SEOUL VIRUS
0 SEPARATION SEE 'DISLOCATION'
309.21 SEPARATION ANXIETY

SEPSIS
038.9 NOS
038.3 ANAEROBIC
038.0 ANAEROBIC STREPTOCOCCAL
022.3 ANTHRAX
038.3 BACTEROIDES
569.61 CECOSTOMY [038.#(#)]

4th or 4th and 5th Digit Code for Organism: 038
.9 NOS
.3 ANAEROBIC
.3 BACTEROIDES
.3 CLOSTRIDIUM
.42 E COLI
.49 ENTEROBACTER AEROGENES
.40 GRAM NEGATIVE
.49 GRAM NEGATIVE OTHER
.41 HEMOPHILUS INFLUENZAE
.2 PNEUMOCOCCAL
.49 PROTEUS
.43 PSEUDOMONAS
.44 SERRATIA
.10 STAPHYLOCOCCAL NOS
.11 STAPHYLOCOCCAL AUREUS
.19 STAPHYLOCOCCAL OTHER
.0 STREPTOCOCCAL (ANAEROBIC)
.49 YERSINIA ENTEROCOLITICA
.8 OTHER SPECIFIED

038.3 CLOSTRIDIUM
569.61 COLOSTOMY [038.#(#)]

4th or 4th and 5th Digit Code for Organism: 038
.9 NOS
.3 ANAEROBIC
.3 BACTEROIDES
.3 CLOSTRIDIUM
.42 E COLI
.49 ENTEROBACTER AEROGENES
.40 GRAM NEGATIVE
.49 GRAM NEGATIVE OTHER
.41 HEMOPHILUS INFLUENZAE
.2 PNEUMOCOCCAL
.49 PROTEUS
.43 PSEUDOMONAS
.44 SERRATIA
.10 STAPHYLOCOCCAL NOS
.11 STAPHYLOCOCCAL AUREUS
.19 STAPHYLOCOCCAL OTHER
.0 STREPTOCOCCAL (ANAEROBIC)
.49 YERSINIA ENTEROCOLITICA
.8 OTHER SPECIFIED

038.42 E COLI
038.49 ENTEROBACTER AEROGENES

SEPSIS (continued)
569.61 ENTEROSTOMY [038.#(#)]

4th or 4th and 5th Digit Code for Organism: 038
.9 NOS
.3 ANAEROBIC
.3 BACTEROIDES
.3 CLOSTRIDIUM
.42 E COLI
.49 ENTEROBACTER AEROGENES
.40 GRAM NEGATIVE
.49 GRAM NEGATIVE OTHER
.41 HEMOPHILUS INFLUENZAE
.2 PNEUMOCOCCAL
.49 PROTEUS
.43 PSEUDOMONAS
.44 SERRATIA
.10 STAPHYLOCOCCAL NOS
.11 STAPHYLOCOCCAL AUREUS
.19 STAPHYLOCOCCAL OTHER
.0 STREPTOCOCCAL (ANAEROBIC)
.49 YERSINIA ENTEROCOLITICA
.8 OTHER SPECIFIED

027.1 ERYSIPELOTHRIX INSIDIOSA (E. RHUSIOPATHIAE)
771.8 FETUS INTRAUTERINE
639.0 FOLLOWING ABORTION / ECTOPIC / MOLAR PREGNANCY
999.3 FOLLOWING INFUSION INJECTION TRANSFUSION OR VACCINATION
536.41 GASTROSTOMY [038.#(#)]

4th or 4th and 5th Digit Code for Organism: 038
.9 NOS
.3 ANAEROBIC
.3 BACTEROIDES
.3 CLOSTRIDIUM
.42 E COLI
.49 ENTEROBACTER AEROGENES
.40 GRAM NEGATIVE
.49 GRAM NEGATIVE OTHER
.41 HEMOPHILUS INFLUENZAE
.2 PNEUMOCOCCAL
.49 PROTEUS
.43 PSEUDOMONAS
.44 SERRATIA
.10 STAPHYLOCOCCAL NOS
.11 STAPHYLOCOCCAL AUREUS
.19 STAPHYLOCOCCAL OTHER
.0 STREPTOCOCCAL (ANAEROBIC)
.49 YERSINIA ENTEROCOLITICA
.8 OTHER SPECIFIED

098.89 GONOCOCCAL
038.40 GRAM NEGATIVE
038.49 GRAM NEGATIVE OTHER
038.41 HEMOPHILUS INFLUENZAE
054.5 HERPES SIMPLEX

SEPSIS (continued)

569.61 ILEOSTOMY **[038.#(#)]**
569.61 JEJUNOSTOMY **[038.#(#)]**

4th or 4th and 5th Digit Code for Organism: 038

- **.9 NOS**
- **.3 ANAEROBIC**
- **.3 BACTEROIDES**
- **.3 CLOSTRIDIUM**
- **.42 E COLI**
- **.49 ENTEROBACTER AEROGENES**
- **.40 GRAM NEGATIVE**
- **.49 GRAM NEGATIVE OTHER**
- **.41 HEMOPHILUS INFLUENZAE**
- **.2 PNEUMOCOCCAL**
- **.49 PROTEUS**
- **.43 PSEUDOMONAS**
- **.44 SERRATIA**
- **.10 STAPHYLOCOCCAL NOS**
- **.11 STAPHYLOCOCCAL AUREUS**
- **.19 STAPHYLOCOCCAL OTHER**
- **.0 STREPTOCOCCAL (ANAEROBIC)**
- **.49 YERSINIA ENTEROCOLITICA**
- **.8 OTHER SPECIFIED**

027.0 LISTERIA MONOCYTOGENES
036.2 MENINGOCOCCAL
038.9 NADIR
038.9 NEUTROPENIC [288.0]
771.8 NEWBORN
771.8 NEWBORN (FETUS) - GONOCOCCAL [098.89]
771.8 NEWBORN (FETUS) - HERPETIC [054.5]
771.8 NEWBORN (FETUS) - SALMONELLA [003.1]
771.8 NEWBORN (FETUS) - VIRAL NOS [079.99]
771.8 NEWBORN (FETUS) - OTHER **[038.#(#)]**

4th or 4th and 5th Digit Code for Organism: 038

- **.9 NOS**
- **.3 ANAEROBIC**
- **.3 BACTEROIDES**
- **.3 CLOSTRIDIUM**
- **.42 E COLI**
- **.49 ENTEROBACTER AEROGENES**
- **.40 GRAM NEGATIVE**
- **.49 GRAM NEGATIVE OTHER**
- **.41 HEMOPHILUS INFLUENZAE**
- **.2 PNEUMOCOCCAL**
- **.49 PROTEUS**
- **.43 PSEUDOMONAS**
- **.44 SERRATIA**
- **.10 STAPHYLOCOCCAL NOS**
- **.11 STAPHYLOCOCCAL AUREUS**
- **.19 STAPHYLOCOCCAL OTHER**
- **.0 STREPTOCOCCAL (ANAEROBIC)**
- **.49 YERSINIA ENTEROCOLITICA**
- **.8 OTHER SPECIFIED**

020.2 PLAGUE
038.2 PNEUMOCOCCAL
999.3 POST TRANSFUSION

SEPSIS (continued)

998.59 POSTOPERATIVE **[038.#(#)]**

4th or 4th and 5th Digit Code for Organism: 038

- **.9 NOS**
- **.3 ANAEROBIC**
- **.3 BACTEROIDES**
- **.3 CLOSTRIDIUM**
- **.42 E COLI**
- **.49 ENTEROBACTER AEROGENES**
- **.40 GRAM NEGATIVE**
- **.49 GRAM NEGATIVE OTHER**
- **.41 HEMOPHILUS INFLUENZAE**
- **.2 PNEUMOCOCCAL**
- **.49 PROTEUS**
- **.43 PSEUDOMONAS**
- **.44 SERRATIA**
- **.10 STAPHYLOCOCCAL NOS**
- **.11 STAPHYLOCOCCAL AUREUS**
- **.19 STAPHYLOCOCCAL OTHER**
- **.0 STREPTOCOCCAL (ANAEROBIC)**
- **.49 YERSINIA ENTEROCOLITICA**
- **.8 OTHER SPECIFIED**

038.49 PROTEUS
038.43 PSEUDOMONAS
999.8 SEPTIC SHOCK DUE TO TRANSFUSION
038.44 SERRATIA
038.1# STAPHYLOCOCCAL

5th Digit: 038.1

- **0. NOS**
- **1. AUREUS**
- **9. OTHER STAPH**

038.0 STREPTOCOCCAL
519.01 TRACHEOSTOMY **[038.#(#)]**

4th or 4th and 5th Digit Code for Organism: 038

- **.9 NOS**
- **.3 ANAEROBIC**
- **.3 BACTEROIDES**
- **.3 CLOSTRIDIUM**
- **.42 E COLI**
- **.49 ENTEROBACTER AEROGENES**
- **.40 GRAM NEGATIVE**
- **.49 GRAM NEGATIVE OTHER**
- **.41 HEMOPHILUS INFLUENZAE**
- **.2 PNEUMOCOCCAL**
- **.49 PROTEUS**
- **.43 PSEUDOMONAS**
- **.44 SERRATIA**
- **.10 STAPHYLOCOCCAL NOS**
- **.11 STAPHYLOCOCCAL AUREUS**
- **.19 STAPHYLOCOCCAL OTHER**
- **.0 STREPTOCOCCAL (ANAEROBIC)**
- **.49 YERSINIA ENTEROCOLITICA**
- **.8 OTHER SPECIFIED**

079.99 VIRAL
038.49 YERSINIA ENTEROCOLITICA
038.8 OTHER SPECIFIED

S

SEPSIS COMPLICATING LABOR, PREGNANCY, PUERPERIUM

771.8 FETUS OR NEWBORN - GONOCOCCAL [098.89]
771.8 FETUS OR NEWBORN - HERPETIC [054.5]
771.8 FETUS OR NEWBORN - SALMONELLA [003.1]
771.8 FETUS OR NEWBORN - VIRAL NOS [079.99]
771.8 FETUS OR NEWBORN - OTHER [**038.#(#)**]

4th or 4th and 5th Digit Code for Organism: 038.#(#)

.9 NOS
.3 ANAEROBIC
.3 BACTEROIDES
.3 CLOSTRIDIUM
.42 E COLI
.49 ENTEROBACTER AEROGENES
.40 GRAM NEGATIVE
.49 GRAM NEGATIVE OTHER
.41 HEMOPHILUS INFLUENZAE
.2 PNEUMOCOCCAL
.49 PROTEUS
.43 PSEUDOMONAS
.44 SERRATIA
.10 STAPHYLOCOCCAL NOS
.11 STAPHYLOCOCCAL AUREUS
.19 STAPHYLOCOCCAL OTHER
.0 STREPTOCOCCAL (ANAEROBIC)
.49 YERSINIA ENTEROCOLITICA
.8 OTHER SPECIFIED

639.0 FOLLOWING ECTOPIC/MOLAR OR ABORTED PREGNANCY
647.8# MATERNAL CURRENT (COEXISTENT) (MAJOR INFECTION)

5th Digit: 647.8
0. EPISODE OF CARE NOS OR N/A
1. DELIVERED
2. DELIVERED WITH POSTPARTUM COMPLICATION
3. ANTEPARTUM COMPLICATION
4. POSTPARTUM COMPLICATION

670.0# MATERNAL DUE TO PREGNANCY POSTPARTUM (PUERPERAL) (MAJOR INFECTION)

5th Digit: 670.0
0. NOS
2. DELIVERED WITH POSTPARTUM COMPLICATION
4. POSTPARTUM COMPLICATION

659.3# MATERNAL DURING LABOR

5th Digit: 659.3
0. EPISODE OF CARE NOS OR N/A
1. DELIVERED
3. ANTEPARTUM COMPLICATION

639.0 POST ABORTION OR ECTOPIC/MOLAR PREGNANCY

0 SEPTAL SEE 'SEPTUM, SEPTAL'

654.7# SEPTATE VAGINA COMPLICATING CHILDBIRTH AND PREGNANCY
660.2# SEPTATE VAGINA OBSTRUCTING LABOR [**654.7#**]

5th Digit: 654.7
0. EPISODE OF CARE NOS OR N/A
1. DELIVERED
2. DELIVERED WITH POSTPARTUM COMPLICATION
3. ANTEPARTUM COMPLICATION
4. POSTPARTUM COMPLICATION

5th Digit: 660.2
0. EPISODE OF CARE NOS OR N/A
1. DELIVERED
3. ANTEPARTUM COMPLICATION

034.0 SEPTIC ANGINA
999.8 SEPTIC SHOCK DUE TO TRANSFUSION
034.0 SEPTIC SORE THROAT
0 SEPTICEMIA SEE 'SEPSIS'

SEPTUM, SEPTAL

745.69 ABSENCE (CONGENITAL) - ATRIAL
745.7 ABSENCE (CONGENITAL) - ATRIAL AND VENTRICULAR
745.0 ABSENCE (CONGENITAL) - BETWEEN AORTA AND PULMONARY ARTERY
745.3 ABSENCE (CONGENITAL) - VENTRICULAR
429.71 DEFECT HEART - ACQUIRED POST MI ACUTE (< 8 WEEKS) [**410.##**]

4th Digit: 410
0. ANTEROLATERAL
1. ANTERIOR (WALL) ANTEROAPICAL ANTEROSEPTAL OTHER ANTERIOR
2. INFEROLATERAL
3. INFEROPOSTERIOR
4. INFERIOR OTHER
5. LATERAL APICAL, BASOLATERAL, POSTEROLATERAL, LATERAL OTHER
6. POSTERIOR (POSTEROBASAL)
7. SUBENDOCARDIAL
8. ATRIUM PAPILLARY OR SEPTUM ALONE
9. UNSPECIFIED

5th Digit: 410
0. EPISODE UNSPECIFIED
1. INITIAL EPISODE
2. SUBSEQUENT EPISODE

429.71 DEFECT HEART - ACQUIRED FOLLOWING MYOCARDIAL INFARCTION (>8 WEEKS) [414.8]
745.9 DEFECT HEART - NOS CONGENITAL
745.8 DEFECT HEART - CLOSURE CONGENITAL
745.4 DEFECT HEART - INTERVENTRICULAR CONGENITAL
745.8 DEFECT HEART - OTHER CONGENITAL

470 NASAL DEVIATED
754.0 NASAL DEVIATED CONGENITAL
0 NASAL SEE ALSO 'NOSE, NASAL', SEPTUM

0 SEQUESTRUM (OF BONE) SEE 'OSTEOMYELITIS'
495.8 SEQUOIOSIS OR RED CEDAR ASTHMA

270.7 SERINE METABOLISM DISTURBANCES
795.6 SEROLOGY FOR SYPHILIS FALSE POSITIVE
0 SEROLOGY FOR SYPHILIS POSITIVE FOLLOW-UP OF LATENT SYPHILIS SEE 'SYPHILIS LATENT'

998.13 SEROMA COMPLICATING A PROCEDURE
998.51 SEROMA POSTOPERATIVE INFECTED

333.99 SEROTONIN SYNDROME
362.42 SEROUS DETACHMENT RETINAL PIGMENT EPITHELIUM
348.2 SEROUS MENINGITIS SYNDROME

370.04 SERPIGINOUS ULCER

041.85 SERRATIA (MARCESCENS) INFECTION OR ORGANISM
038.44 SERRATIA SEPSIS

SERTOLI

186.9 CELL CARCINOMA SITE NOS
0 CELL CARCINOMA SITE SPECIFIED SEE 'CANCER' BY SITE M8640/3
606.0 CELL SYNDROME (GERMINAL APLASIA)
220 LEYDIG CELL TUMOR FEMALE SITE NOS
0 LEYDIG CELL TUMOR FEMALE SITE SPECIFIED SEE 'BENIGN NEOPLASM', BY SITE M8631/0
222.0 LEYDIG CELL TUMOR MALE SITE NOS
0 LEYDIG CELL TUMOR MALE SITE SPECIFIED SEE 'BENIGN NEOPLASM', BY SITE M8631/0

SERUM

V14.7 ALLERGY (HISTORY)
790.99 BLOOD NEC ABNORMAL
999.5 DISEASE NEC
790.5 ENZYMES NEC ABNORMAL
070.3# HEPATITIS
070.2# HEPATITIS WITH COMA

5th Digit: 070.2-3

0. ACUTE OR UNSPECIFIED
1. ACUTE OR UNSPECIFIED WITH DELTA
2. CHRONIC
3. CHRONIC WITH DELTA

790.99 PROTEIN ABNORMAL
790.99 PROTEIN NEC ABNORMAL
790.99 PROTEINS (TOTAL) ABNORMAL
999.5 REACTION
999.5 SICKNESS

733.99 SESAMOIDITIS

V61.10 SEVEN YEAR ITCH

351.8 SEVENTH NERVE ATROPHY
351.9 SEVENTH NERVE DISORDER UNSPECIFIED
767.5 SEVENTH NERVE DISORDER BIRTH TRAUMA
951.4 SEVENTH NERVE INJURY
351.8 SEVENTH NERVE NEURITIS
351.0 SEVENTH NERVE PARALYSIS
997.09 SEVENTH NERVE PARALYSIS POSTOPERATIVE

732.5 SEVER'S DISEASE (OSTEOCHONDROSIS CALCANEUM)

758.81 SEX CHROMOSOME ANOMALIES OTHER CONDITIONS DUE TO SEX CHROMOSOME
758.81 SEX CHROMOSOME MOSAICISM (SYNDROME)
238.9 SEX CORD STROMAL TUMOR SITE NOS
0 SEX CORD STROMAL TUMOR SITE SPECIFIED SEE 'NEOPLASM UNCERTAIN BEHAVIOR' BY SITE M8590/1

SEXUAL

302.72 AROUSAL DISORDER (PSYCHOSEXUAL)
V69.2 BEHAVIOR HIGH RISK
V65.49 COUNSELING NEC
259.0 DEVELOPMENT DELAY NEC
302.9 DEVIATION UNSPECIFIED
302.89 DEVIATION FROTTEURISM
302.89 DEVIATION OTHER SPECIFIED
V62.4 DISCRIMINATION CAUSING ENCOUNTER
302.9 DISORDER (PSYCHOSEXUAL)
0 DYSFUNCTION (PSYCHOLOGICAL) SEE 'PSYCHOSEXUAL DYSFUNCTION'
302.70 FUNCTION DISORDER PSYCHOGENIC
302.79 FUNCTION DISORDER PSYCHOGENIC - SPECIFIED TYPE NEC
V41.7 FUNCTION PROBLEM
302.9 PATHOLOGICAL SEXUALITY
259.1 PRECOCITY (IDIOPATHIC) (CRYPTOGENIC)
255.2 PRECOCITY MALE WITH ADRENAL HYPERPLASIA
0 SEE ALSO 'PSYCHOSEXUAL DYSFUNCTION'
V65.45 TRANSMITTED DISEASE COUNSELING

202.2# SEZARY'S DISEASE OR SYNDROME (RETICULOSIS) M9701/3

5th Digit: 202.2

0. UNSPECIFIED SITE, EXTRANODAL AND SOLID ORGAN SITES
1. LYMPH NODES OF HEAD FACE NECK
2. LYMPH NODES INTRATHORACIC
3. LYMPH NODES ABDOMINAL
4. LYMPH NODES AXILLA AND UPPER LIMB
5. LYMPH NODES INGUINAL REGION AND LOWER LIMB
6. LYMPH NODES INTRAPELVIC
7. SPLEEN
8. LYMPH NODES MULTIPLE SITES

790.4 SGOT ABNORMAL
790.4 SGPT ABNORMAL

995.55 SHAKEN INFANT SYNDROME
503 SHAVER'S DISEASE OR SYNDROME (BAUXITE PNEUMOCONIOSIS)

253.2 SHEEHAN'S SYNDROME (POSTPARTUM PITUITARY NECROSIS)
520.5 SHELL TEETH
V74.3 SHICK TEST

SHIGELLA

004.9 INFECTION NOS
004.2 BOYDII - GROUP C
V02.3 CARRIER
004.0 DYSENTERIAE - GROUP A (SCHMITZ) (SHIGA)
004.1 FLEXNERI - GROUP B
004.3 SONNEI - GROUP D
004.8 OTHER SPECIFIED INFECTIONS

081.2 SHIMAMUSHI DISEASE (SCRUB TYPHUS)
844.9 SHIN SPLINTS
053.9 SHINGLES
077.1 SHIPYARD DISEASE

654.5# SHIRODKAR SUTURE COMPLICATING PREGNANCY
660.2# SHIRODKAR SUTURE OBSTRUCTING LABOR **[654.5#]**

5th Digit: 654.5

0. EPISODE OF CARE NOS OR N/A
1. DELIVERED
2. DELIVERED WITH POSTPARTUM COMPLICATION
3. ANTEPARTUM COMPLICATION
4. POSTPARTUM COMPLICATION

5th Digit: 660.2

0. EPISODE OF CARE NOS OR N/A
1. DELIVERED
3. ANTEPARTUM COMPLICATION

SHOCK

785.50 NOS
995.0 ALLERGIC NOS
995.0 ANAPHYLACTIC
909.9 ANAPHYLACTIC LATE EFFECT
785.51 CARDIOGENIC
250.8# DIABETIC HYPOGLYCEMIC

5th Digit: 250.8

0. TYPE II, ADULT-ONSET, NON-INSULIN DEPENDENT (EVEN IF REQUIRING INSULIN), OR UNSPECIFIED; CONTROLLED
1. TYPE I, JUVENILE-ONSET OR INSULIN-DEPENDENT; CONTROLLED
2. TYPE II, ADULT-ONSET, NON-INSULIN DEPENDENT (EVEN IF REQUIRING INSULIN); UNCONTROLLED
3. TYPE I, JUVENILE-ONSET OR INSULIN-DEPENDENT; UNCONTROLLED

995.4 DUE TO ANESTHESIA
909.9 DUE TO ANESTHESIA LATE EFFECT
995.0 DUE TO DRUG, MEDICINE CORRECTLY ADMINISTERED
909.9 DUE TO DRUG, MEDICINE CORRECTLY ADMINISTERED LATE EFFECT
977.9 DUE TO DRUG, MEDICINE INCORRECTLY ADMINISTERED (OVERDOSE)
909.0 DUE TO DRUG, MEDICINE INCORRECTLY ADMINISTERED (OVERDOSE) LATE EFFECT
995.6# DUE TO NONPOISONOUS FOOD

5th Digit: 995.6

0. UNSPECIFIED FOOD
1. PEANUTS
2. CRUSTACEANS
3. FRUITS AND VEGETABLES
4. TREE NUTS AND SEEDS
5. FISH
6. FOOD ADDITIVES
7. MILK PRODUCTS
8. EGGS
9. OTHER SPECIFIED FOOD

SHOCK (continued)

909.9 DUE TO FOOD LATE EFFECT
995.0 DUE TO NONMEDICAL SUBSTANCE CORRECTLY ADMINISTERED
909.9 DUE TO NONMEDICAL SUBSTANCE CORRECTLY ADMINISTERED LATE EFFECT
994.8 ELECTRIC
909.4 ELECTRIC LATE EFFECT
0 ELECTRIC WITH BURNS SEE 'BURN'
785.59 ENDOTOXIC
639.5 FOLLOWING ABORTION / ECTOPIC / MOLAR PREGNANCY
785.59 GRAM NEGATIVE
785.59 HYPOVOLEMIC (NONTRAUMATIC)
584.5 KIDNEY SYNDROME
958.5 KIDNEY SYNDROME FOLLOWING CRUSH INJURY
518.5 LUNG TRAUMATIC OR POSTSURGICAL (SYNDROME)
998.89 MISADVENTURE THERAPEUTIC
909.3 MISADVENTURE THERAPEUTIC LATE EFFECT
308.9 NEUROGENIC SYNDROME
998.0 POSTOPERATIVE ENDOTOXIC DURING OR RESULTING FROM SURGERY
998.0 POSTOPERATIVE HYPOVOLEMIC DURING OR RESULTING FROM SURGERY
998.0 POSTOPERATIVE SEPTIC DURING OR RESULTING FROM SURGERY
909.3 POSTOPERATIVE LATE EFFECT
308.9 PSYCHIC SYNDROME
785.59 SEPTIC
999.8 SEPTIC DUE TO TRANSFUSION
909.3 SEPTIC DUE TO TRANSFUSION LATE EFFECT
958.4 SYNDROME (TRAUMATIC)
040.89 TOXIC SHOCK SYNDROME
958.4 TRAUMATIC
908.6 TRAUMATIC LATE EFFECT

SHOCK OBSTETRICAL

669.1# OBSTETRIC (L AND D)
5th Digit: 669.1
0. EPISODE OF CARE NOS OR N/A
1. DELIVERED
2. DELIVERED WITH POSTPARTUM COMPLICATION
3. ANTEPARTUM COMPLICATION
4. POSTPARTUM COMPLICATION
639.5 FOLLOWING ABORTION / ECTOPIC / MOLAR PREGNANCY

287.0 SHONLEIN'S PURPURIC DEMATOGRAPHICA
579.3 SHORT BOWEL SYNDROME
426.81 SHORT P-R INTERVAL SYNDROME
783.4 SHORT STATURE
786.05 SHORTNESS OF BREATH

SHOULDER

V49.67 AMPUTATION STATUS
337.9 ARM SYNDROME SEE ALSO 'NEUROPATHY PERIPHERAL' AUTONOMIC
0 BLADE SEE 'SCAPULAR'
736.89 DEFORMITY (ACQUIRED) NEC
718.31 DISLOCATION, RECURRENT
763.1 DYSTOCIA AFFECTING FETUS OR NEWBORN
652.8# DYSTOCIA COMPLICATING PREGNANCY
660.0# DYSTOCIA OBSTRUCTING LABOR [**652.8#**]
660.4# DYSTOCIA (SHOULDER GIRDLE) OBSTRUCTING LABOR
5th Digit: 652.8, 660.0, 4
0. EPISODE OF CARE NOS OR N/A
1. DELIVERED
3. ANTEPARTUM COMPLICATION
755.59 GIRDLE ABSENCE CONGENITAL
723.4 GIRDLE SYNDROME
337.9 HAND SYNDROME SEE ALSO 'NEUROPATHY PERIPHERAL' AUTONOMIC

SHOULDER (continued)

726.2 IMPINGEMENT SYNDROME
959.2 INJURY
912.8 INJURY OTHER AND UNSPECIFIED SUPERFICIAL
912.9 INJURY OTHER AND UNSPECIFIED SUPERFICIAL (INFECTED)
0 JOINT SEE ALSO 'JOINT'
718.81 JOINT INSTABILITY
718.91 JOINT LIGAMENT RELAXATION
0 JOINT LIGAMENT TEAR SEE 'SPRAIN'
719.81 JOINT (REGION) CALCIFICATION
718.11 JOINT (REGION) LOOSE BODY
V43.61 JOINT REPLACEMENT STATUS
726.19 LIGAMENT OR MUSCLE INSTABILITY
726.19 OTHER SPECIFIED DISORDER
763.1 PRESENTATION AFFECTING FETUS OR NEWBORN
840.9 SEPARATION (RUPTURE) (TEAR) (LACERATION) SITE UNSPECIFIED
840.8 SEPARATION (RUPTURE) (TEAR) (LACERATION) OTHER SPECIFIED SITES
840.9 STRAIN (SPRAIN) (AVULSION) (HEMARTHROSIS) SITE UNSPECIFIED
840.8 STRAIN (SPRAIN) (AVULSION) (HEMARTHROSIS) OTHER SPECIFIED SITES

333.93 SHUDDERING ATTACKS (BENIGN)
333.0 SHY-DRAGER SYNDROME (ORTHOSTATIC HYPOTENSION WITH MULTISYSTEM DEGENERATION)
313.21 SHYNESS DISORDER OF CHILDHOOD
527.2 SIALOADENITIS
527.5 SIALOLITHIASIS
527.7 SIALORRHEA
527.8 SIALOSIS
065.4 SIBERIAN HEMORRHAGIC FEVER
082.2 SIBERIAN TICK TYPHUS
313.3 SIBLING JEALOUSY
V61.8 SIBLING RELATIONAL PROBLEM
352.6 SICARD'S SYNDROME
710.2 SICCA SYNDROME (KERATOCONJUNCTIVITIS)
799.9 SICK
276.1 SICK CELL SYNDROME
759.89 SICK CILIA SYNDROME
V61.49 SICK PERSON PROBLEM (IN FAMILY) (IN HOUSEHOLD)
427.81 SICK SINUS SYNDROME

SICKLE CELL

282.60 ANEMIA UNSPECIFIED
282.62 ANEMIA WITH CRISIS
282.61 ANEMIA WITHOUT CRISIS
282.60 ANEMIA WITH RETINOPATHY [362.29]
282.63 HB-C DISEASE
282.69 HB-D DISEASE
282.69 HB-E DISEASE
282.63 HB-S/HB-C DISEASE
282.69 HB-S/HB-D DISEASE
282.69 HB-S/HB-E DISEASE
V78.2 SCREENING FOR DISEASE OR TRAIT
282.60 SPHEROCYTOSIS
282.4 THALASSEMIA
282.5 TRAIT

IF A MANIFESTATION OF AN ADVERSE EFFECT IS KNOWN IT SHOULD BE CODED AS THE PRINCIPAL DIAGNOSIS.

995.2 SIDE EFFECT NOS TO DRUG (CORRECTLY ADMINISTERED SUBSTANCE)
909.9 SIDE EFFECT NOS TO DRUG (CORRECTLY ADMINISTERED SUBSTANCE) LATE EFFECT
280.8 SIDEROPENIC DYSPHAGIA OR SYNDROME

360.23 SIDEROSIS GLOBE
503 SIDEROSIS OCCUPATIONAL
798.0 SIDS (SUDDEN INFANT DEATH SYNDROME)
0 SIDS (SUDDEN INFANT DEATH SYNDROME) NEAR MISS - CODE INDIVIDUAL SYMPTOM(S)
277.3 SIEGAL-CATTAN-MAMOU DISEASE (PERIODIC)
757.31 SIEMENS' ECTODERMAL DYSPLASIA SYNDROME
757.39 SIEMENS' KERATOSIS FOLLICULARIS SPINULOSA (DECALVANS) SYNDROME
V41.0 SIGHT PROBLEM
569.89 SIGMOID COLON LESION
562.10 SIGMOID DIVERTICULA
751.5 SIGMOID DIVERTICULA CONGENITAL
569.89 SIGMOID HYPERTROPHY
560.9 SIGMOID OBSTRUCTION (SEE ALSO INTESTINE, INTESTINAL', OBSTRUCTION)
558.9 SIGMOIDITIS ACUTE NONINFECTIVE

SIGNET RING CELL
199.1 CARCINOMA SITE NOS
0 CARCINOMA SITE SPECIFIED SEE 'CANCER' BY SITE M8490/3
199.1 CARCINOMA METASTATIC SITE NOS
0 CARCINOMA METASTATIC SITE SPECIFIED SEE 'CANCER' BY SITE, METASTATIC M8490/6

756.50 SILFVERSKIOLD'S SYNDROME (OSTEOCHONDRODYSTROPHY, EXTREMITIES)
502 SILICOSIS OCCUPATIONAL
506.9 SILO FILLERS' DISEASE
759.89 SILVER'S SYNDROME (CONGENITAL HEMIHYPERTROPHY AND SHORT STATURE)
282.4 SILVESTRONI-BIANCO SYNDROME (THALASSEMIA MINIMA)
054.3 SIMIAN B DISEASE
253.2 SIMMOND'S DISEASE (PITUITARY CACHEXIA)
272.6 SIMONS' DISEASE (PROGRESSIVE LIPODYSTROPHY)
462 SIMPLE ANGINA - THROAT
079.81 SIN NOMBRE VIRUS
732.4 SINDING-LARSEN DISEASE (JUVENILE OSTEOPATHIA PATELLAE)
478.5 SINGER'S NODES
279.8 SINGLE COMPLEMENT (C1-C9) DISORDER
786.8 SINGULTUS
427.81 SINOATRIAL NODE DYSFUNCTION
426.6 SINUS ARREST

SINUS BRADYCARDIA
427.89 NOS
427.81 PERSISTENT
427.81 SEVERE

959.09 SINUS - NASAL INJURY
473.9 SINUS - NASAL OBSTRUCTION
744.46 SINUS PREAURICULAR CONGENITAL
0 SINUS SEE ALSO 'FISTULA'
686.9 SINUS SKIN INFECTED
707.9 SINUS SKIN NON-INFECTED (SEE ALSO 'ULCER, ULCERATION SKIN')
355.5 SINUS TARSI SYNDROME

SINUSITIS
461.9 ACUTE NOS
461.2 ACUTE ETHMOIDAL
461.1 ACUTE FRONTAL
461.0 ACUTE MAXILLARY
461.3 ACUTE SPHENOIDAL
461.8 ACUTE OTHER OR PANSINUSITIS

SINUSITIS (continued)
759.3 BRONCHIECTASIS-SITUS INVERSUS SYNDROME
473.9 CHRONIC
473.2 CHRONIC ETHMOIDAL
473.1 CHRONIC FRONTAL
473.0 CHRONIC MAXILLARY
473.3 CHRONIC SPHENOIDAL
473.8 CHRONIC OTHER
473.8 CHRONIC OTHER OR PANSINUSITIS
461.8 PANSINUSITIS ACUTE
473.8 PANSINUSITIS CHRONIC
471.1 WOAKES' ETHMOIDITIS

193 SIPPLE'S SYNDROME (MEDULLARY THYROID CARCINOMA-PHEOCHROMOCYTOMA)
992.0 SIRIASIS
909.4 SIRIASIS LATE EFFECT
085.0 SIRKARI'S DISEASE
0 SITUATIONAL ADJUSTMENT REACTION SEE 'ADJUSTMENT REACTION'
308.3 SITUATIONAL REACTION ACUTE DUE TO STRESS

SITUS INVERSUS
759.3 ABDOMINALIS
759.3 SINUSITIS AND BRONCHIECTASIS
759.3 THORACIS

057.8 SIXTH DISEASE (EXANTHEMA SUBITUM)
378.54 SIXTH NERVE ATROPHY
951.3 SIXTH NERVE CRANIAL INJURY
378.54 SIXTH NERVE DISORDER (PALSY)

SJOGREN'S
710.2 DISEASE
710.2 DISEASE WITH LUNG INVOLVEMENT [517.8]
710.2 (-GOUGEROT) SYNDROME (KERATOCONJUNCTIVITIS SICCA)
757.1 LARSSON SYNDROME (ICHTHYOSIS CONGENITA)
710.2 MYOPATHY [359.6]

597.89 SKENE'S ADENITIS
131.02 SKENE'S ADENITIS TRICHOMONAL
989.5 SKEVAS-ZERFUS DISEASE
378.87 SKEW DEVIATION CONJUGATE GAZE

SKIN
757.39 ABSENCE (CONGENITAL)
793.9 ABNORMAL (X-RAY) (ULTRASOUND) (THERMOGRAPHY)
782.3 ANASARCA
782.0 ANESTHESIA
757.39 APLASIA (CONGENITAL)
706.2 ATHEROMA
701.8 ATROPHY (SENILE)
701.3 ATROPHY DEGENERATIVE
782.62 BLUSHING
782.0 BURNING OR PRICKLING SENSATION
709.3 CALCIFICATIONS SUBCUTANEOUS
709.3 CALCINOSIS CIRCUMSCRIPTA
709.3 CALCINOSIS CUTIS
V76.43 CANCER SCREENING
782.4 CHOLEMIA
709.2 CICATRIX
V82.0 CONDITIONS SCREENING
782.5 CYANOSIS
770.8 CYANOSIS NEWBORN
706.2 CYST
692.79 DAMAGE SOLAR NOS
692.72 DAMAGE SOLAR ACUTE
692.74 DAMAGE SOLAR CHRONIC
709.3 DEGENERATION
709.3 DEPOSITS
0 DERMATITIS SEE 'DERMATITIS'
709.3 DERMATOSIS SENILE

SKIN (continued)

709.9	DISORDER
778.9	DISORDER - FETUS OR NEWBORN
778.8	DISORDER - FETUS OR NEWBORN OTHER NEC
306.3	DISORDER (ALLERGIC) (ECZEMATOUS) (PRURITIC) - PSYCHOGENIC
709.1	DISORDER - VASCULAR
709.8	DISORDER - OTHER NEC
V59.1	DONOR NON-AUTOGENOUS
782.3	DROPSY
772.6	ECCHYMOSES NEWBORN
782.7	ECCHYMOSES SPONTANEOUS
782.3	EDEMA LOCALIZED
778.5	EDEMA NEWBORN
782.1	ERUPTION NONSPECIFIC
782.1	EXANTHEM
709.2	FIBROSIS
709.8	FISSURE
686.9	FISSURE STREPTOCOCCAL
782.62	FLUSHING
709.4	FOREIGN BODY GRANULOMA
996.55	GRAFT ARTIFICIAL FAILURE OR REJECTION (DISLODGEMENT) (DISPLACEMENT) (NON-ADHERENCE) (POOR INCORPORATION) (SHEARING)
996.55	GRAFT DECELLULARIZED ALLODERMIS FAILURE OR REJECTION (DISLODGEMENT) (DISPLACEMENT) (NON-ADHERENCE) (POOR INCORPORATION) (SHEARING)
996.52	GRAFT FAILURE OR REJECTION
996.69	GRAFT INFECTION (INFLAMMATION)
V13.3	HISTORY OF SKIN DISEASE
782.0	HYPERESTHESIA
782.0	HYPOESTHESIA
782.4	ICTERUS
782.8	INDURATION
686.9	INFECTION NOS
686.8	INFECTION OTHER
134.9	INFESTATION
0	JAUNDICE SEE 'JAUNDICE'
709.9	LESION
782.2	LUMP SUPERFICIAL
782.2	MASS SUPERFICIAL
782.2	NODULE SUBCUTANEOUS
782.0	NUMBNESS
782.9	OTHER SYMPTOMS
782.61	PALLOR
709.8	PAPULE
134.9	PARASITES
782.0	PARESTHESIA
782.7	PETECHIAE
782.0	PRICKLING
782.1	RASH
782.0	SENSATION DISTURBANCE
686.9	SINUS INFECTED
707.9	SINUS NON-INFECTED (SEE ALSO 'ULCER, ULCERATION SKIN')
782.2	SUBCUTANEOUS NODULES
686.00	SUPPURATION DIFFUSE
782.2	SWELLING SUPERFICIAL
701.9	TAG
757.39	TAG ACCESSORY CONGENITAL
795.79	TEST POSITIVE
795.5	TEST POSITIVE TUBERCULIN (WITHOUT ACTIVE TB)
782.8	TEXTURE CHANGES
782.8	THICKENING
782.0	TINGLING
V42.3	TRANSPLANT (STATUS)
V43.83	TRANSPLANT ARTIFICIAL (STATUS)
707.9	ULCER UNSPECIFIED (SEE ALSO 'ULCER, ULCERATION SKIN')
709.1	VASCULAR LESION
701.8	WRINKLING
709.8	OTHER SPECIFIED LESION
782.9	OTHER SYMPTOMS

SKULL

756.0	BONES ABSENCE
738.19	DEFORMITY (ACQUIRED)
756.0	DEFORMITY CONGENITAL
754.0	DEPRESSIONS CONGENITAL
756.0	IMPERFECT FUSION CONGENITAL
793.0	X-RAY ABNORMAL

286.5 SLE INHIBITOR

0 SLE SEE 'LUPUS', ERYTHEMATOSUS

SLEEP DISORDER / DISTURBANCE

780.50	UNSPECIFIED CAUSE
780.57	APNEA NEC
780.53	APNEA WITH HYPERSOMNIA
780.51	APNEA WITH HYPOSOMNIA
780.51	APNEA WITH INSOMNIA
780.57	APNEA WITH SLEEP DISTURBANCE NEC
780.56	AROUSAL DYSFUNCTION
307.40	CHILD
307.45	CIRCADIAN RHYTHM DISRUPTION
780.55	DISRUPTION OF 24-HOUR SLEEP-WAKE CYCLE CAUSE UNSPECIFIED
307.45	DISRUPTION OF 24-HOUR SLEEP-WAKE CYCLE, PHASE SHIFT, NONORGANIC
307.47	DRUNKENNESS (SLEEP)
780.56	DYSFUNCTION SLEEP STAGES
780.54	HYPERSOMNIA
307.44	HYPERSOMNIA PERSISTENT ASSOCIATED WITH DEPRESSION
307.43	HYPERSOMNIA TRANSIENT DUE TO EMOTIONAL CONFLICT/REACTION
780.53	HYPERSOMNIA WITH SLEEP APNEA
307.42	HYPOSOMNIA PERSISTENT ASSOCIATED WITH ANXIETY, DEPRESSION OR PSYCHOSIS
307.41	HYPOSOMNIA TRANSIENT DUE TO EMOTIONAL CONFLICT/ REACTION
780.52	INSOMNIA (SEE ALSO 'INSOMNIA')
307.48	INTRUSION REPETITIVE, ATYPICAL POLYSOMNOGRAPHIC FEATURES
307.48	INTRUSION REPETITIVE ENVIRONMENTAL DISTURBANCES
307.48	INTRUSION REPETITIVE REM-SLEEP
307.45	JET LAG SYNDROME
347	NARCOLEPSY
307.46	NIGHT TERRORS
307.47	NIGHTMARES
307.40	NONORGANIC
307.40	PSYCHOGENIC
307.41	PSYCHOGENIC, INITIATION OR MAINTENANCE
307.42	PSYCHOGENIC, INITIATION OR MAINTENANCE - PERSISTENT
307.41	PSYCHOGENIC, INITIATION OR MAINTENANCE - TRANSIENT
307.48	REM-SLEEP INTERRUPTIONS, REPEATED
307.47	REM-SLEEP TYPE DYSFUNCTION
780.55	RHYTHM INVERSION
307.49	SHORT SLEEPER
780.56	SLEEP STAGES DYSFUNCTION
780.55	SLEEP-WAKE RHYTHM INVERSION UNDETERMINED CAUSE
780.55	SLEEP-WAKE RHYTHM IRREGULAR UNDETERMINED CAUSE
307.46	SLEEP WALKING
300.13	SLEEP WALKING HYSTERICAL
307.42	SLEEPLESSNESS PERSISTENT ASSOCIATED WITH ANXIETY, DEPRESSION, OR PSYCHOSIS
307.41	SLEEPLESSNESS TRANSIENT DUE TO EMOTIONAL CONFLICT/ REACTION

SLEEP DISORDER / DISTURBANCE (continued)

307.46 SOMNAMBULISM
307.45 TIME-ZONE CHANGE RAPID
307.44 WAKEFULNESS DISORDER PERSISTENT ASSOCIATED WITH DEPRESSION
307.43 WAKEFULNESS DISORDER TRANSIENT DUE TO EMOTIONAL CONFLICT/ REACTION
307.45 WORK-SLEEP SCHEDULE SHIFT
307.49 OTHER DISTURBANCE NONORGANIC NEC
780.59 OTHER DISTURBANCE/DISRUPTION
780.57 OTHER DISTURBANCE/DISRUPTION WITH SLEEP APNEA

347 SLEEPING DISEASE
086.# SLEEPING SICKNESS (SEE ALSO 'TRYPANOSOMIASIS')

4th Digit: 086
0. AMERICAN WITH HEART INVOLVEMENT
1. AMERICAN WITH INVOLVEMENT OF ORGAN OTHER THAN HEART
2. AMERICAN NOS
3. GAMBIAN
4. RHODESIAN
5. AFRICAN NOS
9. NOS

V75.3 SLEEPING SICKNESS SCREENING EXAM
0 SLEEPLESSNESS SEE 'INSOMNIA'
732.2 SLIPPED CAPITAL FEMORAL EPIPHYSIS
255.3 SLOCUMB'S SYNDROME
779.3 SLOW FEEDING NEONATAL
046.9 SLOW VIRUS INFECTION CNS
788.62 SLOWING OF URINARY STREAM
337.0 SLUDER'S SYNDROME
784.5 SLURRED SPEECH

SMALL CELL CARCINOMA

199.1 SITE NOS
0 SITE SPECIFIED SEE 'CANCER' BY SITE M8041/3
199.1 FUSIFORM CELL TYPE SITE NOS
0 FUSIFORM CELL TYPE SITE SPECIFIED SEE 'CANCER' BY SITE M8043/3

656.5# SMALL FOR DATES AFFECTING MANAGEMENT OF MOTHER

5th Digit: 656.5
0. EPISODE OF CARE NOS OR N/A
1. DELIVERED
3. ANTEPARTUM COMPLICATION

0 SMALL FOR DATES PERINATAL SEE 'LIGHT FOR DATES'
115.0 SMALL FORM HISTOPLASMOSIS

SMALL INTESTINE

751.1 ABSENCE CONGENITAL
562.00 DIVERTICULUM
751.5 DIVERTICULUM CONGENITAL
863.3# INJURY WITH OPEN WOUND INTO CAVITY
863.2# INJURY WITHOUT MENTION OF OPEN WOUND INTO CAVITY

5th Digit: 863.2-3
0. UNSPECIFIED SITE
1. DUODENUM
9. OTHER

908.1 INJURY LATE EFFECT
751.1 OBSTRUCTION CONGENITAL
560.81 OBSTRUCTION DUE TO ADHESIONS
560.81 OBSTRUCTION DUE TO ADHESIONS POSTOPERATIVE (POSTINFECTION)
751.1 STENOSIS CONGENITAL
751.1 STRICTURE CONGENITAL

SMALLPOX

050.9 SMALLPOX NOS
050.1 ALASTRIM
V01.3 EXPOSURE
050.0 HEMORRHAGIC (PUSTULAR)
050.0 MALIGNANT
050.2 MODIFIED
V73.1 SCREENING EXAM
V04.1 VACCINATION
050.0 VARIOLA MAJOR
050.1 VARIOLA MINOR

008.64 SMALL ROUND VIRUS NOS ENTERITIS (SRV'S)
443.9 SMALL VESSEL DISEASE
781.1 SMELL AND TASTE DISTURBANCES OF SENSATION
V41.5 SMELL PROBLEM
759.89 SMITH-LEMLI-OPITZ SYNDROME (CEREBROHEPATORENAL SYNDROME)
270.2 SMITH-STRANG DISEASE (OASTHOUSE URINE)
987.9 SMOKE INHALATION
491.0 SMOKERS' COUGH
305.1 SMOKERS' SYNDROME (TOBACCO ABUSE, NONDEPENDENT)
V65.49 SMOKING CESSATION COUNSELING
989.5 SNAKE BITE VENOMOUS
995.0 SNAKE BITE VENOMOUS WITH ANAPHYLAXIS [989.5]
0 SNAKE BITE NONVENOMOUS, SEE 'OPEN WOUND' BY SITE
0 SNAPPING JOINT SEE 'JOINT', SNAPPING
694.1 SNEDDON WILKINSON DISEASE OR SYNDROME (SUBCORNEAL PUSTULAR DERMATOSIS)
784.9 SNEEZING
784.9 SNEEZING UNKNOWN ETIOLOGY
786.09 SNORING
370.24 SNOW BLINDNESS
495.8 SNUFF TAKERS' DISEASE
786.05 SOB (SHORTNESS OF BREATH)
313.22 SOCIAL DISORDER OF CHILDHOOD AND ADOLESCENCE
V62.4 SOCIAL MALADJUSTMENT (REASON FOR ENCOUNTER)
301.7 SOCIOPATHIC PERSONALITY

SODIUM

790.6 ABNORMAL
276.1 DEFICIENCY ABNORMAL FINDINGS
276.1 DEFICIENCY HYPONATREMIA
276.1 DEFICIENCY NUTRITIONAL
276.0 EXCESS ABNORMAL FINDINGS
276.0 EXCESS HYPERNATREMIA
276.9 METABOLISM DISORDER
276.0 OVERLOAD

026.0 SODOKU
366.51 SOEMMERING'S RING
729.9 SOFT TISSUE DISORDER OTHER AND UNSPECIFIED
524.2 SOFT TISSUE IMPINGEMENT

SOLAR

0 DERMATITIS SEE 'DERMATITIS SOLAR'
692.74 ELASTOSIS
702.0 KERATOSIS
363.31 RETINOPATHY
692.79 SKIN DAMAGE NOS
692.72 SKIN DAMAGE NOS ACUTE
692.74 SKIN DAMAGE NOS CHRONIC
692.71 SUNBURN

193 SOLID CARCINOMA SITE NOS
0 SOLID CARCINOMA SITE SPECIFIED SEE 'CANCER' BY SITE M8230/3

238.6 SOLITARY MYELOMA UNCERTAIN BEHAVIOR SITE NOS M9731/1
733.21 SOLITARY CYST BONE
593.2 SOLITARY CYST KIDNEY
312.1# SOLITARY STEALING
5th Digit: 312.1
0. NOS
1. MILD
2. MODERATE
3. SEVERE

SOMATIC DYSFUNCTION
739.8 ABDOMINAL AREA AND OTHER
739.1 CERVICAL REGION
739.0 HEAD REGION
739.6 LOWER EXTREMITIES
739.3 LUMBAR REGION
739.0 OCCIPITOCERVICAL REGION
739.5 PELVIS, HIP PUBIC REGION
739.8 RIB CAGE
739.4 SACRAL REGION
739.2 THORACIC REGION
739.7 UPPER EXTREMITIES

300.81 SOMATIZATION DISORDER
306.9 SOMATIZATION REACTION

300.81 SOMATOFORM DISORDER
300.82 SOMATOFORM DISORDER (ATYPICAL) (UNDIFFERENTIATED)
300.81 SOMATOFORM DISORDER - SEVERE

307.46 SOMNAMBULISM
780.09 SOMNOLENCE

004.3 SONNEI DYSENTERY - GROUP D SHIGELLA

0 SORE THROAT SEE 'PHARYNGITIS'

253.0 SOTO'S SYNDROME (CEREBRAL GIGANTISM)

425.2 SOUTH AFRICAN CARDIOMYOPATHY SYNDROME
133.8 SOUTH AFRICAN CREEPING DISEASE
116.1 SOUTH AMERICAN BLASTOMYCOSIS

784.2 SPACE-OCCUPYING LESION INTRACRANIAL
V60.1 SPACE RESTRICTION (INADEQUATE HOUSING)

754.89 SPADE LIKE HAND CONGENITAL
123.5 SPARGANOSIS
123.5 SPARGANUM MANSONI PROLIFERUM INFECTION

SPASM
781.0 NOS
367.53 ACCOMMODATION
564.6 ANAL
724.8 BACK
306.0 BACK PSYCHOGENIC
564.1 BILE
596.8 BLADDER (SPHINCTER)
306.4 BOWEL PSYCHOGENIC
781.7 CARPOPEDAL
367.53 CILIARY BODY (OF ACCOMMODATION)
378.82 CONJUGATE
378.84 CONVERGENCE
564.89 DUODENAL BULB
564.89 DUODENUM
530.5 ESOPHAGUS
351.8 FACIAL (NERVE)
478.75 GLOTTIS
300.11 GLOTTIS HYSTERICAL
306.1 GLOTTIS PSYCHOGENIC
378.51 INTERNAL OBLIQUE

SPASM (continued)
564.1 INTESTINAL
306.4 INTESTINAL PSYCHOGENIC
478.75 LARYNGEAL
300.11 LARYNGEAL HYSTERICAL
306.1 LARYNGEAL PSYCHOGENIC
333.81 LEVATOR PALBERAE SUPERIORIS
728.85 MUSCLE
378.87 OCULOGYRIC
362.30 OPHTHALMIC ARTERY
723.5 NECK
576.5 SPHINCTER OF ODDI
385.89 STAPEDIUS
593.89 URETER
599.84 URETHRA
625.8 UTERUS
661.4# UTERUS (ABNORMAL) COMPLICATING LABOR
5th Digit: 661.4
0. EPISODE OF CARE UNSPECIFIED OR N/A
1. DELIVERED
2. DELIVERED WITH POSTPARTUM COMPLICATION
3. ANTEPARTUM COMPLICATION
4. POSTPARTUM COMPLICATION

378.82 SPASMODIC UPWARD MOVEMENT, EYE(S) SYNDROME
307.20 SPASMODIC WINKING SYNDROME

307.3 SPASMUS NUTANS

564.1 SPASTIC COLITIS
316 SPASTIC COLON PSYCHOGENIC

V53.1 SPECTACLES FITTING AND ADJUSTMENT

SPEECH
784.5 DISORDER NEC
315.39 DISORDER DEVELOPMENTAL - ARTICULATION
315.31 DISORDER DEVELOPMENTAL - EXPRESSIVE
315.32 DISORDER DEVELOPMENTAL - RECEPTIVE (EXPRESSIVE - RECEPTIVE) MIXED
315.39 DISORDER DEVELOPMENTAL - OTHER
438.1# DISORDER LATE EFFECT OF CEREBROVASCULAR DISEASE
5th Digit: 438.1
0. UNSPECIFIED
1. APHASIA
2. DYSPHASIA
9. OTHER
784.5 IMPEDIMENT
307.9 IMPEDIMENT PSYCHOGENIC
V40.1 PROBLEM
784.5 SLURRED
V57.3 THERAPY

315.09 SPELLING DIFFICULTY SPECIFIC (DELAY IN DEVELOPMENT)
780.39 SPELLS
078.82 SPENCER'S DISEASE (EPIDEMIC VOMITING)
426.9 SPENS' SYNDROME (SYNCOPE WITH HEART BLOCK)

SPERM
792.2 ABNORMAL
606.0 AZOOSPERMIA
V26.2 COUNT FOR FERTILITY EVALUATION
V25.8 COUNT POST VASECTOMY
606.1 OLIGOSPERMIA

SPERMATIC CORD
608.4 ABSCESS (BOIL) (CARBUNCLE) (CELLULITIS)
752.8 ABSENCE (CONGENITAL)
608.89 ATROPHY (FIBROSIS) (HYPERTROPHY) (ULCER)
608.83 HEMATOMA (HEMORRHAGE) NONTRAUMATIC
867.6 INJURY (TRAUMATIC)
867.7 INJURY (TRAUMATIC) WITH OPEN WOUND
608.85 STRICTURE
608.83 THROMBOSIS

608.1 SPERMATOCELE
752.8 SPERMATOCELE CONGENITAL

SPERMATOGENIC
606.0 ARREST COMPLETE
606.0 AZOOSPERMIA
606.1 ARREST INCOMPLETE
606.1 OLIGOSPERMIA

0 SPERMATOZOA SEE 'SPERM'
461.3 SPHENOIDAL SINUS (ABSCESS) (INFECTION) (INFLAMMATION)ACUTE
282.0 SPHEROCYTIC ANEMIA CONGENITAL HEMOLYTIC
282.0 SPHEROCYTOSIS (FAMILIAL)
282.0 SPHEROCYTOSIS HEREDITARY
199.1 SPHEROIDAL CELL CARCINOMA SITE NOS
0 SPHEROIDAL CELL CARCINOMA SITE SPECIFIED SEE 'CANCER' BY SITE M8035/3
759.89 SPHEROPHAKIA-BRACHYMORPHIA SYNDROME CONGENITAL
743.36 SPHEROPHAKIA CONGENITAL
787.6 SPHINCTER ANI INCONTINENCE
576.5 SPHINCTER OF ODDI SPASM
576.2 SPHINCTER OF ODDI STENOSIS
564.89 SPHINCTERAL (DIGESTIVE) ACHALASIA
272.7 SPHINGOLIPIDOSIS CEREBRAL DEGENERATION [330.2]
448.1 SPIDER ANGIOMA
0 SPIDER BITE NONVENOMOUS SEE 'INSECT BITE NONVENOMOUS'
330.1 SPIELMEYER (-VOGT) (-STOCK) DISEASE

SPINA BIFIDA
741.0# CEREBRAL DEGENERATION (HYDROCEPHALIC) [331.7]
5th Digit: 741.0
0. REGION NOS
1. CERVICAL REGION
2. DORSAL (THORACIC REGION)
3. LUMBAR REGION

655.0# FETALIS WITH MYELOMENINGOCELE AFFECTING PREGNANCY MANAGEMENT
5th Digit: 655.0
0. EPISODE OF CARE NOS OR N/A
1. DELIVERED
3. ANTEPARTUM COMPLICATION

756.17 OCCULTA
741.0# WITH HYDROCEPHALUS
741.9# WITHOUT HYDROCEPHALUS
5th Digit: 741.0, 9
0. REGION NOS
1. CERVICAL REGION
2. DORSAL (THORACIC REGION)
3. LUMBAR REGION

SPINAL
442.89 ARTERY (ANEURYSM) (A-V FISTULA) (CIRSOID) (FALSE) (VARICOSE) (RUPTURED)
747.82 ARTERY ANOMALY (ABERRANT) (ABSENCE) (ACCESSORY) (AGENESIS) (ATRESIA)
721.1 ARTERY ANTERIOR - COMPRESSION SYNDROME
433.8# ARTERY ANTERIOR - OBSTRUCTION OR OCCLUSION
433.8# ARTERY ANTERIOR - SYNDROME
433.8# ARTERY ANTERIOR - THROMBOSIS (EMBOLISM) (DEFORMANS)
5th Digit: 433.8
0. WITHOUT CEREBRAL INFARCTION
1. WITH CEREBRAL INFARCTION

336.8 ATROPHY (CORD)
733.99 ATROPHY COLUMN

SPINAL (continued)
335.10 ATROPHY MUSCULAR - NOS
335.19 ATROPHY MUSCULAR - ADULT
335.21 ATROPHY MUSCULAR - ARAN DUCHENNE
335.11 ATROPHY MUSCULAR - FAMILIAL
335.11 ATROPHY MUSCULAR - JUVENILE
335.19 ATROPHY MUSCULAR - OTHER
738.5 DEFORMITY NOS
724.9 DISORDER NEC (NONVERTEBRAL) (NONDISCOGENIC)
336.1 EMBOLISM (THROMBOSIS) (OCCLUSION) (INFARCTION)
720.1 ENTHESOPATHY
792.0 FLUID ABNORMAL
997.09 FLUID LEAKAGE AT LUMBAR PUNCTURE SITE
724.9 JOINT DISORDER (NONVERTEBRAL) (NONDISCOGENIC)
720.1 LIGAMENTOUS OR MUCSCULAR ATTACHMENTS DISORDER - PERIPHERAL
742.59 MENINGES ANOMALY CONGENITAL
355.9 NERVE DISORDER
724.9 NERVE ROOT COMPRESSION OF NEC (NONVERTEBRAL) (NONDISCOGENIC)
907.3 NERVE ROOT(S) SPINAL PLEXUS(ES) AND OTHER NERVES OF TRUNK (INJURY) LATE EFFECT
997.09 PUNCTURE LUMBAR FLUID LEAKAGE
349.0 PUNCTURE REACTION (HEADACHE)
747.82 VEIN ANOMALY (ABERRANT) (ABSENCE) (ACCESSORY) (AGENESIS)
747.82 VESSEL ANOMALY OTHER

SPINAL CORD
742.59 ABSENCE CONGENITAL
742.9 ANOMALY
336.8 ATROPHY (ACUTE)
733.99 ATROPHY COLUMN
335.10 ATROPHY MUSCULAR - NOS
335.19 ATROPHY MUSCULAR - ADULT
335.11 ATROPHY MUSCULAR - FAMILIAL
335.11 ATROPHY MUSCULAR - JUVENILE
335.19 ATROPHY MUSCULAR - OTHER
336.9 COMPRESSION
742.9 DEFORMITY CONGENITAL
266.2 DEGENERATION B12 DEFICIENCY [336.2]
281.1 DEGENERATION B12 DEFICIENCY ANEMIA [336.2]
281.0 DEGENERATION PERNICIOUS ANEMA (DUE TO) [336.2]
742.51 DIASTEMATOMYELIA CONGENITAL
336.9 DISEASE NOS
0 DISEASE COMBINED SYSTEM SEE 'SPINAL CORD', DEGENERATION
742.9 DISEASE CONGENITAL
0 DIVISION SEE 'SPINAL CORD INJURY'
742.53 HYDROMYELIA CONGENITAL
742.53 HYDRORHACHIS CONGENITAL
742.59 HYPOPLASIA CONGENITAL
V53.02 NEUROPACEMAKER FITTING AND ADJUSTMENT
742.59 TETHERED SPINAL CORD SYNDROME

A SPINAL CORD INJURY CAN BE HEMATOMYELIA, PARALYSIS, PARAPLEGIA, QUADRIPLEGIA OR SPINAL CONCUSSION

SPINAL CORD INJURY
952.9 SITE UNSPECIFIED
806.8 SITE UNSPECIFIED WITH FRACTURE CLOSED
806.9 SITE UNSPECIFIED WITH FRACTURE OPEN
767.4 BIRTH TRAUMA
952.4 CAUDA EQUINA
806.6# CAUDA EQUINA WITH FRACTURE CLOSED
806.7# CAUDA EQUINA WITH FRACTURE OPEN
5th Digit: 806.6-7
0. UNSPECIFIED INJURY
1. COMPLETE CAUDA EQUINA INJURY
2. OTHER CAUDA EQUINA INJURY
9. OTHER SPINAL CORD INJURY

SPINAL CORD INJURY (continued)

952.0# CERVICAL
806.0# CERVICAL WITH FRACTURE CLOSED
806.1# CERVICAL WITH FRACTURE OPEN
5th Digit: 806.0-1, 952.0
0. C1-C4 WITH CORD INJURY NOS
1. C1-C4 WITH COMPLETE CORD LESION
2. C1-C4 WITH ANTERIOR CORD SYNDROME
3. C1-C4 WITH CENTRAL CORD LESION
4. C1-C4 WITH INCOMPLETE CORD LESION NOS OR POSTERIOR CORD SYNDROME
5. C5-C7 WITH CORD INJURY NOS
6. C5-C7 COMPLETE LESION OF CORD
7. C5-C7 WITH ANTERIOR CORD SYNDROME
8. C5-C7 WITH CENTRAL CORD SYNDROME
9. C5-C7 WITH INCOMPLETE CORD LESION NOS OR POSTERIOR CORD SYNDROMESPINAL MUSCULAR ATROPHY

952.1# DORSAL
806.2# DORSAL WITH FRACTURE CLOSED
806.3# DORSAL WITH FRACTURE OPEN
5th Digit: 806.2-3, 952.1
0. T1-T6 WITH CORD INJURY NOS
1. T1-T6 WITH COMPLETE LESION OF CORD
2. T1-T6 WITH ANTERIOR CORD SYNDROME
3. T1-T6 WITH CENTRAL CORD SYNDROME
4. T1-T6 WITH INCOMPLETE CORD LESION NOS OR POSTERIOR CORD SYNDROME
5. T7-T12 WITH CORD INJURY NOS
6. T7-T12 WITH COMPLETE LESION OF CORD
7. T7-T12 WITH ANTERIOR CORD SYNDROME
8. T7-T12 WITH CENTRAL CORD SYNDROME
9. T7-T12 WITH SPINAL CORD LESION NOS OR POSTERIOR CORD SYNDROME

331.3 FLUID MALABSORPTION SYNDROME (ACQUIRED) (HYDROCEPHALUS COMMUNICATING)
907.2 LATE EFFECT
952.2 LUMBAR
806.4 LUMBAR WITH FRACTURE CLOSED
806.5 LUMBAR WITH FRACTURE OPEN
952.8 MULTIPLE SITES
952.3 SACRAL
806.6# SACRUM/COCCYX CLOSED
806.7# SACRUM/COCCYX OPEN
5th Digit: 806.6-7
0. UNSPECIFIED INJURY
1. COMPLETE CAUDA EQUINA INJURY
2. OTHER CAUDA EQUINA INJURY
9. OTHER SPINAL CORD INJURY

0 SYNDROME SEE 'SPINAL CORD INJURY', BY SITE
0 THORACIC SEE 'SPINAL CORD INJURY', DORSAL

SPINAL CORD INJURY CAN BE HEMATOMYELIA, PARALYSIS, PARAPLEGIA, QUADRIPLEGIA, OR SPINAL CONCUSSION

SPINAL MUSCULAR ATROPHY

335.10 NOS
335.19 ADULT
335.11 FAMILIAL
335.11 JUVENILE
335.19 OTHER

SPINAL STENOSIS (NONVERTEBRAL) (NONDISCOGENIC)

724.00 NOS
723.0 CERVICAL
724.01 THORACIC (DORSAL)
724.02 LUMBAR
724.09 OTHER

0 SPINAL STENOSIS DISCOGENIC SEE 'HERNIATED DISC (HNP)'

199.1 SPINDLE CELL CARCINOMA SITE NOS
0 SPINDLE CELL CARCINOMA SITE SPECIFIED SEE 'CANCER' BY SITE M8032/3

SPINE

756.13 ABSENCE CONGENITAL
767.4 AND SPINAL CORD INJURY (BIRTH TRAUMA)
756.10 ANOMALY CONGENITAL
738.5 DEFORMITY UNSPECIFIED ACQUIRED
756.15 FUSION CONGENITAL
721.8 OTHER ALLIED DISORDERS

SPINE CURVATURE ABNORMALITY

737.9 CURVATURE UNSPECIFIED
754.2 CURVATURE CONGENITAL
356.1 CHARCOT MARIE TOOTH **[737.4#]**
5th Digit: 737.4
0. CURVATURE UNSPECIFIED
1. KYPHOSIS
2. LORDOSIS
3. SCOLIOSIS

737.9 HUNCHBACK
277.5 MUCOPOLYSACCHARIDOSIS **[737.4#]**
237.7# NEUROFIBROMATOSIS **[737.4#]**
5th Digit: 237.7
0. NOS OR MULTIPLE
1. TYPE I
2. TYPE II

5th Digit: 737.4
0. CURVATURE UNSPECIFIED
1. KYPHOSIS
2. LORDOSIS
3. SCOLIOSIS

731.0 OSTEITIS DEFORMANS **[737.4#]**
252.0 OSTEITIS FIBROSA CYSTICA **[737.4#]**
733.0# OSTEOPOROSIS **[737.4#]**
5th Digit: 733.0
0. UNSPECIFIED
1. SENILE
2. IDIOPATHIC
3. DISUSE
9. OTHER

5th Digit: 737.4
0. CURVATURE UNSPECIFIED
1. KYPHOSIS
2. LORDOSIS
3. SCOLIOSIS

045.9# POLIOMYELITIS **[737.4#]**
5th Digit: 045.9
0. UNSPECIFIED
1. TYPE I
2. TYPE II
3. TYPE III

5th Digit: 737.4
0. CURVATURE UNSPECIFIED
1. KYPHOSIS
2. LORDOSIS
3. SCOLIOSIS

237.7# VON RECKLINGHAUSEN'S DISEASE **[737.4#]**
5th Digit: 237.7
0. NOS OR MULTIPLE
1. TYPE I
2. TYPE II

5th Digit: 737.4
0. CURVATURE UNSPECIFIED
1. KYPHOSIS
2. LORDOSIS
3. SCOLIOSIS

737.8 OTHER SPECIFIED

334.9 SPINOCEREBELLAR DISEASE
334.8 SPINOCEREBELLAR DISEASE OTHER

216.# SPIRADENOMA (ECCRINE) M8403/0

4th Digit: 216

- **0. LIP (SKIN OF)**
- **1. EYELID INCLUDING CANTHUS**
- **2. EAR (EXTERNAL) (AURICLE) (PINNA)**
- **3. FACE (CHEEK) (NOSE) (EYEBROW) (TEMPLE)**
- **4. SCALP NECK**
- **5. TRUNK BACK EXCEPT SCROTUM**
- **6. UPPER LIMB INCLUDING SHOULDER**
- **7. LOWER LIMB INCLUDING HIP**
- **8. OTHER SPECIFIED SITES**
- **9. SKIN NOS**

026.0 SPIRILLARY FEVER

104.9 SPIROCHETAL INFECTION
104.8 SPIROCHETAL INFECTIONS OTHER SPECIFIED NONSYPHILITIC NONRELAPSING FEVER

123.5 SPIROMETRA LARVAE INFECTION
954.1 SPLANCHNIC NERVES INJURY

SPLEEN, SPLENIC

759.0 ABERRANT
289.59 ABSENCE ACQUIRED
759.0 ABSENCE CONGENITAL
759.0 ACCESSORY CONGENITAL
277.3 AMYLOID DISEASE
442.83 ARTERY (ANEURYSM) (A-V FISTULA) (CIRSOID) (FALSE) (VARICOSE) (RUPTURED)
902.23 ARTERY INJURY
908.4 ARTERY INJURY LATE EFFECT
902.23 ARTERY LACERATION (RUPTURE) (HEMATOMA) (AVULSION) (ANEURYSM) TRAUMATIC
908.4 ARTERY LACERATION LATE EFFECT
289.59 ATROPHY
289.59 CALCIFICATION
865.02 CAPSULE TEAR TRAUMATIC
865.12 CAPSULE TEAR TRAUMATIC WITH OPEN WOUND INTO CAVITY
865.01 CONTUSION
865.11 CONTUSION WITH OPEN WOUND INTO CAVITY
289.50 DISEASE (ORGANIC) (POSTINFECTIONAL)
289.59 DISEASE (ORGANIC) (POSTINFECTIONAL) SPECIFIED NEC
120.0 DISEASE WITH BILHARZIAL SPLENIC
759.0 ECTOPIC CONGENITAL
789.2 ENLARGEMENT
289.59 FIBROSIS
569.89 FLEXURE SYNDROME
794.9 FUNCTION STUDY ABNORMAL
865.01 HEMATOMA TRAUMATIC
865.11 HEMATOMA TRAUMATIC WITH OPEN WOUND INTO CAVITY
289.4 HYPERSPLENISM (SYNDROME)
289.59 INFARCTION
865.0# INJURY (TRAUMATIC)
865.1# INJURY (TRAUMATIC) WITH OPEN WOUND INTO CAVITY

5th Digit: 865.0-1

- **0. UNSPECIFIED INJURY**
- **1. HEMATOMA WITHOUT RUPTURE OF CAPSULE**
- **2. CAPSULAR TEARS, WITHOUT MAJOR DISRUPTION OF PARENCHYMA**
- **3. LACERATION EXTENDING INTO PARENCHYMA**
- **4. MASSIVE PARENCHYMAL DISRUPTION**
- **9. OTHER**

908.1 INJURY LATE EFFECT
865.03 LACERATION
865.13 LACERATION WITH OPEN WOUND INTO CAVITY
289.59 LIEN MIGRANS
759.0 LOBULATION CONGENITAL
288.0 NEUTROPENIA SYNDROME
759.0 POLYCYSTIC CONGENITAL

SPLEEN, SPLENIC (continued)

794.9 RADIOISOTOPE STUDY ABNORMAL
767.8 RUPTURE - BIRTH TRAUMA
289.59 RUPTURE - NONTRAUMATIC
865.04 RUPTURE - TRAUMATIC
865.14 RUPTURE - TRAUMATIC WITH OPEN WOUND INTO CAVITY
794.9 SCAN ABNORMAL
282.60 SEQUESTRATION SYNDROME
289.51 SPLENOMEGALY CHRONIC CONGESTIVE
902.34 VEIN INJURY
908.4 VEIN INJURY LATE EFFECT
902.34 VEIN LACERATION (RUPTURE) (HEMATOMA) (AVULSION) (ANEURYSM) TRAUMATIC
908.4 VEIN LACERATION LATE EFFECT
289.59 WANDERING

289.59 SPLENITIS

SPLENOMEGALY

789.2 UNSPECIFIED
289.51 CHRONIC CONGESTIVE
759.0 CONGENITAL
288.0 NEUTROPENIC
789.2 UNKNOWN ETIOLOGY

SPLINT

V54.8 CHANGE (ORTHOPEDIC)
V54.8 EXTERNAL ORTHOPEDIC AFTERCARE
V54.8 REMOVAL (ORTHOPEDIC)

0 SPLINTER SEE 'FOREIGN BODY', BY SITE, SUPERFICIAL
788.61 SPLITTING OF URINARY STREAM

SPONDYLITIS

720.9 NOS
720.0 ANKYLOPOIETICA
720.0 ANKYLOSING (CHRONIC)
720.9 ATROPHIC (LIGAMENTOUS)
721.90 CHRONIC (TRAUMATIC)
721.90 DEFORMANS (CHRONIC)
098.53 GONOCOCCAL
274.0 GOUTY
721.90 HYPERTROPHIC
720.9 INFECTIOUS NEC
720.0 JUVENILE (ADOLESCENT)
721.7 KUMMELL'S
720.0 MARIE STRUMPELL (ANKYLOSING)
720.9 MUSCULARIS
721.6 OSSIFICANS LIGAMENTOSA
721.90 OSTEOARTHRITICA
721.7 POSTTRAUMATIC
720.0 PROLIFERATIVE
720.0 RHEUMATOID
720.0 RHIZOMELICA
720.2 SACROILIAC NEC
721.90 SENESCENT
721.90 SENILE
721.90 STATIC
721.90 TRAUMATIC (CHRONIC)
015.0# TUBERCULOSIS [720.81]

5th Digit: 015.0

- **0. NOS**
- **1. LAB NOT DONE**
- **2. LABS PENDING**
- **3. MICROSCOPY POSITIVE (IN SPUTUM)**
- **4. CULTURE POSITIVE - MICROSCOPY NEGATIVE**
- **5. CULTURE NEGATIVE - MICROSCOPY POSITIVE**
- **6. CULTURE AND MICROSCOPY NEGATIVE CONFIRMED BY OTHER METHODS**

002.0 TYPHOSA [720.81]
0 SEE ALSO 'SPONDYLOSIS'

S

721.1 SPONDYLOGENIC COMPRESSION OF CERVICAL SPINAL CORD
721.91 SPONDYLOGENIC COMPRESSION OF SPINAL CORD

SPONDYLOLISTHESIS
738.4 ACQUIRED
763.1 AFFECTING FETUS OR NEWBORN
756.12 CONGENITAL
738.4 DEGENERATIVE
653.3# MATERNAL WITH FETOPELVIC DISPROPORTION
660.1# MATERNAL WITH FETOPELVIC DISPROPORTION OBSTRUCTING LABOR **[653.3#]**
5th Digit: 653.3, 660.1
0. EPISODE OF CARE NOS OR N/A
1. DELIVERED
3. ANTEPARTUM COMPLICATION
738.4 TRAUMATIC

SPONDYLOLYSIS
738.4 ACQUIRED
763.1 AFFECTING FETUS OR NEWBORN
756.19 CERVICAL CONGENITAL
756.11 CONGENITAL
756.11 LUMBOSACRAL CONGENITAL
653.3# MATERNAL WITH FETOPELVIC DISPROPORTION
660.1# MATERNAL WITH FETOPELVIC DISPROPORTION OBSTRUCTING LABOR **[653.3#]**
5th Digit: 653.3, 660.1
0. EPISODE OF CARE NOS OR N/A
1. DELIVERED
3. ANTEPARTUM COMPLICATION

SPONDYLOPATHIES
720.9 INFLAMMATORY NOS
720.89 INFLAMMATORY OTHER
015.0# TUBERCULOUS [720.81]
5th Digit: 015.0
0. NOS
1. LAB NOT DONE
2. LABS PENDING
3. MICROSCOPY POSITIVE (IN SPUTUM)
4. CULTURE POSITIVE - MICROSCOPY NEGATIVE
5. CULTURE NEGATIVE - MICROSCOPY POSITIVE
6. CULTURE AND MICROSCOPY NEGATIVE CONFIRMED BY OTHER METHODS

SPONDYLOSIS:

WITH OSTEOPOROSIS [733.0#]
721.0 CERVICAL
721.1 CERVICAL WITH MYELOPATHY (CORD COMPRESSION)
721.3 LUMBAR
721.42 LUMBAR WITH MYELOPATHY (CORD COMPRESSION)
721.3 LUMBOSACRAL
721.42 LUMBOSACRAL WITH MYELOPATHY (CORD COMPRESSION)

648.7#: SPECIFY THE MATERNAL SPONDYLOSIS WITH AN ADDITIONAL CODE. .

648.7# MATERNAL CURRENT (CO-EXISTING) IN PREGNANCY
5th Digit: 648.7
0. EPISODE OF CARE NOS OR N/A
1. DELIVERED
2. DELIVERED WITH POSTPARTUM COMPLICATION
3. ANTEPARTUM COMPLICATION
4. POSTPARTUM COMPLICATION
653.3# MATERNAL WITH DISPROPORTION
660.1# MATERNAL WITH DISPROPORTION OBSTRUCTING LABOR **[653.3#]**
5th Digit: 653.3, 660.1
0. EPISODE OF CARE NOS OR N/A
1. DELIVERED
3. ANTEPARTUM COMPLICATION

SPONDYLOSIS: (continued)

WITH OSTEOPOROSIS [733.0#]
721.90 SPINE
721.91 SPINE WITH MYELOPATHY (CORD COMPRESSION)
721.2 THORACIC
721.41 THORACIC WITH MYELOPATHY (CORD COMPRESSION)
721.7 TRAUMATIC
WITH OSTEOPOROSIS [733.0#]
5th Digit: 733.0
0. UNSPECIFIED
1. SENILE
2. IDIOPATHIC
3. DISUSE
9. DRUG INDUCED

989.5 SPONGE DIVERS' DISEASE

SPONGIOBLASTOMA
191.9 SITE NOS
0 SITE SPECIFIED SEE 'CANCER' BY SITE M9422/3
191.9 POLARE SITE NOS
0 POLARE SITE SPECIFIED SEE 'CANCER' BY SITE M9423/3
191.9 PRIMITIVE POLAR SITE NOS
0 PRIMITIVE POLAR SITE SPECIFIED SEE 'CANCER' BY SITE

0 SPONGIOCYTOMA SEE 'CANCER', BY SITE

199.1 SPONGIONEUROBLASTOMA SITE NOS
0 SPONGIONEUROBLASTOMA SITE SPECIFIED SEE 'CANCER' BY SITE M9504/3

0 SPONTANEOUS FRACTURE SEE 'FRACTURE PATHOLOGICAL'

117.1 SPOROTHRIX (SPOROTRICHUM) SCHENCKII INFECTION

SPOROTRICHOSIS
117.1 BONE
117.1 CUTANEOUS
117.1 DISSEMINATED
117.1 LYMPHOCUTANEOUS
117.1 PULMONARY

MEDICALLY, A SPRAIN OCCURS WHEN EXCESSIVE FORCE CAUSES INJURY TO A LIGAMENT, AND A STRAIN OCCURS WHEN EXCESSIVE FORCE CAUSES INJURY TO A MUSCLE OR TENDON. IN ICD-9, THOUGH, SPRAIN IS THE TERM USED TO COVER ALL SPRAINS, STRAINS, AVULSIONS, HEMARTHROSES, TEARS AND RUPTURES. IN EASY CODER YOU'LL FIND THAT CODES FOR ALL OF THE ABOVE CONDITIONS ARE LISTED BY SITE UNDER THE HEADING, SPRAIN.

SPRAIN
848.9 NOS
848.8 ABDOMINAL MUSCLES
845.09 ACHILLES TENDON
840.0 ACROMIOCLAVICULAR (JOINT) (LIGAMENT)
843.8 ADDUCTOR THIGH (MAGNUS)
845.00 ANKLE - NOS
845.02 ANKLE - CALCANEOFIBULAR (LIGAMENT)
845.01 ANKLE - DELTOID (LIGAMENT)
845.01 ANKLE - INTERNAL COLLATERAL (LIGAMENT)
845.03 ANKLE - TIBIOFIBULAR (LIGAMENT) DISTAL
845.09 ANKLE - OTHER SPECIFIED
845.00 ANKLE AND FOOT
844.2 ANTERIOR CRUCIATE LIGAMENT
717.83 ANTERIOR CRUCIATE LIGAMENT OLD
840.9 ARM
840.9 ARM (UPPER) AND SHOULDER UNSPECIFIED
840.8 ARM (UPPER) AND SHOULDER OTHER SPECIFIED
840.4 ARM ROTATOR CUFF
845.00 ASTRAGALUS
847.0 ATLANTO-AXIAL (JOINTS)
847.0 ATLANTO-OCCIPITAL (JOINTS)
847.0 ATLAS
847.0 AXIS

SPRAIN (continued)

847.9	BACK - NOS
847.0	BACK - CERVICAL
847.4	BACK - COCCYX
846.9	BACK - LOW
847.2	BACK - LUMBAR (SPINE)
846.0	BACK - LUMBOSACRAL
724.6	BACK - LUMBOSACRAL (JOINT) (LIGAMENT) CHRONIC (OLD)
846.9	BACK - SACROILIAC (REGION)
846.1	BACK - SACROILIAC LIGAMENT
724.6	BACK - SACROILIAC CHRONIC (OLD)
846.8	BACK - SACROILIAC REGION OTHER SPECIFIED SITES
846.2	BACK - SACROSPINATUS (LIGAMENT)
846.3	BACK - SACROTUBEROUS (LIGAMENT)
847.3	BACK - SACRUM
847.1	BACK - THORACIC
840.8	BICEPS ARM (BRACHII)
843.8	BICEPS LEG (FEMORIS)
848.40	BREAST BONE
843.8	BUTTOCK
845.02	CALCANEOFIBULAR (LIGAMENT)
844.8	CALF
717.85	CAPSULAR LIGAMENT OLD (KNEE)
842.01	CARPAL (JOINT)
842.11	CARPOMETACARPAL (JOINT)
847.0	CERVICAL SPINE ACUTE
848.3	CHEST WALL
848.3	CHONDROCOSTAL
848.42	CHONDROCOSTAL INVOLVING STERNUM
848.42	CHONDROSTERNAL (JOINT)
840.9	CLAVICLE
847.4	COCCYX
840.9	COLLAR BONE
844.0	COLLATERAL LIGAMENTS - LATERAL (KNEE)
844.1	COLLATERAL LIGAMENTS - MEDIAL (KNEE)
717.89	COLLATERAL LIGAMENTS OLD - NOS (KNEE)
717.81	COLLATERAL LIGAMENTS OLD - LATERAL (KNEE)
717.82	COLLATERAL LIGAMENTS OLD - MEDIAL (KNEE)
840.8	CORACOACROMIAL
840.1	CORACOCLAVICULAR (LIGAMENT)
840.2	CORACOHUMERAL (LIGAMENT)
840.9	CORACOID (PROCESS)
844.8	CORONARY KNEE
848.3	COSTAL CARTILAGE
848.42	COSTAL CARTILAGE INVOLVING STERNUM
848.3	COSTOCHONDRAL
848.2	CRICOARYTENOID (JOINT) (LIGAMENT)
848.2	CRICOTHYROID (JOINT) (LIGAMENT)
844.2	CRUCIATE LIGAMENT - ACUTE
717.89	CRUCIATE LIGAMENT - OLD
717.83	CRUCIATE LIGAMENT - ANTERIOR OLD
717.84	CRUCIATE LIGAMENT - POSTERIOR OLD
845.01	DELTOID ANKLE (LIGAMENT)
840.8	DELTOID SHOULDER
847.1	DORSAL SPINE
848.8	EAR CARTILAGE
841.9	ELBOW
841.2	ELBOW RADIOHUMERAL
841.1	ELBOW ULNAR COLLATERAL LIGAMENT
841.3	ELBOW ULNOHUMERAL
841.0	ELBOW RADIAL COLLATERAL LIGAMENT
841.8	ELBOW OTHER SPECIFIED SITES
843.9	FEMUR PROXIMAL
844.9	FEMUR DISTAL
844.9	FIBULA PROXIMAL
845.00	FIBULA DISTAL
842.13	FINGER
842.13	FINGER INTERPHALANGEAL

SPRAIN (continued)

845.10	FOOT - NOS
845.13	FOOT - INTERPHALANGEAL (JOINT) TOE
845.12	FOOT - METATARSOPHALANGEAL (JOINT)
845.11	FOOT - TARSOMETATARSAL (JOINT) (LIGAMENT)
845.19	FOOT - OTHER
845.00	FOOT AND ANKLE
841.9	FOREARM
841.8	FOREARM OTHER SPECIFIED SITES
844.8	GASTROCNEMIUS
840.8	GLENOID (SHOULDER)
843.8	GLUTEUS MAXIMUS
848.8	GROIN
843.8	HAMSTRING
842.10	HAND
842.11	HAND CARPOMETACARPAL
842.13	HAND INTERPHALANGEAL (JOINT)
842.12	HAND METACARPOPHALANGEAL
842.19	HAND MIDCARPAL
842.19	HAND OTHER JOINT
843.9	HIP - NOS
843.0	HIP- ILIOFEMORAL (LIGAMENT)
843.1	HIP- ISCHIOCAPSULAR (LIGAMENT)
843.8	HIP- LIGAMENTUM TERES FEMORIS
843.8	HIP- OTHER SPECIFIED SITES
841.9	HUMERUS DISTAL
840.9	HUMERUS PROXIMAL
843.0	ILIOFEMORAL (LIGAMENT)
840.3	INFRASPINATUS (MUSCLE) (TENDON)
848.8	INGUINAL
843.9	INNOMINATE ACETABULUM
848.5	INNOMINATE PUBIC JUNCTION
846.1	INNOMINATE SACRAL JUNCTION
842.13	INTERPHALANGEAL (JOINT) HAND
843.1	ISCHIOCAPSULAR (LIGAMENT)
848.1	JAW (CARTILAGE) (MENISCUS)
524.69	JAW (CARTILAGE) (MENISCUS) - OLD

KNEE ACUTE (CURRENT INJURY)

844.9	UNSPECIFIED
844.2	CRUCIATE LIGAMENT
844.0	LATERAL COLLATERAL LIGAMENT
844.1	MEDIAL COLLATERAL LIGAMENT
844.8	PATELLAR LIGAMENT
844.3	TIBIOFIBULAR LIGAMENT (JOINT), SUPERIOR
844.8	OTHER SPECIFIED SITES

KNEE OLD

717.89	UNSPECIFIED
717.81	COLLATERAL LIGAMENT LATERAL
717.82	COLLATERAL LIGAMENT MEDIAL
717.83	CRUCIATE LIGAMENT ANTERIOR
717.84	CRUCIATE LIGAMENT POSTERIOR
717.89	PATELLAR LIGAMENT
717.85	OTHER LIGAMENTS

SPRAIN (continued)

905.7	LATE EFFECT
905.8	LATE EFFECT WITH TENDON INJURY
844.0	LATERAL COLLATERAL LIGAMENT KNEE
717.81	LATERAL COLLATERAL LIGAMENT KNEE - OLD
844.9	LEG
843.8	LIGAMENTUM TERES FEMORIS
846.9	LOW BACK
847.2	LUMBAR
846.0	LUMBOSACRAL (JOINT) (LIGAMENT)
724.6	LUMBOSACRAL (JOINT) (LIGAMENT) - OLD
848.1	MANDIBLE
524.69	MANDIBLE - OLD
848.1	MAXILLA

SPRAIN (continued)

844.1 MEDIAL COLLATERAL LIGAMENT KNEE
717.82 MEDIAL COLLATERAL LIGAMENT KNEE - OLD
0 MENISCUS SEE 'MENISCUS', KNEE TEAR
842.10 METACARPAL
842.12 METACARPAL DISTAL
842.11 METACARPAL PROXIMAL
842.12 METACARPOPHALANGEAL (JOINT)
845.10 METATARSAL
845.12 METATARSOPHALANGEAL (JOINT)
842.19 MIDCARPAL (JOINT)
845.19 MIDTARSAL (JOINT)
847.0 NECK
848.0 NOSE SEPTAL CARTILAGE
847.0 OCCIPUT FROM ATLAS
843.8 ORBICULAR HIP
844.8 PATELLAR
717.89 PATELLAR - OLD
848.8 PECTORALS
848.5 PELVIS
0 PHALANX SEE 'SPRAIN', FINGER OR 'SPRAIN', TOE
844.2 POSTERIOR CRUCIATE LIGAMENT
717.84 POSTERIOR CRUCIATE LIGAMENT OLD
843.8 QUADRICEPS
841.0 RADIAL COLLATERAL LIGAMENT
842.02 RADIOCARPAL (JOINT) (LIGAMENT)
841.2 RADIOHUMERAL (JOINT)
841.9 RADIOULNAR
842.09 RADIOULNAR JOINT DISTAL
842.00 RADIUS DISTAL
841.9 RADIUS PROXIMAL
842.09 RADIUS AND ULNA DISTAL
841.9 RADIUS AND ULNA PROXIMAL
841.0 RADIUS COLLATERAL (LIGAMENT)
848.8 RECTUS ABDOMINIS
848.3 RIB
848.42 RIB WITH STERNAL INVOLVEMENT
840.4 ROTATOR CUFF (CAPSULE)
843.8 ROUND LIGAMENT FEMUR
847.3 SACROCOCCYGEAL (LIGAMENT)
846.1 SACROILIAC LIGAMENT
724.6 SACROILIAC LIGAMENT - OLD (CHRONIC)
846.9 SACROILIAC REGION
846.8 SACROILIAC REGION OTHER SPECIFIED SITES
846.2 SACROSPINATUS (LIGAMENT)
846.2 SACROSPINOUS
846.3 SACROTUBEROUS (LIGAMENT)
847.3 SACRUM
845.00 SCAPHOID ANKLE
840.9 SCAPULA
844.8 SEMILUNAR CARTILAGE KNEE
717.5 SEMILUNAR CARTILAGE KNEE - OLD
840.9 SHOULDER
840.9 SHOULDER AND UPPER ARM
840.9 SHOULDER BLADE
840.8 SHOULDER AND UPPER ARM OTHER SPECIFIED SITES
847.9 SPINE
848.41 STERNOCLAVICULAR (JOINT) (LIGAMENT)
848.40 STERNUM NOS
848.49 STERNUM OTHER SPECIFIED
840.8 SUBGLENOID
840.5 SUBSCAPULARIS (MUSCLE)
840.6 SUPRASPINATUS (MUSCLE) (TENDON)
848.1 SYMPHYSIS JAW (MANDIBLE)
524.69 SYMPHYSIS JAW (MANDIBLE) - OLD
848.5 SYMPHYSIS PUBIS
845.09 TALOFIBULAR
845.10 TARSAL
845.11 TARSOMETATARSAL (JOINT) (LIGAMENT)
848.1 TEMPOROMANDIBULAR
524.69 TEMPOROMANDIBULAR - OLD

SPRAIN (continued)

843.8 TERES LIGAMENTUM FEMORIS
840.8 TERES MAJOR OR MINOR
843.9 THIGH NOS
843.9 THIGH AND HIP
844.9 THIGH DISTAL
843.9 THIGH PROXIMAL
847.1 THORACIC SPINE
848.8 THORAX
842.13 THUMB
842.13 THUMB INTERPHALANGEAL
848.2 THYROID REGION CARTILAGE
845.00 TIBIA DISTAL
844.9 TIBIA PROXIMAL
845.03 TIBIOFIBULAR DISTAL
844.3 TIBIOFIBULAR LIGAMENT (JOINT), SUPERIOR
717.85 TIBIOFIBULAR LIGAMENT (OLD)
845.13 TOE
845.13 TOE INTERPHALANGEAL (JOINT)
848.8 TRACHEA
840.8 TRAPEZOID
842.01 TRIANGULAR FIBROCARTILAGE COMPLEX
719.83 TRIANGULAR FIBROCARTILAGE COMPLEX - OLD
840.8 TRICEPS
842.00 ULNAR DISTAL
841.9 ULNAR PROXIMAL
841.1 ULNAR COLLATERAL LIGAMENT
841.3 ULNOHUMERAL (JOINT)
842.00 WRIST
842.01 WRIST CARPAL
842.02 WRIST RADIOCARPAL (JOINT) (LIGAMENT)
842.09 WRIST OTHER
848.49 XIPHOID CARTILAGE
848.8 OTHER SPECIFIED SITES

755.52 SPRENGEL'S DEFORMITY

0 SPROM SEE 'PREMATURE', RUPTURE OF MEMBRANES OBSTETRICAL

SPRUE

579.1 UNSPECIFIED
579.0 NONTROPICAL
579.1 TROPICAL

SPUR

726.91 NOS
726.73 CALCANEUS
726.30 ELBOW
726.73 FOOT
726.4 HAND
726.73 HEEL
726.5 HIP
726.5 ILIAC CREST
726.60 KNEE
726.91 NOSE
726.33 OLECRANON
726.69 PREPATELLAR OR SUBPATELLAR
726.4 WRIST
726.8 OTHER SPECIFIED SITE

756.51 SPURWAY'S SYNDROME (BRITTLE BONES AND BLUE SCLERA)

786.4 SPUTUM ABNORMAL (COLOR) (EXCESS) (ODOR)

795.3 SPUTUM CULTURE POSITIVE

CARCINOMAS AND NEOPLASMS SHOULD BE CODED BY SITE FIRST. IF A SITE IS NOT SPECIFIED THEN CODE BY CELL TYPE. DO NOT TRY TO CODE BY CELL TYPE FIRST. WHENEVER POSSIBLE, EASY CODER ALSO PROVIDES THE SITE MENUS FOR YOUR CONVENIENCE.

SQUAMOUS CELL CARCINOMA

199.1 SITE NOS
0 SITE SPECIFIED SEE 'CANCER' BY SITE M8070/3
180.9 ADENOID SITE NOS
0 ADENOID SITE SPECIFIED SEE 'CANCER' BY SITE M8075/3
234.9 IN SITU SITE NOS
0 IN SITU SITE SPECIFIED SEE 'CARCINOMA IN SITU', BY SITE M8070/2
233.1 IN SITU WITH QUESTIONABLE STROMAL INVASION SITE NOS
0 IN SITU WITH QUESTIONABLE STROMAL INVASION SPECIFIED SITE SEE 'CARCINOMA IN SITU' BY SITE M8076/2
0 INTRAEPIDERMAL BOWEN'S TYPE SEE 'CANCER' SKIN BY SITE M8076/2
180.9 KERATINIZING TYPE SITE NOS
0 KERATINIZING TYPE SITE SPECIFIED SEE 'CANCER' BY SITE M8071/3
180.9 LARGE CELL (NONKERATINIZING TYPE) SITE NOS
0 LARGE CELL (NONKERATINIZING TYPE) SITE SPECIFIED SEE 'CANCER' BY SITE M8072/3
199.1 METASTATIC SITE NOS
0 METASTATIC SITE SPECIFIED SEE 'CANCER' BY SITE, METASTATIC M8070/6
180.9 MICRO INVASIVE SITE NOS
0 MICRO INVASIVE SITE SPECIFIED SEE 'CANCER' BY SITE M8076/3
199.1 PAPILLARY SITE NOS
0 PAPILLARY SITE SPECIFIED SEE 'CANCER' BY SITE M8052/3
180.9 SMALL CELL (NONKERATINIZING TYPE) SITE NOS
0 SMALL CELL (NONKERATINIZING TYPE) SITE SPECIFIED SEE 'CANCER' BY SITE M8073/3
180.9 SPINDLE CELL TYPE SITE NOS
0 SPINDLE CELL TYPE SITE SPECIFIED SEE 'CANCER' BY SITE M8074/3

622.1 SQUAMOUS METAPLASIA CERVIX
754.0 SQUASHED NOSE OR BENT CONGENITAL
008.64 SRV ENTERITIS (SMALL ROUND VIRUS) NOS
427.81 SSS - SICK SINUS SYNDROME
695.1 SSSS - SCALDED SKIN SYNDROME
062.3 ST. LOUIS ENCEPHALITIS
592.0 STAGHORN CALCULUS KIDNEY
371.11 STAHLI'S LINES
307.0 STAMMERING
025 STANTON'S DISEASE (MELIOIDOSIS)
385.22 STAPES FIXED

STAPHYLOCOCCAL

462 ANGINA, THROAT
0 ARTHRITIS SEE 'ARTHRITIS OTHER SPECIFIED', PYOGENIC
V02.59 CARRIER
008.41 GASTROENTERITIS
041.1# INFECTION OR ORGANISM
5th Digit: 041.1
0. NOS
1. AUREUS
9. OTHER STAPH

482.4# PNEUMONIA
5th Digit: 482.4
0. NOS
1. AUREUS
9. OTHER STAPH

695.1 SCALDED SKIN SYNDROME

STAPHYLOCOCCAL (continued)

038.1# SEPSIS
5th Digit: 038.1
0. NOS
1. AUREUS
9. OTHER STAPH

038.1# STAPHYLOCOCCEMIA
5th Digit: 038.1
0. UNSPECIFIED
1. AUREUS
9. OTHER

686.00 STAPHYLODERMA (SKIN)
371.73 STAPHYLOMA CORNEAL

STAPHYLOMA SCLERA

379.11 NOS
379.13 EQUATORIAL
379.14 LOCALIZED (ANTERIOR)
379.12 POSTICUM
379.15 RING

362.75 STARGARDT'S DISEASE
994.2 STARVATION
909.4 STARVATION LATE EFFECT
459.81 STASIS DERMATITIS (VENOUS)
459.81 STASIS DERMATITIS (VENOUS) <u>ULCERATED</u> <u>[707.#]</u>
4th Digit: 707
1. LOWER LIMB EXCEPT DECUBITUS
8. CHRONIC OF OTHER SPECIFIED SITE
9. CHRONIC SITE NOS

454.1 STASIS DERMATITIS VARICOSE
454.2 STASIS DERMATITIS VARICOSE WITH ULCER
459.1 STASIS DERMATITIS VARICOSE DUE TO POSTPHLEBITIC SYNDROME
459.81 STASIS <u>ULCER</u> <u>[707.#]</u>
4th Digit: 707
1. LOWER LIMB EXCEPT DECUBITUS
8. CHRONIC OF OTHER SPECIFIED SITE
9. CHRONIC SITE NOS

454.0 STASIS ULCER VARICOSE - SITE NOS
454.0 STASIS ULCER VARICOSE - LOWER EXTREMITY
454.2 STASIS ULCER VARICOSE - LOWER EXTREMITY INFECTED
783.4 STATURE SHORT

STATUS

V49.7# AMPUTATION LOWER LIMB
5th Digit: V49.7
0. UNSPECIFIED LEVEL
1. GREAT TOE
2. OTHER TOE(S)
3. FOOT
4. ANKLE
5. BELOW KNEE
6. ABOVE KNEE
7. HIP

V49.6# AMPUTATION UPPER LIMB
5th Digit: V49.6
0. UNSPECIFIED LEVEL
1. THUMB
2. OTHER FINGER(S)
3. HAND
4. WRIST
5. BELOW ELBOW
6. ABOVE ELBOW
7. SHOULDER

V45.3 ANASTOMOSIS INTESTINAL BYPASS
V45.82 ANGIOPLASTY (PTCA)
V43.66 ANKLE PROSTHESIS

STATUS (continued)

V45.81	AORTOCORONARY BYPASS
V45.81	AORTOCORONARY SHUNT
V45.1	ARTERIOVENOUS SHUNT FOR DIALYSIS RENAL
V43.4	ARTERY DEVICE
V45.4	ARTHRODESIS
V44.8	ARTIFICIAL OPENING OTHER SPECIFIED
V43.5	BLADDER DEVICE
V42.89	BLOOD VESSEL TRANSPLANT
V42.81	BONE MARROW TRANSPLANT
V42.4	BONE TISSUE TRANSPLANT
V43.82	BREAST IMPLANT
V45.83	BREAST IMPLANT REMOVAL
V45.81	BYPASS CORONARY
V45.02	CARDIAC DEFIBRILLATOR IN SITU
V45.00	CARDIAC DEVICE IN SITU
V45.09	CARDIAC DEVICE OTHER SPECIFIED IN SITU
V45.01	CARDIAC PACEMAKER IN SITU
V45.09	CAROTID SINUS STIMULATOR IN SITU
0	CARRIER OR SUSPECTED CARRIER OF INFECTIOUS DISEASE SEE 'CARRIER'
V45.61	CATARACT EXTRACTION WITH ARTIFICIAL LENS STATUS [V43.1]
V45.2	CEREBROSPINAL FLUID DRAINAGE DEVICE
V45.2	CEREBROSPINAL FLUID SHUNT
V45.4	CERVICAL FUSION
V66.2	CHEMOTHERAPY
V44.3	COLOSTOMY
V45.59	CONTRACEPTIVE DEVICE NEC
V45.51	CONTRACEPTIVE DEVICE INTRAUTERINE
V45.52	CONTRACEPTIVE DEVICE SUBDERMAL
V45.69	CORNEAL SURGERY
V42.5	CORNEAL TRANSPLANT
V45.82	CORONARY ANGIOPLASTY (PTCA)
V45.81	CORONARY BYPASS
V45.89	CORONARY STENT/SHUNT
V44.50	CYSTOSTOMY - NOS
V44.52	CYSTOSTOMY - APPENDICO-VESICOSTOMY
V44.51	CYSTOSTOMY - CUTANEOUS-VESICOSTOMY
V44.59	CYSTOSTOMY - OTHER
V45.1	DIALYSIS RENAL
0	DONOR SEE 'DONOR'
V43.62	ELBOW PROSTHESIS
345.3	EPILEPTICUS
V44.4	ENTEROSTOMY
V43.0	EYE GLOBE REPLACEMENT
V45.69	EYE SURGERY AND ADNEXA
V45.69	FILTERING BLEB EYE (POSTGLAUCOMA)
V43.69	FINGER JOINT PROSTHESIS
V44.1	GASTROSTOMY
V43.2	HEART DEVICE
V43.3	HEART VALVE PROSTHESIS
V43.64	HIP PROSTHESIS
V08	HIV INFECTION (ASYMPTOMATIC)
V45.89	HYSTERECTOMY
V44.2	ILEOSTOMY
0	INFECTION WITH DRUG-RESISTANT ORGANISM SEE 'DRUG RESISTANCE'
V45.3	INTESTINAL BYPASS OR ANASTOMOSIS
V42.89	INTESTINE TRANSPLANT
V43.89	INTESTINE DEVICE
V45.51	INTRAUTERINE CONTRACEPTIVE DEVICE
V45.51	IUD
V44.4	JEJUNOSTOMY
V45.4	JOINT FUSION
V43.60	JOINT PROSTHESIS UNSPECIFIED
V43.69	JOINT PROSTHESIS OTHER SPECIFIED
V43.89	KIDNEY DEVICE
V43.65	KNEE JOINT PROSTHESIS

STATUS (continued)

V43.81	LARYNX DEVICE
V45.61	LENS INTRAOCULAR FOLLOWING CATARACT EXTRACTION [V43.1]
V43.7	LIMB PROSTHESIS
V43.89	LIVER DEVICE
V45.89	LOBECTOMY
V45.4	LUMBAR FUSION
V43.89	LUNG DEVICE
V45.89	NEPHRECTOMY
V44.6	NEPHROSTOMY
V45.89	NEUROPACEMAKER
V45.89	OOPHORECTOMY
V42.89	ORGAN SPECIFIED SITE NEC TRANSPLANT
V43.89	ORGAN TISSUE - OTHER REPLACEMENT (MECHANICAL) (ARTIFICIAL) (PROSTHESIS)
V44.9	OSTOMY NOS
V44.4	OSTOMY GI TRACT (OTHER SPECIFIED)
V44.8	OSTOMY OTHER
V45.89	OTHER SURGERY
V45.89	PACEMAKER BRAIN
V45.89	PACEMAKER SPECIFIED SITE NEC
V42.83	PANCREAS TRANSPLANT
V43.89	PANCREAS DEVICE
V45.82	PERCUTANEOUS TRANSLUMINAL CORONARY ANGIOPLASTY
V42.82	PERIPHERAL STEM CELLS TRANSPLANT
310.2	POSTCOMMOTIO CEREBRI
V24.2	POSTPARTUM NEC
V45.89	POSTSURGICAL NEC
V22.2	PREGNANT STATE (INCIDENTAL)
V45.82	PTCA
V45.1	RENAL DIALYSIS
V43.60	REPLACEMENT - JOINT NOS
V43.66	REPLACEMENT - ANKLE JOINT
V43.62	REPLACEMENT - ELBOW JOINT
V43.69	REPLACEMENT - FINGER JOINT
V43.64	REPLACEMENT - HIP JOINT
V43.65	REPLACEMENT - KNEE JOINT
V43.61	REPLACEMENT - SHOULDER JOINT
V43.63	REPLACEMENT - WRIST JOINT
V43.69	REPLACEMENT - OTHER JOINT
V43.61	SHOULDER PROSTHESIS
V43.83	SKIN ARTIFICIAL REPLACEMENT
V42.82	STEM CELLS PERIPHERAL TRANSPLANT
V45.52	SUBDERMAL CONTRACEPTIVE IMPLANT
V45.89	SURGERY OTHER
V45.4	THORACIC FUSION
V42.89	TISSUE SPECIFIED TYPE NEC TRANSPLANT
V43.89	TISSUE REPLACEMENT NEC
V44.0	TRACHEOSTOMY
V42.#(#)	TRANSPLANT ORGAN
	4th or 4th and 5th Digit: V42
	0. KIDNEY
	1. HEART
	2. HEART VALVE
	3. SKIN
	4. BONE
	5. CORNEA
	6. LUNG
	7. LIVER
	8#. OTHER SPECIFIED
	81. BONE MARROW
	82. PERIPHERAL STEM CELLS
	83. PANCREAS
	89. OTHER SPECIFIED
	9. UNSPECIFIED
V43.83	TRANSPLANT SKIN ARTIFICIAL
V26.51	TUBAL LIGATION

STATUS (continued)

V44.6 URETEROSTOMY
V44.6 URETHROSTOMY
V44.6 URINARY TRACT ARTIFICIAL OPENING OTHER
V44.7 VAGINA ARTIFICIAL
V45.89 VASCULAR SHUNT NEC
V26.52 VASECTOMY
V43.4 VEIN DEVICE
V45.2 VENTRICULAR DEVICE CEREBRAL (COMMUNICATING) FOR DRAINAGE
V42.89 VESSEL BLOOD TRANSPLANT
V43.63 WRIST PROSTHESIS

V65.45 STD COUNSELING

996.73 STEAL SYNDROME, ARTERIOVENOUS
435.2 STEAL SYNDROME, SUBCLAVIAN
312.1# STEALING SOLITARY

5th Digit: 312.1
- **0. NOS**
- **1. MILD**
- **2. MODERATE**
- **3. SEVERE**

987.9 STEAM INHALATION
706.2 STEATOCYSTOMA MULTIPLEX

STEATORRHEA

579.8 CHRONIC
579.0 IDIOPATHIC
579.4 PANCREATIC
579.1 TROPICAL

333.0 STEELE-RICHARDSON (-OLSZEWSKI) SYNDROME
256.4 STEIN (-LEVENTHAL) SYNDROME (POLYCYSTIC OVARY)
359.2 STEINERT'S DISEASE
337.9 STEINBROCKER'S SYNDROME (SEE ALSO 'NEUROPATHY PERIPHERAL', AUTONOMIC)
121.6 STELLANTCHASMUS FALCATUS INFECTION
954.1 STELLATE GANGLION INJURY
V59.02 STEM CELL DONOR NON-AUTOGENOUS
V42.82 STEM CELLS PERIPHERAL TRANSPLANT STATUS

STENOSIS

0 SEE ALSO 'STRICTURE'
576.2 AMPULLA OF VATER
751.61 AMPULLA OF VATER CONGENITAL
0 AMPULLA OF VATER WITH CALCULUS SEE 'CHOLEDOCHOLITHIASIS'
569.2 ANUS
751.2 ANUS CONGENITAL (INFANTILE)
747.10 AORTA - ARCH CONGENITAL
440.0 AORTA - ARTERIOSCLEROTIC
747.22 AORTA - ASCENDING CONGENITAL
440.0 AORTA - CALCIFIED

AORTIC VALVE

424.1 NOS
396.0 ATYPICAL
421.0 BACTERIAL ACUTE
421.0 BACTERIAL CHRONIC
746.3 CONGENITAL
746.7 CONGENITAL IN HYPOPLASTIC LEFT HEART
746.81 CONGENITAL SUBAORTIC
747.22 CONGENITAL SUPRAVALVULAR
425.1 HYPERTROPHIC SUBAORTIC - IDIOPATHIC
395.0 RHEUMATIC
395.2 RHEUMATIC WITH INSUFFICIENCY
093.22 SYPHILITIC
424.1 WITH INSUFFICIENCY
421.0 WITH INSUFFICIENCY BACTERIAL (ACUTE) (CHRONIC)
093.22 WITH INSUFFICIENCY SYPHILITIC

STENOSIS (continued)

AORTIC VALVE (continued)

396.2 WITH MITRAL INSUFFICIENCY
396.2 WITH MITRAL INSUFFICIENCY RHEUMATIC
093.22 WITH MITRAL INSUFFICIENCY SYPHILITIC
396.0 WITH MITRAL STENOSIS
396.0 WITH MITRAL STENOSIS RHEUMATIC
093.22 WITH MITRAL STENOSIS SYPHILITIC
396.8 WITH OTHER VALVE MULTIPLE INVOLVEMENT, STENOSIS/INSUFFICIENCY

STENOSIS (continued)

331.4 AQUEDUCT OF SYLVIUS
742.3 AQUEDUCT OF SYLVIUS CONGENITAL
0 AQUEDUCT OF SYLVIUS CONGENITAL WITH SPINA BIFIDA SEE 'SPINA BIFIDA'
447.1 ARTERY NEC
380.50 AUDITORY CANAL ACQUIRED
433.0# BASILAR ARTERY
433.3# BASILAR ARTERY BILATERAL OR MULTIPLE

5th Digit: 433.0, 3
- **0. WITHOUT CEREBRAL INFARCTION**
- **1. WITH CEREBRAL INFARCTION**

576.2 BILE DUCT
751.61 BILE DUCT CONGENITAL
751.61 BILE DUCT CONGENITAL WITH JAUNDICE [774.5]
0 BILE DUCT WITH CALCULUS SEE 'CHOLEDOCHOLITHIASIS'
596.0 BLADDER NECK
753.6 BLADDER NECK CONGENITAL
0 BLADDER NECK WITH INCONTINENCE SEE 'BLADDER DISORDERS WITH INCONTINENCE'
560.9 BOWEL NOS
751.2 BOWEL CONGENITAL LARGE
751.1 BOWEL CONGENITAL SMALL
0 BOWEL SEE ALSO 'INTESTINE, INTESTINAL', OBSTRUCTION
348.8 BRAIN
519.1 BRONCHUS
748.3 BRONCHUS CONGENITAL
095.8 BRONCHUS SYPHILITIC
537.89 CARDIA (STOMACH)
750.7 CARDIA (STOMACH) CONGENITAL
429.2 CARDIOVASCULAR
433.1# CAROTID ARTERY
433.3# CAROTID ARTERY BILATERAL OR MULTIPLE

5th Digit: 433.1, 3
- **0. WITHOUT CEREBRAL INFARCTION**
- **1. WITH CEREBRAL INFARCTION**

560.9 CECUM NOS
751.2 CECUM CONGENITAL
0 CECUM SEE ALSO 'INTESTINE, INTESTINAL', OBSTRUCTION
447.4 CELIAC ARTERY
437.0 CEREBRAL ARTERY NOS
434.1# CEREBRAL ARTERY DUE TO EMBOLISM
434.0# CEREBRAL ARTERY DUE TO THROMBUS

5th Digit: 434.0, 1
- **0. WITHOUT CEREBRAL INFARCTION**
- **1. WITH CEREBRAL INFARCTION**

622.4 CERVIX
654.6# CERVIX - COMPLICATING PREGNANCY

5th Digit: 654.6
- **0. EPISODE OF CARE UNSPECIFIED OR N/A**
- **1. DELIVERED**
- **2. DELIVERED WITH POSTPARTUM COMPLICATION**
- **3. ANTEPARTUM COMPLICATION**
- **4. POSTPARTUM COMPLICATION**

763.89 CERVIX - COMPLICATING PREGNANCY AFFECTING FETUS OR NEWBORN
752.49 CERVIX - CONGENITAL

STENOSIS (continued)

660.2# CERVIX - OBSTRUCTING LABOR **[654.6#]**

5th Digit: 654.6

- **0. EPISODE OF CARE UNSPECIFIED OR N/A**
- **1. DELIVERED**
- **2. DELIVERED WITH POSTPARTUM COMPLICATION**
- **3. ANTEPARTUM COMPLICATION**
- **4. POSTPARTUM COMPLICATION**

5th Digit: 660.2

- **0. EPISODE OF CARE UNSPECIFIED OR N/A**
- **1. DELIVERED**
- **3. ANTEPARTUM COMPLICATION**

S

763.1 CERVIX - OBSTRUCTING LABOR AFFECTING FETUS OR NEWBORN
560.9 COLON
751.2 COLON CONGENITAL
0 COLON SEE ALSO 'INTESTINE, INTESTINAL', OBSTRUCTION
569.62 COLOSTOMY
576.2 COMMON BILE DUCT
751.61 COMMON BILE DUCT CONGENITAL
751.61 COMMON BILE DUCT CONGENITAL WITH JAUNDICE [774.5]
0 COMMON BILE DUCT WITH CALCULUS SEE 'CHOLEDOCHOLITHIASIS'
0 CORONARY SEE ARTERIOSCLEROSIS, ARTERIOSCLEROTIC', CORONARY
575.2 CYSTIC DUCT
751.61 CYSTIC DUCT CONGENITAL
751.61 CYSTIC DUCT CONGENITAL WITH JAUNDICE [774.5]
0 CYSTIC DUCT WITH CALCULUS SEE 'CHOLELITHIASIS'
0 DUE TO ANY DEVICE, IMPLANT OR GRAFT SEE 'COMPLICATION OF AN INTERNAL PROSTHETIC DEVICE, IMPLANT OR GRAFT - (EMBOLUS) (FIBROSIS) (HEMORRHAGE) (PAIN) (STENOSIS) (THROMBUS)'
537.3 DUODENUM
751.1 DUODENUM CONGENITAL
380.50 EAR CANAL (EXTERNAL) - ACQUIRED NOS
380.53 EAR CANAL (EXTERNAL) - POSTINFLAMMATION
380.52 EAR CANAL (EXTERNAL) - POSTSURGICAL
380.51 EAR CANAL (EXTERNAL) - POSTTRAUMATIC
380.89 EAR CANAL (EXTERNAL) - OTHER ACQUIRED
608.89 EJACULATORY DUCT
622.4 ENDOCERVICAL OS
752.49 ENDOCERVICAL OS CONGENITAL
654.6# ENDOCERVICAL OS COMPLICATING PREGNANCY
660.2# ENDOCERVICAL OS OBSTRUCTING LABOR **[654.6#]**

5th Digit: 654.6

- **0. EPISODE OF CARE UNSPECIFIED OR N/A**
- **1. DELIVERED**
- **2. DELIVERED WITH POSTPARTUM COMPLICATION**
- **3. ANTEPARTUM COMPLICATION**
- **4. POSTPARTUM COMPLICATION**

5th Digit: 660.2

- **0. EPISODE OF CARE UNSPECIFIED OR N/A**
- **1. DELIVERED**
- **3. ANTEPARTUM COMPLICATION**

763.89 ENDOCERVICAL OS COMPLICATING PREGNANCY AFFECTING FETUS OR NEWBORN
763.1 ENDOCERVICAL OS OBSTRUCTING LABOR AFFECTING FETUS OR NEWBORN
569.62 ENTEROSTOMY
530.3 ESOPHAGUS
750.3 ESOPHAGUS - CONGENITAL
095.8 ESOPHAGUS - SYPHILITIC
090.5 ESOPHAGUS - SYPHILITIC CONGENITAL
0 EUSTACHIAN TUBE SEE 'EUSTACHIAN', OBSTRUCTION
628.2 FALLOPIAN TUBE
098.17 FALLOPIAN TUBE GONOCOCCAL ACUTE
098.37 FALLOPIAN TUBE GONOCOCCAL CHRONIC
0 FALLOPIAN TUBE TUBERCULOUS SEE 'TUBERCULOSIS', OOPHORITIS

STENOSIS (continued)

575.2 GALLBLADDER
751.69 GALLBLADDER CONGENITAL
751.69 GALLBLADDER CONGENITAL WITH JAUNDICE [774.5]
0 GALLBLADDER WITH CALCULUS SEE 'CHOLELITHIASIS'
536.42 GASTROSTOMY
478.74 GLOTTIS
424.90 HEART OR CARDIAC VALVE NOS
746.89 HEART OR CARDIAC VALVE NOS CONGENITAL
576.2 HEPATIC DUCT
751.61 HEPATIC DUCT CONGENITAL
751.61 HEPATIC DUCT CONGENITAL WITH JAUNDICE [774.5]
0 HEPATIC DUCT WITH CALCULUS SEE 'CHOLEDOCHOLITHIASIS'
537.6 HOURGLASS, OF STOMACH
623.3 HYMEN
425.1 HYPERTROPHIC SUBAORTIC
569.62 ILEOSTOMY
746.83 INFUNDIBULUM CARDIAC
560.9 INTESTINE NOS
751.2 INTESTINE CONGENITAL LARGE
751.1 INTESTINE CONGENITAL SMALL
0 INTESTINE SEE ALSO 'INTESTINE, INTESTINAL', OBSTRUCTION
569.62 JEJUNOSTOMY
375.53 LACRIMAL CANALICULI
743.65 LACRIMAL CANALICULI CONGENITAL
375.56 LACRIMAL DUCT
743.65 LACRIMAL DUCT CONGENITAL
375.52 LACRIMAL PUNCTUM
743.65 LACRIMAL PUNCTUM CONGENITAL
375.54 LACRIMAL SAC
743.65 LACRIMAL SAC CONGENITAL
375.56 LACRIMONASAL DUCT
743.65 LACRIMONASAL DUCT CONGENITAL
375.55 LACRIMONASAL DUCT NEONATAL
478.74 LARYNX
748.3 LARYNX CONGENITAL
095.8 LARYNX SYPHILITIC
090.5 LARYNX SYPHILITIC CONGENITAL
518.89 LUNG
380.50 MEATUS OSSEOUS ACQUIRED
598.9 MEATUS URINARIUS
753.6 MEATUS URINARIUS CONGENITAL

MITRAL VALVE

394.0 NOS
396.1 AND AORTIC INSUFFICIENCY
396.1 AND AORTIC INSUFFICIENCY RHEUMATIC
396.0 AND AORTIC STENOSIS
396.0 AND AORTIC STENOSIS RHEUMATIC
421.0 BACTERIAL (ACUTE) (CHRONIC)
746.5 CONGENITAL
394.0 RHEUMATIC
093.21 SYPHILITIC
394.2 WITH INSUFFICIENCY
421.0 WITH INSUFFICIENCY BACTERIAL (ACUTE) (CHRONIC)
394.2 WITH INSUFFICIENCY RHEUMATIC
093.21 WITH INSUFFICIENCY SYPHILITIC
394.2 WITH REGURGITATION
424.0 SPECIFIED CAUSE NON RHEUMATIC

STENOSIS (continued)

429.1 MYOCARDIAL NOS
425.1 MYOCARDIAL HYPERTROPHIC SUBAORTIC (IDIOPATHIC)
478.1 NARES
748.0 NARES CONGENITAL
375.56 NASAL DUCT
743.65 NASAL DUCT CONGENITAL
375.55 NASAL DUCT NEONATAL

STENOSIS (continued)

375.56	NASOLACRIMAL DUCT
743.65	NASOLACRIMAL CONGENITAL
375.55	NASOLACRIMAL NEONATAL
095.8	NASOPHARYNX SYPHILITIC
478.1	NOSE
748.0	NOSE CONGENITAL
478.1	NOSTRIL
748.0	NOSTRIL CONGENITAL
380.50	OSSEUS MEATUS ACQUIRED
628.2	OVIDUCT
098.17	OVIDUCT GONOCOCCAL ACUTE
098.37	OVIDUCT GONOCOCCAL CHRONIC
0	OVIDUCT TUBERCULOUS SEE 'TUBERCULOSIS', OOPHORITIS
576.2	PAPILLA OF VATER
751.61	PAPILLA OF VATER CONGENITAL
0	PAPILLA OF VATER WITH CALCULUS SEE 'CHOLEDOCHOLITHIASIS'
593.3	PELVIURETERIC JUNCTION
433.9#	PRECEREBRAL ARTERY UNSPECIFIED
433.3#	PRECEREBRAL ARTERY MULTIPLE OR BILATERAL
433.8#	PRECEREBRAL ARTERY OTHER SPECIFIED

5th Digit: 433.3, 8-9
- **0. WITHOUT CEREBRAL INFARCTION**
- **1. WITH CEREBRAL INFARCTION**

417.8	PULMONARY ARTERY
747.3	PULMONARY ARTERY CONGENITAL
745.2	PULMONARY ARTERY CONGENITAL IN TETRALOGY OF FALLOT
745.2	PULMONARY ARTERY CONGENITAL WITH VENTRICULAR SEPTAL DEFECT, DEXTRAPOSITION OF AORTA AND HYPERTROPHY OF RIGHT VENTRICLE
746.83	PULMONARY INFUNDIBULAR CONGENITAL
746.83	PULMONARY SUBVALVULAR CONGENITAL

PULMONARY VALVE

424.3	NOS
421.0	BACTERIAL (ACUTE) (CHRONIC)
746.02	CONGENITAL
397.1	RHEUMATIC
093.24	SYPHILITIC
424.3	WITH INSUFFICIENCY
421.0	WITH INSUFFICIENCY BACTERIAL (ACUTE) (CHRONIC)
397.1	WITH INSUFFICIENCY RHEUMATIC
093.24	WITH INSUFFICIENCY SYPHILITIC

STENOSIS (continued)

417.8	PULMONARY VEIN OR VESSEL
747.49	PULMONARY VEIN CONGENITAL
537.0	PYLORUS
750.5	PYLORUS CONGENITAL OR INFANTILE
569.2	RECTUM AND ANUS
751.2	RECTUM CONGENITAL
569.2	RECTUM DUE TO IRRADIATION
095.8	RECTUM SYPHILITIC
440.1	RENAL ARTERY
527.8	SALIVARY DUCT
576.2	SPHINCTER OF ODDI
751.61	SPHINCTER OF ODDI CONGENITAL
751.61	SPHINCTER OF ODDI CONGENITAL WITH JAUNDICE [774.5]
0	SPHINCTER OF ODDI WITH CALCULUS SEE 'CHOLEDOCHOLITHIASIS'
724.00	SPINAL - UNSPECIFIED REGION
723.0	SPINAL - CERVICAL
724.02	SPINAL - LUMBAR OR LUMBOSACRAL
724.9	SPINAL - NERVE (ROOT) NEC
724.01	SPINAL - THORACIC OR THORACOLUMBAR
724.09	SPINAL - OTHER SPECIFIED REGION NEC

STENOSIS (continued)

537.89	STOMACH
750.7	STOMACH CONGENITAL
537.6	STOMACH, HOURGLASS
746.81	SUBAORTIC
425.1	SUBAORTIC HYPERTROPHIC (IDIOPATHIC)
433.8#	SUBCLAVIAN ARTERY

5th Digit: 433.8
- **0. WITHOUT CEREBRAL INFARCTION**
- **1. WITH CEREBRAL INFARCTION**

478.74	SUBGLOTTIC
747.22	SUPRA (VALVULAR)-AORTIC
095.8	SYPHILITIC NEC
519.1	TRACHEA
748.3	TRACHEA CONGENITAL
095.8	TRACHEA SYPHILITIC
0	TRACHEA TUBERCULOUS SEE 'TUBERCULOSIS', RESPIRATORY OTHER SPECIFIED
519.02	TRACHEOSTOMY

TRICUSPID VALVE

424.2	NOS
746.1	AND ATRESIA CONGENITAL
421.0	BACTERIAL
746.1	CONGENITAL
397.0	RHEUMATIC
093.23	SYPHILITIC
421.0	WITH INSUFFICIENCY BACTERIAL (ACUTE) (CHRONIC)
093.23	WITH INSUFFICIENCY SYPHILITIC

STENOSIS (continued)

628.2	TUBAL
098.17	TUBAL GONOCOCCAL ACUTE
098.37	TUBAL GONOCOCCAL CHRONIC
0	TUBAL TUBERCULOUS SEE 'TUBERCULOSIS', OOPHORITIS
593.3	URETER
753.29	URETER CONGENITAL
593.3	URETER POSTOPERATIVE
593.3	URETEROPELVIC JUNCTION
753.21	URETEROPELVIC JUNCTION CONGENITAL
593.3	URETEROVESICAL ORIFICE
753.22	URETEROVESICAL ORIFICE CONGENITAL
598.9	URETHRA
753.6	URETHRA - CONGENITAL
753.6	URETHRA - VALVE CONGENITAL
0	URETHRA - WITH INCONTINENCE CONGENITAL SEE 'URETHRA, URETHRAL DISORDERS WITH INCONTINENCE'
598.9	URINARY MEATUS
753.6	URINARY MEATUS CONGENITAL
621.5	UTERUS
623.2	VAGINA
752.49	VAGINA CONGENITAL
654.7#	VAGINA COMPLICATING PREGNANCY

5th Digit: 654.7
- **0. EPISODE OF CARE UNSPECIFIED OR N/A**
- **1. DELIVERED**
- **2. DELIVERED WITH POSTPARTUM COMPLICATION**
- **3. ANTEPARTUM COMPLICATION**
- **4. POSTPARTUM COMPLICATION**

763.89	VAGINA COMPLICATING PREGNANCY AFFECTING FETUS OR NEWBORN
660.2#	VAGINA OBSTRUCTING LABOR [**654.7#**]

5th Digit: 654.7
- **0. EPISODE OF CARE UNSPECIFIED OR N/A**
- **1. DELIVERED**
- **2. DELIVERED WITH POSTPARTUM COMPLICATION**
- **3. ANTEPARTUM COMPLICATION**
- **4. POSTPARTUM COMPLICATION**

5th Digit: 660.2
- **0. EPISODE OF CARE UNSPECIFIED OR N/A**
- **1. DELIVERED**
- **3. ANTEPARTUM COMPLICATION**

STENOSIS (continued)
763.1 VAGINA OBSTRUCTING LABOR AFFECTING FETUS OR NEWBORN
0 VALVE HEART OR CARDIAC SEE BY SPECIFIC VALVE
753.6 VALVE URETHRA CONGENITAL
996.1 VASCULAR GRAFT OR SHUNT-MECHANICAL COMPLICATION
996.74 VASCULAR GRAFT OR SHUNT-EMBOLISM, OCCLUSION OR THROMBUS
459.2 VEIN
459.2 VENA CAVA
747.49 VENA CAVA CONGENITAL
996.2 VENTRICULAR SHUNT-MECHANICAL COMPLICATION
433.2# VERTEBRAL ARTERY
433.3# VERTEBRAL ARTERY BILATERAL OR MULTIPLE

5th Digit: 433.2-3
0. WITHOUT CEREBRAL INFARCTION
1. WITH CEREBRAL INFARCTION

596.0 VESICOURETHRAL ORIFICE
753.6 VESICOURETHRAL ORIFICE CONGENITAL
624.8 VULVA

527.8 STENSEN'S DUCT OBSTRUCTION
543.9 STERCOLITH APPENDIX
368.33 STEREOPSIS DEFECT WITH VISUAL FUSION
307.3 STEREOTYPIES
0 STERILITY SEE 'INFERTILITY'
V26.51 STERILIZATION STATUS - TUBAL LIGATION
V26.52 STERILIZATION STATUS - VASECTOMY
V25.2 STERILIZATION
0 STERNBERG'S DISEASE SEE 'HODGKIN'S DISEASE'
739.8 STERNOCHONDRAL REGION SEGMENTAL OR SOMATIC DYSFUNCTION

STERNOCLAVICULAR
739.7 REGION SEGMENTAL OR SOMATIC DYSFUNCTION
848.41 SEPARATION (RUPTURE) (TEAR) (LACERATION)
848.41 STRAIN (SPRAIN) (AVULSION) (HEMARTHROSIS)

754.1 STERNOCLEIDOMASTOID CONTRACTURE CONGENITAL
754.1 STERNOCLEIDOMASTOID MUSCLE DEFORMITY CONGENITAL
754.1 STERNOMASTOID TORTICOLLIS CONGENITAL
754.1 STERNOMASTOID TUMOR CONGENITAL

STERNUM, STERNAL
756.3 ABSENCE CONGENITAL
756.3 BIFIDUM CONGENITAL
756.3 FISSURE CONGENITAL
786.9 RETRACTION DURING RESPIRATION
848.40 SEPARATION (RUPTURE) (TEAR) (LACERATION)
848.40 STRAIN (SPRAIN) (AVULSION) (HEMARTHROSIS)

255.2 STEROID METABOLISM DISORDER
695.1 STEVENS JOHNSON SYNDROME (ERYTHEMA MULTIFORME EXUDATIVUM)
733.3 STEWART-MOREL SYNDROME (HYPEROSTOSIS FRONTALIS INTERNA)
057.0 STICKER'S DISEASE (ERYTHEMA INFECTIOSUM)
286.9 STICKY PLATELET SYNDROME
726.62 STIEDA'S DISEASE (CALCIFICATION KNEE JOINT)

STIFF, STIFFNESS
724.8 BACK NOS
719.5# JOINT NEC

5th Digit: 719.5
0. SITE NOS
1. SHOULDER REGION
2. UPPER ARM (ELBOW) (HUMERUS)
3. FOREARM (RADIUS) (WRIST) (ULNA)
4. HAND (CARPAL) (METACARPAL) (FINGERS)
5. PELVIC REGION AND THIGH (HIP) (BUTTOCK) (FEMUR)
6. LOWER LEG (FIBULA) (KNEE) (PATELLA) (TIBIA)
7. ANKLE AND/OR FOOT (METATARSALS) (TOES) (TARSALS)
8. OTHER
9. MULTIPLE

724.6 LUMBOSACRAL
333.91 MAN SYNDROME
723.5 NECK
724.6 SACROILIAC
724.9 SPINE

714.30 STILL'S DISEASE (JUVENILE RHEUMATOID ARTHRITIS)
714.1 STILL-FELTY DISEASE OR SYNDROME (JUVENILE RHEUMATOID ARTHRITIS WITH SPLENOMEGALY AND LEUKOPENIA)
779.9 STILLBIRTH NEC
V23.5 STILLBIRTH HISTORY AFFECTING PREGNANCY SUPERVISION
656.4# STILLBORN (FETAL DEATH) AFFECTING MANAGEMENT OF MOTHER

5th Digit: 656.4
0. EPISODE OF CARE NOS OR N/A
1. DELIVERED
3. ANTEPARTUM COMPLICATION

780.79 STILLER'S DISEASE (ASTHENIA)
378.71 STILLING-TURK-DUANE SYNDROME (OCULAR RETRACTION SYNDROME)

STING VENOMOUS
0 SEE ALSO 'BITE VENOMOUS'
989.5 AGUA MALA
995.0 AGUA MALA WITH ANAPHYLAXIS [989.5]
989.5 ANT BITE
995.0 ANT BITE WITH ANAPHYLAXIS [989.5]
989.5 ARTHROPOD NEC
995.0 ARTHROPOD NEC WITH ANAPHYLAXIS [989.5]
989.5 BEE
995.0 BEE WITH ANAPHYLAXIS [989.5]
989.5 CATERPILLAR
995.0 CATERPILLAR WITH ANAPHYLAXIS [989.5]
989.5 CENTIPEDE
995.0 CENTIPEDE WITH ANAPHYLAXIS [989.5]
989.5 CORAL
995.0 CORAL WITH ANAPHYLAXIS [989.5]
989.5 FIRE ANT
995.0 FIRE ANT WITH ANAPHYLAXIS [989.5]
989.5 HORNET
995.0 HORNET WITH ANAPHYLAXIS [989.5]
989.5 INSECT POISONOUS
995.0 INSECT POISONOUS WITH ANAPHYLAXIS [989.5]
989.5 JELLYFISH
995.0 JELLYFISH WITH ANAPHYLAXIS [989.5]
989.5 KRAIT
995.0 KRAIT WITH ANAPHYLAXIS [989.5]
909.1 LATE EFFECT
909.9 LATE EFFECT WITH ANAPHYLAXIS
989.5 MARINE ANIMALS OR PLANTS
995.0 MARINE ANIMALS OR PLANTS WITH ANAPHYLAXIS [989.5]
989.5 MARINE PLANT
995.0 MARINE PLANT WITH ANAPHYLAXIS [989.5]

STING VENOMOUS (continued)
989.5 MILLIPEDE (TROPICAL)
995.0 MILLIPEDE (TROPICAL) WITH ANAPHYLAXIS [989.5]
989.5 NEMATOCYST
995.0 NEMATOCYST WITH ANAPHYLAXIS [989.5]
989.5 SCORPION
995.0 SCORPION WITH ANAPHYLAXIS [989.5]
989.5 SEA ANEMONE
995.0 SEA ANEMONE WITH ANAPHYLAXIS [989.5]
989.5 SEA CUCUMBER
995.0 SEA CUCUMBER WITH ANAPHYLAXIS [989.5]
989.5 SEA URCHIN
995.0 SEA URCHIN WITH ANAPHYLAXIS [989.5]
989.5 SNAKE
995.0 SNAKE WITH ANAPHYLAXIS [989.5]
989.5 WASP
995.0 WASP WITH ANAPHYLAXIS [989.5]

STITCH
998.59 ABSCESS POSTOPERATIVE
998.3 BURST
998.89 GRANULOMA POSTOPERATIVE - EXTERNAL
998.89 GRANULOMA POSTOPERATIVE - INTERNAL
998.4 INADVERTENTLY LEFT IN WOUND
998.89 PAIN (WIRE)
V58.3 REMOVAL

098.86 STOJANO'S (SUBCOSTAL) SYNDROME

242.0# STOKES' DISEASE (EXOPHTHALMIC GOITER)
5th Digit: 242.0
0. WITHOUT MENTION OF THYROTOXIC CRISIS OR STORM
1. WITH MENTION OF THYROTOXIC CRISIS OR STORM

426.9 STOKES-ADAMS SYNDROME (SYNCOPE WITH HEART BLOCK)

289.7 STOKVIS' DISEASE OR SYNDROME (ENTEROGENOUS CYANOSIS)

STOMACH
V45.89 ABSENCE (ACQUIRED) (PARTIAL) (POSTOPERATIVE)
750.7 ABSENCE (ACQUIRED) (PARTIAL) (POSTOPERATIVE) - CONGENITAL
564.2 ABSENCE (ACQUIRED) (PARTIAL) (POSTOPERATIVE) - WITH POSTGASTRIC SURGERY SYNDROME
536.8 ACHE
536.3 ATONY
537.89 ATROPHY
536.8 CONTRACTION
750.7 CONTRACTION CONGENITAL
306.4 CONTRACTION PSYCHOGENIC
789.06 CRAMP
536.1 DILATATION ACUTE
536.1 DISTENTION ACUTE
537.9 DISORDER
536.9 DISORDER (FUNCTIONAL)
306.4 DISORDER (FUNCTIONAL) PSYCHOGENIC
750.7 DISPLACEMENT CONGENITAL
537.1 DIVERTICULUM
750.7 DIVERTICULUM CONGENITAL
750.7 DUPLICATION CONGENITAL
536.8 ENGORGEMENT
793.4 FILLING DEFECT
536.3 GASTROPARESIS
750.7 HOURGLASS ANOMALY CONGENITAL
863.0 INJURY
863.1 INJURY WITH OPEN WOUND
908.1 INJURY LATE EFFECT

STOMACH (continued)
277.3 LARDACEOUS
537.89 OBSTRUCTION
536.1 OBSTRUCTION ACUTE
750.7 OBSTRUCTION CONGENITAL
536.8 SPASM
750.7 TRANSPOSITION CONGENITAL

STOMATITIS
528.0 NOS
101 ACUTE NECROTIZING (ULCERATIVE)
528.2 APHTHOUS
528.9 DENTURE
078.4 EPIZOOTIC
528.1 GANGRENOUS
054.2 HERPES (SIMPLEX)
528.2 HERPETIFORMIS
101 SPIROCHETAL
528.0 ULCERATIVE
528.0 VESICULAR
101 VINCENT'S

282.8 STOMATOCYTOSIS

0 STONE COMMON DUCT SEE 'CHOLEDOCHOLITHIASIS'
0 STONE SEE 'CALCULUS'
428.1 STONE HEART SYNDROME

502 STONEMASONS' DISEASE

STOOL
787.7 ABNORMAL
792.1 ABNORMAL CONTENT
578.1 BLOOD
792.1 BLOOD OCCULT
787.7 BULKY
792.1 COLOR ABNORMAL
792.1 CULTURE POSITIVE
792.1 FAT ELEVATED ABNORMAL
792.1 MUCUS ELEVATED ABNORMAL
792.1 MELENOTIC
772.4 MELENOTIC OF NEWBORN DUE TO FETAL G.I. HEMORRHAGE
777.3 MELENOTIC OF NEWBORN DUE TO SWALLOWED MATERNAL BLOOD
792.1 PUS ELEVATED ABNORMAL

368.01 STRABISMIC AMBLYOPIA

STRABISMUS MECHANICAL
378.60 NOS
378.61 BROWN'S TENDON SYNDROME
378.62 FROM OTHER MUSCULOFACIAL DISORDERS
378.63 ASSOCIATED WITH OTHER CONDITIONS

STRABISMUS OTHER ETIOLOGY OR UNSPECIFIED
378.9 NOS
378.71 DUANE'S SYNDROME
378.72 DUE TO OTHER NEUROMUSCULAR DISORDERS
378.72 DUE TO PROGRESSIVE EXTERNAL OPHTHALMOPLEGIA
378.73 IN OTHER NEUROMUSCULAR DISORDERS
0 SEE ALSO 'ESOTROPIA' OR 'EXOTROPIA'

STRABISMUS PARALYTIC
378.50 NOS
378.51 THIRD NERVE PALSY PARTIAL
378.52 THIRD NERVE PALSY TOTAL
378.53 FOURTH NERVE PALSY
378.54 SIXTH NERVE PALSY
378.55 EXTERNAL (OPHTHALMOPLEGIA)
378.56 TOTAL PARALYSIS (OPHTHALMOPLEGIA)

756.19 STRAIGHT-BACK SYNDROME

MEDICALLY, A SPRAIN OCCURS WHEN EXCESSIVE FORCE CAUSES INJURY TO A LIGAMENT, AND A STRAIN OCCURS WHEN EXCESSIVE FORCE CAUSES INJURY TO A MUSCLE OR TENDON. IN ICD-9, THOUGH, SPRAIN IS THE TERM USED TO COVER ALL SPRAINS, STRAINS, AVULSIONS, HEMARTHROSES, TEARS AND RUPTURES. IN EASY CODER YOU'LL FIND THAT CODES FOR ALL OF THE ABOVE CONDITIONS ARE LISTED BY SITE UNDER THE HEADING, SPRAIN.

S

STRAIN

847.9 BACK - NOS
847.0 BACK - CERVICAL
846.9 BACK - LOW
847.2 BACK - LUMBAR (SPINE)
846.0 BACK - LUMBOSACRAL
724.6 BACK - LUMBOSACRAL (JOINT) (LIGAMENT) CHRONIC (OLD)
846.9 BACK - SACROILIAC (REGION)
846.1 BACK - SACROILIAC LIGAMENT
724.6 BACK - SACROILIAC CHRONIC (OLD)
846.8 BACK - SACROILIAC REGION OTHER SPECIFIED SITES
846.2 BACK - SACROSPINATUS (LIGAMENT)
846.3 BACK - SACROTUBEROUS (LIGAMENT)
368.13 EYE NEC
0 LATE EFFECT SEE 'LATE EFFECT' SPRAIN
V62.89 PHYSICAL
V62.89 PSYCHOLOGICAL NEC
0 SEE ALSO 'SPRAIN'

994.7 STRANGULATION
909.4 STRANGULATION LATE EFFECT
788.1 STRANGURY
757.32 STRAWBERRY NEVUS CONGENITAL
026.1 STREPTOBACILLARY FEVER

STREPTOCOCCAL

034.0 ANGINA
0 ARTHRITIS SEE 'ARTHRITIS OTHER SPECIFIED', PYOGENIC
V02.51 B CARRIER
V28.6 B SCREENING ANTENATAL
V02.51 CARRIER GROUP B
V02.52 CARRIER OTHER
V01.8 EXPOSURE
041.0# INFECTION OR ORGANISM

5th Digit: 041.0

- **0. NOS**
- **1. GROUP A**
- **2. GROUP B**
- **3. GROUP C**
- **4. GROUP D (ENTEROCOCCUS)**
- **5. GROUP G**
- **9. OTHER STREP**

034.0 LARYNGITIS
034.0 PHARYNGITIS
482.3# PNEUMONIA

5th Digit: 482.3

- **0. NOS**
- **1. GROUP A**
- **2. GROUP B**
- **9. OTHER STREPTOCOCCUS**

V03.82 PNEUMONIAE VACCINATION
V06.6 PNEUMONIAE AND INFLUENZA VACCINATION
038.0 SEPSIS
034.0 SORE THROAT
034.0 TONSILLITIS

686.00 STREPTODERMA (SKIN)
0 STREPTOMYCES SEE 'ACTINOMYCOSIS'

309.81 STRESS DISORDER POSTTRAUMATIC PROLONGED
733.1# STRESS FRACTURE

5th Digit: 733.1

- **0. UNSPECIFIED SITE**
- **1. HUMERUS**
- **2. DISTAL RADIUS AND ULNA, WRIST**
- **3. VERTEBRA**
- **4. NECK OF FEMUR, FEMUR NOS, HIP NOS**
- **5. OTHER SPECIFIED PART OF FEMUR**
- **6. TIBIA OR FIBULA, ANKLE**
- **9. OTHER SPECIFIED SITE**

625.6 STRESS INCONTINENCE FEMALE
788.32 STRESS INCONTINENCE MALE

STRESS REACTION

308.9 ACUTE UNSPECIFIED
308.2 ACUTE AGITATION OR STUPOR
308.0 ACUTE ANXIETY
308.1 ACUTE FUGUES
308.2 ACUTE STUPOR
308.4 ACUTE MIXED DISORDER
308.3 ACUTE OR BRIEF POSTTRAUMATIC DISORDER
308.3 ACUTE OTHER
308.9 ACUTE REACTION
308.3 ACUTE SITUATIONAL DISTURBANCES
308.1 ACUTE WITH DISTURBANCES OF CONSCIOUSNESS
308.0 ACUTE WITH PANIC ANXIETY
0 CHRONIC SEE ALSO 'ADJUSTMENT REACTION'
308.0 DEPRESSED
308.3 POSTTRAUMATIC ACUTE (BRIEF)
309.81 POSTTRAUMATIC CHRONIC
309.81 POSTTRAUMATIC PROLONGED
308.2 PSYCHOMOTOR

STRESS - REASON FOR ENCOUNTER

V62.3 EDUCATIONAL
V62.81 INTERPERSONAL
V62.5 LEGAL
V62.89 LIFE CIRCUMSTANCE
V62.82 LOSS OF LOVED ONE
V62.2 OCCUPATIONAL
V62.89 PHYSICAL
V62.89 PSYCHOLOGICAL NEC
V62.4 SOCIAL MALADJUSTMENT
V62.0 UNEMPLOYMENT (DUE TO)
V62.1 WORK

701.3 STRETCH MARK
701.3 STRIAE ATROPHICAE
701.3 STRIAE DISTENSAE
333.0 STRIATONIGRAL ATROPHY OR DEGENERATION BASAL GANGLIA
333.90 STRIATOPALLIDAL SYSTEM DISEASE
333.89 STRIATOPALLIDAL SYSTEM DISEASE SPECIFIED NEC

STRICTURE

0 SEE ALSO 'STENOSIS'
799.8 NOS
576.2 AMPULLA OF VATER
0 AMPULLA OF VATER WITH CALCULUS SEE 'CHOLEDOCHOLITHIASIS'
569.2 ANUS
751.2 ANUS CONGENITAL OR INFANTILE
747.22 AORTA (ASCENDING)
747.10 AORTA ARCH
440.0 AORTA ARTERIOSCLEROTIC OR CALCIFIED
424.1 AORTIC VALVE
746.3 AORTIC VALVE CONGENITAL
331.4 AQUEDUCT OF SYLVIUS
742.3 AQUEDUCT OF SYLVIUS CONGENITAL
0 AQUEDUCT OF SYLVIUS CONGENITAL WITH SPINA BIFIDA SEE 'SPINA BIFIDA'
447.1 ARTERY NEC

STRICTURE (continued)

747.6# ARTERY PERIPHERAL VASCULAR CONGENITAL

5th Digit: 747.6

0. PERIPHERAL VASCULAR UNSPECIFIED SITE
1. GASTROINTESTINAL VESSEL
2. RENAL VESSEL
3. UPPER LIMB VESSEL
4. LOWER LIMB VESSEL
9. OTHER SPECIFIED SITE PERIPHERAL VASCULAR

380.50 AUDITORY CANAL
744.02 AUDITORY CANAL CONGENITAL
433.0# BASILAR ARTERY
433.3# BASILAR ARTERY BILATERAL OR MULTIPLE

5th Digit: 433.0, 3

0. WITHOUT CEREBRAL INFARCTION
1. WITH CEREBRAL INFARCTION

576.2 BILE DUCT
751.61 BILE DUCT CONGENITAL
751.61 BILE DUCT CONGENITAL WITH JAUNDICE [774.5]
0 BILE DUCT WITH CALCULUS SEE 'CHOLEDOCHOLITHIASIS'
596.8 BLADDER
753.6 BLADDER CONGENITAL
596.0 BLADDER NECK
753.6 BLADDER NECK CONGENITAL
0 BLADDER NECK WITH INCONTINENCE SEE 'BLADDER DISORDERS WITH INCONTINENCE'
560.9 BOWEL NOS
751.2 BOWEL CONGENITAL LARGE
751.1 BOWEL CONGENITAL SMALL
0 BOWEL SEE ALSO 'INTESTINE, INTESTINAL', OBSTRUCTION
348.8 BRAIN
519.1 BRONCHUS
095.8 BRONCHUS SYPHILITIC
537.89 CARDIA (STOMACH)
750.7 CARDIA (STOMACH) CONGENITAL
429.2 CARDIOVASCULAR
433.1# CAROTID ARTERY
433.3# CAROTID ARTERY BILATERAL OR MULTIPLE

5th Digit: 433.1, 3

0. WITHOUT CEREBRAL INFARCTION
1. WITH CEREBRAL INFARCTION

560.9 CECUM NOS
751.2 CECUM CONGENITAL
0 CECUM SEE ALSO 'INTESTINE, INTESTINAL', OBSTRUCTION
447.4 CELIAC ARTERY
437.0 CEREBRAL ARTERY NOS
747.81 CEREBRAL ARTERY CONGENITAL
434.1# CEREBRAL ARTERY DUE TO EMBOLISM
434.0# CEREBRAL ARTERY DUE TO THROMBUS

5th Digit: 434.0, 1

0. WITHOUT CEREBRAL INFARCTION
1. WITH CEREBRAL INFARCTION

622.4 CERVIX
654.6# CERVIX - COMPLICATING PREGNANCY

5th Digit: 654.6

0. EPISODE OF CARE UNSPECIFIED OR N/A
1. DELIVERED
2. DELIVERED WITH POSTPARTUM COMPLICATION
3. ANTEPARTUM COMPLICATION
4. POSTPARTUM COMPLICATION

763.89 CERVIX - COMPLICATING PREGNANCY AFFECTING FETUS OR NEWBORN
752.49 CERVIX - CONGENITAL

STRICTURE (continued)

660.2# CERVIX - OBSTRUCTING LABOR **[654.6#]**

5th Digit: 654.6

0. EPISODE OF CARE UNSPECIFIED OR N/A
1. DELIVERED
2. DELIVERED WITH POSTPARTUM COMPLICATION
3. ANTEPARTUM COMPLICATION
4. POSTPARTUM COMPLICATION

5th Digit: 660.2

0. EPISODE OF CARE UNSPECIFIED OR N/A
1. DELIVERED
3. ANTEPARTUM COMPLICATION

763.1 CERVIX - OBSTRUCTING LABOR AFFECTING FETUS OR NEWBORN
560.9 COLON
751.2 COLON CONGENITAL
0 COLON SEE ALSO 'INTESTINE, INTESTINAL', OBSTRUCTION
569.62 COLOSTOMY
576.2 COMMON BILE DUCT
751.61 COMMON BILE DUCT CONGENITAL
751.61 COMMON BILE DUCT CONGENITAL WITH JAUNDICE [774.5]
0 COMMON BILE DUCT WITH CALCULUS SEE 'CHOLEDOCHOLITHIASIS'
746.85 CORONARY ARTERY CONGENITAL
0 CORONARY SEE 'ARTERIOSCLEROSIS, ARTERIOSCLEROTIC', CORONARY
575.2 CYSTIC DUCT
751.61 CYSTIC DUCT CONGENITAL
751.61 CYSTIC DUCT CONGENITAL WITH JAUNDICE [774.5]
0 CYSTIC DUCT WITH CALCULUS SEE 'CHOLELITHIASIS'
0 DUE TO ANY DEVICE, IMPLANT OR GRAFT SEE 'COMPLICATION OF AN INTERNAL PROSTHETIC DEVICE, IMPLANT OR GRAFT - (EMBOLUS) (FIBROSIS) (HEMORRHAGE) (PAIN) (STENOSIS) (THROMBUS)'
997.5 CYSTOSTOMY
751.8 DIGESTIVE ORGANS NEC, CONGENITAL
537.3 DUODENUM
751.1 DUODENUM CONGENITAL
380.50 EAR CANAL
744.02 EAR CANAL - CONGENITAL
380.53 EAR CANAL - POSTINFLAMMATION
380.52 EAR CANAL - POSTSURGICAL
380.51 EAR CANAL - POSTTRAUMATIC
608.85 EJACULATORY DUCT
622.4 ENDOCERVICAL OS
752.49 ENDOCERVICAL OS CONGENITAL
654.6# ENDOCERVICAL OS COMPLICATING PREGNANCY
660.2# ENDOCERVICAL OS OBSTRUCTING LABOR **[654.6#]**

5th Digit: 654.6

0. EPISODE OF CARE UNSPECIFIED OR N/A
1. DELIVERED
2. DELIVERED WITH POSTPARTUM COMPLICATION
3. ANTEPARTUM COMPLICATION
4. POSTPARTUM COMPLICATION

5th Digit: 660.2

0. EPISODE OF CARE UNSPECIFIED OR N/A
1. DELIVERED
3. ANTEPARTUM COMPLICATION

763.89 ENDOCERVICAL OS COMPLICATING PREGNANCY AFFECTING FETUS OR NEWBORN
763.1 ENDOCERVICAL OS OBSTRUCTING LABOR AFFECTING FETUS OR NEWBORN
569.62 ENTEROSTOMY
530.3 ESOPHAGUS
750.3 ESOPHAGUS - CONGENITAL
095.8 ESOPHAGUS - SYPHILITIC
090.5 ESOPHAGUS - SYPHILITIC CONGENITAL
0 EUSTACHIAN TUBE SEE 'EUSTACHIAN', OBSTRUCTION
0 EUSTACHIAN TUBE CONGENITAL SEE 'EUSTACHIAN', ANOMALY

S

STRICTURE (continued)

628.2 FALLOPIAN TUBE
098.17 FALLOPIAN TUBE - GONOCOCCAL ACUTE
098.37 FALLOPIAN TUBE - GONOCOCCAL CHRONIC
0 FALLOPIAN TUBE - TUBERCULOUS SEE 'TUBERCULOSIS', OOPHORITIS
575.2 GALLBLADDER
751.69 GALLBLADDER CONGENITAL
751.69 GALLBLADDER CONGENITAL WITH JAUNDICE [774.5]
0 GALLBLADDER WITH CALCULUS SEE 'CHOLELITHIASIS'
536.42 GASTROSTOMY
478.74 GLOTTIS
746.89 HEART VALVE NOS CONGENITAL
576.2 HEPATIC DUCT
751.61 HEPATIC DUCT - CONGENITAL
751.61 HEPATIC DUCT - CONGENITAL WITH JAUNDICE [774.5]
0 HEPATIC DUCT - WITH CALCULUS SEE 'CHOLEDOCHOLITHIASIS'
537.6 HOURGLASS, OF STOMACH
623.3 HYMEN
425.1 HYPERTROPHIC SUBAORTIC
478.29 HYPOPHARYNX
569.62 ILEOSTOMY
746.83 INFUNDIBULUM CARDIAC
560.9 INTESTINE - NOS
751.2 INTESTINE - CONGENITAL LARGE
751.1 INTESTINE - CONGENITAL SMALL
557.1 INTESTINE - ISCHEMIC
0 INTESTINE - SEE ALSO 'INTESTINE, INTESTINAL', OBSTRUCTION
569.62 JEJUNOSTOMY
375.53 LACRIMAL CANALICULI
743.65 LACRIMAL CANALICULI CONGENITAL
375.56 LACRIMAL DUCT
743.65 LACRIMAL DUCT CONGENITAL
375.52 LACRIMAL PUNCTUM
743.65 LACRIMAL PUNCTUM CONGENITAL
375.54 LACRIMAL SAC
743.65 LACRIMAL SAC CONGENITAL
375.56 LACRIMONASAL DUCT
743.65 LACRIMONASAL DUCT CONGENITAL
375.55 LACRIMONASAL DUCT NEONATAL
478.79 LARYNX
748.3 LARYNX CONGENITAL
095.8 LARYNX SYPHILITIC
090.5 LARYNX SYPHILITIC CONGENITAL
518.89 LUNG
380.50 MEATUS EAR
744.02 MEATUS EAR - CONGENITAL
380.53 MEATUS EAR - POSTINFLAMMATION
380.52 MEATUS EAR - POSTSURGICAL
380.51 MEATUS EAR - POSTTRAUMATIC
380.50 MEATUS OSSEOUS
744.03 MEATUS OSSEOUS CONGENITAL
598.9 MEATUS URINARIUS
753.6 MEATUS URINARIUS CONGENITAL
394.0 MITRAL VALVE NOS
746.5 MITRAL VALVE CONGENITAL
424.0 MITRAL VALVE SPECIFIED CAUSE EXCEPT RHEUMATIC
093.21 MITRAL VALVE SYPHILITIC
429.1 MYOCARDIAL NOS
425.1 MYOCARDIAL HYPERTROPHIC SUBAORTIC (IDIOPATHIC)
478.1 NARES
748.0 NARES CONGENITAL
375.56 NASAL DUCT
743.65 NASAL DUCT CONGENITAL
375.55 NASAL DUCT NEONATAL
375.56 NASOLACRIMAL DUCT
743.65 NASOLACRIMAL CONGENITAL
375.55 NASOLACRIMAL NEONATAL
478.29 NASOPHARYNX
095.8 NASOPHARYNX SYPHILITIC

STRICTURE (continued)

997.5 NEPHROSTOMY
478.1 NOSE, NOSTRIL
748.0 NOSE, NOSTRIL CONGENITAL
622.4 OS UTERI
752.49 OS UTERI CONGENITAL
654.6# OS UTERI COMPLICATING PREGNANCY
660.2# OS UTERI OBSTRUCTING LABOR **[654.6#]**

5th Digit: 654.6

0. EPISODE OF CARE UNSPECIFIED OR N/A
1. DELIVERED
2. DELIVERED WITH POSTPARTUM COMPLICATION
3. ANTEPARTUM COMPLICATION
4. POSTPARTUM COMPLICATION

5th Digit: 660.2

0. EPISODE OF CARE UNSPECIFIED OR N/A
1. DELIVERED
3. ANTEPARTUM COMPLICATION

763.89 OS UTERI COMPLICATING PREGNANCY AFFECTING FETUS OR NEWBORN
763.1 OS UTERI OBSTRUCTING LABOR AFFECTING FETUS OR NEWBORN
380.50 OSSEUS MEATUS
744.03 OSSEUS MEATUS CONGENITAL
628.2 OVIDUCT
098.17 OVIDUCT GONOCOCCAL ACUTE
098.37 OVIDUCT GONOCOCCAL CHRONIC
0 OVIDUCT TUBERCULOUS SEE 'TUBERCULOSIS', OOPHORITIS
576.2 PAPILLA OF VATER
0 PAPILLA OF VATER WITH CALCULUS SEE 'CHOLEDOCHOLITHIASIS'
593.3 PELVIURETERIC JUNCTION
478.29 PHARYNX
433.9# PRECEREBRAL ARTERY UNSPECIFIED
433.3# PRECEREBRAL ARTERY MULTIPLE OR BILATERAL
433.8# PRECEREBRAL ARTERY OTHER SPECIFIED

5th Digit: 433.3, 8-9

0. WITHOUT CEREBRAL INFARCTION
1. WITH CEREBRAL INFARCTION

602.8 PROSTATE
417.8 PULMONARY ARTERY
747.3 PULMONARY ARTERY CONGENITAL
746.83 PULMONARY INFUNDIBULAR CONGENITAL
746.83 PULMONARY SUBVALVULAR CONGENITAL
424.3 PULMONARY VALVE
746.02 PULMONARY VALVE CONGENITAL
417.8 PULMONARY VEIN OR VESSEL
747.49 PULMONARY VEIN CONGENITAL
537.0 PYLORUS
750.5 PYLORUS CONGENITAL OR INFANTILE
569.89 RECTOSIGMOID
569.2 RECTUM
751.2 RECTUM - CONGENITAL
947.3 RECTUM - DUE TO CHEMICAL BURN
569.2 RECTUM - DUE TO IRRADIATION
099.1 RECTUM - DUE TO LYMPHOGRANULOMA VENEREUM
098.7 RECTUM - GONOCOCCAL
099.1 RECTUM - INFLAMMATORY
095.8 RECTUM - SYPHILITIC
0 RECTUM - TUBERCULOUS SEE 'TUBERCULOSIS', RECTUM
440.1 RENAL ARTERY
747.62 RENAL ARTERY CONGENITAL
743.58 RETINAL ARTERY CONGENITAL
527.8 SALIVARY DUCT
608.85 SPERMATIC CORD
576.2 SPHINCTER OF ODDI
751.61 SPHINCTER OF ODDI CONGENITAL
751.61 SPHINCTER OF ODDI CONGENITAL WITH JAUNDICE [774.5]
0 SPHINCTER OF ODDI WITH CALCULUS SEE 'CHOLEDOCHOLITHIASIS'
747.82 SPINAL ARTERY CONGENITAL

S

STRICTURE (continued)

537.89 STOMACH
750.7 STOMACH CONGENITAL
537.6 STOMACH, HOURGLASS
746.81 SUBAORTIC CONGENITAL
425.1 SUBAORTIC HYPERTROPHIC ACQUIRED (IDIOPATHIC)
478.74 SUBGLOTTIC
747.22 SUPRA (VALVULAR)-AORTIC
095.8 SYPHILITIC NEC
727.81 TENDON (SHEATH)
519.1 TRACHEA
748.3 TRACHEA CONGENITAL
095.8 TRACHEA SYPHILITIC
0 TRACHEA TUBERCULOUS SEE 'TUBERCULOSIS', RESPIRATORY OTHER SPECIFIED
519.02 TRACHEOSTOMY
0 TRICUSPID SEE 'TRICUSPID', STENOSIS
628.2 TUBAL
098.17 TUBAL GONOCOCCAL ACUTE
098.37 TUBAL GONOCOCCAL CHRONIC
0 TUBAL TUBERCULOUS SEE 'TUBERCULOSIS', OOPHORITIS
608.85 TUNICA VAGINALIS
747.5 UMBILICAL ARTERY CONGENITAL
593.3 URETER
753.29 URETER CONGENITAL
593.3 URETER POSTOPERATIVE
593.3 URETEROPELVIC JUNCTION
753.21 URETEROPELVIC JUNCTION CONGENITAL
997.5 URETEROSTOMY
593.3 URETEROVESICAL ORIFICE
753.22 URETEROVESICAL ORIFICE CONGENITAL
598.9 URETHRA NOS
753.6 URETHRA CONGENITAL (MEATUS OR BLADDER NECK)
098.2 URETHRA GONOCOCCAL OR GONORRHEAL [598.01]
598.00 URETHRA INFECTION NOS (DUE TO)
598.1 URETHRA LATE EFFECT OF INJURY
615.9 URETHRA MYOMETRITIS (DUE TO) [598.01]
598.2 URETHRA POSTCATHETERIZATION
598.1 URETHRA POSTOBSTETRIC
598.2 URETHRA POSTOPERATIVE
598.1 URETHRA POSTTRAUMATIC
614.2 URETHRA SALPINGO-OOPHORITIS NOS (DUE TO) [598.01]
614.0 URETHRA SALPINGO-OOPHORITIS ACUTE (DUE TO) [598.01]
614.1 URETHRA SALPINGO-OOPHORITIS CHRONIC (DUE TO) [598.01]
120.9 URETHRA SCHISTOSOMAL [598.01]
095.8 URETHRA SYPHILITIC [598.01]
598.8 URETHRA SPECIFIED CAUSE NEC
753.6 URETHRA VALVULAR CONGENITAL
0 URETHRA WITH INCONTINENCE SEE 'URETHRA, URETHRAL DISORDERS WITH INCONTINENCE'
598.9 URINARY MEATUS
753.6 URINARY MEATUS CONGENITAL
621.5 UTERUS
623.2 VAGINA
654.7# VAGINA COMPLICATING PREGNANCY

5th Digit: 654.7

0. EPISODE OF CARE NOS OR N/A
1. DELIVERED
2. DELIVERED WITH POSTPARTUM COMPLICATION
3. ANTEPARTUM COMPLICATION
4. POSTPARTUM COMPLICATION

763.89 VAGINA COMPLICATING PREGNANCY AFFECTING FETUS OR NEWBORN

STRICTURE (continued)

752.49 VAGINA CONGENITAL
660.2# VAGINA OBSTRUCTING LABOR [**654.7#**]

5th Digit: 654.7

0. EPISODE OF CARE NOS OR N/A
1. DELIVERED
2. DELIVERED WITH POSTPARTUM COMPLICATION
3. ANTEPARTUM COMPLICATION
4. POSTPARTUM COMPLICATION

5th Digit: 660.2

0. EPISODE OF CARE NOS OR N/A
1. DELIVERED
3. ANTEPARTUM COMPLICATION

763.1 VAGINA OBSTRUCTING LABOR AFFECTING FETUS OR NEWBORN
424.90 VALVE HEART OR CARDIAC NOS (SEE ALSO 'STENOSIS', BY VALVE)
746.89 VALVE HEART OR CARDIAC NOS CONGENITAL
746.3 VALVE AORTIC CONGENITAL
746.5 VALVE MITRAL CONGENITAL
746.02 VALVE PULMONARY CONGENITAL
746.1 VALVE TRICUSPID CONGENITAL
753.6 VALVE URETHRA CONGENITAL
608.85 VAS DEFERENS
752.8 VAS DEFERENS CONGENITAL
996.1 VASCULAR GRAFT OR SHUNT-MECHANICAL COMPLICATION
996.74 VASCULAR GRAFT OR SHUNT-EMBOLISM, OCCLUSION OR THROMBUS
459.2 VEIN
459.2 VENA CAVA
747.49 VENA CAVA CONGENITAL
996.2 VENTRICULAR SHUNT-MECHANICAL COMPLICATION
433.2# VERTEBRAL ARTERY
433.3# VERTEBRAL ARTERY BILATERAL OR MULTIPLE

5th Digit: 433.2-3

0. WITHOUT CEREBRAL INFARCTION
1. WITH CEREBRAL INFARCTION

596.0 VESICOURETHRAL ORIFICE
753.6 VESICOURETHRAL ORIFICE CONGENITAL
624.8 VULVA

786.1 STRIDOR
748.3 STRIDOR LARYNGEAL CONGENITAL

REMEMBER, CODE 436 FOR CVA IS A NON-SPECIFIC CODE. CODE INSTEAD, IF POSSIBLE, THE INFARCTION, EMBOLUS, OR THROMBUS IF DOCUMENTED IN THE PATIENT'S RECORD.

WHEN USING THE 436 CODE, REMEMBER TO CODE ALSO ANY RESIDUAL EFFECTS DUE TO THE CVA.

STROKE

436 NOS
436 ACUTE
V12.59 HISTORY
V17.1 HISTORY FAMILY
997.02 IATROGENIC
435.9 IMPENDING (TRANSIENT ISCHEMIC ATTACK)
434.91 LACUNAR INFARCT
0 LATE EFFECT SEE 'LATE EFFECT', CEREBROVASCULAR DISEASE
435.9 LITTLE SYNDROME
0 OLD WITH RESIDUAL SEE 'LATE EFFECT', CEREBROVASCULAR DISEASE
V12.59 OLD WITHOUT RESIDUAL
997.02 POSTOPERATIVE

127.2 STRONGYLOIDES STERCORALIS INFECTION
127.2 STRONGYLOIDIASIS
127.6 STRONGYLOIDIASIS TRICHOSTRONGYLIASIS

793.9 STRUCTURE ABNORMAL-BODY (ECHOGRAM) (THERMOGRAM) (ULTRASOUND)(X-RAY)
245.3 STRUMA FIBROSA
245.2 STRUMA LYMPHOMATOSA

STRUMA OVARII
220 SITE NOS
0 SITE SPECIFIED SEE 'BENIGN NEOPLASM', BY SITE M9090/0
183.0 MALIGNANT SITE NOS
0 MALIGNANT SITE SPECIFIED SEE 'CANCER' BY SITE M9090/3

241.9 STRUMA NODOSA (SIMPLEX)
242.3# STRUMA NODOSA TOXIC OR WITH HYPERTHYROIDISM
5th Digit: 242.3
0. WITHOUT STORM
1. WITH STORM

720.0 STRUMPELL-MARIE DISEASE (ANKYLOSING SPONDYLITIS)
286.3 STUART-PROWER DISEASE (CONGENITAL FACTOR X DEFICIENCY)
V70.5 STUDENT EXAM (HEALTH)
478.1 STUFFY NOSE
780.09 STUPOR
308.2 STUPOR, ACUTE REACTION TO STRESS
759.6 STURGE -KALISCHER-WEBER SYNDROME (ENCEPHALOTRIGEMINAL ANGIOMATOSIS)
759.6 STURGE -WEBER (-DIMITRI) SYNDROME (ENCEPHALOCUTANEOUS ANGIOMATOSIS)
307.0 STUTTERING
100.89 STUTTGART DISEASE
373.11 STYE

SUBACUTE
336.1 NECROTIC MYELOPATHY
330.8 NECROTIZING ENCEPHALOPATHY OR ENCEPHALOMYELOPATHY
046.2 SCLEROSING PANENCEPHALITIS
046.1 SPONGIFORM ENCEPHALOPATHY

746.81 SUBAORTIC STENOSIS CONGENITAL

SUBARACHNOID
430 HEMORRHAGE (RUPTURE BERRY ANEURYSM)
094.87 HEMORRHAGE (SYPHILITIC)
674.0# HEMORRHAGE MATERNAL DUE TO PREGNANCY
5th Digit: 674.0
0. EPISODE OF CARE NOS OR N/A
1. DELIVERED
2. DELIVERED WITH POSTPARTUM COMPLICATION
3. ANTEPARTUM COMPLICATION
4. POSTPARTUM COMPLICATION

852.## HEMORRHAGE TRAUMATIC
4th Digit: 852
0. WITHOUT OPEN WOUND
1. WITH OPEN WOUND
5th Digit: 852
0. LEVEL OF CONSCIOUSNESS NOS
1. NO LOC
2. LOC < 1 HR
3. LOC 1 - 24 HRS
4. LOC > 24 HRS WITH RETURN TO PRIOR LEVEL
5. LOC > 24 HRS WITHOUT RETURN TO PRIOR LEVEL: OR DEATH BEFORE REGAINING CONSCIOUSNESS, REGARDLESS OF DURATION OF LOC
6. LOC DURATION NOS
9. WITH CONCUSSION NOS

772.2 HEMORRHAGE PERINATAL CAUSE

SUBCLAVIAN
442.82 ARTERY (ANEURYSM) (A-V FISTULA) (CIRSOID) (FALSE) (VARICOSE) (RUPTURED)
901.1 ARTERY INJURY
908.4 ARTERY INJURY LATE EFFECT
901.1 ARTERY LACERATION (RUPTURE) (HEMATOMA) (AVULSION) (ANEURYSM) TRAUMATIC
908.4 ARTERY LACERATION LATE EFFECT
446.7 CAROTID OBSTRUCTION SYNDROME (CHRONIC)
996.62 LINE COMPLICATION - INFECTION OR INFLAMMATION
996.1 LINE COMPLICATION - MECHANICAL
996.74 LINE COMPLICATION - OTHER
435.2 STEAL SYNDROME (INSUFFICIENCY)

901.3 VEIN INJURY
908.4 VEIN INJURY LATE EFFECT
901.3 VEIN LACERATION (RUPTURE) (HEMATOMA) (AVULSION) (ANEURYSM) TRAUMATIC
908.4 VEIN LACERATION LATE EFFECT
451.89 VEIN PHLEBITIS

372.73 SUBCONJUNCTIVAL EDEMA
372.72 SUBCONJUNCTIVAL HEMORRHAGE
447.8 SUBCORACOID-PECTORALIS MINOR SYNDROME
694.1 SUBCORNEAL PUSTULAR DERMATOSIS
431 SUBCORTICAL HEMORRHAGE (CEREBRAL)
098.86 SUBCOSTAL SYNDROME
354.8 SUBCOSTAL NERVE COMPRESSION SYNDROME

SUBCUTANEOUS
793.9 ABNORMAL FINDING TISSUE (X-RAY) (ULTRASOUND) (THERMOGRAPHY)
701.9 ATROPHY
709.3 CALCIFICATION
998.81 EMPHYSEMA POST OP
909.3 EMPHYSEMA POST OP LATE EFFECT
958.7 EMPHYSEMA TRAUMATIC
908.6 EMPHYSEMA TRAUMATIC LATE EFFECT
782.2 MASS
782.2 NODULES
V13.3 TISSUE DISEASE HISTORY

V25.43 SUBDERMAL CONTRACEPTIVE DEVICE - CHECKING, REINSERTION OR REMOVAL
V45.52 SUBDERMAL CONTRACEPTIVE DEVICE - IN SITU
V25.5 SUBDERMAL CONTRACEPTIVE DEVICE - INSERTION

530.6 SUBDIAPHRAGMATIC DIVERTICULUM (ESOPHAGEAL)

SUBDURAL
432.1 HEMATOMA (HEMORRHAGE)
852.## HEMATOMA (HEMORRHAGE) TRAUMATIC
4th Digit: 852
2. WITHOUT OPEN WOUND
3. WITH OPEN WOUND
5th Digit: 852
0. LEVEL OF CONSCIOUSNESS NOS
1. NO LOC
2. LOC < 1 HR
3. LOC 1 - 24 HRS
4. LOC > 24 HRS WITH RETURN TO PRIOR LEVEL
5. LOC > 24 HRS WITHOUT RETURN TO PRIOR LEVEL: OR DEATH BEFORE REGAINING CONSCIOUSNESS, REGARDLESS OF DURATION OF LOC
6. LOC DURATION NOS
9. WITH CONCUSSION NOS

767.0 HEMORRHAGE (BIRTH TRAUMA)
674.0# HEMORRHAGE MATERNAL DUE TO PREGNANCY
5th Digit: 674.0
0. EPISODE OF CARE NOS OR N/A
1. DELIVERED
2. DELIVERED WITH POSTPARTUM COMPLICATION
3. ANTEPARTUM COMPLICATION
4. POSTPARTUM COMPLICATION

410.7# SUBENDOCARDIAL INFARCTION
5th Digit: 410.7
0. EPISODE UNSPECIFIED
1. INITIAL EPISODE
2. SUBSEQUENT EPISODE

411.89 SUBENDOCARDIAL ISCHEMIA
495.3 SUBEROSIS
478.6 SUBGLOTTIC EDEMA
228.09 SUBGLOTTIC HEMANGIOMA
748.2 SUBGLOTTIC WEBBING OF LARYNX CONGENITAL
286.0 SUBHEMOPHILIA
621.1 SUBINVOLUTION UTERUS
674.8# SUBINVOLUTION UTERUS MATERNAL DUE TO PREGNANCY
5th Digit: 674.8
0. EPISODE OF CARE NOS OR N/A
2. DELIVERED WITH POSTPARTUM COMPLICATION
4. POSTPARTUM COMPLICATION

527.8 SUBLINGUAL DUCT ATRESIA
750.23 SUBLINGUAL DUCT ATRESIA CONGENITAL
527.0 SUBLINGUAL GLAND ATROPHY
456.3 SUBLINGUAL VARICES

SUBLUXATION (SEE ALSO DISLOCATION)
839.0# CERVICAL SPINE (VERTEBRA)
5th Digit: 839.0
0. CERVICAL VERTEBRA UNSPECIFIED
1. FIRST CERVICAL VERTEBRA
2. SECOND CERVICAL VERTEBRA
3. THIRD CERVICAL VERTEBRA
4. FOURTH CERVICAL VERTEBRA
5. FIFTH CERVICAL VERTEBRA
6. SIXTH CERVICAL VERTEBRA
7. SEVENTH CERVICAL VERTEBRA
8. MULTIPLE CERVICAL VERTEBRA

839.41 COCCYX
832.0# ELBOW
5th Digit: 832.0
0. UNSPECIFIED
1. ANTERIOR
2. POSTERIOR
3. MEDIAL
4. LATERAL
9. OTHER

754.33 HIP BILATERAL CONGENITAL
754.32 HIP UNILATERAL CONGENITAL
754.35 HIP WITH DISLOCATION OTHER HIP CONGENITAL
836.5# KNEE
5th Digit: 836.5
0. UNSPECIFIED
1. ANTERIOR
2. POSTERIOR
3. MEDIAL
4. LATERAL END
9. OTHER OR ROTATORY

718.26 KNEE PATHOLOGICAL
718.36 KNEE RECURRENT OLD
379.32 LENS NONSURGICAL
839.20 LUMBAR VERTEBRA
836.3 PATELLA
718.36 PATELLA RECURRENT OLD
839.42 SACROILIAC (JOINT)
839.42 SACRUM
839.21 THORACIC VERTEBRA

527.2 SUBMANDIBULAR GLAND INFECTION

527.8 SUBMAXILLARY DUCT OR GLAND ATRESIA
750.23 SUBMAXILLARY DUCT OR GLAND ATRESIA CONGENITAL
750.21 SUBMAXILLARY GLAND ABSENCE (CONGENITAL)
527.0 SUBMAXILLARY GLAND (DUCT) ATROPHY
527.8 SUBMAXILLARY GLAND (DUCT) DILATATION
527.8 SUBMAXILLARY GLAND (DUCT) OBSTRUCTION
527.5 SUBMAXILLARY GLAND (DUCT) OBSTRUCTION WITH CALCULUS
959.09 SUBMAXILLARY REGION INJURY
959.09 SUBMENTAL INJURY
994.1 SUBMERSION
909.4 SUBMERSION LATE EFFECT
566 SUBMUCOSAL ABSCESS RECTUM
528.8 SUBMUCOSAL FIBROSIS ORAL INCLUDING TONGUE
726.69 SUBPATELLAR BURSITIS
267 SUBPERIOSTEAL HEMATOMA SYNDROME
751.4 SUBPHRENIC INTERPOSITION SYNDROME
362.81 SUBRETINAL HEMORRHAGE
362.16 SUBRETINAL NEOVASCULARIZATION
723.4 SUBSCAPULAR NEURITIS
840.5 SUBSCAPULARIS SEPARATION (RUPTURE) (TEAR) (LACERATION)
840.5 SUBSCAPULARIS STRAIN (SPRAIN) (AVULSION) (HEMARTHROSIS)

SUBSTANCE ABUSE IS THE TERM USED TO DESCRIBE THE PRACTICE OF USING DRUGS OR ALCOHOL TO EXCESS WITHOUT HAVING REACHED A STAGE OF PHYSICAL DEPENDENCE. SUBSTANCE DEPENDENCE IS ADDICTION. DEPENDENCE INVOLVES LOSS OF CONTROL AND JUDGMENT TO USE IN MODERATE AMOUNTS.

SUBSTANCE ABUSE
303.0# ALCOHOL (DEPENDENT) ACUTE DRUNKENNESS
303.9# ALCOHOL (DEPENDENT) CHRONIC
305.0# ALCOHOL (NONDEPENDENT)
5th Digit: 303.0, 9, 305.0
0. NOS
1. CONTINUOUS
2. EPISODIC
3. IN REMISSION

V65.42 COUNSELING
304.## DRUG DEPENDENT - ADDICTION
4th Digit: 304
0. OPIOID
1. BARBITURATE, SEDATIVES, AND TRANQUILIZERS WITH A SIMILAR EFFECT
2. COCAINE
3. CANNABIS
4. AMPHETAMINE TYPE
5. HALLUCINOGENIC
6. OTHER SPECIFIED
7. MIXED WITH OPIOID
8. MIXED
9. NOS
5th Digit: 304
0. NOS
1. CONTINUOUS
2. EPISODIC
3. IN REMISSION

S

SUBSTANCE ABUSE (continued)

305.## DRUG NONDEPENDENT - ABUSE

4th Digit: 305

- **0. ALCOHOL**
- **2. CANNABIS**
- **3. HALLUCINOGEN**
- **4. BARBITURATE, SEDATIVE, OR HYPNOTIC WITH A SIMILAR EFFECT**
- **5. OPIOID**
- **6. COCAINE**
- **7. AMPHETAMINE TYPE**
- **8. ANTIDEPRESSANT TYPE**
- **9. MIXED OR OTHER SPECIFIED**

5th Digit: 305

- **0. NOS**
- **1. CONTINUOUS**
- **2. EPISODIC**
- **3. IN REMISSION**

305.1 TOBACCO NONDEPENDENT

300.11 SUBSTITUTION DISORDER

923.3 SUBUNGUAL HEMATOMA FINGERNAIL (THUMB NAIL)
924.3 SUBUNGUAL HEMATOMA TOENAIL

271.3 SUCROSE ISOMALTOSE INTOLERANCE OR MALABSORPTION
705.1 SUDAMINA

674.9# SUDDEN DEATH (PUERPERAL) MATERNAL DUE TO PREGNANCY

5th Digit: 674.9

- **0. NOS**
- **2. DELIVERED WITH POSTPARTUM COMPLICATION**
- **4. POSTPARTUM COMPLICATION**

798.0 SUDDEN INFANT DEATH SYNDROME (SIDS)
0 SUDDEN INFANT DEATH SYNDROME (SIDS) NEAR MISS - CODE INDIVIDUAL SYMPTOM(S)
798.2 SUDDEN UNEXPLAINED DEATH (SUDS)

368.11 SUDDEN VISUAL LOSS
733.7 SUDECK (-LERICHE) ATROPHY OR SYNDROME
798.2 SUDS

SUFFOCATION

994.7 BEDCLOTHES
994.7 CAVE-IN
994.7 CONSTRICTION
909.4 LATE EFFECT
994.7 MECHANICAL
994.7 PLASTIC BAG
994.7 PRESSURE
994.7 STRANGULATION
0 SEE ALSO 'ASPHYXIATION FOOD, MUCUS, OR FOREIGN BODY INHALATION'

SUICIDE

300.9 ATTEMPT
300.9 IDEATION
V71.8 OBSERVATION FOR ALLEGED ATTEMPT
300.9 RISK (IDEATION)

V14.2 SULFA ALLERGY (HISTORY)
289.7 SULFHEMOGLOBINEMIA
270.0 SULFITE OXIDASE DEFICIENCY
V14.2 SULFONAMIDE ALLERGY (HISTORY)
V09.6 SULFONAMIDES RESISTANT INFECTION (SEE 'DRUG RESISTANCE')
692.72 SUMMER ACNE
692.72 SUMMER PRURIGO

992.0 SUN STROKE
909.4 SUN STROKE LATE EFFECT

692.71 SUNBURN
360.24 SUNFLOWER <u>CATARACT</u> [<u>366.34</u>]

SUPERIOR

0 CEREBELLAR ARTERY SYNDROME SEE 'CEREBROVASCULAR', ACCIDENT
902.25 MESENTERIC ARTERY (TRUNK) LACERATION (RUPTURE) (HEMATOMA) (AVULSION) (ANEURYSM)
908.4 MESENTERIC ARTERY INJURY OR LACERATION LATE EFFECT
557.1 MESENTERIC ARTERY SYNDROME
902.31 MESENTERIC VEIN INJURY (PRIMARY SUBDIVISIONS)
902.31 MESENTERIC VEIN LACERATION (RUPTURE) (HEMATOMA) (AVULSION) (ANEURYSM) TRAUMATIC
908.4 MESENTERIC VEIN INJURY OR LACERATION LATE EFFECT
747.49 VENA CAVA ABSENCE (CONGENITAL)
901.2 VENA CAVA INJURY
908.4 VENA CAVA INJURY LATE EFFECT
459.2 VENA CAVA SYNDROME

SUPERNUMERARY

746.5 CUSPS MITRAL VALVE (CONGENITAL)
755.00 DIGITS
755.01 FINGERS
756.2 RIB CERVICAL REGION
755.02 TOES
520.1 TEETH
756.19 VERTEBRA

SUPERVISION

V20.1 CHILD (HEALTHY)
V25.43 CONTRACEPTIVE (SUBDERMAL IMPLANTABLE)
V20.0 FOUNDLING
V20.1 INFANT (HEALTHY)
V24.1 LACTATING MOTHER

SUPERVISION OF PREGNANCY

V23.7 PRENATAL CARE POOR OR NONE
V22.0 NORMAL (FIRST)
V22.1 NORMAL (OTHER THAN FIRST)
V23.9 HIGH RISK
V23.2 HIGH RISK - ABORTION HISTORY

> *ELDERLY MULTIGRAVIDA: SECOND OR MORE PREGNANCY IN A WOMAN WHO WILL BE 35 YEARS OF AGE OR OLDER AT EXPECTED DATE OF DELIVERY.*

V23.82 HIGH RISK - ELDERLY MULTIGRAVIDA

> *ELDERLY PRIMIGRAVIDA: FIRST PREGNANCY IN A WOMAN WHO WILL BE 35 YEARS OF AGE OR OLDER AT EXPECTED DATE OF DELIVERY.*

V23.81 HIGH RISK - ELDERLY PRIMIGRAVIDA
V23.3 HIGH RISK - GRAND MULTIPARITY
V23.1 HIGH RISK - HYDATIDIFORM MOLE HISTORY
V23.0 HIGH RISK - INFERTILITY HISTORY
V23.89 HIGH RISK - MENTAL DISORDER HISTORY
V23.5 HIGH RISK - NEONATAL DEATH HISTORY
V23.4 HIGH RISK - POOR OBSTETRICAL HISTORY
V23.7 HIGH RISK - PRENATAL CARE POOR OR NONE
V23.5 HIGH RISK - STILLBIRTH HISTORY
V23.1 HIGH RISK - TROPHOBLASTIC DISEASE HISTORY
V23.1 HIGH RISK - VESICULAR MOLE HISTORY

> *YOUNG MULTIGRAVIDA: SECOND OR MORE PREGNANCY IN A FEMALE WHO IS LESS THAN 16 YEARS OLD AT EXPECTED DATE OF DELIVERY.*

V23.84 HIGH RISK - YOUNG MULTIGRAVIDA

> *YOUNG PRIMIGRAVIDA: FIRST PREGNANCY IN A FEMALE WHO IS LESS THAN 16 YEARS OLD AT EXPECTED DATE OF DELIVERY.*

V23.83 HIGH RISK - YOUNG PRIMIGRAVIDA
V23.89 HIGH RISK - OTHER SPECIFIED

788.5 SUPPRESSION OF URINARY SECRETION
738.8 SUPRACLAVICULAR RETRACTION
478.6 SUPRAGLOTTIC EDEMA
333.0 SUPRANUCLEAR OPHTHALMOPLEGIA PROGRESSIVE
333.0 SUPRANUCLEAR PALSY PROGRESSIVE
356.8 SUPRANUCLEAR PARALYSIS
959.09 SUPRAORBITAL INJURY

SUPRARENAL
902.49 ARTERIES LACERATION (RUPTURE) (HEMATOMA)(AVULSION) (ANEURYSM) TRAUMATIC
902.49 ARTERY INJURY
908.4 ARTERY INJURY OR LACERATION LATE EFFECT
255.4 ATROPHY (CAPSULE) (GLAND)
255.4 CALCIFICATION (CAPSULE) (GLAND)
255.3 CORTICAL SYNDROME
255.9 DISEASE
255.3 HYPERFUNCTION
255.8 HYPERPLASIA
255.4 HYPOFUNCTION
868.01 INJURY GLAND (MULTIPLE) TRAUMATIC
868.11 INJURY GLAND (MULTIPLE) TRAUMATIC WITH OPEN WOUND

SUPRASPINATUS
726.10 IMPINGEMENT
840.6 SEPARATION (RUPTURE) (TEAR) (LACERATION)
840.6 STRAIN (SPRAIN) (AVULSION) (HEMARTHROSIS)
726.10 SYNDROME

427.61 SUPRAVENTRICULAR PREMATURE BEATS
427.89 SUPRAVENTRICULAR TACHYCARDIA
427.0 SUPRAVENTRICULAR TACHYCARDIA PAROXYSMAL

919.8 SURFER KNOTS
919.9 SURFER KNOTS INFECTED

WHEN SURGERY IS CANCELLED DUE TO AN UNFORSEEN PROBLEM, CODE THE PREOPERATIVE DIAGNOSIS FIRST, THEN USE A CODE FROM V 64.# TO INDICATE THAT SURGERY WAS NOT CARRIED OUT, AND A THIRD CODE TO INDICATE THE REASON. (SURGERY RE-SCHEDULED, PATIENT ELECTS NOT TO HAVE THE SURGERY, SURGEON HAD AN EMERGENCY, ETC.)

SURGERY
V66.0 CONVALESCENCE
V67.0 FOLLOWUP EXAM
V64.4 LAPAROSCOPIC PROCEDURE CONVERTED TO OPEN PROCEDURE
760.6 MATERNAL AFFECTING FETUS OR NEWBORN
V64.2 NOT CARRIED OUT PATIENT DECISION
V62.6 NOT CARRIED OUT PATIENT DECISION - CONSCIENCE OR RELIGION BASED
V64.1 NOT CARRIED OUT DUE TO CONTRAINDICATION
V64.3 NOT CARRIED OUT FOR OTHER REASONS

SURGERY ELECTIVE
V50.9 UNSPECIFIED
V50.1 BREAST AUGMENTATION
V50.1 BREAST REDUCTION
V50.2 CIRCUMCISION ROUTINE OR RITUAL
V50.1 COSMETIC
V50.3 EAR PIERCING
V50.1 FACE LIFT
V50.0 HAIR TRANSPLANT
V50.8 OTHER

709.09 SUTTON'S DISEASE

SUTURE
998.59 ABSCESS POSTOPERATIVE
998.3 BURST
998.89 GRANULOMA POSTOPERATIVE - EXTERNAL
998.89 GRANULOMA POSTOPERATIVE - INTERNAL
998.4 INADVERTENTLY LEFT IN WOUND
998.89 PAIN (WIRE)
V58.3 REMOVAL

427.89 SVT (SUPRAVENTRICULAR TACHYCARDIA)
427.0 SVT PAROXYSMAL (SUPRAVENTRICULAR TACHYCARDIA PAROXYSMAL)

777.3 SWALLOWED BLOOD SYNDROME
787.2 SWALLOWING DIFFICULTY (DYSPHAGIA)
V41.6 SWALLOWING PROBLEMS

100.89 SWAMP FEVER

736.22 SWAN NECK DEFORMITY FINGER ACQUIRED

SWEAT, SWEATING
705.1 DEFICIENCY (RETENTION)
078.2 DISEASE
780.8 EXCESSIVE
078.2 FEVER
705.9 GLAND DISORDER
705.89 GLAND DISORDER SPECIFIED TYPE NEC
238.2 GLAND TUMOR SITE NOS
0 GLAND TUMOR SITE SPECIFIED SEE 'NEOPLASM UNCERTAIN BEHAVIOR' BY SITE M8400/1
705.1 RETENTION SYNDROME

272.4 SWEELEY-KLIONSKY DISEASE

695.89 SWEET'S SYNDROME (ACUTE FEBRILE NEUTROPHILIC DERMATOSIS)

SWELLING
789.3# ABDOMINAL
5th Digit: 789.3
0. UNSPECIFIED SITE
1. UPPER RIGHT QUADRANT
2. UPPER LEFT QUADRANT
3. LOWER RIGHT QUADRANT
4. LOWER LEFT QUADRANT
5. PERIUMBILIC
6. EPIGASTRIC
7. GENERALIZED
9. OTHER SPECIFIED SITE (MULTIPLE)

789.5 ABDOMINAL DUE TO ASCITES
255.8 ADRENAL GLAND, CLOUDY
0 ANKLE SEE 'SWELLING', JOINT
787.99 ANUS
729.81 ARM
611.72 BREAST
125.2 CALABAR
785.6 CERVICAL GLAND
784.2 CHEEK
786.6 CHEST
388.8 EAR
789.36 EPIGASTRIC
729.81 EXTREMITY (LOWER) (UPPER)
379.92 EYE
625.8 FEMALE GENITAL ORGAN
729.81 FINGER
729.81 FOOT
785.6 GLANDS
784.2 GUM
729.81 HAND
784.2 HEAD
719.0# JOINT
5th Digit: 719.0
0. SITE NOS
1. SHOULDER REGION
2. UPPER ARM (ELBOW) (HUMERUS)
3. FOREARM (RADIUS) (WRIST) (ULNA)
4. HAND (CARPAL) (METACARPAL) (FINGERS)
5. PELVIC REGION AND THIGH (HIP) (BUTTOCK) (FEMUR)
6. LOWER LEG (FIBULA) (KNEE) (PATELLA) (TIBIA)
7. ANKLE AND/OR FOOT (METATARSALS) (TOES) (TARSALS)
8. OTHER
9. MULTIPLE

S

S

SWELLING (continued)

593.89 KIDNEY, CLOUDY
729.81 LEG
729.81 LIMB
573.8 LIVER
786.6 LUNG
785.6 LYMPH NODES
197.6 MALIGNANT
786.6 MEDIASTINAL
784.2 MOUTH
729.81 MUSCLE (LIMB)
784.2 NECK
784.2 NOSE OR SINUS
729.81 OF LIMB
784.2 PALATE
789.39 PELVIS
607.83 PENIS
625.8 PERINEUM
787.99 RECTUM
608.86 SCROTUM
782.2 SKIN
789.2 SPLEEN
786.6 SUBSTERNAL
782.2 SUPERFICIAL (SKIN)
608.86 TESTICLE
784.2 THROAT
729.81 TOE
784.2 TONGUE
593.9 TUBULAR NOS
789.35 UMBILICUS
625.8 UTERUS
625.8 VAGINA
625.8 VULVA

985.0 SWIFT (-FEER) DISEASE

380.12 SWIMMERS' EAR ACUTE
120.3 SWIMMERS' ITCH CUTANEOUS
031.1 SWIMMING POOL BACILLUS
077.0 SWIMMING POOL CONJUNCTIVITIS

100.89 SWINEHERD'S DISEASE

785.6 SWOLLEN GLANDS

752.7 SWYER'S SYNDROME (XY PURE GONADAL DYSGENESIS)
492.8 SWYER-JAMES SYNDROME (UNILATERAL HYPERLUCENT LUNG)

SYCOSIS

704.8 NOS
704.8 BARBAE NOT PARASITIC
704.8 LUPOID
110.0 MYCOTIC
704.8 VULGARIS

392.9 SYDENHAM'S CHOREA
392.0 SYDENHAM'S CHOREA WITH HEART INVOLVEMENT

060.0 SYLVAN YELLOW FEVER
074.1 SYLVEST'S DISEASE (EPIDEMIC PLEURODYNIA)

372.63 SYMBLEPHARON
784.60 SYMBOLIC DYSFUNCTION
202.0# SYMMERS DISEASE (FOLLICULAR LYMPHOMA)

5th Digit: 202.0

0. UNSPECIFIED SITE, EXTRANODAL AND SOLID ORGAN SITES
1. LYMPH NODES OF HEAD FACE NECK
2. LYMPH NODES INTRATHORACIC
3. LYMPH NODES ABDOMINAL
4. LYMPH NODES AXILLA AND UPPER LIMB
5. LYMPH NODES INGUINAL REGION AND LOWER LIMB
6. LYMPH NODES INTRAPELVIC
7. SPLEEN
8. LYMPH NODES MULTIPLE SITES

348.2 SYMOND'S SYNDROME

337.0 SYMPATHETIC CERVICAL PARALYSIS SYNDROME
337.9 SYMPATHETIC NERVE DISORDER NEC
625.5 SYMPATHETIC PELVIC SYNDROME

305.7# SYMPATHOMIMETIC ABUSE NONDEPENDENT

5th Digit: 305.7

0. NOS
1. CONTINUOUS
2. EPISODIC
3. IN REMISSION

0 SYMPHALANGY/SYMPHALANGIA SEE 'SYNDACTYLY, SYNDACTYLIC'

732.1 SYMPHYSIS PUBIS OSTEOCHONDROSIS
665.6# SYMPHYSIS PUBIS SEPARATION (OBSTETRICAL)

5th Digit: 665.6

0. EPISODE OF CARE NOS OR N/A
1. DELIVERED
4. POSTPARTUM COMPLICATION

848.5 SYMPHYSIS PUBIS SPRAIN (STRAIN) (RUPTURE) (TEAR)

0 SYNARTHROSIS SEE 'JOINT', CALCIFICATION'

732.1 SYNCHONDROSIS ISCHIOPUBIC (OF VAN NECK)
379.22 SYNCHYSIS SCINTILLANS

780.2 SYNCOPE (NEAR) (-PRE) AND COLLAPSE UNKNOWN ETIOLOGY
337.0 SYNCOPE CAROTID SINUS

SYNDACTYLY, SYNDACTYLIC

755.10 MULTIPLE AND NOS SITES
755.12 FINGERS WITH FUSION OF BONE
755.11 FINGERS WITHOUT FUSION OF BONE
755.55 OXYCEPHALY
755.14 TOES WITH FUSION OF BONE
755.13 TOES WITHOUT FUSION OF BONE

0 SYNDESMOSIS TIBIOFIBULAR JOINT SEE 'DISLOCATION', ANKLE
0 SYNDROME SEE BY SPECIFIC NAME

SYNECHIAE

364.70 NOS (EYE)
364.72 ANTERIOR (EYE)
621.5 INTRAUTERINE (TRAUMATIC)
364.70 IRIS (EYE)
478.1 NASAL OR INTRANASAL
364.73 PERIPHERAL ANTERIOR (EYE)
364.71 POSTERIOR (EYE)
752.49 VULVA CONGENITAL

0 SYNOVIAL SEE 'SYNOVIUM, SYNOVIAL'
215.# SYNOVIOMA BENIGN M9040/0
171.# SYNOVIOMA MALIGNANT M9040/3

4th Digit: 171, 215

0. HEAD FACE NECK
2. UPPER LIMB SHOULDER
3. LOWER LIMB HIP
4. THORAX
5. ABDOMINAL HYPOCHONDRIUM
6. PELVIS BUTTOCK GROIN INGUINAL REGION PERINEUM
7. TRUNK NOS BACK NOS FLANK NOS
8. OTHER SPECIFIED SITES
9. SITE UNSPECIFIED

SYNOVITIS

727.00 NOS
727.06 ANKLE
275.49 CRYSTAL INDUCED - UNSPECIFIED [712.9#]
0 CRYSTAL INDUCED - CHONDROCALCINOSIS SEE 'CHONDROCALCINOSIS'
274.0 CRYSTAL INDUCED - GOUTY
275.49 CRYSTAL INDUCED - OTHER SPECIFIED [712.8#]

5th Digit: 712.8-9

0. SITE NOS
1. SHOULDER REGION
2. UPPER ARM (ELBOW) (HUMERUS)
3. FOREARM (RADIUS) (WRIST) (ULNA)
4. HAND (CARPAL) (METACARPAL) (FINGERS)
5. PELVIC REGION AND THIGH (HIP) (BUTTOCK) (FEMUR)
6. LOWER LEG (FIBULA) (KNEE) (PATELLA) (TIBIA)
7. ANKLE AND/OR FOOT (METATARSALS) (TOES) (TARSALS)
8. OTHER (HEAD) (NECK) (RIB) (SKULL) (TRUNK) (VERTEBRAE)
9. MULTIPLE

727.05 FINGER
727.06 FOOT AND ANKLE
098.51 GONOCOCCAL
274.0 GOUTY
727.05 HAND AND WRIST
095.7 SYPHILITIC
015.## TUBERCULOUS [727.01]

4th Digit: 015

0. VERTEBRAL COLUMN
1. HIP
2. KNEE
5. LIMB BONES
6. MASTOID
7. OTHER SPECIFIED BONE
8. OTHER SPECIFIED JOINT
9. UNSPECIFIED BONES AND JOINTS

5th Digit: 015

0. NOS
1. LAB NOT DONE
2. LABS PENDING
3. MICROSCOPY POSITIVE (IN SPUTUM)
4. CULTURE POSITIVE - MICROSCOPY NEGATIVE
5. CULTURE NEGATIVE - MICROSCOPY POSITIVE
6. CULTURE AND MICROSCOPY NEGATIVE CONFIRMED BY OTHER METHODS

719.2# VILLONODULAR

5th Digit: 719.2

0. SITE NOS
1. SHOULDER REGION
2. UPPER ARM (ELBOW) (HUMERUS)
3. FOREARM (RADIUS) (WRIST) (ULNA)
4. HAND (CARPAL) (METACARPAL) (FINGERS)
5. PELVIC REGION AND THIGH (HIP) (BUTTOCK) (FEMUR) AND THIGH
6. LOWER LEG (FIBULA) (KNEE) (PATELLA) (TIBIA)
7. ANKLE AND/OR FOOT (METATARSALS) (TOES) (TARSALS)
8. OTHER
9. MULTIPLE

727.05 WRIST
727.2 WRIST OCCUPATIONAL
727.09 OTHER
0 SEE ALSO 'TENOSYNOVITIS'

SYNOVIUM, SYNOVIAL

727.40 CYST
727.51 CYST POPLITEAL (BAKER'S)
0 CYST SEE 'GANGLION'
727.9 DISORDER
727.89 DISORDER OTHER SPECIFIED
792.9 FLUID ABNORMAL
727.89 PLICA
727.50 RUPTURE
727.59 RUPTURE OTHER

SYPHILIS

097.9 NOS
097.9 ACQUIRED
093.9 CARDIOVASCULAR
093.89 CARDIOVASCULAR SYNDROME
093.89 CARDIOVASCULAR OTHER
094.9 CENTRAL NERVOUS SYSTEM
0 COMPLICATING PREGNANCY SEE 'SYPHILIS COMPLICATING PREGNANCY'
V65.45 COUNSELING
090.9 DEATH (FROM) UNSPECIFIED (UNDER TWO YEARS OF AGE)
093.22 ENDOCARDITIS AORTIC VALVE
093.21 ENDOCARDITIS MITRAL VALVE
093.24 ENDOCARDITIS PULMONARY VALVE
093.23 ENDOCARDITIS TRICUSPID VALVE
093.20 ENDOCARDITIS VALVE UNSPECIFIED
V01.6 EXPOSURE
795.6 FALSE POSITIVE SEROLOGICAL TEST
091.0 GENITAL (PRIMARY)
097.0 LATE NOS
096 LATE LATENT
097.1 LATENT NOS
092.9 LATENT EARLY NOS
092.0 LATENT EARLY SEROLOGICAL RELAPSE AFTER TREATMENT
096 LATENT LATE
094.2 MENINGITIS
094.2 MENINGOVASCULAR
093.82 MYOCARDITIS
104.0 NONVENEREAL ENDEMIC
093.20 OSTIAL CORONARY DISEASE
093.81 PERICARDITIS
097.1 POSITIVE SEROLOGICAL REACTION
091.0 VULVA

SYPHILIS COMPLICATING PREGNANCY

655.4# MATERNAL (WITH KNOWN / SUSPECTED DAMAGE TO FETUS)

5th Digit: 655.4

0. EPISODE OF CARE NOS OR N/A
1. DELIVERED
3. ANTEPARTUM COMPLICATION

647.0#: USE AN ADDITIONAL CODE TO IDENTIFY THE MATERNAL SYPHILIS.

647.0# MATERNAL CURRENT (CO-EXISTENT)

5th Digit: 647.0

0. EPISODE OF CARE NOS OR N/A
1. DELIVERED
2. DELIVERED WITH POSTPARTUM COMPLICATION
3. ANTEPARTUM COMPLICATION
4. POSTPARTUM COMPLICATION

SYPHILIS CONGENITAL

090.9 NOS
090.0 CHOROIDITIS
090.0 CORYZA (CHRONIC)
090.1 EARLY LATENT
090.2 EARLY LESS THAN 2 YEARS AFTER BIRTH
090.0 EARLY SYMPTOMATIC
090.41 ENCEPHALITIS
090.0 EPIPHYSITIS
090.0 HEPATOMEGALY

SYPHILIS CONGENITAL (continued)

090.3 KERATITIS INTERSTITIAL
090.3 KERATITIS PARENCHYMATOUS
090.3 KERATITIS PUNCTATA PROFUNDA
090.7 LATE MANIFEST 2 YRS. OR MORE AFTER BIRTH
090.6 LATENT MANIFEST 2 YRS. OR MORE AFTER BIRTH
090.42 MENINGITIS
090.0 MUCOUS PATCHES
090.0 PEMPHIGUS
090.0 PERIOSTITIS
090.0 SPLENOMEGALY
090.49 OTHER
090.5 OTHER LATE SYMPTOMATIC MANIFEST 2 YRS. OR MORE AFTER BIRTH

SYPHILIS PRIMARY

091.1 ANUS
091.2 BREAST
091.2 FINGERS
091.0 GENITAL
091.2 LIP
091.2 TONSILS

SYPHILIS SECONDARY

091.9 NOS
091.4 ADENOPATHY
091.82 ALOPECIA
091.3 ANUS
091.51 CHORIORETINITIS
091.62 HEPATITIS
091.52 IRIDOCYCLITIS
091.62 LIVER
091.4 LYMPHADENITIS
091.81 MENINGITIS ACUTE
091.3 MOUTH
091.3 MUCOUS MEMBRANES
091.61 PERIOSTITIS
091.3 PHARYNX
091.7 RELAPSE
091.3 SKIN
091.3 TONSILS
091.50 UVEITIS
091.69 VISCERA OTHER
091.3 VULVA
091.89 OTHER

SYPHILIS TERTIARY

095.9 NOS
095.5 BONE
095.7 BURSITIS
095.0 EPISCLERITIS
095.4 KIDNEY
095.3 LIVER
095.1 LUNG
095.6 MUSCLE
095.2 PERITONITIS
095.7 SYNOVITIS
095.7 SYNOVIUM TENDON AND BURSA
095.8 OTHER SPECIFIED FORMS

SYPHILITIC

093.9 ANGINA
090.5 ANGINA CONGENITAL
091.51 CHORIORETINITIS SECONDARY
090.41 ENCEPHALITIS CONGENITAL
091.52 IRIDOCYCLITIS SECONDARY
091.4 LYMPHADENITIS (SECONDARY)
090.5 SADDLE NOSE MANIFEST 2 YRS. OR MORE AFTER BIRTH
091.50 UVEITIS SECONDARY

SYPHILITIC CNS

094.86 ACOUSTIC NEURITIS
094.87 CEREBRAL ANEURYSM RUPTURED
094.83 DISSEMINATED RETINOCHOROIDITIS
094.81 ENCEPHALITIS
094.83 NEURORECIDIVE RETINA
094.85 NEURORETINITIS
094.84 OPTIC ATROPHY
094.82 PARKINSONISM
094.85 RETROBULBAR NEURITIS

094.89 SYPHILOMA CENTRAL NERVOUS SYSTEM
216.# SYRINGOADENOMA M8400/0
216.# SYRINGOMA M8407/0

4th Digit: 216

0. LIP (SKIN OF)
1. EYELID INCLUDING CANTHUS
2. EAR (EXTERNAL) (AURICLE) (PINNA)
3. FACE (CHEEK) (NOSE) (EYEBROW) (TEMPLE)
4. SCALP NECK
5. TRUNK BACK EXCEPT SCROTUM
6. UPPER LIMB INCLUDING SHOULDER
7. LOWER LIMB INCLUDING HIP
8. OTHER SPECIFIED SITES
9. SKIN NOS

336.0 SYRINGOMYELIA

SYRINGOMYELOCELE

741.0# WITH HYDROCEPHALUS
741.9# WITHOUT HYDROCEPHALUS

5th Digit: 741.0, 9

0. REGION NOS
1. CERVICAL
2. DORSAL
3. LUMBAR

710.8 SYSTEMIC FIBROSCLEROSING SYNDROME
286.5 SYSTEMIC LUPUS ERYTHEMATOSUS INHIBITOR INCREASE
0 SYSTEMIC LUPUS ERYTHEMATOSUS SEE 'LUPUS', ERYTHEMATOSUS
0 SYSTEMIC SCLEROSIS SEE 'SCLERODERMA'
202.6# SYSTEMIC TISSUE MAST CELL DISEASE M9740/3

5th Digit: 202.6

0. UNSPECIFIED SITE, EXTRANODAL AND SOLID ORGAN SITES
1. LYMPH NODES OF HEAD FACE NECK
2. LYMPH NODES INTRATHORACIC
3. LYMPH NODES ABDOMINAL
4. LYMPH NODES AXILLA AND UPPER LIMB
5. LYMPH NODES INGUINAL REGION AND LOWER LIMB
6. LYMPH NODES INTRAPELVIC
7. SPLEEN
8. LYMPH NODES MULTIPLE SITES

785.2 SYSTOLIC CLICK (-MURMUR) SYNDROME

279.10 T-CELL DEFECT IMMUNODEFICIENCY PREDOMINANT
V03.1 TAB VACCINATION ALONE
305.1 TABAGISM SYNDROME

TABES
094.0 DORSALIS
094.0 DORSALIS WITH CHARCOT'S [713.5]
090.40 JUVENILE

094.1 TABOPARESIS
090.40 TABOPARESIS JUVENILE
427.81 TACHYBRADY SYNDROME

TACHYCARDIA
785.0 NOS
427.89 ATRIAL
427.0 ATRIAL PAROXYSMAL
426.89 AV
427.0 AV PAROXYSMAL
427.81 BRADYCARDIA SYNDROME
659.7# FETAL AFFECTING MANAGEMENT OF MOTHER
5th Digit: 659.7
0. EPISODE OF CARE UNSPECIFIED OR N/A
1. DELIVERED
3. ANTEPARTUM COMPLICATION

427.0 JUNCTIONAL PAROXYSMAL
426.89 NODAL
427.2 PAROXYSMAL
427.89 SINUS
427.0 SUPRAVENTRICULAR PAROXYSMAL
427.42 VENTRICULAR FLUTTER
427.1 VENTRICULAR PAROXYSMAL

TACHYPNEA
786.06 NOS
770.6 IDIOPATHIC NEWBORN
770.6 NEWBORN TRANSITORY

TAENIA
123.3 INFECTION
123.2 SAGINATA INFECTION
123.0 SOLIUM INFECTION INTESTINAL FORM

123.2 TAENIARHYNCHUS SAGINATUS INFECTION
123.3 TAENIASIS
757.4 TAENZER'S DISEASE

TAG (HYPERTROPHIED SKIN) (INFECTED)
701.9 NOS
474.8 ADENOID
474.01 ADENOID INFECTED
455.9 ANUS (SKIN) (HEMORRHOIDAL)
455.9 HEMORRHOIDAL
623.8 HYMEN
624.8 PERINEUM
744.1 PREAURICULAR CONGENITAL
455.9 RECTAL (SKIN) (HEMORRHOIDAL)
455.9 SENTINEL
701.9 SKIN
757.39 SKIN ACCESSORY CONGENITAL
474.8 TONSIL
474.00 TONSIL INFECTED
599.84 URETHRA
624.8 VULVA

062.5 TAHYNA FEVER
0 TAIL BONE SEE 'COCCYX, COCCYGEAL'

446.7 TAKAYASU'S DISEASE OR SYNDROME (PULSELESS)
648.9# TAKAYASU'S DISEASE OR SYNDROME (PULSELESS) MATERNAL CURRENT (CO-EXISTENT) IN PREGNANCY [446.7]
5th Digit: 648.9
0. EPISODE OF NOS OR N/A
1. DELIVERED
2. DELIVERED WITH POSTPARTUM COMPLICATION
3. ANTEPARTUM COMPLICATION
4. POSTPARTUM COMPLICATION

TALIPES
754.70 NOS (CONGENITAL)
736.79 NEC ACQUIRED
754.62 CALCANEOVALGUS (CONGENITAL)
736.76 CALCANEOVALGUS ACQUIRED
754.59 CALCANEOVARUS (CONGENITAL)
736.76 CALCANEOVARUS ACQUIRED
754.79 CALCANEUS (CONGENITAL)
736.76 CALCANEUS ACQUIRED
754.71 CAVUS (CONGENITAL)
736.73 CAVUS ACQUIRED
754.69 EQUINOVALGUS (CONGENITAL)
736.72 EQUINOVALGUS ACQUIRED
754.51 EQUINOVARUS (CONGENITAL)
736.71 EQUINOVARUS ACQUIRED
754.79 EQUINUS (CONGENITAL)
736.72 EQUINUS ACQUIRED NEC
754.69 PLANOVALGUS (CONGENITAL)
736.79 PLANOVALGUS ACQUIRED
734 PLANUS (ACQUIRED)
754.61 PLANUS CONGENITAL
754.60 VALGUS (CONGENITAL)
736.79 VALGUS ACQUIRED
754.50 VARUS (CONGENITAL)
736.79 VARUS ACQUIRED

728.85 TALMA'S DISEASE
755.67 TALONAVICULAR SYNOSTOSIS
423.9 TAMPONADE CARDIAC (HEART)
078.89 TANAPOX
272.5 TANGIER DISEASE (FAMILIAL HIGH-DENSITY LIPOPROTEIN DEFICIENCY)
312.1# TANTRUMS
5th Digit: 312.1
0. NOS
1. MILD
2. MODERATE
3. SEVERE

692.4 TAPE DERMATITIS

TAPEWORM
123.9 NOS
123.2 BEEF
123.1 CYSTICERCIASIS (LARVAE FORM)
123.6 DOG
123.6 DWARF
123.4 FISH
123.9 INFECTION (CESTODE)
123.0 PORK (INTESTINAL)
123.6 RAT
123.5 SPARGANUM (MANSONI) (PROLIFERUM)
123.5 SPIROMETRA
123.3 TAENIA
123.3 TAENIASIS NOS
123.8 OTHER SPECIFIED CESTODE INFECTION

T

352.6 TAPIA'S SYNDROME

747.41 TAPVR (TOTAL ANOMALOUS PULMONARY VENOUS RETURN) (SUBDIAPHRAGMATIC) (SUPRADIAPHRAGMATIC)

297.8 TARANTISM

989.5 TARANTULA BITE

995.0. TARANTULA BITE WITH ANAPHYLAXIS [989.5]

354.2 TARDY ULNAR NERVE PALSY

355.9 TARLOV'S CYST

696.4 TARRAL-BESNIER DISEASE (PITYRIASIS RUBRA PILARIS)

TARSAL

755.38 ABSENCE CONGENITAL WITH ABSENCE INCOMPLETE DISTAL ELEMENTS
755.67 COALITIONS
755.38 OR METATARSALS AGENESIS COMPLETE OR PARTIAL
355.5 TUNNEL SYNDROME

838.03 TARSOMETATARSAL JOINT DISLOCATION CLOSED

838.13 TARSOMETATARSAL JOINT DISLOCATION OPEN

845.11 TARSOMETATARSAL STRAIN (SPRAIN) (AVULSION) (HEMARTHROSIS)

743.66 TARSO-ORBITAL FASCIA ATROPHY CONGENITAL

781.1 TASTE DISTURBANCE OF SENSATION

V41.5 TASTE PROBLEM

709.09 TATOO MARK

745.11 TAUSSIG BING SYNDROME OR DEFECT (TRANSPOSITION AORTA AND OVERRIDING PULMONARY ARTERY)

330.1 TAY SACHS DISEASE

759.89 TAYBI'S SYNDROME (OTOPALATODIGITAL) SYNDROME

701.8 TAYLOR'S DISEASE

625.5 TAYLOR'S SYNDROME

0 TB SEE 'TUBERCULOSIS'

246.8 TBG EXCESS OR DEFICIENCY (THYROID BINDING GLOBULIN)

375.69 TEAR DUCT DISEASE

375.15 TEAR FILM INSUFFICIENCY

0 TEAR INTERNAL ORGAN SEE SPECIFIC ORGAN, INJURY

0 TEAR JOINT, LIGAMENT, MUSCLE OR TENDON SEE 'SPRAIN', BY SITE

0 TEAR LIGAMENT, MUSCLE OR TENDON WITH LACERATION SEE 'LACERATION', BY SITE

767.0 TEAR TENTORIAL BIRTH TRAUMA

375.20 TEARING EXCESSIVE

0 TEETH SEE 'TOOTH'

520.7 TEETHING SYNDROME

344.89 TEGMENTAL SYNDROME

TELANGIECTASIA

448.9 NOS
334.8 ATAXIC (CEREBELLAR)
448.0 FAMILIAL
448.0 HEREDITARY HEMORRHAGIC

648.9#: USE AN ADDITIONAL CODE TO IDENTIFY THE SPECIFIC TELANGIECTASIA.

648.9# MATERNAL CURRENT (CO-EXISTENT) IN PREGNANCY

5th Digit: 648.9

0. EPISODE OF NOS OR N/A
1. DELIVERED
2. DELIVERED WITH POSTPARTUM COMPLICATION
3. ANTEPARTUM COMPLICATION
4. POSTPARTUM COMPLICATION

TELANGIECTASIA (continued)

757.33 PIGMENTATION-CATARACT SYNDROME
362.15 RETINAL
362.15 RETINOPATHY
448.1 SPIDER

709.1 TELANGIECTODES

743.63 TELECANTHUS (CONGENITAL)

704.02 TELOGEN EFFLUVIUM

446.5 TEMPORAL ARTERITIS

310.0 TEMPORAL LOBECTOMY BEHAVIOR SYNDROME

959.09 TEMPORAL REGION INJURY

383.02 TEMPORAL SYNDROME

524.6# TEMPOROMANDIBULAR JOINT DISORDER OR SYNDROME

5th Digit: 524.6

0. UNSPECIFIED
1. ADHESIONS AND ANKYLOSIS
2. ARTHRALGIA
3. ARTICULAR DISC DISORDER(REDUCING OR NON REDUCING)
9. OTHER SPECIFIED JOINT DISORDER (MALOCCLUSION)

TENDINITIS

726.90 SITE NOS
726.71 ACHILLES
726.70 ANKLE AND TARSUS
726.12 BICIPITAL
727.82 CALCIFIC
726.30 ELBOW
726.5 GLUTEAL
726.64 PATELLAR
726.79 PERONEAL
726.61 PES ANSERINUS
726.5 PSOAS
726.11 SHOULDER (CALCIFIC)
726.72 TIBIALIS
726.5 TROCHANTERIC
0 SEE ALSO 'TENOSYNOVITIS', BY SITE

TENDON

756.81 ABSENCE (CONGENITAL)
727.82 CALCIFICATION
727.81 CONTRACTURE (ACHILLES)
727.9 DISORDER NOS
726.10 DISORDER SHOULDER REGION
726.90 INFLAMMATION NEC
905.8 INJURY LATE EFFECT (DUE TO LACERATION, SPRAIN OR STRAIN)
0 LACERATION SEE 'LACERATION', TENDON
726.79 PERONEAL DISLOCATING
727.67 RUPTURE - ACHILLES NONTRAUMATIC
727.62 RUPTURE - BICEPS (LONG HEAD) NONTRAUMATIC
727.68 RUPTURE - FOOT AND ANKLE NONTRAUMATIC
727.60 RUPTURE - NONTRAUMATIC
727.69 RUPTURE - NONTRAUMATIC NEC
727.66 RUPTURE - PATELLAR NONTRAUMATIC
727.65 RUPTURE - QUADRICEPS NONTRAUMATIC
727.61 RUPTURE - ROTATOR CUFF NONTRAUMATIC
0 RUPTURE - TRAUMATIC SEE 'SPRAIN'
0 RUPTURE - TRAUMATIC WITH LACERATION SEE 'LACERATION', TENDON
727.63 RUPTURE - WRIST AND HAND EXTENSOR NONTRAUMATIC
727.64 RUPTURE - WRIST AND HAND FLEXOR NONTRAUMATIC
727.42 SHEATH GANGLION (ANY)
727.82 SHEATH LESION (FOOT) (TOES)
756.89 SHORTENING CONGENITAL
727.89 OTHER DISORDER
0 TEAR SEE 'SPRAIN' BY SITE

787.99 TENESMUS

787.99 TENESMUS RECTAL

788.9 TENESMUS URINARY

726.32 TENNIS ELBOW
376.04 TENONITIS ORBIT

TENOSYNOVITIS
727.00 NOS
726.90 ADHESIVE
727.06 ANKLE
727.09 BUTTOCK
275.49 CRYSTAL INDUCED - UNSPECIFIED [**712.9#**]
0 CRYSTAL INDUCED - CHONDROCALCINOSIS SEE 'CHONDROCALCINOSIS'
274.0 CRYSTAL INDUCED - GOUTY
275.49 CRYSTAL INDUCED - OTHER SPECIFIED [**712.8#**]

5th Digit: 712.8-9
0. SITE NOS
1. SHOULDER REGION
2. UPPER ARM (ELBOW) (HUMERUS)
3. FOREARM (RADIUS) (WRIST) (ULNA)
4. HAND (CARPAL) (METACARPAL) (FINGERS)
5. PELVIC REGION AND THIGH (HIP) (BUTTOCK) (FEMUR)
6. LOWER LEG (FIBULA) (KNEE) (PATELLA) (TIBIA)
7. ANKLE AND/OR FOOT (METATARSALS) (TOES) (TARSALS)
8. OTHER (HEAD) (NECK) (RIB) (SKULL) (TRUNK) (VERTEBRAE)
9. MULTIPLE

727.09 ELBOW
727.05 FINGER
727.06 FOOT AND ANKLE
098.51 GONOCOCCAL
274.0 GOUTY
727.05 HAND AND WRIST
727.09 HIP
727.09 KNEE
727.04 RADIAL STYLOID
726.10 SHOULDER
726.0 SHOULDER ADHESIVE
720.1 SPINE
726.10 SUPRASPINATUS
095.7 SYPHILITIC
727.06 TOE
015.## TUBERCULOUS [727.01]

4th Digit: 015
0. VERTEBRAL COLUMN
1. HIP
2. KNEE
5. LIMB BONES
6. MASTOID
7. OTHER SPECIFIED BONE
8. OTHER SPECIFIED JOINT
9. UNSPECIFIED BONES AND JOINTS

5th Digit: 015
0. NOS
1. LAB NOT DONE
2. LABS PENDING
3. MICROSCOPY POSITIVE (IN SPUTUM)
4. CULTURE POSITIVE - MICROSCOPY NEGATIVE
5. CULTURE NEGATIVE - MICROSCOPY POSITIVE
6. CULTURE AND MICROSCOPY NEGATIVE CONFIRMED BY OTHER METHODS

727.05 WRIST
727.09 OTHER

307.81 TENSION HEADACHE PSYCHOGENIC
0 TENSION PNEUMOTHORAX SEE 'PNEUMOTHORAX'
352.3 TENTH CRANIAL NERVE ATROPHY
352.3 TENTH CRANIAL NERVE DISORDER
951.8 TENTH CRANIAL NERVE INJURY
352.3 TENTH NERVE PNEUMOGASTRIC DISORDERS
767.0 TENTORIAL TEAR BIRTH TRAUMA
199.1 TERATOCARCINOMA SITE NOS
0 TERATOCARCINOMA SITE SPECIFIED SEE 'CANCER' BY SITE M9081/3

TERATOMA
238.9 SITE NOS
0 SITE SPECIFIED SEE 'NEOPLASM UNCERTAIN BEHAVIOR' BY SITE M9080/1
211.5 BENIGN SITE NOS
0 BENIGN SITE SPECIFIED SEE 'BENIGN NEOPLASM', BY SITE M9080/0
155.0 MALIGNANT SITE NOS
0 MALIGNANT SITE SPECIFIED SEE 'CANCER' BY SITE M9080/3
199.1 MALIGNANT INTERMEDIATE TYPE SITE NOS
0 MALIGNANT INTERMEDIATE TYPE SITE SPECIFIED SEE 'CANCER' BY SITE M9083/3
186.9 MALIGNANT TROPHOBLASTIC SITE NOS
0 MALIGNANT TROPHOBLASTIC SITE SPECIFIED SEE 'CANCER' BY SITE M9102/3
199.1 MALIGNANT UNDIFFERENTIATED TYPE SITE NOS
0 MALIGNANT UNDIFFERENTIATED TYPE SITE SPECIFIED SEE 'CANCER' BY SITE M9082/3

WHEN USING CODE V66.7, CODE THE TERMINAL ILLNESS FIRST.

V66.7 TERMINAL CARE ENCOUNTER
127.7 TERNIDENS DIMINUTUS INFECTION
371.48 TERRIEN'S MARGINAL DEGENERATION OF CORNEA
362.21 TERRY'S SYNDROME

TESTIS, TESTICULAR
752.51 ABERRANT (CONGENITAL)
752.51 ABERRATIO (CONGENITAL)
608.89 ABSENCE
752.8 ABSENCE CONGENITAL
257.2 ANDROGEN DEFECTIVE BIOSYNTHESIS
752.9 ANOMALY NOS
752.8 APLASIA CONGENITAL
608.3 ATROPHY
V76.45 CANCER SCREENING
608.4 CELLULITIS (CARBUNCLE) (BOIL)
752.51 DESCENDED IMPERFECTLY
608.89 DISORDER OTHER SPECIFIED
257.9 DYSFUNCTION NOS
752.51 ECTOPIC (CONGENITAL)
257.1 FAILURE IATROGENIC (POST IRRADIATION) (POSTSURGICAL)
257.8 FEMINIZATION SYNDROME
608.89 FIBROSIS (HYPERTROPHY) (ULCER)
752.8 FUSION CONGENITAL
608.83 HEMORRHAGE (THROMBOSIS) (HEMATOMA) NONTRAUMATIC
257.2 HORMONE DEFICIENCY
257.0 HYPERFUNCTION
752.52 HYPERMOBILITY CONGENITAL
257.1 HYPOFUNCTION IATROGENIC
257.1 HYPOFUNCTION POSTABLATIVE
257.1 HYPOFUNCTION POSTIRRADIATION
257.1 HYPOFUNCTION POSTSURGICAL
257.2 HYPOFUNCTION OTHER
257.2 HYPOGONADISM
752.8 HYPOPLASIA CONGENITAL
752.51 INGUINAL (CONGENITAL)
911.8 INJURY OTHER AND UNSPECIFIED SUPERFICIAL
911.9 INJURY OTHER AND UNSPECIFIED SUPERFICIAL INFECTED
752.51 INVERSION (CONGENITAL)
752.51 MALDESCENDED (CONGENITAL)

T

TESTIS, TESTICULAR (continued)

608.89 MASS
752.52 MIGRATORY CONGENITAL
257.8 NONVIRILIZING SYNDROME
608.9 PAIN
752.52 RETRACTILE (CONGENITAL)
752.51 RETROVERSION (CONGENITAL)
016.5# TB [608.81]
5th Digit: 016.5
0. NOS
1. LAB NOT DONE
2. LABS PENDING
3. MICROSCOPY POSITIVE (IN SPUTUM)
4. CULTURE POSITIVE - MICROSCOPY NEGATIVE
5. CULTURE NEGATIVE - MICROSCOPY POSITIVE
6. CULTURE AND MICROSCOPY NEGATIVE CONFIRMED BY OTHER METHODS
608.2 TORSION
752.51 UNDESCENDED CONGENITAL

TETANUS

037 NOS
V07.2 ANTITOXIN ADMINISTRATION
670.0# MATERNAL DUE TO PREGNANCY (PUERPERAL) (MAJOR INFECTION)
5th Digit: 670.0
0. NOS
2. DELIVERED WITH POSTPARTUM COMPLICATION
4. POSTPARTUM COMPLICATION
771.3 NEONATORUM
771.3 OMPHALITIS PERINATAL
V74.8 SCREENING EXAM
V03.7 TOXOID VACCINATION (SINGLE)

TETANY

781.7 NOS
781.7 HYPERKINETIC
300.11 HYSTERICAL
771.3 NEONATORUM
775.4 NEWBORN (HYPOCALCEMIC)
252.1 PARATHYROID
252.1 PARATHYROPRIVAL
306.0 PSYCHOGENIC

742.59 TETHERED SPINAL CORD SYNDROME
V09.3 TETRACYCLINE RESISTANT INFECTION (SEE 'DRUG RESISTANCE', FOR COMPLETE LISTING)
745.2 TETRALOGY FALLOT
348.8 THALAMIC SYNDROME
282.4 THALASSEMIA
282.4 THALASSEMIA HB-S DISEASE
282.4 THALASSEMIA SICKLE CELL
579.0 THAYSEN-GEE DISEASE (NONTROPICAL SPRUE)
183.0 THECA CELL CARCINOMA SITE NOS
0 THECA CELL CARCINOMA SITE SPECIFIED SEE 'CANCER' BY SITE M8600/3
620.2 THECA LUTEIN CYST OF OVARY
220 THECOMA SITE NOS
0 THECOMA SITE SPECIFIED SEE 'BENIGN NEOPLASM', BY SITE M8600/0
259.1 THELARCHE PREMATURE
354.0 THENAR ATROPHY, PARTIAL

THERAPY

V57.9 NOS
V57.0 BREATHING EXERCISE
V57.1 EXERCISE
V57.89 MULTIPLE TYPES
V57.21 OCCUPATIONAL
V57.4 ORTHOPTIC
V57.81 ORTHOTIC OR GAIT
V57.1 PHYSICAL
V58.0 RADIATION
V57.3 SPEECH
V57.22 VOCATIONAL
V57.89 OTHER

793.# THERMOGRAPHY ABNORMAL FINDINGS (NONSPECIFIC)
4th Digit: 793
0. SKULL AND HEAD
1. LUNG FIELD
2. OTHER INTRATHORACIC ORGAN
3. BILIARY TRACT
4. GASTROINTESTINAL TRACT
5. GENITOURINARY ORGANS
6. ABDOMINAL AREA INCLUDING RETROPERITONEUM
7. MUSCULOSKELETAL SYSTEM
8. BREAST
9. OTHER

992.0 THERMOPLEGIA
909.4 THERMOPLEGIA LATE EFFECT
275.40 THESAURISMOSIS CALCIUM
710.1 THIBIERGE-WEISSENBACH SYNDROME (CUTANEOUS SYSTEMIC SCLEROSIS)
724.6 THIELE SYNDROME

THIGH

736.89 ABSENCE ACQUIRED
904.8 BLOOD VESSEL NEC INJURY
904.7 BLOOD VESSEL NEC INJURY MULTIPLE
904.7 BLOOD VESSEL INJURY SPECIFIED NEC
959.6 INJURY
916.8 INJURY OTHER AND UNSPECIFIED SUPERFICIAL
916.9 INJURY OTHER AND UNSPECIFIED SUPERFICIAL (INFECTED)
843.9 SEPARATION (RUPTURE) (TEAR) (LACERATION) UNSPECIFIED SITE
843.9 STRAIN (SPRAIN) (AVULSION) (HEMARTHROSIS) UNSPECIFIED SITE

THIRD

426.0 DEGREE HEART BLOCK
664.2# DEGREE LACERATION (PERINEAL)
5th Digit: 664.2
0. EPISODE OF CARE NOS OR N/A
1. DELIVERED
4. POSTPARTUM COMPLICATION
378.51 NERVE ATROPHY - PARTIAL
378.52 NERVE ATROPHY - TOTAL
951.0 NERVE INJURY
378.51 NERVE PALSY (DISORDER) - PARTIAL
378.52 NERVE PALSY (DISORDER) - TOTAL

994.3 THIRST
783.5 THIRST EXCESSIVE
909.4 THIRST LATE EFFECT
359.2 THOMSEN'S DISEASE
757.33 THOMSON'S DISEASE (CONGENITAL POIKILODERMA)

WHEN CODING BACK DISORDERS DUE TO DEGENERATION, DISPLACEMENT OR HNP OF THE INTERVERTEBRAL DISC, IT IS IMPORTANT TO DISTINGUISH WHETHER THESE CONDITIONS ARE WITH OR WITHOUT MYELOPATHY. MYELOPATHY REFERS TO FUNCTIONAL DISTURBANCES AND/OR PATHOLOGICAL CHANGES IN THE SPINAL CORD THAT RESULT FROM COMPRESSION.

THORACIC

901.0 AORTA INJURY
908.4 AORTA INJURY LATE EFFECT
901.9 BLOOD VESSEL INJURY - NOS
901.83 BLOOD VESSEL INJURY - MULTIPLE
901.89 BLOOD VESSEL INJURY - SPECIFIED NEC
722.92 DISC CALCIFICATION OR DISCITIS
722.51 DISC DISEASE/DEGENERATION
722.72 DISC DISEASE/DEGENERATION - WITH MYELOPATHY
722.92 DISC DISORDER
722.72 DISC DISORDER WITH MYELOPATHY
722.11 DISC DISPLACEMENT
722.72 DISC DISPLACEMENT WITH MYELOPATHY
722.11 DISC HERNIATION
722.72 DISC HERNIATION WITH MYELOPATHY
457.1 DUCT OBSTRUCTION OR OCCLUSION
457.8 DUCT RUPTURE
722.11 NERVE COMPRESSION - DISCOGENIC
722.72 NERVE COMPRESSION - DISCOGENIC WITH MYELOPATHY
724.4 NERVE COMPRESSION - ROOT (BY SCAR TISSUE) NEC
722.82 NERVE COMPRESSION - ROOT POSTOPERATIVE
353.3 NERVE ROOT DISORDER
353.0 OUTLET SYNDROME (NONDISCOGENIC)
724.4 RADICULITIS (NONVERTEBRAL) (NONDISCOGENIC)
739.2 REGION SEGMENTAL OR SOMATIC DYSFUNCTION

353.3 ROOT LESIONS NEC (NONDISCOGENIC)
847.1 SEPARATION (RUPTURE) (TEAR) (LACERATION)
724.1 SPINE PAIN (NONVERTEBRAL) (NONDISCOGENIC)
847.1 STRAIN (SPRAIN) (AVULSION) (HEMARTHROSIS)

THORACIC SPONDYLOSIS:

WITH OSTEOPOROSIS [733.0#]

721.2 THORACIC
721.41 THORACIC WITH MYELOPATHY (CORD COMPRESSION)
721.7 TRAUMATIC
WITH OSTEOPOROSIS [733.0#]
5th Digit: 733.0
0. UNSPECIFIED
1. SENILE
2. IDIOPATHIC
3. DISUSE
9. DRUG INDUCED

0 THORACIC TRAUMA SEE 'CHEST', TRAUMA
0 THORACIC SEE ALSO 'DORSAL'

441.7 THORACOABDOMINAL ANEURYSM AORTIC
441.6 THORACOABDOMINAL ANEURYSM AORTIC RUPTURED

731.2 THORACOGENOUS RHEUMATIC SYNDROME (HYPERTROPHIC PULMONARY OSTEOARTHROPATHY)

722.51 THORACOLUMBAR DISC DISEASE/DEGENERATION
722.72 THORACOLUMBAR DISC DISEASE/DEGENERATION - WITH MYELOPATHY

739.2 THORACOLUMBAR REGION SEGMENTAL OR SOMATIC DYSFUNCTION

759.4 THORACOPAGUS
593.9 THORN'S SYNDROME (RENAL DISEASE)
478.29 THORNWALDT'S DISEASE (PHARYNGEAL BURSITIS)
259.2 THORSON-BIORCK SYNDROME (MALIGNANT CARCINOID)

127.4 THREADWORM INFECTION

644.1# THREATENED LABOR >37 WEEKS
644.0# THREATENED LABOR >22 <37 WEEKS
5th Digit: 644.0-1
0. EPISODE OF CARE NOS OR N/A
3. ANTEPARTUM COMPLICATION

270.7 THREONINE METABOLISM DISTURBANCES

THROAT

478.29 ATROPHY
795.3 CULTURE POSITIVE NEC
478.20 DISEASE NOS
034.0 DISEASE SEPTIC
959.09 INJURY
910.8 INJURY OTHER AND UNSPECIFIED (SUPERFICIAL)
910.9 INJURY OTHER AND UNSPECIFIED (SUPERFICIAL) INFECTED
784.1 PAIN
0 SORE SEE 'PHARYNGITIS'
478.29 ULCER
032.0 ULCER DIPHTHERITIC

287.1 THROMBASTHENIA (HEMORRHAGIC) (HEREDITARY)
443.1 THROMBOANGIITIS OBLITERANS
648.9# THROMBOANGIITIS OBLITERANS (PAROXYSMAL DIGITAL CYANOSIS) MATERNAL CURRENT (CO-EXISTENT) IN PREGNANCY [443.1]
5th Digit: 648.9
0. EPISODE OF NOS OR N/A
1. DELIVERED
2. DELIVERED WITH POSTPARTUM COMPLICATION
3. ANTEPARTUM COMPLICATION
4. POSTPARTUM COMPLICATION

287.1 THROMBOCYTASTHENIA
238.7 THROMBOCYTHEMIA HEMORRHAGIC M9962/1
207.2# THROMBOCYTIC LEUKEMIA M9910/3
5th Digit: 207.2
0. WITHOUT MENTION OF REMISSION
1. IN REMISSION

287.1 THROMBOCYTOPATHY (DYSTROPHIC)

THROMBOCYTOPENIA

287.5 NOS
287.3 CONGENITAL
287.4 DILUTIONAL
287.4 DUE TO DIALYSIS
287.4 DUE TO DRUGS OR TRANSFUSION
287.4 DUE TO PLATELET ALLOIMMUNIZATION
287.3 ESSENTIAL
287.4 EXTRACORPOREAL CIRCULATION OF BLOOD
287.3 HEREDITARY
776.1 NEONATAL TRANSIENT
287.3 PRIMARY
287.4 SECONDARY

289.9 THROMBOCYTOSIS ESSENTIAL
444.9 THROMBOEMBOLIC DISEASE (SEE ALSO 'EMBOLISM')
287.1 THROMBOPATHY (BERNARD-SOULIER)
287.3 THROMBOPENIA-HEMANGIOMA SYNDROME

THROMBOPHLEBITIS LOWER EXTREMITIES

451.2 UNSPECIFIED DEEP OR SUPERFICIAL
451.11 FEMORAL VEIN DEEP
451.11 FEMORAL VEIN SUPERFICIAL
451.19 FEMOROPOPLITEAL (DEEP)
V12.52 HISTORY
451.11 ILIOFEMORAL (DEEP)
453.1 MIGRANS (DEEP)
451.19 POPLITEAL VEIN DEEP
451.0 POPLITEAL VEIN SUPERFICIAL
451.0 SAPHENOUS VEIN (GREATER) (LESSER) SUPERFICIAL
451.0 SUPERFICIAL VESSELS OF LOWER EXTREMITIES
451.19 TIBIAL VEIN (DEEP)
451.19 OTHER VESSELS (DEEP)

THROMBOPHLEBITIS UPPER EXTREMITIES

451.82 ANTECUBITAL VEIN (SUPERFICIAL)
451.84 ARM UNSPECIFIED NEC
451.89 AXILLARY VEIN
451.82 BASILIC VEIN (SUPERFICIAL)
451.83 BRACHIAL VEIN (DEEP)
451.82 CEPHALIC VEIN (SUPERFICIAL)
451.83 DEEP VESSELS
V12.52 HISTORY
451.89 JUGULAR VEIN
451.83 RADIAL VEIN (DEEP)
451.89 SUBCLAVIAN VEIN
451.82 SUPERFICIAL VESSELS
451.83 ULNAR VEIN (DEEP)
451.84 UPPER EXTREMITIES

THROMBOPHLEBITIS OTHER

451.9 SITE UNSPECIFIED
451.89 BREAST
326 CAVERNOUS SINUS PYOGENIC LATE EFFECT
451.89 CHEST WALL SUPERFICIAL
996.61 DUE TO CARDIAC DEVICE, IMPLANT, AND GRAFT
996.62 DUE TO OTHER VASCULAR DEVICE, IMPLANT, AND GRAFT
997.2 DURING OR RESULTING FROM A PROCEDURE
999.2 FOLLOWING INFUSION PERFUSION OR TRANSFUSION
274.89 GOUTY [451.9]
451.89 HEPATIC VEIN
V12.52 HISTORY
451.81 ILIAC VEIN (DEEP)
325 INTRACRANIAL SINUS (ANY)
326 INTRACRANIAL SINUS (ANY) LATE EFFECT
437.6 NONPYOGENIC
572.1 PORTAL VEIN
997.2 POSTOPERATIVE
362.18 RETINA
451.9 VEIN
451.89 VEIN OTHER SPECIFIED SITE
453.2 VENA CAVA
451.89 OTHER SPECIFIED SITE

THROMBOPHLEBITIS COMPLICATING ABORTION, PREGNANCY, OR PUERPERIUM

637.7# ABORTION UNSPECIFIED
638.7 ABORTION FAILED ATTEMPTED
636.7# ABORTION ILLEGALLY INDUCED
635.7# ABORTION LEGALLY INDUCED
634.7# ABORTION SPONTANEOUS
5th Digit: 634.7, 635.7, 636.7, 637.7
0. UNSPECIFIED
1. INCOMPLETE
2. COMPLETE

639.8 FOLLOWING ABORTION, ECTOPIC OR MOLAR PREGNANCY
671.3# MATERNAL DUE TO PREGNANCY ANTEPARTUM - DEEP
5th Digit: 671.3
0. EPISODE OF CARE NOS OR N/A
1. DELIVERED
3. ANTEPARTUM COMPLICATION

671.4# MATERNAL DUE TO PREGNANCY POSTPARTUM - DEEP
5th Digit: 671.4
0. EPISODE OF CARE NOS OR N/A
2. DELIVERED WITH POSTPARTUM COMPLICATION
4. POSTPARTUM COMPLICATION

671.2# MATERNAL DUE TO PREGNANCY - SUPERFICIAL
5th Digit: 671.2
0. EPISODE OF CARE NOS OR N/A
1. DELIVERED
2. DELIVERED WITH POSTPARTUM COMPLICATION
3. ANTEPARTUM COMPLICATION
4. POSTPARTUM COMPLICATION

THROMBOPHLEBITIS COMPLICATING ABORTION, PREGNANCY, OR PUERPERIUM (continued)

648.9#: USE AN ADDITIONAL CODE TO IDENTIFY THE SPECIFIC THROMBOPHLEBITIS.

648.9# MATERNAL IN PREGNANCY AND PUERPERIUM CURRENT (CO-EXISTENT)
5th Digit: 648.9
0. EPISODE OF NOS OR N/A
1. DELIVERED
2. DELIVERED WITH POSTPARTUM COMPLICATION
3. ANTEPARTUM COMPLICATION
4. POSTPARTUM COMPLICATION

THROMBOSIS

453.9 NOS
444.1 AORTA
444.0 AORTA ABDOMINAL
444.0 AORTA BIFURCATION
444.81 AORTA ILIAC
444.0 AORTA SADDLE
444.0 AORTA TERMINAL
444.1 AORTA THORACIC
434.0# APOPLEXY
5th Digit: 434.0
0. WITHOUT CEREBRAL INFARCTION
1. WITH CEREBRAL INFARCTION

0 APPENDIX, SEPTIC SEE 'APPENDICITIS', ACUTE
446.6 ARTERIOLAR-CAPILLARY PLATELET DISSEMINATED
444.9 ARTERY NOS
433.8# ARTERY AUDITORY INTERNAL
5th Digit: 433.8
0. WITHOUT CEREBRAL INFARCTION
1. WITH CEREBRAL INFARCTION

444.22 ARTERY EXTREMITY LOWER
444.21 ARTERY EXTREMITY UPPER
433.3# ARTERY PRECEREBRAL MULTIPLE AND BILATERAL
5th Digit: 433.3
0. WITHOUT CEREBRAL INFARCTION
1. WITH CEREBRAL INFARCTION

415.19 ARTERY PULMONARY
415.11 ARTERY PULMONARY IATROGENIC
415.11 ARTERY PULMONARY POSTOPERATIVE
0 ARTERY TRAUMATIC SEE SPECIFIED BLOOD VESSEL, INJURY
444.89 ARTERY OTHER SPECIFIED NEC
424.90 ATRIAL (ENDOCARDIAL)
093.89 ATRIAL (ENDOCARDIAL) DUE TO SYPHILIS
433.8# AUDITORY ARTERY, INTERNAL
5th Digit: 433.8
0. WITHOUT CEREBRAL INFARCTION
1. WITH CEREBRAL INFARCTION

0 AURICULAR HEART SEE 'MYOCARDIAL INFARCTION ACUTE'
453.8 AXILLARY (VEIN)
433.0# BASILAR ARTERY
433.3# BASILAR ARTERY BILATERAL OR MULTIPLE
5th Digit: 433.0, 3
0. WITHOUT CEREBRAL INFARCTION
1. WITH CEREBRAL INFARCTION

453.9 BLAND NEC
444.21 BRACHIAL ARTERY
434.0# BRAIN (ARTERY) (STEM)
5th Digit: 434.0
0. WITHOUT CEREBRAL INFARCTION
1. WITH CEREBRAL INFARCTION

094.89 BRAIN DUE TO SYPHILIS
997.02 BRAIN IATROGENIC
997.02 BRAIN POSTOPERATIVE
448.9 CAPILLARY
446.6 CAPILLARY ARTERIOLAR, GENERALIZED
0 CARDIAC SEE 'MYOCARDIAL INFARCTION ACUTE'
093.89 CARDIAC DUE TO SYPHILIS

THROMBOSIS (continued)

433.1# CAROTID ARTERY
433.3# CAROTID ARTERY BILATERAL OR MULTIPLE
5th Digit: 433.1, 3
0. WITHOUT CEREBRAL INFARCTION
1. WITH CEREBRAL INFARCTION

437.6 CAVERNOUS SINUS
325 CAVERNOUS SINUS PYOGENIC
433.8# CEREBELLAR ARTERY (ANTERIOR INFERIOR) (POSTERIOR INFERIOR)
434.0# CEREBRAL ARTERY
433.8# CHOROIDAL ARTERY (ANTERIOR)
433.8# COMMUNICATING POSTERIOR ARTERY
5th Digit: 433.8, 434.0
0. WITHOUT CEREBRAL INFARCTION
1. WITH CEREBRAL INFARCTION

093.89 CORONARY ARTERY DUE TO SYPHILIS
0 CORONARY ARTERY OR VEIN WITH INFARCTION SEE 'MYOCARDIAL INFARCTION ACUTE'
411.81 CORONARY ARTERY WITHOUT MI
607.82 CORPUS CAVERNOSUM
434.0# CORTICAL
5th Digit: 434.0
0. WITHOUT CEREBRAL INFARCTION
1. WITH CEREBRAL INFARCTION

0 DUE TO A DEVICE SEE 'COMPLICATION OF A DEVICE, IMPLANT OR GRAFT - OTHER SPECIFIED'
453.8 EFFORT
0 ENDOCARDIAL SEE 'MYOCARDIAL INFARCTION ACUTE'
444.22 EXTREMITY ARTERY NOS
444.22 EXTREMITY ARTERY LOWER
444.21 EXTREMITY ARTERY UPPER
0 EYE SEE 'RETINAL ARTERY OCCLUSION'
444.22 FEMORAL ARTERY
453.8 FEMORAL (VEIN) (DEEP)
451.11 FEMORAL (VEIN) (DEEP) WITH INFLAMMATION OR PHLEBITIS
608.83 GENITALIA MALE
0 HEART SEE 'MYOCARDIAL INFARCTION ACUTE'
444.89 HEPATIC ARTERY
572.1 HEPATIC INFECTIONAL OR SEPTIC
453.0 HEPATIC VEIN
V12.51 HISTORY VEIN
433.8# HYPOPHYSEAL ARTERY
5th Digit: 433.8
0. WITHOUT CEREBRAL INFARCTION
1. WITH CEREBRAL INFARCTION

444.81 ILIAC ARTERY
453.8 ILIAC (VEIN)
451.81 ILIAC (VEIN) WITH INFLAMMATION OR PHLEBITIS
0 INFLAMMATION VEIN SEE 'THROMBOPHLEBITIS LOWER EXTREMITIES' OR 'THROMBOPHLEBITIS UPPER EXTREMITIES'
557.0 INTESTINE (WITH GANGRENE)
434.0# INTRACRANIAL
5th Digit: 434.0
0. WITHOUT CEREBRAL INFARCTION
1. WITH CEREBRAL INFARCTION

325 INTRACRANIAL VENOUS SINUS (ANY)
437.6 INTRACRANIAL VENOUS SINUS (ANY) NONPYOGENIC ORIGIN
326 INTRACRANIAL VENOUS SINUS (ANY) LATE EFFECT
0 INTRAMURAL SEE 'MYOCARDIAL INFARCTION ACUTE'
429.89 INTRAMURAL WITHOUT CARDIAC CONDITION, CORONARY ARTERY DISEASE OR MI
453.8 JUGULAR (BULB)
593.81 KIDNEY (ARTERY)
453.8 LEG VESSELS (DEEP) (SUPERFICIAL)
0 LEG VESSELS (DEEP) (SUPERFICIAL) WITH INFLAMMATION OR PHLEBITIS SEE 'THROMBOPHLEBITIS'
453.0 LIVER (VENOUS)
444.89 LIVER ARTERY
572.1 LIVER INFECTIONAL OR SEPTIC

THROMBOSIS (continued)

444.22 LOWER EXTREMITY ARTERY
415.11 LUNG IATROGENIC
415.19 LUNG OTHER AND UNSPECIFIED
415.11 LUNG POSTOPERATIVE
437.6 MARANTIC, DURAL SINUS
433.8# MENINGEAL ARTERY, ANTERIOR OR POSTERIOR
434.0# MENINGES (BRAIN)
5th Digit: 433.8, 434.0
0. WITHOUT CEREBRAL INFARCTION
1. WITH CEREBRAL INFARCTION

557.0 MESENTERIC ARTERY (WITH GANGRENE)
557.0 MESENTERIC VEIN (WITH GANGRENE)
0 MITRAL SEE 'MITRAL INSUFFICIENCY'
0 MURAL SEE 'MYOCARDIAL INFARCTION ACUTE'
093.89 MURAL DUE TO SYPHILIS
429.79 MURAL ISCHEMIC HEART DISEASE (DUE TO) [414.8]
429.79 MURAL POST INFARCTION [410.90]
429.89 MURAL WITHOUT CARDIAC CONDITION, CORONARY ARTERY DISEASE OR MI
0 OBSTETRIC SEE 'THROMBOSIS COMPLICATING PREGNANCY'
557.0 OMENTUM (WITH GANGRENE)
0 OPHTHALMIC ARTERY SEE 'RETINAL ARTERY OCCLUSION'
620.8 PAMPINIFORM PLEXUS FEMALE
608.83 PAMPINIFORM PLEXUS MALE
0 PARIETAL SEE 'MYOCARDIAL INFARCTION ACUTE'
607.82 PENIS
444.22 PERIPHERAL ARTERIES NOS
444.22 PERIPHERAL ARTERIES LOWER
444.21 PERIPHERAL ARTERIES UPPER
446.6 PLATELET
433.8# PONTINE ARTERY
5th Digit: 433.8
0. WITHOUT CEREBRAL INFARCTION
1. WITH CEREBRAL INFARCTION

444.22 POPLITEAL ARTERY
452 PORTAL
093.89 PORTAL DUE TO SYPHILIS
572.1 PORTAL INFECTIONAL OR SEPTIC
433.9# PRECEREBRAL ARTERY NOS
433.3# PRECEREBRAL ARTERY BILATERAL OR MULTIPLE
433.8# PRECEREBRAL ARTERY NEC
5th Digit: 433.3, 8-9
0. WITHOUT CEREBRAL INFARCTION
1. WITH CEREBRAL INFARCTION

415.19 PULMONARY (ARTERY) (VEIN)
415.11 PULMONARY (ARTERY) (VEIN) IATROGENIC
415.11 PULMONARY (ARTERY) (VEIN) POSTOPERATIVE
446.6 PURPURA
444.21 RADIAL ARTERY
593.81 RENAL (ARTERY)
453.3 RENAL VEIN
0 RETINA (ARTERY) SEE 'RETINAL ARTERY OCCLUSION'
608.83 SCROTUM
608.83 SEMINAL VESICLE
325 SIGMOID (VENOUS) SINUS
437.6 SIGMOID (VENOUS) SINUS NONPYOGENIC ORIGIN
453.9 SILENT NEC
434.0# SOFTENING, BRAIN
5th Digit: 434.0
0. WITHOUT CEREBRAL INFARCTION
1. WITH CEREBRAL INFARCTION

608.83 SPERMATIC CORD
444.89 SPINAL ARTERY
433.8# SPINAL ARTERY, ANTERIOR OR POSTERIOR
5th Digit: 433.8
0. WITHOUT CEREBRAL INFARCTION
1. WITH CEREBRAL INFARCTION

336.1 SPINAL CORD
094.89 SPINAL CORD DUE TO SYPHILIS
324.1 SPINAL CORD PYOGENIC ORIGIN

THROMBOSIS (continued)
289.59 SPLEEN
444.89 SPLEEN ARTERY
608.83 TESTES
608.83 TUNICA VAGINALIS
444.21 ULNAR ARTERY
762.6 UMBILICAL CORD AFFECTING FETUS OR NEWBORN
444.21 UPPER EXTREMITY ARTERY
608.83 VAS DEFERENS
453.9 VEIN UNSPECIFIED
453.8 VEIN OTHER SPECIFIED SITE
453.2 VENA CAVA
433.2# VERTEBRAL ARTERY
433.3# VERTEBRAL ARTERY BILATERAL OR MULTIPLE
5th Digit: 433.2-3
0. WITHOUT CEREBRAL INFARCTION
1. WITH CEREBRAL INFARCTION
453.8 SPECIFIED SITE NEC

THROMBOSIS COMPLICATING PREGNANCY
671.9# NOS MATERNAL DUE TO PREGNANCY
674.0# BRAIN (ARTERY) (STEM) MATERNAL DUE TO PREGNANCY
671.5# BRAIN VENOUS MATERNAL DUE TO PREGNANCY
5th Digit: 671.5, 9, 674.0
0. EPISODE OF CARE NOS OR N/A
1. DELIVERED
2. DELIVERED WITH MENTION OF POSTPARTUM COMPLICATION
3. ANTEPARTUM COMPLICATION
4. POSTPARTUM COMPLICATION

WHEN CODING A MATERNAL CARDIOVASCULAR DISEASE COMPLICATING PREGNANCY, 648.6#, USE AN ADDITIONAL CODE TO IDENTIFY THE CONDITION.

648.6# CARDIAC MATERNAL CURRENT (CO-EXISTENT)
671.5# CEREBRAL VEIN OR VENOUS SINUS MATERNAL DUE TO PREGNANCY
5th Digit: 648.6, 671.5
0. EPISODE OF CARE NOS OR N/A
1. DELIVERED
2. DELIVERED WITH POSTPARTUM COMPLICATION
3. ANTEPARTUM COMPLICATION
4. POSTPARTUM COMPLICATION
671.3# DEEP VEIN ANTEPARTUM MATERNAL DUE TO PREGNANCY
5th Digit: 671.3
0. EPISODE OF CARE NOS OR N/A
1. DELIVERED
3. ANTEPARTUM COMPLICATION
671.4# DEEP VEIN POSTPARTUM MATERNAL DUE TO PREGNANCY
5th Digit: 671.4
0. UNSPECIFIED
2. DELIVERED WITH MENTION OF POSTPARTUM COMPLICATION
4. POSTPARTUM CONDITION OR COMPLICATION
671.5# INTRACRANIAL VENOUS SINUS NONPYOGENIC MATERNAL DUE TO PREGNANCY
5th Digit: 671.5
0. EPISODE OF CARE NOS OR N/A
1. DELIVERED
2. DELIVERED WITH MENTION OF POSTPARTUM COMPLICATION
3. ANTEPARTUM COMPLICATION
4. POSTPARTUM COMPLICATION
671.4# PELVIC MATERNAL DUE TO PREGNANCY
5th Digit: 671.4
0. UNSPECIFIED
2. DELIVERED WITH MENTION OF POSTPARTUM COMPLICATION
4. POSTPARTUM CONDITION OR COMPLICATION

THROMBOSIS COMPLICATING PREGNANCY (continued)
673.2# PULMONARY (ARTERY) (VEIN) MATERNAL DUE TO PREGNANCY
671.5# SPINAL CORD MATERNAL DUE TO PREGNANCY
671.2# SUPERFICIAL (VEIN) MATERNAL DUE TO PREGNANCY
5th Digit: 671.2, 5, 673.2
0. EPISODE OF CARE NOS OR N/A
1. DELIVERED
2. DELIVERED WITH MENTION OF POSTPARTUM COMPLICATION
3. ANTEPARTUM COMPLICATION
4. POSTPARTUM COMPLICATION
663.6# UMBILICAL CORD (VESSELS)
5th Digit: 663.6
0. EPISODE OF CARE NOS OR N/A
1. DELIVERED
3. ANTEPARTUM COMPLICATION
671.5# SPECIFIED SITE NEC MATERNAL DUE TO PREGNACY
5th Digit: 671.5
0. EPISODE OF CARE NOS OR N/A
1. DELIVERED
2. DELIVERED WITH MENTION OF POSTPARTUM COMPLICATION
3. ANTEPARTUM COMPLICATION
4. POSTPARTUM COMPLICATION

0 THROMBOTIC OBSTRUCTION SEE 'THROMBOSIS', BY SITE

446.6 THROMBOTIC PURPURA

446.6 THROMBOTIC THROMBOCYTOPENIC PURPURA
648.9# THROMBOTIC THROMBOCYTOPENIC PURPURA MATERNAL CURRENT (CO-EXISTENT) IN PREGNANCY [446.6]
5th Digit: 648.9
0. EPISODE OF NOS OR N/A
1. DELIVERED
2. DELIVERED WITH POSTPARTUM COMPLICATION
3. ANTEPARTUM COMPLICATION
4. POSTPARTUM COMPLICATION

0 THROMBUS SEE 'THROMBOSIS'

THRUSH
112.9 CANDIDAL UNSPECIFIED SITE
112.0 MOUTH
771.7 NEONATAL
112.0 ORAL

THUMB
755.29 ABSENCE CONGENITAL
V49.61 AMPUTATION STATUS
959.5 INJURY
915.8 INJURY OTHER AND UNSPECIFIED SUPERFICIAL
915.9 INJURY OTHER AND UNSPECIFIED SUPERFICIAL INFECTED
307.9 SUCKING (CHILD)

959.5 THUMBNAIL INJURY

370.21 THYGESON'S SUPERFICIAL PUNCTATE KERATITIS

0 THYMIC SEE 'THYMUS, THYMIC'

THYMOMA
212.6 BENIGN SITE NOS
0 BENIGN SITE SPECIFIED SEE 'BENIGN NEOPLASM', BY SITE M8580/0
164.0 MALIGNANT SITE NOS
0 MALIGNANT SITE SPECIFIED SEE 'CANCER' BY SITE M8580/3

THYMUS, THYMIC
254.1 ABSCESS
759.2 ABSENCE CONGENITAL
279.2 ALYMPHOPLASIA OR DYSPLASIA WITH IMMUNODEFICIENCY
254.8 ATROPHY
254.8 CYST
254.9 DISEASE (GLAND)
254.8 DISEASE (GLAND) SPECIFIED NEC
358.0 DISORDER CAUSING MYASTHENIA GRAVIS
254.8 FIBROSIS
862.29 GLAND INJURY
908.0 GLAND INJURY LATE EFFECT
862.39 GLAND INJURY WITH OPEN WOUND
254.0 HYPERPLASIA PERSISTENT
254.0 HYPERTROPHY
279.11 HYPOPLASIA
279.2 HYPOPLASIA WITH IMMUNODEFICIENCY
862.29 INJURY
862.39 INJURY WITH OPEN WOUND INTO CAVITY
908.0 INJURY LATE EFFECT

246.0 THYROCALCITONIN SECRETION DISORDER

THYROGLOSSAL
759.2 DUCT CYST CONGENITAL
759.2 DUCT FISTULA CONGENITAL
759.2 DUCT PERSISTENT

THYROID
245.0 ABSCESS
748.3 ABSENCE - CARTILAGE CONGENITAL
243 ABSENCE - CONGENITAL (GLAND)
246.8 ABSENCE - SURGICAL
226 ADENOMA
258.1 ADRENOCORTICAL INSUFFICIENCY SYNDROME
246.8 ATROPHY
243 ATROPHY CONGENITAL
246.8 BINDING GLOBULIN ABNORMALITY
748.3 CARTILAGE ANOMALY CONGENITAL
748.3 CARTILAGE CLEFT CONGENITAL
246.2 CYST
226 CYSTADENOMA
246.9 DISORDER (GLAND)
246.8 DISORDER (GLAND) OTHER SPECIFIED
V77.0 DISORDER SCREENING

CODE THE SPECIFIC MATERNAL THYROID DYSFUNCTION IN ADDITION TO THE 648.##

648.1# DYSFUNCTION MATERNAL CURRENT (CO-EXISTENT) IN PREGNANCY

5th Digit: 648.1
- **0. EPISODE OF CARE NOS OR N/A**
- **1. DELIVERED**
- **2. DELIVERED WITH POSTPARTUM COMPLICATION**
- **3. ANTEPARTUM COMPLICATION**
- **4. POSTPARTUM COMPLICATION**

759.2 ECTOPIC
0 ENLARGEMENT SEE 'GOITER'
794.5 FUNCTION ABNORMAL FINDING
759.2 GLAND ACCESSORY CONGENITAL
246.3 HEMORRHAGE
240.9 HYPERPLASIA (SEE ALSO 'GOITER')
242.0# HYPERPLASIA PRIMARY
242.2# HYPERPLASIA SECONDARY

5th Digit: 242.0, 2
- **0. WITHOUT MENTION OF THYROTOXIC CRISIS OR STORM**
- **1. WITH MENTION OF THYROTOXIC CRISIS OR STORM**

246.8 HYPER-TBG-NEMIA
246.8 HYPO-TBG-NEMIA

THYROID (continued)
246.3 INFARCTION OR HEMORRHAGE
959.09 INJURY
243 INSUFFICIENCY CONGENITAL
244.# INSUFFICIENCY

4th Digit: 244
- **0. POSTSURGICAL**
- **1. POSTABLATIVE (IRRADIATION)**
- **2. IODINE INGESTION**
- **3. PAS, PHENYLBUT, RESORCINOL**
- **8. SECONDARY NEC**
- **9. NOS**

0 NODULE SEE 'GOITER'
794.5 SCAN ABNORMAL
848.2 SEPARATION (RUPTURE) (TEAR) (LACERATION)
848.2 STRAIN (SPRAIN) (AVULSION) (HEMARTHROSIS)
794.5 UPTAKE ABNORMAL

THYROIDITIS
245.9 NOS
245.0 ACUTE
245.0 ACUTE NONSUPPURATIVE
245.0 ACUTE PYOGENIC
245.0 ACUTE SUPPURATIVE

245.3 CHRONIC FIBROUS (STRUMAL) (LIGNEOUS) (INVASIVE)
245.2 CHRONIC LYMPHOCYTIC (HASHIMOTO'S) (AUTOIMMUNE) (STRUMAL)
245.8 CHRONIC UNSPECIFIED

245.1 DE QUERVAIN (GIANT CELL) (GRANULOMATOUS) (VIRAL)
245.4 IATROGENIC
245.3 RIEDEL'S
245.1 SUBACUTE

759.2 THYROLINGUAL DUCT PERSISTENT
240.9 THYROMEGALY (SEE ALSO 'GOITER')

THYROTOXICOSIS
775.3 NEONATAL
242.## THYROTOXIC EXOPHTHALMOS [376.21]
242.## WITH MYASTHENIC SYNDROME [358.1]
242.## WITH OR WITHOUT GOITER

4th Digit: 242
- **0. DIFFUSE**
- **1. UNINODULAR**
- **2. MULTINODULAR**
- **3. NODULAR UNSPECIFIED**
- **4. ECTOPIC THYROID NODULE**
- **8. OTHER SPECIFIED**
- **9. NOS**

5th Digit: 242
- **0. WITHOUT MENTION OF THYROTOXIC CRISIS OR STORM**
- **1. WITH MENTION OF THYROTOXIC CRISIS OR STORM**

435.9 TIA TRANSIENT ISCHEMIC ATTACK

TIBIA
755.31 ABSENCE CONGENITAL - WITH ABSENCE COMPLETE DISTAL ELEMENTS
755.36 ABSENCE CONGENITAL - WITH ABSENCE INCOMPLETE DISTAL ELEMENTS
755.35 ABSENCE CONGENITAL - WITH ABSENCE FIBULA WITH ABSENCE INCOMPLETE DISTAL ELEMENTS
755.36 AGENESIS
754.43 AND FIBULA BOWING CONGENITAL
755.69 ANGULATION CONGENITAL
958.8 COMPARTMENT SYNDROME
736.89 DEFORMITY ACQUIRED
733.90 DISORDER
733.29 DISORDER FIBROCYSTIC
733.99 DISORDER OTHER SPECIFIED
755.69 PSEUDOARTHROSIS CONGENITAL
736.89 TORSION ACQUIRED
732.4 VARA LOWER EXTREMITY EXCLUDING FOOT JUVENILE

T

TIBIAL
444.22 ARTERY (EMBOLISM) (THROMBOSIS) (OCCLUSION) (INFARCTION)
904.50 ARTERY INJURY - NOS
904.51 ARTERY INJURY - ANTERIOR
904.53 ARTERY INJURY - POSTERIOR
908.3 ARTERY INJURY - LATE EFFECT (ANTERIOR) (POSTERIOR)

355.5 NERVE POSTERIOR COMPRESSION (DISORDER)
956.2 NERVE POSTERIOR INJURY
907.5 NERVE POSTERIOR INJURY LATE EFFECT

736.89 TORSION

904.50 VEIN INJURY - NOS
904.52 VEIN INJURY - ANTERIOR
904.54 VEIN INJURY - POSTERIOR
908.3 VEIN INJURY - LATE EFFECT (ANTERIOR) (POSTERIOR)

904.50 VESSEL INJURY
908.3 VESSEL INJURY LATE EFFECT
904.50 VESSEL LACERATION (ANEURYSM) (AVULSION) (HEMATOMA) (RUPTURE) TRAUMATIC
908.3 VESSEL LACERATION LATE EFFECT

726.72 TIBIALIS TENDINITIS
844.3 TIBIOFIBULAR (JOINT) (LIGAMENT) SUPERIOR SPRAIN, STRAIN OR TEAR

TIC DISORDER
307.20 NOS
307.21 CHILDHOOD TRANSIENT
307.22 CHRONIC MOTOR OR VOCAL HABIT
307.22 CHRONIC MOTOR OR VOCAL SPASM
307.23 GILLES DE LA TOURETTE'S SYNDROME
307.22 HABIT SPASM
307.23 MOTOR VERBAL
333.3 ORGANIC ORIGIN

350.1 TIC DOULOUREUX
053.12 TIC DOULOUREAUX POSTHERPETIC
333.3 TIC ORGANIC ORIGIN

TICK
087.1 AFRICAN TICK-BITE FEVER
066.1 AMERICAN MOUNTAIN TICK-BORNE FEVER
0 BITE SEE 'INSECT BITE' BY SITE
082.# BORNE RICKETTSIOSES
4th Digit: 082
0. SPOTTED FEVER
1. BOUTONNEUSE FEVER
2. NORTH ASIAN TICK FEVER
3. QUEENSLAND TICK TYPHUS
8. OTHER SPECIFIED TICK - BORNE RICKETTSIOSIS
9. UNSPECIFIED TICK - BORNE RICKETTSIOSIS
066.1 COLORADO (VIRUS) TICK-BITE FEVER
066.1 COLORADO TICK-BORNE FEVER
0 ENCEPHALITIS (TICK-BORNE) SEE 'ENCEPHALITIS'
066.1 FEVER TICK-BORNE NEC
065.3 HEMORRHAGIC TICK-BORNE FEVER NEC
065.0 HEMORRHAGIC CRIMEAN TICK-BORNE FEVER
065.2 HEMORRHAGIC KYASANUR FOREST TICK-BORNE FEVER
065.1 HEMORRHAGIC OMSK TICK-BORNE FEVER
066.1 KEMEROVO TICK-BORNE FEVER
0 LYME DISEASE SEE 'LYME DISEASE'
066.1 MOUNTAIN TICK-BORNE FEVER
066.1 NONEXANTHEMATOUS
989.5 PARALYSIS
066.1 QUARANFIL TICK-BORNE FEVER
082.0 ROCKY MOUNTAIN TICK-BITE FEVER

287.3 TIDAL PLATELET DYSGENESIS
733.6 TIETZE'S DISEASE OR SYNDROME
605 TIGHT FORESKIN
307.45 TIME-ZONE SYNDROME (RAPID)

TINEA
110.9 NOS
111.2 BLANCA
110.# BY SITE
4th Digit: 110
0. SCALP AND BEARD
1. NAIL (UNGUIUM)
2. HAND (MANUUM)
3. GROIN AND PERIANAL (CRURIS)
4. FOOT (PEDIS)
5. BODY (CORPORIS)
6. DEEP SEATED (GRANULOMA TRICHOPHYTICUM)
8. OTHER SPECIFIED SITE
9. UNSPECIFIED SITE

110.0 CAPITIS
110.5 CORPORIS
110.3 CRURIS OF GROIN AND PERIANAL AREA
111.0 FLAVA
110.5 IMBRICATA (TOKELAU)
110.2 MANUUM (OF HAND)
110.9 MICROSPORIC
111.1 NIGRA
110.0 OF SCALP AND BEARD KERION
111.1 PALMARIS NIGRA
110.4 PEDIS OF FOOT ATHLETE'S FOOT
110.0 TRICHOPHYTIC (BLACK DOT TINEA), SCALP
110.1 UNGUIUM OF NAIL
111.0 VERSICOLOR

782.0 TINGLING OF SKIN

TINNITUS
388.30 NOS
388.32 OBJECTIVE
388.31 SUBJECTIVE

780.79 TIREDNESS
524.6# TMJ SYNDROME
5th Digit: 524.6
0. UNSPECIFIED
1. ADHESIONS AND ANKYLOSIS
2. ARTHRALGIA
3. ARTICULAR DISC DISORDER (REDUCING OR NON REDUCING)
9. OTHER SPECIFIED JOINT DISORDER

305.1 TOBACCO ABUSE NONDEPENDENT
V15.82 TOBACCO USE HISTORY
162.3 TOBIAS' SYNDROME (CARCINOMA PULMONARY APEX) M8010/3

TOE
755.39 ABSENCE CONGENITAL
755.31 ABSENCE (ALL TOES) (COMPLETE) CONGENITAL
V49.72 AMPUTATION STATUS
V49.71 AMPUTATION STATUS GREAT TOE
735.# DEFORMITY
4th Digit: 735
0. HALLUX VALGUS (ACQUIRED)
1. HALLUX VARUS (ACQUIRED)
2. HALLUX RIGIDUS
3. HALLUX MALLEUS
4. OTHER HAMMER TOE (ACQUIRED)
5. CLAW TOE (ACQUIRED)
8. OTHER ACQUIRED DEFORMITY
9. NOS
755.66 DEFORMITY CONGENITAL
735.8 DROP
917.8 INJURY OTHER AND UNSPECIFIED SUPERFICIAL
917.9 INJURY OTHER AND UNSPECIFIED SUPERFICIAL INFECTED
718.17 JOINT LOOSE BODY
V43.69 JOINT REPLACEMENT STATUS

TOE (continued)

703.8	NAIL DEFORMITY (HYPERTROPHY)
703.8	NAIL DISCOLORATION
703.8	NAIL DISEASE OTHER SPECIFIED
110.1	NAIL FUNGUS
681.9	NAIL INFECTION
703.0	NAIL INFECTION INGROWING
681.11	NAIL INFECTION ONYCHIA OR PARONYCHIA
703.0	NAIL INGROWN (INFECTED)
959.7	NAIL INJURY
110.1	NAIL MYCOSIS
703.8	NAIL THICKENING
735.8	OVERLAPPING
755.66	OVERLAPPING CONGENITAL
729.5	PAIN
0	SEE ALSO 'DIGITAL'

926.0	TOILET SEAT SYNDROME
378.55	TOLOSA-HUNT SYNDROME

TONGUE

0	SEE ALSO 'GLOTTIS(C)'
529.0	ABSCESS
750.11	ABSENCE (CONGENITAL)
529.8	ATROPHY (HYPERTROPHY) (ENLARGED) (SENILE)
529.4	ATROPHY PAPILLAE (SENILE)
474.00	BASE LYMPHOID TISSUE INFECTION
529.3	COATED
529.9	DISEASE UNSPECIFIED
478.6	EDEMA
528.7	ERYTHROPLAKIA
528.8	FIBROSIS
529.5	FISSURED
529.5	FURROWED
529.1	GEOGRAPHIC
959.09	INJURY
524.5	LIP OR FINGER HABITS CAUSING MALOCCLUSION
529.8	OTHER SPECIFIED CONDITIONS
529.6	PAIN GLOSSODYNIA
529.4	PAPILLAE ATROPHY
529.3	PAPILLAE HYPERTROPHY
529.8	PARALYSIS
529.5	PLICATED
529.5	SCROTAL
529.4	SMOOTH ATROPHIC
478.75	SPASM
306.1	SPASM PSYCHOGENIC
529.4	ULCERATION
529.0	ULCERATION TRAUMATIC

TONGUE CONGENITAL ANOMALY

750.10	UNSPECIFIED
750.12	ADHESIONS
750.13	BIFID
750.13	DOUBLE
750.13	FISSURE
750.15	HYPERTROPHY
750.16	HYPOPLASIA
750.0	TIE
750.19	OTHER SPECIFIED

270.0	TONI-FANCONI SYNDROME (CYSTINOSIS)

TONSIL, TONSILLAR

474.8	AMYGDALOLITH
475	ANGINA
474.8	CALCULUS
474.8	CICATRIX
474.9	DISEASE (CHRONIC)
474.8	DISEASE (CHRONIC) SPECIFIED NEC
474.11	ENLARGEMENT
474.01	ENLARGEMENT WITH CHRONIC ADENOIDITIS
474.02	ENLARGEMENT WITH CHRONIC ADENOIDITIS AND TONSILLITIS
474.00	ENLARGEMENT WITH CHRONIC TONSILLITIS

TONSIL, TONSILLAR (continued)

474.11	HYPERPLASIA (LYMPHOID)
474.10	HYPERPLASIA AND ADENOIDS HYPERPLASIA (LYMPHOID)
474.11	HYPERTROPHY (HYPERPLASIA)
474.10	HYPERTROPHY (HYPERPLASIA) WITH ADENOID HYPERTROPHY
474.01	HYPERTROPHY (HYPERPLASIA) WITH CHRONIC ADENOIDITIS
474.02	HYPERTROPHY (HYPERPLASIA) WITH CHRONIC ADENOIDITIS AND TONSILLITIS
474.00	HYPERTROPHY (HYPERPLASIA) WITH CHRONIC TONSILLITIS
959.09	INJURY
474.8	REMNANT
474.00	REMNANT INFECTED
474.8	TAG
474.00	TAG INFECTED
474.8	ULCER
474.10	WITH ADENOIDS HYPERTROPHY

IF THE DIAGNOSIS IS NOT SPECIFIED AS ACUTE ON THE RECORD, SELECT THE CHRONIC OR NOS CODE. IF THE MEDICAL RECORD INDICATES THAT THE REASON THE PATIENT SOUGHT CARE WAS DUE TO AN EXACERBATION OF A CHRONIC CONDITION, CONSULT THE PHYSICIAN FOR FURTHER DOCUMENTATION.

TONSILLITIS

463	NOS
463	ACUTE
463	ACUTE FOLLICULAR
463	ACUTE INFECTIVE
463	ACUTE PNEUMOCOCCAL
463	ACUTE STAPHYLOCOCCAL
034.0	ACUTE STREPTOCOCCAL
463	ACUTE VIRAL
474.00	CHRONIC
474.02	CHRONIC WITH CHRONIC ADENOIDITIS
474.00	CHRONIC WITH HYPERTROPHY (ADENOIDS) (TONSILS)
474.02	CHRONIC WITH HYPERTROPHY (ADENOIDS) (TONSILS) WITH CHRONIC ADENOIDITIS
475	OPEN PERITONSILLAR ABSCESS

465.8	TONSILLOPHARYNGITIS

TOOTH

520.2	ABNORMAL FORM
520.2	ABNORMAL SIZE
520.0	ABSENCE (COMPLETE) (PARTIAL) (CONGENITAL)
525.1	ABSENCE ACQUIRED
525.1	ABSENCE DUE TO ACCIDENT, TRAUMA OR PERIODONTAL DISEASE
524.3	ABSENCE WITH MALOCCLUSION / ABNORMAL SPACING
523.6	ACCRETIONS
525.9	ACHE
521.0	ACHE DUE TO DENTAL CARIES
520.6	ACHE DUE TO OBSTRUCTED OR IMPACTED TOOTH
524.3	ANOMALIES OF POSITION
525.2	ATROPHY OF EDENTULOUS ALVEOLAR RIDGE
873.63	BROKEN
873.73	BROKEN COMPLICATED
521.7	COLOR CHANGES DUE TO METALS, DRUGS, BLEEDING OR UNSPECIFIED
523.6	COLOR CHANGES DUE TO DEPOSITS ON TEETH
521.7	COLOR CHANGES POST-ERUPTIVE
520.8	COLOR CHANGES PRE-ERUPTIVE
520.2	CONCRESCENCE
520.2	CONICAL
524.3	CROWDING
523.6	DEPOSITS BETEL
523.6	DEPOSITS MATERIA ALBA
523.6	DEPOSITS SOFT
523.6	DEPOSITS TARTAR
523.6	DEPOSITS TOBACCO
524.3	DIASTEMA
520.4	DILACERATION DEVELOPMENTAL DISORDER

T

TOOTH (continued)

520.9 DISORDER - DEVELOPMENT AND ERUPTION NOS
525.9 DISORDER - TEETH AND SUPPORTING STRUCTURES NOS
524.3 DISPLACEMENT
520.6 EMBEDDED
524.3 EMBEDDED DUE TO ABNORMAL POSITION OF SUCH TEETH OR ADJACENT TEETH
520.6 ERUPTION ACCELERATED OR NEONATAL
520.6 ERUPTION INCOMPLETE, DELAYED, DIFFICULT
520.6 ERUPTION LATE OR PREMATURE
520.6 ERUPTION OBSTRUCTED, PERSISTENT, PRIMARY
525.0 EXFOLIATION DUE TO SYSTEMIC CAUSES
520.4 FORMATION DISTURBANCE
520.2 FUSION
520.2 GEMINATION
306.8 GRINDING
520.4 HYPOCALCIFICATION
520.6 IMPACTED
524.3 IMPACTED DUE TO ABNORMAL POSITION OF SUCH TEETH OR ADJACENT TEETH
996.69 IMPLANT COMPLICATION - INFECTION OR INFLAMMATION
996.59 IMPLANT COMPLICATION - MECHANICAL
996.79 IMPLANT COMPLICATION - OTHER
873.63 INJURY
873.73 INJURY COMPLICATED
525.8 LOOSE
525.1 LOSS DUE TO ACCIDENT, EXTRACTION OR PERIODONTAL DISEASE
520.3 MOTTLED
524.2 OCCLUSION
520.2 PEG-SHAPED
525.3 RETAINED DENTAL ROOT
524.3 ROTATION
520.5 SHELL
524.3 SPACING ABNORMAL
520.5 STRUCTURE DISTURBANCE HEREDITARY
520.2 SUPERNUMERARY ROOTS
520.1 SUPERNUMERARY TEETH
520.1 SUPPLEMENTAL
524.3 TRANSPOSITION
520.8 OTHER SPECIFIED DISORDERS OF DEVELOPMENT AND ERUPTION
525.8 OTHER SPECIFIED DISORDERS OF TEETH AND SUPPORTING STRUCTURES

TOOTH DISORDER OF HARD TISSUE

521.9 DISEASE OR DISORDER NOS (HARD TISSUES)
521.2 ABRASION
521.6 ANKYLOSIS

523.6 COLOR CHANGES DUE TO DEPOSITS ON TEETH
521.7 COLOR CHANGES POSTERUPTIVE
521.7 COLOR CHANGES POSTERUPTIVE DUE TO DRUGS
521.7 COLOR CHANGES POSTERUPTIVE DUE TO METALS
521.7 COLOR CHANGES POSTERUPTIVE DUE TO PULPAL BLEEDING
520.8 COLOR CHANGES PRE-ERUPTIVE

521.0 DENTAL CARIES

521.3 EROSION
521.3 EROSION DUE TO MEDICINE
521.3 EROSION DUE TO VOMITING
521.3 EROSION IDIOPATHIC
521.3 EROSION OCCUPATIONAL

521.1 EXCESSIVE WEAR
521.4 GRANULOMA INTERNAL OF PULP
521.5 HYPERCEMENTOSIS
521.8 IRRADIATED ENAMEL
521.4 PATHOLOGICAL RESORPTION

521.8 SENSITIVE DENTIA
521.2 WEDGE DEFECT
521.0 WHITE SPOT LESIONS
521.8 OTHER SPECIFIED DISEASES (HARD TISSUES)

TOOTH PULP AND PERIAPICAL DISORDERS

522.3 ABNORMAL HARD TISSUE FORMATION PULP
522.7 ABSCESS PERIAPICAL WITH SINUS
522.5 ABSCESS PERIAPICAL WITHOUT SINUS
522.0 ABSCESS PULPAL
522.8 CYST APICAL, PERIAPICAL OR RADICULAR
522.2 DEGENERATION OF PULP
522.1 NECROSIS OF PULP
522.4 PERIODONTITIS ACUTE OF PULPAL ORIGIN
523.4 PERIODONTITIS CHRONIC
522.0 POLYP PULPAL
522.0 PULPITIS
522.9 OTHER AND UNSPECIFIED DISEASES OF PULP OR PERIAPICAL TISSUE

TORCH SYNDROME

771.1 CYTOMEGALOVIRUS
771.2 HERPES SIMPLEX
771.2 LISTERIOSIS
771.2 MALARIA
771.0 RUBELLA
771.2 TOXOPLASMOSIS
771.2 TUBERCULOSIS

008.69 TOROVIRUS ENTERITIS

TORSION

333.89 DYSTONIA (FRAGMENTS) (OTHER)
333.7 DYSTONIA SYMPTOMATIC
620.5 HYTADID OF MORGAGNI
560.2 INTESTINE
620.5 OVARY
608.2 TESTIS (EPIDIDYMIS) (SPERMATIC CORD)

TORTICOLLIS

723.5 NOS
754.1 CONGENITAL
767.8 DUE TO BIRTH INJURY
300.11 HYSTERICAL
306.0 PSYCHOGENIC
333.83 SPASMODIC
306.0 SYNDROME
847.0 TRAUMATIC CURRENT

117.5 TORULA

0 TORUS FRACTURE SEE 'FRACTURE', (BONE) CLOSED OR OPEN

526.81 TORUS MANDIBULARIS
526.81 TORUS PALATINUS

747.41 TOTAL ANOMALOUS PULMONARY VENOUS CONNECTION

790.99 TOTAL PROTEINS ABNORMAL

756.89 TOURAINE'S SYNDROME (HEREDITARY OSTEO-ONYCHODYSPLASIA)

757.39 TOURAINE-SOLENTE-GOLE SYNDROME (ACROPACHYDERMA)

307.23 TOURETTE'S DISORDER

756.0 TOWER SKULL

0 TOXEMIA SEE 'ECLAMPSIA' OR 'PREECLAMPSIA'

TOXIC

377.34 AMBLYOPIA
695.1 EPIDERMAL NECROLYSIS
695.0 ERYTHEMA
556.5 MEGACOLON
358.2 MYONEURAL DISORDERS
357.7 NEURITIS
710.5 OIL SYNDROME
040.89 SHOCK SYNDROME

TOXIC (continued)

760.70 SUBSTANCE NOS TRANSMITTED VIA PLACENTA OR BREAST MILK AFFECTING FETUS OR NEWBORN
760.75 SUBSTANCE COCAINE TRANSMITTED VIA PLACENTA OR BREAST MILK AFFECTING FETUS OR NEWBORN
760.79 SUBSTANCE NEC TRANSMITTED VIA PLACENTA OR BREAST MILK AFFECTING FETUS OR NEWBORN

796.0 TOXICITY DRUG - ASYMPTOMATIC
0 TOXICITY DRUG - SYMPTOMATIC SEE DRUGS AND CHEMICALS (APPENDIX B) OR 'POISONING MEDICINAL'
796.0 TOXICOLOGY FINDINGS ABNORMAL
128.0 TOXOCARA CANIS CATI INFECTION
128.0 TOXOCARIASIS
0 TOXOPLASMA GONDII INFECTION SEE 'TOXOPLASMOSIS'

TOXOPLASMOSIS

130.9 NOS
130.2 CHORIORETINITIS
771.2 CONGENITAL OR PERINATAL
130.1 CONJUNCTIVITIS
130.5 HEPATITIS
655.4# MATERNAL WITH SUSPECTED DAMAGE TO FETUS

5th Digit: 655.4
0. EPISODE OF CARE NOS OR N/A
1. DELIVERED
3. ANTEPARTUM COMPLICATION

130.0 MENINGOENCEPHALITIS
130.8 MULTIPLE SITES
130.8 MULTISYSTEMIC DISSEMINATED
130.3 MYOCARDITIS
130.4 PNEUMONIA
130.7 OTHER SPECIFIED SITES

V07.8 TOXOXIFEN ADMINISTRATION DUE TO <u>FAMILY HISTORY CANCER BREAST</u> [<u>V16.3</u>]

TRACHEA

478.9 ABSCESS
519.1 ATROPHY
519.1 CALCIFICATION
478.9 CICATRIX
0 COMPLICATION FOLLOWING TRACHEOSTOMY SEE 'TRACHEOSTOMY'
519.1 DISEASE
519.1 DIVERTICULUM
874.02 LACERATION
874.12 LACERATION COMPLICATED
519.1 OBSTRUCTION
519.1 STENOSIS
519.1 TRACHEOMALACIA
519.1 ULCER

TRACHEA CONGENITAL

748.3 ABSENCE OR AGENESIS
748.3 ATRESIA
748.3 CARTILAGE ANOMALY
748.3 DILATION
748.3 DIVERTICULUM
748.3 STENOSIS
748.3 TRACHEOMALACIA

464.4 TRACHEALIS ANGINA

TRACHEITIS

464.3# NOS
464.1# ACUTE
464.1# ACUTE VIRAL
464.1# ACUTE WITH CATARRH
464.2# ACUTE WITH LARYNGITIS

5th Digit: 464.1-3
1. WITH OBSTRUCTION
0. NOS

034.0 ACUTE STREPTOCOCCAL

TRACHEITIS (continued)

491.8 CHRONIC
476.1 CHRONIC WITH LARYNGITIS
487.1 VIRAL INFLUENZA
0 WITH BRONCHITIS SEE 'BRONCHITIS'

TRACHEOBRONCHITIS

490 BRONCHITIS
466.0 ACUTE
493.## ACUTE ASTHMATIC

4th Digit: 493
0. EXTRINSIC (OR ALLERGIC WITH STATED CAUSE)
1. INTRINSIC
2. CHRONIC OBSTRUCTIVE WITH COPD
9. NOS (OR ALLERGIC CAUSE NOT STATED)

5th Digit: 493
0. WITHOUT MENTION OF STATUS ASTHMATICUS
1. WITH STATUS ASTHMATICUS

460 ACUTE DUE TO <u>RSV</u> (RESPIRATORY SYNCYTIAL VIRUS) [<u>079.6</u>]
491.9 CHRONIC
491.2# CHRONIC ASTHMATIC

5th Digit: 491.2
0.WITHOUT MENTION OF ACUTE EXACERBATION
1.WITH ACUTE EXACERBATION

491.20 CHRONIC OBSTRUCTIVE
491.21 CHRONIC OBSTRUCTIVE WITH EXACERBATION
0 SEE ALSO 'BRONCHITIS'

748.3 TRACHEOCELE CONGENITAL
750.3 TRACHEOESOPHAGEAL FISTULA CONGENITAL
519.1 TRACHEOMALACIA
748.3 TRACHEOMALACIA CONGENITAL

TRACHEOSTOMY

V55.0 CARE
V55.0 CLOSURE
519.00 COMPLICATION NOS
519.02 COMPLICATION MECHANICAL
519.09 COMPLICATION OTHER
519.09 FISTULA
519.09 HEMORRHAGE

WHEN CODING AN INFECTION OF AN OSTOMY, USE AN ADDITIONAL CODE TO SPECIFY THE ORGANISM. SEE 'BACTERIAL INFECTION'

519.01 INFECTION
<u>519.01</u> <u>INFECTION</u> WITH CELLULITIS OF NECK [682.1]
<u>519.01</u> <u>INFECTION</u> WITH SEPSIS [**038.#(#)**]

4th or 4th <u>and</u> 5th Digit Code for Organism: 038
.9 NOS
.3 ANAEROBIC
.3 BACTEROIDES
.3 CLOSTRIDIUM
.42 E COLI
.49 ENTEROBACTER AEROGENES
.40 GRAM NEGATIVE
.49 GRAM NEGATIVE OTHER
.41 HEMOPHILUS INFLUENZAE
.2 PNEUMOCOCCAL
.49 PROTEUS
.43 PSEUDOMONAS
.44 SERRATIA
.10 STAPHYLOCOCCAL NOS
.11 STAPHYLOCOCCAL AUREUS
.19 STAPHYLOCOCCAL OTHER
.0 STREPTOCOCCAL (ANAEROBIC)
.49 YERSINIA ENTEROCOLITICA
.8 OTHER SPECIFIED

519.02 MALFUNCTION
519.09 OBSTRUCTION

T

TRACHEOSTOMY (continued)
V55.0 REMOVAL OR REPLACEMENT
709.2 SCAR (ADHERENT, CONTRACTURE, FIBROSIS)
V44.0 STATUS
519.02 STENOSIS
V55.0 TOILET

TRACHOMA
076.9 NOS
076.1 ACTIVE STAGE
076.0 DUBIUM
076.0 INITIAL STAGE
139.1 LATE EFFECTS
V73.6 SCREENING EXAM

V54.8 TRACTION DEVICE CHECKING CHANGE OR REMOVAL (ORTHOPEDIC)
744.1 TRAGUS ACCESSORY CONGENITAL
V60.0 TRAMP (HOMELESS PERSON)
780.09 TRANCE
305.4# TRANQUILIZER ABUSE (NONDEPENDENT)
304.1# TRANQUILIZER ADDICTION (DEPENDENT)

5th Digit: 304.1, 305.4
0. NOS
1. CONTINUOUS
2. EPISODIC
3. IN REMISSION

763.5 TRANQUILIZER REACTION (MATERNAL) AFFECTING FETUS OR NEWBORN
790.4 TRANSAMINASE ABNORMAL (LEVEL)

TRANSFUSION
V58.2 BLOOD WITHOUT REPORTED DIAGNOSIS
772.0 FETAL-MATERNAL SYNDROME
776.4 MATERNAL FETAL WITH POLYCYTHEMIA
999.8 REACTION
999.6 REACTION ABO INCOMPATIBILITY
999.7 REACTION RH INCOMPATIBILITY
762.3 TWIN <u>DONOR</u> SYNDROME (INFANT) [<u>772.0</u>]
762.3 TWIN <u>RECIPIENT</u> SYNDROME (INFANT) [<u>776.4</u>]
762.3 TWIN TO TWIN SYNDROME (INFANT)

TRANSIENT
780.02 ALTERATION OF CONSCIOUSNESS
368.12 BLINDNESS
388.02 DEAFNESS (ISCHEMIC)
437.7 GLOBAL AMNESIA
435.9 ISCHEMIC ATTACK
V60.0 PERSON (HOMELESS) NEC

CARCINOMAS AND NEOPLASMS SHOULD BE CODED BY SITE FIRST, NOT CELL TYPE. IF A SITE IS NOT SPECIFIED, THEN CODE BY CELL TYPE. CODE THE 'SITE NOS' ONLY IF NO SITE IS MENTIONED. WHEN NO SITE IS GIVEN, THE CODE REVERTS TO THE HISTOLOGICAL ORIGIN.

TRANSITIONAL CELL CARCINOMA
151.9 SITE NOS
0 SITE SPECIFIED SEE 'CANCER' BY SITE M8120/3
234.9 IN SITU SITE NOS
0 IN SITU SITE SPECIFIED SEE 'CA IN SITU' BY SITE M8120/2
199.1 PAPILLARY TYPE SITE NOS
0 PAPILLARY TYPE SITE SPECIFIED SEE 'CANCER' BY SITE M8130/3
199.1 SPINDLE CELL TYPE SITE NOS
0 SPINDLE CELL TYPE SITE SPECIFIED SEE 'CANCER' BY SITE M8122/3

758.4 TRANSLOCATION AUTOSOMAL BALANCED IN NORMAL INDIVIDUAL

TRANSPLANT
996.55 ALLODERMIS DECELLULARIZED FAILURE OR REJECTION (DISLODGEMENT) (DISPLACEMENT) (NON-ADHERENCE) (POOR INCORPORATION) (SHEARING)
996.89 FAILURE ORGAN NEC
996.80 REJECTION (FAILURE) ORGAN UNSPECIFIED
996.89 REJECTION (FAILURE) ORGAN OTHER SPECIFIED
996.55 SKIN ARTIFICIAL FAILURE OR REJECTION (DISLODGEMENT) (DISPLACEMENT) (NON-ADHERENCE) (POOR INCORPORATION) (SHEARING)
996.52 SKIN FAILURE
V42.#(#) STATUS

4th or 4th <u>and</u> 5th Digit: V42
0. KIDNEY
1. HEART
2. HEART VALVE
3. SKIN
4. BONE
5. CORNEA
6. LUNG
7. LIVER
8#. OTHER SPECIFIED
81. BONE MARROW
82. PERIPHERAL STEM CELLS
83. PANCREAS
89. OTHER SPECIFIED
9. UNSPECIFIED

V43.83 STATUS SKIN ARTIFICIAL

TRANSPOSITION
745.11 AORTA (DEXTRA)
751.5 APPENDIX
751.5 COLON
745.10 GREAT VESSELS - CLASSICAL
745.12 GREAT VESSELS - CORRECTED
745.11 GREAT VESSELS - INCOMPLETE
745.19 GREAT VESSELS - OTHER NEC
746.87 HEART
751.5 INTESTINES
747.49 PULMONARY VEINS
750.7 STOMACH
524.3 TEETH
759.3 VISCERA (ABDOMINAL) (THORACIC)

TRANS SEXUALISM
302.50 WITH UNSPECIFIED SEXUAL HISTORY
302.51 WITH ASEXUAL HISTORY
302.53 WITH HETEROSEXUAL HISTORY
302.52 WITH HOMOSEXUAL HISTORY

660.3# TRANSVERSE ARREST OF FETAL HEAD

5th Digit: 660.3
0. EPISODE OF CARE NOS OR N/A
1. DELIVERED
3. ANTEPARTUM COMPLICATION

TRANSVERSE LIE
761.7 AFFECTING FETUS OR NEWBORN - BEFORE LABOR
763.1 AFFECTING FETUS OR NEWBORN - DURING LABOR
652.3# COMPLICATING PREGNANCY
<u>660.0#</u> <u>OBSTRUCTING LABOR</u> **[652.3#]**
652.6# WITH MULTIPLE GESTATION
<u>660.0#</u> WITH MULTIPLE GESTATION <u>OBSTRUCTING LABOR</u> **[652.6#]**
652.1# WITH VERSION
<u>660.0#</u> WITH VERSION <u>OBSTRUCTING LABOR</u> **[652.1#]**

5th Digit: 652.1, 3, 6, 660.0
0. EPISODE OF CARE NOS OR N/A
1. DELIVERED
3. ANTEPARTUM COMPLICATION

302.3 TRANSVESTISM

TRAUMA
0 BLUNT SEE ANATOMICAL SITE, INJURY
958.8 COMPLICATION (EARLY) OTHER SPECIFIED
908.6 LATE EFFECT (COMPLICATIONS OF)
V15.4# PSYCHOLOGICAL HISTORY
5th Digit: V15.4
1. PHYSICAL ABUSE, RAPE
2. EMOTIONAL ABUSE, NEGLECT
9. OTHER
V66.6 TREATMENT CONVALESCENCE COMBINED
V62.6 TREATMENT REFUSAL - RELIGION BASED

756.0 TREACHER COLLINS' SYNDROME (INCOMPLETE MANDIBULOFACIAL DYSOSTOSIS)

V66.6 TREATMENT CONVALESCENCE COMBINED
V62.6 TREATMENT REFUSAL RELIGION BASED (REASON FOR ENCOUNTER)

121.9 TREMATODE INFECTION
121.8 TREMATODE INFECTION OTHER SPECIFIED

TREMOR
781.0 NOS
333.1 BENIGN ESSENTIAL
333.1 FAMILIAL

083.1 TRENCH FEVER
991.4 TRENCH FOOT
909.4 TRENCH FOOT LATE EFFECT
101 TRENCH MOUTH

041.84 TREPONEMA DENTICOLA INFECTION
041.84 TREPONEMA MACRODENTICUM INFECTION
097.9 TREPONEMA PALLIDUM INFECTION

TRICHIASIS
704.2 NOS
704.2 CICATRICAL
374.05 EYELID
374.05 WITHOUT ENTROPION (EYELID)

842.01 TRIANGULAR FIBROCARTILAGE COMPLEX SPRAIN (STRAIN) (TEAR)
719.83 TRIANGULAR FIBROCARTILAGE COMPLEX SPRAIN (STRAIN) (TEAR) - OLD

124 TRICHINELLA SPIRALIS INFECTION
124 TRICHINELLOSIS
124 TRICHINIASIS

124 TRICHINOSIS
127.3 TRICHOCEPHALIASIS

216.# TRICHOEPITHELIOMA M8100/0
216.# TRICHOFOLLICULOMA M8101/0
216.# TRICHOLEMMOMA M8102/0
4th Digit: 216
0. LIP (SKIN OF)
1. EYELID INCLUDING CANTHUS
2. EAR (EXTERNAL) (AURICLE) (PINNA)
3. FACE (CHEEK) (NOSE) (EYEBROW) (TEMPLE)
4. SCALP NECK
5. TRUNK BACK EXCEPT SCROTUM
6. UPPER LIMB INCLUDING SHOULDER
7. LOWER LIMB INCLUDING HIP
8. OTHER SPECIFIED SITES
9. SKIN NOS

TRICHOMONAS
V01.8 EXPOSURE
007.3 GASTROENTERITIS
131.9 INFECTION NOS
007.3 INTESTINAL INFECTION
131.03 PROSTATITIS

TRICHOMONAS (continued)
131.02 URETHRITIS
131.00 UROGENITAL
131.01 VAGINITIS
131.01 VULVOVAGINITIS
131.8 OTHER SPECIFIED NON UROGENITAL SITES
131.09 OTHER UROGENITAL SITE

039.0 TRICHOMYCOSIS AXILLARIS

110.0 TRICHOPHYTIC TINEA
110.6 TRICHOPHYTICUM GRANULOMA
0 TRICHOPHYTON INFECTIONS SEE 'DERMATOPHYTOSIS'

704.2 TRICHORRHEXIS (NODOSA)
111.2 TRICHOSPORON (BEIGELII) CUTANEUM INFECTION

127.6 TRICHOSTRONGYLIASIS
127.6 TRICHOSTRONGYLUS SPECIES INFECTION

312.39 TRICHOTILLOMANIA
127.3 TRICHURIASIS
127.3 TRICHURIS TRICHIURIA INFECTION

TRICUSPID
746.1 ABSENCE CONGENITAL
0 INCOMPETENCE SEE 'TRICUSPID', INSUFFICIENCY
424.2 INSUFFICIENCY
421.0 INSUFFICIENCY - BACTERIAL (ACUTE) (CHRONIC)
397.0 INSUFFICIENCY - RHEUMATIC
093.23 INSUFFICIENCY - SYPHILITIC
0 REGURGITATION SEE 'TRICUSPID', INSUFFICIENCY
424.2 STENOSIS
421.0 STENOSIS - BACTERIAL
746.1 STENOSIS - CONGENITAL
397.0 STENOSIS - RHEUMATIC
093.23 STENOSIS - SYPHILITIC
421.0 STENOSIS - WITH INSUFFICIENCY BACTERIAL (ACUTE) (CHRONIC)
093.23 STENOSIS - WITH INSUFFICIENCY SYPHILITIC
746.1 STENOSIS AND ATRESIA CONGENITAL
746.1 VALVE ATRESIA (CONGENITAL)
424.2 VALVE DISORDER NONRHEUMATIC

426.54 TRIFASCICULAR BLOCK
753.3 TRIFID KIDNEY (PELVIS) CONGENITAL

TRIGEMINAL NERVE
350.8 ATROPHY
350.9 DISORDER
350.8 DISORDERS OTHER SPECIFIED
951.2 INJURY
350.1 NEURALGIA
053.12 NEURALGIA POSTHERPETIC
350.9 PARALYSIS

259.8 TRIGEMINAL PLATE SYNDROME
727.03 TRIGGER FINGER
756.89 TRIGGER FINGER CONGENITAL

272.9 TRIGLYCERIDE ABNORMAL FINDINGS
272.7 TRIGLYCERIDE STORAGE TYPE I, II OR III DISEASE

595.3 TRIGONITIS
756.0 TRIGONOCEPHALY

344.89 TRIPLEGIA

758.81 TRIPLE X (FEMALE) SYNDROME
651.1# TRIPLET GESTATION
651.4# TRIPLET GESTATION WITH ONE OR MORE LOSSES
5th Digit: 651.1,4
0. EPISODE OF CARE NOS OR N/A
1. DELIVERED
3. ANTEPARTUM COMPLICATION

761.5 TRIPLET PREGNANCY AFFECTING FETUS OR NEWBORN
781.0 TRISMUS

TRISOMY
758.5 NOS
758.1 13
758.1 14
758.2 16-18
758.5 20
758.0 21 OR 22 (MONGOLISM)
758.1 D1
758.2 E (3)
758.0 G (MONGOLISM)

368.53 TRITAN DEFECT
368.53 TRITANOMALY
368.53 TRITANOPIA
726.5 TROCHANTERIC BURSITIS
726.5 TROCHANTERIC TENDINITIS

TROCHLEAR NERVE
378.53 ATROPHY
378.53 DISORDER
951.1 INJURY
378.53 PALSY
378.53 PARALYSIS

275.0 TROISIER-HANOT-CHAUFFARD SYNDROME (BRONZE DIABETES)
133.8 TROMBICULA INFESTATION
757.0 TROPHEDEMA HEREDITARY
707.9 TROPHIC ULCER CHRONIC (SKIN) (SEE ALSO 'ULCER, ULCERATION SKIN')

TROPHOBLASTIC DISEASE
630 NOS
630 NOS WITH COMPLICATION DURING TREATMENT [**639.#**]
639.# NOS WITH COMPLICATION FOLLOWING TREATMENT

4th Digit: 639
- **0. GENITAL TRACT AND PELVIC INFECTION**
- **1. DELAYED OR EXCESSIVE HEMORRHAGE**
- **2. DAMAGE TO PELVIC ORGANS AND TISSUE**
- **3. RENAL FAILURE**
- **4. METABOLIC DISORDERS**
- **5. SHOCK**
- **6. EMBOLISM**
- **8. OTHER SPECIFIED COMPLICATION**
- **9. UNSPECIFIED COMPLICATION**

V13.1 HISTORY (NONGRAVID)
V23.1 HISTORY MATERNAL AFFECTING PREGNANCY SUPERVISION
0 SEE ALSO 'HYDATIDIFORM MOLE'

TROPICAL
099.1 BUBO
040.81 PYOMYOSITIS
579.1 SPRUE
579.1 STEATORRHEA
707.9 ULCER CHRONIC (SKIN) (SEE ALSO 'ULCER, ULCERATION SKIN')
991.4 WET FEET SYNDROME

453.1 TROUSSEAU'S SYNDROME (THROMBOPHLEBITIS MIGRANS VISCERAL CANCER)
312.2# TRUANCY (CHILDHOOD) SOCIALIZED
312.1# TRUANCY (CHILDHOOD) UNSOCIALIZED

5th Digit: 312.1-2
- **0. NOS**
- **1. MILD**
- **2. MODERATE**
- **3. SEVERE**

745.0 TRUNCUS ARTERIOSUS PERSISTENT CONGENITAL

TRUNK
V48.1 DEFICIENCY
V48.7 DISFIGUREMENT
959.1 INJURY
911.8 INJURY OTHER AND UNSPECIFIED SUPERFICIAL
911.9 INJURY OTHER AND UNSPECIFIED SUPERFICIAL INFECTED
907.3 INJURY NERVE ROOT(S) LATE EFFECT, (SPINAL PLEXUS AND OTHER NERVES OF TRUNK)
954.9 NERVE INJURY NERVE UNSPECIFIED
954.8 NERVE INJURY OTHER SPECIFIED NERVE
V48.9 PROBLEM
V48.3 PROBLEM (MECHANICAL AND MOTOR)
V48.8 PROBLEM (OTHER)
V48.5 PROBLEM (SENSORY)

0 TRYPANOSOMA INFECTION SEE 'TRYPANOSOMIASIS'

TRYPANOSOMIASIS
086.# NOS
086.# ENCEPHALITIS [323.2]
086.# MENINGITIS [321.3]

4th Digit: 086
- **0. CHAGAS' (AMERICAN) WITH HEART INVOLVEMENT**
- **1. CHAGAS' (AMERICAN) WITH INVOLVEMENT OF ORGAN OTHER THAN HEART**
- **2. CHAGAS' (AMERICAN) NOS**
- **3. GAMBIAN**
- **4. RHODESIAN**
- **5. AFRICAN NOS**
- **9. UNSPECIFIED**

V75.3 SCREENING EXAM - CHAGAS DISEASE (SLEEPING SICKNESS)

270.2 TRYPTOPHAN DISTURBANCES OF METABOLISM
242.8# TSH OVERPRODUCTION

5th Digit: 242.8
- **0. WITHOUT THYROTOXIC CRISIS OR STORM**
- **1. WITH MENTION OF THROTOXIC CRISIS OR STORM**

081.2 TSUTSUGAMUSHI FEVER (SCRUB TYPHUS)

TUBAL
633.1 ABORTION
633.1 ABORTION WITH COMPLICATION DURING TREATMENT [**639.#**]
639.# ABORTION WITH COMPLICATION FOLLOWING TREATMENT

4th Digit: 639
- **0. GENITAL TRACT AND PELVIC INFECTION**
- **1. DELAYED OR EXCESSIVE HEMORRHAGE**
- **2. DAMAGE TO PELVIC ORGANS AND TISSUE**
- **3. RENAL FAILURE**
- **4. METABOLIC DISORDERS**
- **5. SHOCK**
- **6. EMBOLISM**
- **8. OTHER SPECIFIED COMPLICATION**
- **9. UNSPECIFIED COMPLICATION**

V25.2 LIGATION ENCOUNTER
V26.51 LIGATION STATUS

TUBAL (continued)

628.2 OCCLUSION
633.1 PREGNANCY
761.4 PREGNANCY AFFECTING FETUS OR NEWBORN
633.1 PREGNANCY WITH COMPLICATION DURING TREATMENT [639.#]
639.# PREGNANCY WITH COMPLICATION FOLLOWING TREATMENT

4th Digit: 639

0. GENITAL TRACT AND PELVIC INFECTION
1. DELAYED OR EXCESSIVE HEMORRHAGE
2. DAMAGE TO PELVIC ORGANS AND TISSUE
3. RENAL FAILURE
4. METABOLIC DISORDERS
5. SHOCK
6. EMBOLISM
8. OTHER SPECIFIED COMPLICATION
9. UNSPECIFIED COMPLICATION

A POSITIVE TUBERCULIN TEST IS NOT A DIAGNOSIS OF TUBERCULOSIS, AND SHOULD NOT BE CODED AS SUCH.

795.5 TUBERCULIN TEST POSITIVE (WITHOUT TB)
795.5 TUBERCULIN TEST REACTOR (WITHOUT TB)

TUBERCULOSIS

011.9# UNSPECIFIED
013.3# ABSCESS BRAIN
013.5# ABSCESS SPINAL CORD
017.2# ADENITIS
017.6# ADRENAL GLANDS
014.8# ANUS
014.0# ASCITES
016.1# BLADDER
015.7# BONE OTHER SPECIFIED
015.9# BONES AND JOINTS
013.2# BRAIN
013.3# BRAIN ABSCESS
012.2# BRONCHIAL ISOLATED
011.5# BRONCHIECTASIS
011.3# BRONCHUS
013.8# CENTRAL NERVOUS SYSTEM OTHER SPECIFIED
013.9# CENTRAL NERVOUS SYSTEM SITE NOS
016.7# CERVICITIS
014.8# COLON
017.0# COLLIQUATIVA
771.2 CONGENITAL OR PERINATAL
795.5 CONVERTER (WITHOUT TB)
017.0# CUTIS
015.5# DACTYLITIS
018.9# DISSEMINATED
018.0# DISSEMINATED ACUTE
018.8# DISSEMINATED OTHER SPECIFIED
017.4# EAR
012.0# EMPYEMA
013.6# ENCEPHALITIS
013.6# ENCEPHALITIS OR MYELITIS
016.7# ENDOMETRITIS
014.8# ENTERITIS
016.4# EPIDIDYMIS
017.1# ERYTHEMA NODOSUM W/HYPERSENSITIVITY REACTION
017.8# ESOPHAGUS
V01.1 EXPOSURE
017.3# EYE

5th Digit: 011, 012, 013, 014, 015, 016, 017, 018

0. NOS
1. LAB NOT DONE
2. LABS PENDING
3. MICROSCOPY POSITIVE (IN SPUTUM)
4. CULTURE POSITIVE - MICROSCOPY NEGATIVE
5. CULTURE NEGATIVE - MICROSCOPY POSITIVE
6. CULTURE AND MICROSCOPY NEGATIVE CONFIRMED BY OTHER METHODS

TUBERCULOSIS (continued)

795.5 FALSE POSITIVE SEROLOGICAL TEST
014.8# GASTROCOLIC
018.9# GENERALIZED
018.0# GENERALIZED ACUTE
018.8# GENERALIZED OTHER SPECIFIED
016.7# GENITAL ORGANS FEMALE OTHER
016.5# GENITAL ORGANS MALE OTHER
016.9# GENITOURINARY
016.9# GENITOURINARY SITE NOS
012.3# GLOTTIS
015.1# HIP [727.01]
V12.01 HISTORY PERSONAL
012.0# HYDROTHORAX
014.8# ILEUM
017.1# INDURATIVIA
014.8# INTESTINE (LARGE) (SMALL)
015.8# JOINT OTHER SPECIFIED
016.0# KIDNEY
015.2# KNEE [727.01]
012.3# LARYNGITIS

5th Digit: 012, 013, 014, 015, 016, 017, 018

0. NOS
1. LAB NOT DONE
2. LABS PENDING
3. MICROSCOPY POSITIVE (IN SPUTUM)
4. CULTURE POSITIVE - MICROSCOPY NEGATIVE
5. CULTURE NEGATIVE - MICROSCOPY POSITIVE
6. CULTURE AND MICROSCOPY NEGATIVE CONFIRMED BY OTHER METHODS

137.3 LATE EFFECTS BONES AND JOINTS
137.1 LATE EFFECTS CENTRAL NERVOUS SYSTEM
137.2 LATE EFFECTS GENITOURINARY
137.4 LATE EFFECTS OTHER SPECIFIED ORGANS
137.0 LATE EFFECTS RESPIRATORY OR UNSPECIFIED

013.0# LEPTOMENINGITIS
017.0# LICHENOIDES
011.9# LUNG NOS
011.4# LUNG FIBROSIS
011.0# LUNG INFILTRATIVE
011.1# LUNG NODULAR
011.2# LUNG WITH CAVITATION
012.1# LYMPH NODES INTRATHORACIC (HILAR) (MEDIASTINAL) (TRACHEOBRONCHIAL)
014.8# LYMPH NODES MESENTERIC OR RETROPERITONEAL
017.2# LYMPH NODES PERIPHERAL (CERVICAL)
015.6# MASTOID

5th Digit: 011, 012, 013, 014, 015, 017

0. NOS
1. LAB NOT DONE
2. LABS PENDING
3. MICROSCOPY POSITIVE (IN SPUTUM)
4. CULTURE POSITIVE - MICROSCOPY NEGATIVE
5. CULTURE NEGATIVE - MICROSCOPY POSITIVE
6. CULTURE AND MICROSCOPY NEGATIVE CONFIRMED BY OTHER METHODS

647.3#: USE AN ADDITIONAL CODE TO IDENTIFY THE MATERNAL TUBERCULOSIS.

647.3# MATERNAL CURRENT (CO-EXISTENT) IN PREGNANCY

5th Digit: 647.3

0. EPISODE OF CARE NOS OR N/A
1. DELIVERED
2. DELIVERED WITH POSTPARTUM COMPLICATION
3. ANTEPARTUM COMPLICATION
4. POSTPARTUM COMPLICATION

TUBERCULOSIS (continued)

012.8# MEDIASTINUM
013.1# MENINGES - TUBERCULOMA
013.0# MENINGITIS
013.0# MENINGOENCEPHALITIS
014.8# MESENTERIC GLANDS
018.9# MILIARY
018.0# MILIARY ACUTE
018.8# MILIARY OTHER SPECIFIED
013.6# MYELITIS
012.8# NASOPHARYNX
013.9# NERVOUS SYSTEM (CENTRAL)
012.8# NOSE (SEPTUM)
016.6# OOPHORITIS
0 OSTEOMYELITIS SEE 'OSTEOMYELITIS', TUBERCULOUS
010.8# OTHER PRIMARY PROGRESSIVE
017.9# OTHER SPECIFIED ORGANS
017.0# PAPULONECROTICA
014.0# PERITONITIS
012.0# PLEURA
012.0# PLEURISY
010.1# PLEURISY PRIMARY PROGRESSIVE TB
011.6# PNEUMONIA
011.7# PNEUMOTHORAX
018.9# POLYSEROSITIS
018.0# POLYSEROSITIS ACUTE
018.8# POLYSEROSITIS OTHER SPECIFIED
010.0# PRIMARY COMPLEX
010.9# PRIMARY INFECTION
016.5# PROSTATE [601.4]
011.9# PULMONARY
011.8# PULMONARY OTHER SPECIFIED
016.0# PYELONEPHRITIS
014.8# RECTUM
016.0# RENAL
011.9# RESPIRATORY NOS
012.8# RESPIRATORY OTHER SPECIFIED
017.3# RETINALIS (JUVENILIS) [362.18]
014.8# RETROPERITONEAL (LYMPH NODES)
016.6# SALPINGITIS OOPHORITIS
V74.1 SCREENING EXAM
016.5# SEMINAL VESICLE [608.81]
012.8# SINUS [ANY NASAL]
017.0# SKIN AND SUBCUTANEOUS CELLULAR TISSUE
013.4# SPINAL CORD
017.7# SPLEEN
015.0# SPONDYLOPATHY [720.81]
0 SYNOVITIS SEE 'SYNOVITIS', TUBERCULOUS
0 TENOSYNOVITIS SEE 'TENOSYNOVITIS', TUBERCULOUS
795.5 TEST NONSPECIFIC REACTION (WITHOUT ACTIVE TB)
016.5# TESTES [608.81]
017.5# THYROID GLAND
012.2# TRACHEAL ISOLATED
012.2# TRACHEAL OR BRONCHIAL ISOLATED
012.1# TRACHEOBRONCHIAL ADENOPATHY
013.1# TUBERCULOMA MENINGES
016.7# ULCER OF VULVA (NONOBSTETRICAL) [616.51]
016.2# URETER
016.3# URINARY ORGANS OTHER
V03.2 VACCINATION
017.0# VERRUCOSA CUTIS
015.0# VERTEBRAL COLUMN

5th Digit: 010, 011, 012, 013, 014, 015, 016, 017, 018

0. NOS
1. LAB NOT DONE
2. LABS PENDING
3. MICROSCOPY POSITIVE (IN SPUTUM)
4. CULTURE POSITIVE - MICROSCOPY NEGATIVE
5. CULTURE NEGATIVE - MICROSCOPY POSITIVE
6. CULTURE AND MICROSCOPY NEGATIVE CONFIRMED BY OTHER METHODS

759.5 TUBEROUS SCLEROSIS
272.2 TUBO-ERUPTIVE XANTHOMA

TUBO OVARIAN

614.2 ABSCESS
614.0 ABSCESS ACUTE
614.4 ABSCESS CHRONIC
614.6 ADHESIONS (POSTOPERATIVE) (POSTINFECTION)
614.2 DISEASE - INFLAMMATORY
620.9 DISEASE - NONINFLAMMATORY
620.8 DISEASE - NONINFLAMMATORY SPECIFIED NEC

TUBOPLASTY

V25.09 COUNSELING (PROPOSED)
V25.2 ENCOUNTER
V26.0 REVERSAL AFTER PREVIOUS STERILIZATION
V26.51 STATUS

382.1 TUBOTYMPANIC DISEASE CHRONIC (WITH ANTERIOR PERFORATION OF EAR DRUM)

TUBULAR (RENAL)

588.0 DISORDER PHOSPHATE-LOSING
584.5 NECROSIS
584.5 NECROSIS ACUTE
997.5 NECROSIS ACUTE SPECIFIED AS DUE TO PROCEDURE
639.3 NECROSIS FOLLOWING ABORTION / ECTOPIC / MOLAR PREGNANCY

TULAREMIA

021.9 NOS
021.2 BRONCHOPNEUMONIC
021.1 CRYPTOGENIC
021.1 ENTERIC
V01.8 EXPOSURE
021.8 GENERALIZED OR DISSEMINATED
021.8 GLANDULAR
021.1 INTESTINAL
021.3 OCULOGLANDULAR
021.2 PULMONARY
021.1 TYPHOIDAL
021.0 ULCEROGLANDULAR
V03.4 VACCINATION
021.8 OTHER SPECIFIED

TUMOR

239.# NOS (SEE ALSO 'NEOPLASM UNSPECIFIED NATURE') M8001/1

4th Digit: 239

0. DIGESTIVE SYSTEM, ANAL
1. RESPIRATORY SYSTEM
2. BONE, SOFT TISSUE, SKIN, (ANAL SKIN MARGIN)
3. BREAST
4. BLADDER
5. OTHER GENITOURINARY
6. BRAIN
7. ENDOCRINE GLANDS AND OTHER PARTS OF NERVOUS SYSTEM
8. OTHER SPECIFIED SITES
9. SITE UNSPECIFIED

229.9 BENIGN SITE NOS
0 BENIGN SITE SPECIFIED SEE 'BENIGN NEOPLASM', BY SITE M8001/0
237.9 CRANIAL NERVE (CENTRAL)
199.1 FUSIFORM CELL TYPE - MALIGNANT SITE NOS
0 FUSIFORM CELL TYPE - MALIGNANT SITE SPECIFIED SEE 'CANCER' BY SITE M8004/3
0 GLOMUS SEE 'HEMANGIOMA'
238.7 HEMORRHAGIC WITH THROMBOCYTHEMIA M9962/1
199.1 MALIGNANT SITE NOS
0 MALIGNANT SITE SPECIFIED SEE 'CANCER' BY SITE M8001/3
238.5 MAST CELL NOS

TUMOR (continued)

199.1 SMALL CELL TYPE - MALIGNANT SITE NOS
0 SMALL CELL TYPE - MALIGNANT SITE SPECIFIED SEE 'CANCER' BY SITE M8041/3
215.9 SOFT TISSUE - BENIGN SITE NOS
0 SOFT TISSUE - BENIGN SITE SPECIFIED SEE 'BENIGN NEOPLASM', BY SITE M8800/0
654.7# VAGINA COMPLICATING PREGNANCY

5th Digit: 654.7

0. EPISODE OF CARE NOS OR N/A
1. DELIVERED
2. DELIVERED WITH POSTPARTUM COMPLICATION
3. ANTEPARTUM COMPLICATION
4. POSTPARTUM COMPLICATION

238.9 TUMORLET SITE NOS
0 TUMORLET SITE SPECIFIED SEE 'NEOPLASM UNCERTAIN BEHAVIOR' BY SITE M8040/1

134.1 TUNGA PENETRANS INFESTATION
134.1 TUNGIASIS

TUNICA VAGINALIS

608.4 ABSCESS (CELLULITIS) (BOIL) (CARBUNCLE)
608.89 ATROPHY (FIBROSIS) (HYPERTROPHY) (ULCER)
608.84 CHYLOCELE
608.83 HEMORRHAGE (THROMBOSIS) (HEMATOMA) NONTRAUMATIC
778.6 HYDROCELE CONGENITAL
608.4 INFECTIVE
608.85 STRICTURE

733.99 TURBINATES ATROPHY (BONE)
478.0 TURBINATES HYPERTROPHY NASAL
378.71 TURK'S SYNDROME (OCULAR RETRACTION SYNDROME)

758.6 TURNER'S SYNDROME
758.6 TURNER-VARNY SYNDROME
520.4 TURNER'S TOOTH
352.5 TWELFTH CRANIAL NERVE ATROPHY
352.5 TWELFTH CRANIAL NERVE DISORDERS
951.7 TWELFTH CRANIAL NERVE INJURY
352.5 TWELFTH NERVE HYPOGLOSSAL DISORDERS

759.4 TWIN CONJOINED

651.0# TWIN PREGNANCY
651.3# TWIN PREGNANCY WITH ONE FETAL LOSS (ONE RETAINED)

5th Digit: 651.0, 3

0. EPISODE OF CARE NOS OR N/A
1. DELIVERED
3. ANTEPARTUM COMPLICATION

761.5 TWIN PREGNANCY AFFECTING FETUS OR NEWBORN
762.3 TWIN-TO-TWIN TRANSFUSION SYNDROME NOS
762.3 TWIN-TO-TWIN TRANSFUSION SYNDROME-<u>DONOR TWIN</u> [<u>772.0</u>]
762.3 TWIN-TO-TWIN TRANSFUSION SYNDROME-<u>RECIPIENT TWIN</u> [<u>776.4</u>]
651.3# TWIN VANISHING

5th Digit: 651.3

0. EPISODE OF CARE NOS OR N/A
1. DELIVERED
3. ANTEPARTUM COMPLICATION

781.0 TWITCH

TYMPANIC MEMBRANE

744.29 ABSENCE CONGENITAL
384.81 ATROPHIC FLACCID
384.82 ATROPHIC NONFLACCID
384.9 DISORDER
959.09 INJURY
384.82 RETRACTED

TYMPANIC MEMBRANE PERFORATION

384.20 NONTRAUMATIC - NOS
384.22 NONTRAUMATIC - ATTIC
384.21 NONTRAUMATIC - CENTRAL
384.81 NONTRAUMATIC - HEALED
384.24 NONTRAUMATIC - MULTIPLE
384.22 NONTRAUMATIC - PARS FLACCIDA
384.23 NONTRAUMATIC - OTHER MARGINAL
384.25 NONTRAUMATIC (POSTTRAUMATIC) - TOTAL
872.61 TRAUMATIC
872.71 TRAUMATIC COMPLICATED
0 WITH OTITIS MEDIA SEE 'OTITIS MEDIA'

787.3 TYMPANITES (ABDOMINAL) (INTESTINAL)
384.00 TYMPANITIS ACUTE WITHOUT OTITIS MEDIA
384.1 TYMPANITIS CHRONIC WITHOUT OTITIS MEDIA

TYMPANOSCLEROSIS

385.00 NOS
385.09 INVOLVING OTHER COMBINATION STRUCTURES
385.02 INVOLVING TYMPANIC MEMBRANE AND EAR OSSICLES
385.03 INVOLVING TYMPANIC MEMBRANE EAR OSSICLES AND MIDDLE EAR
385.01 INVOLVING TYMPANIC MEMBRANE ONLY

996.69 TYMPANOSTOMY TUBE COMPLICATION - INFECTION OR INFLAMMATION
996.59 TYMPANOSTOMY TUBE COMPLICATION - MECHANICAL
996.79 TYMPANOSTOMY TUBE COMPLICATION - OTHER

385.9 TYMPANUM DISEASE
786.7 TYMPANY CHEST

301.4 TYPE A PERSONALITY DISORDER

TYPHOID

V02.1 CARRIER
002.0 FEVER (INFECTION) (ANY SITE)
002.0 <u>OSTEOMYELITIS</u> [**<u>730.8#</u>**]

5th Digit: 730.8

0. SITE NOS
1. SHOULDER REGION
2. UPPER ARM (ELBOW) (HUMERUS)
3. FOREARM (RADIUS) (WRIST) (ULNA)
4. HAND (CARPAL) (METACARPAL) (FINGERS)
5. PELVIC REGION AND THIGH (HIP) (BUTTOCK) (FEMUR)
6. LOWER LEG (FIBULA) (KNEE) (PATELLA) (TIBIA)
7. ANKLE AND/OR FOOT (METATARSALS) (TOES) (TARSALS)
8. OTHER (HEAD) (NECK) (RIB) (SKULL) (TRUNK) (VERTEBRAE)

002.9 PARATYPHOID
002.1 PARATYPHOID A
002.2 PARATYPHOID B
002.3 PARATYPHOID C
V03.1 PARATYPHOID VACCINATION ALONE

TYPHUS

082.9 TYPHUS
082.1 AFRICAN TICK
081.1 BRILL-ZINSSER DISEASE
080 CLASSICAL
081.0 ENDEMIC
080 EPIDEMIC
080 EXANTHEMATIC
081.9 FEVER
081.0 FLEA BORNE
082.1 INDIA TICK
082.1 KENYA TICK
080 LOUSE BORNE

T

TYPHUS (continued)

081.2 MITE BORNE
081.0 MURINE [ENDEMIC]
081.1 RECRUDESCENT
081.2 SCRUB
082.2 SIBERIAN TICK
082.9 TICK BORNE

300.89 TYPIST'S CRAMP NEUROTIC
333.84 TYPIST'S CRAMP ORGANIC
270.2 TYROSINE DISTURBANCES OF METABOLISM
270.2 TYROSINOSIS
270.2 TYROSINURIA

T

757.39 UEHLINGER'S SYNDROME (ACROPACHYDERMA)

746.84 UHL'S DISEASE

ULCER

707.9 UNSPECIFIED SITE
707.9 UNSPECIFIED SITE WITH GANGRENE [785.4]
526.5 ALVEOLAR PROCESS
006.9 AMEBIC (INTESTINE)
534.## ANASTOMOTIC

4th Digit: 534
0. ACUTE WITH HEMORRHAGE
1. ACUTE WITH PERFORATION
2. ACUTE WITH HEMORRHAGE AND PERFORATION
3. ACUTE
4. CHRONIC OR NOS WITH HEMORRHAGE
5. CHRONIC OR NOS WITH PERFORATION
6. CHRONIC OR NOS WITH HEMORRHAGE AND PERFORATION
7. CHRONIC
9. NOS AS ACUTE OR CHRONIC

5th Digit: 534
0. WITHOUT OBSTRUCTION
1. OBSTRUCTED

0 ANTRAL SEE 'ULCER', PYLORIC
569.41 ANUS
569.41 ANUS STERCORAL
455.8 ANUS VARICOSE
455.5 ANUS VARICOSE EXTERNAL
455.2 ANUS VARICOSE INTERNAL
440.23 ARTERIOSCLEROTIC LOWER LIMB
440.24 ARTERIOSCLEROTIC LOWER LIMB WITH ISCHEMIC GANGRENE
447.2 ARTERY
447.8 ARTERY WITHOUT RUPTURE
576.8 BILE DUCT
596.8 BLADDER
120.9 BLADDER BILHARZIAL [595.4]
595.1 BLADDER SUBMUCOSAL
016.1# BLADDER TUBERCULOUS [596.8]

5th Digit: 016.1
0. NOS
1. LAB NOT DONE
2. LABS PENDING
3. MICROSCOPY POSITIVE (IN SPUTUM)
4. CULTURE POSITIVE - MICROSCOPY NEGATIVE
5. CULTURE NEGATIVE - MICROSCOPY POSITIVE
6. CULTURE AND MICROSCOPY NEGATIVE CONFIRMED BY OTHER METHODS

730.9# BONE

5th Digit: 730.9
0. SITE NOS
1. SHOULDER REGION
2. UPPER ARM (ELBOW) (HUMERUS)
3. FOREARM (RADIUS) (WRIST) (ULNA)
4. HAND (CARPAL) (METACARPAL) (FINGERS)
5. PELVIC REGION AND THIGH (HIP) (BUTTOCK) (FEMUR)
6. LOWER LEG (FIBULA) (KNEE) (PATELLA) (TIBIA)
7. ANKLE AND/OR FOOT (METATARSALS) (TOES) (TARSAL)
8. OTHER (HEAD) (NECK) (RIB) (SKULL) (TRUNK)
9. MULTIPLE

ULCER (continued)

519.1 BRONCHUS
031.1 BURULI
530.2 CARDIO-ESOPHAGEAL (PEPTIC)
622.0 CERVIX
616.0 CERVIX WITH CERVICITIS
099.0 CHANCROIDAL
569.82 COLON
372.00 CONJUNCTIVA

CORNEA
370.00 NOS
370.03 CENTRAL
054.42 DENDRITIC
264.3 DUE TO VITAMIN A DEFICIENCY
370.04 HYPOPYON ULCER
370.01 MARGINAL (CATARRHAL)
370.07 MOOREN'S (RODENT)
370.05 MYCOTIC
370.06 PERFORATED
370.02 RING (ANNULAR)
370.04 SERPIGINOUS
017.3# TUBERCULOUS (PHLYCTENULAR) [370.31]

5th Digit: 017.3
0. NOS
1. LAB NOT DONE
2. LABS PENDING
3. MICROSCOPY POSITIVE (IN SPUTUM)
4. CULTURE POSITIVE - MICROSCOPY NEGATIVE
5. CULTURE NEGATIVE - MICROSCOPY POSITIVE
6. CULTURE AND MICROSCOPY NEGATIVE CONFIRMED BY OTHER METHODS

ULCER (continued)

607.89 CORPUS CAVERNOSUM CHRONIC
595.1 CYSTITIS (INTERSTITIAL)
054.42 DENDRITIC
532.## DUODENAL
532.## DUODENAL DUE TO HELICOBACTER PYLORI [041.86]
316 DUODENAL PSYCHOGENIC [532.##]

4th Digit: 532
0. ACUTE WITH HEMORRHAGE
1. ACUTE WITH PERFORATION
2. ACUTE WITH HEMORRHAGE AND PERFORATION
3. ACUTE
4. CHRONIC OR NOS WITH HEMORRHAGE
5. CHRONIC OR NOS WITH PERFORATION
6. CHRONIC OR NOS WITH HEMORRHAGE AND PERFORATION
7. CHRONIC
9. NOS AS ACUTE OR CHRONIC

5th Digit: 532
0. WITHOUT OBSTRUCTION
1. OBSTRUCTED

595.1 ELUSIVE
478.79 EPIGLOTTIS
530.2 ESOPHAGUS
360.00 EYE NEC
478.29 FAUCES
575.8 GALLBLADDER
576.8 GALL DUCT

ULCER (continued)

531.## GASTRIC
531.## GASTRIC DUE TO HELICOBACTER PYLORI [041.86]
316 GASTRIC PSYCHOGENIC [531.##]
534.## GASTROCOLIC
533.## GASTRODUODENAL
533.## GASTRODUODENAL DUE TO HELICOBACTER PYLORI [041.86]
534.## GASTROINTESTINAL
534.## GASTROJEJUNAL

4th Digit: 531, 533, 534

0. ACUTE WITH HEMORRHAGE
1. ACUTE WITH PERFORATION
2. ACUTE WITH HEMORRHAGE AND PERFORATION
3. ACUTE
4. CHRONIC OR NOS WITH HEMORRHAGE
5. CHRONIC OR NOS WITH PERFORATION
6. CHRONIC OR NOS WITH HEMORRHAGE AND PERFORATION
7. CHRONIC
9. NOS AS ACUTE OR CHRONIC

5th Digit: 531, 533, 534

0. WITHOUT OBSTRUCTION
1. OBSTRUCTED

629.8 GENITAL SITES OTHER FEMALE
616.8 GENITAL SITES OTHER FEMALE APHTHOUS
608.89 GENITAL SITES OTHER MALE (APHTHOUS)
523.8 GINGIVA
523.1 GINGIVITIS
478.79 GLOTTIS
523.8 GUM
595.1 HUNNER'S
478.29 HYPOPHARYNX
370.04 HYPOPYON
569.82 INTESTINE (PRIMARY)
569.83 INTESTINE WITH PERFORATION
528.5 LIP
518.89 LUNG
011.2# LUNG TUBERCULOUS

5th Digit: 011.2

0. NOS
1. LAB NOT DONE
2. LABS PENDING
3. MICROSCOPY POSITIVE (IN SPUTUM)
4. CULTURE POSITIVE - MICROSCOPY NEGATIVE
5. CULTURE NEGATIVE - MICROSCOPY POSITIVE
6. CULTURE AND MICROSCOPY NEGATIVE CONFIRMED BY OTHER METHODS

597.89 MEATUS (URINARIUS)
528.9 MOUTH (TRAUMATIC)
528.2 MOUTH APHTHOUS
031.1 MYCOBACTERIUM
478.1 NASAL SEPTUM
456.8 NASAL SEPTUM VARICOSE
771.4 NAVEL CORD (NEWBORN)
528.9 ORAL MUCOSA (TRAUMATIC)
533.## PEPTIC (SYNDROME)
533.## PEPTIC (SYNDROME) DUE TO HELICOBACTER PYLORI [041.86]

4th Digit: 533

0. ACUTE WITH HEMORRHAGE
1. ACUTE WITH PERFORATION
2. ACUTE WITH HEMORRHAGE AND PERFORATION
3. ACUTE
4. CHRONIC OR NOS WITH HEMORRHAGE
5. CHRONIC OR NOS WITH PERFORATION
6. CHRONIC OR NOS WITH HEMORRHAGE AND PERFORATION
7. CHRONIC
9. NOS AS ACUTE OR CHRONIC

5th Digit: 533

0. WITHOUT OBSTRUCTION
1. OBSTRUCTED

ULCER (continued)

474.8 PERITONSILLAR
601.8 PROSTATE
531.## PYLORIC
531.## PYLORIC DUE TO HELICOBACTER PYLORI [041.86]

4th Digit: 531

0. ACUTE WITH HEMORRHAGE
1. ACUTE WITH PERFORATION
2. ACUTE WITH HEMORRHAGE AND PERFORATION
3. ACUTE
4. CHRONIC OR NOS WITH HEMORRHAGE
5. CHRONIC OR NOS WITH PERFORATION
6. CHRONIC OR NOS WITH HEMORRHAGE AND PERFORATION
7. CHRONIC
9. NOS AS ACUTE OR CHRONIC

5th Digit: 531

0. WITHOUT OBSTRUCTION
1. OBSTRUCTED

569.41 RECTUM
363.20 RETINA (SEE ALSO CHORIORETINITIS)
379.09 SCLERA
608.89 SEMINAL VESICLE
0 SKIN SEE 'ULCER, ULCERATION SKIN'
608.89 SPERMATIC CORD
569.41 STERCORAL ANUS OR RECTUM
534.## STOMAL OR ANASTOMOTIC
533.## STRESS (STRESS ULCER)

4th Digit: 533, 534

0. ACUTE WITH HEMORRHAGE
1. ACUTE WITH PERFORATION
2. ACUTE WITH HEMORRHAGE AND PERFORATION
3. ACUTE
4. CHRONIC OR NOS WITH HEMORRHAGE
5. CHRONIC OR NOS WITH PERFORATION
6. CHRONIC OR NOS WITH HEMORRHAGE AND PERFORATION
7. CHRONIC
9. NOS AS ACUTE OR CHRONIC

5th Digit: 533, 534

0. WITHOUT OBSTRUCTION
1. OBSTRUCTED

608.89 TESTIS
529.0 TONGUE (TRAUMATIC)
519.1 TRACHEA
608.89 TUNICA VAGINALIS
597.89 URETHRAL MEATUS
131.02 URETHRAL MEATUS TRICHOMONAL
621.8 UTERUS
622.0 UTERUS NECK
421.0 VALVE, HEART
454.0 VARICOSE (SKIN)
454.2 VARICOSE (SKIN) WITH INFLAMMATION
608.89 VAS DEFERENS

ULCER (ULCERATION) SKIN

707.9 NOS
707.9 NOS WITH GANGRENE [785.4]
707.8 ABDOMEN (WALL)
006.6 AMEBIC
569.41 ANUS
707.8 ARM
611.0 BREAST
707.8 BUTTOCK
707.0 BUTTOCK DECUBITUS
707.0 BUTTOCK DECUBITUS WITH GANGRENE [785.4]
707.9 CHRONIC NOS
707.8 CHRONIC OTHER SPECIFIED SITE

U-V-W

ULCER (ULCERATION) SKIN (continued)

707.0 DECUBITUS

707.0 DECUBITUS WITH GANGRENE [785.4]

250.8# DIABETIC **[707.#]**

250.6# DIABETIC - NEUROPATHIC **[707.#]**

250.7# DIABETIC - PERIPHERAL VASCULAR **[707.#]**

5th Digit: 250.6-8

- **0. TYPE II, ADULT-ONSET, NON-INSULIN DEPENDENT (EVEN IF REQUIRING INSULIN), OR UNSPECIFIED; CONTROLLED**
- **1. TYPE I, JUVENILE-ONSET OR INSULIN-DEPENDENT; CONTROLLED**
- **2. TYPE II, ADULT-ONSET, NON-INSULIN DEPENDENT (EVEN IF REQUIRING INSULIN); UNCONTROLLED**
- **3. TYPE I, JUVENILE-ONSET OR INSULIN-DEPENDENT; UNCONTROLLED**

4th Digit: 707

- **1. LOWER LIMB EXCEPT DECUBITUS**
- **8. CHRONIC OF OTHER SPECIFIED SITE**
- **9. CHRONIC SITE NOS**

373.01 EYELID (REGION)

707.8 FINGER

707.1 FOOT

629.8 GENITAL SITES OTHER FEMALE

616.8 GENITAL SITES OTHER FEMALE APHTHOUS

608.89 GENITAL SITES OTHER MALE (APHTHOUS)

616.50 LABIUM (MAJUS) (MINUS)

440.23 LOWER LIMB ARTERIOSCLEROTIC

440.24 LOWER LIMB ARTERIOSCLEROTIC WITH ISCHEMIC GANGRENE

707.1 LOWER LIMB CHRONIC

250.8# LOWER LIMB CHRONIC DIABETIC [707.1]

250.6# LOWER LIMB CHRONIC DIABETIC - NEUROPATHIC [707.1]

250.7# LOWER LIMB CHRONIC DIABETIC - PERIPHERAL VASCULAR [707.1]

5th Digit: 250.6-8

- **0. TYPE II, ADULT-ONSET, NON-INSULIN DEPENDENT (EVEN IF REQUIRING INSULIN), OR UNSPECIFIED; CONTROLLED**
- **1. TYPE I, JUVENILE-ONSET OR INSULIN-DEPENDENT; CONTROLLED**
- **2. TYPE II, ADULT-ONSET, NON-INSULIN DEPENDENT (EVEN IF REQUIRING INSULIN); UNCONTROLLED**
- **3. TYPE I, JUVENILE-ONSET OR INSULIN-DEPENDENT; UNCONTROLLED**

707.8 LOWER LIMB CHRONIC NEUROGENIC OTHER SPECIFIED SITES

707.1 LOWER LIMB NEUROGENIC

707.1 LOWER LIMB TROPHIC

707.1 LOWER LIMB WITH GANGRENE [785.4]

686.09 MELENEY'S (CHRONIC UNDERMINING)

031.1 MYCOBACTERIUM

707.8 NEUROGENIC CHRONIC NEC

707.9 NON-HEALING

607.89 PENIS CHRONIC

707.0 PLASTER

607.89 PREPUCE

707.0 PRESSURE

608.89 SCROTUM

016.5# SCROTUM TUBERCULOUS [608.89]

5th Digit: 016.5

- **0. NOS**
- **1. LAB NOT DONE**
- **2. LABS PENDING**
- **3. MICROSCOPY POSITIVE (IN SPUTUM)**
- **4. CULTURE POSITIVE - MICROSCOPY NEGATIVE**
- **5. CULTURE NEGATIVE - MICROSCOPY POSITIVE**
- **6. CULTURE AND MICROSCOPY NEGATIVE CONFIRMED BY OTHER METHODS**

ULCER (ULCERATION) SKIN (continued)

456.4 SCROTUM VARICOSE

707.9 SKIN

459.81 STASIS [707.#]

4th Digit: 707

- **1. LOWER LIMB EXCEPT DECUBITUS**
- **8. CHRONIC OF OTHER SPECIFIED SITE**
- **9. CHRONIC SITE NOS**

454.0 STASIS LOWER EXTREMITY VARICOSE

454.2 STASIS LOWER EXTREMITY VARICOSE - INFECTED

091.3 SYPHILITIC

707.9 TROPHIC CHRONIC

707.9 TROPICAL CHRONIC

707.8 UPPER LIMB

616.8 VAGINAL (INFLAMMATORY) (NONOBSTETRICAL)

454.0 VARICOSE

454.2 VARICOSE WITH INFLAMMATION

616.50 VULVA

136.1 VULVA BEHCET'S [616.51]

098.0 VULVA GONOCOCCAL

054.12 VULVA HERPES SIMPLEX

091.0 VULVA SYPHILITIC (PRIMARY)

016.7# VULVA TUBERCULOUS (NONOBSTETRICAL) [616.51]

5th Digit: 016.7

- **0. NOS**
- **1. LAB NOT DONE**
- **2. LABS PENDING**
- **3. MICROSCOPY POSITIVE (IN SPUTUM)**
- **4. CULTURE POSITIVE - MICROSCOPY NEGATIVE**
- **5. CULTURE NEGATIVE - MICROSCOPY POSITIVE**
- **6. CULTURE AND MICROSCOPY NEGATIVE CONFIRMED BY OTHER METHODS**

616.50 VULVOBUCCAL

707.8 OTHER SPECIFIED SITES CHRONIC (TROPHIC) (NEUROGENIC)

556.# ULCERATIVE COLITIS

316 ULCERATIVE COLITIS PSYCHOGENIC [556.#]

4th Digit: 556

- **0. ENTEROCOLITIS (CHRONIC)**
- **1. ILEOCOLITIS (CHRONIC)**
- **2. PROCTITIS (CHRONIC)**
- **3. PROCTOSIGMOIDITIS (CHRONIC)**
- **4. PSEUDOPOLYPOSIS OF COLON**
- **5. LEFT-SIDED (CHRONIC)**
- **6. UNIVERSAL (CHRONIC)**
- **8. OTHER ULCERATIVE COLITIS**
- **9. ULCERATIVE COLITIS (ENTERITIS) UNSPECIFIED**

099.0 ULCUS MOLLE (CUTIS) (SKIN)

742.4 ULEGYRIA CONGENITAL

758.6 ULLRICH (-BONNEVIE) (-TURNER) SYNDROME

759.89 ULLRICH-FEICHTIGER SYNDROME

755.21 ULNA AGENESIS CONGENITAL - WITH ABSENCE COMPLETE OF DISTAL ELEMENTS

755.27 ULNA AGENESIS CONGENITAL - WITH ABSENCE INCOMPLETE OF DISTAL ELEMENTS

736.00 ULNA DEFORMITY

755.50 ULNA DEFORMITY CONGENITAL

ULNAR

442.0 ARTERY ANEURYSM (RUPTURED) (CIRSOID) (VARIX) (FALSE)

440.2# ARTERY ARTERIOSCLEROSIS (DEGENERATION) (OCCLUSION)

5th Digit: 440.2

0. UNSPECIFIED
1. WITH INTERMITTENT CLAUDICATION
2. WITH REST PAIN, OR REST PAIN AND (INTERMITTENT CLAUDICATION)
3. WITH ULCERATION, OR ULCERATION AND (INTERMITTENT CLAUDICATION) (REST PAIN)
4. WITH ISCHEMIC GANGRENE, OR ISCHEMIC GANGRENE AND (INTERMITTENT CLAUDICATION) (REST PAIN) (ULCERATION)
9. OTHER ATHEROSCLEROSIS EXTREMITIES

440.3# ARTERY BYPASS GRAFT ARTERIOSCLEROSIS

5th Digit: 440.3

0. UNSPECIFIED GRAFT
1. AUTOLOGOUS VEIN BYPASS GRAFT
2. NONAUTOLOGOUS BIOLOGICAL BYPASS GRAFT

444.21 ARTERY EMBOLISM (THROMBOSIS) (OCCLUSION) (INFARCTION)
903.3 ARTERY INJURY
908.3 ARTERY INJURY LATE EFFECT

INJURY TO NERVE INCLUDES LACERATION, TRAUMATIC NEUROMA, OR LESION IN CONTINUITY. USE ANATOMICAL SEARCH (THE NAME OF THE NERVE) TO FIND THE SPECIFIED INJURY.

354.2 NERVE DISORDER
955.2 NERVE INJURY
907.4 NERVE INJURY LATE EFFECT
354.2 NERVE LESION
723.4 NERVE NEURALGIA
723.4 NERVE NEURITIS NON-PARALYTIC
354.2 NERVE NEUROPATHY
354.2 NERVE PALSY (TARDY)
354.2 NERVE PARALYSIS
903.3 VEIN INJURY
908.3 VEIN INJURY LATE EFFECT
451.83 VEIN PHLEBITIS

841.3 ULNOHUMERAL SEPARATION (RUPTURE) (TEAR) (LACERATION)
841.3 ULNOHUMERAL STRAIN (SPRAIN) (AVULSION) (HEMARTHROSIS)

ULTRASOUND STUDIES

793.# ABNORMAL FINDINGS (NONSPECIFIC)

4th Digit: 793

0. SKULL AND HEAD
1. LUNG FIELD
2. OTHER INTRATHORACIC ORGAN
3. BILIARY TRACT
4. GASTROINTESTINAL TRACT
5. GENITOURINARY ORGANS
6. ABDOMINAL AREA INCLUDING RETROPERITONEUM
7. MUSCULOSKELETAL SYSTEM
8. BREAST
9. OTHER

V28.3 ANTENATAL SCREENING FOR MALFORMATION
793.2 CARDIOGRAM ABNORMAL
V28.4 FOR FETAL GROWTH RETARDATION

UMBILICAL

747.5 ARTERY ABSENCE
747.5 ARTERY HYPOPLASIA CONGENITAL
789.9 BLEEDING
762.5 CORD - COMPRESSION (AROUND NECK) (ENTANGLEMENT) (KNOT) (TORSION) AFFECTING FETUS OR NEWBORN
771.4 CORD - INFECTION AFFECTING FETUS OR NEWBORN
772.3 CORD - LIGATURE SLIPPED AFFECTING FETUS OR NEWBORN
762.4 CORD - PROLAPSED (PRESENTATION) AFFECTING FETUS OR NEWBORN
772.0 CORD - RUPTURE AFFECTING FETUS OR NEWBORN
762.5 CORD - OTHER ENTANGLEMENT OF CORD AFFECTING FETUS OR NEWBORN
762.6 CORD - OTHER SPECIFIED CONDITION AFFECTING FETUS OR NEWBORN
789.9 DISCHARGE
779.8 DISEASE NEWBORN NEC
771.4 GRANULOMA NEWBORN
686.1 GRANULOMA PYOGENIC
772.3 HEMORRHAGE AFTER BIRTH
771.4 INFECTION NEWBORN
772.3 LIGATURE SLIPPED
789.05 PAIN
753.7 SINUS PERSISTENT CONGENITAL

UMBILICAL CORD COMPLICATIONS OF DELIVERY - MOTHER'S RECORD

663.9# COMPLICATION NOS
663.9# ABNORMALITY COMPLICATING PREGNANCY
663.1# AROUND NECK WITH COMPRESSION
663.6# BRUISING (HEMATOMA) (THROMBOSIS)
663.3# ENTANGLEMENT NOS
663.2# ENTANGLEMENT NOS - WITH COMPRESSION
663.0# PROLAPSE
663.8# RUPTURE
663.4# SHORT
663.5# VASA PREVIA
663.6# VASCULAR LESIONS OF CORD
663.3# OTHER SPECIFIED ENTANGLEMENT
663.2# OTHER SPECIFIED ENTANGLEMENT - WITH COMPRESSION
663.8# OTHER SPECIFIED COMPLICATIONS

5th Digit: 663.0-6, 8-9

0. EPISODE OF CARE NOS OR N/A
1. DELIVERED
3. ANTEPARTUM COMPLICATION

996.1 UMBRELLA VENA CAVA COMPLICATION (MECHANICAL)
V60.4 UNABLE TO CARE FOR SELF
312.1# UNAGRESSIVE CONDUCT DISORDER

5th Digit: 312.1

0. NOS
1. MILD
2. MODERATE
3. SEVERE

0 UNCINARIASIS SEE 'ANCYLOSTOMA'
780.09 UNCONSCIOUS
313.83 UNDERACHIEVEMENT ACADEMIC DISORDER (CHILDHOOD) (ADOLESCENCE)
868.00 UNDERWATER BLAST INJURY SYNDROME (ABDOMINAL)
0 UNDERWEIGHT INFANT FOR GESTATIONAL AGE SEE 'LIGHT FOR DATES'
778.1 UNDERWOOD'S DISEASE (SCLEREMA NEONATORUM)
752.51 UNDESCENDED TESTIS CONGENITAL
V62.0 UNEMPLOYMENT AS CAUSE OF PROBLEM (REASON FOR ENCOUNTER)

703.0 UNGUIS INCARNATUS
313.1 UNHAPPINESS DISORDER CHILDHOOD AND ADOLESCENCE
620.6 UNIVERSAL JOINT SYNDROME-CERVIX
690.10 UNNA'S DISEASE (SEBORRHEIC DERMATITIS)
411.1 UNSTABLE ANGINA
652.0# UNSTABLE LIE COMPLICATING PREGNANCY
660.0# UNSTABLE LIE WITH OBSTRUCTED LABOR [**652.0#**]
652.6# UNSTABLE LIE WITH MULTIPLE GESTATION
660.0# UNSTABLE LIE WITH MULTIPLE GESTATION OBSTRUCTING LABOR [**652.6#**]

5th Digit: 652.0, 6, 660.0
0. EPISODE OF CARE NOS OR N/A
1. DELIVERED
3. ANTEPARTUM COMPLICATION

301.59 UNSTABLE PERSONALITY DISORDER
333.2 UNVERRICHT (-LUNDBORG) DISEASE OR SYNDROME
710.3 UNVERRICHT-WAGNER SYNDROME (DERMATOMYOSITIS)

UPPER ARM
912.9 INJURY OTHER AND UNSPECIFIED SUPERFICIAL (INFECTED)
912.8 INJURY OTHER AND UNSPECIFIED SUPERFICIAL
840.8 SEPARATION (RUPTURE) (TEAR) (LACERATION) OTHER SPECIFIED SITES
840.8 STRAIN (SPRAIN) (AVULSION) (HEMARTHROSIS)

739.7 UPPER EXTREMITIES SEGMENTAL OR SOMATIC DYSFUNCTION
755.20 UPPER LIMB ECTROMELIA
755.20 UPPER LIMB HEMIMELIA

UPPER RESPIRATORY INFECTION
465.9 ACUTE
487.1 ACUTE INFLUENZAL
465.0 ACUTE LARYNGOPHARYNGITIS
465.8 ACUTE MULTIPLE SITES NEC
034.0 ACUTE STREPTOCOCCAL CHRONIC
519.8 CHRONIC

506.2 UPPER RESPIRATORY INFLAMMATION DUE TO FUMES AND VAPORS
478.9 UPPER RESPIRATORY TRACT ATROPHY
378.81 UPWARD GAZE SYNDROME
753.7 URACHUS CYST CONGENITAL
753.7 URACHUS FISTULA CONGENITAL
753.7 URACHUS PATENT CONGENITAL
250.8# URBACH-OPPENHEIM SYNDROME (NECROBIOSIS LIPOIDICA DIABETICORUM) [709.3]

5th Digit: 250.8
0. TYPE II, ADULT-ONSET, NON-INSULIN DEPENDENT (EVEN IF REQUIRING INSULIN), OR UNSPECIFIED; CONTROLLED
1. TYPE I, JUVENILE-ONSET OR INSULIN-DEPENDENT; CONTROLLED
2. TYPE II, ADULT-ONSET, NON-INSULIN DEPENDENT (EVEN IF REQUIRING INSULIN); UNCONTROLLED
3. TYPE I, JUVENILE-ONSET OR INSULIN-DEPENDENT; UNCONTROLLED

272.8 URBACH-WIETHE DISEASE OR SYNDROME (LIPOID PROTEINOSIS)
270.6 UREA CYCLE METABOLISM DISORDER

UREMIA
586 NOS
584.9 ACUTE
585 CHRONIC (SYNDROME)
779.8 CONGENITAL
788.9 EXTRARENAL
403.91 HYPERTENSIVE

UREMIA (continued)
646.2# MATERNAL ACUTE - WITHOUT HYPERTENSION COMPLICATING PREGNANCY [584.9]
646.2# MATERNAL CHRONIC - WITHOUT HYPERTENSION COMPLICATING PREGNANCY [585]

5th Digit: 646.2
0. EPISODE OF CARE NOS OR N/A
1. DELIVERED
2. DELIVERED WITH POSTPARTUM COMPLICATION
3. ANTEPARTUM COMPLICATION
4. POSTPARTUM COMPLICATION

585 NEUROPATHY [357.4]
585 PERICARDITIS [420.0]
585 POLYNEUROPATHY [357.4]
639.3 POST (ABORTIVE) (ECTOPIC) (MOLAR) PREGNANCY
0 SEE ALSO 'RENAL FAILURE'

URETER, URETERAL
593.89 ABSENT
753.4 ABSENT CONGENITAL
753.4 ACCESSORY CONGENITAL
593.89 ADHESIONS
753.22 ADYNAMIC CONGENITAL
753.4 ANOMALOUS IMPLANTATION OF URETER CONGENITAL
753.9 ANOMALY NOS
753.20 ANOMALY NOS OBSTRUCTIVE
753.4 ANOMALY NEC
753.29 ANOMALY NEC OBSTRUCTIVE
753.29 ATRESIA (CONGENITAL)
593.89 CALCIFICATION
592.1 CALCULUS
788.0 COLIC
753.9 DEFECT CONGENITAL
753.29 DEFECT CONGENITAL OBSTRUCTIVE
753.4 DEVIATION CONGENITAL
593.89 DILATATION (IDIOPATHIC)
753.20 DILATATION CONGENITAL
593.9 DISEASE
593.89 DISORDER NEC
753.4 DISTORTION CONGENITAL
753.20 DISTORTION CONGENITAL OBSTRUCTIVE
593.89 DIVERTICULUM
753.4 DIVERTICULUM CONGENITAL
753.4 DOUBLE CONGENITAL
753.4 ECTOPIC CONGENITAL
593.89 FIBROSIS
793.5 FILLING DEFECT
593.82 FISTULA
593.5 HYDROURETER
753.29 HYPOPLASIA CONGENITAL
753.29 IMPERFORATE (CONGENITAL)
753.29 IMPERVIOUS (CONGENITAL)
867.2 INJURY (TRAUMATIC)
867.3 INJURY (TRAUMATIC) WITH OPEN WOUND INTO CAVITY
908.2 INJURY LATE EFFECT
593.3 KINKING
753.20 KINKING CONGENITAL
593.4 OBSTRUCTION
592.1 OBSTRUCTION CALCULUS
753.20 OBSTRUCTION - DEFECT NOS CONGENITAL
753.29 OBSTRUCTION - DEFECT NEC CONGENITAL
593.4 OBSTRUCTION - URETEROPELVIC JUNCTION
753.21 OBSTRUCTION - URETEROPELVIC JUNCTION CONGENITAL
593.4 OBSTRUCTION - URETEROVESICAL JUNCTION
753.22 OBSTRUCTION - URETEROVESICAL JUNCTION CONGENITAL

URETER, URETERAL (continued)

593.4 OCCLUSION
753.29 OCCLUSION CONGENITAL
753.4 ORIFICE DISPLACED CONGENITAL
593.89 POLYP
593.7# REFLUX

5th Digit: 593.7

0. UNSPECIFIED
1. WITH REFLUX NEPHROPATHY, UNILATERAL
2. WITH REFLUX NEPHROPATHY, BILATERAL
3. WITH REFLUX NEPHROPATHY UNSPECIFIED

753.4 RETROCAVAL CONGENITAL
V53.6 STENT REMOVAL
593.3 STRICTURE (POSTOPERATIVE)
753.29 STRICTURE CONGENITAL
753.29 VALVE FORMATION ANOMALY (CONGENITAL)

753.4 URETERIC ORIFICE DISPLACED CONGENITAL
590.3 URETERITIS CYSTICA
593.89 URETEROCELE
753.23 URETEROCELE CONGENITAL
753.23 URETEROCELE CONGENITAL CAUSING URINARY INCONTINENCE [788.3#]

5th Digit: 788.3

0. UNSPECIFIED
1. URGE INCONTINENCE
3. MIXED URGE AND STRESS (MALE) (FEMALE)
4 WITHOUT SENSORY AWARENESS
5. POST-VOID DRIBBLING
6. NOCTURNAL ENURESIS
7. CONTINUOUS LEAKAGE
9. OTHER

592.1 URETEROLITHIASIS
753.21 URETEROPELVIC JUNCTION STRICTURE (ATRESIA) CONGENITAL

WHEN CODING AN INFECTION OF AN OSTOMY, USE AN ADDITIONAL CODE TO SPECIFY THE ORGANISM. SEE 'BACTERIAL INFECTION'

URETEROSTOMY

V55.6 CARE
V55.6 CATHETER ADJUSTMENT OR REPOSITIONING
V55.6 CATHETER REMOVAL OR REPLACEMENT
V55.6 CLOSURE
996.39 COMPLICATION DEVICE MECHANICAL
997.5 COMPLICATION STOMA
997.5 MALFUNCTION
V55.6 REMOVAL OR CHANGE
V44.6 STATUS
V55.6 TOILET STOMA

753.22 URETEROVESICAL ORIFICE STRICTURE (ATRESIA) CONGENITAL

URETHRA, URETHRAL

594.2 CALCULUS
599.3 CARUNCLE
0 CONGENITAL DISORDER SEE 'URETHRA, URETHRAL CONGENITAL'
599.84 CYST
599.84 DEFORMITY (ACQUIRED)
599.84 DILATATION
788.7 DISCHARGE
599.84 DISCHARGE BLOODY
599.9 DISORDER
599.84 DISORDER SPECIFIED TYPE NEC
0 DISORDERS WITH INCONTINENCE SEE 'URETHRA, URETHRAL DISORDERS WITH INCONTINENCE'
599.2 DIVERTICULUM
599.84 ECTROPION
599.84 EVERSION (MEATUS)

URETHRA, URETHRAL (continued)

599.4 FALSE PASSAGE
599.84 FIBROSIS
599.1 FISTULA
599.84 GRANULOMA
599.84 HEMORRHAGE (NONTRAUMATIC)
599.81 HYPERMOBILITY
599.84 HYPERTROPHY
996.64 INDWELLING CATHETER COMPLICATION - INFECTION OR INFLAMMATION
996.31 INDWELLING CATHETER COMPLICATION - MECHANICAL
996.76 INDWELLING CATHETER COMPLICATION - OTHER
665.5# INJURY (OBSTETRICAL)

5th Digit: 665.5

0. EPISODE OF CARE NOS OR N/A
1. DELIVERED
4. POSTPARTUM COMPLICATION

867.0 INJURY (TRAUMATIC)
867.1 INJURY (TRAUMATIC) WITH OPEN WOUND INTO CAVITY
908.2 INJURY (TRAUMATIC) LATE EFFECT
599.82 INTRINSIC SPHINCTER DEFICIENCY (ISD)
599.83 INSTABILITY
599.84 IRRITABILITY
599.84 LACERATION NONTRAUMATIC NONPUERPERAL
599.84 LEUKOPLAKIA
597.89 MEATITIS
597.89 MEATUS ULCER
131.02 MEATUS ULCER TRICHOMONAL
599.5 MUCOSA PROLAPSED
599.84 OBLITERATION
599.6 OBSTRUCTION
598.9 OCCLUSION (SEE ALSO 'URETHRA', STRICTURE)
599.3 POLYP
599.5 PROLAPSE
599.84 RELAXATION
599.84 RUPTURE NONTRAUMATIC
599.84 SHORT
599.84 SPASM
0 SPHINCTER INCONTINENCE SEE 'URINARY', INCONTINENCE
599.84 SPHINCTER INSUFFICIENCY
598.9 STRICTURE
598.00 STRICTURE DUE TO UNSPECIFIED INFECTION
615.9 STRICTURE MYOMETRITIS (DUE TO) [598.01]
598.2 STRICTURE POSTOPERATIVE
598.1 STRICTURE POSTTRAUMATIC
095.8 STRICTURE SYPHILITIC [598.01]
098.2 STRICTURE GONOCOCCAL [598.01]
614.0 STRICTURE SALPINGO OOPHORITIS (DUE TO) [598.01]
120.9 STRICTURE SCHISTOSOMA [598.01]
598.1 STRICTURE TRAUMATIC
598.8 STRICTURE OTHER SPECIFIED CAUSE
597.81 SYNDROME
599.84 TAG
599.84 TORTUOUS
599.89 VERUMONTANUM
599.84 OTHER SPECIFIED DISORDER URETHRA
599.89 OTHER SPECIFIED DISORDER URINARY TRACT

URETHRA, URETHRAL CONGENITAL

753.8 ABSENCE
753.8 ACCESSORY
753.8 DIVERTICULUM
753.8 DOUBLE
753.6 IMPERVIOUS
753.6 OBSTRUCTION OR OCCLUSION
753.8 PENDULOUS
753.8 PROLAPSE
753.6 STRICTURE (MEATUS OR BLADDER NECK)
0 STRICTURE, OBSTRUCTION, OR IMPERVIOUS URETHRA WITH INCONTINENCE SEE 'URETHRA, URETHRAL DISORDERS WITH INCONTINENCE'
753.6 VALVE FORMATION

*URETHRAL DISORDERS WITH INCONTINENCE (RETENTION): WHEN CODING THE DISORDERS BELOW, CODE THE DISORDER FIRST, THEN ADD THE APPROPRIATE ADDITIONAL CODE FOR THE INCONTINENCE (RETENTION) ; (788.3# OR 625.6) FOR EXAMPLE, THE CODES FOR URETHRAL FIBROSIS WITH STRESS INCONTINENCE, FEMALE WOULD BE; 599.84 (URETHRAL FIBROSIS) AND 625.6, (STRESS INCONTINENCE). **THE DISORDER SEQUENCES BEFORE THE INCONTINENCE (RETENTION).***

URETHRA, URETHRAL DISORDERS:

WITH INCONTINENCE, [788.3#]

WITH STRESS INCONTINENCE, FEMALE [625.6]

WITH URINARY RETENTION [788.2#]

599.84 CYST
599.84 EVERSION (MEATUS)
599.84 FIBROSIS
599.84 GRANULOMA
599.89 HEMORRHAGE GENITOURINARY
599.84 HEMORRHAGE (NONTRAUMATIC)
599.84 HYDROURETHRA
599.81 HYPERMOBILITY
599.89 HYPERPLASIA URETHROVAGINAL
599.84 HYPERTROPHY
599.89 HYPERTROPHY VERUMONTANUM
599.84 INCONTINENCE URETHRAL SPHINCTER
599.83 INSTABILITY
599.82 INTRINSIC SPHINCTER DEFICIENCY (ISD)
599.84 IRRITABILITY
599.82 ISD - INTRINSIC (URETHRAL) SPHINCTER DEFICIENCY
599.84 LACERATION NONPUERPERAL, NONTRAUMATIC
599.84 LEUKOPLAKIA
599.84 LEUKOPLAKIA (POST INFECTIONAL)
599.84 MALACOPLAKIA
599.84 OBLITERATION
599.89 OTHER SPECIFIED DISORDER URINARY TRACT
599.84 PNEUMATURIA
599.84 RELAXATION
599.84 RUPTURE
599.84 SHORT
599.84 SPASM
599.84 SPHINCTER INSUFFICIENCY
599.84 TAG
599.84 TORTUOUS
599.89 URINARY TRACT DISORDER OTHER SPECIFIED
599.89 VERUMONTANUM

WITH INCONTINENCE [788.3#]

5th Digit: 788.3

0. UNSPECIFIED
1. URGE INCONTINENCE
2. STRESS, MALE
3. MIXED URGE AND STRESS (MALE) (FEMALE)
4 WITHOUT SENSORY AWARENESS
5. POST-VOID DRIBBLING
6. NOCTURNAL ENURESIS
7. CONTINUOUS LEAKAGE
9. OTHER

WITH URINARY RETENTION [788.2#]

5th Digit: 788.2

0. UNSPECIFIED
1. INCOMPLETE BLADDER EMPTYING
9. OTHER SPECIFIED RETENTION

URETHRITIS

098.0 ACUTE GONOCOCCAL
098.2 CHRONIC GONOCOCCAL
597.80 NONSPECIFIC (NOT SEXUALLY TRANSMITTED)
099.4# NONGONOCOCCAL

5th Digit: 099.4

0. UNSPECIFIED
1. CHLAMYDIA TRACHOMATIS
9. OTHER SPECIFIED ORGANISM

131.02 TRICHOMONAL

URETHROCELE

599.5 MALE
599.5 MALE WITH URINARY INCONTINENCE **[788.3#]**
618.# FEMALE
618.# FEMALE WITH STRESS INCONTINENCE [625.6]
618.# FEMALE WITH OTHER URINARY INCONTINENCE **[788.3#]**

4th Digit: 618

0. WITHOUT UTERINE PROLAPSE
2. WITH INCOMPLETE UTERINE PROLAPSE
3. WITH COMPLETE UTERINE PROLAPSE
4. UTERINE PROLAPSE UNSPECIFIED

5th Digit: 788.3

0. UNSPECIFIED
1. URGE INCONTINENCE
3. MIXED URGE AND STRESS (MALE) (FEMALE)
4 WITHOUT SENSORY AWARENESS
5. POST-VOID DRIBBLING
6. NOCTURNAL ENURESIS
7. CONTINUOUS LEAKAGE
9. OTHER

099.3 URETHRO-OCULOARTICULAR SYNDROME
099.3 URETHRO-OCULOARTICULAR SYNDROME WITH ARTHROPATHY **[711.1#]**

5th Digit: 711.1

0. SITE NOS
1. SHOULDER REGION
2. UPPER ARM (ELBOW) (HUMERUS)
3. FOREARM (RADIUS) (WRIST) (ULNA)
4. HAND (CARPAL) (METACARPAL) (FINGERS)
5. PELVIC REGION AND THIGH (HIP) (BUTTOCK) (FEMUR)
6. LOWER LEG (FIBULA) (KNEE) (PATELLA) (TIBIA)
7. ANKLE AND/OR FOOT (METATARSALS) (TOES) (TARSALS)
8. OTHER (HEAD) (NECK) (RIB) (SKULL) (TRUNK) (VERTEBRAE)
9. MULTIPLE

099.3 URETHRO-OCULOARTICULAR SYNDROME WITH CONJUNCTIVITIS [372.33]

099.3 URETHRO-OCULOSYNOVIAL SYNDROME
099.3 URETHRO-OCULOSYNOVIAL SYNDROME WITH ARTHROPATHY **[711.1#]**

5th Digit: 711.1

0. SITE NOS
1. SHOULDER REGION
2. UPPER ARM (ELBOW) (HUMERUS)
3. FOREARM (RADIUS) (WRIST) (ULNA)
4. HAND (CARPAL) (METACARPAL) (FINGERS)
5. PELVIC REGION AND THIGH (HIP) (BUTTOCK) (FEMUR)
6. LOWER LEG (FIBULA) (KNEE) (PATELLA) (TIBIA)
7. ANKLE AND/OR FOOT (METATARSALS) (TOES) (TARSALS)
8. OTHER (HEAD) (NECK) (RIB) (SKULL) (TRUNK) (VERTEBRAE)
9. MULTIPLE

099.3 URETHRO-OCULOSYNOVIAL SYNDROME WITH CONJUNCTIVITIS [372.33]

599.1 URETHRORECTAL FISTULA
753.8 URETHRORECTAL FISTULA CONGENITAL

599.84 URETHRORRHAGIA
788.7 URETHRORRHEA

WHEN CODING AN INFECTION OF AN OSTOMY, USE AN ADDITIONAL CODE TO SPECIFY THE ORGANISM. SEE 'BACTERIAL INFECTION'

URETHROSTOMY

V55.6 CARE
V55.6 CATHETER ADJUSTMENT OR REPOSITIONING
V55.6 CATHETER REMOVAL OR REPLACEMENT
V55.6 CLOSURE
996.39 COMPLICATION DEVICE MECHANICAL
997.5 COMPLICATION STOMA
997.5 MALFUNCTION
V55.6 REMOVAL OR CHANGE
V44.6 STATUS
V55.6 TOILET STOMA

599.89 URETHROVAGINAL HYPERPLASIA
705.89 URHIDROSIS

URI

465.9 ACUTE
487.1 ACUTE INFLUENZAL
465.0 ACUTE LARYNGOPHARYNGITIS
465.8 ACUTE (MULTIPLE SITES)
034.0 ACUTE STREPTOCOCCAL
519.8 CHRONIC

790.6 URIC ACID BLOOD ABNORMAL

URINARY

592.9 CALCULUS
V13.01 CALCULUS HISTORY
V53.6 CATHETER (FITTING) (ADJUSTMENT) (REMOVAL) (REPLACEMENT)
0 CATHETER OF AN OSTOMY SEE SPECIFIC OSTOMY
791.9 CONSTITUENTS ABNORMAL
997.5 CYSTITIS DUE TO A PROCEDURE
V53.6 DEVICE FITTING AND ADJUSTMENT
599.9 DISORDER (TRACT)
V13.00 DISORDER HISTORY
760.1 DISORDER MATERNAL AFFECTING FETUS OR NEWBORN
599.89 DISORDER OTHER SPECIFIED
V13.09 DISORDER OTHER SPECIFIED HISTORY
788.41 FREQUENCY
788.43 FREQUENCY NOCTURNAL
788.69 HESITANCY
788.3# INCONTINENCE
753.23 INCONTINENCE WITH URETERROCELE CONGENITAL [788.3#]

5th Digit: 788.3

0. UNSPECIFIED
1. URGE INCONTINENCE
2. STRESS, MALE
3. MIXED URGE AND STRESS (MALE) (FEMALE)
4 .WITHOUT SENSORY AWARENESS
5. POST-VOID DRIBBLING
6. NOCTURNAL ENURESIS
7. CONTINUOUS LEAKAGE
9. OTHER

625.6 INCONTINENCE STRESS (FEMALE)
753.8 MEATUS DOUBLE - STRICTURE CONGENITAL
753.6 MEATUS IMPERFORATE CONGENITAL
599.6 OBSTRUCTION

URINARY (continued)

599.6 OBSTRUCTION WITH INCONTINENCE **[788.3#]**

5th Digit: 788.3

0. UNSPECIFIED
1. URGE INCONTINENCE
2. STRESS, MALE
3. MIXED URGE AND STRESS (MALE) (FEMALE)
4 .WITHOUT SENSORY AWARENESS
5. POST-VOID DRIBBLING
6. NOCTURNAL ENURESIS
7. CONTINUOUS LEAKAGE
9. OTHER

599.6 OBSTRUCTION WITH STRESS INCONTINENCE (FEMALE) [625.6]
752.69 OPENING FALSE - MALE
V47.4 PROBLEM NEC
788.2# RETENTION

5th Digit: 788.2

0. UNSPECIFIED
1. INCOMPLETE BLADDER EMPTYING
9. OTHER SPECIFIED RETENTION

997.5 RETENTION POSTOPERATIVE
306.53 RETENTION PSYCHOGENIC
788.5 SECRETION SUPPRESSION
788.61 STREAM INTERMITTENT
788.62 STREAM SLOWING
788.61 STREAM SPLITTING
788.62 STREAM WEAK
788.69 STREAM ABNORMALITY OTHER
753.8 SYSTEM ABSENCE (PART) CONGENITAL
753.9 SYSTEM ANOMALY CONGENITAL
753.9 SYSTEM DEFORMITY CONGENITAL
V13.00 SYSTEM DISORDER HISTORY
788.9 SYSTEM SYMPTOMS
753.29 TRACT ATRESIA CONGENITAL
760.1 TRACT DISEASES MATERNAL AFFECTING FETUS OR NEWBORN
599.9 TRACT DISORDER
599.89 TRACT DISORDER OTHER SPECIFIED
599.6 TRACT OBSTRUCTION
V44.6 TRACT OTHER ARTIFICIAL OPENING STATUS

URINARY TRACT INFECTION IS A NONSPECIFIC DIAGNOSIS. WHENEVER POSSIBLE, AND IF NOTED ON THE MEDICAL RECORD, BE SURE TO CODE THE SPECIFIC CONDITION. (I.E. CYSTITIS, NEPHRITIS, URETHRITIS, ETC.)

URINARY TRACT INFECTION:

WITH KNOWN ORGANISM [041.]

599.0 SITE NOT SPECIFIED
112.2 CANDIDAL
996.64 DUE TO INDWELLING FOLEY
639.8 FOLLOWING ABORTION / ECTOPIC / MOLAR PREGNANCY
760.1 MATERNAL AFFECTING FETUS OR NEWBORN

646.6#: SPECIFY THE MATERNAL UTI WITH AN ADDITIONAL CODE. (CYSTITIS, URETHRITIS, ETC.)

646.6# MATERNAL COMPLICATING PREGNANCY

5th Digit: 646.6

0. EPISODE OF CARE NOS OR N/A
1. DELIVERED
2. DELIVERED WITH POSTPARTUM COMPLICATION
3. ANTEPARTUM COMPLICATION
4. POSTPARTUM COMPLICATION

771.8 NEONATAL [599.0]
997.5 POSTOPERATIVE
997.5 SPECIFIED AS DUE TO A PROCEDURE

U-V-W

URINARY TRACT INFECTION: (continued)

WITH KNOWN ORGANISM [041.]

4th or 4th and 5th Digit Code for Organism: 041

.85 AEROBACTER AEROGENES
.82 BACILLUS FRAGILIS
.84 BACTEROIDES (FRAGILIS)
.83 CLOSTRIDIUM PERFRINGENS
.4 E. COLI
.81 EATON'S AGENT
.04 ENTEROCOCCUS
.3 FRIEDLANDER'S BACILLUS,
.84 GRAM-NEGATIVE ANAEROBES
.85 GRAM-NEGATIVE BACTERIA NOS
.5 H. INFLUENZAE
.86 H. PYLORI
.3 KLEBSIELLA
.85 MIMA POLYMORPHA
.81 MYCOPLASMA
.81 PLEUROPNEUMONIA LIKE ORGANISMS
.2 PNEUMOCOCCUS
.6 PROTEUS (MIRABILIS) (MORGANII)
.7 PSEUDOMONAS
.85 SERRATIA
.10 STAPHYLOCOCCUS UNSPECIFIED
.11 STAPHYLOCOCCUS AUREUS
.19 STAPHYLOCOCCUS OTHER
.00 STREPTOCOCCUS
.01 STREPTOCOCCUS GROUP A
.02 STREPTOCOCCUS GROUP B
.03 STREPTOCOCCUS GROUP C
.04 STREPTOCOCCUS GROUP D
.05 STREPTOCOCCUS GROUP G
.09 STREPTOCOCCUS OTHER
.84 OTHER ANAEROBES
.89 OTHER SPECIFIED BACTERIA

URINATION

788.4# EXCESSIVE

5th Digit: 788.4
1. URINATION FREQUENCY
2. POLYURIA
3. NOCTURIA

788.1 PAINFUL
788.2# RETENTION

5th Digit: 788.2
0. UNSPECIFIED
1. INCOMPLETE BLADDER EMPTYING
9. OTHER SPECIFIED RETENTION

306.53 RETENTION PSYCHOGENIC
788.6# STREAM ABNORMALITY

5th Digit: 788.6
1. STREAM SPLITTING, INTERMITTENT
2. STREAM SLOWING, WEAK STREAM
9. OTHER ABNORMALITY

URINE

791.6 ACETONE ABNORMAL
791.0 ALBUMIN ABNORMAL
791.9 BACTERIA ABNORMAL FINDINGS
791.9 BACTERIURIA
791.4 BILE ABNORMAL
791.7 CASTS ABNORMAL
791.7 CELLS ABNORMAL
791.1 CHYLURIA ABNORMAL
791.9 CULTURE POSITIVE ABNORMAL FINDINGS
788.5 DEFICIENT SECRETION
788.30 ENURESIS

URINE (continued)

788.8 EXTRAVASATION
788.8 EXTRAVASATION UNKNOWN ETIOLOGY
791.5 GLUCOSE ABNORMAL
791.2 HEMOGLOBIN ABNORMAL
0 INCONTINENCE SEE 'URINARY', INCONTINENCE
791.6 KETONE ABNORMAL
788.37 LEAKAGE CONTINUOUS
791.0 PROTEIN ABNORMAL
788.69 RESIDUAL
788.2# RETENTION

5th Digit: 788.2
0. UNSPECIFIED
1. INCOMPLETE BLADDER EMPTYING
9. OTHER SPECIFIED RETENTION

997.5 RETENTION POSTOPERATIVE
306.53 RETENTION PSYCHOGENIC
788.20 STASIS
791.5 SUGAR ABNORMAL
796.9 TOXICOLOGY ABNORMAL

URINOMA

596.8 BLADDER
998.2 DUE TO ACCIDENTAL PUNCTURE OR LACERATION
593.89 KIDNEY
593.89 URETER
599.84 URETHRA

752.8 UROGENITAL SINUS (CONGENITAL)
572.4 UROHEPATIC SYNDROME
592.9 UROLITHIASIS
599.6 UROPATHY OBSTRUCTIVE
0 UROSEPSIS SEE 'UTI'

URTICARIA

708.9 NOS
708.0 ALLERGIC
708.0 ANGIOEDEMA (ALLERGIC)
277.6 ANGIOEDEMA (HEREDITARY)
995.1 ANGIONEUROTIC EDEMA
909.9 ANGIONEUROTIC EDEMA LATE EFFECT
708.5 CHOLINERGIC
708.8 CHRONIC
708.8 CHRONIC RECURRENT
708.3 DERMATOGRAPHIC
708.2 DUE TO COLD AND HEAT
995.1 DUE TO CORRECTLY ADMINISTERED SUBSTANCE
909.9 DUE TO CORRECTLY ADMINISTERED SUBSTANCE LATE EFFECT
708.0 DUE TO DRUG ALLERGY
999.5 DUE TO SERUM
909.3 DUE TO SERUM LATE EFFECT
708.3 FACTITIAL
708.0 FOOD ALLERGY
995.1 GIANT
909.9 GIANT LATE EFFECT
708.1 IDIOPATHIC
778.8 NEONATORUM
708.1 NONALLERGIC
698.2 PAPULOSA (HEBRA)
757.33 PIGMENTOSA
708.8 PLANT EXPOSURE
316 PSYCHOGENIC [708.8]
995.1 QUINCKE'S
909.9 QUINCKE'S LATE EFFECT
708.8 RECURRENT CHRONIC
692.72 SOLARE
708.2 THERMAL
708.4 VIBRATORY

URTICARIA (ANGIONEUROTIC EDEMA)

995.1 ANGIONEUROTIC EDEMA
909.9 ANGIONEUROTIC EDEMA LATE EFFECT
999.5 DUE TO SERUM
909.3 DUE TO SERUM LATE EFFECT
995.1 GIANT
909.9 GIANT LATE EFFECT
995.1 QUINCKE'S
909.9 QUINCKE'S LATE EFFECT

694.4 USHER-SENEAR DISEASE (PEMPHIGUS ERYTHEMATOSUS)

085.5 UTA

0 UTERINE SEE 'UTERUS, UTERINE'

UTERUS, UTERINE

615.9 ABSCESS
615.0 ABSCESS ACUTE
615.1 ABSCESS CHRONIC
621.8 ABSENCE
752.3 ABSENCE CONGENITAL
621.5 ADHESION
614.6 ADHESION TO ABDOMINAL WALL
752.3 AGENESIS CONGENITAL
621.6 ANTEVERSION
752.3 APLASIA CONGENITAL
902.55 ARTERY INJURY
908.4 ARTERY INJURY LATE EFFECT
902.55 ARTERY LACERATION (RUPTURE) (HEMATOMA) (AVULSION) (ANEURYSM) TRAUMATIC
908.4 ARTERY LACERATION LATE EFFECT
621.8 ATRESIA
752.3 ATRESIA CONGENITAL
621.8 ATROPHY ACQUIRED
621.5 BANDS
752.3 BICORNIS (BICORNUATE) CONGENITAL
752.2 BICORNIS (BICORNUATE) WITH CERVIX CONGENITAL
626.9 BLEEDING (ABNORMAL)
902.59 BLOOD VESSEL NEC INJURY
908.4 BLOOD VESSEL NEC INJURY LATE EFFECT
621.8 CALCIFICATION
621.8 CYST
752.2 DIDELPHIC (CONGENITAL)
615.9 DISORDER INFECTIVE
621.9 DISORDER NONINFLAMMATORY
0 DISORDERS COMPLICATING PREGNANCY SEE 'UTERUS, UTERINE DISORDERS COMPLICATING PREGNANCY'
752.2 DOUBLING CONGENITAL
621.2 ENLARGEMENT
618.1 EVERSION - NOS (SEE ALSO 'UTERUS, UTERINE PROLAPSE'
618.1 EVERSION - WITH STRESS INCONTINENCE [625.6]
618.1 EVERSION - WITH OTHER URINARY INCONTINENCE **[788.3#]**

5th Digit: 788.3

0. UNSPECIFIED
1. URGE INCONTINENCE
3. MIXED URGE AND STRESS
4 WITHOUT SENSORY AWARENESS
5. POST-VOID DRIBBLING
6. NOCTURNAL ENURESIS
7. CONTINUOUS LEAKAGE
9. OTHER

618.1 EXTROVERSION
618.1 EXTROVERSION WITH STRESS INCONTINENCE [625.6]
618.1 EXTROVERSION WITH OTHER URINARY INCONTINENCE **[788.3#]**

5th Digit: 788.3

0. UNSPECIFIED
1. URGE INCONTINENCE
3. MIXED URGE AND STRESS
4 WITHOUT SENSORY AWARENESS
5. POST-VOID DRIBBLING
6. NOCTURNAL ENURESIS
7. CONTINUOUS LEAKAGE
9. OTHER

UTERUS, UTERINE (continued)

218.9 FIBROID - NOS
218.1 FIBROID - INTRAMURAL
218.0 FIBROID - SUBMUCOUS
218.2 FIBROID - SUBSEROUS
621.8 FIBROSIS
621.3 HYPERPLASIA ENDOMETRIUM
621.2 HYPERPLASIA MYOMETRIUM
621.2 HYPERTROPHY
621.8 INCARCERATED
639.2 INJURY POST ABORTION / ECTOPIC / MOLAR PREGNANCY
867.4 INJURY TRAUMATIC
867.5 INJURY TRAUMATIC WITH OPEN WOUND INTO CAVITY
908.2 INJURY TRAUMATIC LATE EFFECT
621.7 INVERSION (CHRONIC)
621.8 LACERATION (POSTPARTUM) OLD
621.6 MALPOSITION
625.8 MASS
621.8 METAPLASIA
621.8 OBSTRUCTION OR OCCLUSION
621.0 POLYP
0 PROLAPSE SEE 'UTERUS, UTERINE PROLAPSE'
621.6 RETROFLEXION
621.6 RETROVERSION
621.8 RUPTURE (NONOBSTETRICAL) (NONTRAUMATIC)
621.1 SUBINVOLUTION (CHRONIC) (NONPUERPERAL)
621.5 SYNECHIAE
621.8 ULCER
752.3 UNICORNIS
902.56 VEIN INJURY
908.4 VEIN INJURY LATE EFFECT
902.56 VEIN LACERATION (RUPTURE) (HEMATOMA) (AVULSION) (ANEURYSM) TRAUMATIC
908.4 VEIN LACERATION LATE EFFECT
752.3 WITH ONE FUNCTIONING HORN

UTERUS, UTERINE PROLAPSE:

WITH INCONTINENCE [788.3#]

WITH STRESS INCONTINENCE [625.6]

618.1 NOS
618.4 AND VAGINA PROLAPSE
618.2 AND VAGINA PROLAPSE INCOMPLETE
618.3 AND VAGINA PROLAPSE COMPLETE
618.1 DEGREE FIRST
618.1 DEGREE SECOND
618.1 DEGREE THIRD
618.1 DESCENSUS (FIRST DEGREE) (SECOND DEGREE) (THIRD DEGREE)
618.1 PROCIDENTIA

WITH INCONTINENCE [788.3#]

5th Digit: 788.3

0. UNSPECIFIED
1. URGE INCONTINENCE
3. MIXED URGE AND STRESS
4 WITHOUT SENSORY AWARENESS
5. POST-VOID DRIBBLING
6. NOCTURNAL ENURESIS
7. CONTINUOUS LEAKAGE
9. OTHER

763.89 ABNORMALITIES SHAPE OR POSITION AFFECTING FETUS OR NEWBORN
654.4# ABNORMALITIES SHAPE OR POSITION COMPLICATING CHILDBIRTH
660.2# ABNORMALITIES SHAPE OR POSITION COMPLICATING CHILDBIRTH OBSTRUCTING LABOR **[654.4#]**

5th Digit: 654.4
0. EPISODE OF CARE NOS OR N/A
1. DELIVERED
2. DELIVERED WITH POSTPARTUM COMPLICATION
3. ANTEPARTUM COMPLICATION
4. POSTPARTUM COMPLICATION

5th Digit: 660.2
0. EPISODE OF CARE NOS OR N/A
1. DELIVERED
3. ANTEPARTUM COMPLICATION

666.1# ATONY (HYPOTONIC) (INERTIA)

5th Digit: 666.1
0. EPISODE OF CARE NOS OR N/A
2. DELIVERED WITH POSTPARTUM COMPLICATION
4. POSTPARTUM COMPLICATION

654.0# BICORNIS COMPLICATING CHILDBIRTH
660.2# BICORNIS COMPLICATING CHILDBIRTH OBSTRUCTING LABOR **[654.0#]**

5th Digit: 654.0
0. EPISODE OF CARE NOS OR N/A
1. DELIVERED
2. DELIVERED WITH POSTPARTUM COMPLICATION
3. ANTEPARTUM COMPLICATION
4. POSTPARTUM COMPLICATION

5th Digit: 660.2
0. EPISODE OF CARE NOS OR N/A
1. DELIVERED
3. ANTEPARTUM COMPLICATION

661.4# CONTRACTIONS HYPERTONIC, INCOORDINATE, PROLONGED OR HOURGLASS IN LABOR
763.7 DYSFUNCTION MATERNAL AFFECTING FETUS OR NEWBORN
661.4# DYSTOCIA NOS IN LABOR

5th Digit: 661.4
0. EPISODE OF CARE NOS OR N/A
1. DELIVERED
3. ANTEPARTUM COMPLICATION

763.89 EVERSION / INVERSION AFFECTING FETUS NEWBORN
665.2# EVERSION / INVERSION COMPLICATING DELIVERY
665.2# EVERSION / INVERSION (OBSTETRICAL TRAUMA)
674.8# EVERSION PUERPERAL, POSTPARTUM MATERNAL DUE TO PREGNANCY

5th Digit: 665.2, 674.8
0. NOS
2. DELIVERED WITH POSTPARTUM COMPLICATION
4. POSTPARTUM COMPLICATION

654.1# FIBROID COMPLICATING PREGNANCY
660.2# FIBROID COMPLICATING PREGNANCY OBSTRUCTING LABOR **[654.1#]**

5th Digit: 654.1
0. EPISODE OF CARE NOS OR N/A
1. DELIVERED
2. DELIVERED WITH POSTPARTUM COMPLICATION
3. ANTEPARTUM COMPLICATION
4. POSTPARTUM COMPLICATION

5th Digit: 660.2
0. EPISODE OF CARE NOS OR N/A
1. DELIVERED
3. ANTEPARTUM COMPLICATION

674.8# HYPERTROPHY POSTPARTUM MATERNAL DUE TO PREGNANCY

5th Digit: 674.8
0. EPISODE OF CARE NOS OR N/A
2. DELIVERED WITH POSTPARTUM COMPLICATION
4. POSTPARTUM COMPLICATION

763.7 HYPOTONIC CONGENITAL AFFECTING FETUS OR NEWBORN
0 HYPOTONIC SEE 'UTERUS, UTERINE DISORDERS COMPLICATING PREGNANCY', INERTIA
654.3# INCARCERATED
660.2# INCARCERATED OBSTRUCTING LABOR **[654.3#]**

5th Digit: 654.3
0. EPISODE OF CARE NOS OR N/A
1. DELIVERED
2. DELIVERED WITH POSTPARTUM COMPLICATION
3. ANTEPARTUM COMPLICATION
4. POSTPARTUM COMPLICATION

5th Digit: 660.2
0. EPISODE OF CARE NOS OR N/A
1. DELIVERED
3. ANTEPARTUM COMPLICATION

763.7 INERTIA - OR DYSFUNCTION AFFECTING FETUS OR NEWBORN
661.0# INERTIA - PRIMARY
661.1# INERTIA - SECONDARY
661.2# INERTIA - OTHER AND NOS

5th Digit: 661.0-2
0. EPISODE OF CARE NOS OR N/A
1. DELIVERED
3. ANTEPARTUM COMPLICATION

644.1# IRRITABILITY >37 WEEKS (THREATENED PREMATURE LABOR)
644.0# IRRITABILITY >22 AND <37 WEEKS (THREATENED PREMATURE LABOR)

5th Digit: 644.0-1
0. EPISODE OF CARE UNSPECIFIED OR N/A
3. ANTEPARTUM COMPLICATION

644.2# IRRITABILITY WITH PREMATURE ONSET OF DELIVERY <37 WEEKS

5th Digit: 644.2
0. EPISODE OF CARE UNSPECIFIED OR N/A
1. DELIVERED

654.4# PROLAPSE COMPLICATING PREGNANCY
660.2# PROLAPSE COMPLICATING PREGNANCY OBSTRUCTING LABOR **[654.4#]**
654.3# RETROVERTED INCARCERATED COMPLICATING CHILDBIRTH
660.2# RETROVERTED INCARCERATED COMPLICATING CHILDBIRTH OBSTRUCTING LABOR **[654.3#]**

5th Digit: 654.3-4
0. EPISODE OF CARE NOS OR N/A
1. DELIVERED
2. DELIVERED WITH POSTPARTUM COMPLICATION
3. ANTEPARTUM COMPLICATION
4. POSTPARTUM COMPLICATION

5th Digit: 660.2
0. EPISODE OF CARE NOS OR N/A
1. DELIVERED
3. ANTEPARTUM COMPLICATION

UTERUS, UTERINE DISORDERS COMPLICATING PREGNANCY (continued)

763.89 RUPTURE AFFECTING FETUS OR NEWBORN
665.0# RUPTURE BEFORE ONSET OF LABOR
5th Digit: 665.0
0. EPISODE OF CARE NOS OR N/A
1. DELIVERED
3. ANTEPARTUM COMPLICATION

665.1# RUPTURE DURING LABOR OR NOS
5th Digit: 665.1
0. EPISODE OF CARE UNSPECIFIED OR N/A
1. DELIVERED

763.1 SACCULATION AFFECTING FETUS OR NEWBORN
654.4# SACCULATION COMPLICATING DELIVERY
660.2# SACCULATION COMPLICATING DELIVERY OBSTRUCTING LABOR [654.4#]
5th Digit: 654.4
0. EPISODE OF CARE NOS OR N/A
1. DELIVERED
2. DELIVERED WITH POSTPARTUM COMPLICATION
3. ANTEPARTUM COMPLICATION
4. POSTPARTUM COMPLICATION

5th Digit: 660.2
0. EPISODE OF CARE NOS OR N/A
1. DELIVERED
3. ANTEPARTUM COMPLICATION

654.2# SCAR FROM PREVIOUS CESAREAN DELIVERY COMPLICATING CHILDBIRTH
660.2# SCAR FROM PREVIOUS CESAREAN DELIVERY COMPLICATING CHILDBIRTH OBSTRUCTING LABOR [654.2#]
655.8# SIZE-DATE DISCREPANCY
661.4# SPASM IN LABOR
5th Digit: 654.2, 655.8, 660.2, 661.4
0. EPISODE OF CARE UNSPECIFIED OR N/A
1. DELIVERED
3. ANTEPARTUM COMPLICATION

674.8# SUBINVOLUTION, POSTPARTUM MATERNAL DUE TO PREGNANCY
5th Digit: 674.8
0. NOS
2. DELIVERED WITH POSTPARTUM COMPLICATION
4. POSTPARTUM COMPLICATION

752.3 UNICORNIS CONGENITAL

URINARY TRACT INFECTION IS A NONSPECIFIC DIAGNOSIS. WHENEVER POSSIBLE, AND IF NOTED ON THE MEDICAL RECORD, BE SURE TO CODE THE SPECIFIC CONDITION. (I.E. CYSTITIS, NEPHRITIS, URETHRITIS, ETC.)

UTI (URINARY TRACT INFECTION):

WITH KNOWN ORGANISM [041.]

599.0 SITE NOT SPECIFIED
112.2 CANDIDAL
996.64 DUE TO INDWELLING FOLEY
639.8 FOLLOWING ABORTION / ECTOPIC / MOLAR PREGNANCY
646.6# MATERNAL COMPLICATING PREGNANCY
5th Digit: 646.6
0. EPISODE OF CARE NOS OR N/A
1. DELIVERED
2. DELIVERED WITH POSTPARTUM COMPLICATION
3. ANTEPARTUM COMPLICATION
4. POSTPARTUM COMPLICATION

771.8 NEONATAL [599.0]
997.5 POSTOPERATIVE
997.5 SPECIFIED AS DUE TO A PROCEDURE

UTI (URINARY TRACT INFECTION): (continued)

WITH KNOWN ORGANISM [041.]
4th or 4th and 5th Digit Code for Organism: 041
.85 AEROBACTER AEROGENES
.82 BACILLUS FRAGILIS
.84 BACTEROIDES (FRAGILIS)
.83 CLOSTRIDIUM PERFRINGENS
.4 E. COLI
.81 EATON'S AGENT
.04 ENTEROCOCCUS
.3 FRIEDLANDER'S BACILLUS,
.84 GRAM-NEGATIVE ANAEROBES
.85 GRAM-NEGATIVE BACTERIA NOS
.5 H. INFLUENZAE
.86 H. PYLORI
.3 KLEBSIELLA
.85 MIMA POLYMORPHA
.81 MYCOPLASMA
.81 PLEUROPNEUMONIA LIKE ORGANISMS
.2 PNEUMOCOCCUS
.6 PROTEUS (MIRABILIS) (MORGANII)
.7 PSEUDOMONAS
.85 SERRATIA
.10 STAPHYLOCOCCUS UNSPECIFIED
.11 STAPHYLOCOCCUS AUREUS
.19 STAPHYLOCOCCUS OTHER
.00 STREPTOCOCCUS
.01 STREPTOCOCCUS GROUP A
.02 STREPTOCOCCUS GROUP B
.03 STREPTOCOCCUS GROUP C
.04 STREPTOCOCCUS GROUP D
.05 STREPTOCOCCUS GROUP G
.09 STREPTOCOCCUS OTHER
.84 OTHER ANAEROBES
.89 OTHER SPECIFIED BACTERIA

364.9 UVEAL TRACT DISEASE - ANTERIOR
363.9 UVEAL TRACT DISEASE - POSTERIOR

UVEITIS
364.3 NOS
364.00 ANTERIOR ACUTE SUBACUTE
364.01 ANTERIOR PRIMARY
364.02 ANTERIOR RECURRENT
364.03 ANTERIOR SECONDARY INFECTIOUS
364.04 ANTERIOR SECONDARY NONINFECTIOUS
098.41 GONOCOCCAL
054.44 HERPES SIMPLEX
053.22 HERPES ZOSTER
363.20 POSTERIOR
360.11 SYMPATHETIC
091.50 SYPHILITIC SECONDARY

364.24 UVEOCUTANEOUS SYNDROME
363.22 UVEOMENINGEAL, UVEOMENINGITIS SYNDROME
135 UVEOPAROTID FEVER
750.26 UVULA ABSENCE CONGENITAL
749.20 UVULA BIFID (WITH CLEFT LIP)
0 UVULA BIFID SEE ALSO 'CLEFT PALATE WITH CLEFT LIP'
749.02 UVULA CLEFT
528.9 UVULA HYPERTROPHY (ELONGATION)
750.26 UVULA HYPERTROPHY (ELONGATION) CONGENITAL
959.09 UVULA INJURY
528.9 UVULITIS
528.3 UVULITIS ABSCESS OR CELLULITIS
462 UVULITIS - SORE THROAT (NOS) (VIRAL)

427.1 V TACH
427.1 V TACH PAROXYSMAL

VACCINATION (NEED FOR)

V03.89 AGAINST OTHER SINGLE BACTERIA
V03.9 BACTERIAL
V03.89 BACTERIAL OTHER SPECIFIED
V03.2 BCG
V05.4 CHICKENPOX
V03.0 CHOLERA
V06.0 CHOLERA WITH TYPHOID PARATYPHOID
V04.7 COLD
V06.9 COMBINATION
V06.8 COMBINATION OTHER SPECIFIED
0 COMPLICATION SEE 'COMPLICATION OF MEDICAL CARE NOT ELSEWHERE CLASSIFIED'
V03.5 DIPHTHERIA
V06.5 DIPHTHERIA-TETANUS (TD)
V06.1 DIPHTHERIA-TETANUS-PERTUSSIS
V06.3 DIPHTHERIA-TETANUS-PERTUSSIS WITH POLIO
V06.2 DIPHTHERIA-TETANUS-PERTUSSIS WITH TAB
V05.9 DISEASE (SINGLE)
V05.8 DISEASE (SINGLE) OTHER SPECIFIED
V06.1 DPT
V06.3 DPT WITH POLIO
V06.2 DPT WITH TAB
V06.1 DTP
V06.3 DTP WITH POLIO
V06.2 DTP WITH TAB
V05.0 ENCEPHALITIS (VIRAL ARTHROPOD BORNE)
V04.8 FLU
V03.81 HEMOPHILUS INFLUENZA, TYPE B (HIB)
V05.3 HEPATITIS VIRAL (B, C, E)
V03.81 HIB (HEMOPHILUS INFLUENZA, TYPE B)
V20.2 INFANT OR CHILD ROUTINE APPROPRIATE FOR AGE
V04.8 INFLUENZA
V05.2 LEISHMANIASIS
V05.1 LYME'S DISEASE
V04.2 MEASLES ALONE
V06.4 MEASLES MUMPS RUBELLA
V06.4 MMR
V04.6 MUMPS (ALONE)
V64.0 NOT CARRIED OUT BECAUSE OF CONTRAINDICATION
V06.8 OTHER COMBINATION (PROPHYLACTIC)
V05.8 OTHER SPECIFIED DISEASE
V03.6 PERTUSSIS
V03.3 PLAGUE
V03.82 PNEUMOCOCCUS
V03.82 PNEUMONIA PNEUMOCOCCAL
V04.0 POLIO
V03.82 PPV (PNEUMOCOCCAL POLYSACCHARIDE VACCINE)
V04.5 RABIES
V04.3 RUBELLA (ALONE)
V04.1 SMALLPOX
V03.82 STREPTOCOCCUS PNEUMONIAE
V06.6 STREPTOCOCCUS PNEUMONIAE AND INFLUENZA
V03.1 TAB
V03.2 TB
V06.5 TD
V06.5 TETANUS - DIPHTHERIA (TD)
V06.1 TETANUS - DIPHTHERIA WITH PERTUSSIS (DTP)
V03.7 TETANUS TOXOID
V03.4 TULAREMIA
V03.1 TYPHOID-PARATYPHOID
V05.4 VARICELLA
V05.0 VIRAL ARTHROPOD BORNE ENCEPHALITIS
V05.1 VIRAL ARTHROPOD BORNE OTHER
V04.4 YELLOW FEVER
V06.8 OTHER SPECIFIED COMBINATION
V05.8 OTHER SPECIFIED SINGLE DISEASE

V14.7 VACCINE ALLERGY (HISTORY)

VACCINIA

999.0 NOS
771.2 CONGENITAL
999.3 CONJUNCTIVA
999.0 EYELIDS [373.5]
051.0 EYELIDS NOT FROM VACCINATION [373.5]
999.3 LOCALIZED
999.3 NOSE
051.0 NOT FROM VACCINATION
051.0 SINE VACCINATIONE
051.0 WITHOUT VACCINATION

0 VACUUM EXTRACTION DELIVERY SEE ALSO 'DELIVERY', FORCEPS OR VACUUM
763.3 VACUUM EXTRACTOR DELIVERY AFFECTING FETUS OR NEWBORN
660.7# VACUUM EXTRACTOR FAILURE

5th Digit: 660.7
0. EPISODE OF CARE NOS OR N/A
1. DELIVERED
3. ANTEPARTUM COMPLICATION

V60.0 VAGABOND (HOMELESS PERSON)
132.1 VAGABOND'S DISEASE

VAGINA, VAGINAL

763.89 ABNORMALITY AFFECTING FETUS OR NEWBORN
654.7# ABNORMALITY COMPLICATING CHILDBIRTH (TUMOR) (SEPTATE)
660.2# ABNORMALITY (TUMOR) (SEPTATE) OBSTRUCTING LABOR [654.7#]

5th Digit: 654.7
0. EPISODE OF CARE NOS OR N/A
1. DELIVERED
2. DELIVERED WITH POSTPARTUM COMPLICATION
3. ANTEPARTUM COMPLICATION
4. POSTPARTUM COMPLICATION

5th Digit: 660.2
0. EPISODE OF CARE NOS OR N/A
1. DELIVERED
3. ANTEPARTUM COMPLICATION

752.49 ABSENCE (AGENESIS) (STRICTURE) CONGENITAL
623.2 ADHESIONS (POSTOP) (POSTRADIATION)
752.40 ANOMALY CONGENITAL
752.49 ANOMALY OTHER SPECIFIED CONGENITAL
V55.7 ARTIFICIAL CARE (CLOSURE) (TOILET) (ATTENTION)
V44.7 ARTIFICIAL STATUS
623.2 ATRESIA
752.49 ATRESIA CONGENITAL
098.2 ATRESIA POSTGONOCOCCAL (OLD)
623.2 ATRESIA POSTINFECTIONAL (SENILE)
627.3 ATROPHY (SENILE)
641.2# BLEEDING ABRUPTIO PLACENTAE IN PREGNANCY
640.9# BLEEDING IN PREGNANCY, ANTEPARTUM (<22 WEEKS)
641.9# BLEEDING IN PREGNANCY, ANTEPARTUM NOS
626.7 BLEEDING IRREGULAR POSTCOITAL
641.1# BLEEDING PLACENTA PREVIA IN PREGNANCY

5th Digit: 640.9, 641.1-2, 9
0. EPISODE OF CARE NOS OR N/A
1. DELIVERED
3. ANTEPARTUM COMPLICATION

626.6 BLEEDING IRREGULAR
623.8 CYST
623.5 DISCHARGE
616.9 DISORDER INFLAMMATORY
616.8 DISORDER INFLAMMATORY - SPECIFIED NEC
623.9 DISORDER NONINFLAMMATORY
623.8 DISORDER NONINFLAMMATORY - SPECIFIED NEC
752.2 DUPLICATION (TOTAL) CONGENITAL
623.0 DYSPLASIA

VAGINA, VAGINAL (continued)

618.6 ENTEROCELE CONGENITAL OR ACQUIRED
618.6 ENTEROCELE CONGENITAL OR ACQUIRED WITH STRESS INCONTINENCE [625.6]
618.6 ENTEROCELE CONGENITAL OR ACQUIRED WITH OTHER URINARY INCONTINENCE **[788.3#]**

5th Digit: 788.3
- **0. UNSPECIFIED**
- **1. URGE INCONTINENCE**
- **3. MIXED URGE AND STRESS**
- **4 WITHOUT SENSORY AWARENESS**
- **5. POST-VOID DRIBBLING**
- **6. NOCTURNAL ENURESIS**
- **7. CONTINUOUS LEAKAGE**
- **9. OTHER**

623.8 FIBROSIS
792.9 FLUID ABNORMAL
623.6 HEMATOMA
665.7# HEMATOMA OBSTETRICAL TRAUMA

5th Digit: 665.7
- **0. EPISODE OF CARE NOS OR N/A**
- **1. DELIVERED**
- **2. DELIVERED WITH POSTPARTUM COMPLICATION**
- **4. POSTPARTUM COMPLICATION**

623.8 HEMORRHAGE
616.9 INFLAMMATORY DISEASE
616.8 INFLAMMATORY DISEASE OTHER
911.8 INJURY OTHER AND UNSPECIFIED SUPERFICIAL
911.9 INJURY OTHER AND UNSPECIFIED SUPERFICIAL INFECTED
639.2 INJURY POST ABORTION / ECTOPIC / MOLAR PREGNANCY

623.1 LEUKOPLAKIA
625.8 MASS
623.9 NONINFLAMMATORY DISORDER
623.2 OBSTRUCTION OR OCCLUSION
623.7 POLYP
618.0 PROLAPSE
618.5 PROLAPSE AFTER HYSTERECTOMY
618.5 PROLAPSE AFTER HYSTERECTOMY WITH STRESS INCONTINENCE [625.6]
618.5 PROLAPSE AFTER HYSTERECTOMY WITH OTHER URINARY INCONTINENCE **[788.3#]**

5th Digit: 788.3
- **0. UNSPECIFIED**
- **1. URGE INCONTINENCE**
- **3. MIXED URGE AND STRESS**
- **4 WITHOUT SENSORY AWARENESS**
- **5. POST-VOID DRIBBLING**
- **6. NOCTURNAL ENURESIS**
- **7. CONTINUOUS LEAKAGE**
- **9. OTHER**

618.4 PROLAPSE WITH UTERINE PROLAPSE - NOS
618.3 PROLAPSE WITH UTERINE PROLAPSE - COMPLETE
618.2 PROLAPSE WITH UTERINE PROLAPSE - INCOMPLETE
654.7# RIGID COMPLICATING PREGNANCY CHILDBIRTH OR PUERPERIUM
660.2# RIGID OBSTRUCTING LABOR **[654.7#]**

5th Digit: 654.7
- **0. EPISODE OF CARE NOS OR N/A**
- **1. DELIVERED**
- **2. DELIVERED WITH POSTPARTUM COMPLICATION**
- **3. ANTEPARTUM COMPLICATION**
- **4. POSTPARTUM COMPLICATION**

5th Digit: 660.2
- **0. EPISODE OF CARE NOS OR N/A**
- **1. DELIVERED**
- **3. ANTEPARTUM COMPLICATION**

623.2 STENOSIS
623.2 STRICTURE OR ATRESIA
752.49 STRICTURE OR ATRESIA CONGENITAL

VAGINA, VAGINAL (continued)

654.7# TUMOR COMPLICATING PREGNANCY
660.2# TUMOR OBSTRUCTING LABOR [654.7]

5th Digit: 654.7
- **0. EPISODE OF CARE NOS OR N/A**
- **1. DELIVERED**
- **2. DELIVERED WITH POSTPARTUM COMPLICATION**
- **3. ANTEPARTUM COMPLICATION**
- **4. POSTPARTUM COMPLICATION**

5th Digit: 660.2
- **0. EPISODE OF CARE NOS OR N/A**
- **1. DELIVERED**
- **3. ANTEPARTUM COMPLICATION**

616.8 ULCER (INFLAMMATORY)

625.1 VAGINISMUS
306.51 VAGINISMUS FUNCTIONAL PSYCHOGENIC
300.11 VAGINISMUS HYSTERICAL
306.51 VAGINISMUS PSYCHOGENIC

VAGINITIS

616.10 NOS
760.8 AFFECTING NEWBORN OR FETUS
616.10 BACTERIAL
112.1 CANDIDAL
099.53 CHLAMYDIAL

646.6#: SPECIFY THE MATERNAL VAGINITIS WITH AN ADDITIONAL CODE.

646.6# COMPLICATING PREGNANCY, CHILDBIRTH, OR PUERPERIUM

5th Digit: 646.6
- **0. EPISODE OF CARE NOS OR N/A**
- **1. DELIVERED**
- **2. DELIVERED WITH POSTPARTUM COMPLICATION**
- **3. ANTEPARTUM COMPLICATION**
- **4. POSTPARTUM COMPLICATION**

616.10 E. COLI [041.4]
639.0 FOLLOWING ECTOPIC MOLAR OR ABORTED PREGNANCY
616.10 GARDNERALLA
098.0 GONOCOCCAL ACUTE
098.2 GONOCOCCAL CHRONIC
616.10 HEMOPHILUS VAGINALIS
054.11 HERPETIC
112.1 MONILIAL
127.4 PINWORM [616.11]
616.10 POSTIRRADIATION
627.3 POSTMENOPAUSAL ATROPHIC VAGINITIS
627.3 SENILE (ATROPHIC)
616.10 STAPHYLOCOCCAL **[041.1#]**

5th Digit: 041.1
- **0. UNSPECIFIED**
- **1. AUREUS**
- **9. OHER**

616.10 STREPTOCOCCAL **[041.0#]**

5th Digit: 041.0
- **0. NOS**
- **1. GROUP A**
- **2. GROUP B**
- **3. GROUP C**
- **4. GROUP D (ENTEROCOCCUS)**
- **5. GROUP G**
- **9. OTHER STREP**

131.01 TRICHOMONAL

0 VAGINOSIS SEE 'VAGINITIS'

352.6 VAGOHYPOGLOSSAL SYNDROME
780.2 VAGOVAGAL SYNDROME

352.3 VAGUS NERVE ATROPHY
951.8 VAGUS NERVE INJURY
352.3 VAGUS NERVE NEURITIS (DISORDER)
352.3 VAGUS NERVE PARALYSIS

736.79 VALGUS DEFORMITY FOOT (ACQUIRED)
754.60 VALGUS DEFORMITY FOOT CONGENITAL
754.69 VALGUS DEFORMITY FOOT CONGENITAL OTHER NEC

270.3 VALINE METABOLISM DISTURBANCES
304.1# VALIUM (VALMID) ADDICTION
5th Digit: 304.1
0. NOS
1. CONTINUOUS
2. EPISODIC
3. IN REMISSION

648.2# VALSUANI'S DISEASE MATERNAL CURRENT (CO-EXISTENT) IN PREGNANCY (PROGRESSIVE PERNICIOUS ANEMIA) [281.#]
5th Digit: 648.2
0. EPISODE OF CARE NOS OR N/A
1. DELIVERED
2. DELIVERED WITH POSTPARTUM COMPLICATION
3. ANTEPARTUM COMPLICATION
4. POSTPARTUM COMPLICATION

4th Digit: 281
0. PERNICIOUS (INTRINSIC FACTOR) (CASTLE'S) DEFICIENCY
1. B12 DEFICIENCY
2. FOLATE DEFICIENCY
3. B12 WITH FOLATE DEFICIENCY
4. PROTEIN OR AMINO ACID DEFICIENCY
8. NUTRITIONAL (SCORBUTIC)
9. NOS

046.2 VAN BOGAERT'S DISEASE (SCLEROSING LEUKOENCEPHALITIS)
330.0 VAN BOGAERT-NIJSSEN (-PFEIFFER) DISEASE (LEUKODYSTROPHY)
733.3 VAN BUCHEM'S SYNDROME (HYPEROSTOSIS CORTICALIS)
271.0 VAN CREVELD-VON GIERKE DISEASE (GLYCOGENOSIS I)
289.7 VAN DEN BERGH'S DISEASE (ENTEROGENOUS CYANOSIS)

756.51 VAN DER HOEVE'S SYNDROME (BRITTLE BONES AND BLUE SCLERA, DEAFNESS)
270.2 VAN DER HOEVE-HALBERTSMA-WAARDENBURG SYNDROME (PTOSIS-EPICANTHUS)
270.2 VAN DER HOEVE-WAARDENBURG-GUALDI SYNDROME (PTOSIS-EPICANTHUS)

791.9 VANILLYLMANDELIC ACID ELEVATION (URINARY)
651.3# VANISHING TWIN
5th Digit: 651.3
0. EPISODE OF CARE UNSPECIFIED OR N/A
1. DELIVERED
3. ANTEPARTUM COMPLICATION

732.1 VAN NECK (-ODELBERG) DISEASE OR SYNDROME (JUVENILE OSTEOCHONDROSIS)
987.9 VAPORS INHALATION (NOXIOUS)
238.4 VAQUEZ (-OSLER) DISEASE (POLYCYTHEMIA VERA) M9950/1
413.1 VARIANT ANGINA

VARICELLA
052.9 NOS
052.7 COMPLICATION OTHER SPECIFIED
052.8 COMPLICATION UNSPECIFIED
052.0 ENCEPHALITIS (POST VARICELLA)
V01.7 EXPOSURE

VARICELLA (continued)
052.7 KERATOCONJUNCTIVITIS [370.44]
647.6# MATERNAL COMPLICATING PREGNANCY **[052.#]**
5th Digit: 647.6
0. EPISODE OF CARE UNSPECIFIED OR N/A
1. DELIVERED
2. DELIVERED WITH POSTPARTUM COMPLICATION
3. ANTEPARTUM COMPLICATION
4. POSTPARTUM COMPLICATION

5th Digit: 052
0. POSTVARICELLA ENCEPHALITIS
1. VARICELLA PNEUMONIA
7. OTHER SPECIFIED COMPLICATIONS
8. UNSPECIFIED COMPLICATION
9. WITHOUT MENTION OF COMPLICATION

052.1 PNEUMONITIS HEMORRHAGIC
V05.4 VACCINATION
052.9 WITHOUT COMPLICATION

VARICES
747.6# ARTERIOVENOUS PERIPHERAL VASCULAR CONGENITAL
5th Digit: 747.6
0. PERIPHERAL VASCULAR UNSPECIFIED SITE
1. GASTROINTESTINAL VESSEL
2. RENAL VESSEL
3. UPPER LIMB VESSEL
4. LOWER LIMB VESSEL
9. OTHER SPECIFIED SITE PERIPHERAL VASCULAR

456.5 BROAD LIGAMENT
456.1 ESOPHAGEAL
456.0 ESOPHAGEAL WITH BLEEDING
747.69 ESOPHAGEAL CONGENITAL
456.8 GASTRIC

648.9#: USE AN ADDITIONAL CODE TO IDENTIFY THE VARICES.

648.9# MATERNAL CURRENT (CO-EXISTENT) IN PREGNANCY
5th Digit: 648.9
0. EPISODE OF NOS OR N/A
1. DELIVERED
2. DELIVERED WITH POSTPARTUM COMPLICATION
3. ANTEPARTUM COMPLICATION
4. POSTPARTUM COMPLICATION

456.8 NASAL SEPTUM
747.69 ORBIT CONGENITAL
456.5 PELVIC
456.6 PERINEUM
656.7# PLACENTAL (AFFECTING MANAGEMENT OF PREGNANCY)
5th Digit: 656.7
0. EPISODE OF CARE NOS OR N/A
1. DELIVERED
3. ANTEPARTUM COMPLICATION

456.8 PROSTATE
362.17 RETINAL
456.4 SCROTAL
456.3 SUBLINGUAL
762.6 UMBILICAL CORD AFFECTING FETUS OR NEWBORN
456.6 VULVAL
456.8 OTHER SITES

456.5 VARICOCELE OVARY
456.4 VARICOCELE SPERMATIC CORD (ULCERATED)

UVW

VARICOSE VEINS
747.6# CONGENITAL (PERIPHERAL) NEC
5th Digit: 747.6
0. PERIPHERAL VASCULAR UNSPECIFIED SITE
1. GASTROINTESTINAL VESSEL
2. RENAL VESSEL
3. UPPER LIMB VESSEL
4. LOWER LIMB VESSEL
9. OTHER SPECIFIED SITE PERIPHERAL VASCULAR

454.9 LOWER EXTREMITIES
454.1 LOWER EXTREMITIES WITH INFLAMMATION
454.0 LOWER EXTREMITIES WITH ULCER
454.2 LOWER EXTREMITIES WITH ULCER AND INFLAMMATION

VARICOSE VEINS COMPLICATING PREGNANCY AND PUERPERIUM
671.0# LEG(S) MATERNAL DUE TO PREGNANCY

648.9#: USE AN ADDITIONAL CODE TO IDENTIFY THE SPECIFIC TYPE OF VARICOSE VEINS.

648.9# MATERNAL CURRENT (CO-EXISTENT)
671.1# VULVA AND PERINEUM MATERNAL DUE TO PREGNANCY
5th Digit: 648.9, 671.0-1
0. EPISODE OF CARE NOS OR N/A
1. DELIVERED
2. DELIVERED WITH POSTPARTUM COMPLICATION
3. ANTEPARTUM COMPLICATION
4. POSTPARTUM COMPLICATION

050.0 VARIOLA MAJOR
050.1 VARIOLA MINOR
050.2 VARIOLOID
747.6# VARIX ARTERY PERIPHERAL VASCULAR CONGENITAL
5th Digit: 747.6
0. PERIPHERAL VASCULAR UNSPECIFIED SITE
1. GASTROINTESTINAL VESSEL
2. RENAL VESSEL
3. UPPER LIMB VESSEL
4. LOWER LIMB VESSEL
9. OTHER SPECIFIED SITE PERIPHERAL VASCULAR

736.79 VARUS DEFORMITY FOOT (ACQUIRED)
754.50 VARUS DEFORMITY FOOT CONGENITAL
754.59 VARUS DEFORMITY FOOT CONGENITAL OTHER NEC

VAS DEFERENS
608.89 ABSENCE
752.8 ABSENCE CONGENITAL
752.8 ATRESIA CONGENITAL
608.89 ATROPHY (FIBROSIS) (HYPERTROPHY) (ULCER)
608.83 HEMORRHAGE (THROMBOSIS) (HEMATOMA) NONTRAUMATIC
867.6 INJURY (TRAUMATIC)
867.7 INJURY WITH OPEN WOUND INTO CAVITY
908.2 INJURY LATE EFFECT
996.65 PROSTHETIC RECONSTRUCTION COMPLICATION - INFECTION OR INFLAMMATION
996.39 PROSTHETIC RECONSTRUCTION COMPLICATION - MECHANICAL
996.76 PROSTHETIC RECONSTRUCTION COMPLICATION - OTHER
608.85 STRICTURE

663.5# VASA PREVIA
5th Digit: 663.5
0. EPISODE OF CARE NOS OR N/A
1. DELIVERED
3. ANTEPARTUM COMPLICATION

762.6 VASA PREVIA AFFECTING FETUS OR NEWBORN

VASCULAR
747.60 ATRESIA NEC
459.89 ATROPHY
V58.81 CATHETER CARE (REMOVAL) (REPLACEMENT) (TOILET) (CLEANSING)
459.9 DISEASE NOS

648.9#: USE AN ADDITIONAL CODE TO IDENTIFY THE SPECIFIC VASCULAR DISEASE.

648.9# DISEASE MATERNAL CURRENT (CO-EXISTENT) IN PREGNANCY
5th Digit: 648.9
0. EPISODE OF NOS OR N/A
1. DELIVERED
2. DELIVERED WITH POSTPARTUM COMPLICATION
3. ANTEPARTUM COMPLICATION
4. POSTPARTUM COMPLICATION

447.1 DISEASE - OBLITERATIVE
443.9 DISEASE - OBLITERATIVE (OCCLUSIVE) PERIPHERAL
459.9 DISEASE - OCCLUSIVE
443.9 DISEASE - PERIPHERAL (OCCLUSIVE)
250.7# DISEASE - PERIPHERAL (OCCLUSIVE) DIABETIC [443.81]
5th Digit: 250.7
0. TYPE II, ADULT-ONSET, NON-INSULIN DEPENDENT (EVEN IF REQUIRING INSULIN), OR UNSPECIFIED; CONTROLLED
1. TYPE I, JUVENILE-ONSET OR INSULIN-DEPENDENT; CONTROLLED
2. TYPE II, ADULT-ONSET, NON-INSULIN DEPENDENT (EVEN IF REQUIRING INSULIN); UNCONTROLLED
3. TYPE I, JUVENILE-ONSET OR INSULIN-DEPENDENT; UNCONTROLLED

443.89 DISEASE - PERIPHERAL (OCCLUSIVE) SPECIFIED TYPE NEC
557.9 INSUFFICIENCY - INTESTINE
557.0 INSUFFICIENCY - INTESTINE ACUTE
557.1 INSUFFICIENCY - INTESTINE CHRONIC

648.9#: USE AN ADDITIONAL CODE TO IDENTIFY THE SPECIFIC VASCULAR INSUFFICIENCY.

648.9# INSUFFICIENCY - MATERNAL CURRENT (CO-EXISTENT) IN PREGNANCY
5th Digit: 648.9
0. EPISODE OF NOS OR N/A
1. DELIVERED
2. DELIVERED WITH POSTPARTUM COMPLICATION
3. ANTEPARTUM COMPLICATION
4. POSTPARTUM COMPLICATION

557.1 INSUFFICIENCY - MESENTERIC
443.9 INSUFFICIENCY - DISEASE PERIPHERAL
996.1 INSUFFICIENCY - GRAFT OBSTRUCTION
286.4 INSUFFICIENCY - HEMOPHILIA
443.89 INSUFFICIENCY - PERIPHERAL DISEASES OTHER SPECIFIED
747.6# INSUFFICIENCY - PERIPHERAL SYSTEM OTHER ANOMALIES CONGENITAL
5th Digit: 747.6
0. PERIPHERAL VASCULAR UNSPECIFIED SITE
1. GASTROINTESTINAL VESSEL
2. RENAL VESSEL
3. UPPER LIMB VESSEL
4. LOWER LIMB VESSEL
9. OTHER SPECIFIED SITE PERIPHERAL VASCULAR

459.9 OCCLUSION
557.0 SPLANCHNIC SYNDROME

VASCULITIS
447.6 NOS
287.0 ALLERGIC
273.2 CRYOGLOBULINEMIC
446.29 LEUKOCLASTIC (LEUKOCYTOCLASTIC)
695.2 NODULAR
362.18 RETINAL

VAS DEFERENS
608.89 ATROPHY
608.9 DISEASE
608.89 DISEASE OTHER SPECIFIED

VASECTOMY
V25.09 COUNSELING (PROPOSED)
V25.2 ENCOUNTER
V26.0 REVERSAL AFTER PREVIOUS STERILIZATION
V26.52 STATUS

443.9 VASOMOTOR DISEASE OR SYNDROME

0 VASOPLASTY SEE 'VASECTOMY'

253.5 VASOPRESSIN DEFICIENCY
588.1 VASOPRESSION DEFICIENCY NEPHROGENIC

443.9 VASOSPASTIC PHENOMENON

780.2 VASOVAGAL ATTACK (SYNDROME)
780.2 VASOVAGAL PHENOMENON (VASOMOTOR)

576.8 VATER SPASM (AMPULLA OF VATER)
759.89 VATER SYNDROME

099.9 VD
V01.6 VD EXPOSURE
V74.5 VD SCREENING EXAM
0 VD SEE ALSO BY SPECIFIC DISEASE OR ORGANISM
0 VD SEE ALSO 'VENEREAL DISEASE'

VECTORCARDIOGRAM (VCG)
V72.85 VECTORCARDIOGRAM
794.39 ABNORMAL
V72.81 PREOPERATIVE
V71.7 SUSPECTED MI

780.03 VEGETATIVE STATE PERSISTENT
041.84 VEILLONELLA INFECTION

VEIN , VENOUS
747.81 ABSENCE CONGENITAL - BRAIN
747.49 ABSENCE (ATRESIA) CONGENITAL - GREAT
747.49 ABSENCE (ATRESIA) CONGENITAL - PORTAL
747.49 ABSENCE (ATRESIA) CONGENITAL - PULMONARY
0 ACCESS LOSS-CODE UNDERLYING DISEASE
747.6# ANOMALY OTHER PERIPHERAL VASCULAR (ABERRANT) (ABSENCE) (AGENESIS) (ACCESSORY) (ANEURYSM) (DEFORMITY) (HYPOPLASIA) (MALPOSITION) (CONGENITAL)

5th Digit: 747.6
0. PERIPHERAL VASCULAR UNSPECIFIED SITE
1. GASTROINTESTINAL VESSEL
2. RENAL VESSEL
3. UPPER LIMB VESSEL
4. LOWER LIMB VESSEL
9. OTHER SPECIFIED SITE PERIPHERAL VASCULAR

648.9#: USE AN ADDITIONAL CODE TO IDENTIFY THE SPECIFIC VEIN DISORDER.

648.9# DISORDER MATERNAL CURRENT (CO-EXISTENT) IN PREGNANCY

5th Digit: 648.9
0. EPISODE OF NOS OR N/A
1. DELIVERED
2. DELIVERED WITH POSTPARTUM COMPLICATION
3. ANTEPARTUM COMPLICATION
4. POSTPARTUM COMPLICATION

459.89 DISORDER OTHER SPECIFIED

VEIN , VENOUS (continued)
0 DIVISION SEE 'BLOOD VESSEL INJURY'
453.9 EMBOLISM (THROMBOSIS)
459.89 FIBROSIS (LOWER EXTREMITIES)
459.89 HYPERTROPHY
459.89 INCREASED PRESSURE
459.81 INSUFFICIENCY NOS (CHRONIC)
459.81 INSUFFICIENCY (CHRONIC) <u>ULCERATED</u> [**<u>707.#</u>**]

4th Digit: 707
1. LOWER LIMB EXCEPT DECUBITUS
8. CHRONIC OF OTHER SPECIFIED SITE
9. CHRONIC SITE NOS

459.2 OBSTRUCTION
0 OBSTRUCTION OR OCCLUSION THROMBOTIC SEE 'THROMBOSIS', BY SITE
459.81 STASIS
459.9 STRICTURE

762.6 VELAMENTOUS INSERTION UMBILICAL CORD AFFECTING FETUS OR NEWBORN

VENA CAVA
902.10 INFERIOR INJURY NOS
902.19 INFERIOR INJURY OTHER SITE
908.4 INFERIOR INJURY LATE EFFECT
902.10 INFERIOR LACERATION SITE UNSPECIFIED (RUPTURE) (HEMATOMA) (AVULSION) (ANEURYSM) TRAUMATIC
908.4 INFERIOR LACERATION LATE EFFECT
459.2 OBSTRUCTION
453.2 OCCLUSION
901.2 SUPERIOR INJURY
908.4 SUPERIOR INJURY LATE EFFECT
901.2 SUPERIOR LACERATION (RUPTURE) (HEMATOMA) (AVULSION) (ANEURYSM) TRAUMATIC
908.4 SUPERIOR LACERATION LATE EFFECT
459.2 SYNDROME (INFERIOR) (SUPERIOR) (OBSTRUCTION)
453.2 THROMBOSIS (EMBOLISM)

VENA CAVA CONGENITAL
747.49 ABSENCE
747.40 ANOMALY
747.49 ATRESIA
747.49 LEFT SUPERIOR PERSISTENT
747.49 STENOSIS

VENEREAL DISEASE
099.9 NOS
V02.8 CARRIER OTHER SPECIFIED
<u>099.54</u> <u>DUE TO CHLAMYDIA TRACHOMATIS</u> PELVIC INFLAMMATORY DISEASE [614.9]
<u>099.54</u> <u>DUE TO CHLAMYDIA TRACHOMATIS</u> ORCHITIS AND EPIDIDYMIS [604.91]
V01.6 EXPOSURE

647.2#: USE AN ADDITIONAL CODE TO IDENTIFY THE MATERNAL VENEREAL DISEASE.

647.2# MATERNAL CURRENT (CO-EXISTENT) IN PREGNANCY

5th Digit: 647.2
0. EPISODE OF CARE NOS OR N/A
1. DELIVERED
2. DELIVERED WITH POSTPARTUM COMPLICATION
3. ANTEPARTUM COMPLICATION
4. POSTPARTUM COMPLICATION

099.8 OTHER SPECIFIED
099.5# OTHER DUE TO CHLAMYDIA TRACHOMATIS

5th Digit: 099.5
0. UNSPECIFIED SITE
1. PHARYNX
2. ANUS AND RECTUM
3. LOWER GENITOURINARY SITES

V74.5 SCREENING EXAM

U-V-W

066.2 VENEZUELAN EQUINE FEVER
459.89 VENOFIBROSIS
0 VENOUS SEE VEIN, VENOUS
495.7 VENTILATION PNEUMONITIS
794.2 VENTILATORY OR VITAL CAPACITY REDUCED

VENTRICLE, VENTRICULAR CARDIAC

414.10 ANEURYSM
745.3 COMMON CONGENITAL
429.9 DYSFUNCTION
428.0 DYSFUNCTION WITH CHF
427.69 ESCAPE BEATS
428.9 FAILURE NOS
402.91 FAILURE HYPERTENSIVE
402.11 FAILURE HYPERTENSIVE BENIGN
402.01 FAILURE HYPERTENSIVE MALIGNANT
428.1 FAILURE LEFT
391.8 FAILURE LEFT ACTIVE
392.0 FAILURE LEFT ACTIVE WITH CHOREA
398.91 FAILURE LEFT INACTIVE OR QUIESCENT
398.91 FAILURE LEFT RHEUMATIC
398.91 FAILURE RHEUMATIC (CHRONIC) (INACTIVE)
391.8 FAILURE RHEUMATIC ACTIVE OR ACUTE
392.0 FAILURE RHEUMATIC WITH ACTIVE OR ACUTE CHOREA
428.0 FAILURE RIGHT WITH CHF
427.41 FIBRILLATION
427.42 FLUTTER
429.3 HYPERTROPHY (LEFT) (RIGHT)
746.89 HYPERTROPHY (LEFT) (RIGHT) CONGENITAL
402.90 HYPERTROPHY HYPERTENSIVE - NOS
402.10 HYPERTROPHY HYPERTENSIVE - BENIGN
402.00 HYPERTROPHY HYPERTENSIVE - MALIGNANT
426.7 PRE-EXCITATION
427.69 PREMATURE BEATS CONTRACTIONS
427.69 PREMATURE CONTRACTIONS
745.3 SEPTAL ABSENCE CONGENITAL
429.71 SEPTAL DEFECT ACQUIRED POST MI ACUTE (< 8 WEEKS) [410.##]

4th Digit: 410

- **0. ANTEROLATERAL**
- **1. ANTERIOR (WALL) ANTEROAPICAL ANTEROSEPTAL OTHER ANTERIOR**
- **2. INFEROLATERAL**
- **3. INFEROPOSTERIOR**
- **4. INFERIOR OTHER**
- **5. LATERAL APICAL, BASOLATERAL, POSTEROLATERAL, LATERAL OTHER**
- **6. POSTERIOR (POSTEROBASAL)**
- **7. SUBENDOCARDIAL**
- **8. ATRIUM PAPILLARY OR SEPTUM ALONE**
- **9. UNSPECIFIED**

5th Digit: 410

- **0. EPISODE UNSPECIFIED**
- **1. INITIAL EPISODE**
- **2. SUBSEQUENT EPISODE**

429.71 SEPTAL DEFECT ACQUIRED FOLLOWING MYOCARDIAL INFARCTION (>8 WEEKS) [414.8]
745.4 SEPTAL DEFECT CONGENITAL
745.69 SEPTAL DEFECT CONGENITAL COMMON ATRIOVENTRICULAR CANAL TYPE
429.71 SEPTAL DEFECT DUE TO ISCHEMIC HEART DISEASE [414.8]
745.2 SEPTAL DEFECT HYPERTROPHY OF RIGHT VENTRICLE
745.2 SEPTAL DEFECT IN TETROLOGY OF FALLOT
745.2 SEPTAL DEFECT WITH PULMONARY STENOSIS DEXTRAPOSITION OF AORTA
745.3 SINGLE CONGENITAL
427.5 STANDSTILL
427.1 TACHYCARDIA
427.1 TACHYCARDIA PAROXYSMAL

VENTRICLE, VENTRICULAR CEREBRAL

431 HEMORRHAGE
331.4 OBSTRUCTION OR OCCLUSION
996.63 SHUNT COMPLICATION - INFECTION OR INFLAMMATION
996.2 SHUNT COMPLICATION - MECHANICAL
996.75 SHUNT COMPLICATION - OTHER
V53.01 SHUNT FITTING AND ADJUSTMENT
V45.2 SHUNT IN SITU
793.0 VENTRICULOGRAM ABNORMAL

793.0 VENTRICULOGRAM (CEREBRAL) ABNORMAL
435.1 VERBIEST'S SYNDROME (CLAUDICATIO INTERMITTENS SPINALIS)
742.2 VERMIS OF CEREBELLUM ABSENCE CONGENITAL
352.6 VERNET'S SYNDROME
095.7 VERNEUIL'S DISEASE (SYPHILITIC BURSITIS)
304.1# VERONAL ADDICTION

5th Digit: 304.1

- **0. NOS**
- **1. CONTINUOUS**
- **2. EPISODIC**
- **3. IN REMISSION**

VERRUCA

078.11 ACUMINATA (ANY SITE)
078.10 VERRUCA
078.19 PLANA JUVENILIS
078.19 PLANTARIS
078.19 VENEREAL
078.10 VIRAL NEC
078.10 VULGARIS

078.10 VERRUCOSITIES SEE 'VERRUCA'
199.1 VERRUCOUS CARCINOMA SITE NOS
0 VERRUCOUS CARCINOMA SITE SPECIFIED SEE 'CANCER' BY SITE M8051/3
088.0 VERRUGA PERUANA
275.49 VERSE'S DISEASE (CALCINOSIS INTERVERTEBRALIS) [722.9#]

5th Digit: 722.9

- **0. UNSPECIFIED**
- **1. CERVICAL**
- **2. THORACIC**
- **3. LUMBAR**

761.7 VERSION EXTERNAL OF MALPRESENTATION BEFORE L&D AFFECTING FETUS OR NEWBORN

VERTEBRA, VERTEBRAL

756.13 ABSENCE CONGENITAL
433.2# ARTERY ARTERIOSCLEROSIS (DEGENERATION) (DEFORMANS) (ARTERITIS)

5th Digit: 433.2

- **0. WITHOUT CEREBRAL INFARCTION**
- **1. WITH CEREBRAL INFARCTION**

721.1 ARTERY COMPRESSION SYNDROME
433.2# ARTERY OCCLUSION (THROMBOSIS) (OBSTRUCTION) (EMBOLISM) (NARR.) (STENOSIS)
433.3# ARTERY OCCLUSION BILATERAL OR WITH BASILAR AND/OR CAROTID

5th Digit: 433.2-3

- **0. WITHOUT CEREBRAL INFARCTION**
- **1. WITH CEREBRAL INFARCTION**

721.1 ARTERY SYNDROME - COMPRESSION
435.1 ARTERY SYNDROME (INSUFFICIENCY)
733.99 ATROPHY
722.90 CALCIFICATION (CARTILAGE) (DISC) - NOS
722.91 CALCIFICATION (CARTILAGE) (DISC) - CERVICAL
722.93 CALCIFICATION (CARTILAGE) (DISC) - LUMBAR (LUMBOSACRAL)
722.92 CALCIFICATION (CARTILAGE) (DISC) - THORACIC (THORACOLUMBAR)
733.13 COLLAPSE PATHOLOGICAL

VERTEBRA, VERTEBRAL (continued)

733.90 DISORDER NEC
0 DISORDER DISC SEE 'INTERVERTEBRAL DISC'
756.15 FUSION CONGENITAL
724.4 LUMBAR SYNDROME
435.1 STEAL SYNDROME
756.19 SUPERNUMERARY
733.00 WEDGING

435.3 VERTEBROBASILAR ARTERY SYNDROME (INSUFFICIENCY) (SPASM)
724.5 VERTEBROGENIC (PAIN) SYNDROME
386.9 VERTIGINOUS SYNDROME (LABYRINTHINE)

VERTIGO

780.4 NOS
386.19 AURAL
386.11 BENIGN PAROXYSMAL POSITIONAL
386.2 CENTRAL ORIGIN
780.4 DIZZINESS AND GIDDINESS
078.81 EPIDEMIC
386.2 MALIGNANT POSITIONAL
386.19 OTOGENIC
386.10 PERIPHERAL
386.12 VESTIBULAR (NEURONITIS)

596.0 VESICAL NECK OBSTRUCTION
753.6 VESICAL NECK OBSTRUCTION CONGENITAL
788.9 VESICAL PAIN
0 VESICAL RETENTION SEE 'URINARY', RETENTION
0 VESICAL SEE ALSO 'BLADDER'
867.0 VESICAL SPHINCTER INJURY TRAUMATIC
867.1 VESICAL SPHINCTER INJURY TRAUMATIC WITH OPEN WOUND
788.9 VESICAL TENESMUS
593.7# VESICOURETERAL REFLUX

5th Digit: 593.7

0. UNSPECIFIED
1. WITH REFLUX NEPHROPATHY, UNILATERAL
2. WITH REFLUX NEPHROPATHY, BILATERAL
3. WITH REFLUX NEPHROPATHY UNSPECIFIED

596.0 VESICOURETHRAL ORIFICE OBSTRUCTION
596.0 VESICOURETHRAL ORIFICE STRICTURE
753.6 VESICOURETHRAL ORIFICE STRICTURE CONGENITAL
0 VESICOURETHRAL ORIFICE STRICTURE WITH INCONTINENCE SEE 'URETHRA, URETHRAL DISORDERS WITH INCONTINENCE'
709.8 VESICULAR ERUPTION
V23.1 VESICULAR MOLE MATERNAL HISTORY AFFECTING PREGNANCY SUPERVISION
083.2 VESICULAR RICKETTSIOSIS
528.0 VESICULAR STOMATITIS
794.16 VESTIBULAR FUNCTION STUDIES ABNORMAL
386.12 VESTIBULAR NEURITIS
386.12 VESTIBULAR NEURONITIS
616.10 VESTIBULITIS VULVAR
994.9 VIBRATION DISEASE
001.0 VIBRIO CHOLERA
001.1 VIBRIO CHOLERAE EL TOR
005.4 VIBRIO PARAHAEMOLYTICUS FOOD POISONING
005.81 VIBRIO VULNIFICUS FOOD POISONING
698.3 VIDAL'S DISEASE (LICHEN SIMPLEX CHRONICUS)
723.8 VIDEO DISPLAY SYNDROME
352.6 VILLARET'S SYNDROME
101 VINCENT'S ANGINA (TRENCH MOUTH)
101 VINCENT'S INFECTION (ANY SITE)
280.8 VINSON-PLUMMER SYNDROME (SIDEROPENIC DYSPHAGIA)

989.5 VIPER BITE
995.0 VIPER BITE WITH ANAPHYLAXIS [989.5]
0 VIRAL SEE 'VIRUS, VIRAL'
733.99 VIRCHOW'S DISEASE
790.8 VIREMIA
256.4 VIRILIZATION (FEMALE) ISOSEXUAL (STEIN LEVENTHAL)
255.2 VIRILIZATION (FEMALE) (SUPRARENAL)
255.2 VIRILIZING ADRENOCORTICAL HYPERPLASIA SYNDROME, CONGENITAL

VIRUS, VIRAL

077.99 CONJUNCTIVITIS NOS
078.89 DISEASE NEC
066.9 DISEASE ARTHROPOD BORNE
049.9 DISEASE CENTRAL NERVOUS SYSTEM NEC
048 DISEASE CENTRAL NERVOUS SYSTEM OTHER ENTEROVIRUS
049.8 DISEASE CENTRAL NERVOUS SYSTEM OTHER SPECIFIED NON ARTHROPOD BORNE
V01.7 DISEASE EXPOSURE OTHER SPECIFIED
655.3# DISEASE MATERNAL (WITH KNOWN / SUSPECTED DAMAGE TO FETUS)

5th Digit: 655.3

0. EPISODE OF CARE NOS OR N/A
1. DELIVERED
3. ANTEPARTUM COMPLICATION

647.6#: USE AN ADDITIONAL CODE TO IDENTIFY THE MATERNAL VIRAL DISEASE.

647.6# DISEASES MATERNAL CURRENT (CO-EXISTENT) IN PREGNANCY

5th Digit: 647.6

0. EPISODE OF CARE NOS OR N/A
1. DELIVERED
2. DELIVERED WITH POSTPARTUM COMPLICATION
3. ANTEPARTUM COMPLICATION
4. POSTPARTUM COMPLICATION

V73.99 DISEASE SCREENING UNSPECIFIED DISEASE
V73.89 DISEASE SCREENING OTHER SPECIFIED DISEASE
049.9 ENCEPHALITIS
139.0 ENCEPHALITIS LATE EFFECT
062.8 ENCEPHALITIS OTHER SPECIFIED MOSQUITO-BORNE
063.9 ENCEPHALITIS TICK BORNE
057.9 EXANTHEM
008.8 GASTROENTERITIS
079.99 INFECTION UNSPECIFIED INFECTING AGENT
046.9 INFECTION CENTRAL NERVOUS SYSTEM - SLOW VIRUS
046.8 INFECTION CENTRAL NERVOUS SYSTEM - OTHER SPECIFIED
079.89 INFECTION OTHER SPECIFIED
047.9 MENINGITIS
047.8 MENINGITIS OTHER SPECIFIED
079.99 SYNDROME

128.0 VISCERAL LARVA MIGRANS SYNDROME
759.3 VISCERAL TRANSPOSITION (ABDOMINAL) (THORACIC) CONGENITAL
569.89 VISCEROPTOSIS INTESTINE
787.4 VISIBLE PERISTALSIS

VISION, VISUAL

368.34 ABNORMAL RETINAL CORRESPONDENCE
368.16 AGNOSIA
368.8 BLURRED

CORTEX

377.73 DISORDER
377.73 DISORDER WITH INFLAMMATORY DISORDERS
377.71 DISORDER WITH NEOPLASMS
377.72 DISORDER WITH VASCULAR DISORDERS
950.3 INJURY

VISION, VISUAL (continued)

368.13	DISCOMFORT
368.30	DISORDER (BINOCULAR)
306.7	DISORDER PSYCHOGENIC
368.16	DISORDER PSYCHOPHYSICAL
368.16	DISORIENTATION SYNDROME
368.14	DISTORTION SHAPE AND SIZE
368.15	DISTORTION OTHER (ENTOPTIC PHENOMENA)
368.9	DISTURBANCE
368.16	DISTURBANCE PSYCHOPHYSICAL
368.10	DISTURBANCE SUBJECTIVE
368.2	DOUBLE
794.13	EVOKED POTENTIAL ABNORMAL
V72.0	EXAM ROUTINE
V20.2	EXAM ROUTINE INFANT OR CHILD
	FIELD DEFECT
368.40	NOS
368.42	ANGIOSCOTOMA ENLARGED
368.41	CENTRAL SCOTOMA
368.41	CENTROCECAL SCOTOMA
368.45	GENERALIZED CONTRACTION OR CONSTRICTION
368.46	HEMIANOPSIA (ALTITUDINAL) (HOMONYMOUS)
368.47	HEMIANOPSIA (BINASAL)
368.47	HETERONYMOUS (BILATERAL)
368.44	NASAL STEP
368.44	PERIPHERAL
368.46	QUADRANT ANOPIA
368.44	SCOTOMA
368.43	SCOTOMA ARCUATE
368.43	SCOTOMA BJERRUM
368.42	SCOTOMA BLIND SPOT AREA
368.42	SCOTOMA PARACECAL
368.41	SCOTOMA PARACENTRAL
368.43	SCOTOMA SEIDEL

VISION, VISUAL (continued)

368.33	FUSION WITH DEFECTIVE STEREOPSIS
368.16	HALLUCINATION PSYCHOPHYSICAL
	LOSS
369.9	NOS
369.3	BOTH EYES UNQUALIFIED
V19.0	FAMILY HISTORY
369.4	LEGAL BLINDNESS AS DEFINED IN U.S.A.
368.11	SUDDEN
V72.0	TEST
368.12	TRANSIENT CONCENTRIC FADING
368.12	TRANSIENT SCINTILLATING SCOTOMA
369.8	UNQUALIFIED ONE EYE
	PATHWAYS
377.9	DISORDER
377.63	DISORDER WITH INFLAMMATORY DISORDERS
377.61	DISORDER WITH NEOPLASMS
377.62	DISORDER WITH VASCULAR DISORDERS

VISION, VISUAL (continued)

V72.0	SCREENING EXAM
368.32	SIMULTANEOUS VISUAL PERCEPTION WITHOUT FUSION
V53.09	SUBSTITUTION DEVICE FITTING AND ADJUSTMENT
368.31	SUPPRESSION OF BINOCULAR VISION

VISION IMPAIRMENT

BETTER EYE

FIRST DIGIT		Snellen Fraction	Visual Field in Degrees
0.	Vision Unspecified	---------	--------
1.	Low Vision NOS	---------	--------
2.	20/10 - 20/25 Normal	2.0 -.80	--------
3.	20/30 - 20/60 Near Normal	.70 -.30	--------
4.	20/70 - 20/160 Moderate	.25 -.12	--------
5.	20/200 - 20/400 Severe	.10 -.05	<=20
6.	20/500 - 20/1000 Profound	04 -.02	<=10
7.	<20/1000 Near Total	<.02	<= 5
8.	Total Blindness	----------	--------
9.	Blind NOS	----------	--------

LESSER EYE

SECOND DIGIT		Snellen Fraction	Visual Field in Degrees
0.	Vision Unspecified	----------	--------
1.	Low Vision NOS	----------	--------
2.	Moderate NOS	----------	--------
3.	Severe NOS	----------	--------
4.	20/70 - 20/400 Moderate	.25 - .12	--------
5.	20/200 - 20/400 Severe	.10 - .05	<=20
6.	20/500 - 20/1000 Profound	.04 - .02	<=10
7.	<20/1000 Near Total	<.02	<= 5
8.	Total	----------	--------
9.	Blind NOS	----------	--------

Select the appropriate digit from the better eye, then select the second digit from the lesser eye. You now have a two digit key code which will correlate with the appropriate ICD-9 code listed in the table below.

KEY CODE	ICD-9 CODE	
01	369.70	VISION LOSS ONE EYE MODERATE OR SEVERE IMPAIRMENT
04	369.74	VISION LOSS ONE EYE MODERATE IMPAIRMENT OTHER EYE NOT SPECIFIED
05	369.71	VISION LOSS ONE EYE SEVERE IMPAIRMENT OTHER EYE NOT SPECIFIED
06	369.67	VISION LOSS ONE EYE PROFOUND IMPAIRMENT OTHER EYE NOT SPECIFIED
07	369.64	VISION LOSS ONE EYE NEAR TOTAL IMPAIRMENT OTHER EYE NOT SPECIFIED
08	369.61	VISION LOSS ONE EYE TOTAL IMPAIRMENT OTHER EYE NOT SPECIFIED
09	369.60	VISION LOSS ONE EYE PROFOUND IMPAIRMENT
11	369.20	VISION LOSS BOTH EYES MODERATE OR SEVERE IMPAIRMENT
19	369.10	BETTER EYE MODERATE OR SEVERE LOW VISION LESSER EYE PROFOUND BLIND NOS
24	369.76	VISION LOSS ONE EYE MODERATE IMPAIRMENT OTHER EYE NORMAL VISION
25	369.73	VISION LOSS ONE EYE SEVERE IMPAIRMENT OTHER EYE NORMAL VISION
26	369.69	VISION LOSS ONE EYE PROFOUND IMPAIRMENT OTHER EYE NORMAL
27	369.66	VISION LOSS ONE EYE NEAR TOTAL IMPAIRMENT OTHER EYE NORMAL VISION
28	369.63	VISION LOSS ONE EYE TOTAL IMPAIRMENT OTHER EYE NORMAL VISION
34	369.75	VISION LOSS ONE EYE MODERATE IMPAIRMENT OTHER EYE NEAR NORMAL VISION
35	369.72	VISION LOSS ONE EYE SEVERE IMPAIRMENT OTHER EYE NEAR NORMAL VISION

36 369.68 VISION LOSS ONE EYE PROFOUND IMPAIRMENT OTHER EYE NEAR NORMAL VISION
37 369.65 VISION LOSS ONE EYE NEAR TOTAL IMPAIRMENT OTHER EYE NEAR NORMAL VISION
38 369.62 VISION LOSS ONE EYE TOTAL IMPAIRMENT OTHER EYE NEAR NORMALVISION
43 369.23 BETTER EYE MODERATE IMPAIRMENT LESSER EYE NOS
44 369.25 BETTER EYE MODERATE IMPAIRMENT LESSER EYE MODERATE IMPAIRMENT
45 369.24 BETTER EYE MODERATE IMPAIRMENT LESSER EYE SEVERE IMPAIRMENT
46 369.18 BETTER EYE MODERATE IMPAIRMENT LESSER EYE PROFOUND IMPAIRMENT
47 369.17 BETTER EYE MODERATE IMPAIRMENT LESSER EYE NEAR TOTAL IMPAIRMENT
48 369.16 BETTER EYE MODERATE IMPAIRMENT LESSER EYE TOTAL IMPAIRMENT
49 369.15 BETTER EYE MODERATE IMPAIRMENT LESSER EYE BLIND NOS
53 369.21 VISION LOSS BETTER EYE SEVERE IMPAIRMENT LESSER EYE NOS
55 369.22 VISION LOSS BETTER EYE SEVERE IMPAIRMENT LESSER EYE SEVERE IMPAIRMENT
56 369.14 BETTER EYE SEVERE IMPAIRMENT LESSER EYE PROFOUND IMPAIRMENT
57 369.13 BETTER EYE SEVERE IMPAIRMENT LESSER EYE NEAR TOTALIMPAIRMENT
58 369.12 BETTER EYE SEVERE IMPAIRMENT LESSER EYE TOTAL IMPAIRMENT
59 369.11 BETTER EYE SEVERE IMPAIRMENT LESSER EYE BLIND NOS
66 369.08 BETTER EYE PROFOUND IMPAIRMENT LESSER EYE PROFOUND IMPAIRMENT
67 369.07 BETTER EYE PROFOUND IMPAIRMENT LESSER EYE NEAR TOTAL IMPAIRMENT
68 369.06 BETTER EYE PROFOUND IMPAIRMENT LESSER EYE TOTAL IMPAIRMENT
69 369.05 BETTER EYE PROFOUND IMPAIRMENT LESSER EYE NOS
77 369.04 BETTER EYE NEAR TOTAL IMPAIRMENT LESSER EYE NEAR TOTAL IMPAIRMENT
78 369.03 BETTER EYE NEAR TOTAL IMPAIRMENT LESSER EYE TOTAL IMPAIRMENT
79 369.02 BETTER EYE NEAR TOTAL IMPAIRMENT LESSER EYE NOS
88 369.01 VISION LOSS BETTER EYE TOTAL IMPAIRMENT LESSER EYE TOTAL IMPAIRMENT
99 369.00 VISION LOSS BLINDNESS BOTH EYES NOS

0 VISUAL SEE 'VISION, VISUAL'

794.13 VISUALLY EVOKED POTENTIAL ABNORMAL
794.2 VITAL CAPACITY REDUCED
780.79 VITALITY, LACK OR WANT OF

VITAMIN A DEFICIENCY

264.9 NOS
264.1 BITOT'S SPOT IN YOUNG CHILD
264.8 FOLLICULAR KERATOSIS
264.7 OTHER OCULAR MANIFESTATIONS
264.0 WITH CONJUNCTIVAL XEROSIS
264.1 WITH CONJUNCTIVAL XEROSIS AND BITOT'S SPOT
264.2 WITH CORNEAL XEROSIS
264.3 WITH CORNEAL ULCERATION AND XEROSIS
264.4 WITH KEROTOMALACIA
264.5 WITH NIGHT BLINDNESS
264.6 WITH XEROPHTHALMIC SCARS OF CORNEA
264.8 XERODERMA

278.2 VITAMIN A EXCESS (HYPERVITAMINOSIS)

VITAMIN B DEFICIENCY

266.9 NOS
266.9 NOS WITH POLYNEUROPATHY [357.4]
265.1 B1
265.0 B1 WITH BERIBERI
266.0 B2
266.1 B6 (SYNDROME)
266.1 B6 WITH POLYNEUROPATHY [357.4]
285.0 B6 WITH VITAMIN B6 RESPONSIVE SIDEROBLASTIC ANEMIA
281.3 B12 AND FOLIC ACID DEFICIENCY ANEMIA
266.2 B12 WITH CEREBRAL DEGENERATION [331.7]
266.2 B12
266.2 B12 WITH POLYNEUROPATHY [357.4]
281.1 B12 WITH ANEMIA (DIETARY)
281.1 B12 MALABSORPTION WITH PROTEINURIA AND ANEMIA

267 VITAMIN C DEFICIENCY
268.9 VITAMIN D DEFICIENCY
275.3 VITAMIN D DEFICIENCY CAUSING RICKETS
278.4 VITAMIN D EXCESS HYPERVITAMINOSIS
269.2 VITAMIN DEFICIENCY NOS
269.2 VITAMIN DEFICIENCY MULTIPLE
269.1 VITAMIN DEFICIENCY OTHER
269.1 VITAMIN E DEFICIENCY
266.0 VITAMIN G DEFICIENCY

VITAMIN K DEFICIENCY

269.0 NOS
286.7 CAUSING DEFICIENCY OF COAGULATION FACTOR
286.7 COAGULATION DEFECT ACQUIRED
286.7 DUE TO LIVER DISEASE
776.0 NEWBORN

269.1 VITAMIN P DEFICIENCY
265.2 VITAMIN PP DEFICIENCY
362.76 VITELLIFORM DYSTROPHY HEREDITARY
751.0 VITELLINE DUCT PERSISTENT CONGENITAL
709.01 VITILIGO
374.53 VITILIGO EYELID
103.2 VITILIGO OF PINTA

VITREOUS

379.29 OTHER DISORDER NOS
360.04 ABSCESS
379.29 CALCIFICATION
379.21 CAVITATION
379.21 DEGENERATION
379.22 DEPOSITS (CRYSTALLINE)
379.21 DETACHMENT
379.24 FLOATERS
379.23 HEMORRHAGE
743.51 HYPERPLASIA (HUMOR) PERSISTENT CONGENITAL
379.29 INFILTRATE (HUMOR)
379.21 LIQUEFACTION
379.25 MEMBRANES AND STRANDS
379.24 OPACITIES
743.51 OPACITY CONGENITAL
379.29 OTHER DISORDERS
379.26 PROLAPSE
379.25 STRANDS
997.99 TOUCH SYNDROME

791.9 VMA ELEVATED
791.9 VMA URINARY ELEVATION

VOCAL CORD

478.5 ABSCESS (CELLULITIS) (GRANULOMA) (LEUKOPLAKIA)
478.5 CHORDITIS
478.5 DISEASE NEC
478.5 NODULE

VOCAL CORD (continued)
478.3# PARALYSIS
5th Digit: 478.3
0. UNSPECIFIED
1. UNILATERAL PARTIAL
2. UNILATERAL COMPLETE
3. BILATERAL PARTIAL
4. BILATERAL COMPLETE

478.4 POLYP
0 SEE ALSO 'LARYNX, LARYNGEAL'

V57.22 VOCATIONAL REHABILITATION
333.7 VOGT'S DISEASE OR SYNDROME (CORPUS STRIATUM)
364.24 VOGT-KOYANAGI SYNDROME
330.1 VOGT-SPIELMEYER DISEASE

VOICE
784.49 CHANGE
784.40 DISTURBANCE
784.41 LOSS
V41.4 PROBLEM (WITH PRODUCTION)

403.00 VOLHARD-FAHR DISEASE (MALIGNANT NEPHROSCLEROSIS)
958.6 VOLKMANN'S ISCHEMIC CONTRACTURE ACQUIRED (SYNDROME)
908.6 VOLKMANN'S ISCHEMIC CONTRACTURE LATE EFFECT
276.5 VOLUME DEHYDRATION DEPLETION

VOLVULUS
560.2 COLON
537.3 DUODENUM
560.2 INTESTINE

VOMITING
787.03 NOS
787.01 NOS WITH NAUSEA
0 BLOOD SEE 'HEMATEMESIS'
779.3 NEONATAL
536.2 PERSISTENT NONPREGNANT
564.3 POST OP GI SURGERY
307.54 PSYCHOGENIC
306.4 PSYCHOGENIC CYCLICAL
536.2 UNCONTROLLABLE

VOMITING IN PREGNANCY
643.9# VOMITING MILD OR NOS
643.0# HYPEREMESIS GRAVIDARUM MILD (<22 WKS.)
643.1# HYPEREMESIS GRAVIDARUM WITH METABOLIC DISTURBANCE (<22 WKS.)
643.2# LATE (>22 WKS.)
643.8# DUE TO DISEASE OR OTHER CAUSE
5th Digit: 643.0-2, 8-9
0. EPISODE OF CARE NOS OR N/A
1. DELIVERED
3. ANTEPARTUM COMPLICATION

720.0 VON BECHTEREW'S (STUMPELL) DISEASE OR SYNDROME (ANKYLOSING SPONDYLITIS)
049.8 VON ECONOMO'S DISEASE (ENCEPHALITIS LETHARGICA)
359.2 VON EULENBURG'S DISEASE (CONGENITAL PARAMYOTONIA)
271.0 VON GIERKE'S DISEASE (GLYCOGENOSIS I)
378.72 VON GRAEFE'S DISEASE OR SYNDROME
759.6 VON HIPPEL-LINDAU SYNDROME (ANGIOMATOSIS RETINOCEREBELLOSA)
285.8 VON JAKSCH'S DISEASE (PSEUDOLEUKEMIA INFANTUM)
237.71 VON RECKLINGHAUSEN'S DISEASE M9540/1
252.0 VON RECKLINGHAUSEN'S DISEASE OF BONE
275.0 VON RECKLINGHAUSEN-APPLEBAUM DISEASE (HEMOCHROMATOSIS)
453.8 VON SCHROETTER'S SYNDROME (INTERMITTENT VENOUS CLAUDICATION)
286.4 VON WILLEBRAND'S (-JURGENS) DISEASE OR SYNDROME (ANGIOHEMOPHILIA)
701.0 VON ZAMBUSCH'S DISEASE (LICHEN SCLEROSUS ET ATROPHICUS)
756.4 VOORHOEVE'S DISEASE (DYSCHONDROPLASIA)
366.21 VOSSIUS' RING TRAUMATIC
302.82 VOYEURISM
756.51 VROLIK'S DISEASE (OSTEOGENESIS IMPERFECTA)
745.4 VSD CONGENITAL
684 VULGARIS IMPETIGO

VULVA, VULVAL
0 ABNORMALITY COMPLICATING PREGNANCY, LABOR OR DELIVERY SEE 'VULVA, VULVAL DISORDERS COMPLICATING CHILDBIRTH'
752.49 ABSENCE (AGENESIS) (STRICTURE) CONGENITAL
624.8 ATRESIA
752.49 ATRESIA CONGENITAL
624.1 ATROPHY
233.3 CARCINOMA IN SITU
624.8 CYST
616.9 DISEASE INFLAMMATORY
616.8 DISEASE INFLAMMATORY - OTHER
0 DISORDER COMPLICATING CHILDBIRTH SEE 'VULVA, VULVAL DISORDERS COMPLICATING CHILDBIRTH'
624.9 DISORDER NONINFLAMMATORY
624.8 DISORDER NONINFLAMMATORY - OTHER
624.8 DYSPLASIA
233.3 DYSPLASIA VIN III
624.0 DYSTROPHY NONINFLAMMATORY
624.8 EDEMA
619.0 FISTULA - URINARY TRACT TO VULVA
619.1 FISTULA - DIGESTIVE TO VULVA
619.2 FISTULA - GENITAL TRACT TO SKIN
619.8 FISTULA - OTHER
624.5 HEMATOMA NONOBSTETRICAL
624.8 HEMORRHAGE
624.3 HYPERPLASIA
624.3 HYPERTROPHY
911.8 INJURY OTHER AND UNSPECIFIED SUPERFICIAL
911.9 INJURY OTHER AND UNSPECIFIED SUPERFICIAL (INFECTED)
624.0 KRAUROSIS
624.4 LACERATION OLD OR SCARRING
624.0 LEUKOPLAKIA
625.8 MASS
624.8 OCCLUSION
624.6 POLYP
0 PREVIOUS SURGERY MATERNAL SEE 'VULVA, VULVAL DISORDERS COMPLICATING CHILDBIRTH', ABNORMALITY
624.4 SCAR (OLD)
624.8 STRICTURE
752.49 STRICTURE CONGENITAL
091.0 SYPHILITIC
616.50 ULCER NOS (NONOBSTETRICAL)
136.1 ULCER - BEHCET'S [616.51]
098.0 ULCER - GONOCOCCAL
054.12 ULCER - HERPES SIMPLEX
091.0 ULCER - SYPHILITIC
016.7# ULCER - TUBERCULOUS [616.51]
5th Digit: 016.7
0. UNSPECIFIED
1. LAB NOT DONE
2. LABS PENDING
3. MICROSCOPY POSITIVE (IN SPUTUM)
4. CULTURE POSITIVE - MICROSCOPY NEGATIVE
5. CULTURE NEGATIVE - MICROSCOPY POSITIVE
6. CULTURE AND MICROSCOPY NEGATIVE CONFIRMED BY OTHER METHODS

456.6 VARICES
625.9 VESTIBULITIS

VULVA, VULVAL DISORDERS COMPLICATING CHILDBIRTH
763.89 ABNORMALITY AFFECTING FETUS OR NEWBORN
654.8# ABNORMALITY COMPLICATING CHILDBIRTH
660.2# ABNORMALITY OBSTRUCTING LABOR **[654.8#]**
654.8# SURGERY PREVIOUS COMPLICATING PREGNANCY CHILDBIRTH OR PUERPERIUM
660.2# SURGERY PREVIOUS OBSTRUCTING LABOR **[654.8#]**
654.8# TUMOR COMPLICATING CHILDBIRTH
660.2# TUMOR OBSTRUCTING LABOR **[654.8#]**

5th Digit: 654.8
0. EPISODE OF CARE NOS OR N/A
1. DELIVERED
2. DELIVERED WITH POSTPARTUM COMPLICATION
3. ANTEPARTUM COMPLICATION
4. POSTPARTUM COMPLICATION

5th Digit: 660.2
0. EPISODE OF CARE NOS OR N/A
1. DELIVERED
3. ANTEPARTUM COMPLICATION

VULVITIS
616.10 NOS
752.49 ADHESIVE CONGENITAL
098.0 BLENNORRHAGIC ACUTE
098.2 BLENNORRHAGIC CHRONIC
099.53 CHLAMYDIAL

646.6#: SPECIFY THE MATERNAL VULVITIS WITH AN ADDITIONAL CODE.

646.6# COMPLICATING PREGNANCY OR PUERPERIUM
5th Digit: 646.6
0. EPISODE OF CARE NOS OR N/A
1. DELIVERED
2. DELIVERED WITH POSTPARTUM COMPLICATION
3. ANTEPARTUM COMPLICATION
4. POSTPARTUM COMPLICATION

098.0 GONOCOCCAL ACUTE
098.2 GONOCOCCAL CHRONIC
054.11 HERPETIC
624.0 LEUKOPLAKIC
112.1 MONILIAL
091.0 SYPHILITIC EARLY
095.8 SYPHILITIC LATE
131.01 TRICHOMONAL

625.9 VULVODYNIA
0 VULVOVAGINITIS SEE 'VAGINITIS'

270.2 WAARDENBURG-KLEIN SYNDROME (PTOSIS EPICANTHUS)
709.3 WAGNER'S DISEASE (COLLOID MILIUM)
710.3 WAGNER (-UNVERRICHT) SYNDROME (DERMATOMYOSITIS)
780.54 WAKEFULNESS DISORDER (SEE ALSO 'HYPERSOMNIA')
732.1 WALDENSTROM'S DISEASE (OSTEOCHONDROSIS CAPITAL FEMORAL)
273.0 WALDENSTROM'S HYPERGAMMAGLOBULINEMIA
273.3 WALDENSTROM'S SYNDROME (MACROGLOBULINEMIA)
280.8 WALDENSTROM-KJELLBERG SYNDROME (SIDEROPENIC DYSPHAGIA)
719.7# WALKING DIFFICULTY
5th Digit: 719.7
0. SITE NOS
5. PELVIC REGION AND THIGH (HIP) (BUTTOCK) (FEMUR)
6. LOWER LEG (FIBULA) (KNEE) (PATELLA) (TIBIA)
7. ANKLE AND/OR FOOT (METATARSALS) (TOES) (TARSALS)
8. OTHER
9. MULTIPLE

436 WALLENBERG'S SYNDROME (POSTERIOR INFERIOR CEREBELLAR ARTERY)
459.89 WALLGREN'S DISEASE (OBSTRUCTION OF SPLENIC VEIN WITH COLLATERAL CIRCULATION)
427.89 WANDERING (ATRIAL) PACEMAKER
681.9 WARDROP'S DISEASE (WITH LYMPHANGITIS)
681.02 WARDROP'S DISEASE (WITH LYMPHANGITIS) - FINGER
681.11 WARDROP'S DISEASE (WITH LYMPHANGITIS) - TOE

WARTS
078.10 NOS
078.11 CONDYLOMA ACUMINATUM
078.19 FIG
078.19 GENITAL
371.41 HASSALL-HENLE'S OF CORNEA
078.10 INFECTIOUS OR VIRAL
078.19 JUVENILE
078.10 MOIST
088.0 PERUVIAN
078.19 PLANTAR
702.0 SENILE
702.1# SEBORRHEIC
5th Digit: 702.1
1. INFLAMED
9. OTHER

078.19 VENEREAL (MALE) (FEMALE)
078.19 VERRUCA (PLANA JUVENILIS) (PLANTARIS)
078.10 VERRUCA VULGARIS
078.10 VIRAL
078.19 OTHER SPECIFIED

989.5 WASP STING
989.5 WASP STING WITH ANAPHYLAXIS [995.0]
097.1 WASSERMANN POSITIVE SCREENING EXAM
795.6 WASSERMANN REACTION FALSE POSITIVE
100.0 WASSILIEFF'S DISEASE (LEPTOSPIRAL JAUNDICE)
799.4 WASTING DISEASE
366.12 WATER CLEFTS
994.3 WATER DEPRIVATION
909.4 WATER DEPRIVATION LATE EFFECT
989.5 WATER MOCCASIN BITE
995.0 WATER MOCCASIN BITE WITH ANAPHYLAXIS [989.5]
276.6 WATER OVERLOAD
276.6 WATER RETENTION SYNDROME
787.1 WATERBRASH
036.3 WATERHOUSE FRIDERICHSEN SYNDROME
380.4 WAX IN EAR
734 WEAK ARCHES (FOOT)
754.61 WEAK ARCHES (FOOT) CONGENITAL
596.59 WEAK BLADDER SPHINCTER
728.9 WEAK MUSCLE
785.9 WEAK PULSE
780.79 WEAKNESS GENERALIZED
991.9 WEATHER EFFECT COLD
992.9 WEATHER EFFECT HEAT
909.4 WEATHER EFFECT LATE EFFECT COLD OR HEAT
692.74 WEATHERED SKIN
748.69 WEBBED ALVEOLI CONGENITAL
0 WEBBING OF DIGITS SEE 'SYNDACTYLY, SYNDACTYLIC'

W-V

729.30 WEBER-CHRISTIAN DISEASE OR SYNDROME (NODULAR NONSUPPURATIVE PANNICULITIS)
757.39 WEBER-COCKAYNE SYNDROME (EPIDERMOLYSIS BULLOSA)
759.6 WEBER-DIMITRI SYNDROME (ENCEPHALOCUTANEOUS ANGIOMATOSIS)
344.89 WEBER-GUBLER SYNDROME
344.89 WEBER-LEYDEN SYNDROME
448.0 WEBER-OSLER SYNDROME (FAMILIAL HEMORRHAGIC TELANGIECTASIA)
733.00 WEDGING OF VERTEBRA NOS
446.4 WEGENER'S SYNDROME (NECROTIZING RESPIRATORY GRANULOMATOSIS)
648.9# WEGENER'S SYNDROME (NECROTIZING RESPIRATORY GRANULOMATOSIS) MATERNAL CURRENT (CO-EXISTENT) IN PREGNANCY [446.4]

5th Digit: 648.9

0. EPISODE OF NOS OR N/A
1. DELIVERED
2. DELIVERED WITH POSTPARTUM COMPLICATION
3. ANTEPARTUM COMPLICATION
4. POSTPARTUM COMPLICATION

090.0 WEGNER'S DISEASE (SYPHILITIC OSTEOCHONDRITIS)

646.##: SPECIFY THE MATERNAL WEIGHT GAIN WITH AN ADDITIONAL CODE FOR THE CONDITION CAUSING THE ABNORMAL WEIGHT.

WEIGHT
783.1 GAIN ABNORMAL
278.00 GAIN ABNORMAL - OBESITY
278.01 GAIN ABNORMAL - OBESITY MORBID
646.1# GAIN EXCESSIVE IN PREGNANCY

5th Digit: 646.1

0. EPISODE OF CARE NOS OR N/A
1. DELIVERED
2. DELIVERED WITH POSTPARTUM COMPLICATION
3. ANTEPARTUM COMPLICATION
4. POSTPARTUM COMPLICATION

642.## GAIN EXCESSIVE WITH PREGNANCY WITH HYPERTENSION

4th Digit: 642

0. BENIGN ESSENTIAL
1. SECONDARY TO RENAL DISEASE
2. OTHER PRE-EXISTING
3. TRANSIENT

5th Digit: 642

0. EPISODE OF CARE NOS OR N/A
1. DELIVERED
2. DELIVERED WITH POSTPARTUM COMPLICATION
3. ANTEPARTUM COMPLICATION
4. POSTPARTUM COMPLICATION

783.4 GAIN FAILURE
646.8# GAIN INSUFFICIENT IN PREGNANCY

5th Digit: 646.8

0. EPISODE OF CARE NOS OR N/A
1. DELIVERED
2. DELIVERED WITH POSTPARTUM COMPLICATION
3. ANTEPARTUM COMPLICATION
4. POSTPARTUM COMPLICATION

783.2 LOSS ABNORMAL

100.0 WEIL'S DISEASE (LEPTOSPIRAL JAUNDICE)
759.89 WEILL-MARCHESANI SYNDROME (BRACHYMORPHISM AND ECTOPIA LENTIS)
518.3 WEINGARTEN'S SYNDROME (TROPICAL EOSINOPHILIA)
443.89 WEIR MITCHELL'S DISEASE (ERYTHROMELALGIA)
337.0 WEISS-BAKER SYNDROME (CAROTID SINUS SYNCOPE)
710.1 WEISSENBACH-THIBIERGE SYNDROME (CUTANEOUS SYSTEMIC SCLEROSIS)

040.0 WELCHII BACILLUS INFECTION
370.24 WELDER'S FLASH
V20.2 WELL BABY CHECK
V20.2 WELL CHILD CHECK
V65.5 WELL-WORRIED EXAM
706.2 WEN
426.13 WENCKEBACK'S HEART BLOCK
335.0 WERDNIG-HOFFMANN DISEASE OR SYNDROME
287.3 WERLHOF-WICHMANN SYNDROME
258.0 WERMER'S SYNDROME (POLYGLANDULAR) (POLYENDOCRINE ADENOMATOSIS)
259.8 WERNER'S SYNDROME (PROGERIA ADULTORUM)
083.1 WERNER HIS DISEASE (TRENCH FEVER)
288.0 WERNER -SCHULTZ DISEASE (AGRANULOCYTOSIS)
291.1 WERNICKE SYNDROME (ALCOHOLIC) ACUTE
265.1 WERNICKE'S ENCEPHALOPATHY (SUPERIOR HEMORRHAGIC POLIOENCEPHALITIS)
291.1 WERNICKE-KORSAKOFF SYNDROME ALCOHOLIC
294.0 WERNICKE-KORSAKOFF SYNDROME NONALCOHOLIC
114.9 WERNICKE-POSADAS DISEASE
066.3 WESSELSBRON FEVER (VIRAL)
066.3 WEST NILE FEVER (VIRAL)
062.1 WESTERN EQUINE ENCEPHALITIS
275.1 WESTPHAL-STRUMPELL SYNDROME (HEPATOLENTICULAR DEGENERATION)
303.9# WET BRAIN SYNDROME (ALCOHOLIC)

5th Digit: 303.9

0. NOS
1. CONTINUOUS
2. EPISODIC
3. IN REMISSION

991.4 WET FEET SYNDROME (MACERATION) (TROPICAL)
518.5 WET LUNG SYNDROME
770.6 WET LUNG SYNDROME NEWBORN
V53.8 WHEELCHAIR FITTING AND ADJUSTMENT
786.07 WHEEZING
0 WHEEZING ASTHMATIC SEE 'ASTHMA, ASTHMATIC'
847.0 WHIPLASH NECK (SYNDROME)
040.2 WHIPPLE'S DISEASE OR SYNDROME (INTESTINAL LIPODYSTROPHY)
127.3 WHIPWORM INFECTION
759.89 WHISTLING FACE SYNDROME (CRANIOCARPOTARSAL DYSTROPHY)
757.39 WHITE'S DISEASE (CONGENITAL) (KERATOSIS FOLLICULARIS)
288.8 WHITE BLOOD CELL COUNT ELEVATED ABNORMAL FINDINGS
288.0 WHITE BLOOD CELL COUNT LOW ABNORMAL FINDINGS
288.9 WHITE BLOOD CELL DIFFERENTIAL ABNORMAL FINDINGS
288.9 WHITE BLOOD CELLS DISEASE
288.8 WHITE BLOOD CELLS GRANULOCYSTIC HYPERPLASIA
288.9 WHITE BLOOD CELL MORPHOLOGY ABNORMAL FINDINGS
288.8 WHITE BLOOD CELLS DISEASE SPECIFIED NEC
518.82 WHITE LUNG SYNDROME
111.2 WHITE PIEDRA
681.01 WHITLOW
054.6 WHITLOW HERPES SIMPLEX
025 WHITMORE'S DISEASE (MELIOIDOSIS)

WHOOPING COUGH
033.9 UNSPECIFIED ORGANISM
033.8 BORDETELLA BRONCHISEPTICA [B. BRONCHISEPTICA]
033.1 BORDETELLA PARAPERTUSSIS [B. PARAPERTUSSIS]
033.0 BORDETELLA PERTUSSIS [B. PERTUSSIS]
033.8 DUE TO OTHER SPECIFIED ORGANISM
033.# PNEUMONIA [484.3]
4th Digit: 033
0. B. PERTUSSIS
1. B. PARAPERTUSSIS
8. B. BRONCHISEPTICA
9. UNSPECIFIED ORGANISM

V74.8 SCREENING EXAM

283.9 WIDAL-ABRAMI DISEASE OR SYNDROME (ACQUIRED HEMOLYTIC JAUNDICE)
557.1 WILKIE'S DISEASE OR SYNDROME
694.1 WILKINSON-SNEDDON DISEASE OR SYNDROME (SUBCORNEAL PUSTULAR DERMATOSIS)
696.1 WILLAN-PLUMBE SYNDROME (PSORIASIS)
286.4 WILLEBRAND (-JURGENS) SYNDROME (ANGIOHEMOPHILIA)
759.81 WILLI-PRADER SYNDROME (HYPOGENITAL DYSTROPHY WITH DIABETIC TENDENCY)
189.0 WILM'S TUMOR M8960/3
695.89 WILSON-BROCQ DISEASE (DERMATITIS EXFOLIATIVA)
275.1 WILSON'S DISEASE OR SYNDROME (HEPATOLENTICULAR DEGENERATION)
275.1 WILSON'S DISEASE OR SYNDROME (HEPATOLENTICULAR DEGENERATION) WITH DEMENTIA [294.1]
770.7 WILSON-MIKITY SYNDROME
380.00 WINKLER'S DISEASE
698.8 WINTER ITCH
078.82 WINTER VOMITING DISEASE
696.2 WISE'S DISEASE
279.12 WISKOTT-ALDRICH SYNDROME (ECZEMA-THROMBOCYTOPENIA)

WITHDRAWAL
291.0 ALCOHOL - DELIRIUM (TREMENS)
291.3 ALCOHOL - HALLUCINOSIS (PSYCHOSIS)
291.81 ALCOHOL - SYMPTOMS OR SYNDROME
760.71 ALCOHOL - SYMPTOMS OR SYNDROME NEWBORN
292.0 DRUG - SYMPTOMS OR SYNDROME
779.5 DRUG - SYMPTOMS OR SYNDROME NEWBORN OR INFANT OF DEPENDENT MOTHER
313.22 REACTION OF CHILDHOOD OR ADOLESCENCE

471.1 WOAKE'S SYNDROME (ETHMOIDITIS)
335.11 WOHLFART-KUGELBERG-WELANDER DISEASE
518.5 WOILLEZ'S DISEASE (ACUTE IDIOPATHIC PULMONARY CONGESTION)
426.7 WOLFF-PARKINSON-WHITE SYNDROME (ANOMALOUS ATRIOVENTRICULAR EXCITATION)
752.8 WOLFFIAN DUCT DISORDER (CONGENITAL)
083.1 WOLHYNIAN FEVER
272.7 WOLMAN'S DISEASE (PRIMARY FAMILIAL XANTHOMATOSIS)
0 WOMB SEE 'UTERUS, UTERINE'
495.8 WOOD ASTHMA
022.1 WOOL SORTER'S DISEASE
315.31 WORD DEAFNESS
V62.1 WORK PROBLEM (ADVERSE EFFECT OF WORK ENVIRONMENT) (REASON FOR ENCOUNTER)
102.3 WORM-EATEN SOLES
128.9 WORMS
127.9 WORMS INTESTINAL
780.79 WORN OUT (EXHAUSTION)
V65.5 WORRIED WELL EXAM

WHEN CODING AN INFECTION, USE AN ADDITIONAL CODE, [041.#], TO IDENTIFY THE ORGANISM. SEE 'BACTERIAL INFECTION'.

WOUND
V58.3 CHECK (LACERATION)
V58.41 CLOSURE POST OP PLANNED
674.3# COMPLICATION POST OP OTHER SPECIFIED MATERNAL DUE TO PREGNANCY
5th Digit: 674.3
0. NOS
2. DELIVERED WITH POSTPARTUM COMPLICATION
4. POSTPARTUM COMPLICATION

795.3 CULTURE ABNORMAL
998.3 DEHISCENCE POST OP
998.3 DEHISCENCE POST OP ABDOMINAL WOUND
674.1# DEHISCENCE POST OP C SECTION
674.1# DEHISCENCE POST OP UTERINE MATERNAL DUE TO PREGNANCY
674.2# DEHISCENCE POST OP PERINEAL MATERNAL DUE TO PREGNANCY
674.2# DEHISCENCE POST OP PERINEAL FIRST DEGREE THROUGH FOURTH DEGREE REPAIR
674.2# DEHISCENCE POST OP EPISIOTOMY
5th Digit: 674.1-2
0. NOS
2. DELIVERED WITH POSTPARTUM COMPLICATION
4. POSTPARTUM COMPLICATION

998.12 HEMATOMA COMPLICATING A PROCEDURE
674.3# HEMATOMA OR HEMORRHAGE POST OP C SECTION OR PERINEAL PROCEDURE
5th Digit: 674.3
0. NOS
2. DELIVERED WITH POSTPARTUM COMPLICATION
4. POSTPARTUM COMPLICATION

998.59 INFECTION POST OP
909.3 INFECTION POST OP LATE EFFECT
674.3# INFECTION POST OP C- SECTION
674.3# INFECTION POST OP PERINEAL PROCEDURE MATERNAL DUE TO PREGNANCY
5th Digit: 674.3
0. NOS
2. DELIVERED WITH POSTPARTUM COMPLICATION
4. POSTPARTUM COMPLICATION

958.3 INFECTION POSTTRAUMATIC NEC
908.6 INFECTION POSTTRAUMATIC NEC LATE EFFECT
998.51 INFECTION SEROMA
0 OPEN SEE 'OPEN WOUND', BY SITE
998.59 OPERATION GRANULOMA
0 SUPERFICIAL SEE 'ABRASION', BY SITE
998.83 SURGICAL NON-HEALING
767.8 SCALPEL WOUND (BIRTH TRAUMA)

447.8 WRIGHT'S SYNDROME (HYPERABDUCTION)
0 WRINGER INJURY SEE 'CRUSH INJURY'
701.8 WRINKLING SKIN

WRIST
V49.64 AMPUTATION STATUS
0 BONES SEE ALSO 'CARPAL'
736.00 DEFORMITY ACQUIRED
736.05 DROP (ACQUIRED)
959.3 INJURY
913.8 INJURY OTHER AND UNSPECIFIED SUPERFICIAL
913.9 INJURY OTHER AND UNSPECIFIED SUPERFICIAL - INFECTED
0 JOINT SEE ALSO 'JOINT'
719.83 JOINT CALCIFICATION
718.93 JOINT LIGAMENT RELAXATION
718.13 JOINT LOOSE BODY
V43.63 JOINT REPLACEMENT STATUS

WRIST (continued)

842.0# SPRAIN (STRAIN) (AVULSION) (HEMARTHROSIS)

5th Digit: 842.0

0. NOS SITE

1. CARPAL (JOINT)

2. RADIOCARPAL (JOINT) (LIGAMENT)

9. OTHER OR RADIOULNAR JOINT (DISTAL)

719.83 TRIANGULAR CARTILAGE COMPLEX

736.03 VALGUS DEFORMITY (ACQUIRED)

736.04 VARUS DEFORMITY (ACQUIRED)

333.84 WRITERS' CRAMP ORGANIC

300.89 WRITERS' CRAMP PSYCHOGENIC

754.1 WRY NECK CONGENITAL

125.0 WUCHERERIASIS BANCROFTI

125.1 WUCHERERIASIS BRUGIA MALAYI

U-V-W

413.9 X SYNDROME

X-RAY STUDIES
793.# ABNORMAL FINDINGS (NONSPECIFIC)
4th Digit: 793
0. SKULL AND HEAD
1. LUNG FIELD
2. OTHER INTRATHORACIC ORGAN
3. BILIARY TRACT
4. GASTROINTESTINAL TRACT
5. GENITOURINARY ORGANS
6. ABDOMINAL AREA INCLUDING RETROPERITONEUM
7. MUSCULOSKELETAL SYSTEM
8. BREAST
9. OTHER
990 ADVERSE EFFECTS
909.2 ADVERSE EFFECTS LATE EFFECT
V71.2 CHEST (FOR TB)
V72.5 CHEST (ROUTINE)
V72.5 ROUTINE NEC

272.2 XANTHELASMA HYPERCHOLESTEROLEMIA [374.51]
272.2 XANTHELASMATOSIS ESSENTIAL
757.33 XANTHELASMOIDEA
277.2 XANTHINURIA
277.2 XANTHINURIA METABOLISM DISORDERS

XANTHOMA
272.7 BONE
277.8 CRANIOHYPOPHYSEAL
272.7 CUTANEOTENDINOUS DISSEMINATION
272.2 EYELID (PLANUM) (TUBEROSUM) [374.51]
272.0 HYPERCHOLESTERINEMIC
272.4 HYPERLIPIDEMIC
272.2 TUBEROSUM

272.7 XANTHOMATOSIS PRIMARY FAMILIAL
709.09 XANTHOSIS
998.81 XANTHOSIS SURGICAL
302.89 XENOPHILIA
300.29 XENOPHOBIA

XERODERMA
701.1 ACQUIRED
757.39 CONGENITAL
373.33 EYELID
757.33 PIGMENTOSUM CONGENITAL
264.8 DUE TO VITAMIN A DEFICIENCY

V72.5 XEROGRAM
V72.5 XEROMAMMAMOGRAPHY
793.8 XEROGRAPHY ABNORMAL
372.53 XEROPHTHALMIA
264.7 XEROPHTHALMIA DUE TO VITAMIN A DEFICIENCY

XEROSIS
372.53 CONJUNCTIVAL
371.40 CORNEA
370.00 CORNEA (WITH ULCERATION)
706.8 CUTIS

527.7 XEROSTOMIA

733.99 XIPHOIDITIS
733.99 XIPHOIDYNIA (XIPHOIDALGIA SYNDROME)
759.4 XIPHOPAGUS
758.6 XO SYNDROME
758.81 XXX SYNDROME (COMPLEMENT)
758.81 XXXXY SYNDROME
758.7 XXY SYNDROME
271.8 XYLOSURIA CARBOHYDRATE TRANSPORT DISORDERS
271.8 XYLULOSURIA CARBOHYDRATE TRANSPORT DISORDERS
758.81 XYY SYNDROME (COMPLEMENT)

306.1 YAWNING PSYCHOGENIC

YAWS
102.9 NOS
102.6 BONE AND JOINT LESIONS
102.1 BUTTER
102.0 CHANCRE (INITIAL LESION)
102.2 CUTANEOUS, LESS THAN FIVE YEARS AFTER INFECTION
102.2 EARLY (CUTANEOUS) (MACULAR) (PAPULAR) (MACULOPAPULAR) (MICROPAPULAR)
102.9 EYELID DERMATITIS [373.4]
102.2 FRAMBESIDE
102.5 GANGOSA
102.4 GUMMATA AND ULCERS
102.3 HYPERKERATOSIS (PALMAR OR PLANTAR)
102.7 JUXTA ARTICULAR NODULES
102.8 LATENT
102.7 MANIFESTATION OTHER
102.0 MOTHER
102.7 MUCOSAL
102.1 MULTIPLE PAPILLOMATA AND WET CRAB
102.4 NODULAR LATE (ULCERATED)
102.1 PALMAR PAPILLOMA
102.1 PLANTAR PAPILLOMA
102.8 POSITIVE SEROLOGY WITHOUT CLINICAL MANIFESTATIONS
V74.6 SCREENING EXAM
102.2 SKIN LESIONS OTHER EARLY

112.9 YEAST INFECTION SITE UNSPECIFIED (SEE ALSO 'CANDIDIASIS')

YELLOW ATROPHY
571.5 HEALED
570 LIVER ACUTE
571.8 LIVER CHRONIC
570 LIVER POSTOP

YELLOW FEVER
060.9 NOS
060.0 JUNGLE
V73.4 SCREENING EXAM
060.0 SYLVATIC
060.1 URBAN
V04.4 VACCINATION

762.2 YELLOW VERNIX SYNDROME (PLACENTAL DYSFUNCTION)
008.44 YERSINIA ENTEROCOLITICA (INTESTINAL INFECTION)
0 YERSINIA (PATEURELLA) PESTIS INFECTION SEE 'PLAGUE'
027.8 YERSINIA SEPTICA
758.7 YXX SYNDROME

527.7 ZAGARI'S DISEASE (XEROSTOMIA)
057.8 ZAHORSKY'S DISEASE (EXANTHEM SUBITUM)
530.6 ZENKER'S DIVERTICULUM
333.6 ZIEHEN-OPPENHEIM (SCHWALBE-) DISEASE
571.1 ZIEVE'S SYNDROME (JAUNDICE, HYPERLIPEMIA AND HEMOLYTIC ANEMIA)
066.3 ZIKA FEVER (VIRAL)
790.6 ZINC ABNORMAL BLOOD LEVEL

251.5	ZOLLINGER-ELLISON SYNDROME (GASTRIC HYPERSECRETION WITH PANCREATIC ISLET CELL TUMOR)
0	ZONA SEE 'HERPES ZOSTER' FOR COMPLICATION
053.9	ZONA
027.9	ZOONOTIC BACTERIAL DISEASE
027.8	ZOONOTIC BACTERIAL DISEASES OTHER SPECIFIED
302.1	ZOOPHILIA
300.29	ZOOPHOBIA
117.4	ZOPFIA LEPTOSPHAERIAL SENEGALENSIS INFECTION
281.2	ZUELZER-OGDEN SYNDROME (NUTRITIONAL MEGALOBLASTIC ANEMIA)
755.10	ZYGODACTYLY
738.11	ZYGOMATIC HYPERPLASIA (ACQUIRED)
738.12	ZYGOMATIC HYPOPLASIA (ACQUIRED)
117.7	ZYGOMYCOSIS

APPENDIX A

E CODE DIRECTORY

ACCIDENT VEHICULAR

IN ORDER TO IDENTIFY VEHICLE ACCIDENTS WHERE A PATIENT IS ACCIDENTALLY STRUCK BY A FALLING OBJECT, USE CODE E916 STRUCK BY FALLING OBJECT AS AN ADDITIONAL CODE.

RAILWAY

0 DUE TO NATURAL CATACLYSM SEE 'NATURAL CATACLYSM'
E800.# COLLISION WITH OTHER MOVING RAILCAR
E801.# COLLISION WITH OTHER OBJECT
E802.# DERAILMENT WITHOUT COLLISION
E803.# EXPLOSION FIRE OR BURNING
E804.# FALL IN, ON, OR FROM
E805.# HIT BY TRAIN
E806.# HIT BY OBJECT SET IN MOTION BY TRAIN OR OTHER SPECIFIED
E807.# UNSPECIFIED

4th Digit: E800 - 807

0. RAILWAY EMPLOYEE
1. PASSENGER ON TRAIN
2. PEDESTRIAN
3. BICYCLIST
8. OTHER SPECIFIED PERSON
9. UNSPECIFIED PERSON

MOTOR VEHICLE ON PUBLIC ROADWAY

0 DUE TO NATURAL CATACLYSM SEE 'NATURAL CATACLYSM'
E810.# WITH TRAIN
E811.# RE-ENTRANT WITH ANOTHER MOTOR VEHICLE
E812.# WITH ANOTHER MOTOR VEHICLE
E813.# WITH ANOTHER VEHICLE
E814.# WITH PEDESTRIAN
E815.# WITH ANOTHER VEHICLE ON HIGHWAY
E816.# LOSS OF CONTROL WITHOUT COLLISION
E817.# GETTING INTO OR OUT OF VEHICLE
E818.# NON COLLISION ACCIDENT (FLYING OBJECTS SET IN MOTION BY VEHICLE)
E819.# UNSPECIFIED NATURE

4th Digit: E810 - 819

0. DRIVER
1. PASSENGER
2. MOTORCYCLIST
3. PASSENGER ON MOTORCYCLE
4. PASSENGER IN STREETCAR
5. RIDER ON ANIMAL OR ANIMAL DRAWN VEHICLE
6. BICYCLIST
7. PEDESTRIAN
8. OTHER SPECIFIED PERSON
9. UNSPECIFIED PERSON

ACCIDENT VEHICULAR (continued)

IN ORDER TO IDENTIFY VEHICLE ACCIDENTS WHERE A PATIENT IS ACCIDENTALLY STRUCK BY A FALLING OBJECT, USE CODE E916 STRUCK BY FALLING OBJECT AS AN ADDITIONAL CODE.

MOTOR VEHICLE NOT ON PUBLIC ROAD

0 DUE TO NATURAL CATACLYSM SEE 'NATURAL CATACLYSM'
E820.# SNOWMOBILE
E821.# OFF ROAD VEHICLE
E822.# COLLISION WITH MOVING OBJECT
E823.# COLLISION WITH STATIONARY OBJECT
E824.# WHILE GETTING ON OR OFF
E825.# OTHER AND UNSPECIFIED (CO) (STRUCK BY OBJECT)

4th Digit: E820 - 825

0. DRIVER
1. PASSENGER
2. MOTORCYCLIST
3. PASSENGER ON MOTORCYCLE
4. OCCUPANT OF STREETCAR
5. RIDER OF ANIMAL OR ANIMAL DRAWN VEHICLE
6. BICYCLIST
7. PEDESTRIAN
8. OTHER SPECIFIED PERSON
9. UNSPECIFIED PERSON

NON MOTOR VEHICLE

E826.# BICYCLE

4th Digit: E826

0. PEDESTRIAN
1. BICYCLIST
2. RIDER OF ANIMAL
3. OCCUPANT OF ANIMAL DRAWN VEHICLE
4. OCCUPANT OF STREETCAR
8. OTHER SPECIFIED PERSON
9. UNSPECIFIED PERSON

E827.# ANIMAL DRAWN
E828.# ANIMAL RIDDEN
E829.# STREETCAR

4th Digit: E827 - 829

0. PEDESTRIAN
2. RIDER OF ANIMAL
3. OCCUPANT OF ANIMAL DRAWN VEHICLE
4. OCCUPANT OF STREETCAR
8. OTHER SPECIFIED PERSON
9. UNSPECIFIED PERSON

ACCIDENT VEHICULAR (continued)

IN ORDER TO IDENTIFY VEHICLE ACCIDENTS WHERE A PATIENT IS ACCIDENTALLY STRUCK BY A FALLING OBJECT, USE CODE E916 STRUCK BY FALLING OBJECT AS AN ADDITIONAL CODE.

WATERCRAFT

E830.# SINKING OR CAPSIZING
E831.# ANY INJURY WHETHER COLLISION OR NOT
E832.# FALLING OVERBOARD WHETHER DROWNED OR NOT
E833.# FALL FROM LADDER
E834.# FALL FROM UPPER LEVEL
E835.# OTHER AND UNSPECIFIED
E836.# MACHINERY ACCIDENT
E837.# EXPLOSION, FIRE, OR BURNING
E838.# OTHER AND UNSPECIFIED (BOAT ACCIDENT) (STRUCK BY BOAT)

4th Digit: E830 - 838

0. OCCUPANT OF SMALL BOAT - UNPOWERED
1. OCCUPANT OF SMALL BOAT - POWERED
2. OCCUPANT OF OTHER CRAFT - CREW
3. OCCUPANT OF OTHER CRAFT - NON CREW
4. WATER SKIER
5. SWIMMER
6. DOCKERS / STEVEDORE
8. OTHER SPECIFIED PERSON
9. UNSPECIFIED PERSON

AIRCRAFT OR SPACECRAFT

E840.# DURING TAKEOFF OR LANDING - POWERED AIRCRAFT
E841.# OTHER AND UNSPECIFIED - POWERED AIRCRAFT

4th Digit: E840 - 841

0. OCCUPANT OF SPACECRAFT
1. OCCUPANT OF MILITARY AIRCRAFT
2. CREW OF COMMERCIAL AIRCRAFT
3. OCCUPANT OF COMMERCIAL AIRCRAFT SURFACE TO SURFACE
4. OCCUPANT OF COMMERCIAL AIRCRAFT SURFACE TO AIR
5. OCCUPANT OF OTHER POWERED AIRCRAFT
6. OCCUPANT OF UNPOWERED AIRCRAFT
7. PARACHUTIST
8. GROUND CREW-AIRLINE EMPLOYEE
9. OTHER PERSON

E842.# UNPOWERED AIRCRAFT

4th Digit: E842

6. OCCUPANT OF UNPOWERED AIRCRAFT
7. PARACHUTIST
8. GROUND CREW-AIRLINE EMPLOYEE
9. OTHER PERSON

ACCIDENT VEHICULAR (continued)

IN ORDER TO IDENTIFY VEHICLE ACCIDENTS WHERE A PATIENT IS ACCIDENTALLY STRUCK BY A FALLING OBJECT, USE CODE E916 STRUCK BY FALLING OBJECT AS AN ADDITIONAL CODE.

AIRCRAFT OR SPACECRAFT (continued)

E843.# FALL IN/OUT OF AIRCRAFT
E844.# OTHER SPECIFIED - AIR TRANSPORT ACCIDENT

4th Digit: E843 - 844

0. OCCUPANT OF SPACECRAFT
1. OCCUPANT OF MILITARY AIRCRAFT
2. CREW OF COMMERCIAL AIRCRAFT
3. OCCUPANT OF COMMERCIAL AIRCRAFT SURFACE TO SURFACE
4. OCCUPANT OF COMMERCIAL AIRCRAFT SURFACE TO AIR
5. OCCUPANT OF OTHER POWERED AIRCRAFT
6. OCCUPANT OF UNPOWERED AIRCRAFT
7. PARACHUTIST
8. GROUND CREW-AIRLINE EMPLOYEE
9. OTHER PERSON

E845.# SPACECRAFT

4th Digit: E845

0. OCCUPANT OF SPACECRAFT
8. GROUND CREW-AIRLINE EMPLOYEE
9. OTHER PERSON

OTHER VEHICLES NEC

E846 POWERED VEHICLES USED SOLELY WITHIN BUILDINGS OR ESTABLISHMENTS
E847 CABLE CARS NOT RUNNING ON RAILS
E848 VEHICLES NEC

PLACE OF OCCURRENCE CODES [E849.#] ARE USED TO INDICATE THE PLACE WHERE THE INJURY OR POISONING OCCURRED.

PLACE OF OCCURRENCE

E849.# PLACE OF OCCURRENCE

4th Digit: E849

0. HOME
1. FARM
2. MINE OR QUARRY
3. INDUSTRIAL PLACE OR PREMISES
4. RECREATIONAL AREA
5. STREET OR HIGHWAY
6. PUBLIC BUILDING
7. INSTITUTION (HOSPITAL, DORM, PRISON, ETC.)
8. OTHER SPECIFIED PLACE
9. UNSPECIFIED PLACE

MISADVENTURES DURING SURGERY / PROCEDURE OR MEDICAL CARE

E870.# ACCIDENTAL CUT, PUNCTURE, PERFORATION, HEMORRHAGE DURING CARE

E870.7 ACCIDENTAL CUT, PUNCTURE, PERFORATION, HEMORRHAGE DURING ADMINISTRATION OF ENEMA

E871.# FOREIGN BODY LEFT IN BODY DURING A PROCEDURE

E871.7 FOREIGN BODY LEFT IN BODY DURING REMOVAL CATHETER / PACKING

E872.# FAILURE OF STERILE PRECAUTIONS DURING PROCEDURE

4th Digit: E870, E871, E872

- **0. SURGICAL OPERATION**
- **1. INFUSION OR TRANSFUSION**
- **2. KIDNEY DIALYSIS / OTHER PERFUSION**
- **3. INJECTION / VACCINATION**
- **4. ENDOSCOPIC EXAMINATION**
- **5. ASPIRATION FLUID OR TISSUE, PUNCTURE, AND CATHETERIZATION**
- **6. HEART CATHETERIZATION**
- **8. OTHER SPECIFIED MEDICAL CARE**
- **9. NOS MEDICAL CARE**

E873.# FAILURE IN DOSAGE

4th Digit: E873

- **0. EXCESSIVE BLOOD OR OTHER FLUID DURING INFUSION / PERFUSION**
- **1. INCORRECT DILUTION OF FLUID DURING INFUSION**
- **2. OVERDOSE OF RADIATION IN THERAPY**
- **3. INADVERTENT EXPOSURE OF PATIENT TO RADIATION**
- **4. FAILURE IN DOSAGE ELECTROSHOCK OR INSULIN-SHOCK THERAPY**
- **5. INAPPROPRIATE TEMPERATURE IN LOCAL APPLICATION AND PACKING**
- **6. NONADMINISTRATION OF NECESSARY DRUG OR MEDICINAL SUBSTANCE**
- **8. OTHER SPECIFIED FAILURE IN DOSAGE**
- **9. NOS FAILURE IN DOSAGE**

E874.# MECHANICAL FAILURE OF INSTRUMENT OR APPARATUS DURING PROCEDURE

4th Digit: E874

- **0. SURGICAL OPERATION**
- **1. INFUSION OR TRANSFUSION**
- **2. KIDNEY DIALYSIS / OTHER PERFUSION**
- **3. ENDOSCOPIC EXAMINATION**
- **4. ASPIRATION FLUID OR TISSUE, PUNCTURE, AND CATHETERIZATION**
- **5. HEART CATHETERIZATION**
- **8. OTHER SPECIFIED MEDICAL CARE**
- **9. NOS MEDICAL CARE**

E875.# CONTAMINATION OR INFECTED BLOOD, OTHER FLUID, DRUG, OR BIOLOGICAL SUBSTANCE

4th Digit: E875

- **0. CONTAMINATED SUBSTANCE TRANSFUSION / INFUSION**
- **1. CONTAMINATED SUBSTANCE INJECTION / VACCINATION**
- **2. CONTAMINATED DRUG / BIOLOGICAL SUBSTANCE ADMINISTERED OTHER MEANS**
- **8. OTHER CONTAMINATED SUBSTANCE**
- **9. UNSPECIFIIED CONTAMINATED SUBSTANCE**

MISADVENTURES DURING SURGERY / PROCEDURE OR MEDICAL CARE (continued)

E876.# OTHER AND UNSPECIFIED MISADVENTURES DURING MEDICAL CARE

4th Digit: E876

- **0. MISMATCHED BLOOD IN TRANSFUSION**
- **1. WRONG FLUID IN INFUSION**
- **2. FAILURE IN SUTURE AND LIGATURE DURING SURGERY**
- **3. ENDOTRACHEAL TUBE WRONGLY PLACED DURING ANESTHESIA**
- **4. FAILURE TO REMOVE TUBE OR OTHER TUBE / INSTRUMENT**
- **5. PERFORMANCE OF INAPPROPRIATE OPERATION**
- **8. OTHER SPECIFIED MISADVENTURES**
- **9. NOS MISADVENTURE**

SURGICAL/MEDICAL PROCEDURES CAUSING ABNORMAL REACTION OF PATIENT OR LATER COMPLICATION

E878.# DUE TO SURGICAL OPERATION

4th Digit: E878

- **0. TRANSPLANT WHOLE ORGAN**
- **1. ARTIFICIAL IMPLANT, DEVICE**
- **2. ANASTOMOSIS, BYPASS, OR GRAFT**
- **3. OSTOMY**
- **4. OTHER RESTORATIVE SURGERY**
- **5. AMPUTATION LIMB(S)**
- **6. ORGAN REMOVAL**
- **8. OTHER SPECIFIED PROCEDURES**
- **9. UNSPECIFIED PROCEDURE**

E879.# DUE TO OTHER PROCEDURE

4th Digit: E879

- **0. CARDIAC CATHETERIZATION**
- **1. KIDNEY DIALYSIS**
- **2. RADIOLOGICAL PROCEDURE**
- **3. SHOCK THERAPY**
- **4. ASPIRATION OF FLUID**
- **5. INSERTION OF GASTRIC OR DUODENAL SOUND**
- **6. URINARY CATHETERIZATION**
- **7. BLOOD SAMPLING**
- **8. OTHER SPECIFIED, BLOOD TRANSFUSION**
- **9. UNSPECIFIED PROCEDURE**

FALLS

FALLS FROM/INTO DIFFERENT LEVELS

E880.0 ESCALATOR
E880.1 CURB/SIDEWALK - NONMOVING
E880.9 STAIRS/STEPS
E881.0 LADDER
E881.1 SCAFFOLDING
E882 BUILDING OR STRUCTURE (FIRE ESCAPE)
E883.0 WATER/SWIMMING POOL
E883.1 WELL
E883.2 STORM DRAIN OR MANHOLE
E883.9 OTHER HOLE
E884.0 PLAYGROUND EQUIPMENT
E884.1 CLIFF
E884.2 CHAIR
E884.3 WHEELCHAIR
E884.4 BED
E884.5 OTHER FURNITURE
E884.6 COMMODE/TOILET
E884.9 FROM ONE LEVEL TO ANOTHER

FALLS FROM/INTO SAME LEVEL

E885 SIDEWALK - MOVING
E885 SLIPPING OR TRIPPING
E886.0 SPORTS (COLLISION)
E886.9 OTHER AND UNSPECIFIED COLLISION

FALLS UNSPECIFIED

E887 FRACTURE CAUSE UNSPECIFIED
E888 OTHER AND UNSPECIFIED FALL

FIRE

CONFLAGRATION/UNCONTROLLED FIRE

IN ORDER TO IDENTIFY A CONFLAGRATION/UNCONTROLLED FIRE IN A BUILDING WHERE A PATIENT IS ACCIDENTALLY STRUCK BY A FALLING OBJECT, USE CODE E916 STRUCK BY FALLING OBJECT AS AN ADDITIONAL CODE.

E890.# PRIVATE DWELLING
E891.# OTHER OR UNSPECIFIED BUILDING OR STRUCTURE
E892 NOT IN BUILDING OR STRUCTURE

4th Digit: E890 - E891

0. EXPLOSION
1. FUMES FROM PVC (POLYVINYLCHLORIDE)
2. OTHER SMOKE AND FUMES
3. BURNING
8. OTHER ACCIDENT (FALL, COLLAPSE, NONTHERMAL INJURY)
9. UNSPECIFIED

CONTROLLED FIRE

E893.# IGNITION OF CLOTHING

4th Digit: E893

0. FIREPLACE, STOVE, FURNACE, ETC. IN PRIVATE DWELLING
1. FIREPLACE, STOVE, FURNACE, ETC. IN OTHER BUILDING OR STRUCTURE
2. BONFIRE, BRAZIER, TRASH FIRE, ETC. NOT IN BUILDING OR STRUCTURE
8. FROM OTHER SPECIFIED SOURCE
9. FROM UNSPECIFIED SOURCE

E894 IGNITION OF HIGHLY FLAMMABLE MATERIAL
E895 PRIVATE DWELLING - FIREPLACE, FURNACE, STOVE, ETC.
E896 OTHER BUILDING OR STRUCTURE - FIREPLACE, FURNACE, STOVE, ETC.
E897 NOT IN BUILDING OR STRUCTURE - BONFIRE, BRAZIER, TRASH FIRE ETC.

FIRE (continued)

OTHER FIRE

E898.0 BURNING OF BEDCLOTHES
E898.1 OTHER FIRE (CIGARETTES, BLOWTORCH, LIGHTER,ETC.)
E899 UNSPECIFIED FIRE

ENVIRONMENTAL-EXPOSURE INJURIES

E900.# HEAT

4th Digit: E900

0. WEATHER
1. MAN MADE ORIGIN
9. UNSPECIFIED ORIGIN

E901.# COLD

4th Digit: E901

0. WEATHER
1. MAN MADE ORIGIN
8. OTHER SPECIFIED ORIGIN
9. UNSPECIFIED ORIGIN

E902.# AIR PRESSURE

4th Digit: E902

0. HIGH ALTITUDE
1. IN AIRCRAFT
2. DIVING
8. OTHER SPECIFIED CAUSES
9. UNSPECIFIED CAUSE

E903 TRAVEL AND MOTION
E904.# HUNGER, THIRST, EXPOSURE, NEGLECT

4th Digit: E904

0. ABANDONMENT/NEGLECT OF INFANT OR HELPLESS
1. LACK OF FOOD
2. LACK OF WATER
3. EXPOSURE TO WEATHER NEC
9. DESTITUTION OR ECONOMIC CIRCUMSTANCE

INJURIES CAUSED BY PLANTS OR ANIMALS

E905.# VENOMOUS

4th Digit: E905

- 0. SNAKES OR LIZARDS
- 1. SPIDERS
- 2. SCORPION
- 3. BEES, WASPS, HORNETS
- 4. CENTIPEDE OR MILLIPEDE
- 5. OTHER ARTHROPODS
- 6. MARINE ANIMALS OR PLANTS
- 7. POISONING OR TOXIC REACTION TO OTHER PLANTS
- 8. OTHER SPECIFIED
- 9. UNSPECIFIED

E906.# NONVENOMOUS

4th Digit: E906

- 0. DOG BITE
- 1. RAT BITE
- 2. SNAKES OR LIZARDS
- 3. ANIMAL-NON INSECT
- 4. ARTHROPOD (INSECT)
- 5. UNSPECIFIED ANIMAL (ANIMAL BITE NOS)
- 8. OTHER SPECIFIED INJURY CAUSED BY ANIMAL (FALL, BUTTED, ETC.)
- 9. UNSPECIFIED INJURY CAUSED BY ANIMAL

NATURAL CATACLYSMS

E907 LIGHTNING

IN ORDER TO IDENTIFY STORMS OR EARTH SURFACE MOVEMENTS WHERE A PATIENT IS ACCIDENTALLY STRUCK BY A FALLING OBJECT, USE CODE E916 STRUCK BY FALLING OBJECT AS AN ADDITIONAL CODE.

E908.# STORM OR FLOOD FROM STORM

4th Digit: E908

- 0. HURRICANE, STORM SURGE, TIDAL WAVE FROM STORM (TROPICAL), TYPHOON
- 1. TORNADO, CYCLONE, TWISTER
- 2. FLOODS, TORRENTIAL RAINFALL, FLASH FLOOD
- 3. BLIZZARD (SNOW) (ICE)
- 4. DUST STORM
- 8. OTHER STORM (CLOUDBURST)
- 9. UNSPECIFIED STORM OR FLOOD FROM STORM

E909.# EARTH SURFACE MOVEMENTS AND ERUPTIONS

4th Digit: E909

- 0. EARTHQUAKES
- 1. VOLCANIC ERUPTIONS, LAVA BURNS, ASH INHALATION
- 2. AVALANCHE (SNOW), LANDSLIDE, MUDSLIDE
- 3. COLLAPSE DAM OR MAN-MADE STRUCTURE CAUSING FLOOD
- 4. TIDALWAVE FROM EATHQUAKE, TIDALWAVE NOS, TSUNAMI
- 8. OTHER SPECIFIED EARTH MOVEMENTS AND ERUPTIONS
- 9. UNSPECIFIED EARTH MOVEMENTS AND ERUPTIONS

NATURAL CATACLYSMS (continued)

E910.# DROWNING SUBMERSION

4th Digit: E910

- 0. WATER SKIING
- 1. SCUBA OR SKIN DIVING (RECREATIONAL)
- 2. SWIMMING, FISHING, ETC.
- 3. SWIMMING/DIVING - COMMERCIALLY
- 4. IN BATHTUB
- 8. OTHER SPECIFIED (SWIMMING POOL OR FALL INTO WATER)
- 9. UNSPECIFIED (DROWNING NOS)

RESPIRATORY OBSTRUCTION

E911 FOOD

E912 OTHER OBJECT INHALED OR ASPIRATED

E913.# MECHANICAL SUFFOCATION

4th Digit: E913

- 0. BED OR CRADLE
- 1. PLASTIC BAG
- 2. ENCLOSURE OR INSUFFICIENT AIR SUPPLY (REFRIGERATOR OR DIVING WITH INSUFFICIENT AIR SUPPLY)
- 3. FALLING EARTH OR CAVE IN
- 8. OTHER MEANS OR HANGING
- 9. UNSPECIFIED (STRANGULATION, SUFFOCATION NOS)

FOREIGN BODY

E914 EYE OR ADNEXA

E915 OTHER ORIFICE

STRUCK BY

WHEN USING CODE [E916] STRUCK BY FALLING OBJECT, CODE FIRST THE REASON FOR THE FALLING OBJECT, IE. COLLAPSE OF BUILDING ON FIRE, NATURAL CATACLYSMS OR OTHER ACCIDENTS.

E916 FALLING OBJECT

OTHER ACCIDENTS

IN ORDER TO IDENTIFY AN ACCIDENT WHERE A PATIENT IS ACCIDENTALLY STRUCK BY A FALLING OBJECT USE CODE E916 STRUCK BY FALLING OBJECT AN AN ADDITIONAL CODE.

E917.# STRIKING AGAINST OR BY PERSONS OR OBJECTS (KICKING, THROWN, ETC.)
4th Digit: E917
- **0. SPORTS**
- **1. CAUSED BY CROWD OR PANIC**
- **2. RUNNING WATER**
- **9. OTHER**

E918 CRUSHED OR CAUGHT BETWEEN OBJECTS

E919.# CAUSED BY MACHINERY
4th Digit: E919
- **0. AGRICULTURAL**
- **1. MINING OR EARTH DRILLING**
- **2. LIFTING MACHINES OR APPLIANCES**
- **3. METALWORKING MACHINES**
- **4. WOODWORKING MACHINES**
- **5. NONELECTRIC MOTORS, TURBINES, OR ENGINES**
- **6. TRANSMISSION MACHINERY (BELTS PULLEYS, GEARS, ETC.)**
- **7. EARTH MOVING EQUIPMENT**
- **8. OTHER SPECIFIED (MACHINES USED IN MANUFACTURING, PRINTING, ETC.)**
- **9. UNSPECIFIED MACHINERY**

E920.# CAUSED BY CUTTING OR PIERCING EQUIPMENT
4th Digit: E920
- **0. POWERED LAWNMOWER**
- **1. POWERED HAND TOOLS**
- **2. HOUSEHOLD APPLIANCES**
- **3. KNIVES, SWORDS, DAGGERS**
- **4. OTHER HAND TOOLS, NEEDLE (SEWING)**
- **5. HYPODERMIC NEEDLE, CONTAMINATED NEEDLE, NEEDLE STICK**
- **8. OTHER SPECIFIED (GLASS, NAIL, THORN, ETC.)**
- **9. UNSPECIFIED CUTTING OR PIERCING INSTRUMENT**

E921.# CAUSED BY EXPLOSION OF PRESSURE VESSEL
4th Digit: E921
- **0. BOILERS**
- **1. GAS OR AIR TANKS**
- **8. OTHER SPECIFIED (AEROSOL CAN, TIRE, PRESSURE COOKER)**
- **9. UNSPECIFIED PRESSURE VESSEL**

E922.# FIREARM AND AIR GUN MISSILE
4th Digit: E922
- **0. HANDGUN**
- **1. SHOTGUN**
- **2. HUNTING RIFLE**
- **3. MILITARY RIFLE**
- **4. AIR GUN, BB GUN, PELLET GUN**
- **8. OTHER SPECIFIED FIREARM (FLAREGUN)**
- **9. UNSPECIFIED (GUNSHOT NOS)**

E923.# EXPLOSIVES
4th Digit: E923
- **0. FIREWORKS**
- **1. BLASTING MATERIALS**
- **2. EXPLOSIVE GASES**
- **8. OTHER SPECIFIED (BOMBS, MINES, ETC.)**
- **9. UNSPECIFIED EXPLOSION (EXPLOSION NOS)**

OTHER ACCIDENTS (continued)

E924.# CAUSED BY CAUSTICS, CORROSIVES, STEAM, HOT OBJECTS
4th Digit: E924
- **0. HOT VAPORS, LIQUIDS, STEAM**
- **1. CAUSTICS, ACIDS, CORROSIVES**
- **2. HOT (BOILING) TAP WATER**
- **8. BURN BY OTHER HOT OBJECT**
- **9. UNSPECIFIED**

E925.# ELECTRICAL
4th Digit: E925
- **0. DOMESTIC WIRING**
- **1. POWER LINES, GENERATORS, POWER STATIONS**
- **2. INDUSTRIAL WIRING, APPLIANCES, ELECTRICAL MACHINERY**
- **8. OTHER ELECTRICAL CURRENT (FARM, RESIDENTIAL, SCHOOL, PUBLIC BUILDINGS)**
- **9. UNSPECIFIED (ELECTROCUTION NOS)**

E926.# RADIATION
4th Digit: E926
- **0. RADIOFREQUENCY (MICROWAVE, RADAR, TRANSMITTERS)**
- **1. INFRARED HEATERS AND LAMPS**
- **2. VISIBLE AND ULTRAVIOLET LIGHT (ARC LAMP, WELDER, SUN)**
- **3. X-RAYS AND IONIZING RADIATION**
- **4. LASERS**
- **5. RADIOACTIVE ISOTOPES**
- **8. OTHER SPECIFIED RADIATION (BETATRONS, SYNCHROTRONS)**
- **9. UNSPECIFIED RADIATION**

E927 OVEREXERTION AND STRENUOUS MOVEMENTS

E928.# OTHER ENVIRONMENTAL CAUSES
4th Digit: E928
- **0. WEIGHTLESSNESS**
- **1. NOISE EXPOSURE**
- **2. VIBRATION**
- **8. OTHER SPECIFIED**
- **9. UNSPECIFIED ACCIDENT (ACCIDENT NOS, NATURAL FACTOR NEC)**

LATE EFFECTS

E929.# LATE EFFECTS OF ACCIDENTAL INJURY
4th Digit: E929
- **0. MVA (MOTOR VEHICLE ACCIDENT)**
- **1. OTHER TRANSPORT**
- **2. POISONING**
- **3. FALL**
- **4. FIRE**
- **5. NATURAL AND ENVIRONMENTAL FACTORS**
- **8. OTHER ACCIDENTS**
- **9. UNSPECIFIED ACCIDENT**

E959 LATE EFFECTS OF SELF INFLICTED INJURY

E969 LATE EFFECTS ASSAULT INJURIES

E977 LATE EFFECTS INJURIES DUE TO LEGAL INTERVENTION

E989 LATE EFFECTS INJURY UNDETERMINED WHETHER SELF INFLICTED OR PURPOSELY

E999 LATE EFFECTS WAR INJURIES

ADVERSE EFFECT (DRUGS, MEDICINAL AND BIOLOGICAL SUBSTANCES - THERAPEUTIC USE)

E930.# ANTIBIOTICS

4th Digit: E930

0. PENICILLINS
1. ANTIFUNGAL ANTIBIOTICS
2. CHLORAMPHENICOL GROUP
3. ERYTHROMYCIN AND OTHER MACROLIDES
4. TETRACYCLINE GROUP
5. CEPHALOSPORIN GROUP
6. ANTIMYCOBACTERIAL ANTIBIOTICS
7. ANTINEOPLASTIC ANTIBIOTICS
8. OTHER SPECIFIED ANTIBIOTICS
9. UNSPECIFIED ANTIBIOTICS

E931.# OTHER ANTI-INFECTIVES

4th Digit: E931

0. SULFONAMIDES
1. ARSENICAL ANTI-INFECTIVES
2. HEAVY METAL ANTI-INFECTIVES
3. QUINOLINE AND HYDROXYQUINOLINE DERIVATIVES
4. ANTIMALARIALS AND DRUGS ACTING ON OTHER BLOOD PROTOZOA
5. OTHER ANTIPROTOZOAL
6. ANTIHELMINTICS
7. ANTIVIRAL DRUGS
8. OTHER ANTIMYCOBACTERIAL DRUGS
9. OTHER AND NOS ANTI-INFECTIVES

E932.# HORMONES AND SYNTHETIC SUBSTITUTES

4th Digit: E932

0. ADRENAL CORTICAL STEROIDS
1. ANDROGENS AND ANABOLIC CONGENERS
2. OVARIAN HORMONES AND SYNTHETIC SUBSTITUTES
3. INSULINS AND ANTIDIABETIC AGENTS
4. ANTERIOR PITUITARY HORMONES
5. POSTERIOR PITUITARY HORMONES
6. PARATHYROID/PARATHYROID DERIVATIVES
7. THYROID/THYROID DERIVATIVES
8. ANTITHYROID AGENTS
9. OTHER AND NOS HORMONES / SYNTHETIC SUBSTITUTES

E933.# SYSTEMIC AGENTS

4th Digit: E933

0. ANTIALLERGIC AND ANTIEMETIC DRUGS
1. ANTINEOPLASTIC AND IMMUNOSUPPRESSIVE DRUGS
2. ACIDIFYING AGENTS
3. ALKALIZING AGENTS
4. ENZYMES NEC
5. VITAMINS NEC
8. OTHER SYSTEMIC AGENTS NEC
9. NOS SYSTEMIC AGENT

ADVERSE EFFECT (DRUGS, MEDICINAL AND BIOLOGICAL SUBSTANCES - THERAPEUTIC USE) (continued)

E934.# AGENTS AFFECTING BLOOD CONSTITUENTS

4th Digit: E934

0. IRON AND ITS COMPOUNDS
1. LIVER PREPARATIONS AND OTHER ANTIANEMIC AGENTS
2. ANTICOAGULANTS
3. VITAMIN K (PHYTONADIONE)
4. FIBRINOLYSIS-AFFECTING DRUGS
5. ANTICOAGULANT ANTAGONISTS AND OTHER COAGULANTS
6. GAMMA GLOBULIN
7. NATURAL BLOOD AND BLOOD PRODUCTS
8. OTHER AGENTS AFFECTING BLOOD CONSTITUENTS
9. NOS AGENT AFFECTING BLOOD CONSTITUENTS

E935.# ANALGESICS, ANTIPYRETICS, ANTIRHEUMATICS

4th Digit: E935

0. HEROIN
1. METHADONE
2. OTHER OPIATES AND RELATED NARCOTICS
3. SALICYLATES
4. AROMATIC ANALGESICS NEC
5. PYRAZOLE DERIVATIVES
6. ANTIRHEUMATICS (ANTIPHLOGISTICS)
7. OTHER NON-NARCOTIC
8. OTHER SPECIFIED
9. UNSPECIFIED

E936.# ANTICONVULSANTS ANTI-PARKINSONISM

4th Digit: E936

0. OXAZOLIDINE
1. HYDANTOIN
2. SUCCINIMIDES
3. OTHER AND NOS ANTICONVULSANTS
4. ANTI-PARKINSONISM

E937.# SEDATIVES AND HYPNOTICS

4th Digit: E937

0. BARBITURATES
1. CHLORAL HYDRATE
2. PARALDEHYDE
3. BROMINE COMPOUNDS
4. METHAQUALONE
5. GLUTETHIMIDE
6. MIXED SEDATIVES
8. OTHER SEDATIVES AND HYPNOTICS
9. UNSPECIFIED SEDATIVES

E938.# OTHER CENTRAL NERVOUS SYSTEM DEPRESSANTS AND ANESTHETICS

4th Digit: E938

0. MUSCLE-TONE DEPRESSANTS
1. HALOTHANE
2. OTHER GASEOUS ANESTHETICS
3. INTRAVENOUS ANESTHETICS
4. OTHER AND NOS GENERAL ANESTHETICS
5. SURFACE AND INFILTRATION ANESTHETICS
6. PERIPHERAL NERVE-PLEXUS BLOCKING ANESTHETICS
7. SPINAL ANESTHETICS
9. OTHER AND NOS LOCAL ANESTHETICS

ADVERSE EFFECT (DRUGS, MEDICINAL AND BIOLOGICAL SUBSTANCES - THERAPEUTIC USE) (continued)

E939.# PSYCHOTROPIC AGENTS

4th Digit: E939

- **0. ANTIDEPRESSANTS**
- **1. PHENOTHIAZINE-BASED TRANQUILIZERS**
- **2. BUTYROPHENONE-BASED TRANQUILIZERS**
- **3. OTHER ANTIPSYCHOTICS, NEUROLEPTICS AND MAJOR TRANQUILIZERS**
- **4. BENZODIAZEPINE-BASED TRANQUILIZERS**
- **5. OTHER TRANQUILIZERS**
- **6. PSYCHODYSLEPTICS (HALLUCINOGENS)**
- **7. PSYCHOSTIMULANTS**
- **8. OTHER PSYCHOTROPIC AGENTS**
- **9. NOS PSYCHOTROPIC AGENT**

E940.# CENTRAL NERVOUS STIMULANTS

4th Digit: E940

- **0. ANALEPTICS**
- **1. OPIATE ANTAGONISTS**
- **8. OTHER SPECIFIED CENTRAL NERVOUS SYSTEM STIMULANTS**
- **9. NOS CENTRAL NERVOUS SYSTEM STIMULANT**

E941.# AUTONOMIC NERVOUS SYSTEM

4th Digit: E941

- **0. PARASYMPATHOMIMETICS (CHOLINERGICS)**
- **1. PARASYMPATHOLYTICS (ANTICHOLINERGICS AND ANTIMUSCARINICS) AND SPASMOLYTICS**
- **2. SYMPATHOMIMETICS (ADRENERGICS)**
- **3. SYMPATHOLYTICS (ANTIADRENERGICS)**
- **9. NOS DRUG AFFECTING THE AUTONOMIC NERVOUS SYSTEM**

E942.# AFFECTING CARDIOVASCULAR SYSTEM

4th Digit: E942

- **0. CARDIAC RHYTHM REGULATOR**
- **1. CARDIOTONIC GLYCOSIDES AND DRUGS OF SIMILAR ACTION**
- **2. ANTILIPEMIC AND ANTIARTERIOSCLEROTIC DRUGS**
- **3. GANGLION-BLOCKING AGENTS**
- **4. CORONARY VASODILATORS**
- **5. OTHER VASODILATORS**
- **6. OTHER ANTIHYPERTENSIVE AGENTS**
- **7. ANTIVARICOSE DRUGS INCLUDING SCLEROSING AGENTS**
- **8. CAPILLARY-ACTIVE DRUGS**
- **9. OTHER AND NOS**

E943.# AGENTS PRIMARILY AFFECTING GASTROINTESTINAL SYSTEM

4th Digit: E943

- **0. ANTACIDS AND ANTIGASTRIC SECRETION DRUGS**
- **1. IRRITANT CATHARTICS**
- **2. EMOLLIENT CATHARTICS**
- **3. OTHER CATHARTICS, INCLUDING INTESTINAL ATONIA DRUGS**
- **4. DIGESTANTS**
- **5. ANTIDIARRHEAL DRUGS**
- **6. EMETICS**
- **8. OTHER SPECIFIED**
- **9. UNSPECIFIED**

ADVERSE EFFECT (DRUGS, MEDICINAL AND BIOLOGICAL SUBSTANCES - THERAPEUTIC USE) (continued)

E944.# WATER, MINERAL, AND URIC ACID METABOLISM DRUGS

4th Digit: E944

- **0. MERCURIAL DIURETICS**
- **1. PURINE DERIVATIVE DIURETICS**
- **2. CARBONIC ACID ANHYDRASE INHIBITORS**
- **3. SALURETICS**
- **4. OTHER DIURETICS**
- **5. ELECTROLYTIC, CALORIC, AND WATER-BALANCE AGENTS**
- **6. OTHER MINERAL SALTS, NEC**
- **7. URIC ACID METABOLISM DRUGS**

E945.# AGENTS PRIMARILY ACTING ON THE SMOOTH AND SKELETAL MUSCLES AND RESPIRATORY SYSTEM

4th Digit: E945

- **0. OXYTOCIC AGENTS**
- **1. SMOOTH MUSCLE RELAXANTS**
- **2. SKELETAL MUSCLE RELAXANTS**
- **3. OTHER AND NOS DRUGS ACTING ON MUSCLES**
- **4. ANTITUSSIVES**
- **5. EXPECTORANTS**
- **6. ANTI-COMMON COLD DRUGS**
- **7. ANTIASTHMATICS**
- **8. OTHER AND NOS RESPIRATORY DRUGS**

E946.# AGENTS PRIMARILY AFFECTING SKIN AND MUCOUS MEMBRANE: OPHTHALMOLOGICAL, DENTAL , AND OTORHINOLARYNGOLOGICAL DRUGS

4th Digit: E946

- **0. LOCAL ANTI-INFECTIVES AND ANTI-INFLAMMATORY DRUGS**
- **1. ANTIPRURITICS**
- **2. LOCAL ASTRINGENTS AND LOCAL DETERGENTS**
- **3. EMOLLIENTS, DEMULCENTS, AND PROTECTANTS**
- **4. KERATOLYTICS, KERATOPLASTICS, OTHER HAIR TREATMENT DRUGS AND PREPARATIONS**
- **5. EYE ANTI-INFECTIVES AND OTHER EYE DRUGS**
- **6. ANTI-INFECTIVES AND OTHER DRUGS AND PREPARATIONS FOR EAR, NOSE, AND THROAT**
- **7. DENTAL DRUGS TOPICALLY APPLIED**
- **8. OTHER AGENTS PRIMARILY AFFECTING SKIN AND MUCOUS MEMBRANE**
- **9. NOS AGENT PRIMARILY AFFECTING SKIN AND MUCOUS MEMBRANE**

E947.# OTHER AND NOS DRUGS AND MEDICINAL SUBSTANCES

4th Digit: E947

- **0. DIETETICS**
- **1. LIPOTROPIC DRUGS**
- **2. ANTIDOTES AND CHELATING AGENTS, NEC**
- **3. ALCOHOL DETERRENTS**
- **4. PHARMACEUTICAL EXCIPIENTS**
- **8. OTHER DRUGS AND MEDICINAL SUBSTANCES**
- **9. NOS DRUG OR MEDICINAL SUBSTANCE**

ADVERSE EFFECT (DRUGS, MEDICINAL AND BIOLOGICAL SUBSTANCES - THERAPEUTIC USE) (continued)

E948.# BACTERIAL VACCINES

4th Digit: E948

0. BCG VACCINE
1. TYPHOID AND PARATYPHOID
2. CHOLERA
3. PLAGUE
4. TETANUS
5. DIPHTHERIA
6. PERTUSSIS VACCINE, INCLUDING COMBINATIONS WITH A PERTUSSIS COMPONENT
8. OTHER AND NOS BACTERIAL VACCINES
9. MIXED BACTERIAL VACCINES, EXCEPT COMBINATIONS WITH A PERTUSSIS COMPONENT

E949.# OTHER VACCINES AND BIOLOGICAL SUBSTANCES

4th Digit: E949

0. SMALLPOX VACCINE
1. RABIES VACCINE
2. TYPHUS VACCINE
3. YELLOW FEVER VACCINE
4. MEASLES VACCINE
5. POLIOMYELITIS VACCINE
6. OTHER AND NOS VIRAL AND RICKETTSIAL VACCINES
7. MIXED VIRAL-RICKETTSIAL AND BACTERIAL VACCINES, EXCEPT COMBINATIONS WITH A PERTUSSIS COMPONENT
9. OTHER AND NOS VACCINES AND BIOLOGICAL SUBSTANCES

SUICIDE AND SELF INFLICTED INJURY

E950.# POISONING BY SOLID OR LIQUID SUBSTANCES

4th Digit: E950

0. ANALGESICS, ANTIPYRETICS, ANTIRHEUMATICS
1. BARBITURATES
2. SEDATIVES HYPNOTICS
3. TRANQUILIZERS OR OTHER PSYCHOTROPICS
4. OTHER DRUGS AND MEDICINE
5. UNSPECIFIED DRUG OR MEDICINE
6. AGRICULTURAL CHEMICALS AND PHARMACEUTICALS OTHER THAN FERTILIZERS AND PLANT FOODS
7. CORROSIVES AND CAUSTICS
8. ARSENIC OR ARSENIC COMPOUNDS
9. OTHER AND UNSPECIFIED SOLID AND LIQUID COMPOUNDS

E951.# POISONING GASES IN DOMESTIC USE

4th Digit: E951

0. DISTRIBUTED BY PIPELINE
1. IN MOBILE CONTAINERS
8. OTHER UTILITY GAS

E952.# POISONING BY OTHER GASES AND VAPORS

4th Digit: E952

0. MOTOR VEHICLE EXHAUST
1. OTHER CARBON MONOXIDE
8. OTHER SPECIFIED GASES AND VAPORS
9. UNSPECIFIED GASES AND VAPORS

E953.# HANGING, STRANGULATION, SUFFOCATION

4th Digit: E953

0. HANGING
1. BY PLASTIC BAG
8. OTHER SPECIFIED MEANS
9. UNSPECIFIED MEANS

E954 DROWNING OR SUBMERSION

E955.# FIREARMS, AIR GUNS OR EXPLOSIVES

4th Digit: E955

0. HANDGUN
1. SHOTGUN
2. HUNTING RIFLE
3. MILITARY FIREARM
4. OTHER AND UNSPECIFIED FIREARM
5. EXPLOSIVES
6. AIR GUN, BB GUN, PELLET GUN
9. UNSPECIFIED

E956 CUTTING OR PIERCING INSTRUMENT

E957.# JUMPING FROM HIGH PLACE

4th Digit: E957

0. RESIDENTIAL
1. OTHER MAN MADE STRUCTURE
2. NATURAL SITES
9. UNSPECIFIED

E958.# OTHER OR UNSPECIFIED MEANS

4th Digit: E958

0. JUMPING BEFORE MOVING OBJECT
1. FIRE
2. SCALD
3. EXTREMES OF COLD
4. ELECTROCUTION
5. CRASHING MOTOR VEHICLE
6. CRASHING AIRCRAFT
7. CAUSTICS (EXCEPT POISONING)
8. OTHER SPECIFIED MEANS
9. UNSPECIFIED MEANS

ASSAULT

E960.0 FIGHT OR BRAWL
E960.1 RAPE OR SODOMY
E961 ASSAULT BY CAUSTIC OR CORROSIVES EXCEPT POISONING
E962.# POISONING
4th Digit: E962
- **0. DRUGS OR MEDICINE**
- **1. OTHER SOLID OR LIQUIDS**
- **2. OTHER GASES OR VAPORS**
- **9. UNSPECIFIED POISONING**

E963 HANGING OR STRANGULATION
E964 DROWNING
E965.# FIREARMS OR EXPLOSIVES
4th Digit: E965
- **0. HANDGUN**
- **1. SHOTGUN**
- **2. HUNTING RIFLE**
- **3. MILITARY FIREARM**
- **4. OTHER AND UNSPECIFIED FIREARM**
- **5. ANTIPERSONNEL BOMB**
- **6. GASOLINE BOMB**
- **7. LETTER BOMB**
- **8. OTHER EXPLOSIVE**
- **9. UNSPECIFIED EXPLOSIVE**

E966 CUTTING OR PIERCING INSTRUMENT
E967.# ADULT OR CHILD ABUSE
4th Digit: E967
- **0. BY FATHER OR STEPFATHER**
- **1. BY OTHER SPECIFIED PERSON**
- **2. BY MOTHER OR STEPMOTHER**
- **3. BY SPOUSE, EX-SPOUSE, PARTNER, OR EX-PARTNER**
- **4. BY CHILD**
- **5. BY SIBLING**
- **6. BY GRANDPARENT**
- **7. BY OTHER RELATIVE (GRANDCHILD)**
- **8. BY NON-RELATED CAREGIVER**
- **9. BY UNSPECIFIED PERSON**

E968.# BY OTHER SPECIFIED MEANS
4th Digit: E968
- **0. FIRE**
- **1. PUSHED FROM HIGH PLACE**
- **2. STRUCK BY BLUNT OR THROWN OBJECT**
- **3. HOT LIQUID**
- **4. CRIMINAL NEGLECT**
- **5. TRANSPORT VEHICLE PUSHED IN FRONT OF, THROWN FROM, DRAGGED OR RUN DOWN BY, OR COLLIDING WITH A MOVING VEHICLE**
- **6. AIR GUN, BB GUN, PELLET GUN**
- **8. OTHER SPECIFIED MEANS (HUMAN BITE)**
- **9. UNSPECIFIED MEANS**

INJURY DUE TO LEGAL INTERVENTION

E970 FIREARMS
E971 EXPLOSIVES
E972 GAS
E973 BLUNT TRAUMA
E974 CUTTING OR PIERCING INSTRUMENT
E975 OTHER SPECIFIED (BLOW OR MANHANDLING)
E976 UNSPECIFIED MEANS
E978 EXECUTION

INJURY UNDETERMINED WHETHER ACCIDENTAL

E980.# POISONING SOLIDS OR LIQUID SUBSTANCES
4th Digit: E980
- **0. ANALGESICS, ANTIPYRETICS, AND ANTIRHEUMATICS**
- **1. BARBITURATES**
- **2. OTHER SEDATIVES AND HYPNOTICS**
- **3. TRANQUILIZERS AND OTHER PSYCHOTROPIC AGENTS**
- **4. OTHER SPECIFIED DRUGS AND MEDICINE**
- **5. NOS DRUG OR MEDICINE**
- **6. CORROSIVE AND CAUSTIC SUBSTANCES**
- **7. AGRICULTURAL CHEMICALS AND PHARMACEUTICALS OTHER THAN FERTILIZERS AND PLANT FOODS**
- **8. ARSENIC AND ITS COMPOUNDS**
- **9. OTHER AND NOS SOLIDS AND LIQUIDS**

E981.# POISONING GASES IN DOMESTIC USE
4th Digit: E981
- **0. PIPELINE GAS**
- **1. LIQUEFIED PETROLEUM GAS DISTRIBUTED IN MOBILE CONTAINERS**
- **8. OTHER UTILITY GAS**

E982.# POISONING OTHER GASES
4th Digit: E982
- **0. MOTOR VEHICLE EXHAUST GAS**
- **1. OTHER CARBON MONOXIDE**
- **8. OTHER SPECIFIED GASES / VAPORS**
- **9. UNSPECIFIED GASES / VAPORS**

E983.# HANGING, STRANGULATION, SUFFOCATION
4th Digit: E983
- **0. HANGING**
- **1. SUFFOCATION BY PLASTIC BAG**
- **8. OTHER SPECIFIED MEANS**
- **9. UNSPECIFIED MEANS**

E984 DROWNING OR SUBMERSION
E985.# FIREARMS, AIR GUNS AND EXPLOSIVES
4th Digit: E985
- **0. HANDGUN**
- **1. SHOTGUN**
- **2. HUNTING RIFLE**
- **3. MILITARY FIREARM**
- **4. OTHER AND UNSPECIFIED FIREARM**
- **5. EXPLOSIVES**
- **6. AIR GUN, BB GUN, PELLET GUN**

E986 CUTTING OR PIERCING INSTRUMENTS
E987.# FALL FROM HIGH PLACE
4th Digit: E987
- **0. RESIDENTIAL**
- **1. OTHER MAN MADE STRUCTURE**
- **2. NATURAL SITES**
- **9. UNSPECIFIED**

E988.# OTHER OR UNSPECIFIED MEANS
4th Digit: E988
- **0. JUMPING BEFORE MOVING OBJECT**
- **1. FIRE**
- **2. SCALD**
- **3. EXTREMES OF COLD**
- **4. ELECTROCUTION**
- **5. CRASHING MOTOR VEHICLE**
- **6. CRASHING AIRCRAFT**
- **7. CAUSTICS (EXCEPT POISONING)**
- **8. OTHER SPECIFIED MEANS**
- **9. UNSPECIFIED MEANS**

WAR, INSURRECTION, MILITARY ACTION

E990.# AS A RESULT OF FIRE
4th Digit: E990
- **0. FROM GASOLINE BOMB**
- **9. FROM OTHER OR UNSPECIFIED SOURCE**

E991.# FROM BULLETS OR FRAGMENTS
4th Digit: E991
- **0. RUBBER BULLETS**
- **1. PELLETS (RIFLE)**
- **2. OTHER BULLETS**
- **3. ANTIPERSONNEL BOMB (FRAGMENTS)**
- **4. OTHER AND NOS FRAGMENTS**

E992 FROM EXPLOSION OF MARINE WEAPONS
E993 OTHER EXPLOSIONS
E994 DESTRUCTION OF AIRCRAFT
E995 OTHER AND UNSPECIFIED CONVENTIONAL WARFARE
E996 NUCLEAR WEAPONS
E997.# OTHER UNCONVENTIONAL WEAPONS
4th Digit: E997
- **0. LASERS**
- **1. BIOLOGICAL**
- **2. GAS OR CHEMICALS**
- **8. OTHER SPECIFIED UNCONVENTIONAL WARFARE**
- **9. UNSPECIFIED UNCONVENTIONAL WARFARE**

E998 INJURIES AFTER CESSATION OF HOSTILITIES

POISONING - ACCIDENTAL

E850.# ANALGESICS, ANTIPYRETICS, AND ANTIRHEUMATICS
4th Digit: E850
- **0. HEROIN**
- **1. METHADONE**
- **2. OTHER OPIATES AND RELATED NARCOTICS**
- **3. SALICYLATES**
- **4. AROMATIC ANALGESICS, NEC**
- **5. PYRAZOLE DERIVATIVES**
- **6. ANTIRHEUMATICS (ANTIPHLOGISTICS)**
- **7. OTHER NON-NARCOTIC ANALGESICS**
- **8. OTHER SPECIFIED ANALGESICS AND ANTIPYRETICS**
- **9. NOS ANALGESICS AND ANTIPYRETICS**

E851 BARBITURATES
E852.# OTHER SEDATIVES / HYPNOTICS
4th Digit: E852
- **0. CHLORAL HYDRATE GROUP**
- **1. PARALDEHYDE**
- **2. BROMINE COMPOUNDS**
- **3. METHAQUALONE COMPOUNDS**
- **4. GLUTETHIMIDE GROUP**
- **5. MIXED SEDATIVES, NEC**
- **8. OTHER SPECIFIED SEDATIVES / HYPNOTICS**
- **9. NOS SEDATIVE / HYPNOTIC**

E853.# TRANQUILIZERS
4th Digit: E853
- **0. PHENOTHIAZINE-BASED TRANQUILIZERS**
- **1. BUTYROPHENONE-BASED TRANQUILIZERS**
- **2. BENZODIAZEPINE-BASED TRANQUILIZERS**
- **8. OTHER SPECIFIED TRANQUILIZERS**
- **9. NOS TRANQUILIZER**

E854.# OTHER PSYCHOTROPIC AGENTS
4th Digit: E854
- **0. ANTIDEPRESSANTS**
- **1. PSYCHODYSLEPTICS (HALLUCINOGENS)**
- **2. PSYCHOSTIMULANTS**
- **3. CENTRAL NERVOUS SYSTEM STIMULANTS**
- **8. OTHER PSYCHOTROPIC AGENTS**

POISONING - ACCIDENTAL (continued)

E855.# OTHER DRUGS ACTING ON CENTRAL AND AUTONOMIC NERVOUS SYSTEM
4th Digit: E855
- **0. ANTICONVULSANT AND ANTI-PARKINSONISM DRUGS**
- **1. OTHER CNS DEPRESSANTS**
- **2. LOCAL ANESTHETICS**
- **3. PARASYMPATHOMIMETICS (CHOLINERGICS)**
- **4. PARASYMPATHOLYTICS (ANTICHOLINERGICS AND ANTIMUSCARINICS) AND SPASMOLYTICS**
- **5. SYMPATHOMIMETICS (ADRENERGICS)**
- **6. SYMPATHOLYTICS (ANTIADRENERGICS)**
- **8. OTHER SPECIFIED DRUGS ACTING ON CENTRAL AND AUTONOMIC NERVOUS SYSTEMS**
- **9. NOS DRUG ACTING ON CENTRAL AND AUTONOMIC NERVOUS SYSTEMS**

E856 ANTIBIOTICS
E857 OTHER ANTI-INFECTIVES
E858.# OTHER DRUGS
4th Digit: E858
- **0. HORMONES AND SYNTHETIC SUBSTITUTES**
- **1. PRIMARILY SYSTEMIC AGENTS**
- **2. AGENTS PRIMARILY AFFECTING BLOOD CONSTITUENTS**
- **3. AGENTS PRIMARILY AFFECTING CARDIOVASCULAR SYSTEM**
- **4. AGENTS PRIMARILY AFFECTING GASTROINTESTINAL SYSTEM**
- **5. WATER, MINERAL, AND URIC ACID MATABOLISM DRUGS**
- **6. AGENTS PRIMARILY ACTING ON THE SMOOTH AND SKELETAL MUSCLES AND RESPIRATORY SYSTEM**
- **7. AGENTS PRIMARILY AFFECTING SKIN AND MUCOUS MEMBRANE OPHTHALMOLOGICAL, OTORHINOLARYNGOLOGICAL, AND DENTAL DRUGS**
- **8. OTHER SPECIFIED DRUGS**
- **9. NOS DRUG**

E860.# ALCOHOL NEC
4th Digit: E860
- **0. ALCOHOLIC BEVERAGES**
- **1. OTHER AND NOS ETHYL ALCOHOL AND ITS PRODUCTS**
- **2. METHYL ALCOHOL**
- **3. ISOPROPYL ALCOHOL**
- **4. FUSEL ALCOHOL**
- **8. OTHER SPECIFIED ALCOHOLS**
- **9. NOS ALCOHOL**

E861.# CLEANSERS, POLISHES, DISINFECTANTS, PAINTS, VARNISHES
4th Digit: E861
- **0. SYNTHETIC DETERGENTS / SHAMPOOS**
- **1. SOAP PRODUCTS**
- **2. POLISHES**
- **3. OTHER CLEANSERS, POLISHES**
- **4. DISINFECTANTS**
- **5. LEAD PAINTS**
- **8. OTHER PAINTS / VARNISHES**
- **9. UNSPECIFIED**

E862.# PETROLEUM PRODUCTS OTHER SOLVENTS AND THEIR VAPORS NEC
4th Digit: E862
- **0. PETROLEUM SOLVENTS**
- **1. PETROLEUM FUELS AND CLEANERS**
- **2. LUBRICATING OILS**
- **3. PETROLEUM SOLIDS**
- **4. OTHER SPECIFIED SOLVENTS**
- **9. UNSPECIFIED SOLVENT**

POISONING - ACCIDENTAL (continued)

E863.# AGRICULTURAL, HORTICULTURAL CHEMICAL AND PHARMACEUTICAL PREPARATIONS OTHER THAN PLANT FOODS AND FERTILIZERS

4th Digit: E863

- **0. INSECTICIDES OF ORGANOCHLORINE COMPOUNDS**
- **1. INSECTICIDES OF ORGANOPHOSPHORUS COMPOUNDS**
- **2. CARBAMATES**
- **3. MIXTURES OF INSECTICIDES**
- **4. OTHER AND NOS INSECTICIDES**
- **5. HERBICIDES**
- **6. FUNGICIDES**
- **7. RODENTICIDES**
- **8. FUMIGANTS**
- **9. OTHER AND NOS**

E864.# CORROSIVES AND CAUSTICS, NEC

4th Digit: E864

- **0. CORROSIVE AROMATICS**
- **1. ACIDS**
- **2. CAUSTIC ALKALIS**
- **3. OTHER SPECIFIED CORROSIVES AND CAUSTICS**
- **4. NOS CORROSIVES AND CAUSTICS**

E865.# POISONOUS FOODSTUFFS AND POISONOUS PLANTS

4th Digit: E865

- **0. MEAT**
- **1. SHELLFISH**
- **2. OTHER FISH**
- **3. BERRIES AND SEEDS**
- **4. OTHER SPECIFIED PLANTS**
- **5. MUSHROOMS AND OTHER FUNGI**
- **8. OTHER SPECIFIED FOODS**
- **9. NOS FOODSTUFF OR POISONOUS PLANT**

E866.# OTHER AND NOS SOLID / LIQUID SUBSTANCES

4th Digit: E866

- **0. LEAD AND ITS COMPOUNDS AND FUMES**
- **1. MERCURY AND ITS COMPOUNDS AND FUMES**
- **2. ANTIMONY AND ITS COMPOUNDS AND FUMES**
- **3. ARSENIC AND ITS COMPOUNDS AND FUMES**
- **4. OTHER METALS AND THEIR COMPOUNDS AND FUMES**
- **5. PLANT FOODS AND FERTILIZERS**
- **6. GLUES AND ADHESIVES**
- **7. COSMETICS**
- **8. OTHER SPECIFIED SOLID OR LIQUID SUBSTANCES**
- **9. NOS SOLID OR LIQUID SUBSTANCE**

E867 GAS DISTRIBUTED BY PIPELINE

E868.# OTHER UTILITY GAS AND OTHER CARBON MONOXIDE

4th Digit: E868

- **0. LIQUEFIED PETROLEUM GAS DISTRIBUTED IN MOBILE CONTAINERS**
- **1. OTHER AND NOS UTILITY GAS**
- **2. MOTOR VEHICLE EXHAUST GAS**
- **3. CARBON MONOXIDE FROM INCOMPLETE COMBUSTION OTHER DOMESTIC FUELS**
- **8. CARBON MONOXIDE OTHER SOURCES**
- **9. NOS CARBON MONOXIDE**

E869.# OTHER GASES AND VAPORS

4th Digit: E869

- **0. NITROGEN OXIDES**
- **1. SULFUR DIOXIDE**
- **2. FREON**
- **3. LACRIMOGENIC GAS (TEAR GAS)**
- **4. TOBACCO SMOKE SECOND-HAND**
- **8. OTHER SPECIFIED GASES AND VAPORS**
- **9. NOS GASES AND VAPORS**

POISONING - ASSAULT

E962.# ASSAULT

4th Digit: E962

- **0. DRUGS OR MEDICINE**
- **1. OTHER SOLID OR LIQUIDS**
- **2. OTHER GASES OR VAPORS**
- **9. UNSPECIFIED POISONING**

POISONING - SUICIDE AND SELF INFLICTED INJURY

E950.# BY SOLID OR LIQUID SUBSTANCES

4th Digit: E950

- **0. ANALGESICS, ANTIPYRETICS, ANTIRHEUMATICS**
- **1. BARBITURATES**
- **2. SEDATIVES / HYPNOTICS**
- **3. TRANQUILIZERS OR OTHER PSYCHOTROPICS**
- **4. OTHER DRUGS AND MEDICINE**
- **5. UNSPECIFIED DRUG OR MEDICINE**
- **6. AGRICULTURAL CHEMICALS AND PHARMACEUTICALS OTHER THAN FERTILIZERS AND PLANT FOODS**
- **7. CORROSIVES AND CAUSTICS**
- **8. ARSENIC OR ARSENIC COMPOUNDS**
- **9. OTHER AND UNSPECIFIED SOLID AND LIQUID COMPOUNDS**

E951.# GASES IN DOMESTIC USE

4th Digit: E951

- **0. DISTRIBUTED BY PIPELINE**
- **1. IN MOBILE CONTAINERS**
- **8. OTHER UTILITY GAS**

E952.# BY OTHER GASES AND VAPORS

4th Digit: E952

- **0. MOTOR VEHICLE EXHAUST**
- **1. OTHER CARBON MONOXIDE**
- **8. OTHER SPECIFIED GASES AND VAPORS**
- **9. UNSPECIFIED GASES AND VAPORS**

POISONING - UNDETERMINED

E980.# SOLIDS OR LIQUID SUBSTANCES

4th Digit: E980

- **0. ANALGESICS, ANTIPYRETICS, AND ANTIRHEUMATICS**
- **1. BARBITURATES**
- **2. OTHER SEDATIVES AND HYPNOTICS**
- **3. TRANQUILIZERS AND OTHER PSYCHOTROPIC AGENTS**
- **4. OTHER SPECIFIED DRUGS AND MEDICINE**
- **5. NOS DRUG OR MEDICINE**
- **6. CORROSIVE AND CAUSTIC SUBSTANCES**
- **7. AGRICULTURAL CHEMICALS AND PHARMACEUTICALS OTHER THAN FERTILIZERS AND PLANT FOODS**
- **8. ARSENIC AND ITS COMPOUNDS**
- **9. OTHER AND NOS SOLIDS AND LIQUIDS**

E981.# GASES IN DOMESTIC USE

4th Digit: E981

- **0. PIPELINE GAS**
- **1. LIQUEFIED PETROLEUM GAS DISTRIBUTED IN MOBILE CONTAINERS**
- **8. OTHER UTILITY GAS**

E982.# OTHER GASES

4th Digit: E982

- **0. MOTOR VEHICLE EXHAUST GAS**
- **1. OTHER CARBON MONOXIDE**
- **8. OTHER SPECIFIED GASES / VAPORS**
- **9. UNSPECIFIED GASES / VAPORS**

APPENDIX B
CODING GUIDELINES

This section of coding guidelines is not intended to be a comprehensive tutorial on ICD-9 coding. This compilation of guidelines covers many of the basic principles of outpatient coding, including many of the topics most frequently requested on the Unicor Medical coding hotline and in our monthly newsletter. The information presented is based on official government and industry publications. We have made every attempt to assure that the information is accurate; however, no warranty or guarantee is given that this information is error-free and we accept no responsibility or liability should an error occur.

ETHICAL STANDARDS OF CODING

In this era of payment based on diagnostic and procedural coding, the professional ethics of health information continue to be challenged. The following standards for ethical coding were developed by the AHIMA (American Health Information Management Association) Council on Coding and Classification and approved by the AHIMA Board of Directors.

I. Diagnoses that are present on admission or diagnoses and procedures that occur during the current encounter are to be abstracted after a thorough review of the entire medical record. Those diagnoses not applicable to the current encounter should not be abstracted.

II. For Inpatient settings, the selection of the principal diagnosis and principal procedure, along with other diagnoses and procedures, must meet the definitions of the Uniform Hospital Discharge Data Set (UHDDS). *

III. Assessment must be made of the documentation in the chart to ensure that it is adequate and appropriate to support the diagnoses and procedures selected to be abstracted.

IV. Medical record coders should use their skills, their knowledge of ICD-9-CM and CPT, and any available resources to select diagnostic and procedural codes.

V. Medical record coders should not change codes or narratives of codes so that the meanings are misrepresented. Nor should diagnoses or procedures be included or excluded because the payment will be affected. Statistical clinical data is an important result of coding, and maintaining a quality database should be a conscientious goal.

VI. Physicians should be consulted for clarification when they enter conflicting or ambiguous documentation in the chart.

VII. The medical record coder is a member of the healthcare team and, as such, should assist physicians who are unfamiliar with ICD-9-CM, CPT, or DRG methodology by suggesting resequencing or inclusion of diagnoses or procedures when needed to more accurately reflect the occurrence of events during the encounter.

VIII. The medical record coder is expected to strive for the optimal payment to which the facility is legally entitled, but it is unethical and illegal to maximize payment by means that contradict regulatory guidelines.

Reprinted with permission from the American Health Information Management Association (AHIMA).

(* Note that for outpatient settings, the reason for the encounter is coded first. If the major work or effort is directed at at another diagnosis, however, that diagnosis may become primary.)

UNDERSTANDING WHAT YOU CODE

"Understand what you are coding" is perhaps one of the most fundamental rules of coding. This doesn't mean being able to diagnose patients or practice medicine, but you need to have some basic understanding of the diagnoses that you are coding. All too frequently the diagnosis the physician has written cannot be found exactly in the code book.

In these cases, it is very helpful to have access to a couple of reference books that can help you get on track and figure out other terminology that you may use to find the code. For starters, invest in comprehensive medical dictionary, The Merck Manual, and a good anatomy and physiology textbook. Make sure you also keep up to date on your reference books, always using the current edition. (And make sure you have a current ICD-9 book! The terminology for code descriptions changes from year to year.)

Remember that as a coder, your job is to accurately reflect what occurred in the encounter and show through coding the reasons for any procedure, and the complexity of any evaluation and management by utilizing proper coding. This requires that you have some basic understanding of the patient's situation along with some knowledge of basic coding rules.

Understanding what you're coding is especially important now that you're required to match your ICD-9 codes with your procedure codes. If you don't understand what the medical problem is or what the test, exam, or treatment is, how are you going to know what procedure was performed for which problem? Your reference books and your growing base of knowledge will prove invaluable resources.

DOCUMENTATION

When the physician does not provide enough information for the coder, the coder cannot provide enough information for the carrier. The physician must clearly and carefully document all diagnoses in detail so the coder can translate the information into specific and accurate codes reflecting as much detail and precision as the documentation and the ICD-9 system allows. Here are some responsibilities the physician has in order for the coder to be able to assign the correct codes:

Write legibly. Illegible handwriting holds up the coding/billing process.

Describe the patient's condition using terminology which includes specific diagnoses as well as symptoms, problems, or reasons for the encounter.

Remember you are submitting code numbers, not narrative descriptions. Somewhere in the patient documentation there must be specific and explicit information about what diagnoses were treated and what services were provided. Be clear and detailed, noting the site, type, cause, etc. that specifies the exact diagnosis-this is the information the coder must use to accurately translate the documentation into code numbers.

You must document all conditions or problems existing at the time of the visit that impact the treatment or management of the patient. The coder needs all this information in order to adequately convey the patient encounter to the carrier and to justify the services provided.

You must clearly denote which diagnosis or diagnoses are related to which procedure or procedures. The coder is required to link at least one diagnosis to each service billed for, and he or she needs some supporting documentation in order to correctly do this.

MEDICAL NECESSITY

Medical necessity is a determination that items or services furnished, or to be furnished, by any health care provider (for which third party payment may be made) are reasonable and medically necessary for the treatment provided for an illness or injury, for the improvement of function of a malformed body member or for prevention of an illness. Remember that medical necessity is determined by the diagnoses you submit. CPT may show the amount being charged, but ICD-9 diagnoses provides the information that determines whether or not payment will be made.

For years, HCFA has warned physicians to be specific and file correctly—this means document records fully, be unfailingly accurate with code assignments, use the correct amount of digits, correctly link your diagnosis code to the correct procedure code, and make sure you adequately show medical necessity with your diagnoses. The grace period is over. You will do it Medicare's way or suffer lowered reimbursement, claims rejection and worse.

CORRECT CODE VERSUS PAYABLE CODE

As health care data is used for more and more purposes, the demand for accuracy and quality continues to increase. Of course, one of the major purposes to providers is reimbursement.

Sometimes it is true that the correct code (the code that most accurately describes the patient encounter) is not necessarily a payable code (a code that a carrier will reimburse the physician for). It is the coder's job to assign the correct code on the patient's record; hopefully the correct code will also be a payable code. But the assignment must be based on what is correct, not what is payable. This rule applies to V-codes, "not elsewhere classified" codes, and "unspecified" codes.

If you submit a bill with an incorrect code, not only can the physician see repercussions (as in downcoding, rejection, inaccurate practice profile, and long-term audit risk), but the patient can, too.

The appropriate course of action is for physicians and coders to work together to correctly document and code each patient encounter. For each encounter, concentrate on choosing the correct code, not just the first similar code you come across, and not necessarily the code you know is payable.

BASIC CODING RULES

Outpatient coders: code first the diagnosis, condition, problem, or other reason for the encounter that is shown in the medical record to be chiefly responsible for the services provided. Then code additional diagnoses and co-existing conditions.

Inpatient coders: Follow UHDDS guidelines on selecting your principal diagnosis.

Code all current conditions and only current conditions that affect the treatment of the patient. Do not code conditions that have previously been treated and no longer exist, even if reference was made to their previous existence in the current record. (An exception to this would be in the case of late effects of previous injury or illness, or appropriate V-codes for history, family history or status codes.)

If a patient has a chronic disease, it can be coded on an ongoing basis as long as the patient is receiving treatment for the condition or it is a complicating factor that contributes to the complexity of the medical decision-making by the physician.

For physician billing, do not code diagnoses documented as suspected, probable, possible, or rule out as if they are established. If the physician does not document a definite diagnosis at the conclusion of a patient visit, you may code the chief complaint as the reason for the encounter.

Be sure to review the chart to get the details you need (cause, site, type, etc.) to assign the exact code. Don't hesitate to refer to a medical dictionary or a medical terminology book to verify the meanings or synonyms if necessary.

Be sure to check the accuracy of information such as patient's age and sex. You don't need this information to find the right codes, but it never hurts to make sure that you're not giving an obstetric code to one of your male patients or some other equally bizarre scenario that will almost assuredly be rejected by a carrier.

AVOID CODING FROM CONDENSED DIAGNOSIS LISTS

Code directly from the medical record. Don't rely solely on a diagnosis list from a superbill. For every diagnosis on the superbill, hundreds, sometimes thousands, are not on there. A condensed list cannot possibly contain the specificity required for accurate coding. Arthritis, for example, can be coded hundreds of different ways. By always coding with the appropriate acuity and specificity you will avoid setting a profile that causes either your treatment protocol or your billing practices to be questioned.

"RULE OUT", "PROBABLE", "POSSIBLE", "SUSPECTED" OR "VERSUS" CONDITIONS

When coding in an outpatient setting, conditions indicated by the terms, "rule out", "probable", "possible", "suspected", or "versus" should never be coded as though they exist. Though allowed in inpatient coding, (with some caveats on certain diseases such as epilepsy and AIDS), coding of these "rule out" conditions is never allowed in the outpatient setting. Assigning a code to these conditions that are unconfirmed permanently affixes these diagnoses to the patient's medical history with potentially serious medicolegal consequences for the physician and patient. Imagine the consequences of an insurance coverage denial for a "pre-existing" condition that was erroneously coded from a "rule out" statement.

ULTIMATE SPECIFICITY

Always code to ultimate specificity, using all the digits available for the code. Use as many digits in the code as there are digits offered. If you can use five digits, use five. If there are only four digits possible for a code, use all four. Only use three digits if there are no fourth or fifth digit options. Take the code to as many digits as you can.

Remember that each digit helps to specify the diagnosis further and explain to the carrier what the patient's situation is. The claim will not be processed by most carriers if it is not at ultimate specificity.

MULTIPLE CODING

The basic rule of multiple coding is this, be sure to fully code the patient's underlying problem(s) that were addressed along with any complications or conditions that contribute to their medical complexity.

Some examples of this would be fluid overload in a patient with CHF, pneumonia in a patient with COPD, influenza in a patient with asthma, fracture in a diabetic patient, a shunt/catheter infection in a dialysis patient in chronic renal failure, an open wound in a diabetic patient, a urinary tract infection in a patient who is pregnant, arm weakness in a patient with hypertension, or chest tightness in a patient who had previously suffered a myocardial infarction.

Multiple coding is also required for certain conditions when a single code does not fully identify the condition being coded. For instance, you need both 250.5# and 362.01 to correctly code diabetic retinopathy. The 250.5# shows the diabetes with ophthalmic manifestation, and the 362.01 shows the background retinopathy due to diabetes. As is customary in multiple coding, the underlying disease or the condition that the manisfestation is "due to" is coded first, (250.5# in this case).

Use multiple coding whenever applicable, but generally you should not code symptoms of a disease or a disorder. For example, if a patient is documented as having abdominal pain due to appendicitis, you code only the appendicitis, not the abdominal pain. Abdominal pain is intrinsic to the appendicitis, and therefore would not be coded.

Multiple coding is divided into three categories: multiple coding for multiple concurrent diagnoses ("due to" , "with" or "secondary to"), mandatory multiple coding, and discretionary multiple coding.

Multiple coding for multiple concurrent diagnoses
The phrase "due to" indicates a cause and effect relationship between the two diagnoses. You should code both the cause and the effect. For example, if a patient was diagnosed with urinary retention due to BPH, you would code both the urinary retention and the BPH.

600 BPH
788.2# urinary retention

When "with" is used in a diagnosis it means that both conditions are present together, so you'll need to use a code for each condition. For example, a diagnosis of neuritis with gout would need a code for neuritis and a code for gout.

274.89 neuritis
357.4 gout

Note that the exception to using multiple codes for multiple concurrent diagnoses is the case in which there is one ICD-9 code that incorporates each of the conditions under one description. One example is 402.91, the code for hypertensive heart disease with CHF. When a combination code exists for a condition with its manifestation/etiology no additional code is required.

Mandatory multiple coding
There are certain codes that will not stand alone. Both the underlying condition (etiology) and the specific manifestation must be coded, with the underlying disease sequenced first. For example, a diagnosis of diabetic gangrene requires a code for the diabetes, as the underlying disease, as well as a code for the gangrene.

250.7# diabetes
785.4 gangrene

GUIDELINES

Discretionary multiple coding
This type of multiple coding is also know as "use additional code, if desired." The additional code should be used if the physician documents on the medical record that it is present. Every essential part of a diagnosis should be coded in order to fully describe a patient encounter.

An example of discretionary multiple coding would be a diagnosis of peritonitis caused by staphylococcus aureus. The most effective coding for this disease would include two codes, one for peritonitis and one for the bacterial organism.

567.2 peritonitis
041.11 staphylococcus aureus

COMBINATION CODES

A combination code is a single code used to classify one of three things:

1. Two diagnoses at once, such as chronic cholecystitis with choledocholelithiasis, 574.40.

2. A diagnosis with an associated secondary process or manifestation, such as hypertensive CHF, 402.91.

3. An associated complication, such as arteriosclerotic gangrene of the extremities, 440.24.

You should assign a combination code only when the code fully identifies both conditions involved. If only one complication is present, do not use the combination code.

"UNSPECIFIED" (NOS) CODES

The NOS (not otherwise specified) or "unspecified" descriptions are used when the information in the record is not as specific as the information in the code book. For example, if you are simply given "osteoporosis" as the diagnosis, you must choose the NOS code for osteoporosis, 733.00, because you are not given enough information to correctly choose from the more specific listings for osteoporosis.
Be careful when choosing an NOS code. If you can follow up with the physician or get more information from the patient's chart so that you can specify the diagnosis more, do so. Carriers are reluctant to accept and/or pay for NOS codes, but if an NOS code is your only option based on the documentation that you have, you must use it.

"NOT ELSEWHERE CLASSIFIED" (NEC) CODES

NEC (not elsewhere classified) codes or "other specified" codes are used when the description you are given for the diagnosis is more specific than the descriptions for the codes in ICD-9. If there is not a specific code number for a particular condition, the coder must generally revert to an "other specified" or "NEC" code number from the category of condition that fits the closest. A diagnosis of breast calcification, for example would be coded to "other specified disorder of breast", or 611.8.

LATE EFFECTS

A late effect is a condition that is related to (but occurs after) an acute illness or injury that has been treated. Late effects are also called sequelae, residual effects or residual conditions. There is no set time period that must elapse before a sequelae becomes a late effect. Some residual conditions may appear immediately following injury or illness, (aphasia following cerebrovascular disease), and others may appear years following the illness or injury, (contractures forming after burns have been treated). Descriptive statements in the record such as "old", "late", "following", or "due to previous..." may be indicative of late effects that must be coded.

When you code a late effect, there are two codes you must use. First, you must use a code for the residual condition itself. This is the same code you usually would use for the current condition, but you do need to show that it is indeed a late effect. This is where the second code comes in. The second code is taken from the "late effect" section of Easy Coder. These codes generally are from 905 to 909, but there are some specific late effect codes that apply only to certain disease processes. Cerebrovascular disease, for example has its own codes that show the general class of residual condition in a combination code, (single number). These combination codes would not require an additional code from the 905 to 909 series of codes.

Following are some examples:

The diagnosis is malunion of a fractured femur shortly following the acute fracture. Code the malunion as a residual (733.81) and then add the code number for late effect of a fracture (905.4). Don't use the code for an acute fracture of the femur (821.00).

The diagnosis of brain damage following cerebral abscess six months earlier. Here are the codes:

348.9 brain damage
326 late effect abscess
intracranial

In almost every case you will sequence the actual residual condition first, followed by the "late effect" code to indicate the previous condition. Note, though, there are exceptions:

1. When the residual condition is not identified, as in "residual of traumatic amputation of arm," you obviously can't use a code for the residual because it is not specified. The only code you can use is the code identifying the previous condition, in this case 905.9 for late effect of a traumatic amputation.

2. When there is no code given in the "late" section that covers the previous condition you're looking for, you only need to use the code for the actual effect or residual condition.

3. If the coding book specifically indicates that the code for the previous condition should be sequenced first followed by the code for the late effect, do it that way.

4. If Easy Coder has a condition that is specified as "late" or "old", then this is considered to be a combination code and should be the only one used.

ADVERSE REACTIONS TO PROPERLY ADMINISTERED SUBSTANCES

One important rule to remember is the fact that an adverse reaction to a properly administered substance always requires two codes: one for the adverse reaction and one for the substance.

An adverse reaction is defined as a reaction to a correct substance properly administered. Adverse reactions are usually indicated in the diagnostic statement by one of the following terms: accumulative effect, intoxication due to, allergic reaction, idiosyncratic reaction, hypersensitivity, side effects, toxicity, synergistic reaction, or interaction between two drugs.

At least two codes are required to correctly code an adverse reaction. First, code the manifestation or condition caused by the drug—the adverse reaction itself. Second, code the substance or substances that caused the reaction; you'll do this using an E-code ranging from E930-E949 (Therapeutic Use) to indicate each substance involved.

Here are a couple of examples of correctly coding adverse reactions:

The diagnosis is dizziness due to valium taken as prescribed.

780.4 dizziness
E939.4 adverse effect of valium, therapeutic use

When the manifestation of an adverse reaction is not identified, use code 995.2. Then use the E-code for the substance as you normally would. Here's an example:

995.2 adverse reaction to drug
E930.0 penicillin–therapeutic use

The basic rule to remember about adverse reactions is to code both the reaction itself as well as the substance that caused the reaction. Use a diagnosis code for the exact adverse reaction, or use code 995.2 if no specific adverse reaction is specified. To identify the substance, use the corresponding E-code from the "therapeutic" column of the table of drugs and chemicals in the back of your ICD-9 book.

POISONINGS

A poisoning is any condition caused by drugs, medicines, or other chemical substances not used in accordance with the physician's instructions. Poisonings are identified in the diagnostic statement by the following terms: intoxication, overdose, poisoning, toxic effect, wrong dosage given in error, wrong dosage taken in error.

Drug interactions are also considered to be poisonings. For example, any condition caused by an interaction between a drug taken with alcohol or between prescribed drugs and nonprescribed drugs (over the counter medications) is considered a poisoning.

Poisonings due to drugs and related substances such as antibiotics, analgesics, and vaccinations are classified to categories 960-979. The table of drugs and chemicals also includes chemical substances that are non-medicinal in categories 980-989. This second category would include substances such as gases, acids, lead materials, and fumes. In both cases, the code you use will identify the type of substance that caused the poisoning.

To code a poisoning, use the table of drugs and chemicals in the back of your ICD-9 book the. First, identify the substance involved by looking it up alphabetically; beside the listing will be a code number for a poisoning due to this substance (960-989). For example, a valium overdose would be coded as follows:

969.4 valium poisoning

When a manifestation of the poisoning is identified, you should list the code for the manifestation in addition to the poison code. Remember that the poison code is always sequenced first and the manifestation code is always sequenced second. For example, here are the codes for a coma due to a valium overdose:

969.4 valium poisoning
780.01 coma

The use of E-codes to identify the external cause of the poisoning is the final step to fully coding poisonings. ICD-9 provides the following E-code categories for poisonings:

E850-869 accidental
E950-959 suicide and self-inflicted injury
E962 assault
E980-989 undetermined

Following are the codes for a patient in a coma due to a suicide attempt by valium overdose:

969.4 valium poisoning
780.01 coma
E950.3 suicide attempt-valium

To code a late effect of a poisoning, apply the same rules you would apply for coding late effects of an injury. The code identifying the residual effect is sequenced first, followed by the code for the late effect of the poisoning, and then the E-code for the late effect.

Here are the E-codes for late effects of poisonings:

E929 accidental
E959 self-inflicted
E969 assault
E989 undetermined

Here's an example of those codes in use for the diagnosis anoxic brain damage due to attempted suicide by barbiturate overdose four years ago:

348.1 anoxic brain damage
909.0 late effect poisoning
E959 late effect self-inflicted injury

V-CODES

The V-codes in ICD-9 CM are provided to identify health service encounters or contact with health services for reasons other than illness or injury. The following circumstances or problems are the primary reason for assigning V-codes:

1. When a person who is not currently sick encounters health services to act as an organ or tissue donor, the need for prophylactic vaccination, to discuss a problem, counseling, or health screenings.

2. When a person with known disease or injury (current, chronic or resolving) encounters health services for specific treatment of that disease or injury including aftercare, cast change, chemotherapy, dialysis, gastrostomy care/closure, or radiotherapy.

3. A. A circumstance or problem is present which influences the person's health status but is not a current illness or injury. Examples include alcoholism, family problems (reason for encounter), divorce estrangement (reason for encounter), and stress/unemployment problems (reason for encounter).

B. A circumstance or problem is present (the person may or may not currently be sick) and the V-code is assigned as an additional code to show a personal or family history of certain diseases or show a person with replacement status, such as heart valve (artificial)(prosthesis).

4. Newborn birth status.

Assignment of V-codes are appropriate both in the inpatient and outpatient setting but are particularly useful in coding ambulatory care encounters. V-codes indicate the reason for an encounter (V55.1 gastrostomy closure) and should not be confused with the procedure code that documents what procedure was actually performed.

Sequencing of V-codes may be first or second depending on the circumstances of the encounter.

V-code categories include:

1. Contact/exposure to communicable diseases

2. Need for inoculation and vaccination

3. Status: Indicates that a patient underwent a procedure that may influence future health or treatment.

4. History codes (personal) (family)
There are two types of history codes, personal and family. Personal history codes are valuable additional codes to denote past medical history of conditions that have been treated and for which no treatment is currently being rendered. However, the potential for recurrence is possible and the condition may need monitoring. History codes will usually be sequenced second. History codes may be assigned as additional codes on any record to provide further information regardless of the reason for the visit or whether the condition is still present or in any way alters the treatment provided.

5. Screening codes
Codes for screening exams are not assigned to individual tests administered to a patient to "screen for" a suspected condition. Screening exams are coded only when exams are used to screen for disease in defined population groups. The code does not in itself apply to any particular test or study.

(Remember, the testing of a person to rule out or confirm a suspected condition is usually done because there are some signs or symptoms to suspect a problem. This is a diagnostic exam, not a screening exam. In this case, do not assign a screening code, assign a code for the sign or symptoms.)

6. Observation codes
There are two categories of observation codes in ICD-9-CM. these codes are used only when a person is being observed for a suspected condition that is ruled out. These observation codes should not be used if an injury, illness, or any sign or symptom related to the suspected condition is present. In such cases, assign the diagnosis or symptom code with appropriate E-code.

7. Aftercare codes
Aftercare codes are codes that are used after the initial treatment of the acute disease or injury is completed and the patient requires continued care during the recovery period or care for long-term consequences of the original disease.

For routine visits for the purpose of changing surgical dressings, checking wound healing, or removing sutures form wounds without mention of complication, use code V58.3, attention to surgical dressings and sutures.

8. Follow-Up codes
V24.# and V67.# are used to explain continuing surveillance following completed treatment of a disease or injury. Follow-up codes denote that the condition has been satisfactorily treated and no longer exist. They are sequenced first and may be used with an additional history code to explain fully the healed condition.

9. Donor codes
V59.# or V59.## are not used for self-donation (autogenous) of tissue or organ, but rather for non-autogenous donation by other living individual who is donating tissue, blood, or other body tissue for person other than self.

10. Counseling codes
Counseling codes are used for counseling of a patient or patient's family member, following illness, injury or other type of family or social crisis. These codes are used when support is needed to assist the person in coping with their problem. Reference these codes under Counseling.

11. Reproduction and Development V-codes
V-codes for obstetric care are used for the following reasons:

V20#	supervision child infant (healthy) well baby check
V22.#	supervision of pregnancy normal
V23.#	supervision of pregnancy high risk
V24.#	postpartum care
V25.#	contraception, contraceptive device/management
V26.#	procreative management
V27.#	outcome of delivery (code on mother's chart) Inpatient only
V28.#	screening antenatal
V29.#	observation newborn /infant suspected condition (undiagnosed)
V30.#	outcome of delivery (code on infant's record) (inpatient only)

13. Examinations Administrative and Routine

14. V-codes miscellaneous
These codes include other health encounters not mentioned as the reason for the encounter and sequence first.

15. V-codes nonspecific
These codes are so nonspecific or redundant that there is little reason for their use in an inpatient setting.

In the outpatient setting, use these codes only when there is insufficient documentation in the chart to select a better diagnosis, and when you have made the physician aware of the lack of documentation. When possible and documentation allows, select any other sign or symptom code as the reason for the encounter rather than the nonspecific V-code.

WHERE CAN I GET CERTIFICATION AS A CODER?

Becoming involved in a professional organization for coders is an ideal way to make contacts, learn more about coding, share problems and solutions, and receive accreditation. Here's a brief rundown of a few professional organizations that you may be interested in joining.

AAPC

The American Academy of Professional Coders is designed to aid healthcare professionals interested in reimbursement and procedural and diagnosis coding.

The AAPC offers an Independent Study Program, which allows participants to work at their own pace as they learn more about CPT coding and reimbursement issues. Through the AAPC, you may earn the certification of Certified Professional Coder (CPC) or Certified Professional Coder-Hospital (CPC-H).

For more information about the AAPC, call 1-800-626-CODE.

AHIMA

AHIMA, the American Health Information Management Association, offers membership to anyone who is interested in the knowledge and understanding of health information issues.

AHIMA has various state and local chapters, and several particular sections and societies that deal with a specific area of health information. Members may be certified as a Registered Records Administrator (RRA), Accredited Records Technician (ART), or Certified Coding Specialist (CCS).

For information about AHIMA, call 312-787-2672 or e-mail info@ahima.org.

PAHCOM

PAHCOM stands for the Professional Association of Health Care Office Managers. It provides support for managers of small group and solo health care practices.

Local chapters routinely meet to discuss relevant issues and educational programs for their communities. PAHCOM offers accreditation as a Certified Medical Manager (CMM).

For information on PAHCOM, call 1-800-451-9311.

NOTES

NOTES

NOTES

NOTES

NOTES